System Vaccinology

System Vaccinology

The History, the Translational Challenges and the Future

Edited by

Vijay Kumar Prajapati
Department of Biochemistry, School of Life Sciences,
Central University of Rajasthan, Ajmer, Rajasthan, India

ELSEVIER

ACADEMIC PRESS
An imprint of Elsevier
elsevier.com/books-and-journals

Academic Press is an imprint of Elsevier
125 London Wall, London EC2Y 5AS, United Kingdom
525 B Street, Suite 1650, San Diego, CA 92101, United States
50 Hampshire Street, 5th Floor, Cambridge, MA 02139, United States
The Boulevard, Langford Lane, Kidlington, Oxford OX5 1GB, United Kingdom

ISBN: 978-0-323-85941-7

For Information on all Academic Press publications visit our website at
https://www.elsevier.com/books-and-journals

Publisher: Stacy Masucci
Acquisitions Editor: Linda Versteeg-Buschman
Editorial Project Manager: Sam W. Young
Production Project Manager: Maria Bernard
Cover Designer: Vicky Pearson

Typeset by Aptara, New Delhi, India

Contents

Part IV
Vaccine future and ethics

Contributors

Raphael T. Aruleba Department of Molecular and Cell Biology, University of Cape Town, Cape Town, South Africa

Hemant Arya Department of Biotechnology, Central University of Rajasthan, Bandarsindri, Ajmer, Rajasthan, India

Derya T. Ata Strathclyde Institute of Pharmacy and Biomedical Sciences, University of Strathclyde, Glasgow, United Kingdom

Aparna Bhardwaj Indian Institute of Technology Mandi, School of Basic Sciences, VPO Kamand, Himachal Pradesh, India

Taniya Bhardwaj Indian Institute of Technology Mandi, School of Basic Sciences, VPO Kamand, Himachal Pradesh, India

Tarun Kumar Bhatt Department of Biotechnology, Central University of Rajasthan, Bandarsindri, Ajmer, Rajasthan, India

Olga Borges Center for Neuroscience and Cell Biology, University of Coimbra, Coimbra, Portugal; Faculty of Pharmacy, University of Coimbra, Coimbra, Portugal

Fabiana A Carneiro Núcleo Multidisciplinar de Pesquisa em Biologia (Numpex-Bio), Campus Duque de Caxias Professor Geraldo Cidade, Universidade Federal do Rio de Janeiro (UFRJ), Rio de Janeiro, Brazil

Katharine C. Carter Strathclyde Institute of Pharmacy and Biomedical Sciences, University of Strathclyde, Glasgow, United Kingdom

Shashi Bhushan Chauhan Department of Medicine, Institute of Medical Sciences, Banaras Hindu University, Varanasi, India

Víctor Chavarria Neuroimmunology and Neuro-Oncology Unit, Instituto Nacional de Neurología y Neurocirugía (INNN), Mexico City, Mexico

Juliana dos Reis Cortines Departamento de Virologia, Instituto de Microbiologia Paulo de Góes, Universidade Federal do Rio de Janeiro, Rio de Janeiro, Brazil

Isis Botelho N da Silva Escola de Química, Instituto de Química, Universidade Federal do Rio de Janeiro, Rio de Janeiro, Brazil

João Lucas Lima Calandrini de Azevedo Department of Bioscience and Technology, Institute of Tropical Pathology and Public Health, Federal University of Goiás, Goiânia, Brazil

Anabel Elisa Rodriguez Instituto de Patobiología (IP), IPVET, INTA-CONICET, Hurlingham, Argentina

Victor Alejandro Essus Departamento de Virologia, Instituto de Microbiologia Paulo de Góes, Universidade Federal do Rio de Janeiro, Rio de Janeiro, Brazil

Rubén Figueroa Neuroimmunology and Neuro-Oncology Unit, Instituto Nacional de Neurología y Neurocirugía (INNN), Mexico City, Mexico

Simone Gonçalves Fonseca Department of Bioscience and Technology, Institute of Tropical Pathology and Public Health, Federal University of Goiás, Goiânia, Brazil

Luiz Gustavo Gardinassi Department of Bioscience and Technology, Institute of Tropical Pathology and Public Health, Federal University of Goiás, Goiânia, Brazil

Vibhav Gautam Centre of Experimental Medicine and Surgery, Institute of Medical Sciences, Banaras Hindu University, Varanasi, India

Varsha Gautam Amity Institute of Advanced Research and Studies (M&D), Amity University, Noida, Uttar Pradesh, India

Rajanish Giri Indian Institute of Technology Mandi, School of Basic Sciences, VPO Kamand, Himachal Pradesh, India

Ramona Hurdayal Department of Molecular and Cell Biology, University of Cape Town, Cape Town, South Africa

Shivani Krishna Kapuganti Indian Institute of Technology Mandi, School of Basic Sciences, VPO Kamand, Himachal Pradesh, India

Prashant Khare Department of Microbiology, All India Institute of Medical Sciences, Bhopal, Madhya Pradesh, India

Prateek Kumar Indian Institute of Technology Mandi, School of Basic Sciences, VPO Kamand, Himachal Pradesh, India

Awnish Kumar Centre of Experimental Medicine and Surgery, Institute of Medical Sciences, Banaras Hindu University, Varanasi, India

Rajiv Kumar Centre of Experimental Medicine and Surgery, Institute of Medical Sciences, Banaras Hindu University, Varanasi, India

Mariela Luján Tomazic Instituto de Patobiología Veterinaria (IPVET), INTA-CONICET. Nicolás Repetto y De los Reseros s/n, Hurlingham, Argentina; Universidad de Buenos Aires, Facultad de Farmacia y Bioquímica, Cátedra de Biotecnología, Ciudad Autónoma de Buenos Aires, Argentina

André Guilherme Costa Martins Department of Clinical and Toxicological Analyses, School of Pharmaceutical Sciences, University of São Paulo, São Paulo, Brazil

Virginia Marugan-Hernandez The Royal Veterinary College, University of London, Hawkshead Lane, United Kingdom

Radheshyam Maurya Department of Animal Biology, School of Life Sciences, University of Hyderabad, Hyderabad, India

Dharmendra Kumar Maurya Department of Biochemistry, Institute of Science, Banaras Hindu University, Varanasi, India

Pawan Kumar Maurya Department of Biochemistry, Central University of Haryana, India

Ram Niwas Meena Department of Surgery, Institute of Medical Sciences, Banaras Hindu University, Varanasi, India

María Maximina Bertha Moreno-Altamirano Laboratorio de Inmunorregulación, Departamento de Inmunología, Escuela Nacional de Ciencias Biológicas, Instituto Politécnico Nacional, Mexico City, Mexico

Shyam Lal Mudavath Infectious Disease Biology Laboratory, Institute of Nano Science & Technology, Mohali, Punjab, India

Helder I Nakaya Department of Clinical and Toxicological Analyses, School of Pharmaceutical Sciences, University of São Paulo, São Paulo, Brazil; Hospital Israelita Albert Einstein, São Paulo, Brazil

Madhulika Namdeo Department of Animal Biology, School of Life Sciences, University of Hyderabad, Hyderabad, India

Namyashree Nayak Indian Institute of Technology Mandi, School of Basic Sciences, VPO Kamand, Himachal Pradesh, India

Rupal Ojha Department of Biochemistry, School of Life Sciences, Central University of Rajasthan, Ajmer, Rajasthan, India

Jacqueline Oliva-Ramírez Translational Molecular Pathology, MD Anderson Cancer Center, Houston, TX, United States

Benjamín Pineda Neuroimmunology and Neuro-Oncology Unit, Instituto Nacional de Neurología y Neurocirugía (INNN), Mexico City, Mexico

Vijay Kumar Prajapati Department of Biochemistry, School of Life Sciences, Central University of Rajasthan, Ajmer, Rajasthan, India

Dhaneswar Prusty Department of Biochemistry, School of Life, Sciences, Central University of Rajasthan, Ajmer, India

Verónica Pérez de la Cruz Neurobiochemistry and Behaviour Laboratory, Instituto Nacional de Neurología y Neurocirugía (INNN), Mexico City, Mexico

Utkarsha Sahu Department of Microbiology, All India Institute of Medical Sciences, Bhopal, Madhya Pradesh, India

Aleli Salazar Neuroimmunology and Neuro-Oncology Unit, Instituto Nacional de Neurología y Neurocirugía (INNN), Mexico City, Mexico

Francisco Javier Sánchez-García Laboratorio de Inmunorregulación, Departamento de Inmunología, Escuela Nacional de Ciencias Biológicas, Instituto Politécnico Nacional, Mexico City, Mexico

Viviane Schuch Department of Clinical and Toxicological Analyses, School of Pharmaceutical Sciences, University of São Paulo, São Paulo, Brazil

Shyamali Department of Biochemistry, Institute of Science, Banaras Hindu University, Varanasi, India

João Marcos Maia Silva Department of Bioscience and Technology, Institute of Tropical Pathology and Public Health, Federal University of Goiás, Goiânia, Brazil

Bhawana Singh Department of Medicine, Institute of Medical Sciences, Banaras Hindu University, Varanasi, India

Om Prakash Singh Department of Biochemistry, Institute of Science, Banaras Hindu University, Varanasi, India

Santosh K Singh Centre of Experimental Medicine and Surgery, Institute of Medical Sciences, Banaras Hindu University, Varanasi, India

Edna Soares Center for Neuroscience and Cell Biology, University of Coimbra, Coimbra, Portugal; Faculty of Pharmacy, University of Coimbra, Coimbra, Portugal

Shyam Sundar Department of Medicine, Institute of Medical Sciences, Banaras Hindu University, Varanasi, India

Rahul Tiwari Centre of Experimental Medicine and Surgery, Institute of Medical Sciences, Banaras Hindu University, Varanasi, India

Adrian Wildfire Director, Scientific and Business, Strategy, hVIVO

Part I

History and introduction

Chapter 1

History of vaccine: from centuries to present

Rupal Ojha, Vijay Kumar Prajapati
Department of Biochemistry, School of Life Sciences, Central University of Rajasthan, Ajmer, Rajasthan, India

1.1 Introduction

Vaccination provides protection and helps our immune system to develop immune responses against pathogens. Since time immemorial, vaccines have been well known for the treatment of various diseases. Edward Jenner has been regarded as the father of vaccination; however, the concept of inoculation/vaccination was initially originated from the Indian peninsula by "Woodiah" Brahmans (Oriya) for ages [1]. Afterward, in 1000 CE, the practice and knowledge were then transferred to China via Chinese scholars visited Indian universities. Finally, in the 17th century (1796), Jenner worked on smallpox disease; he inoculated the pus cells from smallpox blister to a young child James Phipps, infected with cowpox (vaccinia virus), and discovered immunity against smallpox [2]. The method developed by Jenner was recognized with tremendous value, and later, in 1798, the first vaccine for smallpox was developed, and after massive immunization in 1979, the disease was declared eradicated. Though, before Jenner discovered smallpox, the process of vaccination was already revealed by Benjamin Jesty (farmer at Yetminster) in 1774 [3]. He used cowpox material and inoculated it into his wife and two sons; the same statement has been engraved on the tombstone of Benjamin Jesty. Like the discovery of smallpox vaccines, many diseases in the past centuries were eradicated by vaccination, such as anthrax, polio, chickenpox, and measles. In the late 18th century, Louis pasture had developed the vaccine against anthrax and immunize it successfully in animals like cows, sheep, and goats. He weakened the rabies virus, performed the immunization process, and harvested it from the rabbit's spinal cord but failed to develop a vaccine in the laboratory environment [4]. This happened because, comparatively, the replication and mutation rates of viruses are higher than bacteria.

Nevertheless, after several serial passages, he found that the virulence of the virus was decreasing when injected into different species. He started again

System Vaccinology. https://doi.org/10.1016/B978-0-323-85941-7.00018-8

with rabbit immunization and made the rabies strain less virulent; later, with this strategy, he vaccinated several dogs and tested the first human vaccine against rabies in a 9-year-old boy. After these milestones, in 1890, the first serum therapy against diphtheria and tetanus has come into the picture [5]. This therapy transmits the blood sera from a recovered person to the infected one to develop antibodies against the infection and is yet in use as first-line therapy to treat COVID-19 patients. Next, in 1921, the first whole celled live attenuated Bacillus-Calmette Guerin (BCG) vaccine was developed against tuberculosis to protect infants [6]. This vaccine is still in use for tuberculosis treatment, and several studies reported that in many countries, BCG vaccine trials are ongoing to treat COVID-19 patients. The reason behind this approach is still not well known. After the effective development of various kinds of vaccines, the research took a new turn, leading to the efficacy of vaccines. In 1926, Alexander Tomas Glenny (British immunologist) discovered the alum adjuvants that possess immunostimulatory properties and proved to boost the efficacy of the diphtheria toxoid vaccine [7].

After the discovery of adjuvant, in 1938 aluminum adjuvanted vaccine against tetanus toxoid was discovered (https://www.cdc.gov/vaccines/pubs/pinkbook/downloads/tetanus.pdf). Further, in 1951, Max Theiler won the Nobel prize for discovering the yellow fever vaccine 17D [8]. As time passed, new diseases kept encountering, and vaccines discovery has become the foremost preventive measure. Later, in 1974, the World Health Organization had commenced the EPI (Expanded Programme on Immunization); in this program, the worldwide uptake of childhood immunization was performed against diseases like tetanus, measles, tuberculosis, poliomyelitis, pertussis. After the successful immunization, the program is gradually drawn out to cover the immunization for other viral diseases such as rubella and hepatitis B in developing countries. The development of vaccines started progressing over time, and as a result, polysaccharides and recombinant vaccines have come to the fore. The polysaccharide vaccines are the inactivated subunit vaccines and generate B-cell mediated humoral antibody immune responses [9]. In 1980, the first polysaccharide vaccine was developed against Hemophilus influenza type B, a pathogen majorly responsible for causing meningitis and pneumonia in children. Later, in 1986, the first recombinant DNA vaccine, Recombivax HB (composed of hepatitis surface B antigen), was developed against Hepatitis B for human use [10]. When injected in children, this recombinant vaccine generated a tremendous immune response and protected against Hepatitis B infection. In this manner, many milestones were achieved by researchers (Fig. 1.1); in the year 2000, the reverse vaccinology approach takes a knock. Rino Rappoli led this approach by utilizing the genomic information of the MenB strain, and with the help of the bioinformatic servers, the antigenic proteins were identified for the designing of recombinant epitope vaccine against Neisseria meningitidis [11]. Nowadays, the system biology approach has overtaken the development of effective and safe vaccines with extended-lasting immune responses. After a

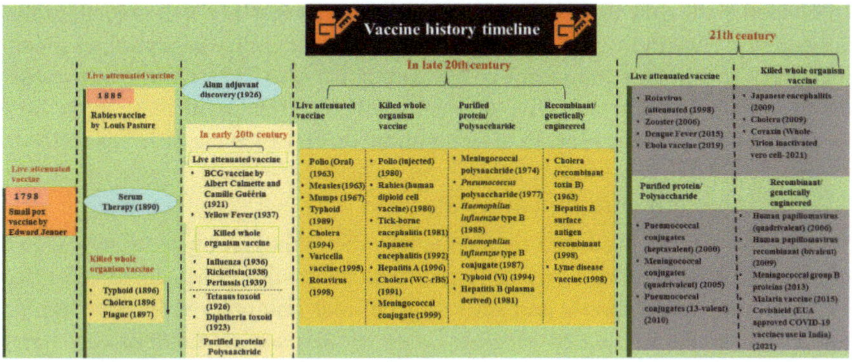

FIG. 1.1 Historic timeline of vaccine discovery.

brief introduction about vaccine evolution, we will discuss the generations and present scenario of the vaccines in the next section.

1.2 Generations of vaccines

Vaccines are categorized into three generations based on components used in the synthesis of vaccine, specific characteristics, and the spectrum covered by the organism (Fig. 1.2).

1.2.1 First-generation vaccines

The first-generation vaccines were traditionally synthesized vaccines that utilize the conventional production approach by employing whole organism or

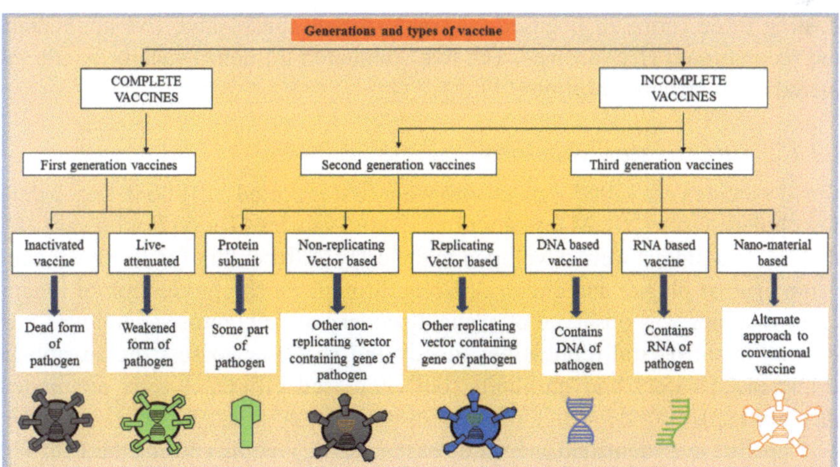

FIG. 1.2 Pictorial representation of various types and generation of vaccines.

attenuated pathogen or inactivated bacterial toxin that possess potent immunogenicity. The traditional vaccines possess a high ability to stimulate innate immunity and induce long-term protection of the host [12]. On the other side, the use of whole organisms (live or attenuated) could induce disease in the host by retrieving virulence [13]. First-generation vaccines are classified as follows.

1.2.1.1 Live attenuated vaccines

These vaccines are produced by attenuating the pathogen by serial passage of the virus to a foreign host species [14] or cold adaptation. They act by inducing efficient antibody response and activating cellular immunity [15]. Here are the few examples of attenuated vaccines, seen in the case of smallpox that dates back to 10,000 BC in Africa, that later evoke an epidemic in Europe in the 18th century, killing 40,000 people annually with a fatality rate ranging from 20% to 60% [16] which was treated by a technique named "variolation" developed by Edward Jenner [17]. Vaccinia was developed by attenuation in the mid-20th century that had eradicated the disease by 1980 (the three original publications on vaccination against smallpox).

Measles, produced by infection of a virus of the family Paramyxoviridae, was noticed in 1912 in the United States with an average of 6000 deaths each year eventually rose to 3-4 million cases by the mid-20th century (https://www.cdc.gov/measles/about/history.html). In 1968, a weaker measles vaccine named "Moraten" (Edmonston-Enders strain) was distributed in the United States. Generally, it is combined with mumps and rubella to produce the MMR vaccine [18].

Influenza belongs to the Orthomyxoviridae family and is a highly infectious disease affecting the respiratory system, often characterized by myalgia, fever, and respiratory symptoms. The "Asian Flu" pandemic that occurred in the late 19th century initiated in Russia and then spread to the West. Later, the H1N1 virus initiated the "Spanish Flu," which led to 40–50 million deaths [19]. The existing three forms of licensed vaccines include inactivated, live attenuated, and recombinant HA vaccines. The live attenuated influenza vaccine is administered as an intranasal spray.

1.2.1.2 Inactivated vaccines

These vaccines are killed viruses that were first reported in 1886 in heat-killed hog cholera virus [20]. Many other inactivated vaccines for typhoid fever [21], cholera, and plague were developed in the early 20th century (protective inoculation against plague and cholera). Breakthrough for the production of inactivated vaccines was observed after the discovery of cell culture techniques that allowed in-vitro viral replication. Inactivated vaccines possess the advantage of increased safety and immunity, but decreased efficiency over attenuated vaccines [22].

Hepatitis was identified as liver disease-causing jaundice during the 17th and 18th centuries in Europe that later in the 19th century was termed as epidemic jaundice [23]. The disease was common in adults with an incubation period of 15–40 days and exhibiting symptoms, such as anorexia, nausea, and diarrhea. The virus exhibited exceptional resistance to attenuation procedures such as heating & chlorination, hence required a novel approach to develop vaccine for this disease. Epaxal, an inactivated form of vaccine is produced by formalin inactivation of HAV (strain RG-SB) adsorbed to the surface of virosomes that replace aluminum hydroxide as adjuvant [22].

Cutaneous leishmaniasis, caused by parasitic flagellates of genus Leishmania, is a zoonotic disease mainly transmitted by *Phlebotomus* sand flies. It is caused by two species, namely *L. major* and *L. aethopica.* This skin disease is observed in the middle-East & the Eastern Mediterranean region, Africa, and Central & South Africa [24]. An inactivated vaccine comprising single dose whole cell autoclave-killed Leishmania major (ALM) mixed with BCG was tested in randomized double-blind trial in Bam, Iran. The leishmanin skin test indicated that ALM+BCG was safe and more immunogenic than BCG alone [25].

1.2.2 Second-generation vaccines

As the first generation vaccines had a possibility of retrieval of virulence by the injected pathogen, researchers solved this problem by synthesizing the second-generation vaccines, which was basically composed of subunit elements, recombinant or synthetic proteins, non-protein antigens [26]. The second-generation vaccines are subdivided into the following.

1.2.2.1 Subunit vaccines

Subunit vaccines are composed of peptide or polysaccharide present on the pathogen surface. The absence of genetic material in the vaccine does not allow the proliferation but initiates an immune response cascade [27]. The bacterial subunit vaccines are categorized into Toxoid vaccines and polysaccharide vaccines. Toxoids are produced by formaldehyde inactivation of toxins to convert into non-toxins employed in vaccines. The toxin neutralization by the antibodies is initiated due to structural resemblance between toxin and toxoid. Some common examples are tetanus, diphtheria, and pertussis toxoid vaccines [28].

The polysaccharide vaccines are produced by polysaccharide capsule of encapsulated bacteria that could enhance the membrane hydrophilicity and antiphagocytic properties. A vaccine for Pneumococcal pneumonia, caused by *Streptococcus pneumoniae* consists of 23 antigenically different capsular polysaccharides that act by forming opsonizing antibodies [29]. Pneumococcal pneumonia is common bacterial pneumonia found in adults, with an estimated number of 90,000 cases recorded annually in the United States. The T-cells are unable to process the polysaccharide antigens, hence follow the B-cell activation resulting in IgM production and development of memory cells (https://www.cdc.gov/pneumococcal/about/facts.html).

1.2.2.2 Conjugated vaccines

Conjugated vaccines generally comprise the polysaccharide antigens, i.e., respective epitopes of the pathogen conjugated to a protein carrier [30]. The polysaccharide-protein conjugate is relatively immunogenic than solo polysaccharide, as the conjugate could activate the TH cells and enable class switching from IgM to IgG. Protein conjugate is added to enhance the immunological memory, as observed in the case of polysaccharide antigen of S. pneumonia type 3 [31]. As observed in case of *Hemophilus influenza B* (HiB), which was the first conjugate vaccine used for bacterial meningitis in children. The HiB conjugate is made of type B capsular polysaccharide covalently linked to carrier proteins such as tetanus toxoid [32], diphtheria toxoid, diphtheria toxin mutant that accounted for increased efficacy of the vaccine.

1.2.2.3 Recombinant vaccines

Advancements in genetic engineering and molecular biology enabled the mass production of pathogenic surface proteins by gene cloning into bacterial, yeast, or mammalian expression vectors. Due to the availability of sequence of antigens, the protein surface antigens are synthetically produced by rDNA technology which is further produced by cloning into expression systems. The first recombinant antigen vaccine approved for human use is hepatitis B vaccine, which is produced by cloning the Hepatitis-surface antigen (HBsAg) into yeast cells. The HBsAg is highly immunogenic and have shown to induce the production of antibodies [33].

1.2.3 Third-generation vaccines

The third-generation vaccines also called as next-generation vaccines or genetic vaccines, developed by administration of plasmid containing the antigen gene into the expression cells [34]. A peculiar feature of next-generation vaccines is they can be developed from the sequence information alone, thus making this procedure highly adaptable and accelerate the vaccine development [35]. These vaccines are classified according to the type of genetic material introduced into the expression cells, i.e., DNA vaccines, RNA (mRNA) vaccines, and plasmid vaccines. DNA vaccines produced by administering the antigen gene containing plasmid into cells with specific promoter that initiates the immune cascade, as observed in the case of vaccinia vector vaccine that utilizes vaccinia promoter inserted in plasmid with antigen gene from pathogen which are co-cultured with vaccinia virus to produce recombinant vaccinia vector vaccine. Following the administration of DNA vaccine, the antigenic gene is translocated into the nucleus that initiates transcription due to the presence of promoter. The expressed protein stimulate both humoral and cell mediated immunity [34]. As DNA vaccines contain the source gene for antigenic diversity, it possess the ability to immunize against several different strains of antigen [36]. Besides the merits, use of DNA vaccines is also associated with a few demerits [37].

1. Can only express protein antigens, unlike the subunit or conjugate vaccines.
2. Induce tumor formation due to joining of DNA with host genome.
3. It can cause autoimmune diseases.

DNA vaccines containing the plasmid with the desired antigen are administered by intramuscular injection mode or gene gun mode of delivery into the epidermis [38]. Development of genetic vaccines is in progress for dreadful diseases such as hepatitis, HIV, influenza and Ebola [39]. In the case of NCDs, an antitumor DNA vaccine was developed against cervical cancer induced by papilloma virus type 16 in mouse model [40]. Vaccines are developed and commercialized for SARS-CoV-2, the seedbed of the 21st-century pandemic. Diverse models of genetic vaccines were developed to acquire resistance for COVID-19 disease, such viral vector based vaccines, DNA vaccines, mRNA vaccines, and APCs [35]. Most DNA vaccines were developed by cloning the Spike (S) & Nucleocapsid (N) genes of SARS-CoV-2 [41]. The INO-4800 vaccine is developed by introducing S protein into plasmid pGX9501 and tested for single immunization in mice and currently in phase 1 clinical trials [42].

mRNA vaccines comprise of mRNA of the antigen and work alike as the DNA vaccines, but evade the nuclear translocation and gene transcription steps. Due to the autonomous replicating ability, RNA vaccines can induce protective immunity at lower dose [43], but require a carrier molecule, such as lipid nanoparticles to facilitate the entry into cells. Despite the mRNA instability, vaccines are developed to increase its stability & translation efficacy to enhance immune response [44]. In the case of HIV mRNA vaccines, dendritic cells are transfected with Gag protein mRNA that result in CD4 & CD8 T-cell immune response in-vitro, thus overcome the requirement for plasmid entry into nucleus prior the protein expression [45]. For Ebola, vaccines with the surface glycoprotein (GP) mRNA were developed using a human IgK signal peptide which displayed improved translocation through intracellular secretory network for subsequent display on the cell surface [46]. mRNA vaccines for COVID-19 were developed by Moderna Inc. in collaboration with Cambridge, MA, USA. & BioNTech, Mainz, Germany. mRNA-1273 (Clinicaltrials.gov number, NCT04470427) developed by Moderna Inc. was the first mRNA vaccine developed against COVID-19 by inserting the mRNA that encodes Spike protein of SARS-CoV-2 encapsulated in lipid nanoparticle which is currently in phase 3 clinical trial [47]. Another mRNA-based vaccine, called BNT162 developed by BioNTech is another LNP encapsulated mRNA vaccine that has four variants, namely a1, b1, b2, and c2. It is currently in the phase 2/3 clinical trial [48]. In contrast to mRNA-1273, BNT162 showed better immune response with high level of neutralizing antibodies. Other mRNA vaccines with inclusion of adjuvant were developed for cancers to increase the vaccine efficacy [49].

An effective adjuvant named TriMix (combination of mRNAs encoding CD70, CD40 & TLR4) enhanced the immunogenicity of vaccines & increased DC maturation and CTL response.

Viral vector-based vaccines were developed for infectious diseases and cancers by utilizing their packaging capacity for foreign genes [50]. The commonly used viral vectors are Adenovirus vectors, Poxvirus vectors, Retrovirus vectors, CMV vectors, and Sendai virus vectors [51]. The poxvirus vectors were used to develop smallpox vaccine that involves the production of highly attenuated vaccinia virus. Modified vaccinia Ankara is derived from vaccinia strain Ankara by attenuation leading to loss of 15% of its genome [52]. Retrovirus vector based therapy was performed on patients with X-linked severe combined immunodeficiency (SCID-X1) [53] or malignant glioma [54]. The adenovirus vectors are double-stranded linear DNA genome, with human Ad serotype 5 (Ad5) being widely employed for gene delivery vector. Ad vectors are replication deficient due to deletion of E1A & E1B viral gene [55]. Recombinant Ad vector based vaccines were examined in clinical trials against HIV-1 [56], influenza [57], and solid tumors [58]. Adenoviruses, specifically Ad5, Ad26, and simian AdChOx1, were utilized for viral vectors developed for SARS-CoV-2. The Sputnik V vaccine developed by Russia based on vaccination with Ad26-SARS-CoV-2 S followed by a booster dose of Ad5-SARS-CoV-2 S displayed good safety and immunogenicity in preclinical studies [59]. Another vaccine developed by Oxford University and AstraZeneca named ChAdOx1 nCoV-19 was developed by expressing Spike protein from chimpanzee Ad vector ChAdOx1 [60]. These intramuscular vaccines have been demonstrated to elicit both humoral and cellular immune responses.

1.3 The present scenario in the field of vaccine development

Vaccines are the only weapon used to defeat any infectious disease, and their development is a very complex process. Vaccine development within a short period is challenging and skillful work. The rapid development of any vaccine under pressure or because of any reason may be dangerous [61]. If we talk about the types of vaccines and techniques used in the current scenario, then we can take a look at the world's largest pandemic, i.e., COVID-19. Nearly all types of vaccines have been used for COVID-19 vaccine development. Different coronavirus vaccines have been authorized for emergency or general use in the last few months. For example (1) Sinopharm, Sinovac (both developed by China), Covaxin (ICMR & Bharat Biotech, India) are inactivated vaccines. The benefit of the inactivated vaccine is that it cannot replicate and infect cells but can activate the immune system. Some other vaccines are licensed under this technology are Rabies, Polio, and Hepatitis A vaccines [62]. (2) Pfizer (BioNTech) and Moderna, these two vaccines are the RNA/mRNA vaccines—this is a newly developed technique for vaccine development, and previously no vaccines have been licensed under this technique;

however, several trials are going on against different pathogens. In this technique, mRNA that codes for the vital part of the protein have been used, like spike GP majorly involved in developing the COVID-19 vaccines (necessary for the coronavirus entry). Immune cells of the body detect these foreign particles and elicit a response against them. mRNA vaccines have proved much safer, as it does not contain any live component of the pathogen. However, the major challenge is to prevent free RNA degradation as it degrades very fast in the body. (3) Next technique used for vaccine development is a non-replicating viral vector; previously licensed vaccine on this technique is Ebola virus vaccine, and currently used vaccines are Covishield (Oxford-AstraZeneca, UK), Sputnik V (Gamaleya Research Institute, Russia). In this technique, the modified virus is used as a vector to transfer the pathogen's genetic material. As the body cells get infected by the modified virus containing the genetic code of antigen, they start producing proteins based on that genetic code, and then our immune system plays its role in triggering an immune response [63]. (4) Protein subunit—this technique is widely used for vaccine development, and different vaccines are licensed under this technique; for example, Hepatitis B, *Shingles* infection, pneumococcal disease, and meningococcal disease. Protein subunit vaccine contains purified protein which is only a part of the pathogen instead of the whole organism, which triggers immune cells to elicit a proper immune response. This type of vaccine is safe compared to other techniques because it contains only a part of the pathogen. Complex manufacturing and the requirement of adjuvants and a booster dose are the significant challenges of this technique [64].

A review by Yatoo et al. mentioned different approaches like examining DNA, protein, or capsular polysaccharides that are utilized to develop a vaccine against Mycoplasma to prevent its infection. The novel approach used to develop vaccine candidates includes subunit vaccines, nanoparticle-based vaccines, cytokine or TLR-based vaccines, plant-based or edible vaccines, and recombinant protein or DNA vaccines [65].

The vaccine development approach that was used for the eradication of river blindness was categorized into three parts. The first approach prevents the establishment of the parasite by using a prophylactic vaccine that is primary immunization and then inoculation of two booster doses. The prophylactic vaccine reduces the chance of transmission and protects a significant part of the population. The second approach was to stop the chances of reinfection in the area due to infected migrant workers and migration of infected black flies, which can be done using immunoprophylaxis at the individual level [66]. Protein subunit vaccine strategy was used to develop a vaccine against *O. volvulus* (responsible for causing river blindness), which was done by expressing Ov-103 and Ov-RAL in two different expression vectors *Pichia Pink* and *Escherichia coli*. After the immunization study in mice and humans, it was confirmed that Ov-103 and Ov-RAL could trigger the immune system and helps to develop immunity against O. volvulus [67].

Lymphatic filariasis parasitic infection caused by *Wuchereria bancrofti*, *Brugia malayi*, and *Brugia timori* responsible for most physical disabilities worldwide, and India alone contributes 40% of global filariasis burden. WHO passed the resolution in 1997 to eliminate filariasis by 2020 with the help of the Mass Drug Administration (MDA), and currently, this is the only step taken by WHO to control this infection. MDA was highly successful in controlling the lymphatic filariasis infection throughout the world, but also there is some case of the reemergence of infection in a few countries. Hence, there was an urgent need for the development of a vaccine. To develop the prophylactic vaccine combined with MDA, Khatri et al., and others isolated some important vaccine candidates against filariasis, but the result shows only 35% protection. Therefore, the authors decided to modify the current formulation in two ways; first, by addition thioredoxin peroxide antigen that helps make the tetravalent vaccine. They have also included an adjuvant AL019 (alum along with glucopyranosyl lipid adjuvant). This adjuvant is previously known to assist and balance Th1/Th2 response [68].

1.4 Conclusion

From time immemorial to now, the treatment of many infectious diseases relies solely on vaccines. Many vaccines have reached milestones and made remarkable history, while some of them faced failures also in the path of their efficacy. The failures in vaccination could be a result of a limited understanding of the immune mechanism or functioning. During the achievement of the first smallpox vaccination by Jenner in the 17th century, in the line, other vaccines are aimed to produce a long-lasting memory response that responds speedily, eliciting protective immunity to future infections. For invading pathogens and eliminating infection, the vaccine must produce both humoral and cell-mediated immunity. By the time, the generation of vaccines has also been evolved as the centuries passed on. The classical vaccines have majorly contributed to eradicating various diseases; however, they are associated with some limitations; hence, for better and long-lasting treatment, the next-generation vaccines platform comes to light. Thus, the comprehensive study for developing potential vaccines becomes needful to fight pandemics and epidemics such as COVID-19, black fungus infection, and many others.

References

[1] Kumar V. Introductory chapter: The journey of vaccines—The Past and the Present. Vaccines- the History and Future. DOI:10.5772/intechopen.86274.

[2] Behbehani AM. The smallpox story: life and death of an old disease. Microbiol Rev 1983;47:455–509.

[3] Pead PJ. Benjamin Jesty: the first vaccinator revealed. The Lancet 2006;368:2202.

[4] Fooks A, Jackson A. Rabies: Scientific Basis of the Disease and Its Management. 4th ed. Elsevier; 2020.

[5] Kaufmann SHE. Remembering Emil von Behring: from tetanus treatment to antibody cooperation with phagocytes. mBio 2017;8:e00117–17.
[6] Luca S, Mihaescu T. History of BCG vaccine. Maedica (Bucur) 2013;8:53–8.
[7] Reed SG, Orr MT, Fox CB. Key roles of adjuvants in modern vaccines. Nature Med 2013;19:1597–608.
[8] Frierson JG. The yellow fever vaccine: a history. Yale J Biol Med 2010;83:77.
[9] Mitchell R, Kelly DF, Pollard AJ, Trück J. Polysaccharide-specific B cell responses to vaccination in humans. Hum Vaccin Immunother 2014;10:1661–8.
[10] Cabral GA, Marciano-Cabral F, Funk GA, Sanchez Y, Hollinger FB, Melnick JL, Dreesman GR. Cellular and humoral immunity in guinea pigs to two major polypeptides derived from hepatitis B surface antigen. J Gen Virol 1978;38:339–50.
[11] Rappuoli R, Bottomley MJ, D'Oro U, Finco O, De Gregorio E. Reverse vaccinology 2.0: Human immunology instructs vaccine antigen design. J Exp Med 2016;213:469–81.
[12] Noazin S, Modabber F, Khamesipour A, Smith PG, Moulton LH, Nasseri K, Sharifi I, Khalil EA, Bernal ID, Antunes CM, Kieny MP, Tanner M. First generation leishmaniasis vaccines: a review of field efficacy trials. Vaccine 2008;26:6759–67.
[13] Huang DB, Wu JJ, Tyring SK. A review of licensed viral vaccines, some of their safety concerns, and the advances in the development of investigational viral vaccines. J Infect 2004;49:179–209.
[14] Jordan I, Sandig V. Matrix and backstage: cellular substrates for viral vaccines. Viruses 2014;6:1672–700.
[15] Clem AS. Fundamentals of vaccine immunology. J Glob Infect Dis 2011;3:73.
[16] Barquet N, Domingo P. Smallpox: the triumph over the most terrible of the ministers of death. Ann Intern Med 1997;127:635–42.
[17] Willis NJ. Edward Jenner and the eradication of smallpox. Scot Med J 1997;42:118–21.
[18] Weibel R, Villarejos V, Hernández G, Stokes Jr J, Buynak E, Hilleman M. Combined live measles-mumps virus vaccine. Arch Dis Child 1973;48:532.
[19] Kuszewski K, Brydak L. The epidemiology and history of influenza. Biomed Pharmacother 2000;54:188–95.
[20] Salmon DE, Smith T. On a new method of producing immunity from contagious diseases. Am Vet Rev 1886;10:63–9.
[21] Wright A, Semple D. Vaccination against typhoid fever. BMJ 1897;1:432.
[22] Bovier PA. Epaxal: a virosomal vaccine to prevent hepatitis A infection. Expert Rev Vaccines 2008;7:1141–50.
[23] Purcell RH. Hepatitis viruses: changing patterns of human disease. Proc Natl Acad Sci USA 1994;91:2401–2406.
[24] Rioux JA, Lanotte G. Leishmania infantum as a cause of cutaneous leishmaniasis. Trans R Soc Trop Med Hyg 1990;84:898.
[25] Sharifi I, FeKri AR, Aflatonian MR, Khamesipour A, Nadim A, Mousavi MR, Momeni AZ, Dowlati Y, Godal T, Zicker F, Smith PG, Modabber F. Randomised vaccine trial of single dose of killed Leishmania major plus BCG against anthroponotic cutaneous leishmaniasis in Bam, Iran. Lancet (London) 1998;351:1540–3.
[26] Plotkin LA. Vaccines: the fourth century. Clin Vaccine Immunol 2009;16:1709–19.
[27] Robinson HL, Amara RR. T cell vaccines for microbial infections. Nat Med 2005;11: S25–32.
[28] O'Hagan DT. Recent developments in vaccine delivery systems. Curr Drug Targets Infect Disord 2001;1:273–86.

[29] Butler JC, Shapiro ED, Carlone GM. Pneumococcal vaccines: history, current status, and future directions. Am J Med 1999;107:69s–76s.

[30] Baker PJ. T cell regulation of the antibody response to bacterial polysaccharide antigens: an examination of some general characteristics and their implications. J Infect Dis 1992;165(Suppl 1):S44–8.

[31] Avery OT, Goebel WF. Chemo-immunological studies on conjugated carbohydrate-proteins: ii. Immunological specificity of synthetic sugar-protein antigens. J Exp Med 1929;50:533–50.

[32] Ward J, Berkowitz C, Pescetti J, Burkart K, Samuelson O, Gordon L. Enhanced immunogenicity in young infants of a new haemophilus influenzae type B(HIB) capsular polysaccharide(PRP)-diphtheria toxoid(D) conjugate vaccine. Pediatr Res 1984;18:287.

[33] Plotkin SA. Vaccines: past, present and future. Nat Med 2005;11:S5–11.

[34] Palatnik-de-Sousa CB. Vaccines for leishmaniasis in the fore coming 25 years. Vaccine 2008;26:1709–24.

[35] van Riel D, de Wit E. Next-generation vaccine platforms for COVID-19. Nat Mater 2020;19:810–2.

[36] Borja-Cabrera GP, Santos FB, Nico D, Gravino AE, Manna L, Palatnik M, Palatnik-de-Sousa CB. The Leishmune®s Nucleoside hydrolase DNA vaccine as an aid in immunotherapy of canine visceral leishmaniasis. Procedia Vaccino 2012;6:64–73.

[37] Smillie C, Garcillán-Barcia MP, Francia MV, Rocha EP, de la Cruz F. Mobility of plasmids. Microbiol Mol Biol Rev 2010;74:434–52.

[38] Arnon A, Levi R. Synthetic recombinant vaccines against viral agents. Int Arch Allergy Immunol. 1995;108:321–6.

[39] Bins AD, van den Berg JH, Oosterhuis K, Haanen JB. Recent advances towards the clinical application of DNA vaccines. Neth J Med 2013;71:109–17.

[40] Tahamtan A, Ghaemi A, Gorji A, Kalhor HR, Sajadian A, Tabarraei A, Moradi A, Atyabi F, Kelishadi M. Antitumor effect of therapeutic HPV DNA vaccines with chitosan-based nanodelivery systems. J Biomed Sci 2014;21:69.

[41] Lan J, Ge J, Yu J, Shan S, Zhou H, Fan S, Zhang Q, Shi X, Wang Q, Zhang L, Wang X. Structure of the SARS-CoV-2 spike receptor-binding domain bound to the ACE2 receptor. Nature 2020;581:215–20.

[42] Smith TRF, Patel A, Ramos S, Elwood D, Zhu X, Yan J, Gary EN, Walker SN, Schultheis K, Purwar M, Xu Z, Walters J, Bhojnagarwala P, Yang M, Chokkalingam N, Pezzoli P, Parzych E, Reuschel EL, Doan A, Tursi N, Vasquez M, Choi J, Tello-Ruiz E, Maricic I, Bah MA, Wu Y, Amante D, Park DH, Dia Y, Ali AR, Zaidi FI, Generotti A, Kim KY, Herring TA, Reeder S, Andrade VM, Buttigieg K, Zhao G, Wu JM, Li D, Bao L, Liu J, Deng W, Qin C, Brown AS, Khoshnejad M, Wang N, Chu J, Wrapp D, McLellan JS, Muthumani K, Wang B, Carroll MW, Kim JJ, Boyer J, Kulp DW, Humeau L, Weiner DB, Broderick KE. Immunogenicity of a DNA vaccine candidate for COVID-19. Nat Commun 2020;11:2601.

[43] Vogel AB, Lambert L, Kinnear E, Busse D, Erbar S, Reuter KC, Wicke L, Perkovic M, Beissert T, Haas H, Reece ST, Sahin U, Tregoning JS. Self-amplifying RNA vaccines give equivalent protection against influenza to mRNA vaccines but at much lower doses. Mol Ther 2018;26:446–55.

[44] Zhang C, Maruggi G, Shan H, Li J. Advances in mRNA vaccines for infectious diseases. Front Immunol 2019;10:594.

[45] Mata M, Paterson Y. Th1 T cell responses to HIV-1 Gag protein delivered by a Listeria monocytogenes vaccine are similar to those induced by endogenous listerial antigens. J Immunol (Baltimore, Md: 1950) 1999;163:1449–56.

[46] Meyer M, Huang E, Yuzhakov O, Ramanathan P, Ciaramella G, Bukreyev A. Modified mRNA-based vaccines elicit robust immune responses and protect guinea pigs from ebola virus disease. J Infect Dis 2018;217:451–5.

[47] Chakraborty R, Parvez S. COVID-19: an overview of the current pharmacological interventions, vaccines, and clinical trials. Biochem Pharmacol 2020;180:114184.

[48] Koirala A, Joo YJ, Khatami A, Chiu C, Britton PN. Vaccines for COVID-19: the current state of play. Paediatr Respir Rev 2020;35:43–9.

[49] Eickhoff CS, Van Aartsen D, Terry FE, Meymandi SK, Traina MM, Hernandez S, Martin WD, Moise L, De Groot AS, Hoft DF. An immunoinformatic approach for identification of Trypanosoma cruzi HLA-A2-restricted CD8(+) T cell epitopes. Hum Vaccin Immunother 2015;11:2322–8.

[50] Schiedner G, Morral N, Parks RJ, Wu Y, Koopmans SC, Langston C, Graham FL, Beaudet AL, Kochanek S. Genomic DNA transfer with a high-capacity adenovirus vector results in improved in vivo gene expression and decreased toxicity. Nat Genet 1998;18:180–3.

[51] Ura T, Okuda K, Shimada M. Developments in viral vector-based vaccines. Vaccines 2014;2:624–41.

[52] Stickl H, Hochstein-Mintzel V, Mayr A, Huber HC, Schäfer H, Holzner A. MVA vaccination against smallpox: clinical tests with an attenuated live vaccinia virus strain (MVA) (author's transl). Dtsch Med Wochenschr (1946) 1974;99:2386–92.

[53] Cavazzana-Calvo M, Hacein-Bey S, Geneviève de Saint B, Gross F, Yvon E, Nusbaum P, Selz F, Hue C, Certain S, Casanova J-L, Bousso P, Le Deist F, Fischer A. Gene therapy of human severe combined immunodeficiency (SCID)-X1 disease. Science 2000;288:669–72.

[54] Soto C, Sigurdsson EM, Morelli L, Kumar RA, Castaño EM, Frangione B. Beta-sheet breaker peptides inhibit fibrillogenesis in a rat brain model of amyloidosis: implications for Alzheimer's therapy. Nat Med 1998;4:822–6.

[55] Sumida SM, Truitt DM, Lemckert AA, Vogels R, Custers JH, Addo MM, Lockman S, Peter T, Peyerl FW, Kishko MG, Jackson SS, Gorgone DA, Lifton MA, Essex M, Walker BD, Goudsmit J, Havenga MJ, Barouch DH. Neutralizing antibodies to adenovirus serotype 5 vaccine vectors are directed primarily against the adenovirus hexon protein. J Immunol (Baltimore, Md: 1950) 2005;174:7179–85.

[56] Hammer SM, Sobieszczyk ME, Janes H, Karuna ST, Mulligan MJ, Grove D, Koblin BA, Buchbinder SP, Keefer MC, Tomaras GD, Frahm N, Hural J, Anude C, Graham BS, Enama ME, Adams E, DeJesus E, Novak RM, Frank I, Bentley C, Ramirez S, Fu R, Koup RA, Mascola JR, Nabel GJ, Montefiori DC, Kublin J, McElrath MJ, Corey L, Gilbert PB. Efficacy trial of a DNA/rAd5 HIV-1 preventive vaccine. N Engl J Med 2013;369:2083–92.

[57] Gurwith M, Lock M, Taylor EM, Ishioka G, Alexander J, Mayall T, Ervin JE, Greenberg RN, Strout C, Treanor JJ, Webby R, Wright PF. Safety and immunogenicity of an oral, replicating adenovirus serotype 4 vector vaccine for H5N1 influenza: a randomised, double-blind, placebo-controlled, phase 1 study. The Lancet (Infectious Diseases) 2013;13: 238–50.

[58] Diaz CM, Chiappori A, Aurisicchio L, Bagchi A, Clark J, Dubey S, Fridman A, Fabregas JC, Marshall J, Scarselli E, La Monica N, Ciliberto G, Montero AJ. Phase 1 studies of the safety and immunogenicity of electroporated HER2/CEA DNA vaccine followed by adenoviral boost immunization in patients with solid tumors. J Transl Med 2013;11:62.

[59] Logunov DY, Dolzhikova IV, Zubkova OV, Tukhvatulin AI, Shcheblyakov DV, Dzharullaeva AS, Grousova DM, Erokhova AS, Kovyrshina AV, Botikov AG, Izhaeva FM, Popova O, Ozharovskaya TA, Esmagambetov IB, Favorskaya IA, Zrelkin DI, Voronina DV, Shcherbinin DN, Semikhin AS, Simakova YV, Tokarskaya EA, Lubenets NL, Egorova DA,

Shmarov MM, Nikitenko NA, Morozova LF, Smolyarchuk EA, Kryukov EV, Babira VF, Borisevich SV, Naroditsky BS, Gintsburg AL. Safety and immunogenicity of an rAd26 and rAd5 vector-based heterologous prime-boost COVID-19 vaccine in two formulations: two open, non-randomised phase 1/2 studies from Russia. Lancet (London, England) 2020;396:887–97.

[60] van Doremalen N, Lambe T, Spencer A, Belij-Rammerstorfer S, Purushotham JN, Port JR, Avanzato VA, Bushmaker T, Flaxman A, Ulaszewska M, Feldmann F, Allen ER, Sharpe H, Schulz J, Holbrook M, Okumura A, Meade-White K, Pérez-Pérez L, Edwards NJ, Wright D, Bissett C, Gilbride C, Williamson BN, Rosenke R, Long D, Ishwarbhai A, Kailath R, Rose L, Morris S, Powers C, Lovaglio J, Hanley PW, Scott D, Saturday G, de Wit E, Gilbert SC, Munster VJ. ChAdOx1 nCoV-19 vaccine prevents SARS-CoV-2 pneumonia in rhesus macaques. Nature 2020;586:578–82.

[61] Badgujar KC, Badgujar VC, Badgujar SB. Vaccine development against coronavirus (2003 to present): an overview, recent advances, current scenario, opportunities and challenges. Diabetes Metab Syndr 2020;14:1361–76.

[62] Rather RA, Islam T, Rehman IU, Pandey D. Development of vaccine against coronavirus disease 2019 (COVID-19) In India. Asian J Adv Med Sci 2021:13–21.

[63] Ikegame S, Siddiquey M, Hung C-T, Haas G, Brambilla L, Oguntuyo K, Kowdle S, Vilardo A, Edelstein A, Perandones C. Neutralizing activity of Sputnik V vaccine sera against SARS-CoV-2 variants. Res Sq 2021;3:rs–400230.

[64] Sharma O, Sultan AA, Ding H, Triggle CR. A review of the progress and challenges of developing a vaccine for COVID-19. Front Immunol 2020;11:2413.

[65] Yatoo MI, Parray OR, Bhat RA, Nazir QU, Haq AU, Malik HU, Fazili MUR, Gopalakrishnan A, Bashir ST, Tiwari R. Novel candidates for vaccine development against Mycoplasma Capricolum subspecies Capripneumoniae (Mccp)—Current knowledge and future prospects. Vaccines (Basel) 2019;7:71.

[66] Makepeace BL, Babayan SA, Lustigman S, Taylor DW. The case for vaccine development in the strategy to eradicate river blindness (onchocerciasis) from Africa. Expert Rev. Vaccines 2015;14:1163–5.

[67] George PJ, Hess JA, Jain S, Patton JB, Zhan T, Tricoche N, Zhan B, Bottazzi ME, Hotez PJ, Abraham D. Antibody responses against the vaccine antigens Ov-103 and Ov-RAL-2 are associated with protective immunity to Onchocerca volvulus infection in both mice and humans. PLoS Negl Trop Dis 2019;13:e0007730.

[68] Khatri V, Chauhan N, Vishnoi K, von Gegerfelt A, Gittens C, Kalyanasundaram R. Prospects of developing a prophylactic vaccine against human lymphatic filariasis–evaluation of protection in non-human primates. Int J Parasitol 2018;48:773–83.

Chapter 2

Evolution and development of vaccines against major human infections

Utkarsha Sahu, Prashant Khare
Department of Microbiology, All India Institute of Medical Sciences, Bhopal, Madhya Pradesh, India

2.1 Introduction

The practice of exposing a person to natural infection for providing immunity against future disease has been practiced for many years for instance, plague, leishmanization (LZ), variolation, etc. [1]. The Chinese practiced the initial trial of vaccines by inoculating the pus from smallpox patients in the nose of a healthy person or scratched on the skin to induce self-limiting infection or causing mild symptoms but give long-term immunity against severe disease. This was also introduced in Europe during the early 18th century. The milkmaids were immune to smallpox due to prior cowpox infection. Well before Jenner, the farmer Benjamin Justy prevented cowpox in his family by inoculating them with cowpox pus [2]. With all this knowledge, Jenner carried out his first human scientific experimentation to investigate the prevention of smallpox in the year 1796. The findings supported the fact that inoculation of cowpox virus prevented smallpox infection lead to the foundations of immunology and vaccine sciences [3]. Edward Jenner's live attenuated vaccine was the only vaccine available for the next 100 years after its discovery. The next vaccine was a chemically attenuated rabies vaccine discovered by Louis Pasteur from the neural tissue. Later on, the work done by American, British, and French researchers resulted in vaccines with killed bacteria. The development of live vaccines started in the 20th century with yellow fever and Bacille de Calmette et Guérin (BCG). Furthermore, Ramon and his co-workers prepared toxoids from inactivated tetanus and diphtheria toxins based on Roux and Behring's findings [4]. Until the 19th century, the cowpox vaccination was practiced worldwide with a major impact in North America and Europe. For approximately the next 150 years, no new vaccine was developed. Later the findings of Louis Pasteur

System Vaccinology. https://doi.org/10.1016/B978-0-323-85941-7.00011-5

disapproving the theory of spontaneous generation and leading to the foundation of the germ theory of disease development were discovered [4,5]. The ending of the 19th century witnessed crucial discoveries in the field of vaccinology mainly contributed by Robert Koch, Louis Pasteur, von Behring, and Ehrlich [4,5]. During this period, the focus was on bacteria, medical applications, and antibody discovery.

The initial work on bacterial vaccines started in 1945 using polysaccharide preparations [1]. With the efforts of Dr. Robert Austrian, the pneumococcal vaccine research was continued in the early 1970s and resulted in the development of 23- and 14-valent vaccines during 1977 and 1984 [6–8]. This was followed by the development of killed whole-cell vaccines, subunit vaccines, and toxoids. Edward Jenner led the foundation of viral vaccines in 1796 with his works on smallpox. The variolation practiced by Jenner was carried forward in large-scale vaccination campaigns that resulted in the eradication of smallpox in 1977 [9]. Similarly, Enders' propagation of poliovirus in non-neural cell cultures ultimately resulted in a polio vaccine that was licensed in 1960 [10]. Similar works were carried out by Hilleman and his workers resulting in a vaccine against severe pediatric diseases such as mumps, measles, rubella, and varicella [5,11]. Hillman and his co-workers also went forward to develop Hepatitis A and B vaccines in the years 1994 and 1986, respectively [12–15]. The protozoans were known even before the virus and bacteria. However, the development of an anti-protozoan vaccine is still neglected. This might be due to the delay in the knowledge of the complete life cycle and involvement of intermediate insect hosts. Malaria causes severe morbidity every year in underdeveloped countries. Still, an effective anti-malaria vaccine is not yet licensed. The initial work of the anti-malaria vaccine was started in 1930 but it did not give promising results [16]. The synthesis of the synthetic anti-malaria vaccine began in the 1980s while the field assays were carried out in the 1990s employing SPf66 subunit of circumsporozoite protein (CSP) and three *P. falciparum* blood-stage antigens [17]. Later in the 1980s, the development of synthetic malaria vaccine was started but even after so many years, they have only reached phase II of clinical trials [18]. Leishmaniasis is another fatal protozoan disease that affects a large set of the population worldwide. The initial practice of inoculative live parasites that caused the mild illness but provided immunity against severe parasitic infection popularly known as LZ, began in the 1970s in Iran and Israel in the 1980s but was later discontinued [19]. This was followed by inoculating the killed parasite and later by using parasite genes cloned in different vectors. These vaccines are the modern-day vaccines being developed against *Leishmania* [20,21]. Recently, due to advancements in biotechnology, cell culture tools and in-vivo studies, different recombinant, subunit, and synthetic vaccines are being developed that might be more effective and immunogenic and safer than the conventional vaccines. In the present book chapter, we have discussed the history of vaccine development against major infectious diseases that caused distress to mankind (Fig. 2.1).

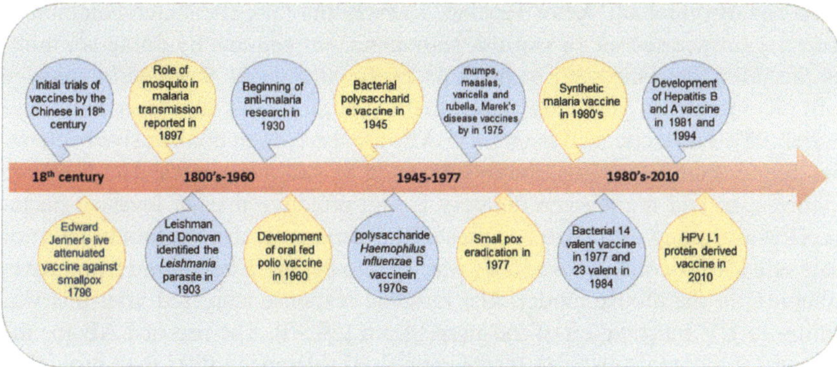

FIG. 2.1 Vaccine development against human infectious diseases.

2.2 Vaccines against major human infections

2.2.1 Bacterial disease vaccines

The research in modern-day, focus on bacterial vaccines started in 1945 employing bacterial polysaccharide preparations. Pneumococcal vaccines, comprising of some serotypes were primarily licensed in 1946 and later withdrawn after the introduction of antibiotics and sulfonamides [1]. These drugs were effective in the clearance of bacterial infections but they did not prevent death in few patients. Due to these reasons and the efforts of Dr. Robert Austrian, the research in pneumococcal vaccines was continued in the early 1970s and lead to the foundation of 23- and 14-valent vaccines during 1977 and 1984 [6–8]. To address the problem of sulfonamide resistance among military recruits, meningococcus vaccines were developed. Different monovalent, bivalent and quadrivalent group vaccines were developed and registered during 1974 and 1982 [22,23]. Currently, the bacterial vaccines are divided into five categories—live attenuated vaccines, killed whole-cell vaccines, subunit vaccines, and toxoids.

Live vaccines comprise living attenuated bacteria. This attenuation could be a targeted or spontaneous mutation of different virulent genes. However, comparatively less pathogenic serotypes or strains could be used to prevent the progression of bacterial disease. The immune response triggered by live bacteria is strong and long-lasting. A major disadvantage of living bacterial vaccine is the regeneration of attenuated bacteria back into the pathogenic form [24]. An example of such vaccine is the Ty21a typhoid vaccine with a number of mutations, including a mutation in polysaccharide gene Vi [25]. The mutation in galE gene causes galactose auxotrophy in bacteria which is present in a limited amount in hosts thus preventing the growth of bacteria outside the laboratory [26]. Another bacterial vaccine, the BCG vaccine against tuberculosis was created from the *Mycobacterium bovis* Calmette-Guérin strain [27]. Another avenue in vaccination is using live attenuated bacteria as a recombinant gene carrier known as recombinant vector vaccine. To carry out this, attenuated commensal bacterial surface secrete or express pathogenic antigen and by doing so, mimics the infection. One such example is of the attenuated *Salmonella enterica* with recombinant *Clostridium tetani* toxin subunit C that was tested in mouse model [28]. The lactic acid bacteria (LAB) are the type of noninvasive bacteria, and due to their safe status, they were tested as vaccine vectors. The LAB are noninvasive, and the antigen delivery is less effective than in invasive bacteria. However, they also have been tested for use as vaccine vectors because of their safe status. *Lactococcus lactis* was used to deliver *Clostridium tetani* toxin subunit C in the mouse model. The immune response triggered after this was similar to UV inactivation of the same strain [29,30]. The use of LAB for the delivery of antigen causes an increased risk of tolerance rather than providing immunity since the commensal bacteria does not induce the host immunity [26].

The inactivated vaccines comprised of killed/inactivated bacteria. This inactivation is carried out by heat, radiation, or chemical treatment of the disease-causing bacteria. Initially, the killed *Vibrio cholera* containing cholera vaccine was administered that provided partial protection for a small period of time after vaccination. The newly developed vaccine is based on the killed *V. cholerae* in combination with the cholera toxin B-subunit [31]. This vaccine induces the production of antigen-specific antibodies that neutralize the cholera toxin and preventing the toxin intermediated diarrhea [32].

Toxoids can be defined as chemically inactivated toxins from bacteria such as *Corynebacterium diphtheria* or *Clostridium tetani*. The infection caused by these bacteria is not harmful, but the exotoxins released by these bacteria cause the illness. The vaccination with toxoids leads to the production of specific antibodies that neutralize the toxins thus providing protection against several diseases [33,34]. Other examples of exotoxin secreting bacteria include *Bacillus anthracis* which secretes exotoxins lethal factor (LF) and edema factor (EF) with common antigen- a protective antigen (PA) crucial for internalizing LF and EF into the host cell [35]. The PA based vaccines protect the cells from LF and EF toxins [36].

The subunit vaccines contain a single antigen. Although, the immune response triggered is comparatively weaker than the whole cell, but the chances of hyperactivation and infection are very less. Polysaccharide vaccines are a type of subunit vaccines that triggers T-cell independent immune response [24]. An example of a polysaccharide vaccine developed in the 1970s against *Haemophilus influenzae type B* (Hib). The Hib infections lead to childhood pneumonia and meningitis. However, the polysaccharide vaccine was not sufficient because T-cell independent immune response only arises in children 16–18 months of age [37,38]. To address this problem, the conjugate vaccines concept was developed with a protein attached to capsular polysaccharide [39]. Three vaccines against Hib are used with different protein conjugates and varying polysaccharide structure and length. These were namely—polyribosyl phosphate outer membrane protein (PRP-OMP), haemophilus conjugate vaccine, and polyribosyl phosphate-T (PRP-T) [40]. Vaccination against *Streptococcus pneumoniae* is carried out by conjugating polysaccharide to diphtheria toxoid, providing immunity to both adults and young children [41,42]. The only disadvantage of this vaccine is that it only provides immunity against only seven serotypes [43,44].

2.2.2 Viral disease vaccines

The initial work of viral vaccines was carried out by the Chinese people who inoculated the pus from smallpox patients into healthy people that caused self-limiting illness with mild symptoms but provided immunity against severe smallpox disease. This work was carried forward by the experiments of Edward Jenner on smallpox in 1796. Jenner was a British physician who variolized himself and inoculated the lesion component from cowpox into an 8-year-old child, who displayed immunity when challenged with the puss from smallpox infected person. At that time Jenner was unaware that he was inoculating a live virus. The work of Edward Jenner later replicated this variolation using the cowpox virus causing minor lesions but providing counter-protection [45]. The major advantage of Jenner's experiment was not only the development of the Variola vaccine but also its universalization [18]. Jenner convinced the government to vaccinate the United States army. The success of this vaccination drive led to large-scale vaccination programs around the world under the campaign of WHO in 1966. Finally, in 1977 smallpox was eradicated [9].

Another major event in the field of viral vaccine development began with Ender's propagation of poliovirus in non-neural cell cultures [10]. The killed Salk polio trivalent vaccine was constructed by culturing virus in renal cells of Macaque, which was licensed in 1955. However, there was a major problem in manufacturing of killed polio vaccine when contamination of live simian virus 40 (SV40) was found in the finished product [46,47]. Various attempts to counter the inconstant potency of the vaccine lead the development of a purified poliomyelitis vaccine- Purivax, that was licensed in 1960 but was discontinued later [2]. A live oral-fed polio vaccine Sabin was developed by using a non-neurotropic poliovirus strain that was licensed in 1960. This vaccine too suffered from SV40 contamination but later was solved [2]. The live polio vaccine remains the paradigm for the eradication of poliomyelitis across the world. The live attenuated vaccines against different pediatric diseases such as mumps, measles, varicella, and rubella were introduced in 1975 by Hilleman and his co-workers [5,11]. They also developed and licensed a vaccine against Marek's disease in the year 1975. Marek's disease causes visceral and neural lymphoma of chickens that affected the economic outcome of the poultry industry [48].

During the 1960s, several efforts were carried out to develop a vaccine against lethal hepatitis A and B virus. The foundation of the hepatitis A vaccine was led in 1973 by isolation of CR326 strain of hepatitis A [49,50]. Complete characterization of hepatitis A virus and disease by Hilleman and his co-workers provided new insights to vaccine development. This later lead to the development of a formaldehyde-killed viral vaccine in 1978 [12]. In 1979, the cell culture and propagation of hepatitis A virus aided the research of the killed virus vaccine against hepatitis A that was licensed in 1994 [12,13]. The discovery of hepatitis B surface antigen in 1965 was a major step in vaccine development against hepatitis B. Till 1968 several trials for purification, yield, inactivation, and efficiency test of different vaccine candidates against hepatitis B were carried out. These resulted in high efficacy vaccine against hepatitis B that came to clinical trials in 1980 and for general use in 1981 [51]. The initial vaccines depended on human carrier plasma however, the amount of adequate carrier human plasma was not sufficient to meet the demand. This helped in developing the recombinant hepatitis B vaccine. The recombinant expression was carried out in yeast and the expression and cultivation were optimized in the laboratory. The hepatitis B vaccine licensed in 1986 was the first recombinant vaccine [14,15]. Another recombinant vaccine was the human papillomavirus (HPV) vaccine with HPC L1 protein-derived virus-like particles that constitute the HPV vaccine came to use in 2010 [52].

2.2.3 Protozoan disease vaccines

Vaccines against bacteria and viruses came to light during 1796 and 1800 by the works of Jenner and Louis Pasteur [53]. However, protozoan diseases like Malaria are known since the 5th century BCE. Hippocrates first described it as a disease associated with bad air [54]. Also, references about malaria disease are also found in Rome, Egypt, and European Renaissance [54]. Even though the first description of parasitic disease came to light 2500 years ago, to date there is no prominent vaccine available against protozoan diseases. The postponement in the development of antiprotozoan vaccines might be due to—(1) the late description of the complete life cycle of protozoans causing Chagas disease, Malaria, and Leishmaniasis and (2) involvement of insects in human transmission. Both of the factors came to light in the 1900s with the work of Ross, Carlos Chagas, Leishman, and Donovan. The role of mosquito in transmission of malaria parasite was reported in 1897 [55]. Carlos Chagas defined that blood-sucking insects spread American Trypanosomiasis also called "Chagas Disease" [56]. In 1903, Leishman and Donovan identified the parasite that causes visceral leishmaniasis (VL) in Indian soldiers [57]. The warm climate of subtropical and tropical countries and poverty exacerbated the protozoan diseases. In India, Leishman and Donovan described Leishmaniasis while Ross explored Malaria. Also, Saul Adler discovered the *Leishmania donovani* vertebrate host in Palestine [58]. Both Leishmaniasis and Malaria are neglected disease and only recently, the active efforts of vaccine development have started against them. These diseases are not endemic in the United States where major vaccine manufacturers are established. The major steps for antiprotozoan vaccines were taken by the United States only after the US troops returned with the *Leishmania* infection from Middle East countries [18]. Since precautionary vaccines are economically less commercial as compared to drug development the pharmaceutical companies have diverted their research toward immunotherapeutic preparations [59,60].

2.2.3.1 Malaria vaccine

About 50% of the world is at threat of malaria disease. In underdeveloped countries, the number of deaths caused by malaria is high mainly among children less than 5 years of age [17,61]. Even though the mortality rates associated with malaria have decreased due to residence-spraying programs, access to combined artemisinin therapy, and insecticide nets, a preventive vaccine is still required [17,61,62]. The anti-malaria vaccine research began in 1930 using dead or inactivated parasites but it provided incomplete protection in ducklings that too after the adjuvant's addition [16]. Later the studies in rodents and ultimately led to the first human vaccine consisting of killed parasites of *Plasmodium falciparum* from mosquito bites [63]. However, this method was not fit for vaccination at a larger scale. Afterward, the use of synthetic peptides of immunogenic parasite proteins started in the 1980s. Several tests of reactogenicity and safety of these vaccines were needed to be performed before introducing it to phase II of clinical trials on children. These tests were time-consuming and difficult and required constant funding and also had a risk of adverse results. To overcome this problem, controlled human malaria infection (CHMI) is used since the 1940s to test Malaria drugs and vaccines [17,64]. In CHMI tests, the sporozoites are inoculated via the bite of the Anopheles mosquito in an optimized environment. Thus, CHMI can be used as an approach for immunization, to regulate the efficacies of drugs and vaccines and study the host immune response against the parasite [64]. The synthesis of the synthetic anti-malaria vaccine began in the 1980s while the field assays were carried out in the 1990s employing SPf66 subunit of CSP and three *P. falciparum* blood-stage antigens [17]. The sequencing of *Plasmodium falciparum* genome was the next step in developing an anti-malaria vaccine [17]. At present, the vaccines against malaria can be classified according to different developmental stages of parasites namely—blood-stage vaccines (BSV), pre-erythrocytic vaccines (PEV), transmission-blocking vaccines, anti-toxic [65], or combination vaccines [61] and anti-pregnancy associated malaria vaccines. However, even after 40 years of study and various clinical trials, the PEV vaccine was the only candidate that reached phase II of clinical trials. The PEV vaccine is reported to be effective against early hepatocyte infection thus, inhibiting the whole parasite life cycle. On the contrary, the BSV vaccine only prevents blood infection and the onset of disease. The TBV vaccine targets the parasite gametocyte stage that infects mosquitoes. The antibodies against the parasite obstruct the binding of parasite gametes to the gut of the vector insect thus inhibiting its development. Hence mosquitoes suckled with TBV- vaccinated blood does not transfer the parasite to another host [65,66]. The basic challenge with developing anti-malaria vaccine is the absence of consistent correlates of protection [17]. The specific antibodies are considered as a key component of an effective immune response against any infection. In the case of malaria, these findings are not consistent in different studies. Even though, 5400 antigens are already identified the precise antigens that trigger the host immune response are still unclear [62].

2.2.3.2 *Leishmania vaccine*

Leishmaniasis is a disease with high morbidity and mortality along with wide geographical distribution [67]. Leishmaniasis has three clinical forms namely, VL, cutaneous leishmaniasis (CL) and muco-cutaneous leishmaniasis. The first generations of anti-leishmanial vaccines comprised of dead parasites with and without adjuvants. These vaccines were oriented against CL. The anti-leishmanial vaccines are broadly divided into the following categories: (1) live parasite with genetically modified constructs, (2) first-generation vaccines with whole killed parasite or fractions of *Leishmania* with or without the adjuvants, (3) second-generation vaccines comprising recombinant DNA and protein vaccines [68]. (4) Third-generation vaccines parasitic antigens cloned in eukaryotic vectors [20,21].

Just like cowpox, the exudates from lesions were injected into healthy children to provide immunity against leishmaniasis. This approach was known as LZ. The live promastigotes isolated from cell-free cultures were replaced by exudates inoculation [19]. In Israel, LZ was used as a prophylactic vaccine during the 1970s and during the 1980s in Iran. LZ was stopped in Israel due to loss of parasite infectivity because of constant subculturing. Also, immunosuppression was reported in people that was evident with decreased responsiveness against pertussis, diphtheria and tetanus vaccine in children after LZ [69]. Presently, there is only a single live prophylactic vaccine comprising of mixture of killed parasite and live virulent *L. major* registered in Uzbekistan [68].

Another approach for the development of anti-leishmanial vaccines was knock-out parasites. Different leishmanial lines were engineered in which various crucial genes required for the survival of parasite in host body were replaced, removed, or blocked. The first construct prepared was a *L. major* knockout of dihydrofolate reductasethymidylate synthase (DHFR-TS) [70]. This construct provided short-term protection in mice but did not provide immunity in monkeys thus the construct was not developed further [71]. Later on, second-generation anti-leishmanial vaccines including genetically modified live/attenuated *Leishmania* parasite and recombinant purified antigen subunits were developed. Finally, the most recent and third-generation vaccines comprise of cloned parasitic antigens in eukaryotic vectors inoculated to host muscles [20,21].

2.3 Discussion

The first trials of vaccination initiated using the live or attenuated organism and later evolved along with the use of live organisms of different species that are not virulent rather provided the host with heterologous protection [1,5]. Recently due to advancements in biotechnology and cell culture tools, different subunit vaccines, recombinant DNA vaccines, and synthetic vaccines are developing [18,45]. Thus, unlike the initial vaccines, the modern-day vaccines gained more safety but mislaid their immunogenicity and effectiveness. However, in some cases, this effect is relapsed by using adjuvants [72]. The first golden era of vaccine development was from the 1800s following the findings of Louis Pasteur. This was followed by the second golden era of vaccine development during 1940–70 [45]. Pasteur introduced a novel approach to vaccination involving isolation, inactivation, and injection of germs that caused the disease [73]. He also discovered the advantages of attenuation in providing immunity and invented an anti-rabies vaccine. Accompanied by Robert Koch, he also developed the anthrax vaccine [73]. Later, Tetanus and Diphtheria causing toxins were discovered. In 1920, Behring and Gaston Ramon described a vaccine for tetanus and diphtheria consisting of inactivated toxins along with alumina as an adjuvant to enhance the vaccine efficacy [74]. In 1924, Camille Guerin and Albert Calmette attenuated *Mycobacterium bovis* and developed BCG vaccine for tuberculosis [75]. In 1949, due to the development of tissue culture technology, vaccines were developed against different viral diseases such as mumps, measles, polio and rubella and against rotavirus, Influenza, and varicella-zoster [76]. Another live attenuated vaccine developed in Cuba in the 1930s was against yellow fever comprising of 17D substrains [77]. The development of the anti-malaria vaccine also began in the 1930s but did not provide satisfactory results [16]. Another attenuated vaccine developed was Sabin vaccine, the first oral vaccine that was used worldwide as of 1962 [78]. The synthesis of the synthetic anti-malaria vaccine began in the 1980s while the field assays were carried out in 1990's employing SPf66 subunit of CSP and three *P. falciparum* blood-stage antigens [17]. In Iran and Israel just like smallpox, the practice of inoculation parasites into humans in order to prove immunity against fatal disease popularly known as LZ was carried out in 1970s–80s [19]. However, this was later discontinued. In addition, during 1970s different polysaccharide vaccines against *Haemophilus influenzae* and pneumococcus were launched [76]. Furthermore, in the late 1900s, advancement in recombinant techniques enabled the production of Hepatitis A and B vaccine and most recently HPV vaccine with HPC L1 protein derived virus like particles that constitute HPV vaccine that came to use in 2010 [12,13,51,52,76]. Here, we have tried to cover the evolutionary and developmental process of vaccines against major infectious agents, and understanding of this process will help to excel the knowledge in the field of vaccinology.

References

[1] Plotkin MSLS PS. A short history of vaccination. In: Plotkin SA, editor. Vaccines. Philadelphia, PA: Saunders; 1988.

[2] Hilleman MR. Vaccines in historic evolution and perspective: a narrative of vaccine discoveries. Vaccine 2000;18(15):1436–47.

[3] Edward J. An enquiry into the causes and effects of the variolae vaccinae. London 1798.
[4] Plotkin SA. Vaccination against the major infectious diseases. C R Acad Sci III 1999; 322(11):943–51.
[5] Hilleman MR. Personal historical chronicle of six decades of basic and applied research in virology, immunology, and vaccinology. Immunol Rev 1999;170:7–27.
[6] Austrian R. Pneumococcus the first 100 years. Rev Infect Dis 1981;3:183–9.
[7] Smit P, et al. Protective efficacy of pneumococcal polysaccharide vaccines. JAMA 1977; 238(24):2613–6.
[8] Hilleman MR, et al. Polyvalent pneumococcal polysaccharide vaccines. Bull World Health Organ 1978;56(3):371–5.
[9] Stockton PL. Smallpox zero: an illustrated history of smallpox and its eradication. Emerg Infect Dis 2010;16(11):1820.
[10] Enders JF, Weller TH, Robbins FC. Cultivation of the Lansing strain of poliomyelitis virus in cultures of various human embryonic tissues. Science 1949;109(2822):85–7.
[11] Hilleman MR. Six decades of vaccine development—a personal history. Nat Med 1998; 4(5 Suppl):507–14.
[12] Provost PJ, Hilleman MR. An inactivated hepatitis A virus vaccine prepared from infected marmoset liver. Proc Soc Exp Biol Med 1978;159(2):201–3.
[13] Provost PJ, Hilleman MR. Propagation of human hepatitis A virus in cell culture in vitro. Proc Soc Exp Biol Med 1979;160(2):213–21.
[14] McAleer WJ, et al. Human hepatitis B vaccine from recombinant yeast. Nature 1984; 307(5947):178–80.
[15] Valenzuela P, et al. Synthesis and assembly of hepatitis B virus surface antigen particles in yeast. Nature 1982;298(5872):347–50.
[16] Freund J, et al. Immunization of Rhesus Monkeys against Malarial Infection (P. Knowlesi) with Killed Parasites and Adjuvants. Science 1945;102(2643):202–4.
[17] Ouattara A, Laurens MB. Vaccines against malaria. Clin Infect Dis 2015;60(6):930–6.
[18] Palatnik-de-Sousa CB, Nico D. The delay in the licensing of protozoal vaccines: a comparative history. Front Immunol 2020;11(204).
[19] Senekji HA, Beattie CP. Artificial infection and immunization of man with cultures of Leishmania tropica. Trans R Soc Trop Med Hyg 1941;34(6):415–9.
[20] Palatnik-de-Sousa CB. Vaccines for leishmaniasis in the fore coming 25 years. Vaccine 2008;26(14):1709–24.
[21] Modabber F. Vaccines against leishmaniasis. Ann Trop Med Parasitol 1995;89(Suppl 1): 83–8.
[22] Gotschlich EC, Liu TY, Artenstein MS. Human immunity to the meningococcus. 3. Preparation and immunochemical properties of the group A, group B, and group C meningococcal polysaccharides. J Exp Med 1969;129(6):1349–65.
[23] Weibel RE, V.V. VPP, Woodhour AF, McLean AA, Hilleman MR. Clinical and laboratory investigations of monovalent and combined meningococcal polysaccharide vaccines Groups A and C. Proc Soc Exp Biol Med 1976;153:436–40.
[24] Giesker K, Hensel M. Types of Bacterial vaccines. In: Sience Direct; 2014, https://www.sciencedirect.com/topics/medicine-and-dentistry/bacterial-vaccine (1) (PDF) Veterinary vaccine development: The helical project. Available from: https://www.researchgate.net/publication/346993577_Veterinary_vaccine_development_The_helical_project [accessed Jan 12 2022].
[25] Germanier R, Füer E. Isolation and characterization of Gal E mutant Ty 21a of Salmonella typhi: a candidate strain for a live, oral typhoid vaccine. J Infect Dis 1975;131(5):553–8.

[26] Detmer A, Glenting J. Live bacterial vaccines—a review and identification of potential hazards. Microb Cell Fact 2006;5:23.

[27] Oettinger T, et al. Development of the Mycobacterium bovis BCG vaccine: review of the historical and biochemical evidence for a genealogical tree. Tuber Lung Dis 1999;79(4): 243–50.

[28] Roberts M, et al. Comparison of abilities of Salmonella enterica serovar typhimurium aroA aroD and aroA htrA mutants to act as live vectors. Infect Immun 2000;68(10):6041–3.

[29] Robinson K, et al. Oral vaccination of mice against tetanus with recombinant Lactococcus lactis. Nat Biotechnol 1997;15(7):653–7.

[30] Norton PM, Le Page RW, Wells JM. Progress in the development of Lactococcus lactis as a recombinant mucosal vaccine delivery system. Folia Microbiol (Praha) 1995; 40(3):225–30.

[31] Black RE, et al. Protective efficacy in humans of killed whole-vibrio oral cholera vaccine with and without the B subunit of cholera toxin. Infect Immun 1987;55(5):1116–20.

[32] D. Sinclair, et al., Oral vaccines for preventing cholera. Cochrane Database Syst Rev, 2011. 2011(3): p. Cd008603.

[33] Marvaud JC, et al. TetR is a positive regulator of the tetanus toxin gene in Clostridium tetani and is homologous to botR. Infect Immun 1998;66(12):5698–702.

[34] Collier RJ. Diphtheria toxin: mode of action and structure. Bacteriol Rev 1975;39(1): 54–85.

[35] Leppla SH. Anthrax toxin edema factor: a bacterial adenylate cyclase that increases cyclic AMP concentrations of eukaryotic cells. Proc Natl Acad Sci USA, 1982;79(10):3162–6.

[36] Reuveny S, et al. Search for correlates of protective immunity conferred by anthrax vaccine. Infect Immun 2001;69(5):2888–93.

[37] Peltola H, et al. Prevention of Hemophilus influenzae type B bacteremic infections with the capsular polysaccharide vaccine. N Engl J Med 1984;310(24):1561–6.

[38] Peltola H, et al. Haemophilus influenzae type B capsular polysaccharide vaccine in children: a double-blind field study of 100,000 vaccinees 3 months to 5 years of age in Finland. Pediatrics 1977;60(5):730–7.

[39] Heath PT, McVernon J. The UK Hib vaccine experience. Arch Dis Child 2002;86(6):396–9.

[40] Griffiths UK, et al. Dose-specific efficacy of Haemophilus influenzae type B conjugate vaccines: a systematic review and meta-analysis of controlled clinical trials. Epidemiol Infect 2012;140(8):1343–55.

[41] Fattom A, et al. Serum antibody response in adult volunteers elicited by injection of Streptococcus pneumoniae type 12F polysaccharide alone or conjugated to diphtheria toxoid. Infect Immun 1990;58(7):2309–12.

[42] Dagan R, et al. Reduction of nasopharyngeal carriage of Streptococcus pneumoniae after administration of a 9-valent pneumococcal conjugate vaccine to toddlers attending day care centers. J Infect Dis 2002;185(7):927–36.

[43] Pittet LF, Posfay-Barbe KM. Pneumococcal vaccines for children: a global public health priority. Clin Microbiol Infect 2012;18(Suppl 5):25–36.

[44] Wolfe RM. Update on adult immunizations. J Am Board Fam Med 2012;25(4):496–510.

[45] D'Amelio E, Salemi S, D'Amelio R. Anti-infectious human vaccination in historical perspective. Int Rev Immunol 2016;35(3):260–90.

[46] Sweet BH, Hilleman MR. The vacuolating virus, S.V. 40. Proc Soc Exp Biol Med 1960;105:420–7.

[47] Hilleman MR. Discovery of simian virus 40 (SV40) and its relationship to poliomyelitis virus vaccines. Dev Biol Stand 1998;94:183–90.

[48] Hilleman MR. Marek's disease vaccine: its implications in biology and medicine. Avian Dis 1972;16(1):191–9.
[49] Mascoli CC, et al. Recovery of hepatitis agents in the marmoset from human cases occurring in Costa Rica. Proc Soc Exp Biol Med 1973;142(1):276–82.
[50] Provost PJ, et al. Etiologic relationship of marmoset-propagated CR326 hepatitis A virus to hepatitis in man. Proc Soc Exp Biol Med 1973;142(4):1257–67.
[51] Szmuness W, et al. A controlled clinical trial of the efficacy of the hepatitis B vaccine (Heptavax B): a final report. Hepatology 1981;1(5):377–85.
[52] Gupta G, Glueck R, Patel PR. HPV vaccines: global perspectives. Hum Vaccin Immunother 2017;13(6):1–4.
[53] Gribanov ED, Potapchuk TB. The classic work of Girolamo Fracastoro (on the 450th anniversary of the publication of his book "De contagione et de contagiosis morbis et curatione"). Voen Med Zh 1996;317(8):74–6.
[54] Nerlich A. Paleopathology and paleomicrobiology of Malaria. Paleomicrobiology of Humans 2016;4(6):155–160.
[55] Ross R. The role of the mosquito in the evolution of the malarial parasite: the recent researches of Surgeon-Major Ronald Ross, I.M.S. 1898. Yale J Biol Med 2002;75(2):103–5.
[56] Steverding D. The history of Chagas disease. Parasit Vectors 2014;7:317.
[57] Ross R. Note on the bodies recently described by leishman and donovan. Br Med J 1903;2(2237):1261–2.
[58] Adler GDS. Pioneer of Tropical Medicine: A Biography, 1st ed. Rehovot Balaban Publishers; 1997.
[59] Kremer M, Snyder CM. Why are drugs more profitable than vaccines? NBER Working Paper Series Reference No. 9833; 2003. Available at: http://www.nber.org/papers/w9833.
[60] Palatnik-de-Sousa CB. Editorial: preventive vaccination. Procedia Vaccinol 2015;9:1–5.
[61] van den Berg M, et al. RTS,S malaria vaccine pilot studies: addressing the human realities in large-scale clinical trials. Trials 2019;20(1):316.
[62] Tuju J, et al. Vaccine candidate discovery for the next generation of malaria vaccines. Immunology 2017;152(2):195–206.
[63] Clyde DF, et al. Immunization of man against sporozite-induced falciparum malaria. Am J Med Sci 1973;266(3):169–77.
[64] Stanisic DI, McCarthy JS, Good MF. Controlled human malaria infection: applications, advances, and challenges. Infect Immun 2017;86(1):e00479–517.
[65] WHO. Guidelines for the evaluation of plasmodium falciparum vaccines in populations exposed to natural infection. https://www.who.int/tdr/publications/training-guideline-publications/evaluation-of-plasmodium-falciparum/en/ (accessed August 22, 2018).
[66] WHO. Malaria transmission blocking vaccines: an ideal public good. https://www.who.int/tdr/publications/tdr-research-publications/malaria-transmission-blocking-vaccines/en/ (accessed August 22, 2018)
[67] Leishmaniasis. https://www.who.int/news-room/fact-sheets/detail/leishmaniasis (accessed September 13, 2019).
[68] Khamesipour A, et al. Leishmaniasis vaccine candidates for development: a global overview. Indian J Med Res 2006;123(3):423–38.
[69] Nadim A, et al. Effectiveness of leishmanization in the control of cutaneous leishmaniasis. Bull Soc Pathol Exot Filiales 1983;76(4):377–83.
[70] Cruz A, Coburn CM, Beverley SM. Double targeted gene replacement for creating null mutants. Proceedings of the National Academy of Sciences of the United States of America, 88; 1991:7170–4.

[71] Titus RG, et al. Development of a safe live Leishmania vaccine line by gene replacement. Proc Natl Acad Sci USA, 1995;92(22):10267–71.

[72] Hilleman MR, Hampil B, Sweet BH. Poliovirus vaccines in mineral oil adjuvant. I. Animal toxicity and serologic response data. J Allergy 1963;34:413–9.

[73] Bordenave G. Louis Pasteur (1822-1895). Microbes Infect 2003;5(6):553–60.

[74] Kaufmann SH. Remembering Emil von Behring: from tetanus treatment to antibody cooperation with phagocytes. mBio 2017;8(1), e00117–17.

[75] Tran V, Liu J, Behr MA. BCG vaccines. Microbiol Spectr 2014;2(1) Mgm2-0028-2013.

[76] De Gregorio E, Rappuoli R. From empiricism to rational design: a personal perspective of the evolution of vaccine development. Nat Rev Immunol 2014;14(7):505–14.

[77] Kleinert RDV, et al. Yellow fever: integrating current knowledge with technological innovations to identify strategies for controlling a re-emerging virus. Viruses 2019;11(10):960.

[78] Van Damme P, et al. The safety and immunogenicity of two novel live attenuated monovalent (serotype 2) oral poliovirus vaccines in healthy adults: a double-blind, single-centre phase 1 study. Lancet 2019;394(10193):148–58.

Part II

Immunology of vaccine designing

Chapter 3

Vaccine Omics: role of bioinformatics in vaccinology

Shivani Krishna Kapuganti, Aparna Bhardwaj, Namyashree Nayak, Taniya Bhardwaj, Prateek Kumar, Rajanish Giri

Indian Institute of Technology Mandi, School of Basic Sciences, VPO Kamand, Himachal Pradesh, India

3.1 History of vaccinology

Vaccination has protected humans from many fatal viral infections and considerably increased their life expectancy. Edward Jenner is credited with the discovery of vaccination. He discovered the mechanism of variolation, now called vaccination, which basically involved using an attenuated organism to prevent infection from a virus. Jenner first used cowpox in 1796, which causes mild infections in humans to prevent infection by the fatal smallpox. Smallpox was completely eradicated by 1979 [1]. The most important steps in completely eradicating a virus involve extensive screening and tracing contacts. The steps become easier to act on assiduously if the infections have visible symptoms; as in the case of, like smallpox and measles. However, in the case of asymptomatic infections, like polio, complete eradication is a tough challenge. Another milestone achieved in this line is the eradication of rinderpest virus, declared by WHO in 2011. Rinderpest causes high mortality in cattle which could badly affect the economy of the countries that depend on animal husbandry [2]. In 1885, Pasteur developed the rabies vaccine by drying the virus particles obtained from the infected rabbit brain. Nowadays, the attenuated virus is grown in tissue culture [3]. In a similar manner, the early vaccine for the Yellow Fever Virus was developed by passaging the virus-infected tissues by M. Theiler in 1938. The viscerotropic virulence of the virus cultivated in tissues for three long years started diminishing such that subcutaneous injection into monkeys produced mild infection [4]. Similar approach was taken for measles and poliomyelitis vaccines developed in the 1950s and 1960s, respectively. Rubella, influenza, rotavirus, tuberculosis, and typhoid vaccines have been developed from attenuated viruses. Such vaccines induce a strong sustained immune response, especially at the mucosal surfaces. A limitation with attenuated vaccines is a reversal to virulence, as seen in some cases of oral polio and tuberculosis vaccines (BCG). Using killed viruses is another method of vaccination. A few examples

System Vaccinology. https://doi.org/10.1016/B978-0-323-85941-7.00012-7

are vaccines for pneumococcus, meningococcus, and typhoid bacillus. Subunit vaccines that use only a part of the virus were also developed. However, whole-unit vaccines offer the advantage of providing multi-epitope antigens [5,6].

WHO established the expanded program on immunization in 1974 because of which, by the 1980s, infectious diseases of children were no longer a significant threat. This had decreased the burden on the health care system. By 2012, a dramatic decrease in childhood tetanus and measles was observed as compared to the 1980s. However, it is still a challenge to reach the underprivileged and isolated communities of the world. Even though vaccination causes severe side effects in some people, the benefits outweigh the risks [7].

Pneumonia and diarrhea are common factors that are responsible for child mortality in underdeveloped countries. They are caused by *Pneumococcus pneumoniae* and rotavirus, respectively. Pneumococcus requires 10–13 components to prepare the subunit vaccine. Vaccines like this are challenging to prepare and are expensive to produce [8]. Moreover, awareness about these diseases and related vaccines is not as high as measles or polio. To address the lack of awareness, the Global alliance for vaccines and immunization (GAVI) was established in 2000. Several international donors support GAVI because of which it was able to subsidize the cost of such vaccines in poor countries. Advanced Market Commitment also contributed to this cause. GAVI established the pneumococcal and rotavirus accelerated development and introduction plans and the Hib initiative, which helped spread local awareness about these infections and conducting vaccine trials in association with academic institutions. Programs like GAVI can help meet the cost of vaccination in underdeveloped countries [9]. In Fig. 3.1, the major milestones achieved in the history of vaccines are shown in a chronological order.

3.2 Immune response involved in vaccination

An organism's immune system protects it from foreign molecules, generally called antigens, that can cause possible harm to the host. For example, when it comes to animals, the immune system offers protection from pathogens such as virus, bacteria, protozoa fungi other parasites, and toxins. It even defends the host from tumors to a certain extent. Rarely the immune system can start attacking self-factors/cells and lead to auto-immune disorders [10].

Immune response to a pathogen or foreign elements can be classified as either innate or acquired. Innate immunity is the first line of defense mechanism inherently present in the host and doesn't require prior exposure to the antigen. It consists mainly of the mononuclear cell lineage such as macrophages, and polymorphonuclear leukocytes. It gives a rapid response and is non-specific, though, capable of distinguishing between self and non-self-antigens [11].

Physiological barriers such as skin, mucosal layers, body secretions, etc., and cells of myeloid lineage such as natural killer cells, which are recruited rapidly to the site of infection upon activation by secreted cytokines, are effectors

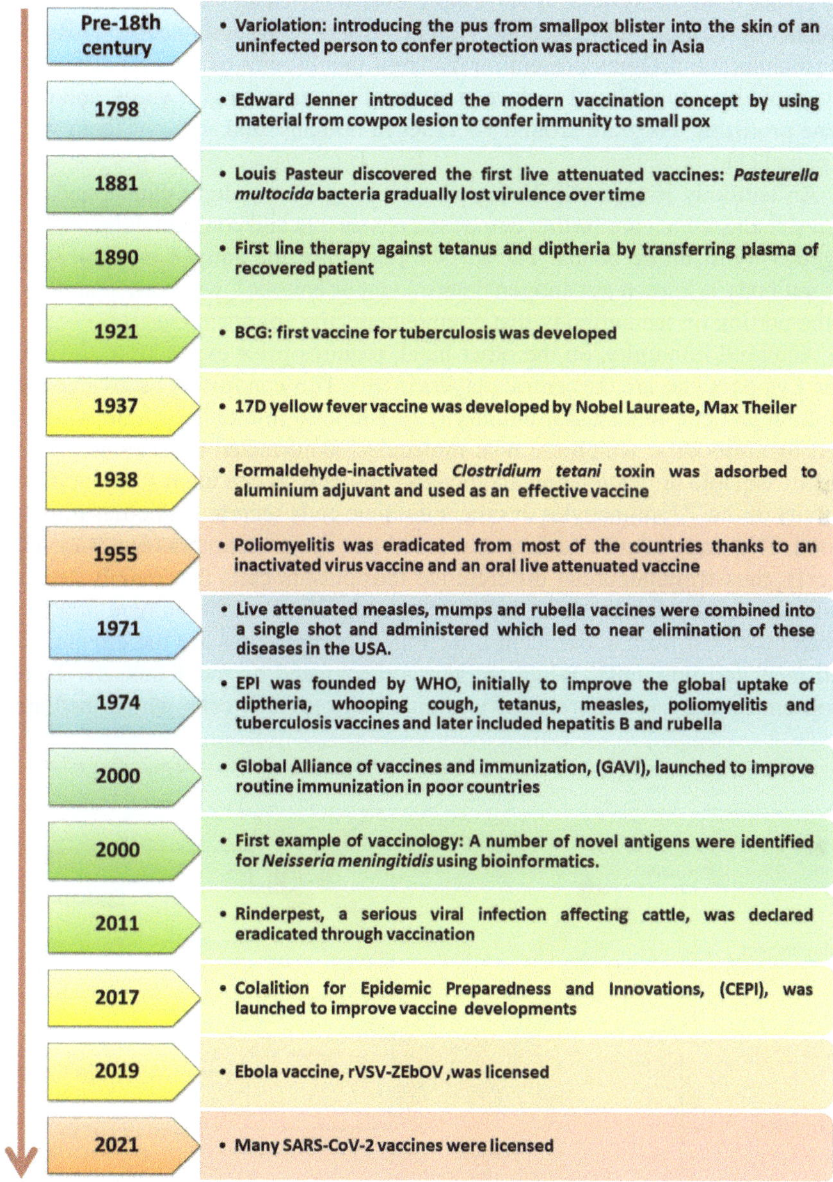

FIG. 3.1 Major milestones achieved in the history of vaccinology.

of innate immunity. The progenitors of this myeloid lineage include phagocytic cells such as monocytes, macrophages, and neutrophils. Apart from phagocytosis, pathogens can also be killed by the action of complement proteins. Interferons (IFNs) and toll-like receptors (TLRs) also play a massive role in the innate immune system. IFNs are proteins secreted by cells that have been infected by viruses and induce antiviral activity in surrounding cells. TLRs are transmembrane proteins present on different membranes of the cell. They can detect and bind to different surface proteins of bacteria, fungi, viruses, and even some protozoa. They are around 10 TLRs in humans, and some of them work in pairs [11].

An antibody is typically Y-shaped consisting of two light chains and two heavy chains which are further composed of variable and constant domains held together by disulfide bonds. The surface portion of the antigen recognized by the antibody is known as "antigen determinant or epitope," whereas, "Paratope" is the portion on the antibody that complements the epitope.

Acquired immunity, on the other hand, requires prior exposure to the antigen. Lymphocytes are the central players in this. This can further be divided into humoral and cell-mediated immunity [12]. Humoral immunity is mainly mediated by antibodies, which are host molecules, synthesized by B lymphocytes and are capable of recognizing and binding antigens. B cell upon stimulation by activity of the T lymphocytes or others immune cells secrete antibodies into the blood. They may also be surface-expressed and act as receptors (Fig. 3.2). The B cells thus stimulated can differentiate into plasma cells that mainly secrete antibodies and memory cells that retain the memory of the antigen and thus protect the host from subsequent infection. T lymphocytes are the effectors of cell-mediated immunity. When antigen is recognized by the T cell, the T cell proliferates and can differentiate into either cytotoxic T cells which mediates

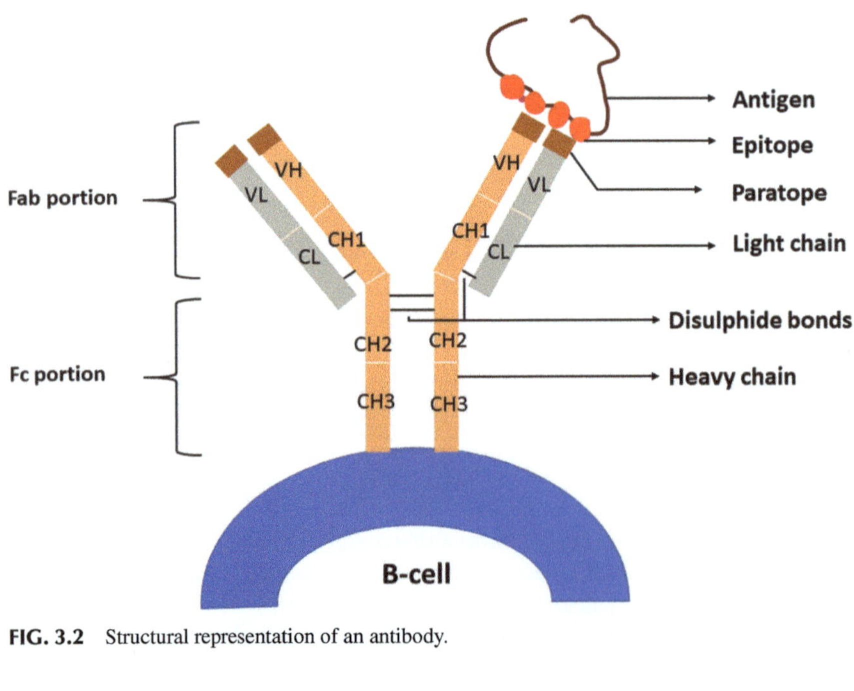

FIG. 3.2 Structural representation of an antibody.

lysis of virus-infected cells or Helper T cells which have a role in both cell-mediated and humoral immune responses. MHC molecules are membrane glycoproteins that are used by host cells to present the antigen to the T cell. Any cell can present intracellular peptide antigens via the class I MHC molecules to cytotoxic T cells which detect the antigen via their CD8 membrane receptor. Macrophages and B cells present fragments of extracellular peptide antigens via the class II MHC molecules to helper T cells which detect the antigen via their CD4 membrane receptor (Fig. 3.3) [12].

Adaptive immunity has four main characteristics: antigen specificity, immunological memory diversity, and self/non-self-recognition ability [13]. The host body produces antibodies and cytotoxic cells to fight pathogens when exposed. Some of these antibody-producing plasma cells and cytotoxic cells are maintained as memory cells to protect the host from subsequent infection by the same pathogen. This is called natural active immunity. When a person is exposed to a pathogen, the antibodies produced can be transferred to another person to offer the person immunity from the same or closely related pathogen. This is called natural passive immunity. Vaccination falls under artificial active immunity where parts of the pathogen are manually introduced into the host, eliciting a prolonged protective immune response [14].

As mentioned earlier, vaccines induce artificial active immunity. A mixture of antigens derived from the pathogen is often used to immunize the host. This is known as vaccination. Live attenuated vaccines such as the Sabin polio vaccine induce secretory IgA in the intestine which defends the host against the naturally acquired virus. Inactivated or killed vaccines are effective but less

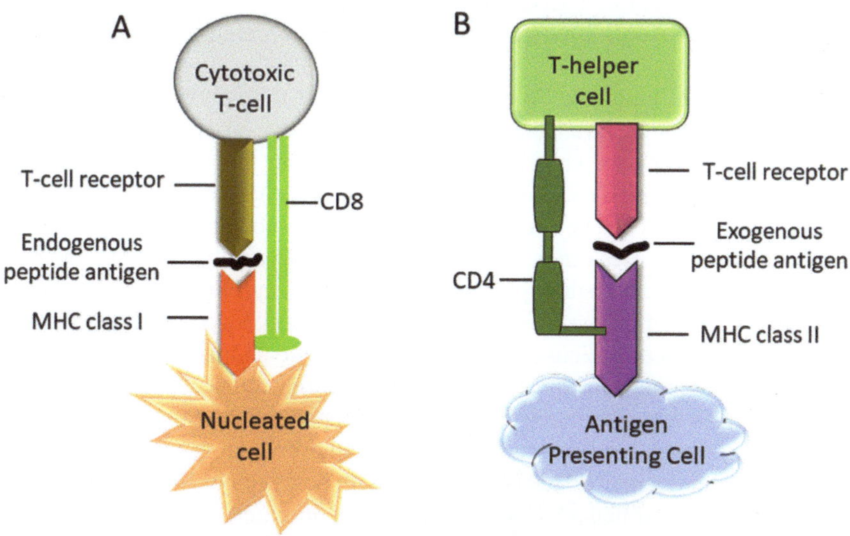

FIG. 3.3 (A) APC presenting MHC-I bound peptide to CD8+ T-cell. (B) APC presenting MHC-II bound peptide to CD4+ T-cell.

immunogenic [14]. Therefore, they require booster doses as they don't stimulate sufficient humoral or cell-mediated immunity. Recombinant antigen vaccine such as the hepatitis B vaccine primarily induces humoral response as the antigens are processed via MHC-II pathway [15]. In DNA vaccines, the fragment/s of the pathogen's genome consisting of coding regions is introduced into the host cells directly where the fragment incorporates into chromosomal DNA or exists as episome and codes for the foreign proteins. These proteins act as immunogenic rather than the viral DNA itself. DNA vaccines induce both humoral and cell-mediated immunity [16].

3.3 Vaccine immunoinformatics and in-silico designing of vaccines

If the knowledge of the genome of a disease-causing organism is known, then it is possible to identify all the possible epitopes (on proteins) that can be produced through bioinformatics tools. These epitopes can be arranged into combinations that elicit a robust immune response and thus predict a possible vaccine construct. This is called reverse vaccinology [17]. This approach has certain advantages, such as it reduces the cost and time of vaccine development. Some proteins of an infectious organism are produced later in its life cycle, but such proteins can act as good allergens or vaccine candidates. With reverse vaccinology, such proteins can be identified early, further, the number of proteins that can be incorporated into the vaccine can be narrowed down efficiently. For this, the knowledge of the genome is an absolute requirement. His method was first applied to develop vaccine for *Neisseria menigitidis* [18]. Lipid and carbohydrate-based vaccines cannot be synthesized using reverse vaccinology. Although, lipids and carbohydrates are being used as adjuvants these days [19].

Bioinformatic tools can be employed to predict the epitopes on a protein. Already databases are available with stored knowledge of epitopes which can be analyzed. Further, the knowledge of all the reactions involved in the immune response to an epitope is required. Infectious proteins can have more than one epitope. These epitopes can be combined to synthesize a subunit vaccine. Even epitopes of different viruses can be combined to synthesize a polyvalent vaccine that could confer immunity to multiple viruses simultaneously. However, modern subunit vaccines sometimes are less immunogenic and need an adjuvant to increase the potential immunogenicity. In such cases, synthetic and natural carbohydrate structures have come a long way as adjuvants and are in clinical trials [19].

There are a few characteristics that the epitopes should have to be considered good vaccine candidates. These include the cellular localization of the viral protein, antigenicity, lack of similarity with host proteins, lower amount of hydrophobicity, and helical structures. Since the immune cells, in most cases, interact with the surface of the infectious organism. As immune cells keep freely circulating in the blood, it will be a better strategy to choose viral proteins that localize to the cell surface [20]. If viral proteins are similar to the host proteins, there is a possibility that antibodies induced against viral proteins can cross-react with host proteins resulting in an autoimmune reaction. Therefore, this should be avoided. Immune factors recognize epitopes present on the surface of the proteins easily. If the proteins are hydrophobic in nature, there is a good chance that these epitopes would be buried in the protein's interior. If the protein is rich in helical structure, it might even form transmembrane domains, thus, becoming unavailable to the immune cells [21].

These are all the criteria that webservers mostly employ for reverse vaccinology and predicting possible epitopes (basic methods are shown in Fig. 3.4). Some examples of such servers are Vaxign, Vacceed, NERVE, and Jenner-predict server. In these servers, the viral protein sequence is required or some servers have a database of certain infectious organisms that can be chosen as an input. Some servers such as VIOLIN and MycobacRV have

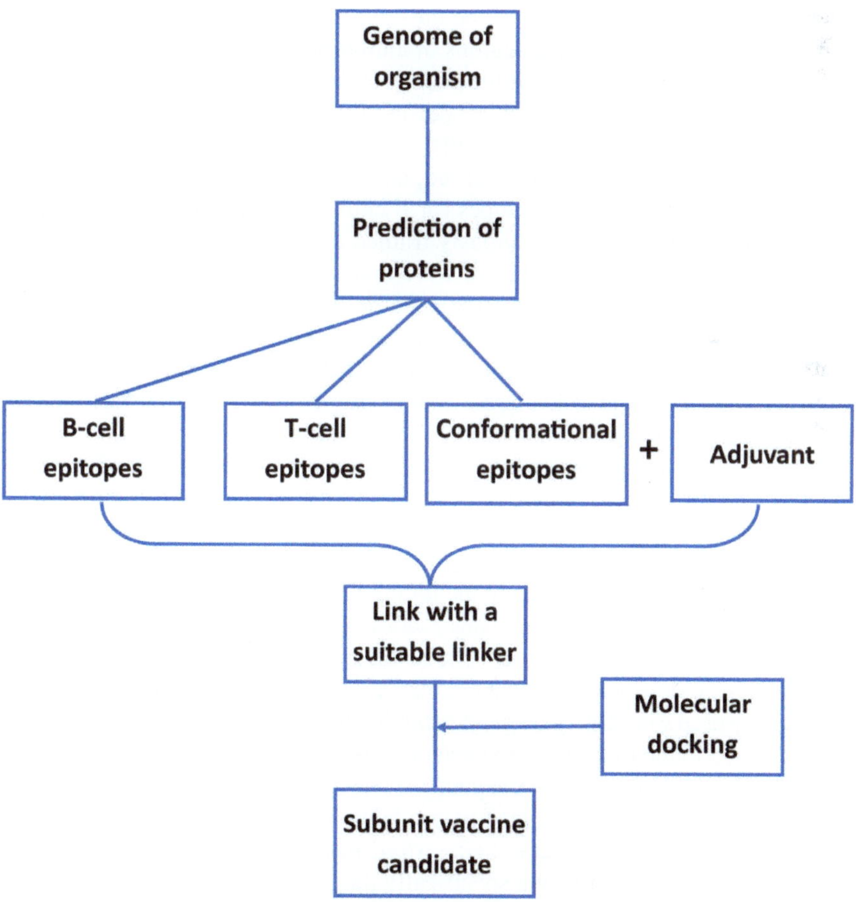

FIG. 3.4 Schematic representation of basic steps involved in reverse vaccinology.

databases for already identified vaccines. Mainly, there are two types of predictors: those that can identify peptide sequences that can bind to the MHC molecules present in the T cells and those that can identify B cell epitopes. Since T-cell epitopes bind to human leukocyte antigen in a linear form, these epitopes can be predicted accurately [12]. The predicted epitope can be tested in-vitro to check for their ability to elicits a T-cell response using ELISA or elispot assay. CD4+ targeting antigens are good candidates as T helper cells are critically important to the development of memory B-cell (antibody) and memory CTL (cytotoxic T-cell) responses and being active against pathogens on their own. Softwares like CTLPred, iVAX, nHLAPred, SVMHC, ProPred-I, GPS-MBA, PREDIVAC, TEpredict, SVMHC, NetMHC, NetCTL, MHC2 Pred, KISS, IEDB, BIMAS, POPI, Epitopemap, FRED2, Rankpep, BIMAS, MAPPP, PickPocket, and MHC2MIL can identify T cell epitopes. MHC binding peptides are presented to the surface of killer T cells. The prediction of epitopes binding to MHC-II is more complicated as MHC-II has the open groove structure instead of the closed groove structure in MHC-I. The complementarity determining regions of antibodies are flexible and recognize 3D epitopes [22]. Therefore, limited tools are available to predict B-cell epitopes as they are challenging to model in silico. Examples of software that predict sequential epitopes for B cells include BCPREDS, BepiPred, BEpro or PEPITO, ABCpred, Bcepred, IgPred, and BCEP. At the same time, servers that predict conformational epitopes for B cells include the CEP, SEPPA, and DiscoTope. Computers are previously trained to with identified epitopes and non-epitopes. Based on this, the software makes predictions on new proteins. Different techniques such as position-specific scoring matrices, artificial neural networks (ANNs), hidden Markov models, and support vector machines (SVMs) are used for this machine learning (ML). Servers such as MHCBN AntiJen, AgAbDb, and IEDB are a few examples that have databases about existing antigens [23].

B-Cell and T-cell epitope predictors are linear epitope predictors. But inside the cells, a viral protein would probably assume a tertiary folded structure to become functional. This would allow different regions of the protein sequence to come together, which may then act as a conformational epitope. Such epitopes are highly flexible, leading to the failure of vaccines if only linear epitopes were considered during vaccine construction. Molecular docking helps calculate the binding affinity between cellular factors and candidate viral proteins, thus helping in designing the best conformational or linear epitope. For example, Kumar et al., in 2021, designed a candidate vaccine against SARS-CoV-2 using bioinformatic tools and a molecular docking approach [24]. This example is covered in detail later in the chapter.

Conventional methods of vaccine production cost a lot of time and money. Reverse vaccinology, as mentioned earlier, has a few advantages over this: targeted immune responses via specifically designed constructs that minimize the side effects and considerable reduction of cost and time. The basic idea in this method recognizes epitopes that can bind with antibodies and T cell receptors. Then the constructs are designed using a combination of these epitopes followed by simulation trials to evaluate vaccine efficiency. The selection of the B cell and T cell epitopes is the most important step, which induces a humoral and cellular immune response, respectively. Then these epitopes are fused with adjuvants using appropriate linkers. Later, simulation helps in identifying the best arrangement of the epitopes. Jenner-predict and VacSol predict vaccine candidates are based on a decision-tree learning algorithm. Vacceed uses ML to predict eukaryotic pathogens. The number of antigens to be validated through experimental assays needs to be determined. This is the limiting step in conventional vaccinology, however, through computational techniques, it is possible to scan the antigens along with cellular defense processes and, therefore, narrow down the antigens to be screened. Adjuvants work to elicit more substantial and prolonged immune responses. They also help in refreshing the immune system in older patients and decrease the required dosage. Therefore, adjuvants are included in vaccine constructs [25]. Once the B-cell and T-cell epitopes are selected, as mentioned earlier, the epitopes and the adjuvants are linked together using linker or spacer sequences. Linkers provide intramolecular flexible regions and also prevent misfolding of proteins. The criteria that one looks for while choosing a linker are its length, amino acid composition, arrangement, hydrophobicity, secondary structure, potential intramolecular interactions, and sensitivity to proteases. SynLinker is a software that one can use to choose suitable linkers based on the input criteria given by the user and model the constructs. The server has a database of around 2150 peptide linkers [26].

After deciding the vaccine sequence, its 3D structure needs to be modeled. The tertiary structure predictors search the PDB to find any matching sequences then give output based on E-value, alignment length, identity, and total score. Based on these values, the best model is selected. The model generating software includes Rosetta, EasyModeller4.0, SWISS-MODEL, Phyre2, I-Tasser, and RaptorX that use different techniques such as matching homology or PDB structures ab-initio folding [27–29]. Then, potential energy minimalization is used to bring down the energy level of the constructed model to a level close to the most stable form. Molecular dynamic simulation is then used to study the movement of atoms and molecules in space to find the best fit, followed by structural validation [30].

An example of the case study is the multiepitope vaccine designed by Kumar et al. against SARS-CoV-2 using in silico approach. The structural proteins spike, envelope, and nucleocapsid of SARS-COV-2 were used to predict highly antigenic B-cell and T-cell epitopes. Available translated protein sequences available on UniProt were used for the study. IEDB and BepiPred were used to predict B-cell epitopes with 49% sensitivity and 75% specificity. IEDB was also utilized to predict MHC-II binders. The top 10 hits based on IC_{50} values were selected. MHC-I binders for supertype A3 were predicted using NetCTL1.2.

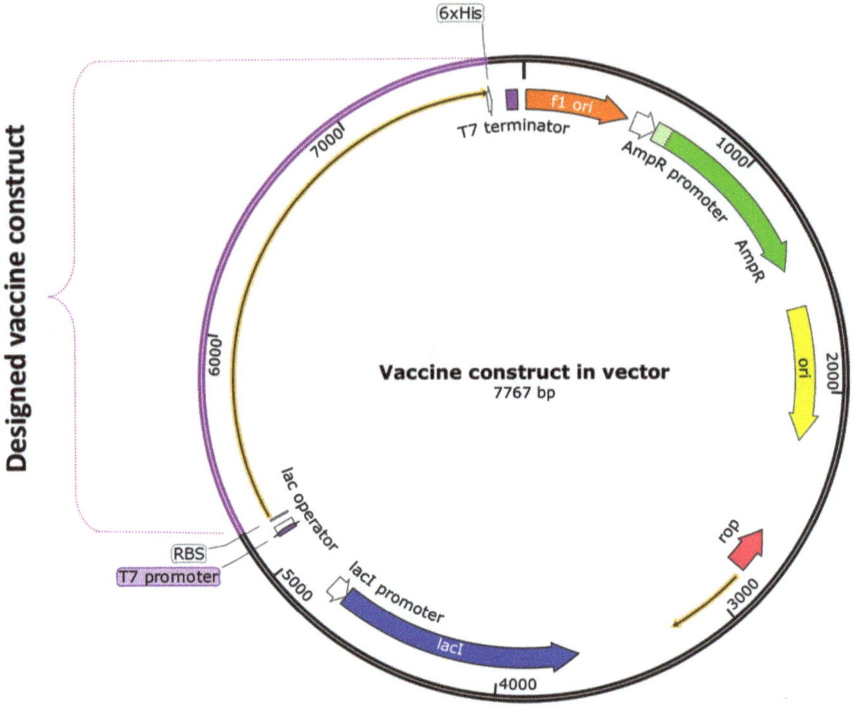

FIG. 3.5 Virtually cloning the designed vaccine construct into pET21a+ vector using snapgene.

Proteasomal cleavage was predicted using ANN, and TAP transport efficiency was predicted using a weight matrix. IFNepitope was used to predict epitopes that can induce cell-mediated immunity. The selected sequences were linked together using CTL linker (AAY), HTL linker (GPGPG), and B epitope linker (KK), and β-defensin 1 was used as the adjuvant. After vaccine sequence construction the antigenicity was predicted using ANTIGENpro and VaxiJen v2.0. The servers AllerTOP v2.0 and AllergenFP were used to predict allergenicity. Physicochemical properties were assayed using ProtParam server. Psipred was used to predict the secondary structure of the coded protein and PONDR and IUPRED 2A were used to generate the disorder profile. I-TASSER was used to generate a tertiary structure, and the construct was evaluated and validated via RAMPAGE and PROCHECK. PIPER program by Schrodinger was used to analyze the docking with TLR3 and TLR5. The stability of this interaction was checked in an aqueous environment for 20ns. Finally, the construct was virtually cloned into pET21a+ vector using SnapGene, and translation was simulated (Fig. 3.5). A moderate amount of disorder was predicted in the cloned product. The adjuvant in the construct showed interaction with TLR3 and TLR5 [24].

3.4 Commonly used epitope predictors

3.4.1 Prediction of B-cell epitopes

The antigenic determinant regions (or epitopes) on the antigens are determined by the complementary determinant regions (CDRs) (or paratopes) on the hypervariable loops of the variable domains of antibodies. Thus antibodies, after activation, recruit immune components and clear the antigen via humoral immunity. This property of the antibody is used as a key basis in the identification of virtual non-self-molecules, which makes it useful in immunodiagnostics, validation of therapeutics like epitope/peptide-based vaccines, antibody production, etc. [31]. There are two types of antigenic sites which were classified as continuous and discontinuous based on accessible amino acid clusters on the surface of the antigen [32]. The main purpose is to identify the specific sites over antigen, leading to structural-functional studies and antibody production for therapeutic means.

Prediction of continuous/linear B-cell epitope (BCE): Linear epitopes consist of amino acid residues present locally in the antigen peptide where antibodies specifically bind. Continuous epitopes are less commonly present than discontinuous epitopes. Predominantly these epitopes are present in the loop regions on the protein's surface and provide the best antigenic sites [33]. Here, we have listed several predictors for the prediction of B-cell epitopes.

- EPMLR: Prediction is based on the amino acid sequence, which predicts linear epitopes. The prediction model was built on multiple linear regression. For training and testing of the model, BEOD (BEOracle dataset) is used. The data from this predictor are 10-fold cross-validated gives average sensitivity of 81.8% and precision of 64.1% [34].
- iBCE-EL: The investigation of the linear B-cell epitope is done by six ML algorithms; SVM, random forest (RF), extremely randomized tree (ERT), AdaBoost (AB), gradient boosting (GB), and k-nearest neighbors (k-NN). It is an ensemble approach as it combines two different ML-based predictors which are ERT and GB. Then, the final prediction combines the amino acid composition and physicochemical properties to give an average final output from these predictors. Two non-redundant datasets are used from the Immune Epitope Database (IEDB), one dataset with 5550 experimentally validated BCEs and the other with 6893 non-BCEs. The data from this predictor is 5-fold cross-validated with 66.7% accuracy of the predicted BCE [35].
- EpiDope: It takes the primary amino acid sequence as input and uses a deep neural network (DNN) for the epitopic region prediction. DNN algorithm makes this predictor better than other linear epitope predictors as it takes into consideration the classification features of the query sequence. Potential prediction is achieved by using context-sensitive embedding of the input amino acids. The local information of the amino acids and the context information are encoded numerically for the considered sliding window from the

whole input protein. The dataset is created from all the verified regions from the IEDB [36].

- BepiPred-2.0: It is a sequence-based B-cell epitope predictor trained from epitopic data from the 3D crystal structure of the IEDB database. The dataset contains 649 antigen-antibody complex crystal structures from PDB. The model is trained by the 5-fold cross-validation approach of the RF regression algorithm. Each centered residue, in a window size of 9, is computed for the hydrophobicity, polarity, relative surface accessibility, and secondary surface [37].

Prediction of discontinuous/conformational B-cell epitopes: These determinants are formed during the folding of the protein into the native structure. The different regions of the antigenic proteins which are distantly located come close to become functional 3D structures. These epitopes are known as discontinuous epitopes, and most of the B-cell epitopes are discontinuous [33].

- DiscoTope: It uses the 3D structure of the query protein for the prediction of discontinuous B-cell epitopes. This method combines the calculated log odd ratios of features such as the amino acid statistical difference between epitope and non-epitope regions, spatial information, and surface accessibility of the residues for prediction. The structure-based methods outperform the sequence-based methods for the epitope prediction. The output from DiscoTope identifies only 15.5% residues from the discontinuous epitope with 95% specificity. But the conventional Parker hydrophilicity scale detects 11% of the total epitopic residues with the same specificity [38].
- PEPITO: The predictor uses the information of propensity scale and side-chain orientation of amino acids. It also combines the concept of solvent accessibility using half-sphere exposure values at a threshold of multiple distances from the target residue. The dataset is derived from DiscoTope and Epitome datasets with different epitope/non-epitope protein and classification rules. The former dataset is having 75 and later has 140 protein chains with different distance criteria of 4Å and 6Å, respectively, of antigen regions from the CDRs of Ab [39].
- ElliPro: This structure-based predictor server identifies discontinuous epitopes from the antigen-antibody complex 3D structures. It can take input in two forms: firstly, it accepts protein with UniProt ID or FASTA format sequence for modeling the 3D structure. The second form asks for the PDB ID or PDB format query protein. Then, the ElliPro uses the minimum residue score or the threshold value (set differently for different queries) for the prediction. Three algorithms used in this server are for protein shape approximation, residual protrusion index (PI), and identification of the neighbor residue cluster based on PI. In addition, for the visualization of the epitopes, a molecular visualization tool, Jmol is used. The testing dataset of the Ellipro contains 39 proteins having epitopes with only one discontinuous epitope [40].

- PEPOP 2.0: Predicts the peptides for discontinuous epitopes, which are experimentally used as an antigen and act as Ag inhibitors or replace the Ag in the Ab-Ag complex. It uses 34 algorithms for giving and output for the prediction of the query protein. It resulted in detecting a peptide sequence that can competitively replace the epitope from its specifically bonded Ab. On average, it identifies about 84% of the total residues in the epitope/antigenic determinant. The PEPOP 2.0 uses three ways for the peptide synthesis from the input 3D structure to facilitate its use in different ways in experimental detections. Three different ways for peptide designing are "one specific peptide design," "paired peptide design," and "peptide bank design." The first and second are for the peptide prediction, which is used to generate anti-protein antibodies. The third is exclusively for peptide designing, which will be used for its antigenic properties [41].

3.4.2 Prediction of T-cell epitopes

The endogenous antigenic peptide of 8–11 residues, presented by the MCH-I on the cell surface of antigen-presenting cells, activates the cytotoxic T-cells. The MHC II molecules express processed peptides of 13–17 residues for the activation of helper T-cells. T-cell epitope predictor aims to identify the antigenic regions within the foreign peptides responsible for the activation of T-cells (T_C/T_H) [12].

- TEpredict: This is an efficient software for T-cell epitope prediction that gives peptide processing information and binds to a specific MHC class. Prediction of peptide binding with MHC I is based on the models from ProPred 1 and nHLAPred, and MHC II binding uses a model from ProPred. The overall model used in this tool is built upon the partial least square regression method trained by the data from the IEDB. Thus, it is beneficial for the polypeptide vaccine development because of its high prediction sensitivity (0.50–0.80) and specificity (0.75–0.99) [42].
- CTLPred: Unlike other indirect T-cell epitope predictors which identify the peptide-MHC binding, CTLPred directly predicts the Cytotoxic T-Lymphocyte (CTL) epitopes from the antigen peptide sequence. To distinguish the CTL epitopes from the peptide pool, this method is based upon the quantitative matrix (QM), SVM, and ANN. These algorithms give a recognition accuracy of about 70.0%, 72.2%, and 75.2%, respectively. The evaluation of this accuracy is done by the leave one out cross-validation, giving a sensitivity of 79.4% and specificity of 88.4%. Training and testing of the combined model are done through the dataset extracted from MHCBN version 1.1, having 1137 CTL epitopes and 1134 non-epitopes [43].
- nHLAPred: It is a hybrid tool based on two algorithms to identify many MHC I alleles. Initially, the QM-based method is developed, having 47 alleles, and 15 binders for all these alleles are available from MHCBN 1.1. Then, the

ANN-based method having 47 alleles is prepared, out of which 30 alleles have 40 binders from the database. Both these methods are combined to improve the accuracy, which gives an average accuracy of about 92.8% for the 30 MHC alleles. The validation for the prediction results is done by the jack-knife method [44].

- ProPred-I: It is used to identify antigen peptide residues that act as binding sites for the MHC II and the prediction of multiple regions on the antigen that binds to different HLA-DR alleles of human MHC II. This server uses a pocket profile database for the development of the matrix of 51 HLA-DR alleles. This web server gives a graphical GDPlot, showing the propensity score for binding from the input primary sequence of the protein. Thus, by identifying promiscuous binders to the HLA-DR, this tool is helpful for subunit vaccine development [45].
- SVMHC: The predictor distinguishes between the peptides that bind to MHC I and MHC II using reference data from protein databases. The MHC I binding peptides analysis model is based on the SVM algorithm. This model is trained by the data from MHCPEP and SYFPEITHI databases which contain natural, synthetic peptides, and natural peptides, respectively. The model for identifying the MHC II binding peptides is based on the matrices of the promiscuous HLA-ligand binding. The result is compiled in tabular format with an ordered summary according to the peptide sequences. The property of SVMHC to analyze the effect of single nucleotide polymorphism on MHC epitope is best for viral epitope prediction [46].
- NetMHC: NetMHC 4.0 is the latest version of the server that applies the ANN in the gapped sequence alignment to predict the binding affinity of peptide-MHC I. The model is trained with the extracted peptide MHC binding dataset from the IEDB. The peptide length preferred by the MHC I is 8–11 residues, but the data of IEDB is biased toward the optimal length of the peptide, i.e., 9-mers. Also, identifying residual insertion and deletion in a peptide will better understand the binding interpretation for longer peptides. Nested cross-validation for avoiding the overlap between the training and test datasets and validation of the model with ligands of the SYFPEITHI database make it a high-performance tool [47].
- POPISK: The tool relies on the fact that the immunogenicity of peptides is based on the binding with the MHC. The physicochemical properties are taken into consideration while predicting give good results for the peptide prediction. Here, to identify induced immunogenicity and analyze the essential peptide residues, the SVM algorithm is used along with string kernels. The IMMA2 dataset compiles the immunogenicity data of MHCPEP, SYFPEITHI, and IEDB and gives a result accuracy of 60%. The 10-fold cross-validated immunogenicity check of POPISK with the HLA-A2 binding peptides gives a precision of 68% [48].

3.5 Bioinformatic tools for analysis of the vaccine construct

3.5.1 Prediction of antigenicity

After the vaccine construction, the final step is to check the antigenicity of the formed peptide to validate the efficiency. This will also give an idea about the immunogenic pathway triggered in the body after the vaccination.

- VaxiJen: First alignment independent web server that predicts novel antigens based on the distinct physiochemical properties of the peptides. Antigen prediction by this method is based on the auto cross-covariance (ACC) transformation of the input peptide into the vectors of uniform lengths. ACC is an extraction method for the structure–activity relationship of the protein and accounts for the transformation of the neighboring effect. Thus, this method predicts the protective antigens and subunit vaccines using z descriptors of amino acids, including hydrophobicity, molecular size, and polarity. Three independent datasets each for bacterial, viral, and tumorigenic antigens train the model and cross-validate it using leave-one-out-cross validation (LOO-CV). Accuracy by compiling the three datasets is ranges between 70% and 89% [20].
- ANTIGENpro: This method scans the whole proteome of the antigen for the generation of significant humoral immunity. It overcomes the limitation of other homology-based methods and results in the prediction of potential protective antigens by using a sequence-based prediction model. The model is trained by a set of protein microarray and gives overall accuracy of 76% after cross-validation. The microarray dataset contains three different subdatasets, with 100 literature antigens and 100 random antigens for each bacterial, viral, and tumor antigens [49].

3.5.2 Prediction of allergenicity

It is one of the essential steps for validating the vaccine construct because the vaccine should be safe and must not be responsible for any allergy inside the body.

- AllerTOP v.2: This is an online tool that distinguishes the allergens based on the physicochemical properties of the amino acid residues. Version 2 of the AllerTOP relies on the model which uses the E-descriptors and ACC transformation of amino acids. Five E-descriptors, hydrophobicity, size, the propensity of helix-formation, and the amino acid abundance and β-strand forming propensity are considered. The ACC transforms all the variable-length inputs with different descriptors into equal-length vectors. Different models are built for allergens' classification based on ML algorithms such as logistic regression, decision tree, RF, multilayer perceptron, and k-NN. A dataset of 2427 allergens and 2427 non-allergens is formed from different allergen databases. The kNN model gives the best results with 85.3% accuracy of prediction [50].

- AllergenFP: This server identifies the allergens from non-allergens based on fingerprints of E-descriptors. The ACC changes strings into uniform vectors; these vectors are further transformed into binary fingerprints for the analysis [51].

3.5.3 Analysis of toxicity, solubility, and physicochemical properties

The vaccine construct must not be toxic to the body and should be readily soluble to show high-efficiency in-vivo. ToxinPred, a tool for toxicity prediction, and SOLpro and Protein-Sol for solubility prediction are discussed here.

- ToxinPred: Web server that allows predicting the extent of toxicity of any peptide and identifying specific toxin regions or residues. The model to distinguish between the toxin and non-toxin peptides is developed on the SVM algorithm. The dataset of 1805 toxic peptides (>35 residues) is collected from different databases such as ATDB, DBETH, BTXpred, NTXpred, Arachno-Server, SwissProt [52].
- SOLpro: Two-tier SVM classification is applied in distinguishing the soluble peptides from insoluble peptides. Primary sequence-based physiochemical features (23 sets) are related to the extent of solubility in the aqueous medium. The training dataset, consisting of 17,408 peptides, is a combination of soluble and insoluble peptides. Tenfold cross-validation of the model gives a significant increase in the accuracy of prediction up to 74% [53].
- Protein-Sol: It processes the amino-acid sequences and gives a solubility profile. A linear model is built upon the 35 features, including amino acid composition. The proteins which are predicted to have transmembrane regions are excluded from the search. Different amino acid combinations are formed to relate the solubility with the complexity of the peptide, like K-R combination gives high solubility. Predictor gives 70.6% solubility with 679 proteins in the dataset and 76.1% solubility with the test set of 200 proteins [54].

The evaluation of physical and chemical parameters is done by using servers to predict vaccines' behavior under different environments.

- ProtParam: It is a protein identification and analysis tool in the Expasy web server. The query sequence can be from Swiss-Prot or TrEMBL or one letter code raw amino acid sequence. It calculates nine parameters for any query protein; molecular weight, theoretical PI, amino acid composition, atomic composition, extinction coefficient, estimated half-life, instability index, aliphatic index, and grand average of hydropathicity (GRAVY) [55].

3.6 Structure modeling of the vaccine construct

The 3D modeled structure of a vaccine is constructed from its primary amino acid sequence to help in predicting the folding of the peptide inside the host cell. In addition, it identifies the atomic spatial arrangement of the amino acids, often essential in elucidating the role of protein. Commonly used modeling servers are RaptorX, I-TASSER, SWISS-MODEL, Phyre2, etc.

- RaptorX: It is best suited for queries with no homologous template or a distantly related template. Thus, RaptorX considers all the available homologs (distant or closely related) for accessing the sequence profile. Further, the running algorithms are conditional neural field and conditional random field for integrating the signals into nonlinear scoring functions. Finally, multiple-template threading is applied for modeling the target signal using multiple templates. It performs secondary and tertiary structure modeling of the input sequence [27].
- I-TASSER: It is a protein structure and function prediction server that relies on the sequence-structure-function relationship. Initially, a query sequence is searched for homologs template using multiple threading alignments, and atomic models are generated through iterative template structure-based assembly. It results in secondary and tertiary structure modeling, and putative function of the model derived from aligned template 3D structure [28].
- SWISS-MODEL: The homomeric and heteromeric protein complexes modeling with their function is possible using this web server. The template is searched in SWISSMODEL template library (SMLT) using BLAST and HHblits. Template selection is based on the ranking done by Global Model Quality Estimation (GMQE) and Quaternary Structure Quality Estimation (QSQE). The latest updated model building and model evaluation methods are ProMod3 and QMEANDisCo, respectively [29].

3.7 Disorder perspective in vaccine construction

Organisms that tend to live in diverse environments such as pathogens tend to have more disorder in their proteomes because disordered proteins have structural and functional flexibility. The abundance of disorder in the pathogen's proteome was first discovered in the causative agent of malaria, *Plasmodium Sp.* Therefore, disordered regions are often important targets for antibodies [56]. MacRaild et al. assembled a dataset using antigens present on the IEDB. They found that predicted disordered regions had a higher likelihood of test positive in antibody binding assay. This could be because disordered regions would likely be exposed to solvents, making it a suitable antigen [57]. Disordered regions can bind with different immune system factors and accordingly assume different conformations called coupled folding and binding. Disordered epitopes are very short in length, therefore, interact with the antibody entirely. Disordered epitopes can adapt to their binding sites on the antibody, which offers a kind of flexibility. Since most of these disordered epitopes are conserved and accessible on the pathogen's surface, they are more likely to elicit an efficient immune response.

An example of a case study is the c-terminal region of MSP2 protein of *Plasmodium falciparum* as a potential component of malaria vaccine this $MSP2_{207\text{-}224}$ region is intrinsically disordered. Different monoclonal antibodies have a differing capacity of recognizing this region as an antigen. 4D11 is a monoclonal antibody that binds to MSP2 as shown by western blot and immunofluorescence. The crystal structure of 4D11 Fc bound to $MSP2_{215\text{-}222}$ was elucidated at 2.2A. It was observed that upon binding $MSP2_{215\text{-}222}$ assumes a B-bend ribbon structure consisting of overlapping B-turns. From this information, it is clear that choosing 4D11 epitopes would be a better strategy for vaccine construction [58].

3.8 Future perspectives

Currently, the world is in turmoil, dealing with the covid-19 pandemic. Initially, there were no vaccines available, but many vaccines were developed and put to use within the past year. The spike protein, which interacts with the host ACE2 receptor, has been explored as an epitope-based vaccine candidate in most examples. However, using bioinformatics tools significantly improves the probability of developing an efficient and safe vaccine and an economical option. Many infections do not have effective or safe vaccines. The cost of clinical trials and the lack of appropriate animal models act as tremendous obstacles. It is challenging to predict personalized immune reactions to vaccines. Complete and thorough knowledge about the immune response to vaccines is required. Although many webservers and bioinformatics tools are available for in-silico vaccine designing, the vaccines need to be designed carefully. The main advantage of using predictors is the possibility of designing vaccines that are immunogenic but not allergenic. Moreover, this method is time and cost-effective. Further, the importance of disordered peptides as good peptide vaccine candidates needs to be explored. Lower organisms employ IDPs to achieve a large number of functions. Tools to predict the conformation of IDPs in the bound state may help in the progress in this direction.

Acknowledgments

All the authors would like to thank IIT Mandi for providing facilities. S.K.K. is grateful to ICMR for SRF funding. A.B. is thankful to MHRD for funding. P.K. is supported by SERB, Government of India (CRG/2019/005603). T.B. is grateful to DST-INSPIRE fellowship. R.G. would like to acknowledge the DBT-IYBA program (BT/11/IYBA/2018/06).

Conflict of Interest

All authors declare that there is no financial competing interest.

References

[1] Strassburg MA. The global eradication of smallpox. Am J Infect Control 1982;10:53–9.

[2] Youde J. Cattle scourge no more: the eradication of rinderpest and its lessons for global health campaigns. Polit Life Sci 2013;32:43–57.

[3] Wu X, Smith TG, Rupprecht CE. From brain passage to cell adaptation: the road of human rabies vaccine development. Expert Rev Vaccines 2011;10:1597–608.

[4] Theiler M, Smith HH. The effect of prolonged cultivation in vitro upon the pathogenicity of yellow fever virus. J Exp Med 1937;65:767.

[5] Nuttall JJC, Eley BS. BCG vaccination in HIV-infected children. Tuberc Res Treat 2011;2011:1–6.

[6] Lu YJ, et al. GMP-grade pneumococcal whole-cell vaccine injected subcutaneously protects mice from nasopharyngeal colonization and fatal aspiration-sepsis. Vaccine 2010;28:7468–75.

[7] Arora NK, Lal AA, Hombach JM, Santos JI, Bhutta ZA, Sow SO, Greenwood B. The need for targeted implementation research to improve coverage of basic vaccines and introduction of new vaccines. Vaccine 2013;31(Suppl 2):B129–36. doi: 10.1016/j.vaccine.2013.01.058.

[8] Berical AC, Harris D, Cruz D, C. S, Possick JD. Pneumococcal vaccination strategies: an update and perspective. Annals Am Thoracic Soc 2016;13:933–44.

[9] Levine OS, et al. The future of immunisation policy, implementation, and financing. Lancet North Am Ed 2011;378:439–48.

[10] Chaplin DD. Overview of the immune response. J Allergy Clin Immunol. 2010;125(2 Suppl 2):S3–23. doi: 10.1016/j.jaci.2009.12.980.

[11] Beutler B. Innate immunity: an overview. Mol Immunol 2004;40:845–59.

[12] Sanchez-Trincado JL, Gomez-Perosanz M, Reche PA. Fundamentals and Methods for T- and B-Cell Epitope Prediction. J Immunol Res. 2017;2017:2680160. doi: 10.1155/2017/2680160. Epub 2017 Dec 28.

[13] Cooper MD, Alder MN. The evolution of adaptive immune systems. Cell 2006;124:815–22.

[14] Clem AS. Fundamentals of vaccine immunology. J Glob Infect Dis 2011;3:73.

[15] Desombere I, Gijbels Y, Verwulgen A, Leroux-Roels G. Characterization of the T cell recognition of hepatitis B surface antigen (HBsAg) by good and poor responders to hepatitis B vaccines. Clin Exp Immunol 2000;122:390.

[16] Zhao L-S, et al. DNA-based vaccination induces humoral and cellular immune responses against hepatitis B virus surface antigen in mice without activation of C-myc. World J Gastroenterol 2000;6:239–43.

[17] Rappuoli R. Reverse vaccinology. Curr Opin Microbiol 2000;3:445–50.

[18] Pizza M, et al. Identification of vaccine candidates against serogroup B meningococcus by whole-genome sequencing. Science (80-) 2000;287:1816–20.

[19] Pifferi C, Fuentes R, Fernández-Tejada A. Natural and synthetic carbohydrate-based vaccine adjuvants and their mechanisms of action. Nature Rev Chem 2021;vol. 5:197–216.

[20] Doytchinova IA, Flower DR. VaxiJen: a server for prediction of protective antigens, tumour antigens and subunit vaccines. BMC Bioinformat 2007;8:4. doi: 10.1186/1471-2105-8-4.

[21] Oli AN, et al. Immunoinformatics and vaccine development: an overview. ImmunoTargets Ther 2020;9:13–30.

[22] Sun P, Ju H, Liu Z, Ning Q, Zhang J, Zhao X, Huang Y, Ma Z, Li Y. Bioinformatics resources and tools for conformational B-cell epitope prediction. Comput Math Methods Med. 2013;2013:943636. doi: 10.1155/2013/943636. Epub 2013 Jul 21.

[23] Soria-Guerra RE, Nieto-Gomez R, Govea-Alonso DO, Rosales-Mendoza S. An overview of bioinformatics tools for epitope prediction: Implications on vaccine development. J Biomed Inform 2015;53:405–14.

[24] Kumar A, et al. Exploring the SARS-CoV-2 structural proteins for multi-epitope vaccine development: an in-silico approach. Expert Rev Vaccines 2020;19:887–98.

[25] Dietrich J, Andreasen LV, Andersen P, Agger EM. Inducing dose sparing with inactivated polio virus formulated in adjuvant CAF01. PLoS One. 2014;9(6):e100879. doi: 10.1371/journal.pone.0100879.

[26] Liu C, Chin JX, Lee DY. SynLinker: an integrated system for designing linkers and synthetic fusion proteins. Bioinformatics 2015;31:3700–2.

[27] Källberg M, Margaryan G, Wang S, Ma J, Xu J. Raptorx server: a resource for template-based protein structure modeling. Methods Mol Biol 2014;1137:17–27.

[28] Roy A, Kucukural A, Zhang YI-T. A unified platform for automated protein structure and function prediction. Nat Protoc 2010;5:725–38.

[29] Waterhouse A, et al. SWISS-MODEL: homology modelling of protein structures and complexes. Nucleic Acids Res 2018;46:W296–303.

[30] Parvizpour S, Pourseif MM, Razmara J, Rafi MA, Omidi Y. Epitope-based vaccine design: a comprehensive overview of bioinformatics approaches. Drug Discov Today 2020;25:1034–42.

[31] Dudek NL, Perlmutter P, Isabel Aguilar M, Croft PN, Purcell WA. Epitope discovery and their use in peptide based vaccines. Curr Pharm Des 2010;16:3149–57.

[32] Atassi MZ, Smith JA. A proposal for the nomenclature of antigenic sites in peptides and proteins. Mol Immunol 1978;15:609–10.

[33] Barlow DJ, Edwards MS, Thornton JM. Continuous and discontinuous protein antigenic determinants. Nature 1986;322:747–8.

[34] Lian Y, Ge M, Pan XM. EPMLR: sequence-based linear B-cell epitope prediction method using multiple linear regression. BMC Bioinformat 2014;15(1):414. doi: 10.1186/s12859-014-0414-y.

[35] Manavalan B, Govindaraj RG, Shin TH, Kim MO, Lee GiBCE-EL. A new ensemble learning framework for improved linear B-cell epitope prediction. Front Immunol 2018;9:1695.

[36] Collatz M, et al. EpiDope: a deep neural network for linear B-cell epitope prediction. Bioinformatics 2021;37:448–55.

[37] Jespersen MC, Peters B, Nielsen M, Marcatili P. BepiPred-2.0: improving sequence-based B-cell epitope prediction using conformational epitopes. Nucleic Acids Res 2017;45:W24–9.

[38] Haste Andersen P, Nielsen M, Lund O. Prediction of residues in discontinuous B-cell epitopes using protein 3D structures. Protein Sci 2006;15:2558–67.

[39] Sweredoski MJ, Baldi PP. Improved discontinuous B-cell epitope prediction using multiple distance thresholds and half sphere exposure. Bioinformatics 2008;24:1459–60.

[40] Ponomarenko J, Bui HH, Li W, Fusseder N, Bourne PE, Sette A, Peters B. ElliPro: a new structure-based tool for the prediction of antibody epitopes. BMC Bioinformat 2008;9:514. doi: 10.1186/1471-2105-9-514.

[41] Demolombe V, de Brevern AG, Felicori L, NGuyen C, Machado de Avila RA, Valera L, Jardin-Watelet B, Lavigne G, Lebreton A, Molina F, Moreau V. PEPOP 2.0: new approaches to mimic non-continuous epitopes. BMC Bioinformat 2019;20(1):387. doi: 10.1186/s12859-019-2867-5.

[42] D V Antonets AZM. [TEpredict: software for T-cell epitope prediction] - PubMed. Mol Biol (Mosk) 2010;44(1):130–9.

[43] Bhasin M, Raghava GPS. Prediction of CTL epitopes using QM, SVM and ANN techniques. Vaccine 2004;22:3195–204.

[44] Bhasin M, Raghava GPS. A hybrid approach for predicting promiscuous MHC class I restricted T cell epitopes. J Biosci 2007;32:31–42.
[45] Singh H, Raghava GPS. ProPred: prediction of HLA-DR binding sites. Bioinformatics 2002;17:1236–7.
[46] Dönnes P, Kohlbacher O. SVMHC: a server for prediction of MHC-binding peptides. Nucleic Acids Res 2006;34.
[47] Andreatta M, Nielsen M. Gapped sequence alignment using artificial neural networks: application to the MHC class i system. Bioinformatics 2016;32:511–7.
[48] Tung CW, Ziehm M, Kämper A, Kohlbacher O, Ho SY. POPISK: T-cell reactivity prediction using support vector machines and string kernels. BMC Bioinformat 2011;12:446. doi: 10.1186/1471-2105-12-446.
[49] Magnan CN, et al. High-throughput prediction of protein antigenicity using protein microarray data. Bioinformatics 2010;26:2936–43.
[50] Dimitrov I, Bangov I, Flower DR, Doytchinova I. AllerTOP v.2: a server for in silico prediction of allergens. J Mol Model 2014;20(6):2278. doi: 10.1007/s00894-014-2278-5. Epub 2014 May 31.
[51] Dimitrov I, Naneva L, Doytchinova I, Bangov I. AllergenFP: Allergenicity prediction by descriptor fingerprints. Bioinformatics 2014;30:846–51.
[52] Gupta S, Kapoor P, Chaudhary K, Gautam A, Kumar R. Open Source Drug Discovery Consortium, Raghava GP. In silico approach for predicting toxicity of peptides and proteins. PLoS One 2013;8(9):e73957. doi: 10.1371/journal.pone.0073957.
[53] Magnan CN, Randall A, Baldi P. Accurate sequence-based prediction of protein solubility. Bioinformatics 2009;25:2200–7.
[54] Hebditch M, Carballo-Amador MA, Charonis S, Curtis R, Warwicker J. Protein-Sol: a web tool for predicting protein solubility from sequence. Bioinformatics 2017;33:3098–100.
[55] Gasteiger E, et al. Protein identification and analysis tools on the ExPASy Server. In: The Proteomics Protocols Handbook Humana Press, Switzerland; 2005. p. 571–607. http://doi.org/10.1385/1-59259-890-0:571.
[56] Aly ASI, Vaughan AM, Kappe SHI. Malaria parasite development in the mosquito and infection of the mammalian host. Annu Rev Microbiol 2009;63:195–221.
[57] MacRaild CA, Seow J, Das SC, Norton RS. Disordered epitopes as peptide vaccines. Pept Sci (Hoboken) 2018;110(3):e24067. doi: 10.1002/pep2.24067. Epub 2018 Apr 14.
[58] Seow J, et al. Structure and characterisation of a key epitope in the conserved C-terminal domain of the malaria vaccine candidate MSP2. J Mol Biol 2017;429:836–46.

Chapter 4

Vaccine engineering & structural vaccinology

Fabiana A Carneiro[a], Juliana dos Reis Cortines[b], Victor Alejandro Essus[b], Isis Botelho N da Silva[c]

[a]Núcleo Multidisciplinar de Pesquisa em Biologia (Numpex-Bio), Campus Duque de Caxias Professor Geraldo Cidade, Universidade Federal do Rio de Janeiro (UFRJ), Rio de Janeiro, Brazil [b]Departamento de Virologia, Instituto de Microbiologia Paulo de Góes, Universidade Federal do Rio de Janeiro, Rio de Janeiro, Brazil [c]Escola de Química, Instituto de Química, Universidade Federal do Rio de Janeiro, Rio de Janeiro, Brazil

4.1 Introduction

Vaccination is one of the most cost-effective ways to control and prevent the spread of infectious diseases. It has proven pivotal against arrays of infectious viral diseases and has considerably reduced morbidity and mortality caused by viruses. However, there are still no effective vaccines against many viruses.

The World Health Organization estimates that vaccines prevent 2–3 million human deaths annually [1]. Only two infectious diseases have been eliminated in human history, both the result of a successful vaccination campaign: smallpox, which was officially declared eliminated from the human population in 1979 [2]; and the livestock disease rinderpest was declared eliminated in 2011 [3]. While other diseases such as measles and polio are also close to elimination, there is still much to be done [2].

Vaccines are ultimately dependent on the development of an effective adaptive immune response. Broadly, adaptive immune responses are divided into two different categories, humoral and cellular. Cells of the adaptive immune system respond to specific regions of infectious agents known as epitopes. One or more humoral responses are dependent on the activity of the antibodies, secreted glycoproteins from B cells that bind to specific epitopes. A naïve B cell contains B cell receptors on its surface, which vary in their specificities [4].

Cellular immune responses are based on the action of T cells. All nucleated cells have on their surface Major Histocompatibility Complex Class I (MHC-I) molecules. When infected with an intracellular infectious agent, cells can present on their surface linear epitopes from those infectious agents complexed with MHC-I to alert the immune system of the infection. Cytotoxic T cells (T_C) that

System Vaccinology. https://doi.org/10.1016/B978-0-323-85941-7.00005-X

contain the matching T cell receptor can bind to the MHC-I presenting specific epitopes leading to the death of the infected cell [4].

One of the most important cell types in vaccine development is T helper cells (T_H). Antigen presenting cells (APCs) such as dendritic cells (DCs), macrophage, and B cells are able to phagocytize, process, and present $CD4^+$ epitopes in complex with Major Histocompatibility Complex Class II (MHC-II) on their surface. These epitopes stimulate $CD4^+$ T cells leading to their maturation into T_H cells. Active T_H cells are able to stimulate cells of both the innate and adaptive immune system through the secretion of cytokines. These cytokines are able to modulate the immune system leading to a stronger and more effective immune response. Based on the profile of the secreted cytokine responses, they are either classified as T helper 1 response (T_{H1}) or T helper 2 response (T_{H2}). T_{H1} responses favor the development of a cellular-based immune response, while T_{H2} responses favor the development of a humoral immune response. Traditionally, vaccine development has focused on the development of strong T_{H2} responses. Currently, a vaccine candidate that has a balanced T_{H1}/T_{H2} response is considered optimal [5].

After activation, B cells, T_H, and T_C undergo proliferation to effectively deal with the infection. In an ideal situation, some of these cells persist after clearance resulting in the development of immunological memory. When a host is previously exposed to an infectious agent again, antigen-specific immune memory cells are activated and proliferate faster and to a greater magnitude, leading to rapid clearance of the infectious agent and mitigation of disease. Strong and effective memory responses protect hosts against subsequent infections leading to lifelong immunity, the hallmark of an effective vaccine [5].

Vaccines not only work on the individual level but also on the population level. In the concept known as herd immunity, if a certain fraction of the population is immune to an infectious agent, the disease will have a very low likelihood of finding another naïve host and of spreading. The number of people who need to be vaccinated for herd immunity varies from disease to disease, normally between 60% and 90%. It is extremely important because, in any given population, some vaccinated individuals will not develop protection based upon genetics; there will be individuals who cannot be vaccinated because of age or disease state, and there will also be unvaccinated individuals [6,7]. Herd immunity is the altruistic side of vaccination that will ultimately lead to the elimination of pathogens from either the human or animal population.

The modern biotechnology revolution was important for the way we can think and produce new vaccines, reflecting on the advances in new antigens, adjuvants, vectors, and delivery systems. Vaccines have been applied over 200 years, and were introduced by Edward Jenner [8] and Louis Pasteur [9,10]. Since then, many kinds of vaccines were produced. They can be classified in three groups: first, second, and third generation. The first generation employs a pathogenic agent in their constitution derived from its attenuated, inactivated, or a portion of the microorganism. This approach is well characterized by BCG (*Mycobacterium bovis*), poliomyelitis, and smallpox vaccines. The second generation is based on antibodies produced by a toxin that causes the symptoms or surface sugars, that allows the host immune system to neutralize bacteria or other pathogens. Examples for such vaccines are the ones against hepatitis B, pneumonia, and meningitis. Lastly, the third generation of vaccines adds an innovative concept employing genetic engineering. They are called DNA vaccines and started to be used in the late 1990s when tests related to genetic therapies were used to substitute defective genetic infringement [11]. Nowadays, DNA vaccines are improved by the biotechnological advances in DNA recombinant techniques, for example as in the vaccine against melanoma and the DNA vaccine expressing different forms of the SARS-CoV-2 spike (S) protein [12].

Traditional production methods, based on technologies developed decades ago, including live attenuated and inactivated vaccines, can induce strong and long-term effective immune responses in host cells [10] and have thus held a prominent position within the vaccine market. Although many traditional vaccines are safe and effective in humans, several inherent risks are associated with certain live attenuated and inactivated vaccines, including incomplete attenuation, unstable toxicity, and risk of mutation, which make it difficult to guarantee the longevity of these formulations.

Besides that, many viruses remain without effective vaccines including dengue viruses, human immunodeficiency virus (HIV), enterovirus A71, and hepatitis C virus [13]. In addition, emerging infectious diseases will continue to threaten public health. Therefore, rapid vaccine development is mandatory to prevent pandemics.

New structural insights into the viral envelope, protein conformation, and antigenic epitopes can guide the design of novel vaccines against challenging viruses, which have received widespread attention, offering greater immunogenicity, and safety.

Therefore, the focus for vaccine development should be based on newer rational vaccine design platforms (Fig. 4.1). This chapter will discuss how structural vaccinology could lead to the discovery of antibodies for passive immunization and provide suggestions on how different vaccinology approaches can be exploited for future vaccine design.

4.2 Methodology used for vaccine production

4.2.1 Attenuated and inactivated microorganisms

An attenuated vaccine is developed by reducing the virulence of the pathogen, which remains replication-competent after administration. Basically, the attenuated virus administered is sufficiently replicated by the host and thus induce an immune response that can protect against infection before the virus is cleared by the immune system. Because the vaccine viral strain is replication-competent, there is a risk of reversion to virulence after administration, albeit small. Despite these potential risks, live attenuated virus vaccines offer considerable advantages over inactivated ("killed") vaccines. More specifically, attenuated

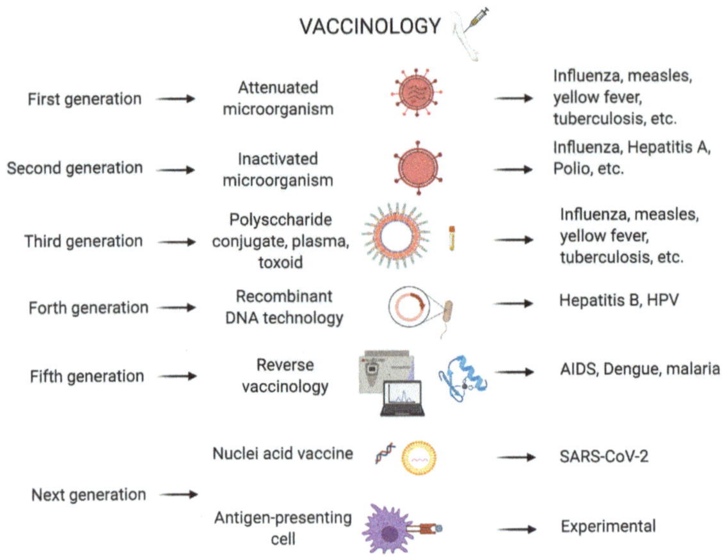

FIG. 4.1 Schematic representation of vaccine generation, instruments used, and disease correlated. *(Figure created with BioRender.com).*

vaccines (1) activate a wide range of immune responses, (2) induce long-lasting and rapid onset of immunity, (3) often reduce the need for booster vaccinations, (4) do not need adjuvants, (5) can be produced at relatively low cost, and (6) can be administered by the oral route. Examples of live attenuated vaccine are the vaccines against influenza [14], measles [15], and SARS-CoV-2 [16].

In order to achieve viral inactivation, it is necessary to perform procedures that will chemically alter the virus in some way. Some of the most widely used processes are solvent/detergent inactivation (chemical inactivation), heating (temperature inactivation), pH acidification, and ultraviolet light inactivation. In all these procedures, the virus remains with structure and is able to be recognized by the immune system.

In the case of inactivated vaccine, the pathogen is not replicated but its presence as an antigen still confers immunogenicity. Inactivated pathogen or subunit vaccines, such as influenza, are generally used for pathogens for which a humoral immune response is considered the primary protective response and as such, would be inadequate for inducing the appropriate forms of cellular immunity needed for certain diseases such as XYZ (examples of diseases).

4.2.2 Vectors

Vaccine vectors deliver the antigen in such a way as to induce a particular arm of immunity or to bias the type of immune response. This technology was developed decades ago using a vaccinia virus vector expressing the hepatitis B surface antigen (HBsAg), which provided protective immunity to chimpanzees exposed to hepatitis B [17]. Most vector vaccines are produced against animal viruses; there is only one with such technology licensed for human use against Ebola virus [18], approved in 2019.

Many kinds of viruses are used to develop vector vaccines, such as poxvirus, adenoviruses, herpesviruses, arenaviruses, retroviruses, paramyxoviruses, and flaviviruses, among others [19]. The main advantage of viral vectors over traditional vaccines is their ability to evoke a robust adaptive immune response in the absence of an adjuvant. However, the tradeoff for enhanced immunogenicity is the concern for potential reversion of the attenuated viral vector to virulence, especially when using a replication-competent vector [20].

4.2.3 Protein conjugate vaccine

An important observation about vaccines is that they were produced to fight against a variety of pathogens. Pneumococcus and meningococcus are bacteria that cause severe diseases such as pneumonia, meningitis, and bacteremia. Conjugate vaccines are developed to induce a robust immune response against bacterial capsular polysaccharides. Glycoconjugate vaccines are vaccines in which a bacterial polysaccharide antigen is conjugated to a carrier protein to enhance immunogenicity by promoting T cell-dependent immune response [21] (Fig. 4.2).

Briefly, after immunization, polysaccharides, or conjugate vaccines are taken up by DCs and transported to lymph nodes where, to induce an immune

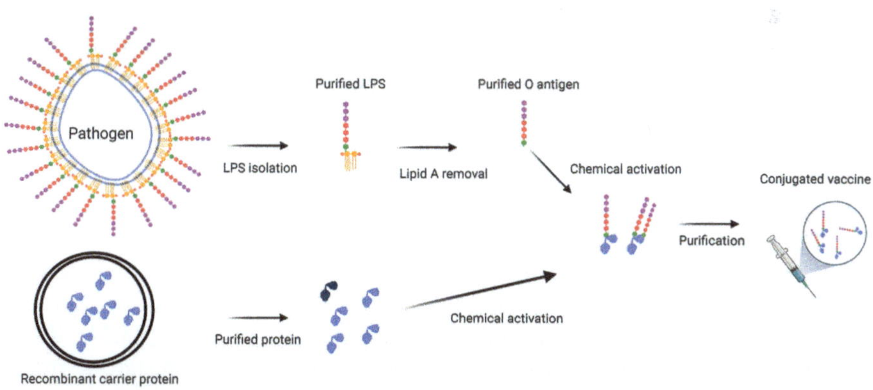

FIG. 4.2 Traditional chemical conjugation method to produce glycoconjugate vaccines. Multiple steps are required whereby the O-antigen must be purified from the pathogen of interest, detoxified, and subject to chemical activation. In parallel, the protein must also be purified and chemically activated before protein and glycan can be conjugated. Following conjugation, further rounds of purification are necessary before vaccine can be administered. *(Figure created with BioRender.com).*

response, they need to engage both B and T cells and start the formation of germinal centers (GCs). GCs are sites within lymph nodes and the spleen where mature B cells proliferate, differentiate, and mutate their antibody genes through somatic hypermutation. To form GCs, three main cells are necessary: the polysaccharide-specific B cells expressing the antibody on their surface as a receptor [B cell receptor (BCR)]; the follicular helper T (Tfh) cells, which recognize the protein carrier antigen presented on the surface of B cells; and follicular dendritic cells, which contain and present the antigen to the B cells. The GC reaction produces higher-affinity antibodies and switches the class of antibodies (e.g., from IgM to IgG) during a normal immune response to an infection or after vaccination [22].

4.3 Reverse vaccinology

The availability of the whole genome has permitted the development of a new strategy called "reverse vaccinology" [22], an improved vaccinological technology that combines genomics, bioinformatics, and proteomic information to predict antigenic epitopes.

The genome represents a list of virtually all the protein antigens that a pathogen can express at any time. It becomes possible to choose potentially surface-exposed proteins in a reverse manner, starting from the genome rather than from the microorganism, with the great advantage that cultivation of dangerous microorganisms is not needed anymore. Consequently, the process can be equally applied to cultivable and non-cultivable microorganisms. This approach, starting from the genomic sequence by computer analysis, predicts those antigens that are most likely to be vaccine candidates [22]. The feasibility of the approach relies heavily on the availability of a high-throughput system to screen protective immunity. This approach permitted the discovery of a novel surface exposed proteins that are able to induce bactericidal or viral antibodies.

Reverse vaccinology can select potential antigenic targets that will be provided through a pipeline (Fig. 4.3). By combining structural vaccinology, comparative genomics, and pan-genomics technologies, novel potential antigen targets can be identified, further analyzed, and screened through computational antigen prediction or expressed as a recombinant protein for a further immunological test.

The other two techniques, proteomics and mass spectrometry, are already playing a central role in the identification and characterization of novel antigens. Proteomics allows for the selection of potential vaccine candidates through the identification of pathogen secreted or surface-exposed proteins [23,24]. This technique complements the reverse vaccinology approach, which starting from pathogen genomes permits the in silico selection of open-reading frames encoding for those antigens.

The first vaccine derived from reverse vaccinology was against meningococcus B (Serruto et al., 2012; O'Ryan et al., 2014) [25,26], but still is not available due to the slow progress in the identification of antigenic targets [27]. By analyzing the

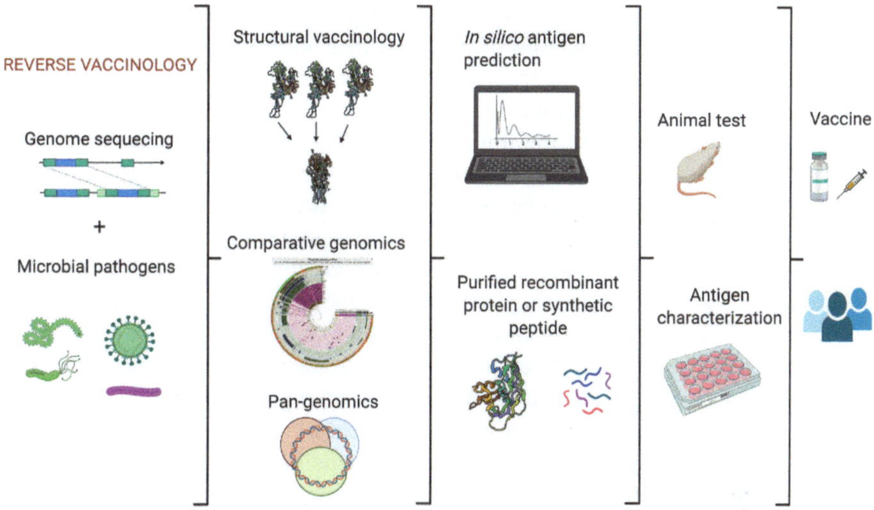

FIG. 4.3 Schematic pipeline of reverse vaccinology. *(Created with BioRender.com).*

whole genome sequence of MenB, the meningococcal factor H-binding protein (fHBP) was found to be an essential protein, which could induce relatively high levels of antibodies in mice [25].

Today, a new wave of technologies in the fields of human immunology and structural biology provide the molecular information that allows for the discovery and design of vaccines against the respiratory syncytial virus [26] and human CMV (HCMV) [28] that have been impossible to tackle thus far and to propose universal vaccines targeting influenza and HIV infections [21].

4.4 Structural vaccinology

Technics that predict molecular structures such as X-ray crystallography and NMR spectroscopy were important for the advance of vaccines, because of the determination of the structure of most antigens and their epitopes. This knowledge would form the basis for structural vaccinology, in which three-dimensional (3D) structural information could be used to design novel and/or improve vaccine antigens [29]. The advancements of genomics, proteomics, and bioinformatics promote the improvement of structural biology, and structural vaccinology comes as the next step of reverse vaccinology.

Structural vaccinology is a genome-based approach combined with structural biology, a revolutionary way to produce vaccine antigens that were not possible before. A tool that makes it possible to design an entire synthetic sequence and one day maybe a universal vaccine, based on the complete understanding of the nature of the antigen epitopes that are recognized by the human immune system.

This technology has been applied to several aspects of the vaccine studies: (1) characterization the 3D structure of proteins, especially the structural epitopes of immunogenic antigens; (2) analysis of the presence and activities of surface-exposed epitopes, which region of the pathogens bind and interact with the host cells; (3) evaluation of the immunogenicity of synthetic antigens or sub-specific antigens; (4) identification of structural variations between wild type and genetically mutated antigens, which help develop more prevalent vaccines [30]. Genetic mutations may not necessarily cause amino acid substitutions, and protein sequence changes may not result in structural or functional alterations. Therefore, structural vaccinology will provide the most direct evidence of the efficiency of vaccine administrations and possible immune responses [31,32].

One of the first structure-based antigen design vaccines was against *N. meningitidis* serogroup A, C, Y, and W135 [33]. Based on the genome sequence of the antigen surface-exposed lipoprotein, factor H-binding protein (fHbp) [34] was discovered. However, this lipoprotein presents more than 500 amino acid variants, which makes it difficult to design a vaccine, as they belong to different groups. To solve this problem, a vaccine created through structure-based epitopes from each of the three fHbp antigenic-variant groups was engineered into a single molecule. An important consideration to engineering this kind of epitope is that not only the key amino acids of each epitope are necessary, but the surface that mimics the 3D structure in the native molecule is also relevant [35].

4.4.1 Multiepitope peptide vaccines

Recombinant DNA technology has created a major breakthrough in biotechnological history, enabling the production of diverse and natural fusion proteins from many organisms. Additionally, the wide availability of genomic information, provided by the advances in cost and speed of DNA sequencing technologies, and the development of novel bioinformatics software and databases, have facilitated a more rational approach for designing and production of vaccines such as the multiple-epitopes-based ones. Multiepitope peptides based vaccines (MEV) are fusion proteins composed of a series of different peptides that together aim to provide protection against a specific infection [36].

In general, the successful construction of recombinant fusion proteins requires two important elements: the proteins/peptides to be fused together and the linkers connecting them [37]. For MEVs, peptides containing B or T cell epitopes are used, connected through linkers, in order to sufficiently elicit an effective immune response.

Recent advancements in bioinformatics have enabled a more systematic approach for MEV in *in silico* design. The first step involves the screening of the most suitable B-cell or T-cell epitopes, generally using immunoinformatics tools, such as those available at the Immune Epitope Database. Those sequences will be evaluated according to their predicted antigenicity, immunogenicity, allergenicity, toxicity, structural stability/flexibility, and physicochemical properties [36]. Then the most promising epitopes will be selected and connected using fusion linkers.

Regarding these linkers, some that are commonly used for vaccine construction are AAY, GPGPG, and EAAAK. They are important elements in MEV design, being responsible for ensuring protein stability, facilitating epitope presentation, and preserving their independent immunogenic activities [36,37]. EAAAK linkers, for example, reduce interaction with other protein regions, promoting efficient separation, and increasing stability. AAY and GPGPG prevent the formation of junctional epitopes, which is a major concern in the design of MEVs [36]. Junctional epitopes are created by the juxtaposition of epitopes, which might cause the redirection of the immune response to less relevant residues in the sequence, in some cases possibly suppressing the induction of the desired immunogenic response [38]. Thus, linkers selection also plays an important role in MEV efficacy.

In addition, molecular docking and dynamics simulations are also conducted to further evaluate the behavior of the MEVs. Ultimately, once validated in silico, the MEV codons are optimized for the desired expression system and the sequence cloned in the appropriate vector so it can be finally introduced in the expressing organism of choice [36].

Compared to classical and single epitope vaccines, MEVs, depending on their design, may have many appealing immunogenic features: they can be composed of MHC-restricted epitopes that can be recognized by T cell receptors (TCRs) of multiple clones from various T-cell subsets; the combination of CTL, Th, and B-cell epitopes can induce both cellular and humoral immune responses simultaneously (Fig. 4.4); MEVs can have in its sequence components with the adjuvant capacity to improve the immunogenicity and generate a long-lasting immune response—as an example, β-defensin, an antimicrobial peptide that also has immunomodulatory functions, has already been included as an adjuvant in MEVs against Dengue [39] and Influenza infections [40]. Besides, during the MEVs design, it is possible to remove elements and components that might trigger either pathological immune responses or adverse effects [36]. Lastly, the customized design of this type of vaccine enables its scaled-up production in cheaper and easier expression platforms such as *Escherichia coli*, avoiding some productivity issues associated with mammalian cell culture, commonly used for conventional vaccines.

In summary, the multiepitope vaccines have a lot of potential to be explored considering its versatility, costs, and time advantages. Despite some MEVs having already reached the phases of the clinical trial, this approach still needs to be further improved, since it heavily depends on the selection of the most suitable epitopes, which is related to the capacity of accurately predicting and evaluating its immunogenic properties. However, it is important to notice that immunoinformatics methods for antigen screening have been advancing so far, which might lead to an enhancement in efficacy for future MEVs. Another challenge for this vaccine strategy is the development of new and more efficient delivery systems, which also play an important role in the vaccine success.

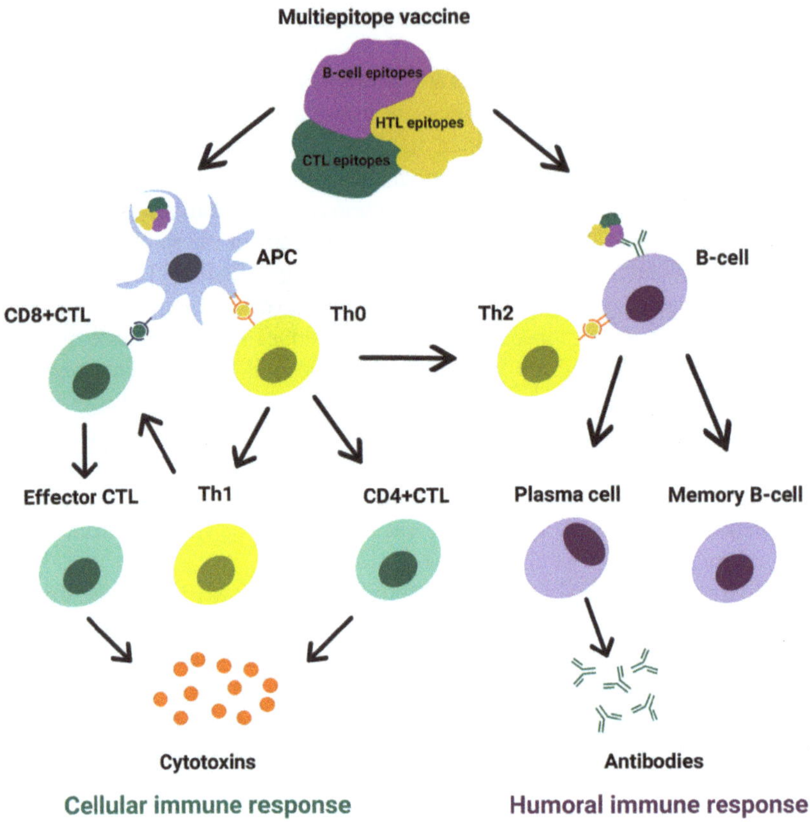

FIG. 4.4 Immune responses induced by a multiepitope vaccine (*MEV*). MEVs can have CTL, T helper (Th), and B-cell epitopes in their structure, which makes them capable of inducing both cellular and humoral immune responses. The B-cells recognize the B epitopes of the MEV, internalize it, and then present the HTL epitopes to the Th2 cells. The Th2 cells induce B cell differentiation to plasma cells, which will then secrete multiepitope vaccine-specific antibodies. The B cells can also differentiate into memory B cells. APCs can internalize the antigen and present the CTL and HTL epitopes to CD8+CTL or Th0 cells, respectively. Th0 cells, in response, can differentiate into Th1, Th2, or CD4+CTL. The Th1 cells stimulate, alongside the CTL epitopes recognition, the CD8+CTL to produce effector CTL cells. Those will then kill the target cells by secreting cytotoxins such as perforin and granzyme, or by activating other cytotoxic pathways. The CD4+CTL can also secrete cytotoxins against the infectious agent.

4.5 Vaccine engineering

Vaccination is the single most successful and cost-effective intervention in medical history. However, many of the vaccines that we know and use were discovered more than 50 years ago. About 2 years ago, cancer vaccination moved from a theoretical concept to actual working intervention. In this context, differents engineering approaches became an essential tool to discover novel antigens, epitopes, and adjuvants that can stimulate and manipulate the immune system, as well as their targeted delivery, for the prevention and treatment of important diseases such as cancer and infectious diseases.

Also, many vaccines are delivered by nanoparticles of specific sizes, degradation characteristics, targeted surface molecules, coatings, and compositions. Another approach is to engineer virus-like particles (VLPs). Both are significant research areas in nanotechnology. Engineering adjuvants are another area where engineering expertise is needed, mainly chemical engineering and formulation science. A third engineering challenge is epitope discovery: tens of thousands of infectious organisms, autoantigens, cancer antigens, and allergens contain millions of epitopes that can be presented to the immune system. Computer engineering challenges exist in curating and standardizing the existing data and aligning them with new data.

4.5.1 Vaccines based on virus-like particles

VLPs are a type of protein cage derived from viruses consisting of capsid-like structures generated by the self-assembly of viral structural components. They are composed mainly of capsid protein subunits, although some also require other structural molecules such as RNA during assembly [41–43]. VLPs have been extensively explored in nanotechnology, especially in medicinal applications as tools for the targeted delivery of cargo. Their application as vehicles to deliver and present epitopes as vaccine platforms have also been considerably studied [41–45].

The VLPs have inherited the architectures of their viral templates making them highly immunogenic due to presenting the antigens in a conformation matching that of the native virus being able to stimulate both cellular and humoral immune responses, which makes them particularly interesting as vaccine models, especially when considering their safety. Because VLPs are made solely with the structural components of their viral counterparts, they don't possess any of the genetic elements necessary for replication and therefore are unable to cause an infection [41,44–47]. On a different note, vaccines based on attenuated viruses are limited by the potential reversion of virulence or incomplete inactivation of the virus, which makes them unsafe to use in young children and immunocompromised individuals [41,48]. They also differ from other recombinant vaccines such as the ones based on subunits that contain either single or multiple antigenic components, since they are able to generate a strong immune response without the supplementation with adjuvants, while also being able to be used as adjuvants themselves [46–48]. As such, they retain most virtues of whole pathogens vaccines such as the high immunogenicity without issues regarding safety due to its non-infectious nature, while also having other virtues such as being easily obtainable through heterologous expression.

VLPs can be obtained by several different heterologous expression systems such as those based on animal, yeast, bacteria, and plant cells [42,47,49]. However, the expression system chosen for VLP production must be considered as each system has its advantages and limitations, with some having limitations that can impede the production of certain VLPs [47,49]. Bacterial-based VLP-production systems, for example, have a high yield and are suitable for the expression of non-enveloped VLPs formed with up to two structural proteins, but it does not support post-translational modifications that may be required to generate a proper immune response [47,49]. Yeast-based systems also have a similarly high yield to bacterial systems and have the advantage of being able to perform some post-translational modification but are not adequate to more complex modifications like protein glycosylation [47]. VLPs that require such modifications can be obtained from mammalian cells at the cost of having a very low yields, the main drawback of this expression system when compared to others [49]. To generate enveloped VLPs, the structural proteins of the virus must be produced in cells to simulate a natural infection, promoting self-assembly of the protein core, and its exit of the cell through a budding process. As an example, to obtain enveloped influenza A VLPs, hemagglutinin (HA), neuraminidase (NA), and matrix proteins (M) from influenza are expressed in the baculovirus/insect cell expression system [47,49]. This system is suitable for the production of vaccines for epidemic viruses whose surface protein can vary between each outbreak [47,49]. The main disadvantage is that enveloped baculoviruses are also produced simultaneously to the VLPs, making purification harder and more expensive [47]. The capacity to heterologously obtain VLPs represents an advantage over conventional vaccine production such as the traditional embryonated egg-based approach that has a high cost, slow development, and low dose yield. Additionally, vaccines derived from egg-based systems could result in allergies in susceptible individuals, a problem does not present in VLPs [48].

The incredible diversity of the virosphere also influences the VLPs development with a considerable library of models having been developed based on bacteria, plant, and animal viruses [41–43]. Due to that, their architecture can vary considerably in terms of size and complexity, with some possessing one to multiple protein layers, and others having an external lipid envelope [47,50]. For vaccine development, the main type of VLP explored is derived from human viruses due to the possibility of harnessing their inherent immunogenicity and natural affinity to our organism as a way to treat their infection, with VLP-based vaccines being commercialized since the 1980s [41,49]. A hepatitis B virus (HBV) vaccine was the first to be commercialized consisting of empty particles of HBV containing the surface antigen (HBsAg) [47,49]. A VLP based on the core protein (HBcAg) of the virus has also been developed [41,50]. Other commercially successful VLP vaccines include hepatitis E virus (HEV) and human papillomavirus (HPV) [49,50]. For the latter, there are two available vaccines, Gardasil and Cervarix, based on the major capsid protein L1 that has the ability to self-assemble inside the expressing cell forming the VLP, and that confer protection against cancer-associated HPV serotypes 16 and 18 [41,47,49,50]. The main advantage of utilizing the VLPs of these viruses as vaccine models is their capacity of inducing a strong immune response.

VLPs can be used in the activation of a series of immune cells through different processing pathways, inducing humoral or cellular immune responses through the recognition of repetitive subunits on the surface of the particle by the immune system [45–47]. After immunization with VLP-based vaccines, they are first recognized and incorporated by APCs such as DCs and macrophages, later being presented to lymphocytes, and inducing the adaptive immune response [41,48]. The size and geometry of VLPs are important aspects for its application as a vaccine platform since both antigens' size and form play an important role in uptake, activation, and presentation to the immune cells [45,49,51]. Since the original architecture of the virus is preserved in the VLP, multiple copies of their antigenic capsid proteins are displayed in a multivalent and repetitive array that is considerably immunogenic, resulting in a presentation similar to that of the native virus [41,45,49]. This structural mimicry permits the VLPs to attach and penetrate host cells because they conserve their receptor binding sites. The particles are sensed by pathogen recognition receptors (PRRs) which are expressed on the surface of APCs, like DCs, allowing the cell to recognize VLPs in the same way they detect wild-type viruses [45,49]. These features enable a stronger induction of immunity than antigens in their soluble forms [41]. VLPs particulate nature helps DC activation since particles are easily taken up by DCs and this event increases the expression of costimulatory molecules. For instance, HCV-VLPs induce overexpression of CD80 and CD86 on DCs after their exposure for 16h while denatured VLPs fail to induce this overexpression, indicating that DC activation is mediated by VLPs and not by protein monomers [49]. PRRs involved in the interaction and captation of VLPs act on the internalization of particulate antigens and include C-type lectin receptors (CLR)s, Toll-like receptors (TLRs), RIG-I-like receptors (RLRs), and NOD-like receptors (NLRs), with phagocytosis and macropinocytosis being the two main mechanisms by which VLPs are taken up by APCs [49,50]. VLPs uptake prompts cell maturation and induce the release of proinflammatory cytokines to recruit more APCs which later elicits an adaptive immune response. An example would be the rabbit hemorrhagic disease virus (RHDV) VLPs that can induce the expression of interferon-γ (IFNγ) and a cytotoxic T-lymphocyte (CTL) response [49]. The activation of the APCs also prompts antigen processing and presentation of peptides loaded into major histocompatibility complex (MHC) class I or class II molecules for inducing CD8+ or CD4+ T cell responses, respectively [41,45,49]. During this process, peptide-MHC complexes are produced and lymphocyte costimulatory molecules are expressed in high quantity on the surface of DCs including CD80, CD83, and CD86, which are necessary for efficient activation of effector B and T cells [49], although the VLPs are also able to go directly to the lymph nodes due to its small size and directly activate B cells.

The size for most VLPs ranges from 20 to 100 nm in diameter which aside from making them particularly susceptible to DC capture at both the injection site and plasma, also allows them to pass directly through lymphatic vessels without the help of any APC and reach the lymph nodes where they are trapped by resident DCs [46,49,51]. There, VLPs also enter in contact with B cells, which they can promote the activation through the extensive crosslinking of their receptors (BCRs) thanks to its multivalent epitope distribution, resulting in robust and long-lasting antibody responses [51]. The stimuli can generate a strong enough response to induce the production of antibodies even without the help of CD4+ T cells [50,51], while also being able to override B cell tolerance mechanisms, allowing the induction of potent antibody responses against self-antigens [51]. B cells can also work as APCs, taking up VLPs, processing and presenting them to T cells prompting their activation [49]. As such, it becomes evident that most VLPs have an immense potential to activate an effective humoral and cellular response, but this potential is not equal among them: while some may favor a stronger immune reponse, other may induce low levels of MHC molecules [49]. However, such limitations can be overcome thanks to VLPs tolerance to structural modifications that allow for the insertion of stronger heterologous antigens, creating a chimeric VLP that is more immunogenic than its native counterpart [45,49–51].

The capability to extensively modify the particle architecture and expand its functionality by the incorporation of exogenous structures has been used to confer specificity toward a target cell type through the conjugation of a ligand, to change the properties of the particle, and/or to load cargo in VLPs [44–46]. In vaccine design, it has been used for the presentation of non-native antigens in VLPs, resulting in the development of chimeric VLPs that can be used to increase the immunogenicity of either the VLP itself or the displayed antigen [47,52,53]. This can be done in several ways, but usually occurs through either genetic modification or chemical conjugation. One of the most common approaches to genetic modification involves the fusion of the foreign antigen to the VLPs components, mainly coat proteins, by incorporating the antigen genes in the VLPs gene sequence resulting in its presentation on the surface of the assembled particle [45,51]. This can be exploited to increase the efficacy of vaccines against highly variable antigens, like influenza A's HA, as it has been reported that VLPs containing simultaneously epitopes from the extracellular domain of M2 protein from human, avian and porcine influenza A viruses showed better protection than the ones containing HA alone [49]. This approach can also be used to present antigens from non-viral pathogens such as bacteria and parasites [46]. An example of a chimeric VLP based vaccine used to present non-viral antigens is RTS,S/AS01 (Mosquirix), used to combat malaria, which consists of HBsAg displaying parts of the secreted circumsporozoite protein from the malaria parasite. Upon expression in yeast cells, the fusion protein forms VLPs with the antigens exposed in its surface, presenting them to the immune system and provoking an efficient response [46,47]. A drawback in the genetic insertion of antigens is that it can destabilize the VLP structure or interfere with protein and/or epitope folding, with positive or highly hydrophobic amino acids and large molecules, like whole proteins domains, being unfavorable to this insertion approach [47]. For such structures, postproduction modifications of VLPs are preferable and can take advantage of naturally occurring sites of conjugation or the VLP can be engineered through to have added functionalities [51]. Besides the development of a recombinant fusion of VLP-antigen, genetic manipulation can also be used to make amino acid residue substitutions and/or insertions on the primary sequence of VLP subunits that can be exploited for chemical conjugation [42,43]. The considerable malleability of the VLPs structure together with the variety of ways that the modifications can be implemented is what has allowed the use of non-animal viruses as a platform for the development of VLP-based vaccines.

VLPs based on non-pathogenic associated viruses include those derived from bacteriophages, such as Q-beta and P22, and plant viruses, like cowpea mosaic virus (CPMV) [48]. They have also shown a remarkable potential to be used in the development of vaccines, mainly developed as heterologous nanoparticle display platforms capable of presenting multivalent antigens, including entire proteins, in a high-density fashion [43,48,50]. The resulting construct is considerably immunogenic being capable of mounting a very effective antigen-specific antibody response for protection against cognate viruses. The VLP derived from bacteriophages P22 has been applied to such an end when the globular head domains of Influenza's HA antigen were covalently conjugated in multiple copies to the surface of preassembled P22 VLPs and immunized in mice [50]. The administration of the construct resulted in the full protection against sublethal doses of homologous influenza challenge, with a faster and more robust antibody response when compared with the soluble HA head alone or with the mixture of P22 VLP and HA head separated. Although both VLPs derived from bacterial and plant viruses have been used for the development of vaccines against infectious disease, the latter has also been applied for immunotherapy. Particularly CPMV VLP has been widely used for immune modulation since they are able to elicit potent antitumor immunity [44,46].

Besides the application of VLPs in the development of vaccines against infectious diseases, they have also been implemented as allergen and cancer vaccines. One particular obstacle that an effective cancer vaccine has to surpass is the immune tolerance for self-antigens, that have an inherently low immunogenicity [41,45]. VLPs are an alluring candidate to the development of such vaccines since they can be used as a platform for the presentation of self-antigens in such disposition that it's capable of breaking the natural tolerance of the immune system and stimulate the immune system to create specific antibodies toward self-proteins [41,45,51]. VLPs capacity of inducing CTL response, either through its inherent properties or through the presentation of exogenous structures, is advantageous to its application as an oncolytic vaccine as CD8+ T lymphocytes have played an important role in the control of tumor growth [45,49]. Plant viruses

VLPs have shown a particular potential to be utilized for cancer therapeutics, as indicated by the CPMV VLPs immunotherapeutic efficacy and capacity to generate potent systemic antitumor immunity. It has been reported that CPMV reprograms the tumoral environment recruiting neutrophils and natural killer cells, while also activates and reprograms tumor-associated macrophages resulting in the innate immune cells attacking and lysing the tumor, allowing the APCs to process tumoral antigens and activate tumor specific T-cell responses [41,44]. Utilizing CPMV as an in situ immunotherapy agent, a favorable therapeutic effect has been verified in models of ovarian tumor, breast cancer, melanoma, and metastatic carcinoma [44]. VLPs also represent a safe platform for the generation of antiallergic vaccines as allergens coupled with them do not promote anaphylactic reactions. Instead, they act as adjuvants facilitating antigen presentation and enhancing the Th1 immune response, which is ideal since molecules from the Th2 response profile are associated with asthmatic problems [41,49]. Q-beta VLP is one of the most explored to this end, with one example reporting that a peptide comprising 16 amino acids of the house dust mite was chemically coupled to its surface and it was observed a rapid humoral immune response based on IgM and IgG against both the 16 amino acid peptide and VLPs; the only side effect observed was a mild skin reaction [49]. Thus, from the literature published so far, it becomes evident that VLPs have remarkable potential as a platform for vaccine development against not only infectious diseases but oncolytic and allergenic as well.

4.5.2 Engineering adjuvants

Adjuvants are exogenous substances that have a wide variety of nature and origin, ranging from mineral salts, oil and water-based emulsions, polymers, microparticles, liposomes, saponins, microbial products, and even cytokines [52]. The term adjuvant comes from the Latin *adjuvare*, which means to help or aid [53]. Adjuvants can be defined as substances that increase the immunogenicity of a vaccine formulation when added/mixed to it. The choice of the adjuvant is of utmost importance as it can stimulate strong humoral and cell-mediated immunity indispensable for protection against some pathogens. In addition, the balance between the adjuvant properties and adverse effects plays a critical role in the selection.

The search for biological structures that could be used as an adjuvant began many years ago, exemplified by the work of Edgar Ribi that characterized the adjuvant activity of lipopolysaccharide (LPS), eliminating its toxic effects, which led to the development of monophosphoryl lipid A (MPL) [54]. Even though the importance of adjuvants in the immune response has been demonstrated, the mechanisms of action by which most adjuvants enhance innate and adaptive immunity need to be understood.

According to the classification of adjuvants, they can be a delivery system type or immunostimulators. Delivery systems, particulates, or emulsions including alum (aluminum salts) [55], water-in-oil, and oil-in-water emulsions (Freund's Complete Adjuvant (CFA) [56] or MF59 [57], were developed to generate a high concentration of antigen at the injection site, which is then slowly released over time. This process leads to greater uptake and presentation of antigens by APCs and to the induction of high titers of antibodies specific to the antigen.

Nowadays, only seven adjuvants are licensed for human vaccine: aluminum salt, virosomes, MF59, R837/R848, AS04, AS03, and metallic nanoparticles (MeNPs); and some still are in a clinical trial (Fig. 4.5).

Immunostimulating substances, on the other hand, increase the immune response through a direct effect on the activation and function of immune cells. These adjuvants induce (1) positive regulation of the levels of surface expression of the main histocompatibility complexes I and II (MHC I and MHC II) in APCs and improved presentation of antigens to the TCR; (2) APC maturation/activation and increased surface expression of costimulatory molecules (CD40, CD80, CD86) necessary for the proper activation of naive T cells; (3) direct and indirect immunomodulation and differentiation of T lymphocytes; (4) recruitment of immune cells at the injection site and migration to draining lymph nodes. In addition, both categories of adjuvants induce immune cell responses mediated by inflammatory cytokines and surface receptors and adhesion molecules. The convergence of events triggered by immune adjuvants leads to increased adaptive immune response and subsequent immune protection, particularly through activation of DCs and T cells [58,59].

Recently, engineered nanoparticles (NPs) have been introduced as novel alternatives to traditional vaccine adjuvant. Metallic nanoparticles (MeNPs) are among the most promising NPs used for vaccine adjuvant as well as the delivery system that can improve immune responses against pathogens. Iron NPs, as an important class of MeNPs, have gained increasing attention as novel vaccine adjuvants [62]. These particles have shown acceptable results in preclinical studies, but it is still important to have a deeper understanding of the

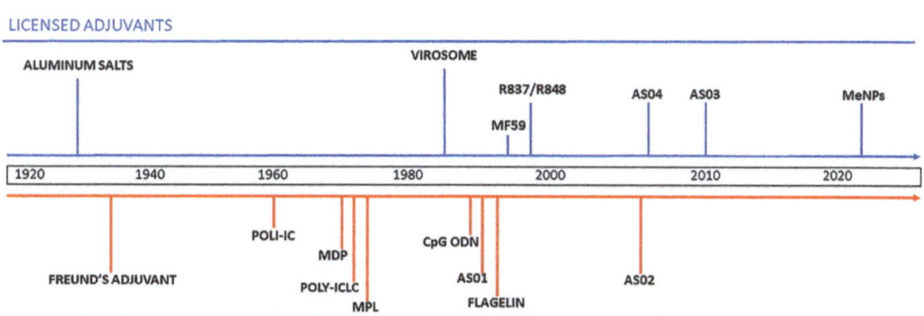

FIG. 4.5 Timetable of adjuvants licensed and in clinical trials. *(Created with BioRender.com).*

physicochemical properties of iron NPs, including size, surface properties, charge, and route of administration, for use in vaccine production [60].

4.6 Immunogenicity

Our planet is inhabited, ultimately, by hosts and pathogens. All life forms thrived and evolved due to the development of an effective collection of defense mechanisms. In mammals, response to pathogen attacks is governed by the innate and adaptive immune responses. These responses have to be "trained" to recognize different antigens, from different branches of life and different biomolecular nature. Therefore, evolution was and always will be dependent on the survival of the species. This, in turn, is dependent on a metastable equilibrium between pathogens and hosts. For the sake of simplicity, this text will focus on human immune responses [61].

Antigens are mainly formed by proteins, polysaccharides, and/or a mixture of both. The kind of immune response will depend on the antigenic biomolecule and the route at which the immunogenic substance is introduced to the organism [63]. The approved vaccines for human use are summarized in Fig. 4.1 and Table 4.1 [65].

4.6.1 Biomolecular origin of antigens and the induced immune response

4.6.1.1 Polysaccharides

Even though polysaccharides are highly immunogenic, they are recognized as T-cell independent responders that induce B cells directly [64]. Therefore, there is a significant drawback: these vaccines are not effective in young children and the elderly [64,65]. The most significant example of polysaccharide-derived vaccine is the one developed in the 1970s against *Streptococcus pneumoniae*, PPSV23 capsular serotypes that induced protection in individuals 2 years and older. This observation led to the need of the creation of novel strategies for vaccine development, since the most affected population was not being protected by this vaccine. In present days, conjugated vaccines overcame this obstacle. Another extremely relevant contribution of anti-bacterial vaccines (as PPSV23) is the reduction in antibiotic drugs used to fight such infections, which ends up resulting in the reduction of antimicrobial resistance [66].

4.6.1.2 Proteins

Vaccine discovery and implementation is an always-evolving field. The most recent findings show that the ease of manipulation and the kind of immune response garnished by protein-based vaccines is responsible for the improvement of immunization success in many cases [67].

TABLE 4.1 Summary of approved vaccines for human use.

Antigen/biomolecule	Age/dosage	Notes
BCG Antigen: Live attenuated bacterial vaccine derived from *M. bovis*	1 dose at birth 1 dose for unvaccinated adolescents and adults in high incidence locations	-Not recommended during pregnancy -Clinically and immunologically stable HIV-infected individuals can be vaccinated -Moderate-to-late preterm infants (gestational age > 31 weeks) and low birth weight infants (<2500 g) can be vaccinated
Hepatites B Antigen: Viral protein antigen as a monovalent vaccine or combined with other infant vaccines	3–4 doses, 1 dose at birth (monovalent) followed by 2–3 doses (monovalent or combined) in the first year 3 doses (monovalent) for unvaccinated adolescents and adults	-The second and third doses can be applied in combination with DTP-vaccine first and third doses -4 weeks interval between doses is recommended -Low birth weight and premature infants can be vaccinated -Vaccination of high-risk groups individuals recommended
Polio Antigen: Vaccines based on live attenuated pathogens containing two (bivalent) or three (trivalent) serotypes	4-5 doses; 1 oral vaccine (bivalent) dose at birth in high-risk countries; 3 oral doses after the 6th week and at least 1 intramuscular vaccine (trivalent) dose after the 14th week	-4 weeks interval between doses is recommended -Can be coadministrated with other infant vaccines -Lower dose schedules are available for low-incidence countries

(*Continued*)

TABLE 4.1 (Cont'd)

Antigen/biomolecule	Age/dosage	Notes
Difteria-Tetanus-Pertussis (DTP) Antigen: Combination vaccine of protein toxoids of Tetanus and Diptheria with either the inactivated pathogen or protein antigens of Pertussis	3 doses; 1 dose after the 6th week followed by 2 doses ideally until 6 months of age 1 booster dose of DPT-vaccine should be provided at 12–23 months of age, followed by 2 booster doses of diphtheria and tetanus toxoid-containing vaccine at 4–7 years of age, and 9–15 years of age	-4 years interval between booster doses is recommended -Tetanus vaccine confers maternal immunization to newborn infants against birth-associated tetanus and can be applied in immunocompromised individuals
Haemophylus influenza B Antigen: Bacterial polysaccharide conjugated to a carrier protein	2-3 doses starting after the 6th week followed by a booster 6 months after the last dose, or 3 doses with DTP co-administration	-Single-dose recommended for children over 12 months of age -Vaccination not recommended for children older than 5 years old -Can be coadministrated with DTP-vaccine -The conjugate vaccine is contraindicated in people with known allergies to any component of the vaccine
Pneumococcal Antigen: Vaccine based on bacterial polysaccharide conjugated to a carrier protein	3 doses starting at 6 weeks of age; can be applied as 3 sequential doses or 2 primary doses with a booster dose at 9–18 months of age	-Can be co-administrated with DTP-vaccine -4 weeks interval between doses is recommended -There are two types of vaccines available, PCV10 and PCV13 -HIV positive individuals and preterm neonate may require a booster dosage -Application not recommended in individuals over 5 years of age

Antigen/biomolecule	Age/dosage	Notes
Rotavirus Antigen: Two oral vaccines one monovalent, based on the live attenuated pathogen, and one pentavalent, based on the reassortant rotaviruses developed from human and bovine strains	3 doses starting at 6 weeks of age, applied together with DTP vaccine	-Can be co-administrated with DTP-vaccine -Application in children over 24 months of age is not recommended -Can be coadministrated with other infant vaccines -Allergic reactions after dosing and immunodeficiency are contraindications of use
MMR (measles, mumps, rubella) Antigen: A combined vaccine based on live attenuated pathogens	2 doses, 1st at 9 months of age and the 2nd between 15-18 months 1 dose of rubella vaccine may be given to unvaccinated adolescents and women at child-bearing age	-In epidemic or high-risk situations, vaccines may be given to children over 6 months -Vaccination in asymptomatic HIV infected individuals may be applied - Should be avoided during pregnancy and by allergenic and immunosuppressed individuals -Vaccinated persons are not eligible to donate blood for 1 month after vaccination
HPV Antigen: Three vaccines (bivalent, quadrivalent, and nonavalent) available based on protein antigen	2 doses to females aged 9–14 years, prior to becoming sexually active 3 doses should be used for all vaccinations initiated after 15 years of age, and in those known to be immunocompromised and/or HIV infected	-All three HPV vaccines can be co-administered with other vaccines using separate syringes and different injection sites - Should be avoided during pregnancy -Vaccination of secondary target populations, like. females aged over 15 years or males, is recommended in viable conditions

(*Continued*)

TABLE 4.1 (Cont'd)

Antigen/biomolecule	Age/dosage	Notes
Japanese encephalitis Antigen: One vaccine based on the inactivated pathogen (the inactivated Vero cell-derived vaccines), and two based on the live attenuated pathogen (the live attenuated vaccines and the live recombinant vaccines) are the main classes used	2 doses of the inactivated Vero cell-derived vaccine, 1st at 6 months of age and the 2nd 4 weeks later in endemic situations 1 dose of the live attenuated vaccine; administered at 8 months of age 1 dose of the recombinant attenuated vaccine; administered at 8 months of age	-Inactivated JE vaccine can be used in immunocompromised persons including inactivated Vero cell-derived vaccines should be preferentially used -Should it be necessary, vaccination of pregnant women with inactivated Vero cell-derived vaccines can be applied
Yellow Fever Antigen: Vaccines based on the live attenuated pathogen	1 dose, given to children at age 9–12 months together with the measles vaccine	-Single does is enough to confer life-long protective immunity -May be applied together with other vaccines -Not recommended to children younger than 8 months, individuals hypersensitivity to egg antigens, or that suffer severe immunodeficiency
Tick-borne encephalitis Antigen: Four vaccines (TBE-Moscow, EnceVir, FSME-Immun, and Encepur) based on inactivated pathogen	3 doses for all age groups, starting from 1(FSME-Immun and Encepur) and 3(TBE-Moscow and EnceVir) years old, in highly endemic regions 3 doses for individuals over 50 years old in medium-low incident areas Booster doses may be required in intervals of close to 3 years	-There are four vaccines currently utilized, one fabricated in Austria (FSME-Immun), another in Germany (Encepur) and two in Russia (TBE-Moscow and EnceVir) -Dosage highly dependant on regional and epidemic conditions

Antigen/biomolecule	Age/dosage	Notes
Typhoid Antigen: Three vaccines are available, one vaccine based on bacterial polysaccharide conjugated to protein (typhoid conjugate vaccine-TCV), one based on unconjugated bacterial polysaccharide (unconjugated Vi polysaccharide-ViPS), and one based on the live attenuated pathogen (Ty21a vaccines)	1 dose at all ages groups for TCV 1 dose for children from 2 years of age for ViPS 3–4 doses for children from 6 years of age Ty21a live oral vaccine Revaccination for ViPS and Ty21a every 3–7 years	-Catch-up vaccination with TCV up to 15 years of age is recommended when feasible -Use during pregnancy should be avoided -Vaccination is a viable response for outbreaks
Cholera Antigen: Two types of oral cholera vaccines are currently available both based on the inactivated pathogen, but one is a monovalent recombinant vaccine (WC-rBS) while the other is a bivalent vaccine (WC) without the recombinant subunit	3 doses at 2-5 years of age for WC-rBS, with a booster every 6 months, and 2 doses for children over 6 years and adults, with a booster every 2nd year 2 doses for children over 1 year for WC, with a booster dose after 2 years	-WC vaccines should be given 14 days apart, while WC-rBS need an interval of 1-6 weeks between doses -Can be applied during gestation and HIV-positive individuals
Meningococcal Antigen: Three vaccines are currently used all based on bacterial polysaccharide conjugated to protein, two monovalent (MenA and MenC), and one quadrivalent (Quadrivalent conjugate)	1 dose of MenA vaccine at 9-18 months of age. 2 doses can be applied to individuals younger than 9 months if necessary 1 dose of the MenC vaccine is recommended for individuals aged over 12 months, teenagers, and adults. 2 doses are administered to children 2–11 months at an interval of a least 2 months and a booster about 1 year after 1 dose of quadrivalent conjugate vaccines should be administered to individuals over 2 years, but one type can also be used for children 9-23 months of age, and given as a 2-dose series, 3 months apart beginning at age 9 months	-Conjugate vaccines are preferred over polysaccharide vaccines due to eliciting herd protection -All vaccines require intramuscular injection -Meningococcal polysaccharide vaccines are less, or not, immunogenic in children under 2 years of age, but can be used in older children in case of outbreaks in countries with limited resources

(Continued)

TABLE 4.1 (Cont'd)

Antigen/biomolecule	Age/dosage	Notes
Hepatites A Antigen: Two types of vaccines are applied, one based on the live attenuated pathogen and one based on the inactivated pathogen	1 dose of the live attenuated HAV vaccine can be applied after the first year of birth A 2 dose schedule with the intramuscular administration of inactivated HAV vaccine may be used for susceptible or immunocompromised individuals	-Vaccination not recommended in endemic countries where most of the population is asymptomatically infected -Intervals between dose range from 6-18 months -Live attenuated vaccines should not be used on severely immunocompromised patients nor during pregnancy
Rabies Antigen: Vaccine based on the inactivated patogen	2 doses of intradermal injection or 1 dose of intramuscular injection at days 0 and 7, for PrEP	-Application consists of two strategies, either post-exposure prophylaxis (PEP) or pre-exposure prophylaxis (PrEP) - PEP which includes extensive and thorough wound washing at the exposure site, and the administration of a course of several doses of rabies vaccine -PrEP consists of the application of several doses of rabies vaccine before exposure and is recommended for individuals at high risk of RABV exposure
Dengue (CYD-TDV) Antigen: The vaccine utilized is CYD-TDV, a live attenuated recombinant tetravalent vaccine	3 doses to individuals with more than 9 years and up to 45 years	-Ideal age for immunization depends on the disease incidence on the population -Pre-vaccination screening is the recommended strategy -Not recommended during pregnancy or nursing, nor to immunocompromised individuals

Antigen/biomolecule	Age/dosage	Notes
Seasonal Influenza Antigen: Two vaccines are available, one trivalent vaccine derived from the inactivated influenza(TIV) and one trivalent vaccine based on the live attenuated influenza (LAIV)	2 doses (TIV) for children 6-59 months old; 1 dose of revaccination applied yearly 1 dose (LAIV) for individuals older than 9 years old	-Pregnant women, children between 6-59 months old, individuals with chronic medical conditions, and the elderly over 65 years compose the priority group -Maternal immunization is the only way to confer protection to children under 6 month old -Annual vaccination or revaccination is necessary
Varicella Antigen: Vaccines based on live attenuated pathogens	2 doses, with the 1st at 12–23 months of age, and the 2nd from 4 weeks to 3 months after the 1st dose 2 doses in adolescents and adults old in countries with a high incidence in older (over 15 years) populations	-Can be administered concomitantly with other live vaccines -Not recommended during pregnancy

There are several advantages in having protein-based antigens (PBA). Among them, the first is the fact that the response for PBAs is T-cell dependent, which in turn can induce B-cell long-lasting response mediated by the production of specific antibodies [67]. Detailed immune responses on protein-based vaccines are well described in Section 4.5.1. In summary, APCs generate proteolyzed antigenic linear peptides that bind avidly to MHC to then induce T cell-dependent response. From these, antibodies will be specific to one or a small number of such peptides (immunodominant). The sequences of immunodominant antigens can be derived using bioinformatics and are being used, for example, to predict epitopes that trigger immune response against SARS-CoV-2 [68]. In the case of B-cells, a conformational-dependent antigen is recognized [69].

Additionally, protein-based carriers have been developed in order to increase immunogenicity in polysaccharide vaccines [70]. A great advantage to use protein as costimulants is the fact that the manipulation, production, and synthesis of such biomolecules are, to a great extent, understood by our current knowledge in protein biochemistry, especially considering the advances in high-resolution structure determination. A direct result of these advances is the production of glycoconjugates: the vaccines that use such technology are very important for immunization of young children, where immune response to polysaccharides is not yet matured as later in life but can be induced by this strategy [67].

4.6.2 Vaccine administration site and immune response determination

The immune response against diseases requires action from mucosal or systemic antibodies. A simple way of manipulating these reactions is to carefully choose the vaccination site [62]. In simplicity, diseases that affect the mucosa have greater protection if vaccines are introduced through a mucosa. One of the most classical examples is the oral polio vaccine. It is noteworthy that these vaccines can also elicit humoral response, as is the case of adeno-derived H1N1 aerosol vaccine under study [62].

On the other hand, parenteral vaccines are given via intradermal, subcutaneous, or intramuscular injections, with intradermal being the most efficient from the three in inducing and immune response. Most of the available vaccines nowadays use this route of administration.

An important difference between the two kinds of administration routes is the need for a specialized workforce to vaccinate with mucosal or parenteral solutions, with the first being more costly and less accessible in remote areas.

In any case, as it has been mentioned throughout this chapter, the main goal in vaccination campaigns is to protect humanity against the burn of vaccine-preventable diseases by achieving successful levels of herd immunity.

4.7 Challenges in mass vaccination

Besides the constant mutation and development of pathogens, a new obstacle to the efficacy of vaccines has risen in recent years in the form of the anti-vaxxers, or anti-vaccine, movement. This movement is heterogeneous in nature, headed by groups of people from different backgrounds and occurring in different locales, but shares the opposition, either partial or total, to the application of vaccines. It justifies itself with arguments that range from the fear of possible side effects of vaccines to issues regarding individual freedom [71]. Even with the plethora of evidence of vaccine safety, these ideas have been gaining momentum recently and threaten to cause serious harm to public health.

Anti-vaccine tendencies have been present in different moments throughout the long history of vaccines, with the current trend apparently starting due to an article published that alleged a correlation between autism and measles vaccination [71,72]. Later, it was spread that vaccine components such as adjuvants, mainly mercury, would be responsible for causing autism in vaccinated children [72]. These false allegations caused temerity at the prospect that vaccination could cause irreparable harm to children resulting in a number of parents opting to not vaccinate theirs.

Although the original allegations have already been extensively disproven [72], and the scientific community has time and again reaffirmed the efficacy and safety of vaccines, the fear instilled from this misinformation had already taken deep roots in certain parcels of society. Though, far from the majority of the population, the more radical groups tend to be very vocal about their beliefs of the presumed dangers of vaccines and can do considerable damage to vaccination efforts, especially when individuals in power echo and validate such claims. Thanks to the instantaneous nature of modern communication, it becomes very easy to spread false information in large quantities, to such a point that it is easy for the average individual to be drowned in this sea of information and become unable to distinguish truth from lies [73].

This dissemination of misinformation fuels fears, ignorance, and an anti-science sentiment that propels vaccination boycotts which can have disastrous consequences as vaccination not only protects the immunized individual but, due to the herd immunity protection, also affects those that remain unvaccinated. This is important in order to protect children too young to be vaccinated or immunocompromised individuals. Consequently, unvaccinated individuals represent a threat as they can act as reservoirs for the pathogens, allowing them to remain present among the population enabling its infection of non-vaccinated individuals. In a worst-case scenario, if enough people are susceptible to the pathogen it can reenter a previously cleared population causing an epidemics and undoing the progress obtained through vaccination. A tragic example is Brazil, in which a resurgence of measles, which had been recently eliminated from the country thanks to an efficient vaccination program [74], has been observed. Due to a rise in the anti-vaccine ideas, the program was undermined and an outbreak occurred. This behavior can cause further harm as we are currently dealing with a global pandemic of SARS-CoV-2, and such mentality could severely hinder vaccination efforts resulting in an unprecedented loss of lives [75].

All in all, vaccines have brought unmeasurable benefits for humanity and through them, we have achieved feats that seemed impossible, such as the complete eradication of smallpox. As such, it is paramount that vaccine development continues, effective vaccination programs and campaigns still be implemented, and that the scientific community sustains the effort of elucidating the unprecedented value of vaccines to the wider population.

References

[1] Andre FE, Booy R, Bock HL, Clemens J, Datta SK, John TJ, et al. Vaccination greatly reduces disease, disability, death and inequity worldwide. Bull World Health Organ 2008;86:140–6.

[2] Greenwood B. The contribution of vaccination to global health: past, present and future. Philos Trans R Soc Lond, B, Biol Sci 2014;369(1645):20130433.

[3] Morens DM, Holmes EC, Davis AS, Taubenberger JK. Global Rinderpest eradication: lessons learned and why humans should celebrate too. J Infect Dis 2011;204:502–5.

[4] Karch CP, Burkhard P. Vaccine technologies: from whole organisms to rationally designed protein assemblies. Biochem Pharmacol 2016;120:1–14.

[5] Siegrist C-A. Vaccine immunology. In: Vaccines, 48, Amsterdam, Elsevier; 2013. p. 14–32.

[6] Fine P, Eames K, Heymann DL. "Herd immunity": a rough guide. Clin Infectious Disease 2011;52:911–6.

[7] Rashid H, Khandaker G, Booy R. Vaccination and herd immunity. Curr Opin Infect Dis 2012;25:243–9.

[8] Beale N, FRCGP MD, Beale E. Evidence-based medicine in the eighteenth century: the Ingen Housz–Jenner correspondence revisited. Med Hist 2005;49(1):79–98.

[9] Pasteur L, Chamberland C, Roux E. Compte rendu sommaire des experiences faites a Pouilly-Le-Fort, pres de Melun, sur la vaccination charbonneuse. CR Acad Sci 1881;92:1378–83.

[10] Pasteur L, Chamberland C, Roux E. De l'attenuation des virus et de leur retour a la virulence. CR Acad Sci 1881;92:430–5.

[11] Graham BS, Sullivan NJ. Emerging viral diseases from a vaccinology perspective: preparing for the next pandemic. Nat Immunol 2018;19(1):20–8.

[12] Xue-Liang P, et al. Advances in the design and development of SARS-CoV-2 vaccines. Mil Med Res 2021;8(1):67–98. doi:10.1186/s40779-021-00360-1.

[13] Diniz MO, Ferreira LCS. Biotecnologia aplicada ao desenvolvimento de vacinas. Estudos Avançados 2010;24(70):19–30.

[14] Anasir MI, Poh CL. Structural vaccinology for viral vaccine design. Front Microbiol 2019;10:738.

[15] Center of Disease Control and Prevention (CDC). https://www.cdc.gov/flu/prevent/nasalspray.htm (accessed November 1, 2021)

[16] Tangy F, Naim HY. Live attenuated measles vaccine as a potential multivalent pediatric vaccination vector. Viral Immunol 2005;18(2):317–26.

[17] Zhang Y, Zeng G, Pan H, Li C, Hu Y, Chu K, et al. Safety, tolerability, and immunogenicity of an inactivated SARS-CoV-2 vaccine in healthy adults aged 18-59 years: a randomised, double-blind, placebo-controlled, phase 1/2 clinical trial. Lancet Infect Dis 2020;S1473-S3099(20):30843–4.

[18] Moss B, Smith GL, Gerin JL, Purcell RH. Live recombinant vaccinia virus protects chimpanzees against hepatitis B. Nature 1884;311(5981):67–9.

[19] Tell JG, Coller BG, Dubey SA, Jenal U, Lapps W, Wang L, et al. Environmental risk assessment for rVSVdeltaG-ZEBOV-GP, a genetically 8Live vaccine for Ebola virus disease. Vaccines, Basel 2020;8(4):779.

[20] Draper SJ, Heeney JL. Viruses as vaccine vectors for infectious diseases and cancer. Nat Rev Microbiol 2010;8(1):62–73.

[21] Condit RC, Williamson AL, Sheets R, Seligman SJ, Monath TP, Excler JL, et al. Unique safety issues associated with virus-vectored vaccines: potential for and theoretical consequences of recombination with wild type virus strains. Brighton Collaboration Viral Vector Vaccines Safety Working Group (V3SWG). Vaccine 2016;34(51):6610–6.

[22] Rappuoli R. Glycoconjugate vaccines: principles and mechanisms. Sci Transl Med 2018;10:4615.

[23] Rappuoli R, Gregorio ED, Costantino P. On the mechanisms of conjugate vaccines. PNAS 2019;116(1):14–6.

[24] Rappuoli R. Reverse vaccinology. Curr Opin Microbiol 2020;3:445–50.

[25] Serruto D, Bottomley MJ, Ram S, Giuliani MM, Rappuoli R. The new multicomponent vaccine against meningococcal serogroup B, 4CMenB: immunological, functional and structural characterization of the antigens. Vaccine 2012;30(Suppl 2):B87–97 2012.

[26] O'Ryan M, Stoddard J, Toneatto D, Wassil J, Dull PM. A multi-component meningococcal serogroup B vaccine (4CMenB): the clinical development program. Drugs 2014;74(1): 15–30.

[27] Doro F, Liberatori S, Rodriguez-Ortega MJ. Surfome analysis as a fast track to vaccine discovery: identification of a novel protective antigen for Group B Streptococcus hypervirulent strain COH1. Mol Cell Proteomics 2009;8(7):1728–37.

[28] Giuliani MM, Adu-Bobie J, Comanducci M, Arico B, Savino S, Santini L, et al. A universal vaccine for serogroup B meningococcus. PNAS 2006;103(29):10834–9.

[29] Green CA, Scarselli E, Voysey M, Capone S, Vitelli A, Nicosia A, et al. Safety and immunogenicity of novel respiratory syncytial virus (RSV) vaccines based on the RSV viral proteins F, N and M2-1 encoded by simian adenovirus (PanAd3-RSV) and MVA (MVA-RSV); protocol for an open-label, dose-escalation, single-centre, phase 1 clinical trial in healthy adults. BMJ Open 2015;5:e008748.

[30] Adler SP, Lewis N, Conlon A, Christiansen MP, Al-Ibrahim M, Rupp R. Phase 1 clinical trial of a conditionally replication-defective human cytomegalovirus (CMV) vaccine in CMV-seronegative subjects. J Infect Dis 2019;220(3):411–9.

[31] Dormitzer PR, Ulmer JB, Rappuoli R. Structure-based antigen design: a strategy for next generation vaccines. Trends Biotechnol 2008;26:659–67.

[32] Cozzi R, Scarselli M, Ferlenghi I. Structural vaccinology: a three-dimensional view for vaccine development. Curr Top Med Chem 2013;13(20):2629–37.

[33] Lundstrom K. Structural genomics and drug discovery. J Cell Mol Med 2007;11(2):224–38.

[34] Anderson WF. Structural genomics and drug discovery for infectious diseases. Infect Disord Drug Target 2009;9(5):507–17.

[35] Schneider MC, Prosser BE, Caesar JJE, Kugelberg E, Li S, Zhang Q, et al. *Neisseria meningitidis* recruits factor H using protein mimicry of host carbohydrates. Nature 2009;458: 890–3.

[36] Jiang HQ, Hoiseth SK, Harris SL, McNeil LK, Zhu D, Tan C, Scott AA, et al. Broad vaccine coverage predicted for a bivalent recombinant factor H binding protein based vaccine to prevent serogroup B meningococcal disease. Vaccine 2010;28:6086–93.

[37] Sanchez-Trincado JL, Gomez-Perosanz M, Reche PA. Fundamentals and methods for T- and B-Cell epitope prediction. J Immunol Res, Peptide-Based Immunotherapeutics Vaccines 2017. doi:10.1155/2017/2680160 ID 2680160.

[38] Zhang L. Multi-epitope vaccines: a promising strategy against tumors and viral infections. Cell Mol Immunol 2018;15(2):182–4.

[39] Chen X, Zaro JL, W-C S. Fusion protein linkers: property, design and functionality. Adv Drug Deliv Ver, 2013;65(10):1357–69.

[40] Livingston B, Crimi C, Newman M, et al. A rational strategy to design multiepitope immunogens based on multiple Th lymphocyte epitopes. J Immunol 2002;168(11):5499–506.

[41] Ali M, Pandey RK, Khatoon N, Narula A, Mishra A, Prajapati VK. Exploring dengue genome to construct a multi-epitope based subunit vaccine by utilizing immunoinformatics approach to battle against dengue infection. Sci Rep 2017;7(1):1–13.

[42] Kalenik BM, Góra-Sochacka A, Sirko A. B-defensins – underestimated peptides in influenza combat. Virus Res 2018;247:10–4.

[43] Chung YH, Cai H, Steinmetz NF. Viral nanoparticles for drug delivery, imaging, immunotherapy, and theranostic applications. Adv Drug Deliv Rev 2020;156:214–35.

[44] Rohovie MJ, Nagasawa M, Swartz JR. Virus-like particles: next-generation nanoparticles for targeted therapeutic delivery. Bioeng Transl Med 2017;2(1):43–57.

[45] Rother M, Nussbaumer MG, Renggli K, Bruns N. Protein cages and synthetic polymers: a fruitful symbiosis for drug delivery applications, bionanotechnology and materials science. Chem Soc Rev 2016;45(22):6213–49.

[46] Wu J, Wu H, Nakagawa S, Gao J. Virus-derived materials: bury the hatchet with old foes. Biomater Sci 2020;8(4):1058–72.

[47] Yan D, Wei YQ, Guo HC, Sun SQ. The application of virus-like particles as vaccines and biological vehicles. Appl Microbiol Biotechnol 2015;99(24):10415–32.

[48] Butkovich N, Li E, Ramirez A, Burkhardt AM, Wang SW. Advancements in protein nanoparticle vaccine platforms to combat infectious disease. Wiley Interdiscip Rev Nanomed Nanobiotechnol 2020:e1681 Advance online publication.

[49] Fuenmayor J, Gòdia F, Cervera L. Production of virus-like particles for vaccines. New Biotechnol 2017;39(Pt B):174–80.

[50] Sharma J, Shepardson K, Johns LL, Wellham J, Avera J, Schwarz B, Rynda-Apple A, Douglas T. A self-adjuvanted, modular, antigenic VLP for rapid response to influenza virus variability. ACS Appl Mater Interfaces 2020;12(16):18211–24.

[51] Zepeda-Cervantes J, Ramírez-Jarquín JO, Vaca L. Interaction between virus-like particles (VLPs) and pattern recognition receptors (PRRs) from dendritic cells (DCs): toward better engineering of VLPs. Front Immunol 2020;11:1100.

[52] Donaldson B, Lateef Z, Walker GF, Young SL, Ward VK. Virus-like particle vaccines: immunology and formulation for clinical translation. Expert Rev Vaccines 2018;17(9): 833–49.

[53] Frietze KM, Peabody DS, Chackerian B. Engineering virus-like particles as vaccine platforms. Curr Opin Virol 2016;18:44–9.

[54] Apostólico JS, Lunardelli VAS, Coirada FC, Boscardin SB, Rosa DS. Adjuvants: classification, modus operandi, and licensing. J Immunol Res 2016;2016:16 Article ID 1459394.

[55] Cox JC, Coulter AR. Adjuvants—a classification and review of their modes of action. Vaccine 1997;3(15):248–56.

[56] Ribi E. Beneficial modification of the endotoxin molecule. J Biol Response Mod 1984;3(1):1–9.

[57] Glenny AT. Immunological notes: antigenic value of toxoid precipitated by potassium alum. J Pathol Bacteriol 1926;29:38–9.
[58] Freund J. The mode of action of immunologic adjuvants. Bibl Tuberc 1956;10:130–48.
[59] Calabro S, Tritto E, Pezzotti A, Taccone M, Muzzi A, Bertholet S, et al. The adjuvant effect of MF59 is due to the oil-in-water emulsion formulation, none of the individual components induce a comparable adjuvant effect. Vaccine 2013;31:3363–9.
[60] Janeway Jr. CA. Immunogenecity: Signal 1,2,3…and 0. Immunol Today 1989;10:283–7.
[61] Awate LAB, Mutwiri G. Mechanisms of action of adjuvants. Front Immunol 2013;4:114 http://doi.org/10.3389/fimmu.2013.00114 eCollection.
[62] Behzadi M, Vakili B, Ebrahiminezhad A, Nezafat N. Iron nanoparticles as novel vaccine adjuvants. Eur J Pharm Sci 2021;16:105718.
[63] Pollard AJ, Bijker EM. A guide to vaccinology: from basic principles to new developments. Nat Rev Immunol 2021;21:83–100.
[64] Zhang L, Wang W, Wang S. Effect of vaccine administration modality on immunogenicity and efficacy. Expert Rev Vaccines 2015;14(11):1509–23.
[65] World Health Organization https://www.who.int/health-topics/vaccines-and-immunization #tab=tab_1 2020 (accessed November 1, 2021)
[66] Mitchell R, Kelly DF, Pollard AJ, Trück J. Polysaccharide-specific B cell responses to vaccination in humans. Hum Vaccin Immunother 2014;10(6):1661–8.
[67] Heilmann C. Human B and T lymphocyte responses to vaccination with pneumococcal polysaccharides. APMIS Suppl 1990;15:1–23.
[68] Bloom DE, Black S, Salisbury D, Rappuoli R. Antimicrobial resistance and the role of vaccines. Proc Natl Acad Sci USA 2018;115(51):12868–71.
[69] Saylor K, Gillam F, Lohneis T, Zhang C. Designs of antigen structure and composition for improved protein-based vaccine efficacy. Front Immunol 2020;11:283.
[70] Grifoni A, Sidney J, Zhang Y, Scheuermann RH, Peters B, Sette A. A sequence homology and bioinformatic approach can predict candidate targets for immune responses to SARS-CoV-2. Cell Host Microbe 2020;27(4):671–680.e2.
[71] Sun P, Ju H, Liu Z, Ning Q, Zhang J, Zhao X, Huang Y, Ma Z, Li Y. Bioinformatics resources and tools for conformational B-cell epitope prediction. Comput Math Methods Med 2013:943636. doi:10.1155/2013/943636.
[72] Micoli F, Adamo R, Costantino P. Protein carriers for glycoconjugate vaccines: history, selection criteria, characterization and new trends. Molecules 2018;23(6):1451.
[73] Stolle LB, Nalamasu R, Pergolizzi Jr. JV, Varrassi G, Magnusson P, LeQuang J, Breve F. Fact vs fallacy—the anti-vaccine discussion reloaded. Adis J Media 2020;37 https://doi.org/10.6084/m9.figshare.12927965.
[74] Baker JP. Mercury, vaccines, and autism: one controversy, three histories. Am J Public Health 2008;98(2):244–53 https://doi.org/10.2105/AJPH.2007.113159.
[75] Burki T. The online anti-vaccine movement in the age of COVID-19. The Lancet Digital Health 2020;2(10):e504–5 http://doi.org/10.1016/s2589-7500(20)30227-2.

Chapter 5

Infection, immunity, and vaccine development

Bhawana Singh[a,#], Awnish Kumar[b,#], Rahul Tiwari[b], Shashi Bhushan Chauhan[a], Om Prakash Singh[c], Santosh K Singh[b], Vibhav Gautam[b], Shyam Sundar[a], Rajiv Kumar[b]

[a]Department of Medicine, Institute of Medical Sciences, Banaras Hindu University, Varanasi, India [b]Centre of Experimental Medicine and Surgery, Institute of Medical Sciences, Banaras Hindu University, Varanasi, India [c]Department of Biochemistry, Institute of Science, Banaras Hindu University, Varanasi, India

#Joint 1st author.

5.1 Introduction

Our surrounding environment contains a variety of microorganisms, such as bacteria, viruses, protozoa, and other parasites that causes different diseases. Infectious diseases have been a challenge to the healthcare sector, with devastating consequences under certain disease conditions. The human body has evolved an immune system to fight against invading pathogens. Each pathogen possesses unique proteins/peptides called antigens which mark their identity and distinguish them from host (self) molecules. When the immune system encounters a new antigen, it prepares to eliminate the foreign pathogen and developing immunological memory. Subsequent encounters with the same antigen trigger these memory cells, which in turn, induces a quick and robust immune response to control the invading microorganism.

Before the advent of vaccines and their widespread deployment, infectious diseases topped the list of killers for the world community. Many infectious diseases have now been contained, especially in developed countries due to the use of vaccines. Indeed, the development of safe and effective vaccines is one of the main ways for conferring protection against infections by and saving lives of millions.

Individuals in a population can be categorized into three groups, depending upon their immune status: first, susceptible to infection; secondly, infected/infectious, and third, recovered from infection/immune. Upon encountering a pathogen, our body elicits immune responses in the form of inflammation. The inflamed tissue/site triggers the release of chemical mediators that increases the blood flow to the affected area and attracts white blood cells (WBCs).

System Vaccinology. https://doi.org/10.1016/B978-0-323-85941-7.00006-1

A subset of WBCs called phagocytes, engulfs the target pathogen, kill them, and then digest them into smaller molecules, prior to traveling to the local lymph nodes. In the lymph nodes, the phagocytes present the antigen to the other cells of immune system to induce heightened and antigen-specific T cell immune responses. The production of antigen-specific antibodies by B cells is also initiated and these can bind the circulating pathogens and lead to the development of a cell-mediated immune response (adaptive immunity; CMI). The entire duration from the first encounter with the pathogen to the development of adaptive immunity takes several days. Once the antigen-specific T- and B-cells are activated, they expand leading to pathogen clearance, followed by development of immunological memory for subsequent pathogen encounters. Memory against infection persists for extended periods, but over time, immunity (memory) wanes. However, memory can be boosted by asymptomatic re-exposure to pathogens, as in the case of measles [1] and pertussis [2]. Secondary immune responses prevent disease resurgence because the pathogen is detected, attacked, and destroyed before the symptoms reappear. Adults have a more rapid and strong memory responses as compared to children; this accounts for the increased likelihood of children getting sick as compared to the adults. Natural infections and/or vaccinations are crucial players in shaping the overall immune status of the host. As immunity wanes over time after exposure to the pathogen, there is a need for boosting, otherwise the individual will be susceptible to reinfection. The generation of vaccine-induced memory cells without disease is the basis for the effectiveness of many vaccines. Vaccines are estimated to have prevented more than 100 million disease cases in the last century (in the United States alone) [3]. Immunization/vaccination programs have saved millions of lives throughout the world by improving the immune system. Variolation is one of the most ancient forms of vaccination, used many centuries before Edward Jenner tested its use with cowpox as a safer alternative to variola virus. Jenner's work laid the foundation for modern vaccinology (using attenuated, killed pathogens or their components to induce adaptive immunity) for protecting against pathogens. Therefore, vaccines prime the immune system so that the body is ready to fight against particular invading pathogens and subvert disease manifestations, as well as its spread in a population. In this chapter, we provide an insight into the clinical research aimed at understanding the immunology behind our defense against infections and how vaccines can be used to stimulate these protective responses.

5.2 Basic concept of vaccine immunology

As discussed previously, the immune system is a well-orchestrated system that remembers a pathogenic encounter for several decades and/or even lifetime. This property of the immune system has formed the basis for vaccine development and for inducing lifelong protection against pathogens. Most licensed vaccines have targeted microbes that cause acute infections, including diphtheria, tetanus, pneumococcal, MMR vaccine, etc. Earlier vaccines relied on the development of humoral (antibody) arm of the immune response. However, after the HIV pandemic in late 1980s, vaccine development programs pivoted and tried to stimulate both the cell-mediated and humoral arms of the immune system [4], generating effective vaccine against diseases such as hepatitis A [5], hepatitis B [6], influenza [7], varicella [8] and typhoid [9], etc.

A successful vaccine is the one that induces strong memory T-cell responses. However, there are different facets of generating optimal immunological memory. In this chapter, we will shed light on these different immunological aspects for a better understanding of the immune mechanisms needed for the maintenance of different effector arms of immunity in a vaccination strategy for combating infections.

5.2.1 Innate immunity

Innate immunity is the non-specific arm of immune system that reacts rapidly to the invading pathogen due to its multilayered nature: physical barriers (lysozyme rich mucosa, respiratory cilia), antimicrobials, surfactants, defensins, and mannose binding lectin. Principally, the innate immune system recognizes the molecular patterns of the invading pathogens (PAMPs) and helps to initiate the adaptive arm of immune machinery (i.e., T- and B-cells), that persists for a longer periods of time than innate immune cells. Indeed, the nature of immune responses against a pathogen and its duration is determined by the initial encounter with pattern recognition receptors (PRR) on innate cells (macrophages, NK cells and dendritic cells (DCs)) [10]. A series of innate receptors trigger responses to these initial pathogen encounters, including the nucleotide binding oligomerization domain (NOD) like receptors and toll-like receptors (TLR). This leads to a cascade of events manifesting in the form of production of innate cytokines, activation of NK cells and other innate lymphoid cells (ILCs), production of mannose binding lectins, interferons, neutrophil chemotaxis, phagocytosis, deployment of neutrophil extracellular traps (NETs) and generation of reactive oxygen species. Apart from its role as the first-line, non-specific arm of the immune system, innate immune cells, and responses play key roles in amplification of the T- and B-cell responses. The concept of trained innate immunity is emerging, whereby innate immune cells change their phenotype after a pathogen encounter to be better able to respond to a second encounter. The major innate immune cells (i.e., the monocytes/macrophages and NK cells) have lower turnover rates compared to the neutrophils (short life and terminally differentiated population), which may allow them to serve as trained memory cells for a limited period of time.

Recent research has highlighted the importance of reprogramming innate cells after previous pathogenic exposures, leading to increased production of cytokines and improved pathogen clearance following a second exposure [11]. This reprogramming of the innate cells in response to a previous pathogenic insult is termed trained immunity or innate immune memory. Compared to the classical immunological memory involving T and B cells, innate memory involves different cell subsets (NK cells, myeloid cells, and ILCs or innate lymphoid cells) that recognize PRRs and cytokines (different from classical memory cells). Innate memory cells responses are not specific for a particular pathogen but instead are mediated through epigenetic changes that do not cause permanent physiological changes, as seen in mutations or genetic recombination events. Furthermore, innate memory depends on the altered functional state of the innate cells (existing for weeks to months rather than for years as seen in classical immunological memory), in the absence of initial stimulus [12]. Recent investigations have highlighted important roles for trained immunity in different infectious diseases. The trained innate leukocytes respond to secondary encounters with the same or unrelated microorganisms. Trained immunity has been successfully induced by mycobacterial components upon treatment with BCG/PPD, muramyl dipeptide, and Freund's complete adjuvant against candidiasis, Klebsiella and FMDV (Foot and Mouth disease virus), respectively [13–15]. Conversely, BCG-mediated cross-protection effectively controlled *Schistosoma manosni* infection. It was also found to induce heterologous protection against gastrointestinal infections [16], sepsis [17], respiratory tract pathogens [18], and yellow fever [19]. Studies using *ex vivo* stimulation reported the duration of innate memory cells for up to three months [20,21]. Thus, BCG induced non-specific protection against unrelated pathogens.

Innate immune cell signaling has been known to be associated with metabolic alterations and epigenetic changes that significantly affect innate memory responses. Histone methylation is one of the most important effector pathways of epigenetic manipulation in monocytes; the innate memory induced by epigenetic reprogramming provided protection against Candidiasis in *Rag1*-deficient mice [22]. Histone modification (acetylation of H3K9) epigenetic changes can provide trans-generational transmission of disease resistance [23]. In addition to epigenetic reprogramming, gene recombination is employed by NK cells for triggering memory responses. Innate immune responses decline rapidly after clearance of infection and the functionality of innate immune responses does not return to steady state due to the epigenetic alterations in innate cells. Immune ontological studies have demonstrated TLR-induced changes in cytokine production profiles as an indicator of the maturation of innate immune responses and their ability to reduce the severity of subsequent infections [24]. Memory NK cells are known to mediate protection after cytomegalovirus infection, independent of T and B cells. $CXCR6^+$ NK cells are the main mediators of memory responses in T and B cell-deficient mice [25,26]. This NK cell-based memory response is mainly driven by a set of cytokines, including IL-12, IL-15, and IL-18 in humans and mice [27]. Thus, trained immunity appears to have potential therapeutic applications.

In terms of vaccine design and development, non-specific side effects of vaccines can have life-threatening consequences. However, this can be reduced by managing the sequence and/or timing of vaccination. Non-specific side effects can also be abrogated by using adjuvants that trigger PRR-induced innate memory. However, non-specific immunity can induce herd immunity and improve immune responses against different pathogens. Therefore, a better understanding of innate memory regulation would help in designing vaccines to take advantage of trained immunity.

5.2.2 Adaptive immunity

Once the innate immune system is alerted by the presence of a pathogen, it activates the adaptive immune system. T-cells and B-cells mediate specific immune responses are termed adaptive immunity. Although these responses are slow to develop *de novo*, due to the time lag from the priming of the immune system to response against the pathogen, a second encounter with the same antigen (pathogen), elicits a stronger and more rapid immune response to destroy the invading pathogen. It relies on the generation of memory T-and B-cells that take a few weeks, but these lasts much longer than innate trained immune responses. This property of adaptive immunity has been utilized for vaccine development. Vaccines utilize adaptive immunity and immunological memory to abrogate disease, thus understanding the immunological responses that underlie effective vaccines is critical.

5.2.2.1 T-cells responses

T and B cells arise from progenitors in the bone marrow, but T-cells need to develop in the thymus where they undergo selection so that the T-cell receptor (TCR) they express can recognize MHC molecules (positive selection), but do not recognize self-antigens (negative selection). After maturation in the thymus, T cells express a unique TCR capable of recognizing peptide antigens in the context of MHC classes I and II for $CD8^+$ and $CD4^+$ T cells, respectively. The activation, clonal expansion and differentiation of $CD8^+$ and $CD4^+$ T cells are similar. Following infection, $CD8^+$ T cell activation occurs following the recognition of a reactive peptide associated with an MHC I molecule on the surface of a DC. DC-mediated T-cell activation is essential for optimal development of immunological responses. In this context, the antigen specific interaction between the T-cells and DCs is for a relative shorter duration (up to 12 hours), however, T-cells receive all necessary triggers for activation in this time [28,29]. These signals include the activation signals (signal-1), costimulation (signal-2), and appropriate signals from pro-inflammatory cytokines (signal-3) [30]. Chemokine receptors CCL19 and CCL21 are also known to amplify immune responses by stimulating the interaction between the T-cells and DCs [31,32]. Additionally, chemokines secreted by activated DCs and $CD4^+$ T-cells increase $CD8^+$ T-cell accumulation that can help their activation. Overall, activation of T-cells modulates the expression of several integrins, selectins, and chemokine receptors that effect chemokine and cytokine expressions, leading to the proliferation, migration, and differentiation of T-cells to fight against invading pathogens. After the infection resolves, the majority of these cells (90-95%) dies by apoptosis, while a small fraction of cells differentiates into memory cells [33]. Memory cells can further be classified on the basis of their proliferation, phenotype and homing potential into effector memory T cells (T_{EM}) expressing surface markers- KLRG1^{hi}CD44^{hi}CD127^{hi} CD62L^{lo}, central memory T cells (T_{CM}) expressing KLRG1^{lo}CD44^{hi}CD127^{hi} CD62L^{hi} and tissue-resident memory T cells (T_{RM}) that mainly expresse CD69^{hi}CD62L^{lo} CD44^{hi} [34]; there are other minor memory cells population including stem cell like memory cells (T_{SCM}), virtual memory cells (T_{VM}) and terminally differentiated memory (T_{EMRA}) [35]. T_{CM} are directed toward the secondary lymphoid organs, exhibit superior proliferation and produce IL-2 for better secondary expansion. On the contrary, T_{EM} reside in non-lymphoid tissue and exhibits limited proliferation potential upon TCR stimulation, but rapidly produce effector cytokines (IFN-γ, TNF). Both T_{EM} and T_{CM} can be found in the circulation whereas T_{RM} lack migratory capacity and reside in the peripheral tissues [36,37]. Given these various fates for T-cells in response to infection, there has been a lot of interest in the factors that regulate these processes. Apart from different transcription factors, the role of cytokines in regulating these signaling pathways has been extensively investigated. IL-7 and IL-15 are important cytokines for the homeostasis of memory CD8$^+$ T cell populations [38]. Differentiated CD4$^+$ and CD8$^+$ T cells can also be divided into several types based on their cytokine-producing profiles—Th1, Th2, and Th17 cells (subclasses of CD4$^+$ T cells) and Tc1 and Tc2, and more recently Tc17 cells (subclasses of CD8$^+$ T cells). In addition to T cell effector and memory subsets, there are also T cells with immunosuppressive characteristics [39,40]. These regulatory T (Treg) cells can belong to either CD4$^+$ and /or CD8$^+$ class and express the FOXP3 transcription factor. They represent approximately 0.4 and 0.1% of peripheral blood T-cells in healthy humans and mice, respectively. In mice, their frequencies are quite similar in lymph nodes (LNs) and the spleen, but two to threefold higher in Peyer patches and mesenteric LNs. Identification of Tregs remains a tedious task since the markers used for their identification are generally T-cell activation markers (CD25, CTLA4, GITR, LAG3, CD127, and Foxp3). CD8$^+$ Treg cells express low levels of CD127, but higher levels of activation and proliferation markers, such as CTLA-4, ICOS and Ki-67, compared with other CD8$^+$ T-cells [41]. They also express high levels of CD25, and as a result, are 20- to 40-fold more sensitive to IL-2 stimulation in vitro than CD8$^+$ effector T-cells, but 2–4 times less sensitive than CD4$^+$ Treg cells [42]. Overall, this subset of T-cells is known to negatively regulate the immune responses; however, their roles are still not fully understood.

T follicular helper cells (Tfh) are another specialized cell subset of CD4$^+$ T-cell that works hand in hand with B-cells to generate humoral immune responses. As compared to other T-cell subsets, they are unique, as their differentiation is multi-step and relies on the interaction with DCs and B-cells [43,44].

Unlike conventional T-cell differentiation, Tfh cells play crucial roles in germinal center (GC) development and function [45]. The GC is the primary site for antibody isotype switching and affinity maturation. These cells are important players in controlling pathogens and commensal microbiota and production of IgE in allergic reactions [46,47]. Autoimmune diseases are associated with increased frequencies of Tfh-like cells (CXCR5+ and $PD1^{hi}$ or $ICOS^{hi}$) leading to excessive autoantibody production and disease pathology [48,49]. Thus, Tfh cells are a crucial determinant for generating humoral responses after immunization. Indeed, boosting the Tfh cell numbers by vaccines is important in several diseases. Thus, T-cells are well-defined controllers of immunity and the study of them is critical for developing effective vaccines.

5.2.2.2 B-cells responses

The adaptive immune system relies on antigen presenting cells (APCs) and lymphocytes to fight against immune challenges. B-cells serve dual function by acting as APCs, supporting other mononuclear cells functions, participating directly in triggering inflammatory reactions and producing antibodies. B-cell mediated humoral responses are triggered upon the encounter of antigen reactive B-cells with the antigen, in the secondary lymphoid tissue (lymph node, Peyer's patches, spleen). A sub-capsular region that captures antigens from lymph and mediates directional transport to contact the follicular B-cell, another specialized compartment called lymphoid follicles has follicular DCs (FDC) that is non-phagocytic and efficiently captures as well as presents the opsonized antigen on its surface for weeks. B-cell migration to the follicles is guided by CXCL13 and other follicle associated stromal cells. B-cells migrate non-directionally scanning the sub capsular macrophages and FDCs, to determine if they display surface antigens or soluble antigens in the circulation they are reactive against. After several hours of surveillance, if B-cells do not encounter antigen then they exit the lymphoid tissue and travel to other lymphoid tissues to scan the tissue for the presence of foreign antigens [50,51]. On the contrary, if they encounter antigen, the cascade of B-cell receptor (BCR) signaling is triggered and this leads to B-cell activation *via.* clustering of the BCR on the membrane to begin signaling [52]; alternatively, the BCR clusters before pathogen exposure and upon encountering the antigen these clusters dismantle and enable the signaling to begin [53]. Other models for B-cell activation have also been proposed [52,53].

Naïve B-cells express immunoglobulins (IgM and/or IgD) that are deficient in intracellular domains, relying on other intracellular molecules for signal transduction, particularly Igα and Igβ that contain ITAM motifs which are phosphorylated by tyrosine kinases [53,54]. This leads to a downstream cascade of events culminating in B-cells activation *via.* changes in the expression of numerous genes. This includes the upregulation in expression of cell cycle related molecules, survival factors, migration molecules, costimulatory molecules (CD80, CD86), and adhesion molecules. In addition to the BCR, coreceptors such as

TLRs or complement receptors amplify BCR signaling and reduce the antigenic threshold for B-cells activation [55,56]. B-cells also express several ITIM containing receptors (FcγRIIb, CD22), that recruit phosphatases such as SHIP1 and SHP1 that dampen BCR signals [57].

Once the BCR is triggered, it internalizes bound antigen that travels *via.* the endosomal pathway to the lysosomes for antigen processing and upon docking onto the MHC-II these are then presented to $CD4^+$ T-cells [58]. Clonal expansion of B-cells is triggered in response to helper T-cell derived signals called the T-cell dependent pathway, while the T-cell independent pathway utilizes cytokine derived signals (BAFF and APRIL) from innate cells for proliferation followed by differentiation and class switching. B-cells terminally differentiate into plasma cells that secrete antibodies [59]. Memory B-cells are another subset, which remains quiescent, however, following antigenic re-exposure, these differentiate into the GC B-cells or plasma cells as well as the subsets of IgM and IgG memory B cells. Memory B-cells also undergo class switch recombination and exhibit characteristic transcriptional or epigenetic profiles that play essential roles in determining the ability to respond to antigenic re-exposure [60,61]. Atypical memory B-cells constitutes another important cell subset, recently studied in infectious diseases. Immune activation or inflammation drives the expansion of these cells. The peculiar feature of these cells is their un-/ hypo-responsiveness to stimulation through BCRs, and subsequent inability to secrete cytokines or antibodies [62].

Regulatory B-cells (Breg) are another important subset that exerts immunomodulatory effects by producing IL-10 and TGF-β. These cytokines exert immunoregulatory effects on antigen-presenting DCs or support the survival and differentiation of other immune cells. IL-10 and other anti-inflammatory mediators are involved in maintaining tolerance and immune homeostasis [63–65]. Reduced frequencies and functions of Breg cells cause chronic inflammation. Furthermore, the cellular microenvironment also plays crucial role in their induction. Breg cell activation is enhanced by CD40, TLR, and BCR signaling, and exposure to pro-inflammatory cytokines (IL-1β, IL-6, IL-21, IFNβ, IFNα) [66–68]. Immunomodulatory therapies targeting Breg cells hold potential for different diseases, however, the stability, plasticity, and efficacy of transferred Breg cells are a major concern for use in clinical settings. Efforts are now being directed more toward vaccine design for disease eradication aims to trigger B-cells activation and generate broadly neutralizing antibody responses.

5.3 Immunological memory

The adaptive immune system is critical for protection against life-threatening infections. Following clearance of infection, a proportion of T and B cells differentiate to form the memory pool, which provides long-lasting protection against previously exposed pathogens. Immunological memory is characterized by the ability of our immune system to respond with greater speed and intensity toward re-encounters with pathogens. It is the basis for the vaccine-mediated protection against disease, whereby individuals who survived a disease rarely developed more severe disease a second time. The concept of modern vaccination, started in the 17th century with Jenner recognizing immunological memory in cured cowpox cases against smallpox [69].

Despite much research directed toward understanding the key components of immunological memory, there is still an incomplete understanding about how immunological memory is generated and maintained. As previously discussed, much effort has been made to understand the diversity in lymphocyte subsets, however, research regarding different memory types of memory T and B cells is still in its infancy. To date, three subsets of memory cells ($CD4^+$ T, $CD8^+$ T, and B cells) have been identified. However, novel subpopulations are starting to be recognized (as discussed in the previous section). The use of transgenic mouse models, adoptive transfer strategies, and technological advances have facilitated cellular studies on trafficking, homeostasis, and lineage commitment of memory T and B cells.

5.3.1 T-cells memory

In recent years, much research has focused on differentiation patterns of memory cells and it has been assumed to be multifaceted. One model postulated that memory cells arise during the immune contraction phase from effector cells, meaning that effector cells either die or differentiate into memory cell subsets depending on the survival signals they receive. Another model for memory cells suggests formation by linear differentiation from effector cells [70]. This theory fits equally well for $CD4^+$ and $CD8^+$ T-cells, where multiple cytokine-producing $CD4^+$ T-cells transits to form memory cell subsets [71,72]. Another model suggests stepwise or bifurcated differentiation of activated T-cells that leads to the gradual loss of memory potential of the cells, while acquiring a terminally differentiated phenotype, depending activation signals they receive during infection (antigen dose, affinity, cytokine milieu, TCR-MHC II affinity, and costimulatory signals) [71,72]. An additional theory postulated a multidimensional pattern of differentiation into memory cells (Fig. 5.1). The development of antigen-specific T-cells into memory or effector cells is pre-determined based on the numeric differences and diversified nature of TCR clonal (inter- and intra-clonal diversifications) precursors [73]. These models of memory development are further characterized by compartmentalization patterns of memory cells. For example, T_{CM} reside in lymphoid tissue, T_{EM} in circulation, and T_{RM} in peripheral tissues [74]. Additionally, differences have been noted between $CD4^+$ and $CD8^+$ T-cells, whereby $CD4^+$ T-cells have multifunctional "helper cell" subsets that have diverse regulatory pathways not found in $CD8^+$ T cells [75,76]. Through viral disease model, it has been established that activated T-cells are converted into central memory cells over time however, this process depends on several factors including tissue-specific responses that varies in lymphoid and

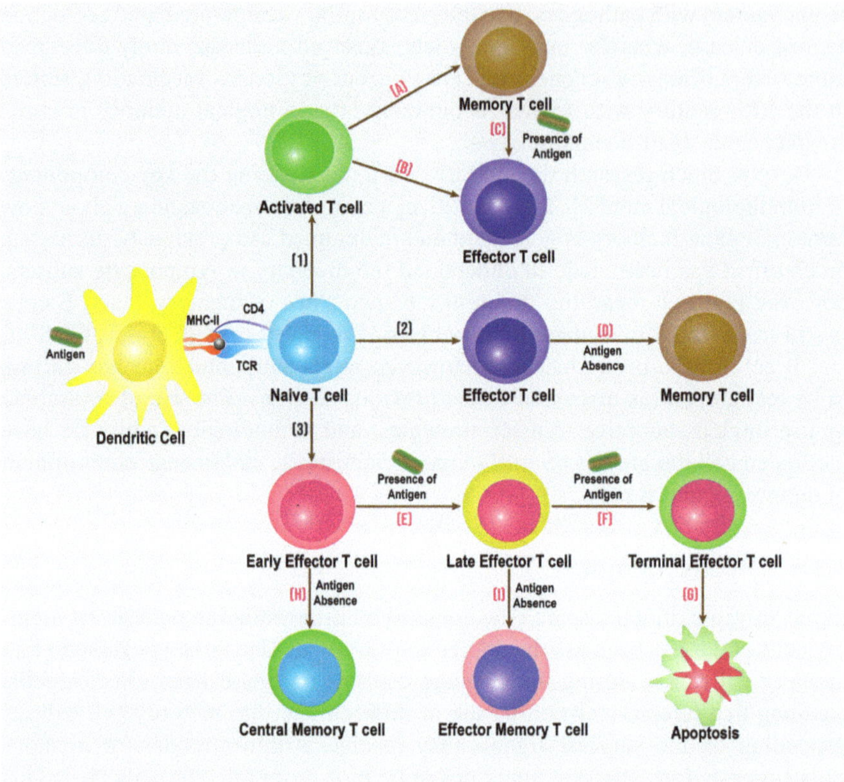

FIG. 5.1 Generation of memory T cells: T cells can follow divergent, linear development, or decreasing potential pathway for memory generation. In divergent model (1), in presence of antigen and costimulatory signals, T cells becomes activated and depending upon inflammatory signals and stimuli, either form memory T cells (A) or effector T cells (B). Memory T cells on further antigen encounter can convert to effector T cells (C). During linear development model (2), after antigen encounter and costimulation, naïve T cells become activated to form effector T cells which in absence of antigen stimulation is converted to memory Cells (D). In decreasing potential model, naïve T cells in presence of antigen and costimulatory signals are driven to early effector cells (3) to late effector cells (E) and finally to terminal effector cells (F) which undergo apoptosis (G). However, in absence of antigen, early effector cells can give rise to central memory T cells (H) while late effector cells can form effector memory T cells (I).

non-lymphoid tissues [77], peptide specificity [78], initial frequency of naïve precursors [79], and longevity of immune responsiveness [80].

Inflammatory cytokines are drivers of terminal differentiation of CD8+ T-cells, rather than promoting the memory cell development. There is evidence for the requirement of prolonged antigenic stimulation in CD4+ T cells for the cellular programming to differentiate into memory cell subsets and the longevity depends on the strength of TCR signals during primary response to antigen [81]. Likewise, inflammatory cytokines, particularly IFN-γ and IL-2 signaling, remains a key regulator for driving the transcriptional program for differentiation of CD4+ and CD8+ T-cells into effector and memory cell phenotypes [81]. IL-2 signaling remains key determinant whether T-cells would adopt terminally differentiated phenotype or switch toward the generation of memory cells. Conversely, in the absence of IL-2 signaling results in normal expansion of T-cells and memory generation but causes faults in recall responses [82]. By contrast, low/short-term IL-2 signals results in incomplete effector differentiation and increased generation of memory cells with high recall ability. High/long term IL-2 signals trigger effector differentiation at the expense of memory generation. IL-2 and inflammation together trigger distinct transcriptional program that determines the differentiation fate of the T-cells [83]. Therefore, IL-2 has an important role to drive the development of memory cells, this could be exploited as immunotherapeutic strategy aiming to boost vaccine-induced memory responses for conferring protection against subsequent reinfections.

Another cytokine driver, IL-12, increases Tbet expression that promotes CD4+ T cell differentiation into TH1, as well as stimulating CD8+ T-cells to acquire cytolytic effector functions [84]. Conversely, decreasing IL-12 levels cause a decline in Tbet expression that can be compensated by another transcription factor called EOMES, that promotes IL-2Rβ and IL-15R expression, as well as IL-7R mediated STAT6 signaling to induce CD8+ T-cells migration to infection sites. Conversely, IFN-γ blockade has been shown to prevent effector/memory cell death and induced secondary cytotoxic T-cells responses [84,85]. Indeed, cumulative signals received by antigen specific T-cells play vital roles in clonal expansion and synchronizing the diversified patterns of effector and memory cells that develop after infection resolves. Immune cells entering immune responses during later phases of infection also synchronizes with similar diversification patterns, thereby forming a heterogeneous population of multifunctional cells that are essential for determining the quality and amplitude of memory cell responses in reaction to vaccine or antigenic exposure [1].

5.3.2 B-cells memory

Surviving infection often provides life-long immunity against the invading pathogen. This immunity is often conferred by the memory B-cells, including the long-lived plasma cells and memory B-cells that are an important part of immunological memory in many infectious diseases [86]. Antigen driven differentiation of naïve B-cells into long-lived plasma and memory cells occurs in secondary lymphoid organs in two phases: first, the antigenic stimulation of BCR drives naïve cell differentiation into short-lived plasma cells, and in the second phase, antigens drive GC B-cells into long-lived plasma and memory cells (Fig. 5.2). During a secondary immune response, memory B cells respond to antigen and differentiate into long lived plasma cells or GC B-cells that undergo somatic hypermutation [87,88]. The decision regarding the developmental fate of B-cells depends on multiple factors including the strength of

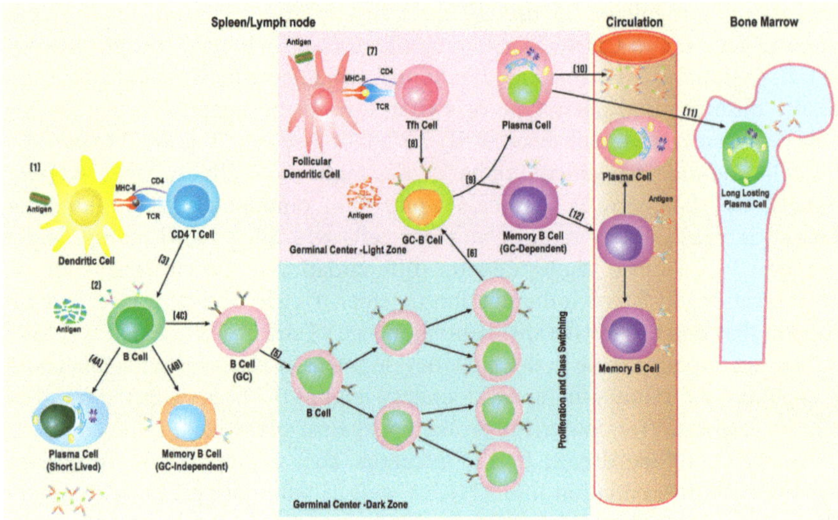

FIG. 5.2 Generation of memory B cells: in secondary lymphoid organ, antigen captured by antigen presenting cell is presented to helper CD4$^+$ T cells to kick off the activation signal (1); B cells also encounter the antigen to become activated B cells (2) and in response to activation signal received from CD4$^+$ T cells (3), it differentiates in to short lived plasma cells (4A), germinal center (*GC*) independent memory B cells (4B) and GC-B cells. In dark zone, GC-B cells proliferate and undergo class switching (5) and then enter in to light zone (6). In light zone, follicular dendritic cells activate the specialized CD4$^+$ T cells called T-follicular/Tfh Cells (7) which further provide the survival signal to antigen encountered GC-B cells (8) to differentiate in to plasma cells (9) which secrete antibody in circulation (10) or move to bone marrow to form long lasting plasma cells (11). There is also generation of GC dependent memory B cells (12) which come in circulation and upon further antigen encounter form antibody secreting plasma cells as well as new batch of memory cells.

BCR signaling by naïve B-cells, signaling strength of co-stimulatory molecules (CD21, CD40, CD80, and CD86), serum complement component C3, cytokines, B-cell activating factor (BAFF), a proliferation inducing ligand (APRIL), exposure to environmental antigens, duration of follicular DCs maturation. The ultimate fate of antigen-specific naïve B-cells is determined by early B-cell activation signals [81]. High-affinity B-cells are directed toward the plasma cell pool while moderate affinity B-cells develop into memory B-cells. Therefore, decreased initial BCR affinity maturation may decrease the strength of the signal and favors memory differentiation. Generation of memory B-cells is also determined by lowered expression of CD21 (in infants), CD40-mediated signaling, cytokines (IL-21), BAFF, APRIL that eventually impairs the development of plasma cells [89,90]. Furthermore, T-cell activation and DCs activation signals can serve as additional triggers for B-cells differentiation and hence, set of factors are essential for driving the differentiation program toward memory and/or long-lived plasma cells phenotype. Memory B-cells possess low affinity and lesser number of mutations than plasma cells gave evidence regarding the development of former before affinity maturation-based development of high-affinity BCRs. Memory B-cells differentiation requires Bach-2 and T-cell help *via* CD40-CD40L interaction represses Bach2 in GC B-cells [91]. By contrast, relatively weak T-cell help, in case of low-affinity B-cells maintained relatively higher Bach2 expression that is believed to act as suppressor of Blimp-1 and pro-apoptotic factors (Bim and Puma) [86,92,93] therefore, lack of strong signaling and instructions driving plasma cells differentiation forces the activated B-cells to adopt memory phenotype.

It is well known that signaling through the BCR or TCR, cytokine production and costimulatory molecule expression all play vital roles in determining lymphocyte activation and memory cell development. Apart from B- and T-cells, maternal antibodies and microbiome have also been shown to have an important role in regulating memory immune cell responses by modulating cytokine microenvironments. Thus, better understanding of the different parameters affecting the memory cell responses is still needed for the design of effective vaccines. In summary, antigen-specific memory B- and T-cells are essential for the long-lasting immunity and protection against reinfection or low levels of persisting pathogens.

5.4 Vaccine development

Vaccine development is a tedious process including selection of a proper vaccine candidate, an adjuvant, stable formation, pre-clinical studies, clinical trial, and finally licensing (Fig. 5.3). As vaccines are generally derived from pathogen gene products or synthetic analogues, it serves as triggers for the immune system without causing the disease. Different immunization approaches have helped in the elimination/control of several diseases, including polio, smallpox, mumps, measles, rubella, tetanus, pertussis, and diphtheria [94]. These vaccines were developed by traditional approaches of heat-, chemical-, or irradiation-based inactivation to produce killed organism vaccines. Immunization approaches using serologically related pathogens that undergo tissue culture passage-based attenuation was also used to produce live attenuated vaccines. Recent technological advances are aimed at improving these conventional approaches and enhance the immunogenicity of vaccine candidates. Judiciously designed immunogens will typically be in soluble form, in combination with an adjuvant for an effective vaccination strategy. The immunogenicity can further be enhanced by using the protein in a multivalent format with liposomes, virus-like particles or nanoparticles.

Most licensed vaccines are available in injectable form and elicit strong humoral responses, while weaker T-cell and mucosal responses are generally achieved [88]. One problem with many vaccines is the requirement of specified storage and transportation conditions that limit their use in resource-poor settings. In addition, most vaccine requires administration by trained people.

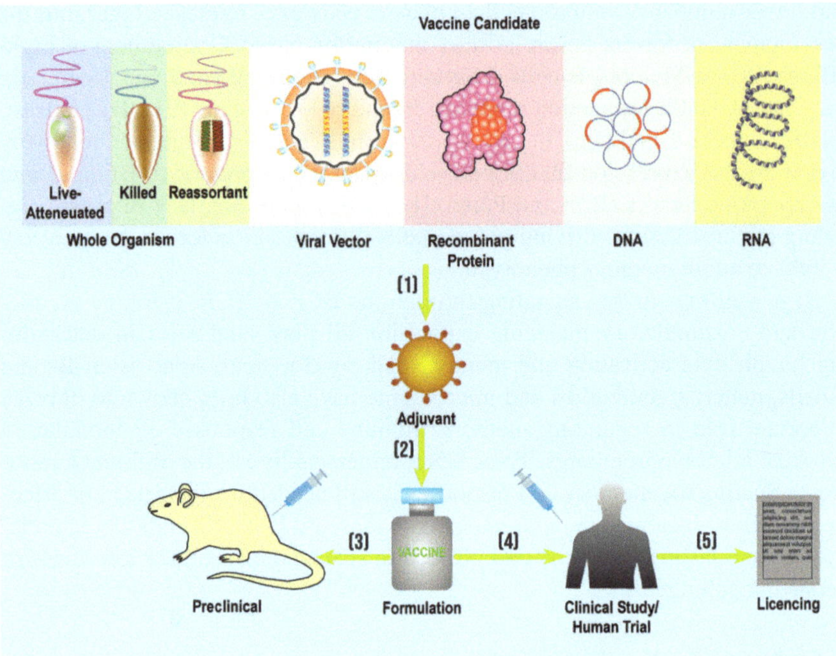

FIG. 5.3 Vaccine development strategy: during vaccine development, an ideal vaccine candidate is selected and mixed with an adjuvant to enhance the immunogenicity (1). A stable vaccine formulation is made (2) which undergoes first to preclinical studies (3) and then to different stages of clinical studies and human trials (4). Based on safety and efficacy data, finally vaccine is licensed for public use (5).

These issues have directed research efforts to identify alternate routes of administration. An ideal vaccine should be the one that can be produced efficiently and delivered to recipients in acceptable forms. Earlier vaccines were based on whole organism preparations using live, attenuated (or related less pathogenic strains that induced cross-reactive immunity without causing the disease) or killed organisms. Although these preparations are considered to be highly immunogenic, there is a risk of development of disease pathology similar to natural infection. Furthermore, whole organism preparations are complex mixtures of lipids, proteins, and carbohydrates that makes their production and quality control a tedious task. Additionally, these types of vaccines are not appropriate where natural infection does not generate protective immunity. This has prompted alternative strategies based on specific antigens, termed purified antigenic preparations, where a particular antigen induces strong immune responses with minimal reactogenicity. Subunit vaccines are vaccines that include only the proteins or epitopes from a pathogen to which antibodies or T cells are generated to initiate protective immune responses (for example hepatitis B vaccine). Conjugate vaccines are a type of subunit vaccine where antigens are linked to polysaccharides (from the outer coat of microbes) to stimulate immunity. Toxoid vaccines are produced by formalin-based inactivation of bacterial toxins (e.g., diphtheria and tetanus toxins). Naked DNA vaccines use DNA from microbes to stimulate immunity. RNA vaccines have recently gained popularity in the COVID-19 era, mRNA vaccines against Zika, flu, rabies, cytomegalovirus (CMV) although there have been ongoing researches since early 1990s. mRNA vaccines use mRNA encoding for an antigen for eliciting immune responses, in short it is the technology that brings together molecular biology and immunology. Although the vaccine approach is closely related to the gene therapy, however, the mRNA instability, high immunogenicity and lack of delivery platform remained the major pitfall for limiting its commercial use (in the early 1990s). Later, several researches led to substantial improvement in the safety and efficacy of these vaccines. RNA vaccines utilize a small piece of mRNA that codes for bacterial or viral protein is transfected into the host immune cells. Once inside the host cell, the vaccine RNA is recognized as the mRNA and gets translated into bacterial/viral protein. The host immune system recognizes the foreign protein and elicits immune responses (humoral and cell-mediated immunity). Once produced the immune system keeps the memory of the encounter and quickly responds to the subsequent encounters. In other words, once the individual is exposed to virus after receiving mRNA vaccination specific to that virus, host immune system recognizes it and clears off the infection before it can result in serious pathological consequences. Usually, the production of mRNA vaccines is far easier than the protein-based or attenuated vaccines and it does not affect the host DNA and the synthetic RNA (after translation) is destroyed by the host cellular machinery [95].

Purified antigenic preparations can be poorly immunogenic. Therefore, efficacy has been improved by using vaccine delivery modalities that enhance immunogenicity [96]. Improving vaccine delivery modalities can include changing route of administration (intravenous, mucosal, intradermal, subcutaneous), number of doses or vaccination strategy (e.g., a prime-boost approach). However, these changes can increase the complexity of the vaccination process. Also, different routes of administration may result in unanticipated outcomes, such as altered antigen availability, different epitope recognition patterns [97,98]. These issues have led to the use of adjuvants that exhibit safety, but trigger humoral responses or cellular immune responses.

There are different types of adjuvants depending on their component, physiochemical properties, or mechanism of action into two types: immunostimulants (TLR ligands, cytokines, saponins, bacterial exotoxins; that boosts immune responses to antigens) and vehicle (liposomes, mineral salts, emulsions, virosomes, polymeric microspheres; that present the antigens to the immune system). Adjuvants presently approved for human vaccines include alum, oil-in-water emulsion and TLR ligand. Alum has been widely used in several licensed vaccines including diptheria-pertussis-tetanus (DPT), diptheria-tetatnus (DT), inactivated polio vaccine, DT with hepatitis B, hepatitis A, human papilloma virus, Streptococcus pneumoniae, meningococcal infection. Alum is thought to trigger immune responses in three ways: (1) mediating continuous antigen release by depot formation, (2) promoting phagocytosis by APCs by forming particulate structures and finally, by increasing the antigen presentation, MHC-II expression, chemokines secretion and thereby recruiting monocytes to the site of injection.

Conversely, oil-in-water adjuvants (MF 59, AS03 etc.) are most commonly used adjuvants that have been tested in herpes simplex (HSV), hepatitis B and HIV [99]. MF59 is known to elicit strong immune activation, efficient antigen uptake properties, and increased number of antigen-loaded APCs as compared to alum [96]. The best example of TLR ligand-based adjuvant is MPL, derived from lipopolysaccharide (LPS), MPL is strong stimulator of T-cells, and antibody responses. It has been first TLR ligand to be used in licensed human vaccines. Thus, adjuvants can be used as immune potentiators the maximizes immunological effects while minimizing the side effects by altering the pharmacokinetic properties, facilitating the immune-stimulation by inducing higher quality of immune responses for improving therapeutic and vaccination outcomes.

In addition to adjuvants, Chiron scientists developed microparticles with positive or negative charges to carry proteins or DNA respectively [100,101]. The potency of protein-loaded particles was further enhanced by combining with of CpG oligodeoxynucleotide (TLR7 activator) that significantly enhanced antibody production, as compared to the protein loaded with Freund's adjuvant or protein loaded with alum. Microparticles can also enhance the potency of DNA vaccines in viral disease models, compared to DNA alone [100,102].

Immunogenicity is intricately linked with immunological memory. Immune memory is a feature of the adaptive immune response. The immunogenicity of an antigen can determine the outcome of immune responses, its strength, duration, efficacy, and the robustness of recall responses. The kinetics of transition from effector cells into long-lived memory cells is also determined by different types of infections, vectors, and immunization approaches. These issues need to be considered for vaccination that aims to activate antigen-specific T-cells for clonal expansion, pro-inflammatory cytokine production, and later development into a memory T cell response.

The strategy of repeated immunization with the same immunogen is not as effective as sequential immunization with an antigen mixture, since, it would fail to induce a broadly neutralizing antibody response [103]. Several vaccine programs have highlighted the need for an immune boost for teenagers or young adults because of waning long-term immunity. This concept gave rise to the strategy of prime-boost that has been successfully adopted for vaccine approaches against several infectious diseases. This approach has been extensively used by employing DNA, live viral vectors, and recombinant proteins. The outcome is primarily determined by type of vaccine. For example, a subunit vaccine induces a humoral response, while recombinant vectors and attenuated viral vaccines stimulate cell-mediated immune responses [104].

Antibody-mediated neutralization is the major goal of vaccines. However, newer vaccination approaches targeting complex pathogens also aim to enhance cellular and innate immune responses. Thus, the collective contribution of innate immune cells, antibodies, CD4+ T and CD8+ T cells is often needed to confer protection against primary and subsequent reinfections.

Any challenge to the immune system alerts the body and triggers the release of chemicals (cytokines and chemokines), inflammatory mediators, and causes alterations to the blood supply that attracts helps infiltration to sites of infection by leucocytes. This initial recognition of foreign antigen is performed by innate cells *via*. PRR. Multiple innate cells and molecules are needed to eliminate pathogens, including opsonization that facilitates their intake by the APCs (monocytes, macrophages, and DCs). APCs digest antigen into smaller pieces and present them onto their cell surface with MHC-II molecules to CD4+ T cells (in the case of viral antigens, these are processed and presented with MHC-I molecules to CD8+ T cells) triggering cell mediated immune responses. If antigen is derived from bacteria or parasites, it is likely to be presented by APCs to CD4+ T cells that can help generate an antibody-mediated immune response. Unlike T-cells, B-cells recognize antigens in a native state without the need for antigen processing and presentation. B-cells activation with T-cell help results in a better immune response and generates robust memory, a prerequisite for vaccine-mediated protection. Following antigen binding to the BCR and help from helper T-cells, somatic hypermutation is initiated and B-cell maturation into antibody-producing plasma cells occurs. The differentiation of these stimulated B-cells into plasma cells and memory cells that reside in secondary lymphoid tissues is important for pathogen clearance. This is mediated following clonal selection and expansion to produce IgM (first antibody to be produced), followed by IgG, IgA, IgD and IgE (during a primary infection). Memory cells produced during primary infection generally produce IgG during subsequent infections, leading to effective and robust immune responses that are crucial for vaccine efficacy [97].

Although antibodies are important for vaccine-induced protection, the involvement of T-cells cannot be discounted, as documented in different disease models [98,101,105]. Vaccination-induced T-cell activation is a prerequisite for conferring robust protection and preventing disease reactivation [103,106,107]. Vaccine-induced T-cells differentiate into diverse subsets (TH1, TH2, TH17, TH21, TFH, TH22 or TH9, Tc1, Tc2, etc.) with different pathways of protection against different pathogens [104].

5.5 Concluding remarks

A variety of vaccines are currently used or under development for preventing infectious diseases. Ideally, a vaccine is expected to trigger innate, as well as both arms of the adaptive immune system. However, current vaccines have their limitations for inducing long-term protection.

Live attenuated vaccines are easy to prepare, however, the requirement for refrigeration and risk of reversion of virulence limits their use for immune-compromised populations, since it may lead to development of disease pathology. Many other vaccines using killed pathogens elicit strong immune responses and protect against future infections without risk of pathogenic reversion. DNA and live recombinant vaccines have relatively easy production and the stability of DNA promotes its use. However, they are often not potent enough to elicit robust immune responses. The potency of vaccination has been a challenge for vaccinologists, leading to innovations in the field of vaccine delivery platforms. Apart from conventional approaches using needle and syringe, newer approaches include edible vaccines and inhaled vaccines that facilitate the use of the vaccines in remote areas without the help of trained medical professionals. Current research focuses on overcoming the need for cold chain system for storage, making vaccine use feasible in resource poor settings. Researchers have also tried to improve vaccine delivery by incorporating powder and solution in a syringe for simultaneous reconstitution and administration at the time of use. These efforts are aimed at improving vaccine delivery to those in need and stable during transportation, without the need for refrigeration. New technological approaches such as reverse vaccinology [108], has greatly accelerated vaccine development programs by facilitating the identification of candidate antigens and providing a targeted approach for vaccine programs. The success of vaccination in controlling different infectious diseases stimulates further research to combat diseases for which no vaccines are available.

Acknowledgments

Authors would like to acknowledge scholars and scientist of Infectious Disease Research Laboratory, Department of Medicine, Institute of Medical Sciences, Banaras Hindu University for their comments. Finally, this work was made possible with the support of Institute of Eminence (IoE) grant of Banaras Hindu University and ad-hoc grant of Indian Council of Medical Research (ICMR), India.

References

[1] Whittle HC, et al. Effect of subclinical infection on maintaining immunity against measles in vaccinated children in West Africa. Lancet 1999;353(9147):98–102.

[2] Cattaneo LA, et al. The seroepidemiology of Bordetella pertussis infections: a study of persons ages 1-65 years. J Infect Dis 1996;173(5):1256–9.

[3] van Panhuis WG, et al. Contagious diseases in the United States from 1888 to the present. N Engl J Med 2013;369(22):2152–8.

[4] Nabel GJ. Challenges and opportunities for development of an AIDS vaccine. Nature 2001;410(6831):1002–7.

[5] Schmidtke P, et al. Cell mediated and antibody immune response to inactivated hepatitis A vaccine. Vaccine 2005;23(44):5127–32.

[6] Wieland SF, Chisari FV. Stealth and cunning: hepatitis B and hepatitis C viruses. J Virol 2005;79(15):9369–80.

[7] Okamoto S, et al. Influenza hemagglutinin vaccine with poly(gamma-glutamic acid) nanoparticles enhances the protection against influenza virus infection through both humoral and cell-mediated immunity. Vaccine 2007;25(49):8270–8.
[8] Arvin A. Aging, immunity, and the varicella-zoster virus. N Engl J Med 2005;352(22):2266–7.
[9] Salerno-Goncalves R, Wahid R, Sztein MB. Immunization of volunteers with Salmonella enterica serovar Typhi strain Ty21a elicits the oligoclonal expansion of CD8+ T cells with predominant Vbeta repertoires. Infect Immun 2005;73(6):3521–30.
[10] Hajishengallis G, Lambris JD. Microbial manipulation of receptor crosstalk in innate immunity. Nat Rev Immunol 2011;11(3):187–200.
[11] Arts RJ, et al. Glutaminolysis and fumarate accumulation integrate immunometabolic and epigenetic programs in trained immunity. Cell Metab 2016;24(6):807–19.
[12] Netea MG, et al. Trained immunity: a program of innate immune memory in health and disease. Science 2016;352(6284):aaf1098.
[13] van 't Wout JW, Poell R, van Furth R. The role of BCG/PPD-activated macrophages in resistance against systemic candidiasis in mice. Scand J Immunol 1992;36(5):713–9.
[14] Chedid L, et al. Enhancement of nonspecific immunity to Klebsiella pneumoniae infection by a synthetic immunoadjuvant (N-acetylmuramyl-L-alanyl-D-isoglutamine) and several analogs. Proc Natl Acad Sci USA 1977;74(5):2089–93.
[15] Gorhe DS. Inhibition of multiplication of foot and mouth disease virus in adult mice pretreated with Freund's complete adjuvant. Nature 1967;216(5121):1242–4.
[16] Elliott AM, et al. Inverse association between BCG immunisation and intestinal nematode infestation among HIV-1-positive individuals in Uganda. Lancet 1999;354(9183):1000–1.
[17] de Castro MJ, Pardo-Seco J, Martinon-Torres F. Nonspecific (Heterologous) protection of neonatal BCG vaccination against hospitalization due to respiratory infection and sepsis. Clin Infect Dis 2015;60(11):1611–9.
[18] Hollm-Delgado MG, Stuart EA, Black RE. Acute lower respiratory infection among Bacille Calmette-Guerin (BCG)-vaccinated children. Pediatrics 2014;133(1):e73–81.
[19] Arts RJW, et al. BCG vaccination protects against experimental viral infection in humans through the induction of cytokines associated with trained immunity. Cell Host Microbe 2018;23(1):89–100 e5.
[20] Kleinnijenhuis J, et al. Bacille Calmette-Guerin induces NOD2-dependent nonspecific protection from reinfection via epigenetic reprogramming of monocytes. Proc Natl Acad Sci USA 2012;109(43):17537–42.
[21] Kleinnijenhuis J, et al. BCG-induced trained immunity in NK cells: Role for non-specific protection to infection. Clin Immunol 2014;155(2):213–9.
[22] Quintin J, et al. Candida albicans infection affords protection against reinfection via functional reprogramming of monocytes. Cell Host Microbe 2012;12(2):223–32.
[23] Slaughter A, et al. Descendants of primed Arabidopsis plants exhibit resistance to biotic stress. Plant Physiol 2012;158(2):835–43.
[24] Philbin VJ, et al. Imidazoquinoline Toll-like receptor 8 agonists activate human newborn monocytes and dendritic cells through adenosine-refractory and caspase-1-dependent pathways. J Allergy Clin Immunol 2012;130(1):195–204.e9.
[25] Paust S, et al. Critical role for the chemokine receptor CXCR6 in NK cell-mediated antigen-specific memory of haptens and viruses. Nat Immunol 2010;11(12):1127–35.
[26] Lopez-Verges S, et al. Expansion of a unique CD57(+)NKG2Chi natural killer cell subset during acute human cytomegalovirus infection. Proc Natl Acad Sci USA 2011;108(36):14725–32.

[27] Peng H, Tiang Z. Natural killer cells memory: progress and implications. Front Immunol 2017. https://doi.org/10.3389/fimmu.2017.01143.

[28] Fooksman DR, et al. Functional anatomy of T cell activation and synapse formation. Annu Rev Immunol 2010;28:79–105.

[29] Mempel TR, Henrickson SE, Von Andrian UH. T-cell priming by dendritic cells in lymph nodes occurs in three distinct phases. Nature 2004;427(6970):154–9.

[30] Curtsinger JM, Mescher MF. Inflammatory cytokines as a third signal for T cell activation. Curr Opin Immunol 2010;22(3):333–40.

[31] Marsland BJ, et al. CCL19 and CCL21 induce a potent proinflammatory differentiation program in licensed dendritic cells. Immunity 2005;22(4):493–505.

[32] Kaiser A, et al. CC chemokine ligand 19 secreted by mature dendritic cells increases naive T cell scanning behavior and their response to rare cognate antigen. J Immunol 2005;175(4):2349–56.

[33] Zhang M, et al. Differential survival of cytotoxic T cells and memory cell precursors. J Immunol 2007;178(6):3483–91.

[34] Sallusto F, et al. Two subsets of memory T lymphocytes with distinct homing potentials and effector functions. Nature 1999;401(6754):708–12.

[35] Mahnke YD, et al. The who's who of T-cell differentiation: human memory T-cell subsets. Eur J Immunol 2013;43(11):2797–809.

[36] Masopust D, Schenkel JM. The integration of T cell migration, differentiation and function. Nat Rev Immunol 2013;13(5):309–20.

[37] Pepper M, Jenkins MK. Origins of CD4(+) effector and central memory T cells. Nat Immunol 2011;12(6):467–71.

[38] Kaech SM, et al. Selective expression of the interleukin 7 receptor identifies effector CD8 T cells that give rise to long-lived memory cells. Nat Immunol 2003;4(12):1191–8.

[39] Jandinski J, et al. Separation of helper T cells from suppressor T cells expressing different Ly components. I. Polyclonal activation: suppressor and helper activities are inherent properties of distinct T-cell subclasses. J Exp Med 1976;143(6):1382–90.

[40] Swain SL, et al. Monoclonal antibody to L3T4 blocks the function of T cells specific for class 2 major histocompatibility complex antigens. J Immunol 1984;132(3):1118–23.

[41] Sojka DK, Huang YH, Fowell DJ. Mechanisms of regulatory T-cell suppression—a diverse arsenal for a moving target. Immunology 2008;124(1):13–22.

[42] Churlaud G, et al. Human and mouse CD8(+)CD25(+)FOXP3(+) regulatory T cells at steady state and during Interleukin-2 therapy. Front Immunol 2015;6:171.

[43] Goenka R, et al. Cutting edge: dendritic cell-restricted antigen presentation initiates the follicular helper T cell program but cannot complete ultimate effector differentiation. J Immunol 2011;187(3):1091–5.

[44] Xu H, et al. Follicular T-helper cell recruitment governed by bystander B cells and ICOS-driven motility. Nature 2013;496(7446):523–7.

[45] Crotty S. Follicular helper CD4 T cells (TFH). Annu Rev Immunol 2011;29:621–63.

[46] Wei M, et al. Mice carrying a knock-in mutation of Aicda resulting in a defect in somatic hypermutation have impaired gut homeostasis and compromised mucosal defense. Nat Immunol 2011;12(3):264–70.

[47] Liang HE, et al. Divergent expression patterns of IL-4 and IL-13 define unique functions in allergic immunity. Nat Immunol 2011;13(1):58–66.

[48] Simpson N, et al. Expansion of circulating T cells resembling follicular helper T cells is a fixed phenotype that identifies a subset of severe systemic lupus erythematosus. Arthritis Rheum 2010;62(1):234–44.

[49] Szabo K, et al. Follicular helper T cells may play an important role in the severity of primary Sjogren's syndrome. Clin Immunol 2013;147(2):95–104.
[50] Batista FD, Harwood NE. The who, how and where of antigen presentation to B cells. Nat Rev Immunol 2009;9(1):15–27.
[51] Cyster JG. B cell follicles and antigen encounters of the third kind. Nat Immunol 2010;11(11):989–96.
[52] Liu W, Wang H, Xu C. Antigen receptor nanoclusters: small units with big functions. Trends Immunol 2016;37(10):680–9.
[53] Yang J, Reth M. Receptor dissociation and B-Cell activation. Curr Top Microbiol Immunol 2016;393:27–43.
[54] Kurosaki T, Shinohara H, Baba Y. B cell signaling and fate decision. Annu Rev Immunol 2010;28:21–55.
[55] Suthers AN, Sarantopoulos S. TLR7/TLR9- and B cell receptor-signaling crosstalk: promotion of potentially dangerous B cells. Front Immunol 2017;8:775.
[56] Carroll MC, Isenman DE. Regulation of humoral immunity by complement. Immunity 2012;37(2):199–207.
[57] Tsubata T. Ligand recognition determines the role of inhibitory B cell co-receptors in the regulation of B cell homeostasis and autoimmunity. Front Immunol 2018;9:2276.
[58] Hoogeboom R, Tolar P. Molecular mechanisms of B cell antigen gathering and endocytosis. Curr Top Microbiol Immunol 2016;393:45–63.
[59] Nutt SL, et al. The generation of antibody-secreting plasma cells. Nat Rev Immunol 2015;15(3):160–71.
[60] He JS, et al. Biology of IgE production: IgE cell differentiation and the memory of IgE responses. Curr Top Microbiol Immunol 2015;388:1–19.
[61] Kurosaki T, Kometani K, Ise W. Memory B cells. Nat Rev Immunol 2015;15(3):149–59.
[62] Portugal S, et al. Atypical memory B cells in human chronic infectious diseases: an interim report. Cell Immunol 2017;321:18–25.
[63] Blair PA, et al. CD19(+)CD24(hi)CD38(hi) B cells exhibit regulatory capacity in healthy individuals but are functionally impaired in systemic Lupus Erythematosus patients. Immunity 2010;32(1):129–40.
[64] Carter NA, et al. Mice lacking endogenous IL-10-producing regulatory B cells develop exacerbated diease and present with an increased frequency of Th1/Th17 but a decrease in regulatory T cells. J Immunol 2011;186(10):5569–79.
[65] Flores-Borja F, et al. CD19+CD24hiCD38hi B cells maintain regulatory T cells while limiting TH1 and TH17 differentiation. Sci Transl Med 2013;5(173):173ra23.
[66] Rosser EC, et al. Regulatory B cells are induced by gut microbiota-driven interleukin-1beta and interleukin-6 production. Nat Med 2014;20(11):1334–9.
[67] Menon M, et al. A regulatory feedback between plasmacytoid dendritic cells and regulatory B cells is aberrant in systemic lupus erythematosus. Immunity 2016;44(3):683–97.
[68] Yoshizaki A, et al. Regulatory B cells control T-cell autoimmunity through IL-21-dependent cognate interactions. Nature 2012;491(7423):264–8.
[69] Ahmed R, Gray D. Immunological memory and protective immunity: understanding their relation. Science 1996;272(5258):54–60.
[70] Kaech SM, et al. Molecular and functional profiling of memory CD8 T cell differentiation. Cell 2002;111(6):837–51.
[71] Lohning M, et al. Long-lived virus-reactive memory T cells generated from purified cytokine-secreting T helper type 1 and type 2 effectors. J Exp Med 2008;205(1):53–61.

[72] Harrington LE, et al. Memory CD4 T cells emerge from effector T-cell progenitors. Nature 2008;452(7185):356–60.

[73] Touvrey C, et al. Dominant human CD8 T cell clonotypes persist simultaneously as memory and effector cells in memory phase. J Immunol 2009;182(11):6718–26.

[74] Thome JJ, et al. Spatial map of human T cell compartmentalization and maintenance over decades of life. Cell 2014;159(4):814–28.

[75] D'Souza WN, Hedrick SM. Cutting edge: latecomer CD8 T cells are imprinted with a unique differentiation program. J Immunol 2006;177(2):777–81.

[76] Catron DM, et al. CD4+ T cells that enter the draining lymph nodes after antigen injection participate in the primary response and become central-memory cells. J Exp Med 2006;203(4):1045–54.

[77] Hogan RJ, et al. Activated antigen-specific CD8+ T cells persist in the lungs following recovery from respiratory virus infections. J Immunol 2001;166(3):1813–22.

[78] Sierro S, Rothkopf R, Klenerman P. Evolution of diverse antiviral CD8+ T cell populations after murine cytomegalovirus infection. Eur J Immunol 2005;35(4):1113–23.

[79] Marzo AL, et al. Initial T cell frequency dictates memory CD8+ T cell lineage commitment. Nat Immunol 2005;6(8):793–9.

[80] Roberts AD, Ely KH, Woodland DL. Differential contributions of central and effector memory T cells to recall responses. J Exp Med 2005;202(1):123–33.

[81] Snook JP, Kim C, Williams MA, et al. TCR signal strength controls the differentiation of CD4 + effector and memory T cells. Sci. Immunol. 2018;3(25). doi:10.1126/sciimmunol.aas9103.

[82] Williams MA, Tyznik AJ, Bevan MJ. Interleukin-2 signals during priming are required for secondary expansion of CD8+ memory T cells. Nature 2006;441(7095):890–3.

[83] Pipkin ME, et al. Interleukin-2 and inflammation induce distinct transcriptional programs that promote the differentiation of effector cytolytic T cells. Immunity 2010;32(1):79–90.

[84] Takemoto N, Intelekofer AM, et al. Cutting Edge: IL-12 inversely regulates T-bet and eomesodermin expression during pathogen-induced CD8+ T cell differentiation. J Immunol 2006;177(11):7515–19. doi:10.4049/jimmunol.177.11.7515.

[85] Keppler SJ, Rosenits K. Signal 3 cytokines as modulators of primary immune responses during infections: the interplay of type I IFN and IL-12 in CD8 T cell responses. Plos One 2012;7(7):e40865. doi:10.1371/journal.pone.0040865.

[86] Clybouw C, et al. Regulation of memory B-cell survival by the BH3-only protein Puma. Blood 2011;118(15):4120–8.

[87] Meffre E, Catalan N, et al. Somatic hypermutation shapes the antibody repertoire of memory B cells in humans. J Exp Med 2001;194(3):375–8. doi:10.1084/jem.194.3.375.

[88] Amanna IJ, Slifka MK. Contribution of humoral and cellular immunity to vaccine induced protection in humans. Virology 2011;411(2):206–15.

[89] Bryant VL, et al. Cytokine-mediated regulation of human B cell differentiation into Ig-secreting cells: predominant role of IL-21 produced by CXCR5+ T follicular helper cells. J Immunol 2007;179(12):8180–90.

[90] Benson MJ, et al. Affinity of antigen encounter and other early B-cell signals determine B-cell fate. Curr Opin Immunol 2007;19(3):275–80.

[91] Weisel FJ, et al. A temporal switch in the germinal center determines differential output of memory B and plasma cells. Immunity, 2016;44(1):116–30.

[92] Muto A, et al. The transcriptional programme of antibody class switching involves the repressor Bach2. Nature 2004;429(6991):566–71.

[93] Fischer SF, et al. Proapoptotic BH3-only protein Bim is essential for developmentally programmed death of germinal center-derived memory B cells and antibody-forming cells. Blood 2007;110(12):3978–84.

[94] Bonanni P, Picazo JJ, Remy V. The intangible benefits of vaccination—what is the true economic value of vaccination? J Mark Access Health Policy 2015;3.
[95] Park JW, et al. mRNA vaccines for COVID-19: what, why and how. Int J Biol Sci 2021;17(6):1446–60.
[96] Calabro S, et al. Vaccine adjuvants alum and MF59 induce rapid recruitment of neutrophils and monocytes that participate in antigen transport to draining lymph nodes. Vaccine 2011;29(9):1812–23.
[97] Nossal GJ. Current concepts: immunology. The basic components of the immune system. N Engl J Med 1987;316(21):1320–5.
[98] Arvin AM. Humoral and cellular immunity to varicella-zoster virus: an overview. J Infect Dis 2008;197(Suppl 2):S58–60.
[99] Barnett SW, et al. Antibody-mediated protection against mucosal simian-human immunodeficiency virus challenge of macaques immunized with alphavirus replicon particles and boosted with trimeric envelope glycoprotein in MF59 adjuvant. J Virol 2010;84(12):5975–85.
[100] O'Hagan DT, et al. Recent advances in the discovery and delivery of vaccine adjuvants. Nat Rev Drug Discov 2003;2(9):727–35. doi:10.1038/nrd1176.
[101] Bunde T, et al. Protection from cytomegalovirus after transplantation is correlated with immediate early 1-specific CD8 T cells. J Exp Med 2005;201(7):1031–6.
[102] Kazzaz J, et al. Novel anionic microparticles are a potent adjuvant for the induction of cytotoxic T lymphocytes against recombinant p55 gag from HIV-1. J Control Release 2000;67(2–3):347–56.
[103] Pantaleo G, Koup RA. Correlates of immune protection in HIV-1 infection: what we know, what we don't know, what we should know. Nat Med 2004;10(8):806–10.
[104] Margolick JB, Markham RB, Scott AL. The immune system and host defense against infections. In: Infectious Disease Epidemiology: Theory and Practice. 2nd ed. Sudbury, USA: Jones and Bartlett Publishers; 2007. pp. 317–43.
[105] Sester M, et al. Levels of virus-specific CD4 T cells correlate with cytomegalovirus control and predict virus-induced disease after renal transplantation. Transplantation 2001;71(9):1287–94.
[106] Reyes-Sandoval A, et al. Potency assays for novel T-cell-inducing vaccines against malaria. Curr Opin Mol Ther 2009;11(1):72–80.
[107] Hoft DF. Tuberculosis vaccine development: goals, immunological design, and evaluation. Lancet 2008;372(9633):164–75.
[108] Rappuoli R. Reverse vaccinology, a genome-based approach to vaccine development. Vaccine 2001;19(17–19):2688–91.

Further reading

Pennock ND, White JT. T cell responses: naïve to memory and everything in between. Adv Physiol Educ 2013;37(4):273–83. doi:10.1152/advan.00066.2013.

Chapter 6

Immune responses to vaccines: from classical to systems approaches

João Lucas Lima Calandrini de Azevedo[a], Viviane Schuch[b], João Marcos Maia Silva[a], André Guilherme Costa Martins[b], Luiz Gustavo Gardinassi[a], Helder I Nakaya[b,c], Simone Gonçalves Fonseca[a]

[a]*Department of Bioscience and Technology, Institute of Tropical Pathology and Public Health, Federal University of Goiás, Goiânia, Brazil,* [b]*Department of Clinical and Toxicological Analyses, School of Pharmaceutical Sciences, University of São Paulo, São Paulo, Brazil,* [c]*Hospital Israelita Albert Einstein, São Paulo, Brazil*

6.1 Introduction

The scientific community and the vaccine industry were imbued with the mission of responding, as a matter of urgency, to various emergency scenarios in public health, such as the H1N1, Zika, and Ebola outbreaks. Nowadays, these alarming scenarios are in evidence due to the pandemic caused by SARS-CoV-2, which has already had severe economic and social impacts around the world [1].

Effective and safe therapies, such as vaccines, require research and time, and need to be safe to be widely distributed [2]. It was estimated that an average period of 5–10 years is needed for the conception, testing, and distribution of a new vaccine; however, the period between the first sequencing of SARS-CoV-2 and the clinical trials of efficacy of the first vaccine is less than 300 days [2,3].

Thanks to the commitment of the scientific community and the prior knowledge acquired through similar scenarios, several vaccines are already in use against COVID-19. Methodologies involving the use of mRNA, non-replicating adenoviruses, subunit vaccines—mainly through the use of spike (S) protein, in addition to SARS-CoV-2 itself, inactivated—allowed the use of a wide range of vaccines that, until now, has reflected positive impacts in the reduction of severe cases and concomitant hospitalization of infected individuals [1,4,5].

The development of vaccines requires a series of events that will allow, based on a hypothesis, the vaccine to be designed, synthesized, tested, and distributed, as shown in Fig. 6.1. Vaccines are an important scientific breakthrough and one of the main factors responsible for increasing the quality and life expectancy of the population through the search of correlates of protection [6].

System Vaccinology. https://doi.org/10.1016/B978-0-323-85941-7.00008-5

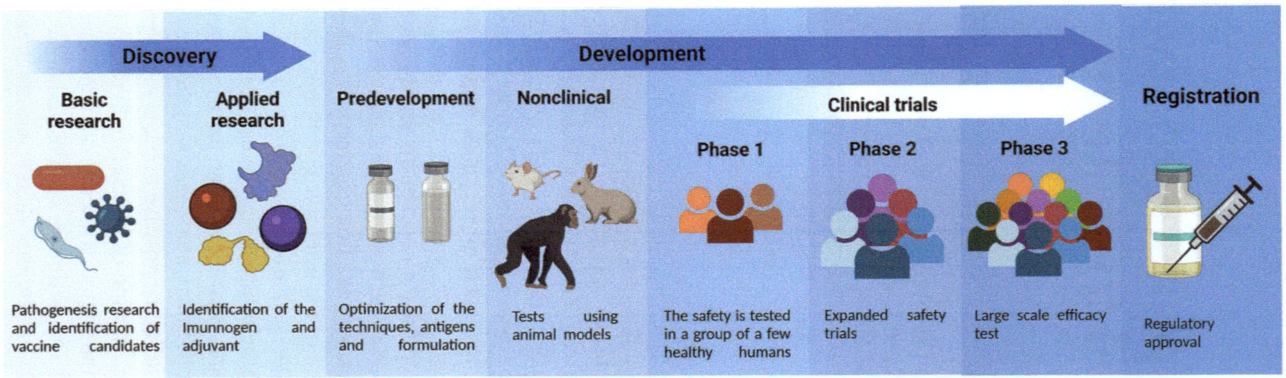

FIG. 6.1 Visual representation of the stages commonly applied in the development of new vaccines. There is a representation of the early stages, including discovery of antigens and target sites, achieving the preclinical stages in order to prove the safety of the vaccine formulation before its application in human subjects. The clinical trials must have three phases (phases I, II, and III), which are applied to increasing numbers of individuals, in order to observe their effects in heterogeneous populations and their effectiveness. Only after all the tests, the vaccine is approved to be widely distributed to the population. *(Created with BioRender.com).*

Correlates of protection are defined as a specific immune response to an infection or vaccine that is closely related to protection against an infection or disease or some other defined endpoint. Antibodies, for example, are one of the best-known correlates of protection, since they are closely associated with the seroprotection of individuals responding to an immunization [7].

Correlates of protection are increasingly important for vaccine development and validation. Over the years, studies of the correlates of protection were focused in the verification of molecules and/or immunological functions that guarantee the efficacy of vaccine candidates [8]. With the advent and constant evolution of omics tools, it is possible to obtain a systemic overview of the correlates of protection thanks to the holistic approach of omics methodologies [9].

The use of omics tools provides insights into the body's response to a given vaccine. Transcriptome studies provide relevant insights into the differential gene expression that occurs in peripheral whole blood, peripheral blood mononuclear cells (PBMCs), and/or specific cell subsets. This allows for a detailed monitoring of the physiological and cellular processes of the response promoted by the immunized individual to the administered vaccine candidates [10,11]. In addition, markers of inflammation and immune system regulators can be quantified by analyzing the proteomics, metabolomics profiles, and cell phenotype and function at different time points to verify the immune response and the generation of immunological memory [12].

Integrating knowledge at a systemic level through the application of systems biology to monitoring vaccine metrics is one of the great promises of a field called immunomonitoring, which refers to approaches applied to monitor and characterize the immune responses of individuals after infection or vaccination [13]. The integration initiative has already provided relevant insights into predictive biomarkers of immune system mechanisms against infections and vaccination. Thus, it is possible to envision collaborative actions through biobanks, meta-analyses, and operational procedures that allow the rapid development of vaccines that can prevent future threats to public health.

6.2 Immune response to vaccines

The stimulation of both the innate and adaptive immune responses is essential to achieve effective immunization when vaccinating. This mechanism must enable humoral and cell-mediated stimulation and the consequent generation and maintenance of memory and effector cells [14].

Humoral and cellular immune responses are essential factors for promoting an individual's protection against an infection and may act as correlates of protection. In this sense, vaccines are one of the most widely applied methods to allow an individual who has had no direct contact with an infection to express factors that protect him/her from the pathogen and its associated symptoms [15].

6.2.1 Innate immune response

Innate immune response is defined as a fast and nonspecific response that is capable of identify and interact with a large number of pathogens and stimuli through the expression of receptors on innate immune cells that can recognize conserved molecular patterns expressed by most microorganisms [16–18].

The innate immune system relies on physical barriers (e.g., the skin and internal walls, such as those of the lungs and stomach), constituted of highly interconnected cells—through GAP-type junctions—and which are generally able to prevent the entry of microorganisms into tissues and the bloodstream. These internal physical barriers can count on the presence of mucous membranes, which are able to protect the tissue against mechanical, chemical, and microbiological insults [16]. In addition, the production and presence of peptides, such as lysozyme, may result in antimicrobial activity on the surface of epithelial cells and body fluids [19].

The most common method of vaccination is through the intramuscular route, into the deltoid muscle or in the thigh. This method is capable of overcoming the physical barriers of the innate immune system, such as the skin, and is able to maximize the immunogenicity of the vaccine, avoiding most side effects [20].

Once the antigen is inoculated through the vaccine, the next step is its recognition by the innate immune system cells. The recognition of the antigen occurs because the innate immune system cells present pattern recognition receptors (PRRs), which are able to identify pathogen-associated molecular patterns or PAMPs [19,21–23]. PAMPs are vital molecular components of the microorganism constitution and since they are essential, these patterns usually remain unchanged, even in the face of mutations of the infectious agent [19,21].

Aiming the PAMP recognition, mammals are able to express several distinct classes of PRRs, such as toll-like receptors (TLRs), nucleotide-binding oligomerization domain-like receptors (NOD-like receptors or NLRs), retinoic acid-inducible gene-I-like receptors (RIG-I-like receptors or RLRs), C-type lectin receptors (CLRs), and many others. The TLRs were the first to be identified and remain the best characterized [21,24,25]. TLRs are transmembrane proteins that present a leucine-rich repeat on the outside of the membrane and may be found on the surface of the cell or in intracellular compartments. These proteins compose the superfamily of Toll/interleukin-1 (TIR), which includes the interleukine-1 (IL-1) receptors (IL-1Rs). There are 10 known and characterized variations of TLRs in humans (TLR1–TLR10) and each one is able to recognize different PAMPs such as proteins, lipids, and nucleic acids [25–27].

The signaling observed after an interaction between an antigen and a receptor is able to activate the transcription of factors. NF-κB, which is able to regulate the expression of pro-inflammatory cytokines, and interferon regulatory factor 3 (IRF3) pathway, an important anti-viral mechanism. Also, the production of type 1 interferon (IFN-α and IFN-β), being a primary focus on formulations that seek an effective response against this type of infectious agent [28,29].

Due to their abundance, high mobility, distribution, and versatility, macrophages are able to influence the development and outcome of an immune response [30]. These cells are able to release cytokines, such as tumor necrosis factor (TNFα), and mediators, such as reactive oxygen species [30–32]. Some studies involving the development of vaccines propose increasing the amount or activation of macrophages, such as the study developed by Yang and collaborators and published in 2020. In this project, they performed a test of a recombinant Bacillus Calmette-Guérin (BCG) vaccine against *Mycobacterium tuberculosis* in mice. The researchers demonstrated that the vaccine increased the number of macrophages in the animals' lungs. This can be considered a long-term protective factor, bearing in mind the role of this cell in the elimination of bacteria [33].

Another important function of macrophages in the development of an effective immune response is the ability to present antigens, since this is one of the key mechanisms for the initiation and persistence of the adaptive immune response [34,35]. It is established that for the presentation of the antigens, the endocytosis of the infectious agent is necessary, along with the consequent processing of the material in endosomal vesicles, which culminates in the dissociation of the pathogen in subunits (peptides) that will be displayed on the cell surface [36]. The process of displaying peptides to be presented to T cells, in mammals, is performed by the major histocompatibility complex (MHC) molecules. MHC is a highly polymorphic region of the genome, which has a wide range of loci that are capable of encoding functional molecules. $CD8^+$ T cells recognize peptide presented by class I MHC and $CD4^+$ T cells recognize peptide presented by class II MHC [37,38].

MHC also represents an important factor to consider when developing a vaccine. In another study involving *M. tuberculosis*, researchers used liquid chromatography tandem mass spectrometry to identify 43 peptides belonging to the bacterium that was presented by MHC I, as well as 94 presented by MHC II. These findings suggest ways to discover new antigens that can be used in the development of increasingly effective and specific vaccines [39].

Although there is a group of cells capable of effectively presenting antigens (antigen-presenting cells or APCs), dendritic cells (DCs) are known to be the most specialized in this mechanism, being able to demonstrate a capacity up to 100 times more powerful than other APCs [35,40–42]; its mechanism of action is represented in Fig. 6.2. Due to its high capacity in the presentation of antigens associated with the ability to sensitize naive T cells in vivo, this cell type has been the target of studies aiming to sensitize T cells against a wide range of antigens [41,43–45].

Recently, it has been shown that the innate immune system could develop a type of non-specific immune memory known as "trained immunity" or "innate memory" [46]. Trained immunity is developed by innate immune cells, such as monocytes, macrophages, and natural killer (NK) cells, after an infection or vaccination [47]. Trained immunity can be induced by β-glucan [48], *Candida*

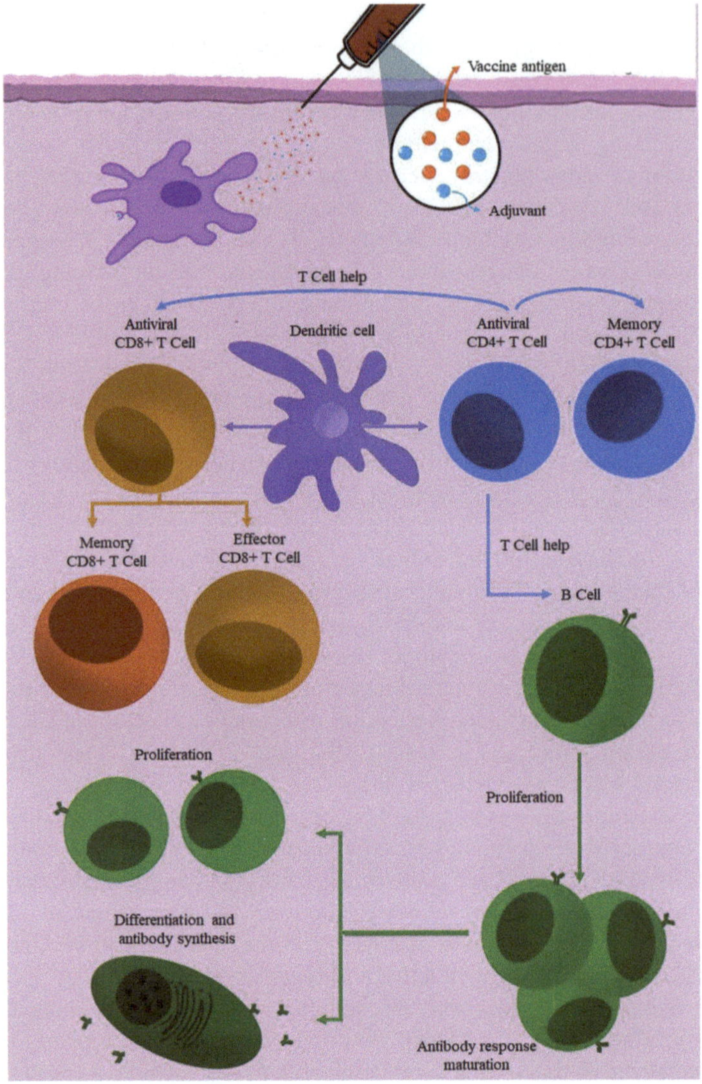

FIG. 6.2 Schematic representation of the mechanism of action of vaccines—cellular and humoral immune responses. Starting with the inoculation of the antigens and adjuvant, sequentially the antigens will be recognized by dendritic cells, whose function is to present these antigens to cells of the adaptive immune system, capable of specific response, and memory development. Dendritic cells, through MHC molecules, are able to present these antigens to the naive CD4+ T cells, which will undergo differentiation into CD4+ T Helper. Helper CD4+ T cells are able to stimulate CD8+ T lymphocytes—which is also capable of recognize the antigen through dendritic cells—and B lymphocytes. CD8+ T cells will differentiate into effector cells, whose capacity is the cytotoxic activity, or memory cells. B cells, through the recognition of antigens, will undergo a process of intense proliferation, and after they will experience the differentiation into cells with larger cytoplasm that are capable of increased antibody synthesis.

albicans [49], and live vaccines such as BCG [50]. Innate immune cells exposed to an infectious pathogen can undergo epigenetic modifications such as methylation of histones in some proinflammatory genes (e.g., TNF-α, IL-1β, IL-6), yielding to a trained immunity. In this context, the cells respond in a faster and stronger manner to an infection [50]. The non-specific protection promoted by the trained immunity can be a strategy to protect against many infectious pathogens, especially the BCG vaccine, that is already used to protect children against tuberculosis.

6.2.2 Adaptive immune response

While the innate immune system uses a series of powerful, but not very specific, tools to stop infection, the adaptive immune system is considered a much more sophisticated and specific-defense response. The adaptive response is mediated by two cell types, T and B lymphocytes, which are responsible for cellular and humoral immune responses, through the cytokine production, synthesis, and release of antibodies, respectively [51]. T and B lymphocyte interactions and functions are represented in Fig. 6.2.

The role of the adaptive immune response begins with the presentation of a small fraction of the pathogen (peptides) to T lymphocytes [52]. T lymphocytes can be classified into T $CD4^+$ or T $CD8^+$, based on the expression of specific receptors on their surface. Both $CD4^+$ and $CD8^+$ T lymphocytes are capable of proliferation and differentiation in the face of antigen identification [53–56], as represented in Fig. 6.2.

As a reaction to the presence of the pathogen, $CD8^+$ T cells undergo massive clonal expansion, acquiring cytotoxic capacity and migrating to more diverse areas of the body [57]. Since $CD8^+$ T lymphocyte activity is a cytotoxic response, its function is important to fight intracellular infections, such as those caused by viruses. For this reason, studies aiming at the development of new vaccines against viral agents, such as the human immunodeficiency virus (HIV), the hepatitis B virus (HBV), and the hepatitis C virus, understand the importance of generating an effective and potent $CD8^+$ T cell response [58].

The main mechanism by which cytotoxic cells are able to promote the death of an infected cell is through the release of perforin and granzyme, capable of interacting with the target cell and inducing its death. The mechanism of action of granzyme and perforin is through the opening of pores in the plasma membrane of the target cell, leading to its disruption and posterior destruction by apoptosis. Furthermore, the cytotoxicity can be mediated by the interaction of Fas on cell surface of target cells and Fas-ligand on $CD8^+$ T cells leading to apoptosis [59].

Focused on smallpox immunization, Rock and colleagues investigated, using flow cytometry, the activation of $CD8^+$ T lymphocytes with effector phenotype in vaccinated patients. It was possible to observe the expression of granzyme A and B, as well as perforin, which highlights the importance of these factors in combating viral agents through infection and vaccination [60].

$CD4^+$ T cells have a vast capacity, being capable of triggering the activation of cells belonging to the innate immune system, B lymphocytes, and cytotoxic $CD8^+$ T cells, as well as mediating inflammatory and anti-inflammatory responses during this process. These functions will be exercised by the different subtypes in which these cells are able to differentiate, such as T-helper 1 (Th1), T-helper 2 (Th2), T-helper 17 (Th17), follicular helper T cell (Tfh), and T-regulatory cells (Treg) [61].

Epigenetic alterations during the differentiation of $CD4^+$ T cells can define the course of an immune response against a pathogen or some compound that mimics it. Transcription factors such as T-bet, GATA3, RORγt, FOXP3, and BCL6, which are present during the development of $CD4^+$ T cells, favor the acquisition of specific effector functions, mediated by Th1, Th2, Th17, Treg, and Tfh, respectively [62]. These phenotypes are crucial for the cellular immune responses to pathogens. $CD4^+$ T cells have already been reported as a protective correlate for vaccines, such as the herpes zoster virus vaccine [63].

During an infection or after a vaccination, there is an increase in the activation and proliferation of $CD4^+$ T cells, which, through stimuli, must differentiate into effector $CD4^+$ T cells. These effector cells are able to perform their function acting against the vaccine antigen, until the infectious focus is eliminated and most of these cells die; however, some survive and become $CD4^+$ T cells of memory [64–66]. These memory cells are capable of providing an enhanced and quicker response when they come in contact with the antigen in the future [66]. This response may provide protection, as it happens much more quickly than is seen in the primary contact with the antigen [67,68].

Memory T lymphocytes can be classified into different subtypes: stem cell memory T cell (T_{SCM}), central memory T cell (T_{CM}), effector memory T Cell (T_{EM}), and the terminally differentiated effector memory T cell (T_{EMRA}) depending on the expression of certain markers, as shown in Fig. 6.3. T_{SCM} cells have the ability to self-renew, making them capable of renewing the entire population of memory as well as effector cells [69]. T_{CM} cells have little or no effector capacity, but they can easily proliferate, generating effector cells. T_{EM} cells, on the other hand, are able to migrate to the tissues where the infection is taking place and generate an effector response [70].

The generation of memory cells is essential for any vaccine, because in addition to providing a long-term immune response, it can enable an improved response when compared to the first exposure to the antigen [66].

6.2.3 Humoral immune response

B lymphocytes originate from the bone marrow and are of vital importance in the immune response, due to their ability to synthesize and release antibodies. These cells are able to recognize antigens through their B cell receptor (BCR) and become activated. $CD4^+$ T cells can interact with B cells through the interaction of costimulatory molecules, such as CD40 and inducible T-cell co-stimulator (ICOS), and the production of cytokines. Memory $CD4^+$ T cells are able to

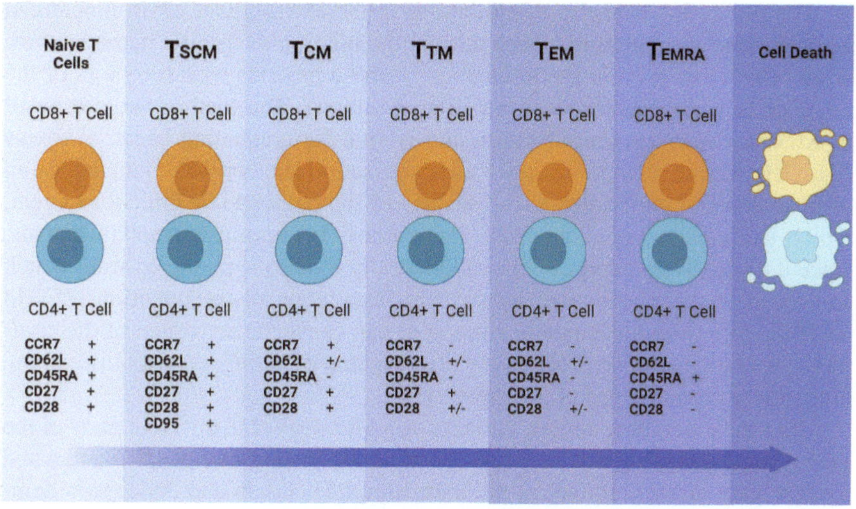

FIG. 6.3 Representation of memory T-cell subsets and their main cell markers—CCR7, CD62L, CD45RA, CD27, and CD28—, according to their expression. From left to right, there is naive T cells, before antigen presentation; the memory subpopulations: T Memory Stem Cells (T_{SCM}), Central Memory T Cells (T_{CM}), Transitional Memory T Cells (T_{TM}), Effector Memory T Cells (T_{EM}), and terminally differentiated effector memory T cell (T_{EMRA}). *(Created with BioRender.com).*

trigger most of the initial responses of B lymphocytes; this allows the formation of germinal centers in the secondary lymphoid organs, undergo immunoglobulin (Ig) class switch, recombination and affinity maturation and differentiate in antibody-secreting plasma cells [66,71].

Antibodies or immunoglobulins are glycosylated proteins that can be found on the surface of B cells acting as BCRs, or can be secreted into the extracellular medium where they perform their function as antibodies [72]. These molecules are heterodimeric proteins made up of two light and two heavy chains, functionally distinguished into variable domains, which bind antigens, and constant domains, which assume effector functions, such as the activation of the complement system or binding to the Fc receptor. Each variable region is generated through successive events of gene recombination and somatic hypermutation after the first exposure to an antigen for maturation of the immunoglobulin affinity to this one [73].

Each variable domain can be subdivided into three regions of sequence variability, termed complementarity-determining regions (CDR) and four regions of relatively constant sequences. These regions of variability are called framework regions. To constitute the antigen-binding site, the light-chain CDRs join the heavy-chain CDRs [73].

Mature B cells express IgM and IgD, while class-switched B cells express IgA, IgE, or IgG. Secreted antibodies are capable of destroying pathological agents or suspending the spread of an intracellular infection [74]. The antigen recognition, proliferation, and differentiation of B cells is shown in Fig. 6.2.

The protection capacity of antibodies in the extracellular environment can be performed through three mechanisms: the binding to specific pathogen proteins, which can prevent the interaction of these proteins with receptors of the target cells, and the subsequent infection of this cell. This method is represented in what is known as neutralization and is vital for combating bacterial toxins [74]. The second method is known as opsonization and consists of the adhesion of opsonins and antibodies to the surface of the pathogen or infectious agent, which facilitates its phagocytosis. This process is important for phagocytosis, since the negatively charged cell wall naturally repels the pathogen wall, which can result in the evasion and subsequent installation of the infection [75]. In addition, as a third mechanism, antibodies can cause the activation of the complement system, whose proteins are also capable of acting as opsonins and are able to lyse certain types of pathogens [74].

With the emergence of new variants of SARS-CoV-2 in different parts of the globe, some studies aimed to assess the antibody response of people vaccinated against such viruses. In results published in 2021, Edara and colleagues demonstrated that 3 months after vaccination with an mRNA vaccine or after the second dose, all patient sera were able to neutralize the new viral variants, such as the delta variation [76]. These results highlight the importance of vaccination and antibodies in protecting individuals.

To maintain antigen recognition activities, but with distinct effector functions, the heavy chain domains of the immunoglobulin can be exchanged, which guarantees antigen specificity. The heavy portions of Igs can be classified into 5: IgM, IgG, IgA, IgD, and IgE. While IgG can be divided into four subclasses (IgG1–IgG4), IgA can be subdivided into IgA1 and IgA2, each one of them with an specific biological activity [73].

6.2.3.1 *Immunoglobulin M*

IgM immunoglobulins are produced by plasma cells as part of the body's adaptive humoral immune response against a foreign pathogen. Resting mature yet naïve, B lymphocytes express IgM as a transmembrane antigen receptor that functions as part of the BCR. B cell activation in response to antigen binding to the BCR results in rapid cell division and clonal expansion of the activated B lymphocyte, producing many progeny cells that can differentiate into either antibody-secreting plasma cells or memory B lymphocytes. IgM is the first antibody secreted by the adaptive immune system in response to a foreign antigen; however, the secreted form of IgM exists predominantly in a pentameric con [73].

IgM antibodies participate in both neutralization and clearance of pathogens in addition to initiating inflammatory reactions against pathogens through the complement pathway. IgM is the predominant antibody during a primary challenge to an antigen, and for some non-peptide antigens, IgM may be the only isotype of antibody secreted on subsequent encounters with the antigen. The primary humoral immune response to a novel pathogen typically requires a time period of close to a week before substantial amounts of IgM appear in the blood, and the innate immune response is necessary to fight the infection until the response of T cells and the clonal expansion of antibody-secreting plasma cells against the pathogen in sufficient numbers. IgM can neutralize pathogens, though not as effectively as IgG or IgA isotypes; this is most likely due to the increased flexibility of these isotypes provided by a hinge region [77].

6.2.3.2 Immunoglobulin G

As one of the main molecules responsible for activating the complement system, IgG has 4 well-defined subclasses in humans. Ranging from IgG1–IgG4, that have a positive correlation with chronic immune responses, among other biological activities. One of these biological activities is placental transfer, in which the four IgG subclasses favor the initial construction of the fetus' immune system through vertical transmission from the mother, allowing it to be trained against several pathogens during its development. Furthermore, IgGs also had reported cytophilic activity, which allows interaction with cells of the monocyte/macrophage lineage; this is a key and highly specific function of IgG's in humans and other mammalian species. In addition to these, the ability to interact with lymphocytes through their Fc portion was also reported [78].

IgG also has potent antiviral neutralizing activity, as demonstrated by Klingler et al. (2020) in a study in which practically all of the in convalescent and acute plasma/sera of SARS-CoV-2 infected individuals involved had detectable levels of IgG1 in plasma; this antibody was marked by anti-spike and anti-RBD (receptor-binding domain) coronavirus activity [79]. As well as IgG, other studies have also identified IgA as molecules with neutralizing capacity against viral pathogens [80,81].

6.2.3.3 Immunoglobulin A

IgA is the predominant antibody isotype in the mucosal immune system, participating extensively in the defense of the body's mucous membranes. These promote immune exclusion, binding to pathogens in a hydrophilic shell conformation, thus being repelled from the mucosal surface. Other functions involve the neutralization of bacterial products, agglutination of microorganisms, and reduction in their ability to move them. IgA has two isomeric forms: IgA1 (90% prevalence in circulation) and IgA2 (<10% prevalence in circulation) [82,83].

Other functions of IgA include activation of complement proteins, concurrent with the activation of alternative pathways of this system through the induction of the mannan-binding lectin [84]. IgA can also bind to and activate multiple receptors such as CD71, known as the transferrin receptor [85]. With regard to vaccination (Pfizer BNT162b2) against COVID-19, IgA levels underwent a considerable increase in their plasma titers in individuals infected with SARS-CoV-2 when collected 9 months after the onset of symptoms. After the vaccination of previously infected individuals as well as of COVID-19-naïve patients, in the third week, there was a new boost in the titration of this immunoglobulin; this boost was positively correlated with the response of $CD4^+$ T cells and circulating follicular helper T cells (cTfh). This is indicative that prevaccination, $CD4^+$ T cells may aid in a better IgA response, regardless of whether there is a previous SARS-CoV-2 infection [86].

6.3 Approaches for assessing the immune response following the vaccination

Nowadays, vaccines are one of the best tools used to fight infections, preventing millions of cases of infection and deaths annually [87]. However, after vaccination, it is important to prove that vaccinated subjects are able to develop an immune response to the infectious agent, as well as to understand how this response works. The way in which the vaccine will be validated depends on the sample choice for the analysis, as shown in Fig. 6.4. For this purpose, the following methods can be applied.

6.3.1 Neutralizing antibody assay

Neutralizing antibodies or NAbs may be able to block the infectivity or pathogenesis of viruses, bacteria, fungi, or parasites by neutralizing receptors important for binding the pathogen to the host [88], as represented in Fig. 6.5.

The neutralizing antibodies are able to prevent viruses from entering their target cells, through their interaction with key receptors in the pathogen's entry mechanism. Thus, NAbs have been seen as potential protective correlates that can be vital in the development of vaccines for several diseases, such as the acquired immunodeficiency syndrome (AIDS) caused by the HIV-1 virus [7,89–91]. NAbs can also be observed with high specificity for virus glycoproteins, being considered essential in the construction of protection against the infectious agent, as observed in the immune response against the rabies virus [92,93].

In this way, a cell-based assay for neutralizing antibodies is a type of assay performed in vitro using cell cultures that are capable of interacting or responding to the stimulus being studied. Through this method, the detection of NAbs is made based on the assumption that the presence of this type of antibody must be able to extinguish any biological responses or activities associated with the pathogen or toxin [94].

The plaque reduction neutralization test (PRNT) is considered the gold standard method for detecting neutralizing antibodies, especially for application in viral diseases [95]. This method was first described in 1950 and is based on the assessment of the individual's serum capacity to neutralize viral particles through antibodies. Usually, PRNT is developed in tubes or plates with constant volumes of virus particles, which will be exposed to the patient's serum in different dilutions. The presence of neutralizing specific antibodies in the serum can neutralize the virus, preventing the virus from causing the formation of

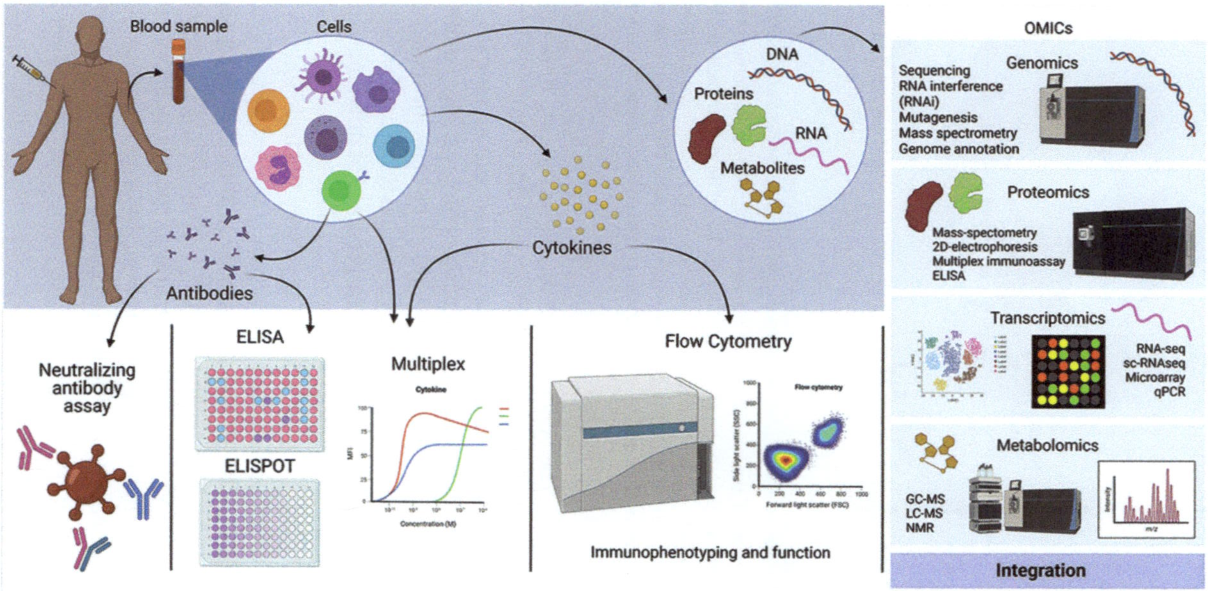

FIG. 6.4 Methods of assessing immune response provide by vaccines. There are several ways to validate the action of vaccines in an organism, depending on the mechanisms by which the vaccine will perform its activity. For cellular investigation, methods such as flow cytometry are able to identify and separate the target cells. In cases where the interest is in produced antibodies or cytokines, flow cytometry may be used to; however, ELISA and ELISPOT are also capable of identify the cytokines. If the vaccine is focused in humoral response, neutralizing antibodies assays may be applied to identify the neutralizing capacity of the patient's sample. However, nowadays it is also possible to use "omics" methodologies in order to assess responses through DNA, mRNA, proteins, and metabolites, through genomics, transcriptomics, proteomics, and metabolomics, respectively. *(Created with BioRender.com).*

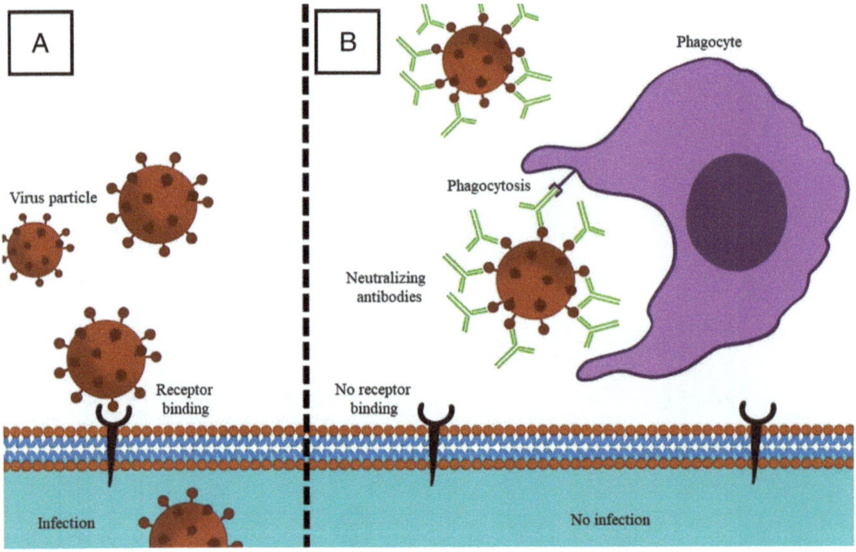

FIG. 6.5 Visual representation of the mechanism of action of neutralizing antibodies. On the A side, the entry of viral particles into the target cell is outlined, based on the interaction of viral surface proteins with cell receptors. On the B side, there is the representation of viral particles surrounded by antibodies that bind to viral surface proteins, preventing their interaction with target cells and allowing the phagocytosis of viruses by phagocytes, represented by the macrophage.

plaques in a cell monolayer. The concentration of plaque forming units can be determined by the number of plaques formed after a few days [96].

A viral neutralizing test (VNT) is a technique based on adding samples from the patient in a solution where there is a known amount of virus. This solution is mixed with a known number of cells—usually Vero cells—and incubated for a couple of days. Finally, in order to identify antigen-antibody interaction, there is an analysis of the neutralizing virus growth in the presence of different dilution of the sample containing the antibodies. A cytopathic effect based virus neutralization test is evaluated [97]. This test is based on a very old technique, which meant that it was considered outdated for a long time; however, with the latest developments involving COVID-19 and the interest in therapies using serum from convalescent patients, this technique was revived [98,99]. Regarding SARS-CoV-2 infection, the VNT presented 99.93% of specificity and sensitivity between 95% and 100% in two large cohorts from different countries, being, therefore, widely used for detection of neutralizing antibodies and validation of vaccines in this context [100].

6.3.2 Effector functions of antibodies

In addition to their neutralizing activity, antibodies can also play other important roles during an insult. Through their constant domain (Fc), antibodies are able to induce responses from the innate and adaptive immune system, which can make a difference in a situation in which the organism fights an infectious process [101].

Currently, only pneumococcal conjugate vaccines recognize the activities performed by the Fc portion of antibodies as a correlate of protection; however, there is growing evidence that the effector function of antibodies is of vital importance for the response to viruses, bacteria, fungi, and parasites [102,103].

In this context, the advent of systems serology, which deals with the objective of identifying new correlates of protection against infections and in the postvaccination/immunization process, has been considered as a tool for evaluating antibody functions after vaccination [102]. System serology is an integrative approach based on the use of high-throughput experimental techniques that aim to understand the morphological and functional aspects of antibodies, so that these data are confronted using computer programs [104]. Using systems serology, several antibody functions mediated by the Fc portion can be evaluated, such as Ab-dependent cellular phagocytosis (ADCP), Ab-dependent NK cell degranulation, and cytokine/chemokine secretion [101,102].

In trials using the RV144 trial vaccine (ALVAC and AIDSVAX B/E) against HIV in humans, a study was able to confirm the increased IgG3 response, highlighting the importance of systems serology in understanding the mechanisms behind the effectiveness of vaccines [105,106].

6.3.3 Enzyme-linked immunosorbent assay

The enzyme-linked immunosorbent assay (ELISA) is the gold standard of immunoassays. Being a sensitive test, it is capable of identifying and quantifying several substances, such as antigens, antibodies, enzymes, proteins, and hormones [107–110].

This assay is usually performed in a polystyrene 96-well plate. This plate is normally coated by attaching highly specific antibodies or antigens to the bottom of the wells. Through this specificity, it is possible to diagnose diseases or identify the presence of antibodies in the serum of patients using the interaction between the molecules present in the serum and the proteins attached to the plate [107,109–111].

Thus, in order to evaluate the immunogenicity of vaccines during testing periods in animals or in clinical trials in humans, ELISA has been used to measure antibody titers in the serum. In addition to this method being able to generate extremely reliable responses, it is one of the easiest methods to apply and reproduce to detect antibody titers during vaccine development and testing [112].

6.3.4 Enzyme-linked immunospot (ELISPOT)

The enzyme-linked immunospot or ELISPOT is an assay that measures the frequency of cytokine-secreting cells at the single-cell level, and is able to detect antigen-specific T cells [113,114]. This method is functional, has a wide detection range, and is applicable in quantitative investigations, turning it into a widely applicable assay in vaccine research [114].

ELISPOT was initiated under very similar conditions to those observed in the ELISA method, where a 96-well plate is coated with a specific capture antibodies and cells are cultured on that surface in the presence or absence of stimuli. Cytokines that are secreted by the cells will be captured by the specific antibodies on the surface. The detection antibody is either biotinylated and followed by a streptavidin-enzyme conjugate or the antibody is directly conjugated to an enzyme. Substrate are added and the formed spots are visible on the surface. Each spot corresponds to an individual cytokine-secreting cell.

ELISPOT were initially uses to detect antibody-producing cells, and the surface is coated with protein or antibody. Later, this technique was adapted to observe T cell specificity and cytokine synthesis, and was used to identify responses from developing vaccines (phases I and II) [114,115].

6.3.5 Cytokine multiplex

Cytokines are responsible for the homeostasis of cells of the immune system, because of the ability to coordinate signal-dependent responses [116]. These proteins are essential for effector immune responses of pro-inflammatory and anti-inflammatory immunological processes. For this reason, the detection of the cytokine context in a post-vaccine situation provides valuable information about the immune response [117]. The multiplex technology allows the simultaneous quantification of several cytokines, chemokines, or growth factors in samples of body fluids (serum, plasma, liquor, etc.) and supernatants of cell culture, using a smaller number of samples than traditional ELISA.

The multiplex method is based on the detection of cytokines at the protein level, so several techniques can be applied; however the most applied methods are membrane-based assay and flow cytometry [117]. Membrane-based methodologies can be developed in 96-well plates, as in the case of the ELISA protocol. There is a chemiluminescence-based methodology that is capable of reading up to 16 proteins in each of the 96 wells of the plate, allowing for broad detection of cytokines. The cytometric bead array (CBA), on the other hand, is based on the use of a cytometer for its reading. This is a particle-based immunoassay that is derived from the measurement of soluble analytes. The number of results depends on the range of the kit used and, mainly, on the range of reading of the device [117].

Currently, the methodologies that are used most commonly are those that allow the analysis of hundreds of variants in a single sample, such as xMap Luminex and the MesoScale Discovery platform, which use beads marked with different colors combinations, specific for each microsphere. Reading and interpreting results share steps common to flow cytometry, involving lasers, passing the sample through a flow, and also optics. Due to the versatility of marking the beads, it is possible to measure a profile of up to 500 analytes in a single sample. The MesoScale Discovery detection system has some advantages, which include a high sensitivity and range of detection, in addition to being less influenced by factors inherent to the matrix. This is possible due to its similarity to the multiplexed ELISA, being based on reactions between antigen and antibody; this is evidenced by electrochemiluminescent signals, measured later in the device [118].

Methodologies such as those described above, aimed at quantifying cytokines and chemokines have a well-founded potential for vaccine evaluation. Several studies have been published, evaluating the fluctuations of these biomarkers after immunization against the human papillomavirus (HPV), *M. tuberculosis*, influenza, and yellow fever, through the YF-17D vaccine [119–121].

In a study that used the Multiplex method to assess the T cell response to immunization against the influenza virus in humans, Skibinski et al. (2018) found that immunization induced antiviral responses from both $CD4^+$ T cells and $CD8^+$ T cells. Furthermore, it was possible to notice an increase in the synthesis of the cytokines such as interferon-γ (IFN-γ), interleukin-17A (IL-17A), interleukin-17F (IL-17F), interleukin-5 (IL-5), interleukin-13 (IL-13), interleukin-9 (IL-9), interleukin-10 (IL-10), and interleukin-21 (IL-21). Emphasizing the importance of IFN-y in a viral context makes the effectiveness of the immunizing compound indisputable [122].

6.3.6 Multiparametric flow cytometry—cell phenotype and cytokine production

Flow cytometry is frequently used as a technology to detect surface or intracellular cell proteins using antibodies conjugated with fluorophores. In the field of vaccine research, flow cytometry is widely used to identify T cells activated by the immunization, as well as those that can serve to characterize T and B cell subsets. Therefore, it is a widely used method for evaluating clinical trials during vaccine development [123].

Cytokine flow cytometry is also a method that can be used to measure the specificity of T cells against the antigen through the identification of cytokine synthesis, as observed using ELISPOT. This method is based on the stimulation of cells; so, the cells are able to produce the cytokines, the stimulated cells are fixated and permeabilized, which allows the entry of specific antibodies attached to fluorochromes that will bind to the molecules of interest, so that they can be identified. Then, these cells containing labeled cytokines are subjected to a reading through the flow cytometer, which allows for the cell-to-cell visualization of one or more markers [124].

Activated T lymphocytes have some receptors on their surface, such as CD137, a highly sensitive marker for antigen stimulation; CD69, a fast-appearing activation marker; and CD134/OX40, an activation marker that is directly linked to the survival and proliferation of lymphohematopoietic cells [125–127]. In addition, these cells can also express molecules known as co-stimulators on their surface, including CD26, CD27, CD28, and CD154 [128]. After vaccination, innate and adaptive immune responses can be evaluated by flow cytometry. T cells differentiate into effectors or memory cells, expressing several markers that will enable to identify the memory cell subtypes. CCR7 and CD62L receptors, for example, are tissue-dependent and act as markers of where the cell resides. There are also signaling molecules such as CD27, CD28, and CD45RA [129–132]. All these markers are important for the differentiation of memory T lymphocytes between T_{SCM}, T_{CM}, T_{EM}, and T_{EMRA}, as shown in Fig. 6.3.

Multiparametric flow cytometry is particularly appropriate for deep analysis of immune responses after vaccination, as it permits the measurement of the frequency, the phenotype, and the functional status of antigen-specific cells. The multiparametric flow cytometry allows the staining of several makers in the same time, depending on the capacity of the flow cytometer used. T cell memory phenotype and/or T cell subsets can be combined with functional markers such as cytokine and cytotoxicity markers (i.e., perforin and granzymes), by intracellular staining with antibodies with distinct fluorophores. T cell proliferation can be evaluated using fluorescent dyes such as carboxyfluorescein succinimidyl ester and analyzed by flow cytometry. The simultaneous staining for several functional markers such as cytokines (IFN-γ, TNF-α, IL-2, IL-10, MIP-1α among others), perforin, granzymes, and proliferation allow for the characterization of the polyfunctionality of the antigen-specific T cells after infection or vaccination [143,144]. Different stages of memory B cells as well as monocyte subsets can be also identified by flow cytometry.

The fluorescence-activated cell sorting method, or FACS, is a subtype of flow cytometry that allows the separation of cells based on their surface proteins [133,134]. Considering the context of vaccinology, the cell sorting is important to separate subpopulations of cells, such as vaccine-induced T cells and B cells, for further evaluation through genomic and transcriptomic methods.

6.3.6.1 Activation-induced marks (AIM)

The detection of antigen-specific T cells is one of the key points for the validation of vaccine-induced responses and immunogenicity [135,136]. Most of the methods used to identify and quantify T cells that are expressing an antigen-specific response after immunization are based on the use of methods such as conventional flow cytometry and ELISA, which have limitations as they are normally dependent on cytokines produced by the target cells. The production of cytokines is usually heterogeneous among cells, so the use of this method for the detection of specific response of T cells tends to relativize the real capacity of the antigen-specific immune response of these cells [136–138].

For this reason, the cytokine-independent activation-induced marker (AIM) method has gained much notoriety. In this methodology, cells are exposed for a few hours to the presence of antigens capable of inducing cell activation. After this period, which can vary from one method to another, the cells are acquired in a flow cytometer [139]. The ultimate goal is to identify markers that indicate the activation of these cells, such as CD137, CD69, and OX40.

In a study published in 2018, Bowyer and colleagues used the AIM method to assess the antigen-specific response of $CD4^+$ and $CD8^+$ T cells from healthy UK adults who had undergone candidate vaccines against EBOLA (ChAd3-EBO-Z and MVA-EBO-Z). Using the markers CD25, CD134 (OX40), CD274 (PDL1), and CD107a, the group was able to demonstrate that the vaccines generated a satisfactory antigen-specific response, also validating the AIM method as one of the methods that can be used to assess the post-immunization response [135].

A much more recent study was able to demonstrate through the AIM method that in recovered individuals, after the first dose of vaccine against SARS-CoV-2, the cells were already able to express an effective response against the virus spike protein. This result was observed through the identification of $CD69^+$ and $CD137^+$ markers of antigen-specific $CD8^+$ T cells and CD137+ and OX40+ markers of antigen-specific $CD4^+$ T cells [140].

6.3.7 Time-of-flight mass cytometry—CyTOF

To overcome the limitations presented by flow cytometry, such as the low number of parameters analyzed per panel, the need for a larger volume of samples, and the redundancy of lineage markers for identification in different stains, the use of high-dimensional time-of-flight mass cytometry (CyTOF) has been implemented in several studies [141,142].

CyTOF's ability to combine multiple parameters in a single panel allows the detection of over 40 analytical variables. Unlike flow cytometry, the CyTOF methodology marks cells with antibodies conjugated to heavy metals. Once marked, the cells have their time of flight analyzed in an atomic mass cytometer [143]. Since each atom has its time of flight determined by its mass, the composition of the atoms in each cell can be accurately analyzed as they flow through. In contrast to flow cytometry, whose label overlapping is frequently observed (5%–100%) due to the redundancy of the labels, this event is reduced to <2% with the use of CyTOF, in addition to a drastic reduction of background in the samples; this is because cells do not naturally present heavy metals [144].

However, it is necessary to emphasize that, despite having advantages, the CyTOF methodology provides data with a much higher density; this is one of the direct consequences of its analytical breadth [143].

6.4 Other factors that influence the immune response to a vaccine

Many factors are linked to alterations in vaccine activity. Factors such as age, gender, ethnic factors, body mass index, smoking, and even route of administration are able to increase or decrease vaccine capacity to provide protection

[145–150]. Factors that can compromise the vaccine's efficacy can be divided into three categories: (1) factors that are intrinsic to the formulation, such as the dosage, the selected antigen and adjuvant, and the type of vaccine developed; (2) variation among vaccine recipients; or (3) factors linked to vaccine administration, such as route of administration [151].

6.5 Systems vaccinology

Due to the genomic revolution that has taken place in the last 20 years, several technologies and tools have emerged to study different "layers" of biological systems at high-throughput scales. These include next-generation sequencing (NGS) of DNA (DNA-seq) and RNA (RNA-seq), high-resolution mass spectrometry of proteomics/metabolomics, as well as CyTOF to study the profile of cellular immune responses, among others. This progress has renewed the interest to understand biology at a systemic level. To accomplish this task, large amounts of data are generated and integrated to predict the behavior of the interactions between components of a biological system under varying conditions [152,153].

Systems immunology is an emerging research field that aims to understand the dynamics of the immune system during health and disease [154]. When applied to vaccinology, system immunology approaches can help to understand the mechanisms by which vaccines stimulate protective immune responses, and also to identify predictors of vaccine-induced immunity and efficacy [155]. This strategy often initiates with high-throughput measurements to profile the transcriptome, proteome, or metabolomes from cells, biological fluids, and tissues, which are later analyzed and integrated via computational models and interaction networks that explain the perturbations induced by vaccines in humans [156]. Both low- and high-throughput technologies can be used by systems vaccinologists to investigate the mechanisms of vaccines. The integration or association of the data obtained from omics tools with the data obtained from conventional immunological assays, such as ELISA, ELISpot, FACS, and neutralization assays, allow for the quantitative and qualitative assessment of the immune status and responses and, therefore, can be useful to determine outcomes in the predictive analysis [157].

Systems vaccinology studies have allowed for broad descriptions of the response to vaccines. Examples include the discovery of early gene expression signatures that predict adaptive immune outcomes, like neutralizing antibody response and $CD8^+$ T cell activity after vaccination against yellow fever [158] and influenza [159]. Systems vaccinology also revealed new insights related to the molecular mechanisms responsible for the vaccine response. Indeed, the observation that CaMK4 gene expression is negatively associated with antibody production to the inactivated influenza vaccine provided the basis to identify this gene as a critical regulator of antibody production, both in vitro and in animal models [159]. Another important discovery was the observation that the expression of TLR5 on days 3–7 after the influenza vaccination is correlated with the magnitude of the antibody response on day 28. The impact of this finding stems from the fact that TLR5, a bacterial flagellin receptor, was not previously associated with the viral response [160]. Vaccination of mice deficient in this molecule indicated a significant role of the intestinal microbiota in regulating vaccine immunity [160].

Considering the urgency with which new vaccines need to be implemented to address the pandemic caused by SARS-CoV-2, systems vaccinology shall reveal the molecular mechanism they induce. Through systems vaccinology, Arunachalam and colleagues were able to map the innate and adaptive immune response profile of 56 healthy patients immunized with the Pfizer-BioNTech mRNA vaccine. They reported a satisfactory neutralizing antibody and cellular response, as evidenced by the presence of polyfunctional $CD4^+$ T and $CD8^+$ T cells [161]. These findings reinforce the importance of systems vaccinology in understanding the efficacy of vaccines and open the door for vaccines to be developed and tested even more rapidly in the future.

6.5.1 Transcriptomics

Transcriptome is the complete set of transcripts (messenger RNAs and non-coding RNAs, such as ribosomal RNAs, transporter RNAs, and lncRNAs and microRNAs) from a given cell line or tissue. Investigating the transcriptome has been a successful approach to interpret biological responses and reveal the cellular and molecular constituents in the response to vaccination [162].

High-throughput tools for the screening of whole transcriptomes include oligonucleotide microarrays and RNA-seq. These technologies can be used to measure the expression of thousands of genes at the same time, which are used to investigate the changes in the transcriptome in response to a particular perturbation, including vaccination.

DNA microarrays are microscope slides that are printed with thousands of spots in defined positions. It works under the principle of hybridization of complementary strands of DNA. Each spot contains a known DNA sequence or gene that acts as probes to detect the set of transcripts expressed from both an experimental sample and a reference sample. However, by allowing for a more quantitatively accurate measurement and in order to obtain absolute transcript abundance, RNA-Seq has become the favored technique.

Meanwhile, bulk tissue RNA-seq is a widely adopted method to understand genome-wide transcriptomic variations under different conditions [163]. The problem is that bulk analysis measures transcription of different cells in a samples, while cell frequency changes between each individual or condition, resulting in a loss of signal from lowly abundant cell types [164]. Recently, the single-cell RNA-seq (scRNA-seq) technology emerged to overcome such limitations.

Essentially, RNA-seq methodologies can be done in 5 steps: (1) extraction, fragmentation, and conversion of RNA samples into cDNA; (2) mapping of these cDNA molecules for a given transcriptome or genome; (3) estimation of each gene expression level; (4) normalization and statistical treatment of the obtained data, resulting in the selection of differentially expressed genes (DEGs); and (5), performing of the functional analysis to evaluate the relevance of those genes on a biological context [165].

Factors such as the levels of gene expression and their kinetics are able to provide important information, especially due to immunizations, in order to understand its effects in situ and systemically [159,166–169]. For these reasons, the use of transcriptomics in the development of vaccines is of vital importance and can be used for several purposes, including the validation of adjuvants [170]. However, mRNA often does not act as an effector molecule in response to the infection or vaccination, and may generate a response that does not reflect these cases, since not all mRNA converts to proteins. In these situations, other techniques can be applied, such as proteomics [166].

6.5.1.1 Whole blood and peripheral blood mononuclear cell

The evaluation of the transcriptomic profile of whole blood and PBMCs has been important for understanding the mechanisms involved in the inflammatory response to vaccination [171–173]. Through the evaluation of the transcript, it is possible to make a survey about the efficiency of new candidates for adjuvants and even about the effectiveness of vaccines [174].

In contrast to whole blood, PBMCs consist predominantly of monocytes and lymphocytes, which are separated from whole blood using density gradients and centrifugation. Both whole blood and PBMC transcriptomics have been compared in immunological and physiopathological studies of inflammatory diseases [175,176]. One of the main applications of these methods is the identification of transcriptional signatures, innate immunity and adaptive immunity, after vaccination or infection, that may lead to the de-development of protective responses [177]. Another important use of these techniques is the interpretation of the reasons why some people do not develop an immune response against an infectious agent or vaccine, as demonstrated in studies involving vaccines against yellow fever and hepatitis B [10,178].

Bartholomeus et al. (2018) selected 34 healthy individuals with no history of infection and use of vaccines against HBV (Hepatitis B Virus), to administer a vaccine against this pathogen, in order to understand its low efficacy. Whole blood samples were collected at four-time points (0, 3, 7, and 60 days after vaccination); on days 0, 3, and 7, RNA was extracted for whole blood transcriptomic analysis. Among patients who responded adequately to the vaccine (59%), there was an increase in the expression of genes related to myeloid lineage, immune system effectors, neutrophil degranulation, antigen processing and presentation, and type 1 interferon. Interestingly, among the non-responders, an upregulation of CD81 and immune regulator interactions, such as lectin-like receptors present on NK cells, was observed. On the other hand, in some, there was a downregulation of CD22, IRF2, and signaling through the Fc receptor, pointing to the modulation of the immune system [11].

Gene coexpression analysis is widely applied to transcriptomic data from PBMCs extracted before and after vaccine administration to cluster genes into several modules based on the correlation estimation [179–181]. The derived modules allow researchers to understand how genes are interacting with one another and to predict their possible roles; this is because genes with similar biological functions tend to exhibit a strong correlation in expression levels [182]. Voigt et al. (2018) investigated the use of co-expression analysis to identify vaccine response-related genes in PBMC transcriptomic datasets collected from 138 healthy older adults (aged 50–74) before and after seasonal trivalent influenza vaccination. Fifteen gene clusters were identified based on observed gene expression patterns across subjects, and eight clusters were strongly enriched for genes involved in specific immune cell types and processes, such as B cells, T cells, NK cells, monocytes, and antiviral signaling [171]. The availability of this information in public databases is also of major importance for the construction of solid and accessible knowledge about the validation of vaccine platforms [183].

6.5.1.2 Single-cell RNA sequencing

In recent years, scRNA-Seq has been used in vaccination studies for transcriptional evaluation at the cellular level, bringing to light systemic aspects linked to the study of cell heterogeneity and development [184]. To date, more than 25 techniques have been developed for the application of the scRNA-Seq method. All these techniques are based on the same sequence of steps, which correspond to cell isolation and lysis and RNA capture, and use of reverse transcriptase to synthetize a molecule of cDNA, which will be amplified and sequenced using next-generation techniques. Through the application of these methodologies associated with computational resources for detailed analysis, it is possible to identify response profiles that would not be detected using methods at the systemic level, and may allow the application of other omics tools [185].

The main differences among the methods used for scRNA-Seq analysis are the specificity, sensitivity, and accuracy of the methods; in addition, they differ in the techniques used for cell isolation and the platform used to develop the sequencing [184,186]. For this reason, these methodologies can be used aiming at different results, such as studies of genomes and surface proteins, through single-cell genome and transcriptome sequencing (G&T-seq) and cellular indexing of transcriptomes and epitopes by sequencing (CITE-seq), respectively [184,187,188]. Its application is essential for the identification and validation of correlates of protection, due to the ability to identify the global expression of genes and the specificity of different cell types and different antigens from the same pathogen [184]. When studying diseases whose infection does not guarantee the subject's complete protection, as observed in influenza and malaria, the evaluation of the immune response using scRNA-Seq can demonstrate which barriers need to be overcome by the vaccination process [184,189,190].

In vaccinology, the use of scRNA-Seq can help to understand different transcriptional signatures of T cells after activation and after their clonal expansion. Through the study of TAK-003, a recombinant, tetravalent DENV vaccine [191,192], the implementation of scRNA-Seq allowed the identification of transcriptional signatures that enabled the identification of $CD8^+$ T cell precursors with most durable vaccine-reactive memory in PBMC samples [193]. Moreover, through spec-seq of human plasmablasts, it was possible to observe the transcriptional differences between vaccine-negative and vaccine-positive IgA plasmablasts [194]. This study also highlights the importance of this finding, since the induction of an increased number of these IgA plasmablasts in the peripheral blood would provide greater mucosal protection.

6.5.2 Proteomics

Proteomics is based on the study of the multi-proteins of a system, aiming at the identification of its role and its properties within that system [195]. The visualization of changes caused by infection and vaccination in proteins is one of the mechanisms used for the development of new vaccines. In this sense, proteomics is capable of making a global mapping of all proteins in a cell, which allows for a broad assessment, capable of understanding their interactions and functions in the face of the immunization process [12,196].

In the sense of vaccinology, immunoproteomics is essential for understanding the functioning of vaccines [166,197]. Immunoproteomics is a combination of the proteomics technique with the detection of immunoreactive proteins/antigens during infection in the serum of patients, making it possible to identify potential target candidates for future vaccines [198]. This method can also be performed by identifying the epitopes expressed by T cells or by identifying the antibodies that are expressed, measuring their specificity [199,200]. Through the evaluation of the serum of vaccinated, infected, or after-recovery patients, it has already helped in the identification of several pathogen-specific antigens [198].

The presence of differentially abundant proteins in response to vaccination has already been reported in a study by Galassie et al. (2018), in which a set of protein families was detected by a proteomics method, whose activity was positively correlated with the phenotype of seroprotection against H5N1. Proteins associated with inflammation, oxidative stress, immunoproteasome subunits (PSME1 and PSME2), and HLA class I proteins were detected in the innate immunity cells, such as neutrophils and monocytes. In the first 24 hours after vaccination, proteins such as granzyme B and neutrophil cytosolic factor were identified. On the third day postvaccination, signaling through the B cell receptor was significantly enriched in neutrophils and monocytes. Proteins with functionality for antigen presentation, interferon signaling, phagosomes, and class 1 MHC were also abundantly detected [12].

Aiming to assess the efficacy of the BCG vaccine, 307 individuals received a BCG vaccine dose in a study. Markers such as interleukin-17C, tumor necrosis factor-like weak inducer of apoptosis (TWEAK), neurotrophin-3 (NT-3), adenosine deaminase (ADA), and delta/notch-like epidermal growth factor-related receptor (DNER) were detected throughout the study period with their concentration peaks between the second and fourth week after administration, and found to decrease after this period. Once all these markers are indicative of activation of the immune system after vaccination, the data demonstrate the ability of a vaccination to downregulate inflammatory markers of relevance in modulating the immune system [201].

Some methodologies can be used to identify immunoproteomics, such as ELISA and liquid chromatography-mass spectrometry (LC-MS), which can be associated with the Western blotting method [166]. The LC-MS technique has been widely used due to its high sensitivity, specificity, and versatility, since it can be applied to several biological materials and to several analyses in a single experimental process, with only a small increase in costs [202]. This method consists of the enzymatic cleavage of the proteins of interest, which will later be evaluated according to the physical or biochemical properties of their by-products, identified through a mass spectrometer [195,203].

6.5.3 Metabolomics

As the name suggests, the metabolome is a methodology that seeks to survey all metabolites in a system, which comprises a wide variety of molecules [204]. Its application can also be used to identify new protection correlates, which can be decisive in the development of a vaccine formulation; there is also an application to confirm the effects generated after immunization/vaccination[205].

Metabolites have been used more as specialized agents in the identification of disease, as they often have a direct relation with the type of pathogen being diagnosed or studied, acting as biomarkers [206]. Metabolites are disturbed in abnormal situations for the body, both when it comes to infections and when it comes to vaccination. During an infection, for example, changes in the metabolism of lipids and amino acids can be observed, while postvaccine, there are changes in the carbohydrate and bile acid pathways [207].

Hemorrhagic fever with renal syndrome currently has an inactivated virus vaccine known as Hantavax. Although efficient, the mechanisms by which the vaccine provides protection are not fully elucidated. Using metabolomic profile, it was possible to observe and increase the expression of cholesteryl nitrolinoleate, octanoyl-carnitine, tyrosine, ubiquinone-9, and benzoate in high responders, while in other pathways, such as chenodeoxycholic acid and methyl palmitate were upregulated in low responders and non-responders [208].

Through the use of LC-MS aiming at a metabolomic analysis, it was possible to comprehend, for example, that the infection caused by the SARS-CoV-2 causes disturbance in several metabolic pathways, including the bile acid, diacylglycerols, free fatty acid, triglycerides, and tryptophan pathways [209–212].

For this reason, its use as a tool for identifying potential targets for vaccine development is just as important [205]. To put this methodology into practice, techniques such as spectroscopy and spectrometry techniques can be performed in association with high-resolution mass spectrometry [213].

6.5.4 Data integration

The first step in the analysis of biological systems via omics tools often consists of a description of its parts (transcriptome, proteome, metabolome). However, it is critical to understand the nature of the interactions between these components [159] (Fig. 6.6). Data integration aim to determine biological insights that cannot be identified, analyzing only one dataset or only one component of the system. This approach has emerged to improve predictions of response variables and provide a better understanding of the biology itself, often resulting in high-quality mechanistic hypothesis [214].

The challenge relies in integrating multiple datasets from the same type of data (transcriptomics x transcriptomics) to different layers of orthogonal information

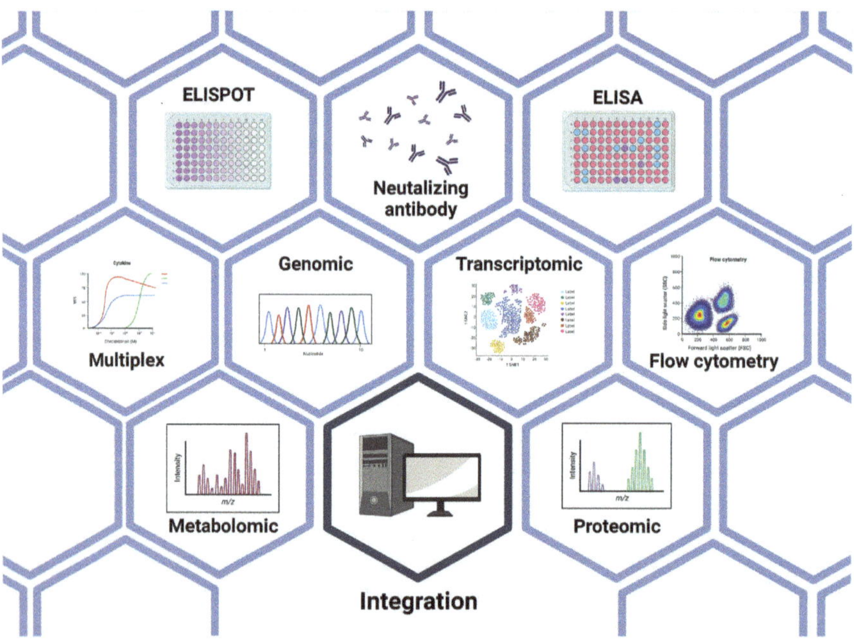

FIG. 6.6 Visual representation of data integration. This is an important step in vaccinology, once it allows the integration between different data in order to generate a realistic representation of the immunization consequences, generating broad and reliable results. The integration aims to connect the "omic" evaluations—genomic, transcriptomic, proteomic and metabolomic—as well as other methods such as ELISA, ELISPOT, neutralizing antibodies, flow cytometry, and cytokine multiplex. *(Created with BioRender.com).*

(transcriptomics x metabolomics). Therefore, combinations of experimental and computational approaches have been formulated to solve these issues [152,159].

The measurement of how gene expression changes under different biological conditions has offered important insights about genes and pathways involved on the immune response to vaccines [215]. Of interest, transcriptomics data are publicly available in several databases, including the Gene Expression Omnibus database (https://www.ncbi.nlm.nih.gov/geo/). Thus, one can integrate several datasets from the same data type to investigate how vaccines work in different populations, using meta-analysis methods. However, the identification of DEGs in vaccinees can be challenging, since a there are wide varieties of data types (RNA-seq or microarrays), platforms, and normalization methods [216]. Other parameters need to be considered, such as the quality of study design, the sample size, and the immune status of the subjects (i.e., age, overall health, or treatments) [217]. De Lima et al. (2019) used a meta-analysis approach and public data to create co-expression gene modules from the blood of hundreds of individuals vaccinated with the influenza or yellow fever vaccine, identifying that long noncoding RNAs are involved in multiple immunological pathways in response to vaccination [218].

More than concatenating different datasets from the same type of data, the integration of omics data derived from distinct technologies (NGS vs LC-MS) has been particularly challenging. Data integration methods include those relying only on prior knowledge (enzyme X catalyzes reaction of metabolite Y), and thus, consists of a conceptual correlation, which has been used particularly when datasets are acquired from limited samples or different populations. However, this approach lacks the robustness of statistical testing and determination of significant associations. To overcome this issue, statistical methods rely on data-driven associations, which include univariate correlations between individual features of each type of omics data. However, this and other similar approaches result in large and complex correlation matrices that can be highly redundant and where the underlying biology can be difficult to interpret. Therefore, effective integration needs to address dimension reduction, redundancy, and different variance structures generated by distinct technologies [219]. The hierarchical community networks (HiCoNet, https://github.com/shuzhao-li/hiconet) approach was developed to overcome such challenges and has been applied to understand the human responses to infection [220] and vaccines. Indeed, it was first applied to integrate metabolomics, transcriptomics, cell populations, and cytokine data upon response to the herpes zoster vaccine, which revealed that inositol phosphate, glycerophospholipids, and sterol metabolism are critical regulators of adaptive immune responses [221]. More recently, the HiCoNet approach was applied to understand the impact of antibiotic-driven dysbiosis in human immune responses to influenza vaccine [222]. This study demonstrated that gut microbiomes have a direct impact on the development of effective antibody responses to influenza, while also affecting inflammatory signaling via metabolism of secondary bile acids.

6.5.5 Network analysis in vaccinology

Network analysis offers a new way to categorize systems of very different origins under a single framework. It has been used to identify patterns between the organization of various complex systems [223,224]. By integrating the vast knowledge already generated about different types of vaccines, adjuvants, and routes of administration with molecular and immunological data, we can better understand how vaccines work [225].

A biological network is a set of nodes and edges connecting them, as represented in Fig. 6.7. They are similar to a map that allows the visualization of how

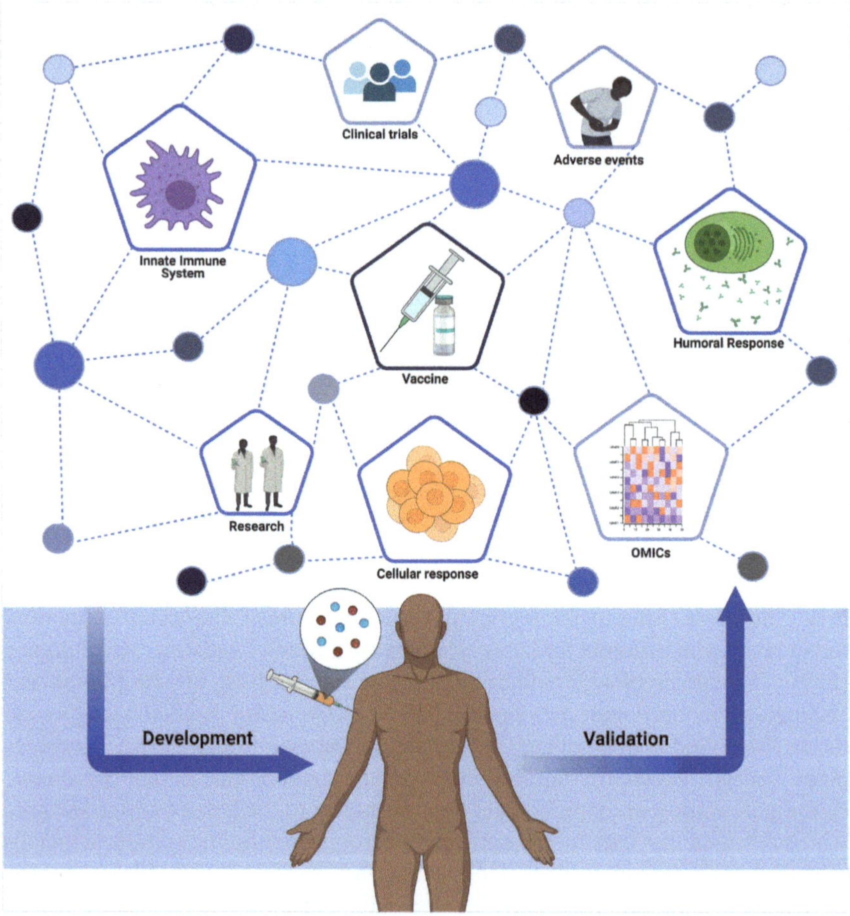

FIG. 6.7 Schematic demonstration of Biological Network in vaccinology. Different aspects are important during the design and production of a new vaccine. The aspects related to innate, cellular, and humoral responses, adverse events and omics—genomic, transcriptomic, proteomic, and metabolomic—are important to the construction of the vaccine, its antigens and adjuvants and after the distribution aiming validation of the results and security of the formulation. *(Created with BioRender.com).*

complex systems operate inside and between cells. They are complex; their components are highly connected and are governed by a series of basic principles in their structure and evolution that distinguish them from random networks [226]. The biological components are represented as nodes in the network, and they can be gene sequences, RNA and protein expression levels, phenotypes, signaling pathways, or biological processes. The edges represent the connections between the nodes, which also may be defined in numerous ways depending on the data, such as physical protein–protein interactions, regulatory processes, gene coexpression, or co-occurrent terms in scientific papers [226–229].

Network theory methods have the ability to improve predictive models of immune response, identifying important nodes that act as hubs and determine the structure of the network, for example, genes or sets of genes, based on their connectivity with other nodes [226]. Degree centrality, which gives the number of links the node has to other nodes, and betweenness centrality, which illustrates the degree to which a node is directly connected to others nodes that are not connected to each other, are the most elementary network measures; they allow the identification of the most important components of the biological network [230].

In topological analysis of biological networks, three concepts are important: location, neighborhood, and distance [227]. Location is important because central nodes that are highly connected can participate in essential molecular processes, while the nodes that are located on the periphery are less connected and have a less profound effect [224]. Neighborhood is crucial because different nodes associated with the same disease or vaccine are not randomly spread out but occupy well-defined places in the network [226]; this is useful because identifying that a certain neighborhood is important helps one to find other nodes in this same neighborhood that may also be important for the same context. For example, genes or proteins that are closer in the human interactome tend to have common biological functions, such as participating in the same metabolic or signaling pathways, and tend to be involved in similar diseases [231]. Finally, physical distance is important, because two nodes are connected if they share one or several links. In the human disease network, two diseases that are closely related are located next to each other in the network, for example, obesity and diabetes [226].

Most biological networks show a high degree of clustering, implying the existence of topological modules that represent highly interlinked local regions in the network [226]. Genes associated with the same disease in a gene x disease network form connected subgraphs, called disease modules, and disease pairs with overlapping modules, have some phenotype similarities and high comorbidity [226,231–233].

So, how do we apply network medicine to directly help people? It is very difficult to find the genetic variations responsible for a disease or an adverse effect of a vaccine, because we all have thousands of small variations in our DNA, which result in our individuality. The challenge is to find the right variations in patients' DNA. Network medicine can help us to map all the variations found in an individual and check which ones follow a pattern of expression found in similar diseases or phenotypes. Therefore, this will tell us which neighborhood in the network most likely has the variation that is causing this phenotype. Once we find the location of the genetic variations, we have a molecular diagnosis [234].

6.6 Concluding remarks

When designing vaccines, several factors need to be taken in consideration, starting with the type of pathogen that will be investigated, passing through the type of immune response it triggers, and the ideal one to fight its infection, reaching on the implication of these factors in the population that will be immunized. Aiming for this objective, the omics sciences and classical methods, through systems vaccinology, are able to amplify the study of all factors linked to a vaccine, allowing a broader view on its mechanisms of action, side effects, and systemic effects in the population. The systemic evaluation capacity of a vaccine is an important factor, since its effects are not restricted to a cell or organ and the functioning of the organism as a whole can influence what is seen in vitro and in vivo.

For this reason, the advancement of systems vaccinology, especially nowadays, is an ally in the validation and better understanding of new vaccines, which is reflected in better efficacy and the greater speed in their widespread distribution.

Acknowledgments

We would to thank the Graduate Program in Tropical Medicine and Public Health at the Federal University of Goiás (UFG/Brazil), for the support throughout the graduate program and the writing of this chapter. We would also like to thank Coordenação de Aperfeiçoamento de Pessoal de Nível Superior (CAPES), the funding agency responsible for postgraduate scholarships for students involved in this chapter. Finally, we would like to thank BioRender for providing an accessible platform for developing intuitive scientific figures.

References

[1] Lurie N, Saville M, Hatchett R, Halton J. Developing Covid-19 vaccines at pandemic speed, 2020;382 (21):1969–73. doi:10.1056/NEJMP2005630.

[2] Excler J-L, Saville M, Berkley S, Kim JH. Vaccine development for emerging infectious diseases. Nat Med 2021;274(27):591–600. doi:10.1038/s41591-021-01301-0.

[3] Ball P. The lightning-fast quest for COVID vaccines—and what it means for other diseases. Nature 2021;589(7840):16–8. doi:10.1038/D41586-020-03626-1.

[4] Su S, Du L, Jiang S. Learning from the past: development of safe and effective COVID-19 vaccines. Nat Rev Microbiol 2020;193(3):211–9. doi:10.1038/s41579-020-00462-y.

[5] Forni G, Mantovani A. COVID-19 vaccines: where we stand and challenges ahead. Cell Death & Differentiation 2021;282(28):626–39. doi:10.1038/s41418-020-00720-9.

[6] Plotkin S. History of vaccination Proceedings of the National Academy of Sciences of the United States of America. Natl Acad Sci 2014;111(34):12283–7. doi:10.1073/pnas.1400472111.

[7] Plotkin SA. Correlates of vaccine-induced immunity. Clin Infect Dis 2008;47(3):401–9. doi:10.1086/589862.

[8] Plotkin SA. Updates on immunologic correlates of vaccine-induced protection. Vaccine 2020;38(9):2250–7. doi:10.1016/J.VACCINE.2019.10.046.

[9] Sharma M, Krammer F, García-Sastre A, Tripathi S. Moving from empirical to rational vaccine design in the 'Omics' Era. Vaccines 2019;7(7):89. doi:10.3390/VACCINES7030089.

[10] Qiu S, et al. Significant transcriptome and cytokine changes in hepatitis B vaccine non-responders revealed by genome-wide comparative analysis. Hum Vaccines Immunother 2018;14(7):1763–72. doi:10.1080/21645515.2018.1450122.

[11] E B, et al. Transcriptome profiling in blood before and after hepatitis B vaccination shows significant differences in gene expression between responders and non-responders. Vaccine 2018;36(42):6282–9. doi:10.1016/J.VACCINE.2018.09.001.

[12] Galassie AC, Link AJ. Proteomic contributions to our understanding of vaccine and immune responses. Proteomics—Clinical Applications 2015;9(11-12):972–89. doi:10.1002/prca.201500054.

[13] Duffy D. Standardized immunomonitoring: separating the signals from the noise. Trends Biotechnol 2018;36(11):1107–15. doi:10.1016/J.TIBTECH.2018.06.002.

[14] Clem AS. Fundamentals of vaccine immunology. J Glob Infect Dis 2011;3(1):73–8. doi:10.4103/0974-777X.77299.

[15] Krammer F. A correlate of protection for SARS-CoV-2 vaccines is urgently needed. Nat Med 2021:1–2. doi:10.1038/s41591-021-01432-4.

[16] Alberts B, Johnson A, Lewis J, Raff M, Roberts K, Walter P. Biochemistry and Molecular Biology Education. Molecular Biology of the Cell, 4th ed. New York: Garland Science; 2002.

[17] de Melo Cruvinel W, et al. Immune system-Part I fundamentals of innate immunity with emphasis on molecular and cellular mechanisms of inflammatory response. Revista Brasileira de Reumatologia 2010;50(4). doi:10.1590/S0482-50042010000400008.

[18] Medzhitov R, Janeway CA. Innate immune recognition and control of adaptive immune responses. Semin Immunol 1998;10(5):351–3. doi:10.1006/smim.1998.0136.

[19] Medzhitov R, Janeway C. Innate immune recognition: Mechanisms and pathways. Immunol Rev 2000;173(1):89–97. doi:10.1034/j.1600-065X.2000.917309.x.

[20] Zuckerman JN. The importance of injecting vaccines into muscle. British Medical Journal 2000;321(7271):1237–8. doi:10.1136/bmj.321.7271.1237.

[21] Kawai T, Akira S. Innate immune recognition of viral infection. Nat Immunol 2006;7(2): 131–7. doi:10.1038/ni1303.

[22] Mogensen TH. Pathogen recognition and inflammatory signaling in innate immune defenses. Clin Microbiol Rev 2009;22(2):240–73. doi:10.1128/CMR.00046-08.

[23] Janeway CA. Approaching the asymptote? Evolution and revolution in immunology. Cold Spring Harb Symp Quant Biol 1989;55(1):1–13. doi:10.1101/sqb.1989.054.01.003.

[24] Cai X, Chiu YH, Chen ZJ. The cGAS-cGAMP-STING pathway of cytosolic DNA sensing and signaling. Mol Cell 2014;54(2):289–96. doi:10.1016/j.molcel.2014.03.040.

[25] Kawasaki T, Kawai T. Toll-like receptor signaling pathways. Front Immunol 2014;5:461. doi:10.3389/fimmu.2014.00461.

[26] Schuster JM, Nelson PS. Toll receptors: an expanding role in our understanding of human disease. J Leukoc Biol 2000;67(6):767–73. doi:10.1002/jlb.67.6.767.

[27] Dowling JK, Mansell A. Toll-like receptors: the swiss army knife of immunity and vaccine development. Clin Transl Immunol 2016;20(5). doi:10.1038/cti.2016.22.

[28] Akira S, Takeda K. Toll-like receptor signalling. Nat Rev Immunol 2004;4(7):499–511. doi:10.1038/nri1391.

[29] Pashine A, Valiante NM, Ulmer JB. Targeting the innate immune response with improved vaccine adjuvants. Nat Med 2005;11(4S):S63. doi:10.1038/nm1210.

[30] Nathan CF. Secretory products of macrophages. J Clin Investig 1987;79(2):319–26. doi:10.1172/JCI112815.

[31] Billack B. Macrophage activation: Role of Toll-like receptors, nitric oxide, and nuclear factor kappa B. Am J Pharm Educ 2006;70(5). doi:10.5688/aj7005102.

[32] Janeway CA, Medzhitov R. Innate immune recognition. Annu Rev Immunol 2002;20: 197–216. doi:10.1146/annurev.immunol.20.083001.084359.

[33] Yang S-J, et al. Activation of M1 Macrophages in Response to recombinant TB vaccines with enhanced antimycobacterial activity. Front Immunol 2020;11:1298. doi:10.3389/FIMMU.2020.01298.

[34] Guedj K, et al. M1 macrophages act as LTβR-independent lymphoid tissue inducer cells during atherosclerosis-related lymphoid neogenesis. Cardiovasc Res 2014;101(3):434–43. doi:10.1093/cvr/cvt263.

[35] Hughes CE, Benson RA, Bedaj M, Maffia P. Antigen-presenting cells and antigen presentation in tertiary lymphoid organs. Front Immunol 2016;7:481. doi:10.3389/fimmu.2016.00481.

[36] Jost S, Altfeld M, Chang JJ. Harnessing innate and adaptive immunity for viral vaccine design. Expert Rev Vaccines 2012;11(7):775–7. doi:10.1586/erv.12.48.

[37] Dausset J. The Birth of MAC. Vox Sanguinis 1984;46(4):235–7. doi:10.1111/j.1423-0410.1984.tb00080.x.

[38] Erickson RP. Natural history of the major histocompatibility complex. Am J Hum Genet 1987;40(5):469.

[39] Bettencourt P, et al. Identification of antigens presented by MHC for vaccines against tuberculosis. Vaccines 2020;5(1). doi:10.1038/s41541-019-0148-y.

[40] Kambayashi T, Laufer TM. Atypical MHC class II-expressing antigen-presenting cells: can anything replace a dendritic cell? Nat Rev Immunol 2014;14(11):719–30. doi:10.1038/nri3754.

[41] Fong L, Engleman EG. Dendritic cells in cancer immunotherapy. Annu Rev Immunol 2000;18(1):245–73. doi:10.1146/annurev.immunol.18.1.245.

[42] Inaba K, Romani N, Steinman RM. An antigen-independent contact mechanism as an early step in T cell-proliferative responses to dendritic cells. J Exp Med 1989;170(2):527–42. doi:10.1084/jem.170.2.527.

[43] Mehta-Damani A, Markowicz S, Engleman EG. Generation of antigen-specific CD4+ T cell lines from naive precursors. Eur J Immunol 1995;25(5):1206–11. doi:10.1002/eji.1830250511.

[44] Mehta-Damani A, Markowicz S, Engleman EG. Generation of antigen-specific CD8+ CTLs from naive precursors. J Immunol 1994;153(3).

[45] Guéry JC, Ria F, Adorini L. Dendritic cells but not B cells present antigenic complexes to class II-restricted T cells after administration of protein in adjuvant. J Exp Med 1996;183(3):751–7. doi:10.1084/jem.183.3.751.

[46] MG N, J Q, van der JW M. Trained immunity: a memory for innate host defense. Cell Host Microbe 2011;9(5):355–61. doi:10.1016/J.CHOM.2011.04.006.

[47] Sun JC, Lopez-Verges S, Kim CC, DeRisi JL, Lanier LL. NK cells and immune 'memory,'. J Immunol 2011;186(4):1891. doi:10.4049/JIMMUNOL.1003035.

[48] JC DS, et al. β-glucan-induced trained immunity protects against leishmania braziliensis infection: a crucial role for IL-32. Cell Rep 2019;28(10):2659–72. doi:10.1016/J.CELREP.2019.08.004.

[49] J Q, et al. Candida albicans infection affords protection against reinfection via functional reprogramming of monocytes. Cell Host Microbe 2012;12(2):223–32. doi:10.1016/J.CHOM.2012.06.006.

[50] RJ A, et al. Long-term in vitro and in vivo effects of γ-irradiated BCG on innate and adaptive immunity. J Leukoc Biol 2015;98(6):995–1001. doi:10.1189/JLB.4MA0215-059R.

[51] Alberts B, Johnson A, Lewis J, Raff M, Roberts K, Walter P. The Adaptive Immune System in Molecular Biology of The Cell, 4th ed. New York: Garland Science; 2002.

[52] Charles A Janeway J, Travers P, Walport M, Shlomchik MJ. Immunobiology: the immune system in health and disease, 5th ed. New York: Garland Science; 2001.

[53] Van Stipdonk MJB, Lemmens EE, Schoenberger SP. Naïve CTLs require a single brief period of antigenic stimulation for clonal expansion and differentiation. Nat Immunol 2001;2(5):423–9. doi:10.1038/87730.

[54] Lee WT, Pasos G, Cecchini L, Mittler JN. Continued antigen stimulation is not required during CD4 + T cell clonal expansion. J Immunol 2002;168(4):1682–9. doi:10.4049/jimmunol.168.4.1682.

[55] Wong P, Pamer EG. Proliferation cutting edge: antigen-independent CD8 T Cell. J Immunol 2015;166:5864–8. doi:10.4049/jimmunol.166.10.5864.

[56] Kaech SM, Ahmed R. Memory CD8+ T cell differentiation: initial antigen encounter triggers a developmental program in naïve cells. Nat Immunol 2001;2(5):415–22. doi:10.1038/87720.

[57] Zhang N, Bevan MJ. CD8+ T Cells: foot soldiers of the immune system. Immunity 2011;35(2):161–8. doi:10.1016/j.immuni.2011.07.010.

[58] Koup RA, Douek DC. Vaccine design for CD8 T lymphocyte responses. Cold Spring Harb Perspect Med 2011;1(1). doi:10.1101/cshperspect.a007252.

[59] Charles A Janeway J, Travers P, Walport M, Shlomchik MJ. T Cell-mediated Cytotoxicity in Immunobiology. Immunobiology: the immune system in health and disease, 5th ed. New York: Garland Science; 2001.

[60] Rock MT, Yoder SM, Wright PF, Talbot TR, Edwards KM, Crowe JE. Differential regulation of granzyme and perforin in effector and memory T cells following smallpox immunization 1. J Immunol 2005;174:3757–64.

[61] Luckheeram RV, Zhou R, Verma AD, Xia B. CD4 +T cells: Differentiation and functions. Clin Dev Immunol 2012. doi:10.1155/2012/925135.

[62] Youngblood B, Hale JS, Ahmed R. T-cell memory differentiation: insights from transcriptional signatures and epigenetics. Immunology 2013;139(3):277–84. doi:10.1111/IMM.12074.

[63] Plotkin SA, Gilbert PB. Nomenclature for immune correlates of protection after vaccination. Clin Infect Dis 2012;54(11):1615–7. doi:10.1093/CID/CIS238.

[64] Sprent J, Surh CD. T cell memory. Annu Rev Immunol 2002;20:551–79. doi:10.1146/annurev.immunol.20.100101.151926.

[65] Ahmed R, Gray D. Immunological memory and protective immunity: understanding their relation. Science 1996;272:54–60. doi:10.1126/science.272.5258.54.

[66] MacLeod MKL, Clambey ET, Kappler JW, Marrack P. CD4 memory T cells: What are they and what can they do? Semin Immunol 2009;21(2):53–61. doi:10.1016/j.smim.2009.02.006.

[67] SL S, et al. CD4+ T-cell memory: generation and multi-faceted roles for CD4+ T cells in protective immunity to influenza. Immunol Rev 2006;211:8–22. doi:10.1111/J.0105-2896.2006.00388.X.

[68] Berard M, Tough DF. Qualitative differences between naïve and memory T cells. Immunology 2002;106(2):127–38. doi:10.1046/J.1365-2567.2002.01447.X.

[69] Gattinoni L, Speiser DE, Lichterfeld M, Bonini C. T memory stem cells in health and disease. Nat Med 2017;23(1):18. doi:10.1038/NM.4241.

[70] Sallusto F, Geginat J, Lanzavecchia A. Central memory and effector memory T cell subsets: function, generation, and maintenance. Annu Rev Immunol 2004;22:745–63. doi:10.1146/annurev.immunol.22.012703.104702.

[71] MacLennan ICM, et al. The changing preference of T and B cells for partners as T-dependent antibody responses develop. Immunol Rev 1997;156:53–66. doi:10.1111/j.1600-065X.1997.tb00958.x.

[72] Hoffman W, Lakkis FG, Chalasani G. B cells, antibodies, and more. Clin J Am Soc Nephrol 2016;11(1):137–54. doi:10.2215/CJN.09430915.

[73] HW S, L C. Structure and function of immunoglobulins. J Allergy Clin Immunol 2010;125(2). doi:10.1016/J.JACI.2009.09.046.

[74] Charles A Janeway J, Travers P, Walport M, Shlomchik MJ. The humoral immune response. Immunobiology: the immune system in health and disease, 5th ed. New York: Garland Science; 2001.

[75] Thau L, Mahajan K. Physiology, Opsonization. StatPearls Publishing; 2019.

[76] Edara V-V, et al. Infection and vaccine-induced neutralizing-antibody responses to the SARS-CoV-2 B.1.617 variants. New England J Med 2021;385:664–6. doi:10.1056/NEJMC2107799.

[77] Sathe A, Cusick JK. Biochemistry, Immunoglobulin M, Treasure Island: StatPearls; 2021.

[78] Shakib F, Stanworth DR. Human IgG subclasses in health and disease (A review) Part II. Ric Clin e Lab 1980;104(10):561–80. doi:10.1007/BF02906696.

[79] Klingler J, et al. Role of IgM and IgA antibodies in the neutralization of SARS-CoV-2, medRxiv (2020). doi:10.1101/2020.08.18.20177303.

[80] Suzuki T, et al. Relationship of the quaternary structure of human secretory IgA to neutralization of influenza virus. Proc Natl Acad Sci 2015;112(25):7809–14. doi:10.1073/PNAS.1503885112.

[81] Renegar KB, Small PA, Boykins LG, Wright PF. Role of IgA versus IgG in the control of influenza viral infection in the murine respiratory tract. J Immunol 2004;173(3):1978–86. doi:10.4049/JIMMUNOL.173.3.1978.

[82] Woof JM, Kerr MA. The function of immunoglobulin A in immunity. J Pathol 2006;208(2):270–82. doi:10.1002/PATH.1877.

[83] Aleyd E, Heineke MH, van Egmond M. The era of the immunoglobulin A Fc receptor FcαRI; its function and potential as target in disease. Immunol Rev 2015;268(1):123–38. doi:10.1111/IMR.12337.

[84] Hiemstra PS, Gorter A, Stuurman ME, Van Es LA, Daha MR. Activation of the alternative pathway of complement by human serum IgA. Eur J Immunol 1987;17(3):321–6. doi:10.1002/EJI.1830170304.

[85] IC M, et al. Identification of the transferrin receptor as a novel immunoglobulin (Ig)A1 receptor and its enhanced expression on mesangial cells in IgA nephropathy. J Exp Med 2001;194(4):417–25. doi:10.1084/JEM.194.4.417.

[86] Tauzin A, et al. A single dose of the SARS-CoV-2 vaccine BNT162b2 elicits Fc-mediated antibody effector functions and T cell responses. Cell Host Microbe 2021;29(7):1137–50. doi:10.1016/J.CHOM.2021.06.001.

[87] Clements CJ, Lawrence G, Safety V. Vaccine Safety. Encyclopedia of Virology. Los Angeles: Elsevier Ltd; 2008, pp. 226–35.

[88] Forthal DN. Functions of antibodies, Antibodies for Infectious Diseases 2014;2(4):25–48.

[89] Haynes BF, Montefiori DC. Aiming to induce broadly reactive neutralizing antibody responses with HIV-1 vaccine candidates. Expert Rev Vaccines 2006;5(3):347–63. doi:10.1586/14760584.5.3.347.

[90] Mascola J. Defining the protective antibody response for HIV-1. Curr Mol Med 2005;3(3):209–16. doi:10.2174/1566524033479799.

[91] Montefiori DC, Morris L, Ferrari G, Mascola JR. Neutralizing and other antiviral antibodies in HIV-1 infection and vaccination. Current Opinion in HIV and AIDS 2007;2(3):169–76. doi:10.1097/COH.0b013e3280ef691e.

[92] Wiktor TJ, Clark HF. Application of the plaque assay technique to the study of rabies virus-neutralizing antibody interactions—PubMed. Ann Microbiol 1973;124(2):271–82.

[93] Bordignon J, Comin F, Ferreira SCP, Caporale GMM, Lima Filho JHC, Zanetti CR. Calculating rabies virus neutralizing antibodies titres by flow cytometry. Revista do Instituto de Medicina Tropical de São Paulo 2002;44(3):151–4. doi:10.1590/S0036-46652002000300007.

[94] Gupta S, et al. Recommendations for the design, optimization, and qualification of cell-based assays used for the detection of neutralizing antibody responses elicited to biological therapeutics. J Immunol Methods 2007;321(1-2):1–18. doi:10.1016/j.jim.2006.12.004.

[95] Bewley KR, et al. Quantification of SARS-CoV-2 neutralizing antibody by wild-type plaque reduction neutralization, microneutralization and pseudotyped virus neutralization assays. Nat Protoc 2021;166(16):3114–40. doi:10.1038/s41596-021-00536-y.

[96] Roehrig JT, Hombach J, Barrett ADT. Guidelines for plaque-reduction neutralization testing of human antibodies to dengue viruses. Viral Immunol 2008;21(2):123–32. doi:10.1089/VIM.2008.0007.

[97] Olitsky PK, Casals J. Neutralization tests for diagnosis of human virus encephalitides. Journal of the American Medical Association 1947;134(15):1224–8. doi:10.1001/JAMA.1947.02880320014004.

[98] Wendel S, et al. Screening for SARS-CoV-2 antibodies in convalescent plasma in Brazil: preliminary lessons from a voluntary convalescent donor program. Transfusion 2020;60(12): 2938–51. doi:10.1111/TRF.16065.

[99] Focosi D, Maggi F, Mazzetti P, Pistello M. Viral infection neutralization tests: a focus on severe acute respiratory syndrome-coronavirus-2 with implications for convalescent plasma therapy. Rev Med Virol 2021;31(2). doi:10.1002/RMV.2170.

[100] Tan CW, et al. A SARS-CoV-2 surrogate virus neutralization test based on antibody-mediated blockage of ACE2–spike protein–protein interaction. Nat Biotechnol 2020;389(9):1073–8. doi:10.1038/s41587-020-0631-z.

[101] Lu LL, Suscovich TJ, Fortune SM, Alter G. Beyond binding: antibody effector functions in infectious diseases. Nat Rev Immunol 2017;181(18):46–61. doi:10.1038/nri.2017.106.

[102] Arnold KB, Chung AW. Prospects from systems serology research. Immunology 2018;153(3):279. doi:10.1111/IMM.12861.

[103] Lee LH, Frash CE, Falk LA, Klein DL, Deal CD. Correlates of immunity for pneumococcal conjugate vaccines. Vaccine 2003;21(17-18):2190–6. doi:10.1016/S0264-410X(03)00025-2.

[104] Chung AW, Alter G. Systems serology: profiling vaccine induced humoral immunity against HIV. Retrovirology 2017;14(1):1. doi:10.1186/S12977-017-0380-3.

[105] Supachai R-N, et al. Vaccination with ALVAC and AIDSVAX to prevent HIV-1 infection in Thailand. New England J Med 2009;361(23):2209–20. doi:10.1056/NEJMOA0908492.

[106] Chung AW, et al. Polyfunctional Fc-effector profiles mediated by IgG subclass selection distinguish RV144 and VAX003 vaccines. Sci Transl Med 2014;6(228). doi:10.1126/SCITRANSLMED.3007736.

[107] Alhajj M, Farhana A. Enzyme Linked Immunosorbent Assay, Treasure Island: StatPearls Publishing; 2020.

[108] Aydin S. A short history, principles, and types of ELISA, and our laboratory experience with peptide/protein analyses using ELISA. Peptides 2015;72:4–15. doi:10.1016/j.peptides.2015.04.012.

[109] Shah K, Maghsoudlou P. Enzyme-linked immunosorbent assay (ELISA): the basics. Br J Hosp Med 2016;77(7):98–101. doi:10.12968/hmed.2016.77.7.C98.

[110] Konstantinou GN. Enzyme-linked immunosorbent assay (ELISA). In: Methods in Molecular Biology, vol. 1592. New York: Humana Press Inc.; 2017, pp. 79–94.

[111] Engvall E, Perlmann P. Enzyme-linked immunosorbent assay (ELISA) quantitative assay of immunoglobulin G. Immunochemistry 1971;8(9):871–4. doi:10.1016/0019-2791(71)90454-X.

[112] Miura K, Orcutt AC, Muratova OV, Miller LH, Saul A, Long CA. Development and characterization of a standardized ELISA including a reference serum on each plate to detect antibodies induced by experimental malaria vaccines. Vaccine 2008;26(2):193–200. doi:10.1016/j.vaccine.2007.10.064.

[113] Haslinger C, Sommergruber W, Voss T, Schreiber M. Chapter 1: Identification of tumor-specific genes. In: Handbook of Immunohistochemistry and in Situ Hybridization of Human Carcinomas., 4. Cambridge, MA, USA: Academic Press; 2006, pp. 3–21.

[114] Slota M, Lim JB, Dang Y, Disis ML. ELISpot for measuring human immune responses to vaccines. Expert Rev Vaccines 2011;10(3):299–306. doi:10.1586/erv.10.169.

[115] Kalyuzhny AE. Chemistry and biology of the ELISPOT assay immunohistochemistry for non-experts view project. Methods in Molecular Biology 2005. doi:10.1385/1-59259-903-6:015.

[116] Cytokines in the balance. Nat Immunol 2019;20(12):1557. doi:10.1038/s41590-019-0557-0.

[117] Young HA. Cytokine multiplex analysis. Methods Mol Biol 2009;511:85. doi:10.1007/978-1-59745-447-6_4.

[118] Furman D, Davis MM. New approaches to understanding the immune response to vaccination and infection. Vaccine 2015;33(40):5271–81. doi:10.1016/J.VACCINE.2015.06.117.

[119] James EA, LaFond RE, Gates TJ, Mai DT, Malhotra U, Kwok WW. Yellow fever vaccination elicits broad functional CD4+ T cell responses that recognize structural and nonstructural proteins. J Virol 2013;87(23):12794–804. doi:10.1128/JVI.01160-13.

[120] Eriksson JC, Cox RJ, Szyszko E, Davidsson A, Brokstad KA. Local and systemic cytokine and chemokine responses after parenteral influenza vaccination. Influenza and Other Respiratory Viruses 2007;1(4):139–46. doi:10.1111/J.1750-2659.2007.00019.X.

[121] Smith SG, Lecher S, Blitz R, Locht C, Dockrell HM. Broad heparin-binding haemagglutinin-specific cytokine and chemokine response in infants following Mycobacterium bovis BCG vaccination. Eur. J Immunol 2012;42(9):2511–22. doi:10.1002/EJI.201142297.

[122] Skibinski DAG, et al. Induction of human T-cell and cytokine responses following vaccination with a novel influenza vaccine. Sci Rep 2018;81(8):1–12. doi:10.1038/s41598-018-36703-7.

[123] De Rosa SC. Vaccine applications of flow cytometry. Methods 2012;57(3):383–91. doi:10.1016/j.ymeth.2012.01.001.

[124] Qiu JG, Mei XL, Chen ZS, Shi Z. Cytokine detection by flow cytometry. Methods Mol Biol 2014;1172:235–42. doi:10.1007/978-1-4939-0928-5_21.

[125] Cibrián D, Sánchez-Madrid F. CD69: from activation marker to metabolic gatekeeper. Eur J Immunol 2017;47(6):946–53. doi:10.1002/EJI.201646837.

[126] Yan Z-h, et al. CD137 is a useful marker for identifying CD4+ T cell responses to mycobacterium tuberculosis. Scand J Immunol 2017;85(5):372–80. doi:10.1111/SJI.12541.

[127] Gniadecki R, Rossen K. Expression of T-cell activation marker CD134 (OX40) in lymphomatoid papulosis. Br J Dermatol 2003;148(5):885–91. doi:10.1046/J.1365-2133.2003.05286.X.

[128] E. Wieland, Markers of lymphocyte activation and proliferation, Personalized Immunosuppression in transplantation: role of biomarker monitoring and therapeutic drug monitoring (2016) 227–257. doi:10.1016/B978-0-12-800885-0.00010-2.

[129] Sallusto F, Lenig D, Förster R, Lipp M, Lanzavecchia A. Two subsets of memory T lymphocytes with distinct homing potentials and effector functions. Nature 1999;401:708–12. doi:10.1038/44385.

[130] Sallusto F, Geginat J, Lanzavecchia A. Central memory and effector memory T cell subsets: function, generation, and maintenance. Annu Rev Immunol 2004;22:745–63. doi:10.1146/ANNUREV.IMMUNOL.22.012703.104702.

[131] Zanetti M, Franchini G. T cell memory and protective immunity by vaccination: is more better? Trends Immunol 2006;27(11):511–7. doi:10.1016/J.IT.2006.09.004.

[132] Fonseca SG, Procopio FA, Goulet JP, Yassine-Diab B, Ancuta P, Sékaly RP. Unique features of memory T cells in HIV elite controllers: a systems biology perspective. Current Opinion in HIV and AIDS 2011;6(3):188–96. doi:10.1097/COH.0B013E32834589A1.

[133] G. Choudhary, Cell sorting and its significance in stem cell research. https://www.drugdiscoveryonline.com/doc/cell-sorting-and-its-significance-in-stem-cell-research-0001. (Accessed July 13, 2021).

[134] Liao X, Makris M, Luo XM. Fluorescence-activated cell sorting for purification of plasmacytoid dendritic cells from the mouse bone marrow. JoVE 2016;117:54641. doi:10.3791/54641.

[135] Bowyer G, et al. Activation-induced Markers detect vaccine-specific CD4+ T cell responses not measured by assays conventionally used in clinical trials. Vaccines 2018;6(3). doi:10.3390/VACCINES6030050.

[136] Reiss S, et al. Comparative analysis of activation induced marker (AIM) assays for sensitive identification of antigen-specific CD4 T cells. PLoS One 2017;12(10):e0186998. doi:10.1371/JOURNAL.PONE.0186998.

[137] Sallusto F, Cassotta A, Hoces D, Foglierini M, Lanzavecchia A. Do memory CD4 T cells keep their cell-type programming: plasticity versus fate commitment? T-Cell heterogeneity, plasticity, and selection in humans. Cold Spring Harb Perspect Biol 2018;10(3). doi:10.1101/CSHPERSPECT.A029421.

[138] Crotty S. Do memory CD4 T cells keep their cell-type programming: plasticity versus fate commitment? Complexities of interpretation due to the heterogeneity of memory CD4 T Cells, Including T Follicular Helper Cells. Cold Spring Harb Perspect Biol 2018;10(3). doi:10.1101/CSHPERSPECT.A032102.

[139] Dan JM, et al. A cytokine-independent approach to identify antigen-specific human germinal center T follicular helper cells and rare antigen-specific CD4+ T cells in blood. J Immunol 2016;197(3):983–93. doi:10.4049/JIMMUNOL.1600318.

[140] Geers D, et al. SARS-CoV-2 variants of concern partially escape humoral but not T-cell responses in COVID-19 convalescent donors and vaccinees. Sci Immunol 2021;6(59). doi:10.1126/SCIIMMUNOL.ABJ1750.

[141] Nair N, et al. Mass cytometry as a platform for the discovery of cellular biomarkers to guide effective rheumatic disease therapy. Arthritis Res Ther 2015;171(17):1–9. doi:10.1186/S13075-015-0644-Z.

[142] Ornatsky OI, et al. Study of cell antigens and intracellular DNA by identification of element-containing labels and metallointercalators using inductively coupled plasma mass spectrometry. Anal Chem 2008;80(7):2539–47. doi:10.1021/AC702128M.
[143] Gadalla R, et al. Validation of CyTOF against flow cytometry for immunological studies and monitoring of human cancer clinical trials. Front Oncol 2019:415. doi:10.3389/FONC.2019.00415.
[144] Leipold MD, Newell EW, Maecker HT. Multiparameter phenotyping of human PBMCs using mass cytometry. Methods Mol Biol 2015;1343:81–95. doi:10.1007/978-1-4939-2963-4_7.
[145] Siegrist C-A, Aspinall R. B-cell responses to vaccination at the extremes of age. Nat Rev Immunol 2009;93(9):185–94. doi:10.1038/nri2508.
[146] SL K, I M, EN F. Sex-based differences in immune function and responses to vaccination. Trans R Soc Trop Med Hygiene 2015;109(1):9–15. doi:10.1093/TRSTMH/TRU167.
[147] LC H, et al. Ethnic differences in immune responses to hepatitis B vaccine. Am J Epidemiol 1996;143(7):718–24. doi:10.1093/OXFORDJOURNALS.AJE.A008805.
[148] T H, et al. Differential genetic determination of immune responsiveness to hepatitis B surface antigen and to hepatitis A virus: a vaccination study in twins. Lancet 2002;360:991–5. doi:10.1016/S0140-6736(02)11083-X.
[149] SM L, DL T. Vaccines to prevent viral hepatitis. New England J Med 1997;336(3):196–204. doi:10.1056/NEJM199701163360307.
[150] KK S, et al. Age of recipient and number of doses differentially impact human B and T cell immune memory responses to HPV vaccination. Vaccine 2012;30(24):3572–9. doi:10.1016/J.VACCINE.2012.03.051.
[151] Zhang L, Wang W, Wang S. Effect of vaccine administration modality on immunogenicity and efficacy. Expert Rev Vaccines 2015;14(11):1509. doi:10.1586/14760584.2015.1081067.
[152] Kitano H. Computational systems biology. Nature 2002;420:206–10. doi:10.1038/nature01254.
[153] Kitano H. Systems biology: a brief overview. Science 2002;295(5560):1662–4. doi:10.1126/SCIENCE.1069492.
[154] Arazi A, Pendergraft WF, Ribeiro RM, Perelson AS, Hacohen N. Human systems immunology: hypothesis-based modeling and unbiased data-driven approaches. Semin Immunol 2013;25(3):193–200. doi:10.1016/J.SMIM.2012.11.003.
[155] HI N, S L, B P. Systems vaccinology: learning to compute the behavior of vaccine induced immunity. Wiley Interdisciplinary Rev Syst Biol Med 2012;4(2):193–205. doi:10.1002/WSBM.163.
[156] Pezeshki A, Ovsyannikova IG, McKinney BA, Poland GA, Kennedy RB. The role of systems biology approaches in determining molecular signatures for the development of more effective vaccines. Expert Rev Vaccines 2019;18(3):253–67. doi:10.1080/14760584.2019.1575208.
[157] Nakaya HI, et al. Systems analysis of immunity to influenza vaccination across multiple years and in diverse populations reveals shared molecular signatures. Immunity 2015;43(6):1186. doi:10.1016/J.IMMUNI.2015.11.012.
[158] Querec TD, et al. Systems biology approach predicts immunogenicity of the yellow fever vaccine in humans. Nat Immunol 2008;101(10):116–25. doi:10.1038/ni.1688.
[159] Nakaya HI, et al. Systems biology of vaccination for seasonal influenza in humans. Nat Immunol 2011;12(8):786–95. doi:10.1038/ni.2067.
[160] JZ O, et al. TLR5-mediated sensing of gut microbiota is necessary for antibody responses to seasonal influenza vaccination. Immunity 2014;41(3):478–92. doi:10.1016/J.IMMUNI.2014.08.009.

[161] Arunachalam PS, et al. Systems vaccinology of the BNT162b2 mRNA vaccine in humans. Nature 2021:1–10. doi:10.1038/s41586-021-03791-x.

[162] Bachem CWB, Oomen RJFJ, Visser RGF. Transcript Imaging with cDNA-AFLP: A Step-by-Step Protocol. Plant Mol Biol Rep 1998;16.

[163] Luecken MD, Theis FJ. Current best practices in single-cell RNA-seq analysis: a tutorial. Mol Syst Biol 2019;15(6):e8746. doi:10.15252/MSB.20188746.

[164] Schuch V, et al. Systems immunology of flavivirus infection. Zika Virus Biology, Transmission, and Pathology 2021:221–34.

[165] Li P, Piao Y, Shon HS, Ryu KH. Comparing the normalization methods for the differential analysis of Illumina high-throughput RNA-Seq data. BMC Bioinformatics 2015;161(16): 1–9. doi:10.1186/S12859-015-0778-7.

[166] Raeven RHM, van Riet E, Meiring HD, Metz B, Kersten GFA. Systems vaccinology and big data in the vaccine development chain. Immunology 2019;156(1). doi:10.1111/imm.13012.

[167] Raeven RHM, et al. Molecular and cellular signatures underlying superior immunity against Bordetella pertussis upon pulmonary vaccination. Mucosal Immunol 2018;11(3):979–93. doi:10.1038/mi.2017.81.

[168] Raeven RHM, et al. Molecular signatures of the evolving immune response in mice following a Bordetella pertussis infection. PLoS One 2014;9(8). doi:10.1371/journal.pone.0104548.

[169] Mosca F, et al. Molecular and cellular signatures of human vaccine adjuvants. Proc Natl Acad Sci 2008;105(30).

[170] Santoro F, et al. Transcriptomics of the vaccine immune response: priming with adjuvant modulates recall innate responses after boosting. Front Immunol 2018;9. doi:10.3389/fimmu.2018.01248.

[171] Voigt EA, et al. Transcriptomic signatures of cellular and humoral immune responses in older adults after seasonal influenza vaccination identified by data-driven clustering. Sci Rep 2018;8(1):739. doi:10.1038/s41598-017-17735-x.

[172] Tran TM, et al. Whole-blood transcriptomic signatures induced during immunization by chloroquine prophylaxis and Plasmodium falciparum sporozoites. Sci Rep 2019;9(1). doi:10.1038/s41598-019-44924-7.

[173] Munyaka PM, et al. Characterization of whole blood transcriptome and early-life fecal microbiota in high and low responder pigs before, and after vaccination for Mycoplasma hyopneumoniae. Vaccine 2019;37(13):1743–55. doi:10.1016/j.vaccine.2019.02.016.

[174] Chaussabel D. Assessment of immune status using blood transcriptomics and potential implications for global health. Semin Immunol 2015;27(1):58–66. doi:10.1016/j.smim.2015.03.002.

[175] G B, et al. Comparison of whole blood and peripheral blood mononuclear cell gene expression for evaluation of the perioperative inflammatory response in patients with advanced heart failure. PLoS One 2014;9(12). doi:10.1371/JOURNAL.PONE.0115097.

[176] D H, et al. Whole blood vs PBMC: compartmental differences in gene expression profiling exemplified in asthma. Allergy Asthma Clin Immunol 2019;15(1). doi:10.1186/S13223-019-0382-X.

[177] Obermoser G, et al. Systems scale interactive exploration reveals quantitative and qualitative differences in response to influenza and pneumococcal vaccines. Immunity 2013;38(4):831–44. doi:10.1016/j.immuni.2012.12.008.

[178] Gaucher D, et al. Yellow fever vaccine induces integrated multilineage and polyfunctional immune responses. J Exp Med 2008;205(13):3119–31. doi:10.1084/jem.20082292.

[179] Eisen MB, Spellman PT, Brown PO, Botstein D. Cluster analysis and display of genome-wide expression patterns. Proc Natl Acad Sci 1998;95(25).

[180] Langfelder P, Horvath S. WGCNA: an R package for weighted correlation network analysis. BMC Bioinformatics 2008;9(1):1–13. doi:10.1186/1471-2105-9-559.

[181] Russo PST, et al. CEMiTool: a bioconductor package for performing comprehensive modular co-expression analyses. BMC Bioinformatics 2018;19(1):1–13. doi:10.1186/S12859-018-2053-1.

[182] CW C, DJ B, SB W. Advantages of CEMiTool for gene co-expression analysis of RNA-seq data. Comput Biol Med 2020;125. doi:10.1016/J.COMPBIOMED.2020.103975.

[183] Voigt EA, et al. Transcriptomic signatures of cellular and humoral immune responses in older adults after seasonal influenza vaccination identified by data-driven clustering. Sci Rep 2018;8(1):1–16. doi:10.1038/s41598-017-17735-x.

[184] Noé A, Cargill TN, Nielsen CM, Russell AJC, Barnes E. The application of single-cell RNA sequencing in vaccinology. J Immunol Res 2020. doi:10.1155/2020/8624963.

[185] A H, J E, SA T, T L. A practical guide to single-cell RNA-sequencing for biomedical research and clinical applications. Genome Med 2017;9(1). doi:10.1186/S13073-017-0467-4.

[186] AA K, JK K, V S, JC M, SA T. The technology and biology of single-cell RNA sequencing. Mol Cell 2015;58(4):610–20. doi:10.1016/J.MOLCEL.2015.04.005.

[187] Macaulay IC, Teng MJ, Haerty W, Kumar P, Ponting CP, Voet T. Separation and parallel sequencing of the genomes and transcriptomes of single cells using G&T-seq. Nat Protoc 2016;11(11):2081–103. doi:10.1038/nprot.2016.138.

[188] Macaulay IC, et al. G&T-seq: parallel sequencing of single-cell genomes and transcriptomes. Nat Methods 2015;12(6):519–22. doi:10.1038/nmeth.3370.

[189] F K. The human antibody response to influenza A virus infection and vaccination. Nat Rev Immunol 2019;19(6):383–97. doi:10.1038/S41577-019-0143-6.

[190] AF C, J H, D M, K M. Malaria: biology and disease. Cell 2016;167(3):610–24. doi:10.1016/J.CELL.2016.07.055.

[191] JE O, et al. Efficacy of a tetravalent chimeric dengue vaccine (DENVax) in Cynomolgus macaques. Am J Trop Med Hyg 2011;84(6):978–87. doi:10.4269/AJTMH.2011.10-0592.

[192] A S, et al. Safety and immunogenicity of tetravalent live-attenuated dengue vaccines in Thai adult volunteers: role of serotype concentration, ratio, and multiple doses. Am J Trop Med Hyg 2002;66(3):264–72. doi:10.4269/AJTMH.2002.66.264.

[193] Waickman AT, et al. Dissecting the heterogeneity of DENV vaccine-elicited cellular immunity using single-cell RNA sequencing and metabolic profiling. Nat Commun 2019;101(10):1–16. doi:10.1038/s41467-019-11634-7.

[194] KE N, et al. Spec-seq unveils transcriptional subpopulations of antibody-secreting cells following influenza vaccination. J Clin Investig 2019;129(1). doi:10.1172/JCI121341.

[195] Karpievitch YV, Polpitiya AD, Anderson GA, Smith RD, Dabney AR. Liquid chromatography mass spectrometry-based proteomics: biological and technological aspects. Ann Appl Stat 2010;4(4):1797–823. doi:10.1214/10-AOAS341.

[196] Yates JR, Ruse CI, Nakorchevsky A. Proteomics by mass spectrometry: approaches, advances, and applications. Annu Rev Biomed Eng 2009;11:49–79. doi:10.1146/annurev-bioeng-061008-124934.

[197] Purcell AW, Gorman JJ. Immunoproteomics: mass spectrometry-based methods to study the targets of the immune response. Mol Cell Proteom 2004;3(3):193–208. doi:10.1074/mcp.R300013-MCP200.

[198] Dennehy R, McClean S. Immunoproteomics: the key to discovery of new vaccine antigens against bacterial respiratory infections. Curr Protein Pept Sci 2013;13(8):807–15. doi:10.2174/138920312804871184.

[199] Raeven RHM, et al. Immunoproteomic profiling of bordetella pertussis outer membrane vesicle vaccine reveals broad and balanced humoral immunogenicity. J Proteome Res 2015;14(7):2929–42. doi:10.1021/acs.jproteome.5b00258.

[200] Hunt DF, et al. Pillars article: characterization of peptides bound to the class I MHC molecule HLA-A2.1 by mass spectrometry. Science 1992. 255: 1261-1263. J Immunol 2007;179(5):2669–71.

[201] Koeken VACM, et al. BCG vaccination in humans inhibits systemic inflammation in a sex-dependent manner. J Clin Investig 2020;130(10):5591–602. doi:10.1172/JCI133935.

[202] Pitt JJ. Principles and applications of liquid chromatography-mass spectrometry in clinical biochemistry. Clin Biochem Rev 2009;30(1):19–34.

[203] Han X, Aslanian A, Yates JR. Mass spectrometry for proteomics. Curr Opin Chem Biol 2008;12(5):483–90. doi:10.1016/j.cbpa.2008.07.024.

[204] Zamboni N, Saghatelian A, Patti GJ. Defining the Metabolome: Size, Flux, and Regulation. Molecular Cell 2015;58(4):699–706. doi:10.1016/j.molcel.2015.04.021.

[205] Gray DW, et al. Identification of systemic immune response markers through metabolomic profiling of plasma from calves given an intra-nasally delivered respiratory vaccine. Vet Res 2015;46(1):7. doi:10.1186/s13567-014-0138-z.

[206] Gerszten RE, Wang TJ. The search for new cardiovascular biomarkers. Nature 2008;451(7181):949–52. doi:10.1038/nature06802.

[207] Diray-Arce J, Conti M-G, Petrova B, Kanarek N, Angelidou A, Levy O. Integrative metabolomics to identify molecular signatures of responses to vaccines and infections. Metabolites 2020;10(12). doi:10.20944/PREPRINTS202009.0004.V1.

[208] Khan A, et al. A systems vaccinology approach reveals the mechanisms of immunogenic responses to hantavax vaccination in humans. Sci Rep 2019;9(1):1–14. doi:10.1038/s41598-019-41205-1.

[209] B S, et al. Proteomic and metabolomic characterization of COVID-19 patient sera. Cell 2020;182(1):59–72. doi:10.1016/J.CELL.2020.05.032.

[210] P M, DF M, M B, E S, RS T, JJ M. COVID-19: consider cytokine storm syndromes and immunosuppression. Lancet 2020;395:1033–4. doi:10.1016/S0140-6736(20)30628-0.

[211] T T, et al. COVID-19 infection alters kynurenine and fatty acid metabolism, correlating with IL-6 levels and renal status. JCI insight 2020;5(4). doi:10.1172/JCI.INSIGHT.140327.

[212] JW S, et al. Omics-driven systems interrogation of metabolic dysregulation in COVID-19 pathogenesis. Cell Metab 2020;32(2):188–202. doi:10.1016/J.CMET.2020.06.016.

[213] Segers K, Declerck S, Mangelings D, Vander Heyden Y, Van Eeckhaut A. Analytical techniques for metabolomic studies: a review. Bioanalysis 2019;11(24):2297–318. doi:10.4155/bio-2019-0014.

[214] Gardinassi LG, Xia J, Safo SE, Li S. Bioinformatics tools for the interpretation of metabolomics data. Curr Pharmacol Rep 2017;3(6):374–83. doi:10.1007/S40495-017-0107-0.

[215] Miller GE, et al. A functional genomic fingerprint of chronic stress in humans: blunted glucocorticoid and increased NF-κB signaling. Biol Psychiatry 2008;64(4):266. doi:10.1016/J.BIOPSYCH.2008.03.017.

[216] A C, et al. A survey of best practices for RNA-seq data analysis. Genome Biol 2016;17(1). doi:10.1186/S13059-016-0881-8.

[217] P Z, N C. Factors that influence the immune response to vaccination. Clin Microbiol Rev 2019;32(2). doi:10.1128/CMR.00084-18.

[218] CL G, et al. Influence of burnout on patient safety: systematic review and meta-analysis. Medicina 2019;55(9). doi:10.3390/MEDICINA55090553.

[219] G Z, S L, J X. Network-based approaches for multi-omics integration. Methods Mol Biol 2020;2104:469–87. doi:10.1007/978-1-0716-0239-3_23.
[220] LG G, et al. Integrative metabolomics and transcriptomics signatures of clinical tolerance to Plasmodium vivax reveal activation of innate cell immunity and T cell signaling. Redox Biol 2018;17:158–70. doi:10.1016/J.REDOX.2018.04.011.
[221] S L, et al. Metabolic phenotypes of response to vaccination in humans. Cell 2017;169(5): 862–77. doi:10.1016/J.CELL.2017.04.026.
[222] T H, et al. Antibiotics-driven gut microbiome perturbation alters immunity to vaccines in humans. Cell 2019;178(6):1313–28. doi:10.1016/J.CELL.2019.08.010.
[223] Wuchty S, Ravasz E, Barabási A-L. The architecture of biological networks. Complex Syst Sci Biomedicine 2006:165–81. doi:10.1007/978-0-387-33532-2_5.
[224] M C, et al. A global genetic interaction network maps a wiring diagram of cellular function. Science 2016;353. doi:10.1126/SCIENCE.AAF1420.
[225] Creighton R, Schuch V, Urbanski AH, Giddaluru J, Costa-Martins AG, Nakaya HI. Network vaccinology. Semin Immunol 2020;50:101420. doi:10.1016/J.SMIM.2020.101420.
[226] AL B, N G, J L. Network medicine: a network-based approach to human disease. Nat Rev Genet 2011;12(1):56–68. doi:10.1038/NRG2918.
[227] GA P, et al. Using graph theory to analyze biological networks. BioData Min 2011;4(1). doi:10.1186/1756-0381-4-10.
[228] Pezeshki Z, Mazinani SM. Comparison of artificial neural networks, fuzzy logic and neuro fuzzy for predicting optimization of building thermal consumption: a survey. Artif Intell 2019;52(1):495–525. doi:10.1007/S10462-018-9630-6.
[229] T LD, et al. Drug repositioning for psychiatric and neurological disorders through a network medicine approach. Transl Psychiatry 2020;10(1):141. doi:10.1038/S41398-020-0827-5.
[230] Newman MEJ. Modularity and community structure in networks. Proc Natl Acad Sci 2006;103(23):8577–82. doi:10.1073/PNAS.0601602103.
[231] Menche J, et al. Uncovering disease-disease relationships through the incomplete human interactome. Science 2015;347(6224). doi:10.1126/SCIENCE.1257601.
[232] Cho D-Y, Kim Y-A, Przytycka TM. Chapter 5: Network Biology Approach to Complex Diseases. PLOS Comput Biol 2012;8(12). doi:10.1371/JOURNAL.PCBI.1002820.
[233] M V, ME C, AL B. Interactome networks and human disease. Cell 2011;144(6):986–98. doi:10.1016/J.CELL.2011.02.016.
[234] Barabási A-L. Network science. Philos Trans Royal Soc A 2013;371. doi:10.1098/RSTA.2012.0375.

Chapter 7

Leptin: an immunological adjuvant to improve vaccine response in infectious diseases

Radheshyam Maurya, Madhulika Namdeo
Department of Animal Biology, School of Life Sciences, University of Hyderabad, Hyderabad, India

7.1 Introduction

Leptin is a hormone secreted from adipocyte cells of adipose tissue in response to the individual nutritional status and body mass. The primary task of leptin is to maintain metabolic homeostasis. Leptin was initially identified as a key molecule in regulating food intake and body fat mass by delivering a piece of information to the hypothalamus [1,2]. Subsequently, alter the CNS function by inducing the food intake & energy balance and regulates glucocorticoids and insulin hormone production [3,4]. The circulating plasma leptin level is directly proportional to the amount of energy hoard in the adipose tissue in the form of body fat mass ratio as well as metabolic hormone and gender. Individuals with obesity typically produce a more significant amount of leptin than lean people [5–7]. In general, women have a larger amount of circulating leptin than men [8]. The deficiency of leptin in the host can cause susceptibility to several inflammatory stimuli produced by infectious agents that can be the leading cause for immune suppression and cytokine dysregulation in the host [9]. Leptin incites the macrophage phagocytic activity, controls the apoptosis of macrophages and other immune cells, which are involved in various different aspects of innate and adaptive immunity. Leptin regulates the apoptosis by controlling the cleavage of Bid and Bax transcription factors and activation of both caspase-3 and 8 in leptin-activated immune cells [10].

Leptin elicits the dendritic cells and monocyte/macrophages by regulating the thymic homeostasis. Subsequently, it polarizes the inflammatory cytokine response described as oozing of IFN-γ and TNF-α cytokines leading to Th1 responses [11]. Furthermore, leptin is recognized as the central molecule that controls immunity and acts as pro-inflammatory cytokines such as interleukin (IL)-1, IL-6, IL-8, IL-18, and TNF-α, and its lack enhanced the sensitivity to

System Vaccinology. https://doi.org/10.1016/B978-0-323-85941-7.00004-8

infectious disease [12,13]. Leptin signaling impairment blocks the intercommunication between neuroendocrinologic, metabolic, and immunological processes that are required to mount the protective immune responses toward various infectious diseases, such as influenza [14], human immunodeficiency virus (HIV) [15], tuberculosis [16], and parasitic diseases like Leishmaniasis [17], Malaria [18] and Amebeosis [19], etc. Obesity is one of the well-known risk factors in severe influenza A/ H1N1 infection [14], and it displays the poor turnout from influenza vaccine immunogenicity [20]. Although, the cause of the abnormal response of vaccine-induced immunological dysfunctions is unknown. In concordance, its deficiency in humans is linked with a polarization of Th2 immune response marked by increased generation of IL-10 and IL-4, and decrease of Th1 cytokines production such as TNF-α, IFN-γ, IL-2, IL-12 [21]. The reduction of leptin signaling limits the live attenuated and inactivated viral vaccines response due to thymic atrophy and reduced natural killer (NK) cell function [13]. This condition might be due to nutritional fitness, which is intricately associated with host immunity [2]. Therefore, Leptin might be having a strong correlation between metabolic and immunological homeostasis.

The chapter will discuss the existing knowledge of leptin and possible mechanisms to explore how to improve leptin-based immunotherapy and vaccine response. The chapter will also concisely analyses the genesis of leptin as well as its receptors & signal transduction. Next, the role of leptin in host immunity and infectious diseases. Finally, to explore the prospective use of leptin as an immunological adjuvant to improve the vaccine response.

7.2 Fundamentals of leptin

The ob gene of adipocytes encodes leptin protein. It is a non-glycosylated protein that consists of 167 amino acids with a mass of 16 kDa. Leptin potentially shared a high degree of homology within the species for its various physiological functions like hormones and immunological action like cytokine [1]. Leptin consists of four anti-parallel α-helices interconnected with each other. The structure is prominently similar to the family of long-chain helical cytokines (IL-6, IL-11, IL-12), oncostatin M (OSM), leukemia inhibitory factor, ciliary neurotrophic factor, and granulocyte-colony stimulating factor (G-CSF) [22,23]. A structural similarity of leptin with cytokine is inferring its function in controlling the protective response. Leptin is synthesized predominantly in adipose tissue and is considered an endocrine hormone. However, in certain conditions, it is also produced by the brain, placenta, mammary gland, intestinal cells, gastric fundic epithelium cells, and skeletal muscle [24,25].

The circulating leptin is found in two forms, biologically active free form binds with the soluble leptin receptor isoform Lep-Re and inactive form bind with plasma proteins [5,26]. Hormones and inflammatory mediators regulate the expression of leptin. Leptin-deficient (ob/ob) mice and leptin receptor-deficient (db/db) mice both have shown a distinct functions of leptin, such as marked abnormalities in neuroendocrine function [27,28], angiogenesis [29], reproduction [30,31], insulin secretion [32], wound healing [33], hematopoiesis and lymphopoiesis [34].

7.3 Leptin receptor and leptin signaling

Leptin transduces the signal through leptin receptor (LepR), which is widely expressed on majority tissue and cells [23,35,36]. The Leptin receptor is referred to as the class I cytokine receptor superfamily (such as IL-1, IL-2, IL-6, and growth hormone) and contain a single-transmembrane-domain unit. This kind of receptor does not carry an intrinsic tyrosine enzymatic function. However, signals are transduced through the tyrosine kinase protein of the Janus kinase family (JAK). A single transcript of LepR produces six variants of alternatively spliced forms of the Lep-R gene, such as LepRa, LepRb, LepRc, LepRd, LepRe, and LepRf [36–38]. LepRb is the only long-isoform, contains both an extracellular and an intracellular domain. LepRb isoform is responsible for transducing the signal through JAKs and activates the transcription (STAT) binding sites, leading to transducing downstream leptin signals through the JAK-STAT pathway [22,39–42]. The four short isoforms of LepR are also transmembrane domains but lack all the signal motifs. These isoforms are distributed in almost all peripheral tissues involved in helping leptin actions in peripheral organs and the brain. LepRe is a soluble isoform the lack of cytoplasmic or transmembrane parts involve in the regulation of plasma leptin concentration by binding with leptin without transducing intracellular signals and regulates its bioavailability by removing it from circulation [38,43,44] (Fig. 7.1).

Leptin binding to LepRb induces homo-oligomerization of JAKs which leads to activates and promotes autophosphorylation of JAK2 and in turn phosphorylates three tyrosine residues of LepRb (Tyr985, Tyr1077, and Tyr1138) on intracellular domains. The phosphorylated tyrosine residues of the leptin receptor activate the downstream signal transducers and activator of transcription factors (STATS) comprising STAT1, STAT3, STAT5, and STAT6 in a various cell [41,45]. The activated STATs are further dimerize and translocate into the nucleus, resulting in specific gene response stimulation [23,46].

The phosphorylation of Tyr1138 is crucial in JAK2–dependent pathway for the recruitment of STAT proteins, resulting in transcription activation of target genes such as the suppressor of cytokine signaling (SOCS)3 protein [41,47,48]. SOCS3 negatively regulates when it binds to Tyr985 and/or JAK2 to block the phosphorylation of SHP-2 (src homology 2-containing tyrosine phosphatase), kicking off the SHP-2 signaling [49]. Furthermore, Protein tyrosine phosphatase 1B (PTP1B) also inhibits leptin dependent signaling by dephosphorylating JAK2 protein [50]. In addition, STAT3 can positively regulate the expression of SOCS3 protein, which subsequently

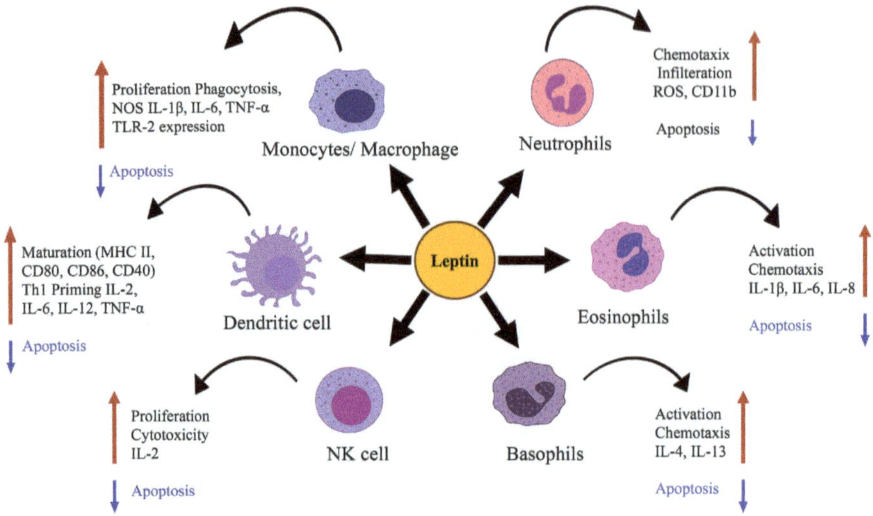

FIG. 7.1 Effect of leptin on innate immune cells: leptin positively regulates the various immune cell functions involved in innate immunity (monocytes, macrophages, dendritic cells, neutrophils, and natural killer (*NK*) cells) in favor of animals. It primes and stimulates their proliferation and phagocytosis activities and increases pro-inflammatory cytokines response. Leptin also induces the chemotaxis properties of cells and increases ROS-dependent cytotoxicity.

inhibits the phosphorylation of tyrosine residues (Tyr 985, Tyr 1077, and Tyr 1138) on the downstream of leptin receptor to suppress the leptin signaling through negative-feedback regulation [51,52]. Phospho-Tyr985 activates the ERK signaling pathway and also serves as a docking site for the inhibitory activity of SOCS-3 [41,47] While phospho-Tyr1077 promotes recruitment and activation of STAT-5, which also activates target gene transcription after dimerization [53].

LepRb also shows two distinct signaling pathways that include phosphatidylinositol 3-kinase (PI3K)/Akt, mitogen-activated protein kinase (MAPK) as well as extracellular signal-regulated kinase (ERK) pathways [54]. The ERK/MAPK pathway can be activated by long-form (Lep-Rb) and short-form (Lep-Ra, LepRc, LepRd, and LepRf) leptin receptors. JAK2 phosphorylation of Tyr985 (dependent or independent) drives to recruit and phosphorylates SHP-2 [55,56]. The phosphorylated SHP-2 initiates the recruitment of growth factor receptor binding-2 (GRB-2) protein, leading to ERK signaling pathway [41,44,57]. In addition, leptin signaling activates phosphoinositide 3 kinases (PI-3K) through autophosphorylation of JAK2, which is extending the autophosphorylation of insulin receptor substrate (IRS) [58,59]. Inclusively, JAK/STAT pathway is a key signaling pathway driven by leptin through LepRb, resulting in downstream signaling of gene expression in the cells [60–62] (Fig. 7.1).

7.4 Leptin signaling in immune cells

The LepR is present in all types of white blood cells involved in innate and cell mediates immunity and precursors of CD34+ hematopoietic cells produced from bone marrow [12,13,63]. In general, LepR signaling in immune cells is activated through STATs pathways. STAT3 protein mediates the downstream leptin signaling to initiates the activation and survival of peripheral blood mononuclear cells such as monocytes/lymphocytes [54,64–66]. In addition, STAT3 also regulates the expression of suppressors of cytokine signaling 3 (SOCS-3) protein. SOCS-3 is recognized as anti-inflammatory cytokines that regulate the cellular responses against inflammatory cytokines by binding to the inhibitory feedback loop of leptin signaling [67]. The high expression of SOCS3 protein due to increased leptin level and its downstream signaling may be a partial explanation of it why an individual with obesity has unresponsiveness to leptin signaling [47,68]. The PI3K/Akt pathway represents an important signaling cascade that influences the pro-inflammatory cytokines during bacterial and viral infections by various immune cells. Leptin also activates insulin receptor substrate (IRS)1/2 via autophosphorylation of JAK2, leading to activation of downstream signaling of the PI3K/Akt pathway. The activation of PI3K-dependent pathways might be helping to the uptake of glucose during starvation and restore the impairment of T-cell function [2]. On the other hand, MAPK and PI3K signaling cascade have been shown to be activated by leptin in peripheral blood mononuclear cells [69,70]. Therefore, the JAK2–PI3K, JAK2-Tyr 985–ERK1/2/MAPK, and JAK2-Tyr 1138–STAT3 pathways are appeared to be major leptin signaling pathways by which leptin can boost activation of immune cell and their proliferation [60,61] (Fig. 7.1).

7.5 Leptin and innate immunity

Leptin can directly activate the immune cells that are involved in innate immunity, such as monocytes, macrophages, neutrophils, dendritic cells (DC), and natural killer (NK) cells through its receptors present on the cells [44,60]. Leptin arouses circulating monocytes by inducing the secretion of the proinflammatory cytokines (TNF-α, IL-6, and IL-12). Subsequently, it promotes the production of reactive oxygen species (ROS), and chemotactic response mediates by inflammatory stimuli [21,71]. Polymorphonuclear cells such as neutrophils, eosinophils, and basophils, also express leptin receptors on their membrane. Leptin activates the neutrophils by inducing the generation of IL-1β, intracellular adhesion molecule-1, and chemokines that promote their chemotaxis nature and migration toward infection sites [72]. Subsequently, activated neutrophil produces ROS that is necessary for effective bacterial killing [10,73,74]. In addition, leptin controls the apoptosis of neutrophils by activating PI3K and MAPK-dependent signaling, which is subsequently delaying the cleavage of Bid and Bax complex and releasing cytochrome c from mitochondria to activate caspases signaling [10,75].

Exogenous leptin treatment was shown to induce DC maturation and survival by activating the downstream signaling (NF)κB and PI3K-AKT pathways for the CD40 expression [56], following the expansion and migration of dendritic cells (DCs) [11]. However, lack of leptin signaling, DC secrets a Th2 type of cytokines while leptin treatment reverses the cytokine response toward a Th1 type [11,56]. The subsequent study revealed that immature DCs upon leptin treatment licensed to skew the immune response toward the Th1 phenotype. Leptin-activated DCs can directly influence the autologous CD8+ T cell's function by regulating the perforin and IFN-γ production [63]. Human NK cells also display LepR receptors on their membrane. Leptin signaling is inevitable for the normal function of NK cells, such as cell activation, proliferation, differentiation, and cytotoxicity [76] and increased IL-12 cytokine production [77]. The primary function of leptin in NK cells is to enhanced immunological activity, cell proliferation and control the apoptotic rate of NK cells [78,79]. Additionally, Mast cells are also considered innate immune cells. Mast cells act as paracrine/autocrine cells due to the expression of leptin and its receptors. Hence leptin treatment provokes the immunomodulatory performance of mast cells [80]. Finally, the leptin-mediated release of TNF-α from monocytes able to activate neutrophils shows the capability of leptin to stimulate the cross-cellular communication among the innate immune cells [73] (Fig. 7.2).

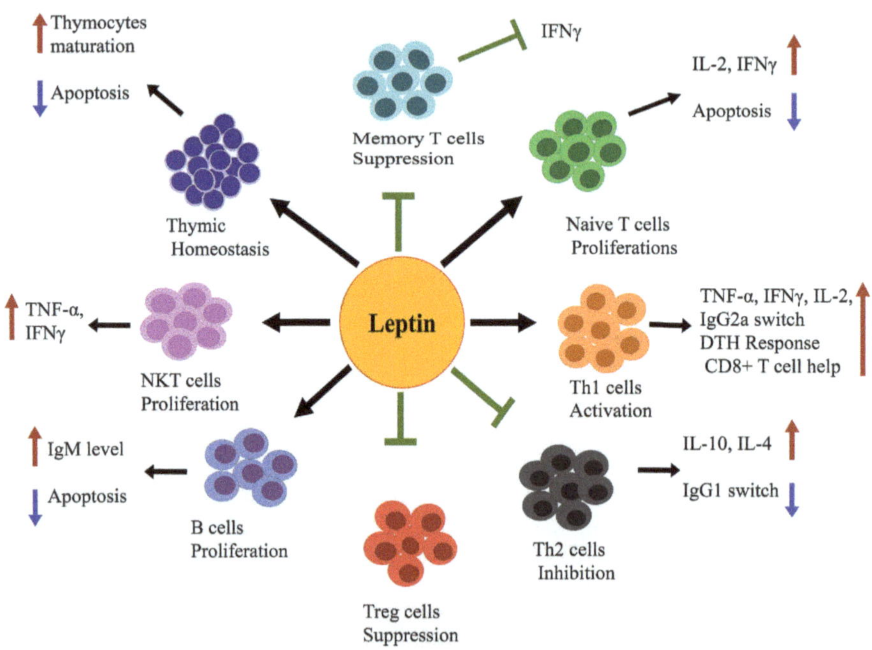

FIG. 7.2 Multiple functions of leptin in the cells that are involved in adaptive immunity. Leptin has positively regulated thymic homeostasis, naive T cells proliferation, Th1 cells activation, B cells proliferation, and NKT cells proliferation. Leptin has negatively regulated memory T cells, Th2 cells, and Treg cells for the action. Leptin primed Th1 cells while downregulating Th2 cells functions by switching on IgG2a and switching off IgG1 production.

7.6 Leptin in adoptive immunity

The roles of leptin in the driving of proinflammatory cytokine generation by tissue macrophages that are involved in innate immunity might indirectly modulate adaptive immunity. Adaptive immunity is primarily classified into T helper 1, and 2 (Th1 & Th2) phenotypes based on cytokine response [44,60]. Th1 lymphocyte promotes mainly proinflammatory cytokine, which is essential for the activation of antigen-presenting cells and the cell-mediated immune response. At the same time, Th2 lymphocyte is covering anti-inflammatory cytokine, which is necessary for B cells and basophils stimulation [78]. Leptin plays a direct role in cell-mediated immunity by controlling T cell-mediated immune function and signaling. Besides, leptin also modulates the cross-talk between innate and adaptive immunity by inciting dendritic cell number, maturation, cytokine production, and capacity to license naïve CD4+ T cells proliferation for Th1 priming [11,81,82].

The T cell subpopulations and B lymphocytes are consistently expressed functional LepRb receptors. Leptin signaling promotes lymphocyte survival, and its functions indicate the role of leptin in adaptive immunity [64,79]. Leptin influences the differential impressions on the multiplication of naïve T cells (CD4+CD45RA+) compared to memory T cells (CD4+CD45RO+) [12,83]. Leptin augments naïve T proliferation and survival by increasing the secretion of proinflammatory cytokine (IFN-γ and IL-2), which further directs the differentiation of Th1 cells and inhibiting the differentiation of Th2 cells [84]. During the Th1 response, leptin also enhances the TNF-α and IFN-γ secretion and switching of IgG2a production by B cells. However, leptin exerts adverse effects on Th2 cells by dipping IgG1 production. Furthermore, studies indicate the leptin regulates the maturation of double-positive CD4+/CD8+ T cells during starvation-induced thymic atrophy. Leptin also reduces the thymic apoptosis and prevents glucocorticoid-induced apoptosis in thymocytes [84,85]. A mutant mice lacking with leptin expression upon leptin treatment restores the T-cell function by augmenting the production of the proinflammatory cytokines. Thus, leptin can polarize the Th1 cells by stimulating the production of IL-2, IL-12, and IFN-γ and the restraint the generation of IL-4, IL-8, and IL-10 cytokines [21,86].

Besides this, Lep-Rb signaling in T cells prolongs proinflammatory Th17 cell differentiation, promoting the expression of the master regulator transcription factor [87]. At the same time, leptin neutralization inhibits Th17 responses, which have a prime role in promoting and maintaining inflammation and autoimmunity [88,89]. Leptin directly controls the regulatory T cells (Treg) function and serves as a negative signal during Treg cell development [83]. Blocking of leptin signaling has shown increased Treg cell proliferation and loss of autoimmune response in mice [83]. Hence, ob/ob and db/db mice represent a high number of Tregs [83]. Furthermore, leptin also activates the mTOR pathway by repressing rapamycin-induced propagation of Treg cells [90]. Leptin also elevates the IgG2a antibody production and abates IgG1 secretion from B cells [2]. Conclusively, the role of leptin on the T cell populations includes many ways to strengthens the immune functions by maintaining the polarization of naive helper T cells to a Th1 phenotype [91,92].

B lymphocytes have also emerged as a key player in controlling inflammation in visceral adipose tissue by presenting antigens to helper T cells. In addition, they also produce proinflammatory cytokines and antibodies against specific pathogens [93] as well as contributing in local and systemic inflammation [94]. B lymphocyte are also express the long form of LepR receptor. Thus, leptin seems to play a major function in the modulation and activation of the B lymphocytes [95]. Moreover, leptin controls the excretion of proinflammatory cytokines (TNF and IL-6) and immunoregulatory cytokine IL-10 by B lymphocytes via downstream signaling of JAK-STAT and p38MAPK–ERK1/2 pathways. Conclusively, leptin is essential for B lymphocyte maturation and expansion by inducing proliferation and lessening apoptotic rate [96] (Fig. 7.3).

JNK pathway; leptin also activates phospholipase C (PLC) via JAK-2 autophosphorylation leading to the downstream stimulation of c-jun N-terminal protein kinase (JNK) via protein kinase C (PKC). Protein tyrosine phosphatase 1B (PTP1B); JAK2 activation is negatively regulated by PTP1B protein.

(IRS1/2: insulin receptor substrate 1/2; PI3K: phosphatidylinositol-3-kinase; SHP-2: src-homology-2 containing phosphotyrosine phosphatase; GRB-2: growth factor receptor-bound-protein 2; RAS: Ras-family of small GTPase; RAF: Raf proto-oncogene serine/threonine-protein kinase; MAPK-mitogen-activated-protein-kinase; MEK: mitogen-activated kinase; PDK-1: phosphoinositide-dependent kinase-1; AKT: ak strain transforming/protein kinase; ERK1/2: extracellular signal-regulated kinase 1/2; STAT-3: signaling transducer and activator of transcription 3; SOCS-3: suppressor of cytokine signaling-3 and FOXO-1: forkhead box protein O1).

7.7 Leptin deficiency and infection diseases

Leptin controls immune response by balancing the Th1/Th2 dichotomy both in mice and humans. Thus, leptin dysregulation is associated with immune dysfunctions, resulting in increased susceptibility to infectious disease. Various studies have confirmed that leptin supplementation abbreviated the pathogenicity by increasing the function of innate and adoptive immunity in several infectious diseases such as tuberculosis [97], pneumonia [98], sepsis [99], colitis [100], viral infection [101,102], leishmaniasis [103], trypanosomiasis [104], amoebiasis [19], and malaria [18] due to defective cytokine production [42,92] (Table 7.1).

Patients with active pulmonary tuberculosis are marked with a reduced lymphocyte stimulation and Th1 cytokines such as IL-2, IFN-γ, and TNF-α response, which are mostly linked with cachexia, weight loss, and low serum leptin levels [105–107]. Thus, the low circulating leptin and an increased adiponectin level in serum might be considered a reliable biomarker for the prognosis of the disease progression [108,109]. Leptin-deficient (ob/ob) mice or

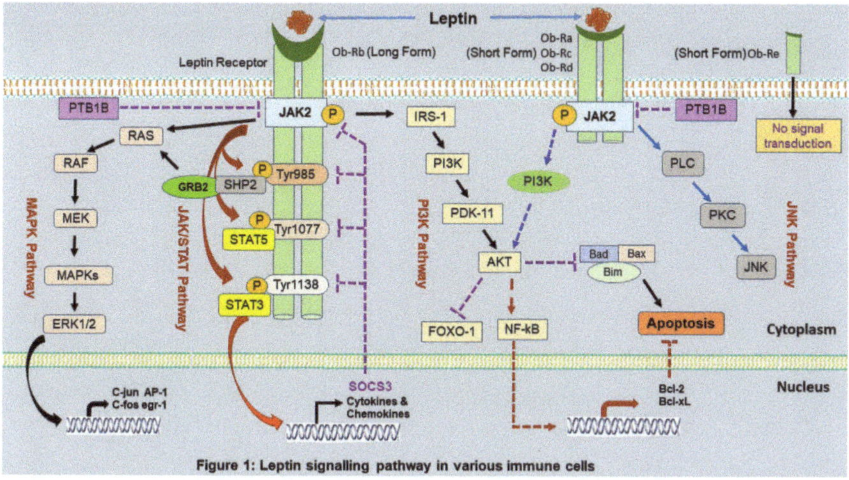

FIG. 7.3 Schematic diagram of the leptin receptors and leptin signaling pathways: immune cells express two types of leptin receptor (LepR) long and short isoforms. Long isoform (Ob-Rb) has an extended intracellular domain in the cytoplasm containing JAK-2 and three basic tyrosine residues (Tyr985, Tyr1077, Tyr1138) of the leptin receptor. The short isoforms of LepR (Ob-Ra, Ob-Rc, and Ob-Rd) comprise only the JAK-2 signaling domain in the cytoplasm. Ob-Re is a soluble isoform. The leptin binding to the long isoform of LepR auto-phosphorylates the JAK-2 and subsequently extended the auto-phosphorylation of the cytoplasmatic domain of tyrosine residues (Tyr985, Tyr1077, Tyr1138) in the intracellular tail of LepR for the activation of specific downstream signaling. Leptin can activate all four major pathways (MAPK Pathways, JAK/STAT pathway, PI3K pathway, and JNK pathways) independently. MAPK pathway; leptin directly activates the auto-phosphorylation JAK-2 or Tyr985 residue to recruits the SHP-2 and GRB-2 adopter protein which activates the RAS/RAF/MAPK signaling molecules that culminates in ERK1/2 activation resulting in expression of the transcription of the c-jun, c-fos, erg-1 genes, and AP-1. JAK/STAT pathways; leptin autophosphorylates JAK-2 leading to autophosphorylation of all three tyrosine residues in the downstream of the leptin receptor and then autophosphorylates STAT3 and STAT5 signaling molecules, which is finally translocated in nucleus to activate target gene transcription such as cytokines, chemokines, and SOCS-3. SOCS-3 negatively regulates signal transduction of leptin by dephosphorylating the JAK-2 and tyrosine residues. PI3K Pathway; Autophophorylation of JAK-2 also activates the IRS1/2 molecules, leading to the activation of PI3K/AKT-dependent signaling pathways, which mediates leptin dependent anti-apoptotic and proliferative effects via downregulating pro-apoptotic factors (Bad, Bim, and Bax) while upregulating anti-apoptotic/survival factors (Bcl-2 and Bcl-XL) via the NF-κB activation.

starvation-induced leptin-deficient mice display impaired bacterial clearance during pulmonary infection and higher mortality during pulmonary tuberculosis, bacterial pneumonia, and sepsis [98,99,110]. *Mycobacterium* infection in ob/ob mice showed a defective granulomas formation, DTH response, and CD4+ and CD8+ T cells functions. Ob/ob mice infected with *Klebsiella pneumoniae* were shown to reduce leukotriene synthesis in alveolar macrophages, reduce phagocytosis, and decrease H_2O_2 synthesis in neutrophils (PMNs) [111,112]. Restoration of leptin at physiological levels in starvation-induced and ob/ob mice displayed notably increased bacterial clearance and survival.

TABLE 7.1 The distinctive immune response of leptin in various infectious diseases.

Infectious group	Infectious species	Effect of leptin on the Immune response	Model used	References
Bacterial disease (Pulmonary infections)	*Mycobacterium tuberculosis, Klebsiella pneumonia, Streptococcus pneumonia*	Positive response: ✓ Increases IFNγ & TNF-α levels and PMN cells & H_2O_2 production. ✓ Induces T helper CD4 T cells & CD8 T cells activity. ✓ Induces Ag- specific antibody response. ✓ Increases DTH response and Granuloma formation. ✓ Promotes phagocytosis index and Leukotriene synthesis ✓ Induces defective alveolar macrophage phagocytosis activity ✓ Increases CD11b expression level. Negative response; ✓ Decreases IL-6 cytokine and reduce mortality. ✓ Reduced TNF-α, MIP-2, PGE2 in the lung. ✓ Improves pulmonary bacterial clearance and survival.	Mice and Human	[107, 110–113]
Bacterial disease (other infections)	*Clostridium difficile Listeria monocytogenes* and *Sepsis*	Positive response: ✓ Improve the Neutrophil function. ✓ inflammation, chemokine expression, and cellular recruitment. Induce CD11b expression on neutrophils. ✓ Induce effective bacterial phagocytosis and lymphocytic apoptosis in sever immune-deficiency. ✓ Improvement of anti-listerial resistance and the MCP-1 mRNA expression. ✓ Increase the phosphorylation of p38 MAP kinase. Negative response; ✓ Control sepsis-induced organ damage. ✓ Supresses IL-6 and MCP-1 level. ✓ Control the bacteraemia load and improve the bacterial clearance.	Mice and Human	[100, 114–116]

Infectious group	Infectious species	Effect of leptin on the Immune response	Model used	References
Viral disease	Influenza A/H1N1 pneumonia Respiratory Syncytial Virus HIV	Positive response: ✓ Promoted Th17 subset differentiation ✓ Increased phosphorylation of ERK1/2 in peripheral Lymphocytes. ✓ Serum leptin level positively correlated with CD4+ T lymphocyte during antiviral therapy in HIV patients Negative response; ✓ Proinflammatory cytokines IL-6 and IL-1β level and increase the INF-γ levels. ✓ Suppressed Th2 subset differentiation. ✓ Leptin inhibits ROS and control oxidative burst mechanism in HIV+ monocyte patients. ✓ Supresses SOCS3 & mTOR expression and Th2 subset differentiation. ✓ Reduced viral load.	Mice and Human	[15,101, 117–121]
Parasitic disease	*Leishmania major / Leishmania donovani* *Trypanosoma cruzi* *Entameoba histolytica* *Plasmodium berghei ANKA parasite*	Positive response: ✓ Activates macrophage phagocytosis and ROS induction. ✓ the phosphorylation of Erk1/2 & Akt in macrophages. ✓ IFN-γ, IL12, IL-1β secretion in macrophage. ✓ Improve IFN-γ/IL-10 ratio, GrzA and Th1 cytokine response. ✓ Activate CD8+ T-cell compartment and improve IgG2a levels and IgG2a/IgG1 ratio. ✓ Improve granuloma formation and neutrophil infiltration to the site of infection. ✓ mTORC1 (Mechanistic target of rapamycin complex 1) activity in CD4+ and CD8+ T cells during malaria. ✓ TNF-α and INF-γ in the regulatory cascade controlling inflammatory responses in malaria. Negative response; ✓ PD-1 & CTLA-4 expression in CD8 T cells in leishmaniasis ✓ Damping down TNF-induced pathology in cerebral malaria. ✓ Th1: Th2 ratio in malaria. ✓ Intestinal parasites deregulate the secretion of leptin and play a role in enteric parasitosis by modulating body immunity. ✓ Reduced parasite load in visceral organs	Mice and Human	[17–19, 104, 122–130, 132]

Leptin reconstitution increased the phagocytic activity of alveolar macrophage and enhanced H_2O_2 production resulting in reduced bacterial load and increased the killing of *S. pneumonia* in vitro [113]. Leptin treatment improves the phagocytic activity of neutrophils more efficiently during *L. monocytogenes* infection [114], and it extends the production of monocyte chemoattractant protein-1 (MCP-1) and MIP-2 in leptin-deficient mice [115]. Clostridium difficile colitis is a bacterium, which causes colitis and bacterial peritonitis in humans as well as in mice. Mice treated with leptin restored the inflammatory immune response, reduced bacterial load, and increased the survival rate of mice [100,116].

Leptin receptor-deficient mice are characterized as high viral load in the lung and decreased IFNγ levels, a leading cause of reduced survival rate from pneumonia during influenza-A infections [117]. Leptin-resistant obese mice have shown increased viral titer, infiltration and are highly susceptible to influenza A infection by inhibiting the T cell function in mice [118]. The lack of effective leptin receptors in T cells (LepRT−/−) decreases pH1N1 influenza infection severity and mortality of ob/ob mice [119]. In the case of human bronchial epithelial cells (hBECs) infected with respiratory syncytial virus (RSV), leptin significantly induced the upregulation of the Th17 subset and downregulates the Th2 subset differentiation through the activation of ERK1/2 pathways [120]. The blood mononuclear cells of a patient infected with the Human immunodeficiency virus (HIV) have shown high expression of leptin receptors on their cell membrane. At the same time, low circulating leptin levels in their serum increased the disease severity of these patients [15]. Furthermore, leptin can change the redox status of monocytes by inhibiting the ROS generation, stating that leptin controls immunological remodeling in HIV infection [101]. Notably, leptin therapy has shown novel strategies of the clinical trial to correct metabolic complications linked with HIV-associated lipodystrophy syndrome [121].

Leishmaniasis is a protozoan disease caused by a parasite belongs to the genus Leishmania. Leptin induced the phagocytosis of macrophages by increasing ROS-dependent oxidative killing of the parasite during *Leishmania donovani* infection. In addition, it activates the macrophage via Erk1/2 and Akt signaling pathways leading to Th1 cytokine responses [103]. Leptin induced the Th1 immune response by increasing the secretion of IFN-γ from CD4+ and CD8+ T cells [122]. Antigen-presenting DCs derived from the bone marrow of leptin-treated normal mice showed an increase of IFN-γ, IL-12, and IL1β cytokine and nitric oxide in response to soluble leishmania antigen (SLA). However, ob/ob mice DCs botched to restore the above response to SLA, predicting that leptin signaling is differentially regulated in these mice [122]. Moreover, leptin also induced the CD8+ T-cell activity by up-regulating the Granzyme A (GrzA) and downregulating the cytotoxic T lymphocyte-associated protein 4 (CTLA-4), and Programmed death-1 (PD-1) in malnutrition coupled *L. donovani* infection [17]. Miltefosine is a conventional antileishmanial drug. In-vitro studies showed that leptin plus miltefosine treatment induced the mouse macrophage activity against *L. donovani* infection [123]. Therefore, leptin therapy may augment the renew the normal function of immune cell via leptin signaling to suppresses the parasite load in leishmaniasis coupled with malnutrition [92]. Trypanosomiasis is another protozoan disease caused by *Trypanosoma* species. *Trypanosoma cruzi* infects all nucleated cells, including adipocyte cells that are the primary source of leptin. *T. cruzi* uses adipocytes as a reservoir and might be playing a significant role in establishing chronic infection of the disease [124]. However, *T. cruzi* infection in mice showed low leptin levels in their serum, suggesting that it may be due to the involvement of adipocytes in disease progression [125]. Trypanosomiasis displays a higher expression of Toll-like receptor (TLR)-2 and 9 and an increased level of pro-inflammatory cytokine and chemokine response in mice [104,126]. Metabolically challenged mice due to defective leptin receptors infected with *T. cruzi* showed a high mortality rate [104].

Amoebiasis is caused by a protozoan parasite called *Entameba histolytica*. Low serum leptin displays a critical role in disease pathogenesis and is the leading cause of diarrheal illness and liver injury by *E. histolytica* [127]. Mice deficient with leptin signaling either by gene deletion or mutation (ob/ob or db/db mice) are highly susceptible to infection. In contrast, wild-type mice are resistant to *E. histolytica* infection. Furthermore, mice with homozygous or heterozygous for the 223R allele of leptin receptor are considerably more likely to get an amoebic infection [128]. A mutation in leptin receptor at position 233 changes from glutamine to arginine is likely to add-on four times more vulnerability to *E. histolytica* infection [129]. In gut mucosal epithelial cells, leptin aids the activation of STAT3 and ERK or Akt signaling pathways extend more protection against *E. histolytica* infection [130,131]. Thus, the above observations reveal the potential role of leptin in controlling systemic immunity and therapeutics role in infectious disease [99]. Importantly, serum leptin level may be used as a prognostic or diagnostic marker in acute infections triggered by bacteria, viruses, fungi, or parasites [132] (Table 7.1).

7.8 Leptin as an immunological adjuvant

Leptin deficient (ob/ob) mice showed a higher bacterial burden than WT mice. Vaccination of these mice with an attenuated *Streptococcus pneumoniae* strain reduced pulmonary bacterial loads in WT but not in ob/ob mice after being challenged with virulence *S. pneumoniae*. Compared with the non-vaccinated WT, vaccination increased the recruitment of pulmonary CD4+ and CD8+ T cells, DCs, NK cells, and exudative macrophages (ExM) after infection in WT but not ob/ob mice. Interestingly, exogenous leptin administered in ob/ob mice reconstituted the ability of vaccination to reduce pulmonary bacterial loads and increase the recruitment of CD4+ and CD8+ T cells, DCs, NK cells as well as ExM to the lungs of ob/ob mice [98,133]. The above finding suggests that leptin performs a critical task in vaccination against *S. pneumoniae* by inducing Th1 specific immune cells and vaccine-induced anti-pneumococcal antibody production against *Pneumococcal pneumonia* infection [111,134]. Mice vaccinated with Ovalbumin (OVA) combined with polyphosphazene (PCEP) or Curdlan + Leptin as adjuvants boost a Th17-type of adaptive immune response in mice. Mice immunized with OVA+PCEP and OVA+Curdlan+Leptin displayed a considerably high quantity of antigen-specific CD4+ T cells secreting IL-17 cytokine comparative to only in OVA-vaccinated mice. High IL-6 and TGF-β with a decreased amount of IL-12 in the cytokine milieu are associated with advancing the immunity by differentiation of Th17-type of cells [135]. Several other studies have also shown that Th17 differentiation of murine splenocytes requires the presence of TGF-β and IL-6 or decreased level of IL- 12 cytokine [136,137]. PCEP increased a significant amount of IL-6 and diminished IL-12 production in muscle. However, it did not increase the TGF-β level in mice. Curdlan+Leptin inoculated intramuscular produced a substantial amount of TGF-β and IL-17 but failed to induce IL-6 or IL-12 cytokines. However, splenocytes stimulated with PCEP could not increase the IL-6, IL-12, TGF-β, or IL-17 levels. Likewise, splenocytes were induced with Curdlan+Leptin (+/−PCEP) failed to increased IL-6, TGF-β, or decreased IL-12, although they made splenic IL-17 production alone [135]. Conclusively, Leptin signaling seems very important for Th1 or Th17 differentiation in immunized mice [79]. Thus, Curdlan+Leptin might act as adjuvants on the Th17 cells directly or indirectly by inducing Th17-type immune responses.

Leptin has been used as a mucosal vaccine adjuvant to improve immunity against *Rhodococcus equi* in foals [138]. *R. equi* causes severe pneumonia-like infection in foals and patients with immunocompromised conditions such as AIDS, cancer, diabetes, malnutrition. The co-immunization with recombinant Lactococcus lactis strain that produces leptin (LL-leptin) and virulence-associated protein A (LL-VapA) from *R. equi* were able to provide a protective immunity against *R. equi* in challenged mice [134]. Mice immunized with *Helicobacter pylori* cell lysate showed a high titer of *H. pylori*-specific antibody in normal mice. In contrast, mice with receptor-deficient were failed to induce the antibody response following *H. pylori* vaccination, suggesting that leptin signaling is needed for an effective immune response in these mice [139]. Leptin is further identified as a suitable adjuvant for dendritic cell-based vaccines to treat patients with cancers and HIV. Ultimately, leptin has the ability to promotes dendritic cell survival, maturation and improves dendritic cell activation to prime helper T cells to enhanced the Th1 type of immune response [63].

In summary, leptin plays a vital role in various metabolic and immunologic processes. Impairment of leptin signaling seems to offer a non-specific immune response and probably contributes to weakened vaccine-induced immunity. Therefore, administering a recombinant leptin as adjuvant or improved leptin signaling may enhance vaccine response in vulnerable populations affected by various infectious diseases. Thus, future considerations to use leptin-based adjuvant therapy alone or in combination with other immunological adjuvants to enhanced cell-mediated immunity in the host is a worthy investigation (Table 7.2).

TABLE 7.2 Effect of Leptin: an immunological adjuvant in vaccination of mice.

Disease	Pathogen	Immune response	Animal	References
Pneumonia	*Streptococcus. pneumoniae*	Increase the recruitment of CD4+ and CD8+ T cells, mDCs, NK cells and macrophage functions. Induces the anti-pneumococcal antibody production. Enhance the effectiveness of pneumococcal vaccine response.	Mice	[111] [134]
	Pneumococcal pneumonia	Th17-type adaptive immune response: significantly higher quantity of antigen-specific CD4+ T cells secreting IL-17. Elevated IL-6 and TGF-β with a decreased secretion of IL-12 in cytokine milieu is known to promote differentiation of Th17-type of immunity	Mice	[79], 136–137
	Rhodococcus equi	Provide a protective immune response associated with a Th1/Th2 cytokine responses such as IFN-γ and IL-4.	Mice	[138]
Peptic ulcers	*Helicobacter pylori*	Induces the infiltration of T lymphocytes in the gastric mucosa. Induces the higher antibody titers against *H. pylori*-specific antigen resulting in developing an effective protective response.	Mice	[139]
AIDS	HIV	Promotes dendritic cell survival, maturation and improves dendritic cell activation. Enhance migratory CD8+ T cell and induce the CD4 + T cells towards Th1 type of immune responses.	Dendritic cell based vaccine	[63]

References

[1] Zhang Y, Proenca R, Maffei M, Barone M, Leopold L, Friedman JM. Positional cloning of the mouse obese gene and its human homologue. Nature 1994;372:425–32. https://doi.org/10.1038/372425a0.

[2] Cava ALa, Matarese G. The weight of leptin in immunity. Nat Rev Immunol 2004;4:371–9. https://doi.org/10.1038/nri1350.

[3] Mantzoros CS, Magkos F, Brinkoetter M, Sienkiewicz E, Dardeno TA, Kim SY, Hamnvik OPR, Koniaris A. Leptin in human physiology and pathophysiology. Am J Physiol - Endocrinol Metab 2011:301. doi:10.1152/ajpendo.00315.2011.

[4] Dardeno TA, Chou SH, Moon H-S, Chamberland JP, Fiorenza CG, Mantzoros CS. Leptin in human physiology and therapeutics. Front Neuroendocrinol 2010;31:377–93. https://doi.org/10.1016/j.yfrne.2010.06.002.

[5] Considine RV, Sinha MK, Heiman ML, Kriauciunas A, Stephens TW, Nyce MR, Ohannesian JP, Marco CC, McKee LJ, Bauer TL. Serum immunoreactive-leptin concentrations in normal-weight and obese humans. N Engl J Med 1996;334:292–5. https://doi.org/10.1056/NEJM199602013340503.

[6] Frederich RC, Lollmann B, Hamann A, Napolitano-Rosen A, Kahn BB, Lowell BB, Flier JS. Expression of ob mRNA and its encoded protein in rodents. Impact of nutrition and obesity. J Clin Invest 1995;96:1658–63. https://doi.org/10.1172/JCI118206.

[7] Maffei M, Fei H, Lee GH, Dani C, Leroy P, Zhang Y, Proenca R, Negrel R, Ailhaud G, Friedman JM. Increased expression in adipocytes of ob RNA in mice with lesions of the hypothalamus and with mutations at the db locus. Proc Natl Acad Sci USA 1995;92:6957–60. https://doi.org/10.1073/pnas.92.15.6957.

[8] Tuan RS, Wildenburg G, Eschbach ML, Tawe W, Zipfel P, Walter RD. Localization and functional analysis of the cytosolic and extracellular CuZn superoxide dismutases in the human parasitic nematode Onchocerca 6 ol 6 ulus, 1997;88:187–202.

[9] Faggioni R, Feingold KR, Grunfeld C. Leptin regulation of the immune response and the immunodeficiency of malnutrition 1. FASEB J 2001;15:2565–71. https://doi.org/10.1096/fj.01-0431rev.

[10] Bruno A, Conus S, Schmid I, Simon H-U. Apoptotic pathways are inhibited by leptin receptor activation in neutrophils. J Immunol 2005;174:8090–6. https://doi.org/10.4049/jimmunol.174.12.8090.

[11] Mattioli B, Straface E, Quaranta MG, Giordani L, Viora M. Leptin promotes differentiation and survival of human dendritic cells and licenses them for Th1 priming. J Immunol 2005;174:6820–8. https://doi.org/10.4049/jimmunol.174.11.6820.

[12] Procaccini C, Jirillo E, Matarese G. Leptin as an immunomodulator. Mol Aspects Med 2012;33:35–45. https://doi.org/10.1016/j.mam.2011.10.012.

[13] Sánchez-Margalet V, Fernández-Riejos P, Najib S, Santos-Alvarez J, Martín-Romero C, Pérez-Pérez A, González-Yanes C. Role of leptin in the activation of immune cells. Mediators Inflamm 2010;2010. doi:10.1155/2010/568343.

[14] Morgan OW, Bramley A, Fowlkes A, Freedman DS, Taylor TH, Gargiullo P, Belay B, Jain S, Cox C, Kamimoto L, Fiore A, Finelli L, Olsen SJ, Fry AM. Morbid obesity as a risk factor for hospitalization and death due to 2009 pandemic influenza A(H1N1) disease. PLoS One 2010;5:1–6. https://doi.org/10.1371/journal.pone.0009694.

[15] Azzoni L, Crowther NJ, Firnhaber C, Foulkes AS, Yin X, Glencross D, Gross R, Kaplan MD, Papasavvas E, Schulze D, Stevens W, Van Der Merwe T, Waisberg R, Sanne I, Montaner LJ. Association between HIV replication and serum leptin levels: an observational

study of a cohort of HIV-1-infected South African women. J Int AIDS Soc 2010;13:1–8. https://doi.org/10.1186/1758-2652-13-33.
[16] Buyukoglan H, Gulmez I, Kelestimur F, Kart L, Oymak FS, Demir R, Ozesmi M. Leptin levels in various manifestations of pulmonary tuberculosis. Mediators Inflamm 2007;2007. doi:10.1155/2007/64859.
[17] Dayakar A, Chandrasekaran S, Veronica J, Bharadwaja V, Maurya R. Leptin regulates Granzyme-A, PD-1 and CTLA-4 expression in T cell to control visceral leishmaniasis in BALB/c Mice. Sci Rep 2017;7:1–12. https://doi.org/10.1038/s41598-017-15288-7.
[18] Pulido-Mendez M, De Sanctis J, Rodríguez-Acosta A. Leptin and leptin receptors during malaria infection in mice. Folia Parasitol (Praha) 2002;49:249–51. https://doi.org/10.14411/fp.2002.046.
[19] Vedantam G, Viswanathan VK. Leptin signaling protects the gut from Entamoeba histolytica infection. Gut Microbes 2012;3:2–4. https://doi.org/10.4161/gmic.19424.
[20] Sheridan PA, Paich HA, Handy J, Karlsson EA, Hudgens MG, Sammon AB, Holland LA, Weir S, Noah TL, Beck MA. Obesity is associated with impaired immune response to influenza vaccination in humans. Int J Obes 2012;36:1072–7. https://doi.org/10.1038/ijo.2011.208.
[21] Napoleone E, Santo ADI, Amore C, Baccante G, Febbo CDI, Porreca E. Leptin induces tissue factor expression in human peripheral blood mononuclear cells : a possible link between obesity and cardiovascular risk? 2007:1462–8.
[22] Baumann H, Morella KK, White DW, Dembski M, Bailon PS, Kim H, Lai CF, Tartaglia LA. The full-length leptin receptor has signaling capabilities of interleukin 6-type cytokine receptors. Proc Natl Acad Sci USA 1996;93:8374–8. https://doi.org/10.1073/pnas.93.16.8374.
[23] Tartaglia LA. The leptin receptor. J Biol Chem 1997;272:6093–6. https://doi.org/10.1074/jbc.272.10.6093.
[24] Ahima RS, Flier JS. Adipose tissue as an endocrine organ. Trends Endocrinol Metab. 2000 Oct;11(8):327–332. doi: 10.1016/s1043-2760(00)00301-5.
[25] Kershaw EE, Flier JS. Adipose tissue as an endocrine organ. J Clin Endocrinol Metab 2004;89:2548–56. https://doi.org/10.1210/jc.2004-0395.
[26] Ogier V, Ziegler O, Méjean L, Nicolas JP, Stricker-Krongrad A. Obesity is associated with decreasing levels of the circulating soluble leptin receptor in humans. Int J Obes Relat Metab Disord. 2002 Apr;26(4):496–503. doi: 10.1038/sj.ijo.0801951.
[27] Yu WH, Kimura M, Walczewska A, Karanth S, McCann SM. Role of leptin in hypothalamic-pituitary function. Proc Natl Acad Sci USA 1997;94:1023–8. https://doi.org/10.1073/pnas.94.3.1023.
[28] Elmquist JK, Ahima RS, Maratos-Flier E, Flier JS, Saper CB. Leptin activates neurons in ventrobasal hypothalamus and brainstem. Endocrinology 1997;138:839–42. https://doi.org/10.1210/endo.138.2.5033.
[29] Bouloumie A, Drexler HC, Lafontan M, Busse R. Leptin, the Product of Ob Gene, Promotes Angiogenesis. Circ Res. 1998 Nov 16;83(10):1059–1066. doi: 10.1161/01.res.83.10.1059.
[30] Chehab FF, Lim ME, Lu R. Correction of the sterility defect in homozygous obese female mice by treatment with the human recombinant leptin. Nat Genet 1996;12:318–20. https://doi.org/10.1038/ng0396-318.
[31] Ahima RS, Dushay J, Flier SN, Prabakaran D, Flier JS. Leptin accelerates the onset of puberty in normal female mice. J Clin Invest 1997;99:391–5. https://doi.org/10.1172/JCI119172.
[32] Friedman JM, Halaas JL. Leptin and the regulation of body weight in mammals. Nature. 1998 Oct 22;395(6704):763–770. doi: 10.1038/27376.

[33] Goren I, Kämpfer H, Podda M, Pfeilschifter J, Frank S. Leptin and wound inflammation in diabetic ob/ob mice: differential regulation of neutrophil and macrophage influx and a potential role for the scab as a sink for inflammatory cells and mediators. Diabetes 2003;52:2821–32. https://doi.org/10.2337/diabetes.52.11.2821.

[34] Bennett BD, Solar GP, Yuan JQ, Mathias J, Thomas GR, Matthews W. A role for leptin and its cognate receptor in hematopoiesis. Curr Biol 1996;6:1170–80. https://doi.org/10.1016/s0960-9822(02)70684-2.

[35] Lee GH, Proenca R, Montez J, et al. Abnormal splicing of the leptin receptor in diabetic mice. Nature 1996;379:632–635. https://doi.org/10.1038/379632a0.

[36] Myers MG. Leptin receptor signaling and the regulation of mammalian physiology. Recent Prog Horm Res 2004;59:287–304. https://doi.org/10.1210/rp.59.1.287.

[37] Dinarello CA, Simon A, van der Meer JWM. Treating inflammation by blocking interleukin-1 in a broad spectrum of diseases. Nat Rev Drug Discov 2012;11:633–52. https://doi.org/10.1038/nrd3800.

[38] Pérez-Pérez A, Vilariño-García T, Fernández-Riejos P, Martín-González J, Segura-Egea JJ, Sánchez-Margalet V. Role of leptin as a link between metabolism and the immune system. Cytokine Growth Factor Rev 2017;35:71–84. https://doi.org/10.1016/j.cytogfr.2017.03.001.

[39] Frühbeck G. Intracellular signalling pathways activated by leptin. Biochem J 2006;393:7–20. https://doi.org/10.1042/BJ20051578.

[40] Bjørbæk C, Uotani S, Silva B, Flier JS. Divergent signaling capacities of the long and short isoforms of the leptin receptor *, 1997;272:32686–95. https://doi.org/10.1074/jbc.272.51.32686.

[41] Banks AS, Davis SM, Bates SH, Myers MG. Activation of downstream signals by the long form of the leptin receptor. J Biol Chem 2000;275:14563–72. https://doi.org/10.1074/jbc.275.19.14563.

[42] Procaccini C, Lourenço E, Matarese G, Cava A. Leptin signaling: a key pathway in immune responses. Curr Signal Transduct Ther 2009;4:22–30. https://doi.org/10.2174/157436209787048711.

[43] Chan JL, Blüher S, Yiannakouris N, Suchard MA, Kratzsch J, Mantzoros CS. Regulation of circulating soluble leptin receptor levels by gender, adiposity, sex steroids, and leptin observational and interventional studies in humans. Diabetes 2002;51:2105–12. https://doi.org/10.2337/diabetes.51.7.2105.

[44] Paz-Filho G, Mastronardi C, Franco CB, Wang KB, Wong M-L, Licinio J. Leptin: molecular mechanisms, systemic pro-inflammatory effects, and clinical implications. Arq Bras Endocrinol Metabol 2012;56:597–607. https://doi.org/10.1590/s0004-27302012000900001.

[45] Kloek C, Haq AK, Dunn SL, Lavery HJ, Banks AS, Myers MG. Regulation of jak kinases by intracellular leptin receptor sequences*. J Biol Chem 2002;277:41547–55. https://doi.org/10.1074/jbc.M205148200.

[46] Gualillo O, Eiras S, White DW, Diéguez C, Casanueva FF. Leptin promotes the tyrosine phosphorylation of SHC proteins and SHC association with GRB2. Mol Cell Endocrinol. 2002 Apr 25;190(1–2):83–89. doi: 10.1016/s0303-7207(02)00012-6.

[47] Bjørbaek C, El-Haschimi K, Frantz JD, Flier JS. The role of SOCS-3 in leptin signaling and leptin resistance. J Biol Chem. 1999 Oct 15;274(42):30059–30065. doi: 10.1074/jbc.274.42.30059.

[48] Vaisse C, Halaas JL, Horvath CM, Darnell JEJ, Stoffel M, Friedman JM. Leptin activation of Stat3 in the hypothalamus of wild-type and ob/ob mice but not db/db mice. Nat Genet 1996;14:95–7. https://doi.org/10.1038/ng0996-95.

[49] Bjørbæk C, Lavery HJ, Bates SH, Olson RK, Davis SM, Flier JS, Myers MG. SOCS3 mediates feedback inhibition of the leptin receptor via Tyr 985 *, 2000;275:40649–57. https://doi.org/10.1074/jbc.M007577200.

[50] Zabolotny JM, Bence-Hanulec KK, Stricker-Krongrad A, Haj F, Wang Y, Minokoshi Y, Kim Y-B, Elmquist JK, Tartaglia LA, Kahn BB, Neel BG. PTP1B Regulates leptin signal transduction in vivo. Dev Cell 2002;2:489–95. https://doi.org/10.1016/S1534-5807(02)00148-X.

[51] Eyckerman S, Broekaert D, Verhee A, Vandekerckhove J, Tavernier J. Identification of the Y985 and Y1077 motifs as SOCS3 recruitment sites in the murine leptin receptor. FEBS Lett. 2000 Dec 1;486(1):33–37. doi: 10.1016/s0014-5793(00)02205-5.

[52] Dunn SL, Björnholm M, Bates SH, Chen Z, Seifert M, Myers J, Martin G. Feedback inhibition of leptin receptor/Jak2 signaling via Tyr1138 of the leptin receptor and suppressor of cytokine signaling 3. Mol Endocrinol 2005;19:925–38. https://doi.org/10.1210/me.2004-0353.

[53] Gong Y, Ishida-Takahashi R, Villanueva EC, Fingar DC, Münzberg H, Myers MG. The long form of the leptin receptor regulates STAT5 and ribosomal protein S6 via alternate mechanisms*. J Biol Chem 2007;282:31019–27. https://doi.org/10.1074/jbc.M702838200.

[54] Martı C. Human leptin activates PI3K and MAPK pathways in human peripheral blood mononuclear cells: possible role of Sam68, 2001;91:83–91. https://doi.org/10.1006/cimm.2001.1851.

[55] Münzberg H, Myers MG. Molecular and anatomical determinants of central leptin resistance, 2005;8:566–70. https://doi.org/10.1038/nn1454.

[56] Lam QLK, Lu L. Role of leptin in immunity. Cell Mol Immunol 2007;4:1–13.

[57] Yin N, Wang D, Zhang H, Yi X, Sun X, Shi B, Wu H, Wu G, Wang X, Shang Y. Molecular mechanisms involved in the growth stimulation of breast cancer cells by leptin. Cancer Res. 2004 Aug 15;64(16):5870–5875. doi: 10.1158/0008-5472.CAN-04-0655.

[58] Tong K, Shieh D, Chen C, Tzeng C, Wang S, Huang K, Chiu Y, Fong Y, Tang C. Leptin induces IL-8 expression via leptin receptor, IRS-1, PI3K, Akt cascade and promotion of NF- κ B /p300 binding in human synovial fibroblasts, 2008;20:1478–1488. https://doi.org/10.1016/j.cellsig.2008.04.003.

[59] Donato J, Frazão R, Elias CF. The PI3K signaling pathway mediates the biological effects of leptin. Arq Bras Endocrinol Metabol 2010;54:591–602. https://doi.org/10.1590/s0004-27302010000700002.

[60] Francisco V, Pino J, Campos-Cabaleiro V, Ruiz-Fernández C, Mera A, Gonzalez-Gay MA, Gómez R, Gualillo O. Obesity, fat mass and immune system: role for leptin. Front Physiol 2018;9:640. https://doi.org/10.3389/fphys.2018.00640.

[61] Ramos-Lobo AM, Donato J. The role of leptin in health and disease, Temperature. 2017;4:258–91. https://doi.org/10.1080/23328940.2017.1327003.

[62] Walduck AK, Becher D. Leptin, CD4(+) T(reg) and the prospects for vaccination against H. pylori infection. Front Immunol 2012;3:316. https://doi.org/10.3389/fimmu.2012.00316.

[63] Mattioli B, Straface E, Matarrese P, Quaranta MG, Giordani L, Malorni W, Viora M. Leptin as an immunological adjuvant: enhanced migratory and CD8 + T cell stimulatory capacity of human dendritic cells exposed to leptin. FASEB J 2008;22:2012–22. https://doi.org/10.1096/fj.07-098095.

[64] Papathanassoglou E, El-Haschimi K, Li XC, Matarese G, Strom T, Mantzoros C. Leptin receptor expression and signaling in lymphocytes: kinetics during lymphocyte activation, role in lymphocyte survival, and response to high fat diet in mice. J Immunol 2006;176:7745–52. https://doi.org/10.4049/jimmunol.176.12.7745.

[65] Cui H, Cai F, Belsham DD, Cui H, Cai F, Belsham DD. Leptin signaling in neurotensin neurons involves STAT, MAP kinases ERK1/2, and p38 through c-Fos and ATF1. FASEB J 2006;20:2654–6. https://doi.org/10.1096/fj.06-5989fje.

[66] Mansour E, Pereira FG, Araújo EP, Amaral MEC, Morari J, Ferraroni NR, Ferreira DS, Lorand-Metze I, Velloso LA. Leptin inhibits apoptosis in thymus through a janus

kinase-2-independent, insulin receptor substrate-1/phosphatidylinositol-3 kinase-dependent pathway. Endocrinology 2006;147:5470–9. https://doi.org/10.1210/en.2006-0223.

[67] Bjørbaek C, Elmquist JK, Michl P, Ahima RS, van Bueren A, McCall AL, Flier JS. Expression of leptin receptor isoforms in rat brain microvessels. Endocrinology. 1998 Aug;139(8):3485–3491. doi:10.1210/endo.139.8.6154.

[68] Kaszubska W, Falls HD, Schaefer VG, Haasch D, Frost L, Hessler P, Kroeger PE, White DW, Jirousek MR, Trevillyan JM. Protein tyrosine phosphatase 1B negatively regulates leptin signaling in a hypothalamic cell line. Mol Cell Endocrinol. 2002 Sep 30;195(1–2): 109–118. doi:10.1016/s0303-7207(02)00178-8.

[69] Najib S, Sánchez-Margalet V. Human leptin promotes survival of human circulating blood monocytes prone to apoptosis by activation of p42/44 MAPK pathway. Cell Immunol 2002;220:143–9. https://doi.org/10.1016/s0008-8749(03)00027-3.

[70] Santos-Alvarez J, Goberna R, Sánchez-Margalet V. Human leptin stimulates proliferation and activation of human circulating monocytes. Cell Immunol 1999;194:6–11. https://doi.org/10.1006/cimm.1999.1490.

[71] Conde J, Scotece M, Gómez R, Gómez-Reino JJ, Lago F, Gualillo O. At the crossroad between immunity and metabolism: focus on leptin. Expert Rev Clin Immunol. 2010 Sep;6(5):801–808. doi:10.1586/eci.10.48.

[72] Rummel C, Inoue W, Poole S, Luheshi GN. Leptin regulates leukocyte recruitment into the brain following systemic LPS-induced inflammation. Mol Psychiatry 2010:523–34. doi:10.1038/mp.2009.98.

[73] Zarkesh-Esfahani H, Pockley AG, Wu Z, Hellewell PG, Weetman AP, Ross RJM. Leptin indirectly activates human neutrophils via induction of TNF-alpha. J Immunol 2004;172:1809–14. https://doi.org/10.4049/jimmunol.172.3.1809.

[74] Fantuzzi G. Adipose tissue, adipokines, and inflammation. J Allergy Clin Immunol 2005;115:911–9. https://doi.org/10.1016/j.jaci.2005.02.023.

[75] Bjørbæk C, Uotani S, Da Silva B, Flier JS. Divergent signaling capacities of the long and short isoforms of the leptin receptor. J Biol Chem 1997;272:32686–95. https://doi.org/10.1074/jbc.272.51.32686.

[76] Zhao Y, Sun R, You L, Gao C, Tian Z. Expression of leptin receptors and response to leptin stimulation of human natural killer cell lines. Biochem Biophys Res Commun 2003;300:247–52. https://doi.org/10.1016/S0006-291X(02)02838-3.

[77] Al-hassi HO, Bernardo D, Murugananthan AU, Mann ER, English NR, Jones A, Kamm MA, Arebi N, Hart AL, Blakemore AIF, Stagg AJ, Knight SC. ARTICLES A mechanistic role for leptin in human dendritic cell migration: differences between ileum and colon in health and Crohn's disease. Mucosal Immunol 2012;6:751–61. https://doi.org/10.1038/mi.2012.113.

[78] Pérez-Pérez A, Sánchez-Jiménez F, Vilariño-García T, Sánchez-Margalet V. Role of leptin in inflammation and vice versa. Int J Mol Sci 2020;21:1–24. https://doi.org/10.3390/ijms21165887.

[79] La Cava A. Leptin in inflammation and autoimmunity. Cytokine 2017;98:51–8. https://doi.org/10.1016/j.cyto.2016.10.011.

[80] Caldefie-Chezet F, Poulin A, Tridon A, Sion B, Vasson MP. Leptin: a potential regulator of polymorphonuclear neutrophil bactericidal action? J Leukoc Biol 2001;69:414–8.

[81] Macia L, Delacre M, Abboud G, Ouk T-S, Delanoye A, Verwaerde C, Saule P, Wolowczuk I. Impairment of dendritic cell functionality and steady-state number in obese mice. J Immunol 2006;177:5997–6006. https://doi.org/10.4049/jimmunol.177.9.5997.

[82] Moraes-Vieira PMM, Larocca RA, Bassi EJ, Peron JPS, Andrade-Oliveira V, Wasinski F, Araujo R, Thornley T, Quintana FJ, Basso AS, Strom TB, Câmara NOS. Leptin deficiency

impairs maturation of dendritic cells and enhances induction of regulatory T and Th17 cells. Eur J Immunol 2014;44:794–806. https://doi.org/10.1002/eji.201343592.

[83] De Rosa V, Procaccini C, Calì G, Pirozzi G, Fontana S, Zappacosta S, La Cava A, Matarese G. A key role of leptin in the control of regulatory T cell proliferation. Immunity 2007;26:241–55. https://doi.org/10.1016/j.immuni.2007.01.011.

[84] Lord GM, Matarese G, Howard JK, Baker RJ, Bloom SR, Lechler RI. Leptin modulates the T-cell immune response and reverses starvation-induced immunosuppression. Nature 1998;394:897–901. https://doi.org/10.1038/29795.

[85] Howard JK, Lord GM, Matarese G, Vendetti S, Ghatei MA, Ritter MA, Lechler RI, Bloom SR. Leptin protects mice from starvation-induced lymphoid atrophy and increases thymic cellularity in ob/ob mice. J Clin Invest 1999;104:1051–9. https://doi.org/10.1172/JCI6762.

[86] Martín-Romero C, Santos-Alvarez J, Goberna R, Sánchez-Margalet V. Human leptin enhances activation and proliferation of human circulating T lymphocytes. Cell Immunol 2000;199:15–24. https://doi.org/10.1006/cimm.1999.1594.

[87] Reis BS, Lee K, Fanok MH, Mascaraque C, Amoury M, Cohn LB, Rogoz A, Dallner OS, Moraes-Vieira PM, Domingos AI, Mucida D. Leptin receptor signaling in T cells is required for Th17 differentiation. J Immunol 2015;194:5253–60. https://doi.org/10.4049/jimmunol.1402996.

[88] Yu Y, Liu Y, Shi F-D, Zou H, Matarese G, Cava ALa. Cutting edge: Leptin-induced RORγt expression in CD4+ T cells promotes Th17 responses in systemic lupus erythematosus. J Immunol 2013;190:3054–8. https://doi.org/10.4049/jimmunol.1203275.

[89] Fujita Y, Fujii T, Mimori T, Sato T, Nakamura T, Iwao H, Nakajima A, Miki M, Sakai T, Kawanami T, Tanaka M, Masaki Y, Fukushima T, Okazaki T, Umehara H. Deficient leptin signaling ameliorates systemic lupus erythematosus lesions in MRL/Mp- Fas lpr mice. J Immunol 2014;192:979–84. https://doi.org/10.4049/jimmunol.1301685.

[90] Procaccini C, Galgani M, De Rosa V, Carbone F, La Rocca C, Ranucci G, Iorio R, Matarese G. Leptin: the prototypic adipocytokine and its role in NAFLD. Curr Pharm Des 2010;16:1902–12. https://doi.org/10.2174/138161210791208884.

[91] de Candia P, Matarese G. Leptin and ghrelin: Sewing metabolism onto neurodegeneration. Neuropharmacology 2018;136:307–16. https://doi.org/10.1016/j.neuropharm.2017.12.025.

[92] Maurya R, Bhattacharya P, Dey R, Nakhasi HL. Leptin functions in infectious diseases. Front Immunol 2018;9:1–15. https://doi.org/10.3389/fimmu.2018.02741.

[93] Kim SY, Lim JH, Choi SW, Kim M, Kim ST, Kim MS, Cho YS, Chun E, Lee KY. Preferential effects of leptin on CD4 T cells in central and peripheral immune system are critically linked to the expression of leptin receptor. Biochem Biophys Res Commun 2010;394:562–8. https://doi.org/10.1016/j.bbrc.2010.03.019.

[94] Matarese G, Procaccini C, De Rosa V, Horvath TL, La Cava A. Regulatory T cells in obesity: the leptin connection. Trends Mol Med 2010;16:247–56. https://doi.org/10.1016/j.molmed.2010.04.002.

[95] Claycombe K, King LE, Fraker PJ. A role for leptin in sustaining lymphopoiesis and myelopoiesis. Proc Natl Acad Sci USA 2008;105:2017–21. https://doi.org/10.1073/pnas.0712053105.

[96] Agrawal S, Gollapudi S, Su H, Gupta S. Leptin activates human B cells to secrete TNF-α, IL-6, and IL-10 via JAK2/STAT3 and p38MAPK/ERK1/2 signaling pathway. J Clin Immunol 2011;31:472–8. https://doi.org/10.1007/s10875-010-9507-1.

[97] Wieland CW, Florquin S, Chan ED, Leemans JC, Weijer S, Verbon A, Fantuzzi G, van der Poll T. Pulmonary Mycobacterium tuberculosis infection in leptin-deficient ob/ob mice. Int Immunol 2005;17:1399–408. https://doi.org/10.1093/intimm/dxh317.

[98] Hsu A, Aronoff DM, Phipps J, Goel D, Mancuso P. Leptin improves pulmonary bacterial clearance and survival in ob/ob mice during pneumococcal pneumonia. Clin Exp Immunol 2007;150:332–9. https://doi.org/10.1111/j.1365-2249.2007.03491.x.

[99] Tschöp J, Nogueiras R, Haas-Lockie S, Kasten KR, Castañeda TR, Huber N, Guanciale K, Perez-Tilve D, Habegger K, Ottaway N, Woods SC, Oldfield B, Clarke I, Chua SJ, Farooqi IS, O'Rahilly S, Caldwell CC, Tschöp MH. CNS leptin action modulates immune response and survival in sepsis. J Neurosci 2010;30:6036–47. https://doi.org/10.1523/JNEUROSCI.4875-09.2010.

[100] Madan R, Guo X, Naylor C, Buonomo EL, Mackay D, Noor Z, Concannon P, Scully KW, Pramoonjago P, Kolling GL, Warren CA, Duggal P, Petri WA. Role of leptin-mediated colonic inflammation in defense against Clostridium difficile colitis. Infect Immun 2014;82:341–9. https://doi.org/10.1128/IAI.00972-13.

[101] Sánchez-Pozo C, Rodriguez-Baño J, Domínguez-Castellano A, Muniain MA, Goberna R, Sánchez-Margalet V. Leptin stimulates the oxidative burst in control monocytes but attenuates the oxidative burst in monocytes from HIV-infected patients. Clin Exp Immunol 2003;134:464–9. https://doi.org/10.1111/j.1365-2249.2003.02321.x.

[102] Zhang AJX, To KKW, Li C, Lau CCY, Poon VKM, Chan CCS, Zheng BJ, Hung IFN, Lam KSL, Xu A, Yuen KY. Leptin mediates the pathogenesis of severe 2009 pandemic influenza A(H1N1) infection associated with cytokine dysregulation in mice with diet-induced obesity. J Infect Dis 2013;207:1270–80. https://doi.org/10.1093/infdis/jit031.

[103] Dayakar A, Chandrasekaran S, Veronica J, Maurya R. Leptin induces the phagocytosis and protective immune response in Leishmania donovani infected THP-1 cell line and human PBMCs. Exp Parasitol 2016;160:54–9. https://doi.org/10.1016/j.exppara.2015.12.002.

[104] Nagajyothi F, Zhao D, Machado FS, Weiss LM, Schwartz GJ, Desruisseaux MS, Zhao Y, Factor SM, Huang H, Albanese C, Teixeira MM, Scherer PE, Chua SCJ, Tanowitz HB. Crucial role of the central leptin receptor in murine Trypanosoma cruzi (Brazil strain) infection. J Infect Dis 2010;202:1104–13. https://doi.org/10.1086/656189.

[105] Çakir B, Yönem A, Güler S, Odabaşi E, Demirbaş B, Gürsoy G, Aral Y. Relation of leptin and tumor necrosis factor α to body weight changes in patients with pulmonary tuberculosis. Horm Res 1999;52:279–83. https://doi.org/10.1159/000023495.

[106] Schwenk A, Hodgson L, Rayner CFJ, Griffin GE, Macallan DC. Leptin and energy metabolism in pulmonary tuberculosis. Am J Clin Nutr 2003;77:392–8. https://doi.org/10.1093/ajcn/77.2.392.

[107] van Crevel R, Karyadi E, Netea MG, Verhoef H, Nelwan RHH, West CE, van der Meer JWM. Decreased plasma leptin concentrations in tuberculosis patients are associated with wasting and inflammation. J Clin Endocrinol Metab 2002;87:758–63. https://doi.org/10.1210/jcem.87.2.8228.

[108] Ye M, Bian L-F. Association of serum leptin levels and pulmonary tuberculosis: a meta-analysis. J Thorac Dis 2018;10:1027–36. https://doi.org/10.21037/jtd.2018.01.70.

[109] Elnemr GM, Elnashar MA, Elmargoushy NM. Adiponectin levels as a marker of inflammation in pulmonary tuberculosis. Egypt J Hosp Med 2015;59:208–13. https://doi.org/10.12816/0012177.

[110] Wieland CW, Florquin S, Chan ED, Leemans JC, Weijer S, Verbon A, Fantuzzi G, van der Poll T. Pulmonary mycobacterium tuberculosis infection in leptin-deficient ob/ob mice. Int Immunol 2005;17:1399–408. https://doi.org/10.1093/intimm/dxh317.

[111] Mancuso P, Huffnagle GB, Olszewski MA, Phipps J, Peters-Golden M. Leptin corrects host defense defects after acute starvation in murine pneumococcal pneumonia. Am J Respir Crit Care Med 2006;173:212–8. https://doi.org/10.1164/rccm.200506-909OC.

[112] Moore SI, Huffnagle GB, Chen GH, White ES, Mancuso P. Leptin modulates neutrophil phagocytosis of Klebsiella pneumoniae. Infect Immun 2003;71:4182–5. https://doi.org/10.1128/IAI.71.7.4182-4185.2003.

[113] Koca C, Şahin Kavakli H, Alici Ö. Leptin tedavisinin deneysel sepsis modelinde immunmodulator rolü. Turkish J Med Sci 2011;41:251–8. https://doi.org/10.3906/sag-1009-1109.

[114] Morshedi A, Zarkesh-Esfahani SH, Behjati M. Effect of leptin on neutrophils phagocytosis and lymphocytes apoptosis challenge by Listeria monocytogenes and Escherichia coli. Jundishapur J Microbiol 2013;6:1–8. https://doi.org/10.5812/jjm.6389.

[115] Ikejima S, Sasaki S, Sashinami H, Mori F, Ogawa Y, Nakamura T, Abe Y, Wakabayashi K, Suda T, Nakane A. Impairment of host resistance to Listeria monocytogenes infection in liver of db/db and ob/ob mice. Diabetes 2005;54:182–9. https://doi.org/10.2337/diabetes.54.1.182.

[116] Moshyedi AK, Josephs MD, Abdalla EK, Mackay SL, Edwards CK, Copeland EM, Moldawer LL. Increased leptin expression in mice with bacterial peritonitis is partially regulated by tumor necrosis factor alpha. Infect Immun 1998;66:1800–2. https://doi.org/10.1128/iai.66.4.1800-1802.1998.

[117] Taylor AK, Cao W, Vora KP, De La Cruz J, Shieh W-J, Zaki SR, Katz JM, Sambhara S, Gangappa S. Protein energy malnutrition decreases immunity and increases susceptibility to influenza infection in mice. J Infect Dis 2013;207:501–10. https://doi.org/10.1093/infdis/jis527.

[118] Hur SJ, Kim DH, Chun SC, Lee SK. Effect of adenovirus and influenza virus infection on obesity. Life Sci 2013;93:531–5. https://doi.org/10.1016/j.lfs.2013.08.016.

[119] Milner JJ, Wang J, Sheridan PA, Ebbels T, Beck MA, Saric J. 1H NMR-based profiling reveals differential immune-metabolic networks during influenza virus infection in obese mice. PLoS One 2014;9:e97238. https://doi.org/10.1371/journal.pone.0097238.

[120] Qin L, Tan YR, Hu CP, Liu XA, He RX. Leptin is oversecreted by respiratory syncytial virus-infected bronchial epithelial cells and regulates Th2 and Th17 cell differentiation. Int Arch Allergy Immunol 2015;167:65–71. https://doi.org/10.1159/000436966.

[121] Sinha U, Sinharay K, Sengupta N, Mukhopadhyay P. Benefits of leptin therapy in HIV patients. Indian J Endocrinol Metab 2012;16:S637–S43. https://doi.org/10.4103/2230-8210.105583.

[122] Maurya R, Bhattacharya P, Ismail N, Dagur PK, Joshi AB, Razdan K, McCoy JP, Ascher J, Dey R, Nakhasi HL. Differential role of leptin as an immunomodulator in controlling visceral leishmaniasis in normal and leptin-deficient mice. Am J Trop Med Hyg 2016;95:109–19. https://doi.org/10.4269/ajtmh.15-0804.

[123] Shivahare R, Ali W, Vishwakarma P, Natu SM, Puri SK, Gupta S. Leptin augments protective immune responses in murine macrophages and enhances potential of miltefosine against experimental visceral leishmaniasis. Acta Trop 2015;150:35–41. https://doi.org/10.1016/j.actatropica.2015.06.024.

[124] Combs TP, Nagajyothi SM, de Almeida CJG, Jelicks LA, Schubert W, Lin Y, Jayabalan DS, Zhao D, Braunstein VL, Landskroner-Eiger S, Cordero A, Factor SM, Weiss LM, Lisanti MP, Tanowitz HB, Scherer PE. The adipocyte as an important target cell for Trypanosoma cruzi infection. J Biol Chem 2005;280:24085–94. https://doi.org/10.1074/jbc.M412802200.

[125] Ferreira AVM, Segatto M, Menezes Z, Macedo AM, Gelape C, de Oliveira Andrade L, Nagajyothi F, Scherer PE, Teixeira MM, Tanowitz HB. Evidence for Trypanosoma cruzi in adipose tissue in human chronic Chagas disease. Microbes Infect 2011;13:1002–5. https://doi.org/10.1016/j.micinf.2011.06.002.

[126] Rodrigues CM, Valadares HMS, Francisco AF, Arantes JM, Campos CF, Teixeira-Carvalho A, Martins-Filho OA, Araujo MSS, Arantes RME, Chiari E, Franco GR, Machado CR, Pena SDJ, Faria AMC, Macedo AM. Coinfection with different Trypanosoma cruzi strains

interferes with the host immune response to infection. PLoS Negl Trop Dis 2010;4:5–10. https://doi.org/10.1371/journal.pntd.0000846.
[127] Alam F, Salam A, Mahmood I, Kabir M, Chowdhury S, Haque R. Amebic liver abscess is associated with malnutrition and low serum leptin level. J Infect Dis Ther 2016;4. doi:10.4172/2332-0877.1000298.
[128] Guo X, Roberts MR, Becker SM, Podd B, Zhang Y, Chua SC, Myers MG, Duggal P, Houpt ER, Petri WA. Leptin signaling in intestinal epithelium mediates resistance to enteric infection by Entamoeba histolytica. Mucosal Immunol 2011;4:294–303. https://doi.org/10.1038/mi.2010.76.
[129] Naylor C, Burgess S, Madan R, Buonomo E, Razzaq K, Ralston K, Petri WA. Leptin receptor mutation results in defective neutrophil recruitment to the colon during Entamoeba histolytica infection. MBio 2014;5:1–8. https://doi.org/10.1128/mBio.02046-14.
[130] Marie CS, Verkerke HP, Paul SN, Mackey AJ, Petri WA. Leptin protects host cells from Entamoeba histolytica cytotoxicity by a STAT3-dependent mechanism. Infect Immun 2012;80:1934–43. https://doi.org/10.1128/IAI.06140-11.
[131] Mackey-Lawrence NM, Petri WA. Leptin and mucosal immunity. Mucosal Immunol 2012;5:472–9. https://doi.org/10.1038/mi.2012.40.
[132] Chen M, Wang B, Xu Y, Deng Z, Xue H, Wang L, He L. Diagnostic value of serum leptin and a promising novel diagnostic model for sepsis. Exp Ther Med 2014;7:881–6. https://doi.org/10.3892/etm.2014.1506.
[133] Mancuso P, Gottschalk A, Phare SM, Peters-Golden M, Lukacs NW, Huffnagle GB. Leptin-deficient mice exhibit impaired host defense in gram-negative pneumonia. J Immunol 2002;168:4018–24. https://doi.org/10.4049/jimmunol.168.8.4018.
[134] White SJ, Taylor MJ, Hurt RT, Jensen MD, Poland GA. Leptin-based adjuvants: an innovative approach to improve vaccine response. Vaccine 2013;31:1666–72. https://doi.org/10.1016/j.vaccine.2013.01.032.
[135] Chaffey A, Hamonic G, Chand D, Mutwiri GK, Wilson HL. The adjuvants polyphosphazene (PCEP) and a combination of curdlan plus leptin promote a Th17-Type immune response to an intramuscular vaccine in mice. Vaccines 2021;9. doi:10.3390/vaccines9050507.
[136] Korn T, Bettelli E, Oukka M, Kuchroo VK. IL-17 and Th17 Cells. Annu Rev Immunol 2009;27:485–517. https://doi.org/10.1146/annurev.immunol.021908.132710.
[137] Veldhoen M, Hocking RJ, Atkins CJ, Locksley RM, Stockinger B. TGFbeta in the context of an inflammatory cytokine milieu supports de novo differentiation of IL-17-producing T cells. Immunity 2006;24:179–89. https://doi.org/10.1016/j.immuni.2006.01.001.
[138] Cauchard S, Bermúdez-Humarán LG, Blugeon S, Laugier C, Langella P, Cauchard J. Mucosal co-immunization of mice with recombinant lactococci secreting VapA antigen and leptin elicits a protective immune response against Rhodococcus equi infection. Vaccine 2011;30:95–102. https://doi.org/10.1016/j.vaccine.2011.10.026.
[139] Wehrens A, Aebischer T, Meyer TF, Walduck AK. Leptin receptor signaling is required for vaccine-induced protection against Helicobacter pylori. Helicobacter 2008;13:94–102. https://doi.org/10.1111/j.1523-5378.2008.00591.x.

Chapter 8

Polymer-based adjuvant requirements for vaccines

Edna Soares[a,b], **Olga Borges**[a,b]
[a]*Center for Neuroscience and Cell Biology, University of Coimbra, Coimbra, Portugal,* [b]*Faculty of Pharmacy, University of Coimbra, Coimbra, Portugal*

8.1 Introduction

The immune system is typically divided into two arms: the innate and adaptive immune systems. The cells from both immunity arms are key players in the process of developing an immune response during vaccination or after an infection. Danger signals usually activate the innate immunity, a quick first line of defense, to stimulate and mobilize antiviral activities of innate immune cells (granulocytes, monocytes, eosinophils, macrophages, dendritic cells (DCs), mast cells, and natural killer cells) that usually involve the ingestion of extracellular particulate materials by phagocytosis. Innate immune cells express Pattern recognition receptors (PRRs) that recognize pathogen-associated molecular patterns (PAMPs) present on microorganisms and damage-associated molecular patterns (DAMPs) released after cellular damage or stress, leading to the activation of transcription factors and expression of small proteins important in cell signaling, the cytokines. The adaptive immune response is slower to develop but is highly specific and establishes an immunological memory which ensures a more rapid and effective response on a subsequent encounter with the same pathogen. Major adaptive immune cells include antibody-secreting B cells and effector T cells, including CD8+ (also called T-cytotoxic cells) and CD4+ (also called T-helper cells) cells that ultimately promote viral clearance. The innate and adaptive immune systems do not operate independently, they rather function as a highly interactive and synergistic system more effective than either branch by itself. The main link between innate and adaptive immune system are established by antigen-presenting cells (APCs) and although macrophages and B cells are important APCs, DCs are recognized as the professional ones. So, DCs represent the main link between innate and adaptive immunity [1]. Consistently, immature DCs reside in peripheral tissues and serve as sentinels for foreign antigens and microbial pathogens. Following vaccine capture and antigen processing, these antigen-capturing cells undergo maturation and migrate to the

System Vaccinology. https://doi.org/10.1016/B978-0-323-85941-7.00009-7

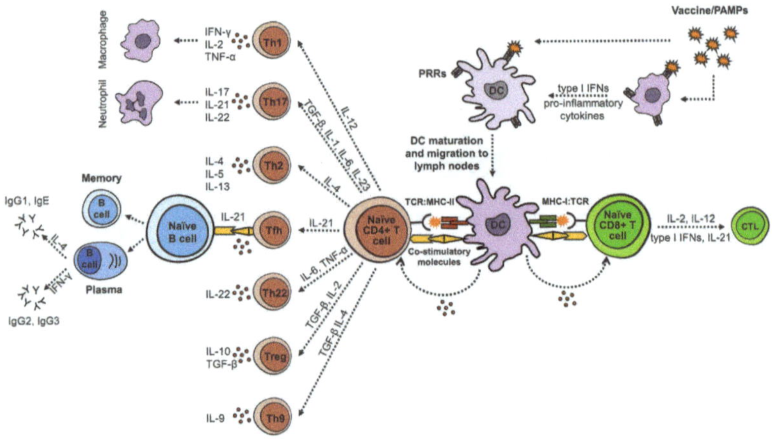

FIG. 8.1 Adaptive immune response to vaccines/PAMPs. Vaccines may contain pathogen-associated molecular patterns (*PAMPs*) as adjuvants. These PAMPs are directly detected by pattern-recognition receptors (PRRs) expressed by dendritic cells (*DCs*), leading to DCs activation, maturation, and migration to the lymph nodes. PRRs are also expressed by macrophages that may cooperate in the activation and orientation of the DC response through the release of cytokines. In the lymph nodes, activated DCs present the antigen to T cells, providing co-stimulatory signals and cytokine-mediated stimulation for CD4+ and CD8+ T cells differentiation via MHC-II and MHC-I, respectively. Depending on the cytokine milieu, CD4+ T cells may differentiate into different T helper (Th) cell subtypes, such as Th1, Th2, Th9, Th17, Th22, Treg, or Tfh cells. In turn, these subsets release distinct cytokines that mediate different functions, such as B cell isotype switching following B cell activation by Tfh cells. CD8+ T cells differentiate into memory and effector CD8+ T cells (*CTLs*). *Adapted from [8].*

draining lymph nodes for T cell presentation, illustrated in Fig. 8.1. As DCs mature, they evolve for processing and transporting antigens to the cell surface. This mechanism coincides with increased expression of costimulatory molecules (e.g., CD40, CD80, and CD86) and release cytokines that will amplify T cell receptor signaling and promote T cell activation and polarization. DCs are capable to process both endogenous and exogenous antigens and present them to naïve T cells in the context of major histocompatibility complex molecules class I (MHC-I) or class II (MHC-II), eliciting antigen-specific CD8+ or CD4+ T cell differentiation, respectively [1,2].

Typically, exogenous processed antigens are presented in the context of MHC-II molecules and result in helper T (Th) cell differentiation. These CD4+ T cells secrete cytokines that provide help to other cells of the immune system. Depending on the activation mechanism and the surrounding cytokine milieu naïve CD4+ T cells can differentiate into different subsets that have unique cytokine profiles and functional properties. Since the discovery of the Th1/Th2 dichotomy, several additional Th subsets were discovered and include Th17 cells, regulatory T cells (Treg), and most recently Th9 cells, Th22 cells, and follicular Th cells (Tfh) (Fig. 8.1) [3,4]. Th1 cells are primarily associated with cell-mediated immunity particularly important against intracellular pathogens. These cells are mainly characterized by IFN-γ and TNF-α secretion that will activate CD8+ T cells and macrophages to kill both the pathogen and infected cells. IFN-γ is a potent proinflammatory cytokine linked with increased phagocytosis and antigen presentations, B cells stimulation to secrete immunoglobulin G2 (IgG2) or IgG3 subclasses of IgG antibodies, generally associated to opsonization and virus neutralization. Th2 cells lineage is associated with host defense against extracellular parasites. It is responsible for the production of IL-4, IL-5, and IL-13 and the co-stimulation of B cells to originate short-lived plasma cells inducing a strong humoral immune response characterized by IgG1 and IgE production. Activated B cells can also differentiate into memory B cells that represent the specific immunologic memory maintenance after vaccination, able to induce a rapid specific immune response following a further pathogen exposition, preventing the establishment of infection [5]. Th17 subset comprises potent inflammatory mediators involved in host defense against infectious diseases, particularly at mucosal sites. The secretion of IL-17, IL-21, and IL-22, responsible for neutrophil recruitment and B cell functions enhancement, is the major contributor. Although strongly associated with immunopathology, mainly serious inflammatory and autoimmune reactions, IL-17 has been recently considered a chief orchestrator of immunity. It is shown to have only modest activity on its own, but has a synergistic action with other factors such as the IFN-γ, serving as an important adjunct to Th1 responses [6]. Conversely, Th17 cell lineage is negatively regulated by Th1 and Th2 cytokines [4,6].

On the other side, endogenously produced viral proteins or exogenous antigens processed by a phenomenon called cross-presentation are presented in the context of MHC-I molecules and result in cytotoxic T lymphocytes (CD8+ T cells, CTLs) differentiation [1]. These CD8+ T cells are mainly involved in the clearance of intracellular pathogens as they can recognize and destroy infected cells. Antigen cross-presentation is a process mainly carried out by DCs and believed to be vital for immunity against viruses that do not readily infect APCs. It is highly dependent on DCs maturation stimuli, influenced by the internalization route, the pathway of endocytic trafficking, and the simultaneous activation through PRRs [7].

8.2 Vaccine design for viral infections

Acquired immunity for a specific organism can result from either an actual infection or a preventive immunization. Indeed, vaccination is one of the great successes of public health, efficiently avoiding a variety of infectious diseases. It is amongst the most cost-effective measures to prevent mortality, the second, after clean water [9]. Since Edward Jenner developed the first vaccine in the 18th century great advances have been made. The field has moved from traditional vaccines that are expensive to produce (inactivated or live-attenuated pathogens) since it is required a high biosafety level for production plant facilities, to RNA vaccines that are faster and cheaper to produce.

Moreover, traditional vaccines have major problems related to safety issues and adverse host reactions which contrast with second and third-generation vaccines which are normally extremely safer options. Advancing technology and the desire for harmless and cost-effective alternatives led to development of subunit vaccines that contain a protective antigen of the pathogen that can be expressed by an attenuated bacterial or virus vector (recombinant vaccines) or encoded by DNA or RNA (DNA or RNA vaccines). Subunit vaccines in general are poorly immunogenic and require the addition of immunostimulatory agents to induce strong and long-lasting protective immune responses. While the generation of a strong antibody-based immune response has demonstrated to be sufficient, at least in some cases, for prophylactic vaccines, a robust antigen specific T cell immune response is required for their use for therapeutic interventions of viral infections. The stimulation of both arms of the adaptive immune system are dependent of the immunostimulatory compounds, also known as adjuvants. So, vaccinology has still some challenges to solve when designing new vaccines, on the one hand, the choice of the antigen and on the other the choice or development of the most suitable adjuvant for a particular antigen.

For instance, the T cell function restoration is commonly recognized as the best immunotherapeutic approach for a functional Hepatitis B cure. Thus, the induction of cell-mediated immunity (based on the action of T cells) is vital for the development of a Hepatitis B therapeutic vaccine and would be, by analogy, for other vaccines for viral diseases. Thus, DCs are key targets to modulate the vaccine-elicited immune response. Specifically, DCs activation to induce antigen-specific CD8+ T cells differentiation is a central factor for the controlled destruction of persisting HBV-producing hepatocytes [1,2].

Design vaccines that mimic pathogen properties, categorizing the microbial features responsible for immunity is a valuable strategy to promote that [10–12].

8.3 Mimicking pathogens

In fact, traditional live-attenuated or inactivated whole-cell vaccines usually do not require additional immunostimulatory components since they contain some naturally occurring adjuvants such as nucleic acids, lipids, and cell membrane components [13]. The repetitive surface molecule organization, the particulate nature and the ability to stimulate both innate and adaptive immune responses are some of the key parameters responsible for their superb immunogenicity. These parameters may serve as the paradigms to successful development of safe and potent modern vaccines that may embrace DNA vaccines and the development and selection of novel vaccine adjuvants, primarily acting via DCs activation [14–17].

8.4 The case of DNA vaccines

The immune response following DNA vaccination suggests that it follows a complex pathway mimicking natural viral infections. The use of DNA as the immunogen will lead to uptake and expression/translation of the transgene using the host cell's replication machinery [18] linked with MHC-I presentation and CTLs differentiation in addition to humoral immunity [1,14,16,18]. Once DNA plasmid (pDNA) is administered through common injectable routes (e.g. subcutaneous (SC) or intramuscular (IM)) the two main cell types that become transfected are myocytes and APCs, ideal targets to trigger and modulate immunity. Other advantages include the low cost of production, transport and storage as DNA vaccines are highly stable and do not require refrigeration. Cold storage is necessary for current available recombinant vaccines to remain antigenically active, a struggle in developing countries where viral diseases is a major problem. Nevertheless, poor transfection, transient antigen expression, and immunological tolerance are the main hurdles of current DNA vaccines research seeking in vivo immunogenicity and efficacy [14,19,20].

A variety of non-viral DNA delivery vehicles have been investigated including physical (e.g. 'gene guns', electroporation) and chemical (e.g., cationic molecules) approaches. Complexation with cationic lipids and cationic polymers to condense pDNA and deliver it to target cells is highly valuable and may shape the future of DNA vaccination [19,20]. Improving cellular internalization, endosomal escape, and enhancing their delivery to cell nucleus are some of the main advantages conferred [21]. Synthetic polymers that have gained some attention in last years include poly(β-amino ester) (PβAE) [20,22] and poly[2-(dimethylamino)ethylmethacrylate] (PDMAEMA) [20,23]. In addition, particles based on PβAEs were recently characterized for their intrinsic immunogenicity, activating DCs, antigen presentation, and enhancing T cell proliferation [24]. PDMAEMA-based polyplexes were also previously considered a potential delivery vehicle for the HBsAg-encoding DNA vaccination [25]. Heterologous prime-boost regimens have also provided significant contributions to DNA vaccine immunogenicity. Again, vaccine targeting to APCs is also a possibility to overcome such limitations [26]. Co-delivery with adjuvants can also enhance vaccine-induced immunity. Therefore, there remains the opportunity for DNA vaccine design improvement to achieve viral clearance not achieved yet by the therapeutic DNA vaccines that entered clinical trials.

8.5 The importance of new adjuvant development

The word adjuvant comes from the Latin word *adiuvare*, which means to help. Adjuvants were first described by Gaston Ramon in the 1920s [27] and consist of substances capable of enhancing, modulating, or prolonging antigen-specific immune responses. To sensitize the immune system against infectious

TABLE 8.1 Adjuvant properties.

Elevate antigen processing and presentation by APCs
Induce cell-mediated immunity (like CTLs)
Facilitate mucosal responses (protecting the antigen from the harsh GI tract)
Increase antigen potency (enabling dose sparing)
Ensure a rapid response
Induce long-lasting adaptive immune responses
Induce antigen-specific clonal expansion
Induce broad and high specific antibody production
Good immunomodulatory capacity
Induce secretion of cytokines that control T and B cell responses
Function as effective innate immune signals
Make vaccine more cost effective (less doses required)
Enhance vaccine efficacy in infants, elderly and immunocompromised people
Facilitate continuous antigen release (depot effect)

APCs, antigen presenting cells; CTLs, cytotoxic T lymphocytes; GI, gastrointestinal tract. Adapted from [28].

agents and induce long-lasting memory response, vaccine adjuvants usually have some properties extensively reviewed by others [17,28,29] and summarized in Table 8.1. Adjuvants have diverse modes of action and are divided into delivery systems and immunomodulators. Antigens and adjuvants are usually formulated for enhanced presentation by APCs as emulsions or particulate delivery systems such as liposomes, virosomes, immune-stimulating complexes (ISCOMs), virus-like particles (VLPs), and polymeric particles. Immunomodulators comprise any substance that activates, suppresses or changes immune responses and generally enhance vaccine efficacy primarily, by stimulating innate immunity. They can modulate cytokine and chemokine secretion and include compounds like toll-like receptor (TLRs) ligands, CpG oligodeoxynucleotides (ONDs), galactosylceramides, and bacterial toxins, among others. Nevertheless, this classification is not static since some particulate delivery systems such as liposomes and polymeric particles also have intrinsic immunomodulatory properties.

Despite the great advance in the field, few adjuvants are currently licensed for human use (see examples in Table 8.2). The reasons are mainly associated with the toxic properties of some materials with adjuvant potential and considerable increase in regulatory demands since the initial approval of aluminum

TABLE 8.2 Examples of licensed adjuvants for human vaccines, approved by FDA and/or EMA.

Adjuvant	Type	Trade name (disease)	Year
Alum	Mineral salt	Various	1926
MF59	Squalene-based oil-in-water emulsion	Fluad, Optaflu (s. influenza) Focetria, Aflunov (p. influenza)	1997
Virosomes	Liposome	Inflexal (seasonal influenza) Epaxal (hepatitis A)	2000
CTB	Non-toxic enterotoxin derivative	Dukoral (cholera)	2004
AS04	Alum adsorbed monophosphoryl lipid A	Fendrix (hepatitis B) Cervarix (human papilloma virus)	2005
AS03	Squalene-based oil-in-water emulsion	Pandremix (s., p. influenza) Prepandrix (pre-pandemic. influenza)	2009
AS01	Combination of liposome, monophosphoryl lipid A and saponin QS-21	Mosquirix (malaria) Shingrix (herpes zoster)	2015

salts (e.g., alum). The European Medicines Agency released a guideline in 2005 [30], in order to obtain the necessary information to apply for the licensing of new or established adjuvants in vaccines. This guideline addresses adjuvant quality, non-clinical, and clinical issues.

Although aluminum salts are the most widely utilized adjuvant in human vaccines since 1926 [31], they are poor inducers of T cell responses and have some inherent complications including local reactions, augmentation of IgE antibody responses, and the occurrence of granulomas [28,32]. For human administrations, adjuvant choice is based on the balance between higher adjuvanticity and lesser side effects. Furthermore, a new-generation of adjuvants is very desired to design new vaccines or improve the existing ones with the capacity to stimulate both, the innate and adaptive immunity and to induce robust cell-mediated immune responses including Th cells and CTLs differentiation, with reduced toxicity [17,28]. In that regard, the rapid increase of knowledge on how the immune system interacts with pathogens means that there is increased understanding of the role of adjuvants and how the formulation of modern vaccines can be better tailored, contrasting from early adjuvants that were used empirically. Depending on the mode of action, each adjuvant can have unique immunological properties (Table 8.1) and should be selected according to the target pathogen and the desired clinical outcome [28]. Nevertheless, many challenges are being experienced including preparation in suboptimal conditions, confinement in adjuvanticity, safety concerns, and biological dissimilarity [29].

Therefore, careful and rational design is mandatory to succeed and in the next subsection, it will be explained why the combination of a particulate form and PAMPs comprise the most rational design of "pathogen-mimicking" adjuvants with the ability to enhance recognition and uptake by APCs, leading to enhanced immune responses with reduced side effects.

8.6 Adjuvant particulate form

The importance of a particulate form is a consistent principle for enhanced immunity, mimicking the particulate nature of a pathogen. In fact, Gaston Ramon has already observed in the 1920s that horses injected with inactivated toxin and starch, breadcrumbs, or tapioca induced local sterile abscesses resulting in increasing anti-sera production [27]. Consistently, particulate antigens are generally more immunogenic than soluble ones. For instance, virus-like-particles (VLPs) particulate structure and size facilitate their uptake into APCs and efficient cross-presentation on MHC-I molecules, an additional advantage for therapeutic approaches for infectious diseases [33]. A perfect example is the surface hepatitis B antigen (HBsAg) that can self-assemble into 22 nm VLP about 1000 times more immunogenic than non-assembled HBsAg [34]. Still, although HBsAg intrinsic immunogenicity it often requires the concomitant use of adjuvants for an efficient vaccination, like the commercially available vaccines that include aluminum hydroxide (Engerix-B) or alum (Recombivax HB).

Moreover, particulate materials often create a proinflammatory environment that recruit immune cells and prolong particle-cell interactions [35]. Beyond the adjuvant characteristic properties described in Table 8.1 and the fact that they can act both as immunomodulators and delivery systems, particulate adjuvants have the potential to be specifically tailored in order to regulate the type of innate immune responses induced, offering significant opportunities in terms of designing systems with increased immune-mediated efficacy [35]. They permit size and surface properties control and the co-delivery of multiple molecules in the same structure (e.g., antigen, adjuvant, targeting molecules) enabling a local, simultaneous and possible synergistic effect usually valuable for the vaccine efficacy and potency [11,36,37]. In fact, the combination of two adjuvants in the same vaccine formulation can be highly beneficial to enhance, but mostly to modulate the type of immune response desired [38]. For instance, Adjuvants from GlaxoSmithKline (AS01, AS02, and AS03) are an example of successful adjuvant combination in the same formulation for enhanced immunogenicity and modulation of the immune response. Particularly for AS04, the addition of MPL to aluminum salts enhanced cell-mediated immunity to human papilloma virus vaccine by rapidly triggering a local cytokine response favorable for APCs activation [39]. Most approaches combine a delivery system with an immunopotentiator, because they have the potential to act synergistically to enhance antigen-specific immunity and increase vaccine safety, reducing the adjuvant-related side effects. The reduction of systemic distribution of the immunopotentiator preventing systemic cytokine-mediated inflammatory toxicity was demonstrated by Illyinskii et al. with the association of TLR agonists R848 and CpG ODN with polymeric nanoparticles [40]. Several particulate platforms have been explored and include VLPs, liposomes, ISCOMs, nanoemulsions, and polymeric-based particles [11,29].

These new adjuvants will be crucial in future clinical development of safer and more effective therapeutic vaccination against intracellular infections, such as the hepatitis B. Nanotechnology has been playing an important role in the design and development of those formulations, giving the appropriate features to particulate systems [11,12], resulting in some successful achievements that already reached the market (e.g., emulsions and liposomes—Table 8.2).

8.7 Pathogen-associated molecular patterns (PAMPs) as immunopotentiators

One of the most exciting areas of adjuvant development is the use of pattern recognition receptors (PRRs) targeting pathogen-associated molecular patterns (PAMPs) present on microorganisms, able to control and shape the subsequent adaptive immune activities specific to the invading pathogen [17,41]. PRRs are central to stimulate innate immunity and are considered key targets to drive the desired T cell responses. PRRs stimulation can promote DCs activation toward polyfunctional Th1 cells, T cell memory and CTL responses [11,17,41]. The generated immune response may differ depending on the PRRs activated that will be translated in a specific cytokine production with distinct T cell polarizing effect. TLRs, C-type lectin receptors (CLRs), nucleotide oligomerization domain (NOD)-Like Receptors (also known NLRs) and gene-I (RIG-I)-Like Receptors (RLRs) are the four main groups of PRRs. In fact, most of the molecular adjuvants currently under evaluation are PRRs ligands, with the most extensively studied being TLRs agonists [36]. TLRs activation may induce the mitogen-activated protein kinase (MAPK), nuclear factor-(NF-κβ) or IFN regulatory factors pathways inducing the expression of cytokines that modulate adaptive immunity [42]. In that regard, several TLRs agonists have been evaluated for their adjuvant properties in vaccines for infectious diseases: (1) TLR-3 ligand polyinosinic:polycytidylic acid (poly (I:C)); (2) TLR4 ligands monophosphoryl lipid A (MPL) (already licensed for use in human vaccines) and lipopolysaccharide (LPS); (3) TLR-5 ligand flagellin; (4) TLR7/8 ligand imiquimod (already has FDA approval for use in actinic keratosis, external genital warts and recently superficial basal carcinoma—Aldara topical cream); and (5) TLR9 ligand CpG ODNs [11]. LPS, also known as endotoxin, is a component of the gram-negative bacteria's outer cell wall that can lead to septic shock or endotoxin tolerance, depending on the dose. CpG ODNs are known to induce the production of Th1 proinflammatory cytokines and increased innate and adaptive immune response, with effects ranging from increased antibody production, faster memory response, or a change in the cytokine profile of the vaccine leading to a stronger immune response. Single stranded RNA from infecting microorganisms stimulates TLR7 and TLR8 leading to the production of proinflammatory cytokines. However, the short half-life of RNA difficult the development of long-lasting vaccine formulations [12]. All these adjuvants work very well by traditional injectable routes of vaccine administration. One of the great challenges of vaccinology is to find good adjuvants for the mucosal routes of administration as well, since it would be desirable to have a greater number of oral and intranasal vaccines on the market.

8.8 The case of oral administration of vaccines

Most infectious agents enter the body through mucosal surfaces, the largest body areas that separate the external milieu from the internal sterile environment. Mucosal surfaces are physical barriers of epithelial and immune cells, representing the body's first line of defense, commonly referred to as mucosal-associated lymphoid tissue (MALT). The MALT mainly comprises B and T cells, but APCs like DCs and macrophages also play a major role in mucosal immunity [43–45]. MALT immune organization usually enables to tolerate the continuous stimulation of a vast variety of commensal microorganisms and to initiate a specific immune response against the plethora of potential pathogens [44], thus being hopeful candidate sites for vaccination [46]. The most attractive feature of mucosal vaccines (e.g., oral, rectal, vaginal, nasal, pulmonary) is the provided double layer of protection characterized by antigen-specific antibody responses in the bloodstream and the local production and secretion of antigen-specific secretory IgA (sIgA), fundamental for virus neutralization and opsonization [47–51]. Additionally, safety, convenience of administration, lower risk of infection transmission, the non-requirement of trained personnel, and simplified manufacturing, transporting, and storing are among the major vantages compared to injectable vaccines, that can benefit vaccination in developing countries. Despite the extensive research regarding needle-free vaccination, it is such a demanding accomplishment owing to physical barriers (e.g., mucus, epithelium) and poor immunogenicity mostly related to degradation of vaccine materials in the harsh stomach environment, rich in enzymes or with a very low pH. Indeed, few mucosal vaccines are currently licensed for human use and none of the options includes subunit antigens (Table 8.3). The induction of immune tolerance frequently occurs in the absence of potent adjuvants.

A winning approach for mucosal vaccination is the oral delivery to the gut associated lymphoid tissue (GALT), mimicking pathogens entry pathways. For instance, new immunotherapies for HBV treatment are being developed for oral administration as they will be absorbed through the intestine and delivered to the liver via the portal vein. Specially, drugs that target PRRs will stimulate

TABLE 8.3 **Examples of licensed mucosal vaccines for human use, approved by FDA and/or EMA.**

Pathogen	Trade name	Route	Vaccine type
Influenza virus	FluMist, Fluenz Tetra, Nasovac-S	Nasal	Live attenuated monovalent or not influenza virus
Poliovirus	Orimune, OPV, etc.	Oral	Live attenuated trivalent, bivalent and monovalent polioviruses
Rotavirus	Rotarix, RotaTeq	Oral	Live attenuated, monovalent or pentavalent rotaviruses
Vibrio cholerae	Dukoral, Orochol, Shanchol	Oral	Inactivated V. cholera with or without CTB
Salmonella Typhi	Vivotif	Oral	Live attenuated *S. Typhi*

the production of antiviral and environment-modifying cytokines (e.g. IFN-α, IFN-γ, TNF-a, IL-6, and IL-12) both in the intestinal tract and in the liver [52]. The GALT is reviewed by Lamichhane as the "command center" for mucosal immunity [46]. It can be subdivided into two immunological distinct regions: (1) highly organized lymphoid tissues such as the Peyer's patches (PPs) that serve as inductive sites for antigen presentation; and (2) poorly organized regions constituted by diffusely distributed lymphoid and plasma cells that serve as effector sites for sIgA synthesis and T cell responses [53,54]. The PPs are referred to as "the immune sensors of the intestine" by Jung and coworkers [55] and consist of macroscopic lymphoid aggregates found in submucosa along the small intestine. PPs, and other lymphoid areas, are separated from the intestinal lumen by a single layer of columnar epithelial cells, known as the follicle associated epithelium. The subepithelial dome (SED) is located underneath and is a more diffuse area of B cells, T cells, macrophages and DCs. The follicular areas are mainly composed by germinal centers (GCs) containing proliferating B cells, follicular DCs and macrophages spaced by interfollicular T cell regions [55,56]. PPs GCs exhibit unique conditions totally different from those in peripheral nodes with a special ability to start, expand and synchronize gut IgA B cell responses [57] (Fig. 8.2). The most notable feature of PPs is the presence of microfold (M) cells, enterocytes specialized to take up antigens, particles and microorganisms from the intestinal lumen by vesicular transport, delivering them to the underlying mucosal immune system [55,58–60]. Interestingly, at basal side, M cell plasma membrane is deeply invaginated to form a large sac-like structure ("M cell pocket"), where DCs and lymphocytes can move in and take up residence [60], providing the ability to start, expand and synchronize gut IgA B cell responses [57]. Additionally, M cells express IgA receptors on their apical plasma membrane and transport sIgA-bound antigens to PPs [50,60].

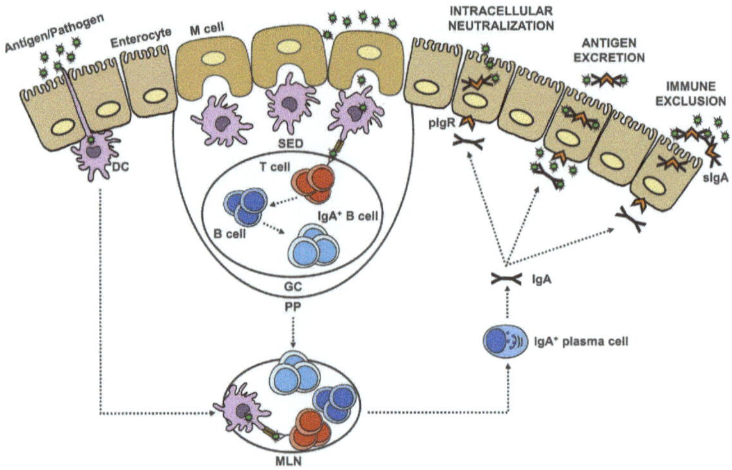

FIG. 8.2 Gut-associated lymphoid tissue IgA production in response to antigens/pathogens. Dendritic cells (*DCs*) can sample antigens both located in the subepithelial dome (*SED*) of Peyer's patches (*PPs*) or in the lamina propria by extending their dendrites between the epithelial cells to reach the external milieu. Then, depending on the case, activated DCs can present the antigen locally on PPs germinal centre (GC) or migrate to the mesenteric lymph nodes (*MLNs*) where they induce B cells to differentiate into IgA+ plasma cells. IgA+ plasma cells home to the lamina propria and secrete dimeric IgA that is transcytozed across the mucosal epithelial cell layer via a polymeric Ig receptor (pIgR), giving rise to the secretory IgA (sIgA). IgA can protect mucosal surfaces by: (1) antigen excretion, through the binding of sIgA to antigens removing them from lamina propria; (2) immune exclusion, by sIgA interaction with antigens blocking their attachment to epithelial cells; and (3) intracellular antigen neutralization, by neutralizing and eventually removing the pathogenic antigens inside the cells. *Adapted from [74,75].*

The production of IgA directed against intestinal antigens depends on resident mucosal APCs, mostly DCs, that sample antigens at various mucosal sites and is illustrated in Fig. 8.2.

8.9 Polymer-based particulate adjuvants in oral vaccine formulation

Surely, to obtain a good immune response, the key strategy is to protect antigens and enhance vaccine uptake by PPs, which can be obtained throughout antigen encapsulation in polymer-based particles [61]. Antigen encapsulation in polymeric particles can be an important tool to ensure that oral tolerance does not develop, reducing the rate of dilution and degradation of antigen. In fact, particulate antigens are generally more immunogenic at mucosal surfaces, where soluble antigens are more prone to induce mucosal tolerance [62,63]. Targeting the antigen to PPs will play a major role in the development of a rapid and potent immune response. Multiple studies demonstrated the ability of polymeric delivery systems to reach PPs, associated or not with M cell ligands (Table 8.4).

TABLE 8.4 Peyer's patches uptake of particulate delivery systems in animal models.

Study type	Delivery system	Size	Charge	M cell ligand	Observations	References
OA	Thiolated HPMCP particles	3.7 μm	–	M cell HP	Thiolation improved mucoadhesive properties; M cell HP improved antigen delivery to PPs.	[76]
ILoop/ OA	Thiolated Eudragit particles	1–10 μm	–	M cell HP	Thiolation resulted in higher residence time; M cell HP induced higher transcytosis to PPs through M cells.	[67]
OA	PLGA particles	166 nm	−20 mV	–	Effective PPs uptake	[73]
OA	Guar gum particles	900 nm	–	–	Targeting potential to PP	[64]
In vitro/ ex vivo	Polystyrene/BSA/ MTBCL microspheres	–	–	AAL	Lectin-coupled microspheres preferentially bind M cells	[77]
ILoop	OVA-AlexaFluor loaded GPs	4 μm	−6 mV	–	Intraepithelial or intraluminal GPs localized in the SED region	[78]
OA	HPMCAS + Eudragit FS 30D particles	0.35 – 2 μm	+16 mV	AAL	Increased particulate uptake in PPs	[79]
OA	HPMCAS + Eudragit FS 30D + BSA particles	1.5 μm	+16 mV	AAL	Prolonged release	[80]
ILoop	PLA particles	200 – 250 nm	−40 mV	–	Uptake exclusively through M cells; PLA interaction with SED B cells and DCs.	[68]
ILoop	Alginate coated chito-san particles	300–600 nm	−34 mV	–	Effective PPs uptake	[69]

AAL, aleuria aurantia lectin; BSA, bovine serum albumin; DCs, dendritic cells; GPs, glucan particles; HP, homing peptide; HPMCAS, hydroxyl propyl methyl cellulose acetate succinate; ILoop, ileal loop; MTBCL, mycobacterium TB cell lysate microspheres; OA, oral administration. OVA, ovalbumin; PLA, poly(lactic acid); PLGA, poly(lactic-co-glycolide); PPs, Peyer's patches; Ref., references; SED, subepithelial dome. Adapted from [61].

In some cases, they generated long-lasting immunological memory, not only at the site of antigen exposure but also systemically or in other mucosal compartments due to antigen-sensitized precursor B and T cells dissemination [44,49,50,54,55,64–73].

Once again, a combination of particle size and surface properties could directly influence interaction with the intestinal mucosa and consequently PPs uptake, better reviewed elsewhere [61]. However, general rules are difficult to draw due to the impossibility to evaluate one exclusive factor and not a multitude of parameters. In fact, polymeric particles with a wide range of size and various surface properties were successfully internalized by PPs, as shown in Table 8.4.

Nevertheless, the literature points out some directions. Size is undoubtedly a key feature, as it will not only determine the efficiency of PPs uptake but also the internalization route through PPs epithelium: the transcellular pathway for smaller particles (<100 nm) and the paracellular pathway for larger particles (>100 nm). Smaller particles (<500 nm) have good probability to be internalized by APCs and transported to the lymph nodes. Oppositely, bigger particles will be retained into PPs and so, mucosal and systemic specific immune responses will not be efficiently induced. In fact, IgA intestinal immune responses were found to be size dependent and favorable for smaller particles.

Regarding the optimal surface properties, the picture is not so clear, but a combination of moderate mucoadhesive properties to improve intestinal residence time, and the incorporation of M cell specific ligands for a targeted particulate delivery seems to be the winning approach. Finally, it is also not clear if the particles should be positively charged. Positively charged particles interact with the mucosa sialic acid and thus their retention time is increased which can be a good feature on the nasal mucosa. However, on GALT, when the interaction is very strong, this can cause particle entrapment in the mucus and so particles would have difficulty to reach PPs. Summarizing, three main factors should be taken into account for particles design toward mucosal vaccine efficacy: (1) particle modification to increase interaction with the mucosa and enhance antigen bioavailability; (2) particles coating with specific targeting agents to increase M cells mediated uptake (e.g., lectins); and (3) include polymers that promote DCs activation and enhance innate and adaptive immunity following uptake [81]. The challenge remains to identify the best combination of adjuvants and/or targeting agents to promote optimal immune activation without the induction of adverse reactions.

8.10 Biodegradable polymer-based particles

Biodegradable polymers have a great potential in medicine simply because they can be degraded in vivo by enzymatic processes and the degradation products further eliminated by the normal metabolic pathways. Thus, regarding the previously described and desired characteristics, biodegradable polymer-based particles arise as a great choice for the development of "pathogen-like" adjuvant candidates for vaccine formulations against infectious diseases. First, they display a particulate form. Second, they can be formulated using PAMPs in its composition. Third, bioactive molecules can be easily trapped in the particles by encapsulation to be released during particle degradation, or simply adsorbed on particle surface by electrostatic or hydrophobic interactions (e.g., immunomodulators, antigens, ligands for specific cells or tissues). Interestingly, the association of immunopotentiators with polymer-based vaccines can potentiate the immune effect and reduce its toxicity by directing the immunopotentiator to appropriate compartments (e.g., lymph nodes), enabling local immune responses rather than clearance to the bloodstream and the induction of a cytokine storm, as can occur with soluble adjuvants. Also, vaccine accumulation in lymph nodes will promote superior antigen-specific humoral immunity due to prolonged exposure to immune cells. Antigen formulation into polymeric nanoparticles allows the process of cross-presentation leading to the induction of cytotoxic immune responses, essential to fight against intracellular pathogens [36]. Additionally, biopolymers can enhance the shelf-life of antigens and display immunostimulatory properties improving antigenicity of conjugated antigens, highly influenced by the polymer chemistry, format, charge and fine balance between hydrophobicity and hydrophilicity [29,36,82].

Overall, particle size and surface composition are the main influencers of the outcome immune response. Several parameters can be controlled to tailor the desired particle size, recently reviewed as an intrinsic characteristic that affects the generation of long-last adaptive immunity, namely through the impact of particle size on the polymer half-life in vivo and the influence of that in the duration and type of the innate and adaptive immune responses generated [29,35]. The effect of particle size on the immune response is not often consensual. Size-dependent immune responses are usually favorable for smaller particles directing to a more balanced Th1/Th2 immune responses [83]. Some authors associated particles with less than 1000 nm to a better uptake profile and an enhanced capacity to induce cell-mediated immunity [84,85]. Even though, there is an ever-increasing obsession with the nanoscale, micro-sized particles also have many advantages as adjuvants. In fact, particulate vaccines typically within 0.1 μm and 10 μm range, resemble the dimensions of common bacteria and viruses, and are therefore recognized by the immune system [86]. Chitosan-based particles of 1 μm had favorable antigen delivery, upregulation of surface activation markers, and cytokine release from macrophages when compared to similar 300 nm and 3 μm particles [87]. Surface composition is the other significant factor for immunomodulation. Hydrophobic domains of polymers are favorable for protein adsorption and APCs recruitment and activation [82]. Particle hydrophobicity was also demonstrated to initiate and enhance immune responses since many PRRs have evolved to recognize and react with hydrophobic molecular structures [88]. On the other side, hydrophilic moieties are also detrimental to determine polymer's adjuvant potential, preventing non-specific interactions of proteins with cells. That is why amphiphilic particles are referred by many authors as the best approach for vaccine delivery [89,90]. A variety of other factors such as the surface chemistry are deeply involved and depend on the biopolymer used, or the use of targeting molecules for surface functionalization, such as PRRs agonists. It affects particle charge, mainly determinant for mucosal vaccination where positively charged particles revealed improved immune responses than anionic particles [91].

Both synthetic and natural biodegradable polymers may be used. However, to date, the most popular biodegradable polymers used in vaccine applications include poly(epsilon-caprolactone) (PCL), poly(lactic acid) (PLA) or poly(lactic-co-glycolic acid) (PLGA), three synthetic polymers [12,92]. PLGA is the most well studied and has been approved by the FDA for use as a drug delivery system since 1969. PLGA particles have been utilized to deliver a wide range of peptide antigens inducing potent immune responses [37]. One of the major drawbacks is the potential exposure of antigens to harsh organic solvents since the conventional antigen loading technique to PLGA particles involves the formation of single or double emulsions and solvent evaporation [37].

8.11 Natural occurring polymers—polysaccharides

Natural occurring polymers, in particular polysaccharides, have attracted attention in the mid-1990s as promising platforms for antigen delivery, representing one of the main tendencies on the field of vaccine adjuvants for infectious diseases and cancer [11,28,41,93]. Polysaccharides are a very diverse group of polymeric carbohydrate structures formed by long chains of monosaccharide units bound by glycosidic linkages and may differ in structure, conformation, length of the chain and the number of branches in it [94]. The natural and ubiquitous character of polysaccharides, together with their intrinsic biocompatibility, biodegradability and low reactogenicity justify their interest in the engineering of nanovaccines [11]. An advantage comparing to the synthetic polymers is that the technologies used to produce particulate systems rely on milder and simpler conditions, which minimize the use of solvents and high-energy sources, easy to scale-up and most importantly suitable for the association of labile biomolecules. These techniques usually rely on physicochemical processes such as ionic gelation, complexation and solvent displacement, among others [11].

Some polysaccharides are natural PAMPs found in the cell walls of bacteria or yeasts that activate PRRs, thus playing a vital role in both innate and adaptive immunity [8,11,17]. This is a characteristic that provides them intrinsic targeting abilities to APCs [11,36] or PPs M cells that express a variety of immunosurveillance receptors on their apical surface enabling them to be modulated through chemokines, interleukins, amines, TLRs activating molecules [95], highly benefic for a potential vaccine adjuvant candidate. As they are present in most of the whole pathogen-based vaccines, the stimulation of PRRs has been unwittingly used in vaccines for years [36]. Actually, most innate responses are directed against three classes of fungal cell wall conserved carbohydrate components: β-glucans, mannans, and chitin/chitosan [93]. In that regard, some authors have proposed the use of those polysaccharides for vaccine applications, with the caution that the natural origin of these materials is related to high variability that may lead to variable results concerning their adjuvant activity [11,41]. The potential of these biomaterials for the vaccine adjuvant field deserves further attention. It is expected that the next few years will bring deeper knowledge in terms of mechanisms of action [11].

8.11.1 Chitosan

Chitosan is a copolymer of β-(1-4)-linked D-glucosamine (deacetylated unit) and N-acetyl-D-glucosamine (acetylated unit) monomers obtained by deacetylation of chitin present in the exoskeletons of crustaceans and cell walls of fungi (e.g., *Mucor* and *Cryptococcus*) or yeast spores (e.g., *Saccharomyces cerevisiae*). When more than 60 % of acetylated units are removed from chitin it is usually considered chitosan and, once solubilized in acidic milieu, normally exhibits a strong positive electrical charge [96]. The degree of deacetylation and, consequently, the number of amino groups, together with molecular weight are known factors that influence chitosan physical and biological properties [97]. Water-solubility (mostly aqueous acidic solutions with a pH ratio lower than 6.5) [98], allowing particle formulation and antigen encapsulation without the use of organic solvents, preserving antigens immunogenicity along with the strong affinity to negatively charged molecules represent the key to the chitosan great interest [37,41,97–99]. Chitosan functional groups (amine and hydroxyl) allow facile chemical modification into chitosan derivatives (e.g. N-trimethyl-chitosan and carboxymethyl chitosan) to enhance solubility and mucoadhesivity [97,100]. Chitosan intrinsic mucoadhesivity is conferred by the presence of amino groups that promote interaction with negatively charged mucins facilitating adherence to mucosal membranes [100]. Additionally, chitosan is able to reversible open epithelial tight junctions promoting penetration through the mucosa [101,102], an attractive feature for mucosal drug delivery [103,104]. Indeed, chitosan was widely used for mucosal vaccination in vivo with some good results achieved. For instance, feeding mice with porcine circovirus type 2 (PCV2) virus-like particles loaded into positively charged chitosan microparticles induced the proliferation of PCV2-specific splenic CD4+/CD8+ T-lymphocytes and the subsequent production of IFN-γ to levels comparable with those induced by an injectable commercial formulation [105]. It is also worth mentioning that chitosan is "generally recognized as safe" (GRAS) by the FDA.

Therefore, chitosan is the most described polysaccharide regarding polymeric particles for vaccine delivery of protein antigens [106,107] and pDNA [108,109], among other biomedical applications. Chitosan-based particles were developed for the first time in the 1990s [110] and have been extensively studied ever since. Notably, although mainly used for formulation of delivery systems, chitosan-based formulations have been shown to enhance antigen uptake and presentation and to possess intrinsic immunomodulatory activities against pathogenic agents enhancing both cellular and humoral immune responses [93,97,99,103,111,112], namely through the activation of the NRLP-3 inflammasome [113]. As an example, antigen-loaded chitosan particles significantly enhanced upregulation of surface activation markers MHC-I, MHC-II, and costimulatory cytokines CD40, CD80, CD86, and CD54 and the release of pro-inflammatory cytokines (e.g., IL-1β, IL-6, TNF-α) as well as the proliferation of CD4+ and CD8+ T cells compared with soluble antigen [87]. Fewer studies evaluated the outcome following oral vaccination [66,114,115], mostly after particles coating with sodium alginate to provide increased stability in the acidic gastric lumen [66,115], resulting in serum anti-HBsAg and mucosal secretions anti-HBsAg sIgA in most of the cases. Overall, chitosan is considered as one of the most advanced polymers in the regulatory path for the indication of vaccination, present in new nasal vaccine formulations against meningitis and norovirus [116–118] and in an IM vaccine hydrogel (ViscoGel) formulation against influenza that already reached clinical trials.

8.11.2 β-glucans

β-glucans are a group of β-D-glucose polysaccharides found in the cell walls of many organisms such as bacteria, yeasts, and even some species of seaweed [119]. The most common forms are those comprising D-glucose units with β-1,3 type glycosidic bonds, from which yeast and fungal β-glucans usually contain β-1,6 side branches and cereal β-glucans contain both β-1,3 and β-1,4 backbone bonds. β-glucans have no charged functional groups and usually need to be modified to favor water solubility or to promote interaction with other molecules. Chemical alterations in the structure through derivatization may include sulfonylation, carboxymethylation, phosphorylation, and acetylation, and may alter the biological activity [120]. Consistently, β-glucans from different sources are differential in their structure, branching frequency, location and length, molecular weight and shape, affecting both solubility and biological activity [121]. Additionally, the conformation also plays a crucial role on β-glucan biological activities [120]. Some β-glucans, such as the ones from *Saccharomyces cerevisiae*, *Ganoderma lucidum mycelium,* and *Aureobasidium pullulans* are GRAS by the FDA and are used as food ingredients.

The β-glucans have been reported to possess immunological, anti-tumor, and anti-infection activities mostly relevant for vaccination purposes. Although the immunostimulatory properties were recognized long before the discovery of PPRs, stimulation of those receptors is the most recognized biological effect. β-glucans are PAMPs recognized by TLR2/6, Dectin-1, CR3 (complement receptor 3), scavenger (scav) and lactosylceramide (LacCer), triggering intracellular signaling activation followed by expression of immune-related molecules that regulate innate and adaptive immunity (Fig. 8.3) [11,122,123].

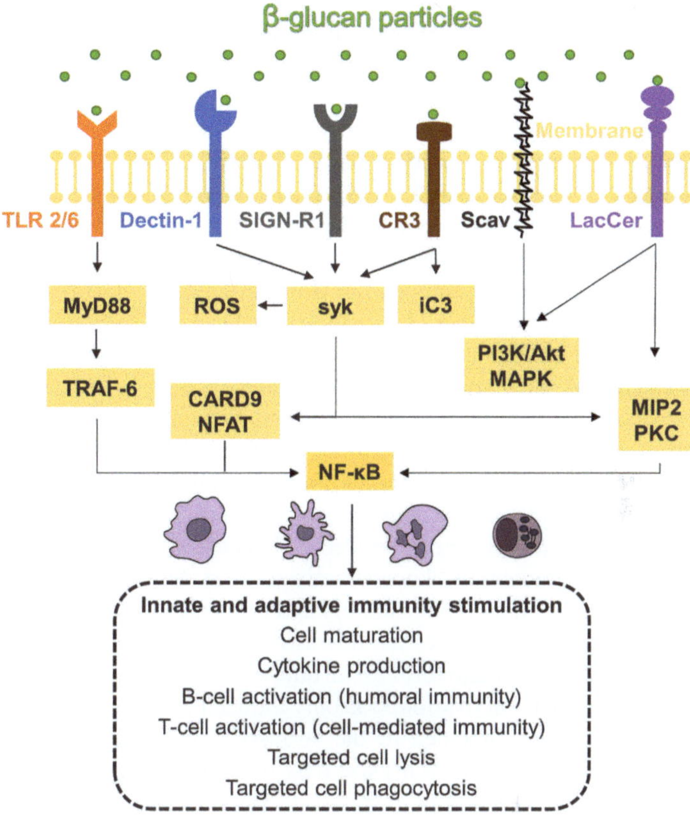

FIG. 8.3 Receptor mediated immune cell activation by β-glucan particles. Particulate β-glucans can activate a variety of membrane receptors found in immune cells (e.g. macrophages, dendritic cells, natural killer cells and neutrophils) that commonly include TLR2/6, Dectin-1, CR3 (complement receptor 3), scavenger (scav), dendritic cell-specific intercellular adhesion molecule-3-grabbing non-integrin -related 1 (SIGN-R1); and lactosylceramide (LacCer). The activation of those receptors will trigger intracellular signaling activation followed by the expression of immune-related molecules (e.g., TNF-α), cell maturation, B and T cell activation, and targeted cells phagocytosis and lysis that collectively regulate both innate and adaptive immunity. Akt, protein kinase B; CARD9, caspase-associated recruitment domain 9; iC3, third intracellular loop; MAPK, mitogen-activated protein kinase; MIP-2, macrophage inflammatory protein 2; MyD88, myeloid differentiation primary response 88; NFAT, nuclear factor of activated T-cells; NF-κβ, nuclear factor-κβ; PI3K, phosphoinositide 3-kinase; PKC, protein kinase C; ROS, reactive oxygen species; syk, spleen tyrosine kinase; TRAF-6, TNF receptor associated factor 6. *Adapted from [123].*

CR3 activation, although not yet fully understood, leads to complement activation resulting in fungal opsonization and the generation of chemotaxins which can recruit inflammatory cells, followed by internalization of the structures [119]. On the other hand, signaling through Dectin-1, the most studied β-glucan receptor, mediates processes such as reactive oxygen species (ROS), cytokine production, and pathogens internalization via phagocytosis [119,124,125].

Additionally, interaction mediated by CLRs (e.g., Dectin-1) is known to facilitate further cross-presentation of the antigen in MHC-I [1]. Dectin-1 receptor is widely expressed by immune cells including monocytes, macrophages, and DCs [126]. Thus, Dectin-1 recognition gives β-glucans interesting targeting capacities to enhance specific immune responses, through the modulation of both innate and adaptive immunity, usually promoting Th17 cell differentiation and cytotoxic T cell responses [127–129]. Indeed, several approaches have been successfully tested using β-glucans for Dectin-1 targeting. Dube et al. reported increased intracellular delivery of the encapsulated anti-tuberculosis drug and enhanced proinflammatory reaction after chitosan-coated PLGA particles functionalization with 1,3-β-glucan [130]. Targeting Dectin-1 receptor augmented and modulated the elicited immune response as demonstrated by Lipinski and coworkers [125]. A tricomponent mannan tetanus toxoid laminarin conjugate vaccine resulted in enhanced IgG antibody titers recognizing *candida albicans* and broad subclass distribution, comparing to the same formulation without the laminarin, after IP or SC administration. Moreover, these authors showed that this new conjugate antigen promoted receptor-based DCs uptake mediated by the interaction of laminarin with the Dectin-1 receptor, resulting in enhanced IL-6 and TGF-β production, known activators of Th17 cells. Concerning Dectin-1 activation, although both soluble and particulate β-glucans bind to the receptor, only the latter activates the downstream signaling [124], confirming the importance of a particulate form for an adjuvant. Coherently, TNF-α release, the hallmark of Dectin-1 activation, was only induced by a soluble β-1,3-glucan when it was covalently attached to the surface of polystyrene beads [131]. Additionally, β-glucan particle (GP) size may be critically important in orchestrating the nature of the immune response to fungi, influencing the secretion of cytokines from DCs. It was recently showed that large β-glucan-stimulated human DCs generate significantly more IL-1β, IL-6, and IL-23 compared to those stimulated with the smaller β-glucans [132].

Most research in terms of immunomodulatory properties has been done with β-1,3 or β-1,6-glucans such as curdlan (from *Alcaligenes faecalis*), laminarin (from *Laminaria digitata*), lentinan (from *Lentinus edodes*), pleuran (from *Pleurotus ostreatus*) and zymosan (from *Saccharomyces cerevisiae*) [93,119]. The use of the commonly designated GPs as a particulate delivery system of a payload molecule, optionally, but typically including a payload trapping molecule was firstly described by Gary Ostroff [133] and extensively explored since then. GPs are highly purified hollow porous cell wall shells derived from *Saccharomyces cerevisiae* (baker's yeast) following a series of hot alkali and organic extractions, primarily composed of β-1,3-glucan free of mannans and proteins, containing some chitin and β-1,6-glucans. The extracted GPs are readily available, biodegradable, substantially spherical particles about 2-4 μm in diameter targeted to phagocytic cells, such as macrophages and cells of lymphoid tissue primarily due to their β-glucan content as an effective vaccine platform [133]. In fact, polymer-complexed cores can be constructed within the hollow GPs, enabling the delivery to DCs and macrophages of a wide variety of "payload" classes including proteins, siRNA, DNA, and other small molecules [128,134–137]. The β-1,3-glucan outer shell provides a Dectin-1 mediated delivery and GPs were early designated as a macrophage targeted delivery system [134,136,138]. In addition, GPs stimulate macrophages to secrete cytokines such as TNF-α, monocyte chemotactic protein-1 (MCP-1), and IL-6 [139]. These proinflammatory cytokines can potentially link the activation of both innate and adaptive immunity.

The potential adjuvant effect was extensively studied using ovalbumin (OVA) trapped with yeast RNA through electrostatic interactions within GPs following repeated SC administrations in mice [128,129,135] which showed robust and long-lasting antigen-specific humoral and T cell responses were consistently observed. Specifically, GP-OVA induced secretion of Th1-associated IgG2c anti-OVA antibodies and induced strong humoral and Th1- and Th17-biased CD4+ T cell responses. In contrast, mice that received OVA admixed with alum predominantly exhibited IgG1 antibody responses [140], consistent with alum being a poor stimulator of T cell responses. Consistently, heat-killed *Saccharomyces cerevisiae* genetically engineered to express antigens are undergoing clinical trials as immunotherapeutic vaccines for chronic infections such as HBV [141–143]. However, because yeast proteins, lipids, and nucleic acids are not eliminated, concerns regarding reactogenicity and autoimmunity could limit the appeal of this platform as a preventive vaccine given to predominantly healthy people [93]. GlobeImmune's Tarmogen immunotherapy platform consists of intact, heat-inactivated yeast containing a target protein. Those vaccines elicit immune-mediated killing of target cells expressing viral and cancer antigens *in vivo* via a CD8+ mediated mechanism. Tarmogens are not neutralized by host immune responses and can be administered repeatedly to boost antigen-specific immunity. Tarmogens are a versatile technology for the treatment of chronic hepatitis B and C and showed to be well tolerated and immunogenic in phase 1 and 2 clinical trials encompassing >600 subjects [144]. Overall, β-glucans intrinsic properties increased the interest of their use for vaccine development as better demonstrated elsewhere [11].

8.12 Summary

The development of novel vaccine adjuvants, together with an optimized antigen delivery platform is becoming as important as the discovery of novel antigens for new vaccines. This idea is especially true for the new generation of antigens, including those identified through genomic screening of microorganisms (recombinant purified proteins, mRNA, and DNA) but often poorly immunogenic. Additionally, increasingly scientific evidence of the advantages associated with the production of antigen-specific sIgA, especially for the microorganisms that invade the body through mucosal surfaces, strongly supports the necessity to have new adjuvants to use in oral and intranasal vaccines.

Among the numerous examples being studies by the scientific community, this text highlights the particulate adjuvants produced with carbohydrate biopolymers, the chitosan, and the glucan. Due to its unique properties, the use of these polymers in vaccinology became and is being a research subject of considerable interest.

References

[1] van Montfoort N, van der Aa E, Woltman AM. Understanding MHC class I presentation of viral antigens by human dendritic cells as a basis for rational design of therapeutic vaccines. Front Immunol 2014;5:182.

[2] McNeela EA, Mills KH. Manipulating the immune system: humoral versus cell-mediated immunity. Adv Drug Deliv Rev 2001;51(1-3):43–54.

[3] Kara EE, et al. Tailored immune responses: novel effector helper T cell subsets in protective immunity. PLoS Pathog 2014;10(2):e1003905.

[4] Raphael I, et al. T cell subsets and their signature cytokines in autoimmune and inflammatory diseases. Cytokine 2015;74(1):5–17.

[5] Lambert PH, Liu M, Siegrist CA. Can successful vaccines teach us how to induce efficient protective immune responses? Nat Med 2005;11(4 Suppl):S54–62.

[6] Veldhoen M. Interleukin 17 is a chief orchestrator of immunity. Nat Immunol 2017;18(6):612–21.

[7] Fehres CM, et al. Understanding the biology of antigen cross-presentation for the design of vaccines against cancer. Front Immunol 2014;5:149.

[8] Desmet CJ, Ishii KJ. Nucleic acid sensing at the interface between innate and adaptive immunity in vaccination. Nat Rev Immunol 2012;12(7):479–91.

[9] WHO. Health topics—immunization. 2017. http://www.who.int/topics/immunization/en/.

[10] Moyle PM, Toth I. Modern subunit vaccines: development, components, and research opportunities. ChemMedChem, 2013;8(3):360–76.

[11] Cordeiro AS, Alonso MJ, de la Fuente M. Nanoengineering of vaccines using natural polysaccharides. Biotechnol Adv 2015;33(6 Pt 3):1279–93.

[12] Karch CP, Burkhard P. Vaccine technologies: from whole organisms to rationally designed protein assemblies. Biochem Pharmacol, 2016;120:1–14.

[13] Reed SG, et al. New horizons in adjuvants for vaccine development. Trends Immunol 2009;30(1):23–32.

[14] Khan KH. DNA vaccines: roles against diseases. Germs 2013;3(1):26–35.

[15] Hasson SSAA, Al-Busaidi JKZ, Sallam TA. The past, current and future trends in DNA vaccine immunisations. Asian Pacific J Trop Biomed 2015;5(5):344–53.

[16] Saade F, Petrovsky N. Technologies for enhanced efficacy of DNA vaccines. Expert Rev Vaccines 2012;11(2):189–209.

[17] Bonam SR, et al. An overview of novel adjuvants designed for improving vaccine efficacy. Trends Pharmacol Sci 2017;38(9):771–93.

[18] Ingolotti M, et al. DNA vaccines for targeting bacterial infections. Expert Rev Vaccines 2010;9(7):747–63.

[19] Hardee CL, et al. Advances in non-viral DNA vectors for gene therapy. Genes (Basel) 2017;8(2):65.

[20] Zhang M, et al. Polymers for DNA vaccine delivery. ACS Biomater Sci Eng 2017;3(2):108–25.

[21] Yin H, et al. Non-viral vectors for gene-based therapy. Nat Rev Genet 2014;15(8):541–55.

[22] Gao Y, et al. Highly branched Poly(beta-amino esters) for non-viral gene delivery: high transfection efficiency and low toxicity achieved by increasing molecular weight. Biomacromolecules 2016;17(11):3640–7.
[23] Agarwal S, et al. PDMAEMA based gene delivery materials. Materials Today 2012;15(9):388–393.
[24] Andorko JI, et al. Intrinsic immunogenicity of rapidly-degradable polymers evolves during degradation. Acta Biomater 2016;32:24–34.
[25] Bos GW, et al. Cationic polymers that enhance the performance of HbsAg DNA in vivo. Vaccine 2004;23(4):460–9.
[26] Qu C, et al. Monocyte-derived dendritic cells: targets as potent antigen-presenting cells for the design of vaccines against infectious diseases. Int J Infect Dis 2014;19:1–5.
[27] Ramon G. Sur l'augmentation anormale de l'antitoxine chez les chevaux producteurs de sérum antidiphtérique. Bull Soc Centr Med Vet 1925;101:227–34.
[28] Lee S, Nguyen MT. Recent advances of vaccine adjuvants for infectious diseases. Immune Netw 2015;15(2):51–7.
[29] Chauhan N, et al. An overview of adjuvants utilized in prophylactic vaccine formulation as immunomodulators. Expert Rev Vaccines 2017;16(5):491–502.
[30] EMEA. Guideline On Adjuvants in Vaccines For Human Use. London, UK: EMEA; 2005. C.F.M.P.F.H. USE and [CHMP], Editors.
[31] Glenny AT, et al. The antigenic value of toxoid precipitated by potassium-alum. J Pathol Bacteriol 1926;29:38–4510.
[32] Powell BS, Andrianov AK, Fusco PC. Polyionic vaccine adjuvants: another look at aluminum salts and polyelectrolytes. Clin Exp Vaccine Res 2015;4(1):23–45.
[33] Mohsen MO, et al. Major findings and recent advances in virus-like particle (VLP)-based vaccines. Semin Immunol 2017;34:123–32.
[34] Cabral GA, et al. Cellular and humoral immunity in guinea pigs to two major polypeptides derived from hepatitis B surface antigen. J Gen Virol 1978;38(2):339–50.
[35] Lebre F, Hearnden CH, Lavelle EC. Modulation of immune responses by particulate materials. Adv Mater 2016;28(27):5525–41.
[36] Gutjahr A, et al. Biodegradable polymeric nanoparticles-based vaccine adjuvants for lymph nodes targeting. Vaccines (Basel) 2016;4(4):34.
[37] Sahdev P, Ochyl LJ, Moon JJ. Biomaterials for nanoparticle vaccine delivery systems. Pharm Res 2014;31(10):2563–82.
[38] Mutwiri G, et al. Combination adjuvants: the next generation of adjuvants?. Expert Rev Vaccines 2011;10(1):95–107.
[39] Didierlaurent AM, et al. AS04, an aluminum salt- and TLR4 agonist-based adjuvant system, induces a transient localized innate immune response leading to enhanced adaptive immunity. J Immunol 2009;183(10):6186–97.
[40] Ilyinskii PO, et al. Adjuvant-carrying synthetic vaccine particles augment the immune response to encapsulated antigen and exhibit strong local immune activation without inducing systemic cytokine release. Vaccine 2014;32(24):2882–95.
[41] Li P, Wang F. Polysaccharides: candidates of promising vaccine adjuvants. Drug Discov Ther 2015;9(2):88–93.
[42] Dalod M, et al. Dendritic cell maturation: functional specialization through signaling specificity and transcriptional programming. Embo J 2014;33(10):1104–16.
[43] Janeway Jr CA. How the immune system works to protect the host from infection: a personal view. Proc Natl Acad Sci U S A 2001;98(13):7461–8.

[44] Neutra MR, Kozlowski PA. Mucosal vaccines: the promise and the challenge. Nat Rev Immunol 2006;6(2):148–58.
[45] Bekiaris V, Persson EK, Agace WW. Intestinal dendritic cells in the regulation of mucosal immunity. Immunol Rev 2014;260(1):86–101.
[46] Lamichhane A, Azegami T, Kiyono H. The mucosal immune system for vaccine development. Vaccine 2014;32(49):6711–23.
[47] Holmgren J, Czerkinsky C. Mucosal immunity and vaccines. Nat Med 2005;11(4 Suppl): S45–53.
[48] Tokuhara D, et al. Secretory IgA-mediated protection against V. cholerae and heat-labile enterotoxin-producing enterotoxigenic Escherichia coli by rice-based vaccine. Proc Natl Acad Sci U S A, 2010;107(19):8794–9.
[49] Azizi A, et al. Enhancing oral vaccine potency by targeting intestinal M cells. PLoS Pathog 2010;6(11):e1001147.
[50] Czerkinsky C, Holmgren J. Mucosal delivery routes for optimal immunization: targeting immunity to the right tissues. Mucosal Vaccines: Modern Concepts, Strategies Challenges 2012;354:1–18.
[51] Shima H, et al. A novel mucosal vaccine targeting Peyer's patch M cells induces protective antigen-specific IgA responses. Int Immunol 2014;26(11):619–25.
[52] Gehring AJ. New treatments to reach functional cure: Rationale and challenges for emerging immune-based therapies. Best Pract Res Clin Gastroenterol 2017;31(3):337–45.
[53] McGhee JR, Fujihashi K. Inside the mucosal immune system. PLoS Biol 2012;10(9):e1001397.
[54] Kim SH, Jang YS. Antigen targeting to M cells for enhancing the efficacy of mucosal vaccines. Exp Mol Med 2014;46:e85.
[55] Jung C, Hugot JP, Barreau F. Peyer's patches: the immune sensors of the intestine. Int J Inflam 2010;2010:823710.
[56] Montilla NA, et al. Mucosal immune system: a brief review. Inmunología 2004;23(2):9.
[57] Lycke NY, Bemark M. The role of Peyer's patches in synchronizing gut IgA responses. Front Immunol 2012;3:329.
[58] Mabbott NA, et al. Microfold (M) cells: important immunosurveillance posts in the intestinal epithelium. Mucosal Immunol 2013;6(4):666–77.
[59] Wang M, et al. Roles of M cells in infection and mucosal vaccines. Hum Vaccin Immunother 2014;10(12):3544–51.
[60] Ohno H. Intestinal M cells. J Biochem 2016;159(2):151–60.
[61] Soares E, Borges O. Oral vaccination through Peyer's Patches: update on particle uptake. Curr Drug Deliv 2017;15(3):321–330.
[62] Lycke N. Recent progress in mucosal vaccine development: potential and limitations. Nat Rev Immunol 2012;12(8):592–605.
[63] Rice-Ficht AC, et al. Polymeric particles in vaccine delivery. Curr Opin Microbiol 2010;13(1):106–12.
[64] Kaur M, et al. Development and characterization of guar gum nanoparticles for oral immunization against tuberculosis. Drug Deliv 2014;22(3):328–334.
[65] Lee WJ, et al. Efficacy of thiolated eudragit microspheres as an oral vaccine delivery system to induce mucosal immunity against enterotoxigenic Escherichia coli in mice. Eur J Pharm Biopharm 2012;81(1):43–8.
[66] Borges O, et al. Evaluation of the immune response following a short oral vaccination schedule with hepatitis B antigen encapsulated into alginate-coated chitosan nanoparticles. Eur J Pharm Sci 2007;32(4-5):278–90.

[67] Singh B, et al. Combinatorial approach of antigen delivery using m cell-homing peptide and mucoadhesive vehicle to enhance the efficacy of oral vaccine. Mol Pharm 2015;12(11):3816–28.

[68] Primard C, et al. Traffic of poly(lactic acid) nanoparticulate vaccine vehicle from intestinal mucus to sub-epithelial immune competent cells. Biomaterials 2010;31(23):6060–8.

[69] Borges O, et al. Uptake studies in rat Peyer's patches, cytotoxicity and release studies of alginate coated chitosan nanoparticles for mucosal vaccination. J Control Release 2006;114(3):348–58.

[70] Garinot M, et al. PEGylated PLGA-based nanoparticles targeting M cells for oral vaccination. J Control Release 2007;120(3):195–204.

[71] Shakweh M, et al. Poly (lactide-co-glycolide) particles of different physicochemical properties and their uptake by peyer's patches in mice. Eur J Pharm Biopharm 2005;61(1-2):1–13.

[72] van der Lubben IM, et al. Chitosan microparticles for oral vaccination: preparation, characterization and preliminary in vivo uptake studies in murine Peyer's patches. Biomaterials 2001;22(7):687–94.

[73] Joshi G, Kumar A, Sawant K. Enhanced bioavailability and intestinal uptake of Gemcitabine HCl loaded PLGA nanoparticles after oral delivery. Eur J Pharm Sci 2014;60:80–9.

[74] Hooper LV, Macpherson AJ. Immune adaptations that maintain homeostasis with the intestinal microbiota. Nat Rev Immunol 2010;10(3):159–69.

]75] Kim SH, Jang YS. The development of mucosal vaccines for both mucosal and systemic immune induction and the roles played by adjuvants. Clin Exp Vaccine Res 2017;6(1):15–21.

[76] Singh B, et al. Attuning hydroxypropyl methylcellulose phthalate to oral delivery vehicle for effective and selective delivery of protein vaccine in ileum. Biomaterials 2015;59:144–59.

[77] Yeboah KG, et al. In vitro and ex vivo characterization of lectin-labeled Mycobacterium tuberculosis antigen-containing microspheres for enhanced oral delivery. J Drug Target 2014;22(1):34–47.

[78] De Smet R, et al. Beta-Glucan microparticles are good candidates for mucosal antigen delivery in oral vaccination. J Control Release 2013;172(3):671–8.

[79] Akalkotkar A, et al. Oral delivery of particulate prostate cancer vaccine: in vitro and in vivo evaluation. J Drug Target 2012;20(4):338–46.

[80] Chablani L, Tawde SA, D'Souza MJ. Spray-dried microparticles: a potential vehicle for oral delivery of vaccines. J Microencapsul 2012;29(4):388–97.

[81] McNeela EA, Lavelle EC. Recent advances in microparticle and nanoparticle delivery vehicles for mucosal vaccination. Curr Top Microbiol Immunol 2012;354:75–99.

[82] Shakya A, Nandakumar K. Polymers as immunological adjuvants: an update on recent developments. J BioSci Biotech 2012;1(3):199–210.

[83] Mottram PL, et al. Type 1 and 2 immunity following vaccination is influenced by nanoparticle size: formulation of a model vaccine for respiratory syncytial virus. Mol Pharm 2007;4(1):73–84.

[84] Shah RR, et al. The impact of size on particulate vaccine adjuvants. Nanomedicine (Lond) 2014;9(17):2671–81.

[85] Oyewumi MO, Kumar A, Cui Z. Nano-microparticles as immune adjuvants: correlating particle sizes and the resultant immune responses. Expert Rev Vaccines 2010;9(9):1095–107.

[86] De Smet R, Allais L, Cuvelier CA. Recent advances in oral vaccine development: yeast-derived beta-glucan particles. Hum Vaccin Immunother 2014;10(5):1309–18.

[87] Koppolu B, Zaharoff DA. The effect of antigen encapsulation in chitosan particles on uptake, activation and presentation by antigen presenting cells. Biomaterials 2013;34(9):2359–69.

[88] Shima F, Akagi T, Akashi M. Effect of hydrophobic side chains in the induction of immune responses by nanoparticle adjuvants consisting of amphiphilic Poly(gamma-glutamic acid). Bioconjug Chem 2015;26(5):890–8.

[89] Ulery BD, et al. Rational design of pathogen-mimicking amphiphilic materials as nanoadjuvants. Sci Rep 2011;1:198.

[90] Petersen LK, et al. Activation of innate immune responses in a pathogen-mimicking manner by amphiphilic polyanhydride nanoparticle adjuvants. Biomaterials 2011;32(28):6815–22.

[91] Fromen CA, et al. Controlled analysis of nanoparticle charge on mucosal and systemic antibody responses following pulmonary immunization. Proc Natl Acad Sci U S A 2015;112(2):488–93.

[92] Lebre F, Hearnden CH, Lavelle EC. Modulation of Immune Responses by Particulate Materials. Adv Mater 2016;28(27):5525–5541.

[93] Levitz SM, et al. Exploiting fungal cell wall components in vaccines. Semin Immunopathol 2015;37(2):199–207.

[94] Vilar G, Tulla-Puche J, Albericio F. Polymers and drug delivery systems. Curr Drug Deliv 2012;9(4):367–94.

[95] Migalovich-Sheikhet H, et al. Novel identified receptors on mast cells. Front Immunol 2012;3:238.

[96] Bueter CL, Specht CA, Levitz SM. Innate sensing of chitin and chitosan. PLoS Pathog 2013;9(1):e1003080.

[97] Vasiliev YM. Chitosan-based vaccine adjuvants: incomplete characterization complicates preclinical and clinical evaluation. Expert Rev Vaccines 2015;14(1):37–53.

[98] Periayah MH, Halim AS, Saad AZ. Chitosan: a promising marine polysaccharide for biomedical research. Pharmacogn Rev 2016;10(19):39–42.

[99] Bernkop-Schnurch A, Dunnhaupt S. Chitosan-based drug delivery systems. Eur J Pharm Biopharm 2012;81(3):463–9.

[100] Jabbal-Gill I, Watts P, Smith A. Chitosan-based delivery systems for mucosal vaccines. Expert Opin Drug Deliv 2012;9(9):1051–67.

[101] Artursson P, et al. Effect of chitosan on the permeability of monolayers of intestinal epithelial cells (Caco-2). Pharm Res 1994;11(9):1358–61.

[102] Sonaje K, et al. Opening of epithelial tight junctions and enhancement of paracellular permeation by chitosan: microscopic, ultrastructural, and computed-tomographic observations. Mol Pharm 2012;9(5):1271–9.

[103] Xia Y, et al. Chitosan-based mucosal adjuvants: Sunrise on the ocean. Vaccine 2015; 33(44):5997–6010.

[104] Wang S, et al. Intranasal and oral vaccination with protein-based antigens: advantages, challenges and formulation strategies. Protein Cell 2015;6(7):480–503.

[105] Bucarey SA, et al. Chitosan microparticles loaded with yeast-derived PCV2 virus-like particles elicit antigen-specific cellular immune response in mice after oral administration. Virol J 2014;11:149.

[106] Garcia-Fuentes M, Alonso MJ. Chitosan-based drug nanocarriers: where do we stand? J Control Release 2012;161(2):496–504.

[107] Lebre F, et al. Progress towards a needle-free hepatitis B vaccine. Pharm Res 2011;28(5):986–1012.

[108] Picola IPD, et al. Effect of ionic strength solution on the stability of chitosan–DNA nanoparticles. J Exp Nanosci 2012;8(5):703–16.

[109] Amaduzzi F, et al. Chitosan-DNA complexes: charge inversion and DNA condensation. Colloids Surf B Biointerfaces 2014;114:1–10.

[110] Calvo P, et al. Chitosan and chitosan/ethylene oxide-propylene oxide block copolymer nanoparticles as novel carriers for proteins and vaccines. Pharm Res 1997;14(10):1431–6.
[111] Borges O, et al. Induction of lymphocytes activated marker CD69 following exposure to chitosan and alginate biopolymers. Int J Pharm 2007;337(1-2):254–64.
[112] Bakhru SH, et al. Oral delivery of proteins by biodegradable nanoparticles. Adv Drug Deliv Rev 2013;65(6):811–21.
[113] Neumann S, et al. Activation of the NLRP3 inflammasome is not a feature of all particulate vaccine adjuvants. Immunol Cell Biol 2014;92(6):535–42.
[114] Premaletha K, et al. Formulation, characterization and optimization of hepatitis B surface antigen (HBsAg)-loaded chitosan microspheres for oral delivery. Pharm Dev Technol 2012;17(2):251–8.
[115] Verma AK, et al. Vitamin B12 grafted layer-by-layer liposomes bearing HBsAg facilitate oral immunization: effect of modulated biomechanical properties. Mol Pharm 2016;13(7):2531–42.
[116] Huo Z, et al. Induction of protective serum meningococcal bactericidal and diphtheria-neutralizing antibodies and mucosal immunoglobulin A in volunteers by nasal insufflations of the Neisseria meningitidis serogroup C polysaccharide-CRM197 conjugate vaccine mixed with chitosan. Infect Immun 2005;73(12):8256–65.
[117] Atmar RL, et al. Norovirus vaccine against experimental human Norwalk Virus illness. N Engl J Med 2011;365(23):2178–87.
[118] Neimert-Andersson T, et al. Evaluation of safety and efficacy as an adjuvant for the chitosan-based vaccine delivery vehicle ViscoGel in a single-blind randomised Phase I/IIa clinical trial. Vaccine 2014;32(45):5967–74.
[119] Goodridge HS, Wolf AJ, Underhill DM. Beta-glucan recognition by the innate immune system. Immunol Rev 2009;230(1):38–50.
[120] Wang Q, et al. Beta-Glucans: relationships between modification, conformation and functional activities. Molecules 2017;22(2).
[121] Sonck E, et al. Varying effects of different beta-glucans on the maturation of porcine monocyte-derived dendritic cells. Clin Vaccine Immunol 2011;18(9):1441–6.
[122] Devi KS, et al. Heteroglucan-dendrimer glycoconjugate: a modulated construct with augmented immune responses and signaling phenomena. Biochim Biophys Acta 2014;1840(9):2794–805.
[123] Chan GC, Chan WK, Sze DM. The effects of beta-glucan on human immune and cancer cells. J Hematol Oncol 2009;2:25.
[124] Goodridge HS, et al. Activation of the innate immune receptor Dectin-1 upon formation of a 'phagocytic synapse'. Nature 2011;472(7344):471–5.
[125] Lipinski T, et al. Enhanced immunogenicity of a tricomponent mannan tetanus toxoid conjugate vaccine targeted to dendritic cells via Dectin-1 by incorporating beta-glucan. J Immunol 2013;190(8):4116–28.
[126] Willment JA, et al. The human beta-glucan receptor is widely expressed and functionally equivalent to murine Dectin-1 on primary cells. Eur J Immunol 2005;35(5):1539–47.
[127] Carter RW, et al. Preferential induction of CD4+ T cell responses through in vivo targeting of antigen to dendritic cell-associated C-type lectin-1. J Immunol 2006;177(4):2276–84.
[128] Huang H, et al. Robust stimulation of humoral and cellular immune responses following vaccination with antigen-loaded beta-glucan particles. MBio 2010;1(3):e00164–10.
[129] Huang H, et al. Characterization and optimization of the glucan particle-based vaccine platform. Clin Vaccine Immunol 2013;20(10):1585–91.

[130] Dube A, et al. Multimodal nanoparticles that provide immunomodulation and intracellular drug delivery for infectious diseases. Nanomedicine 2014;10(4):831–8.
[131] Tam JM, et al. Use of fungal derived polysaccharide-conjugated particles to probe Dectin-1 responses in innate immunity. Integr Biol (Camb) 2012;4(2):220–7.
[132] Elder MJ, et al. Beta-glucan size controls dectin-1-mediated immune responses in human dendritic cells by regulating IL-1beta production. Front Immunol 2017;8:791.
[133] Ostroff GR., Drug delivery product and methods (International Patent No. WO/2006/007372A2). International Bureau 19.01.2006.
[134] Aouadi M, et al. Orally delivered siRNA targeting macrophage Map4k4 suppresses systemic inflammation. Nature 2009;458(7242):1180–4.
[135] Huang H, et al. Relative contributions of dectin-1 and complement to immune responses to particulate beta-glucans. J Immunol 2012;189(1):312–7.
[136] Soto ER, et al. Glucan particles for macrophage targeted delivery of nanoparticles. J Drug Deliv 2012;2012:143524.
[137] Soto ER, Ostroff GR. Characterization of multilayered nanoparticles encapsulated in yeast cell wall particles for DNA delivery. Bioconjug Chem 2008;19(4):840–8.
[138] Soto E, Ostroff GR. Oral macrophage targeted gene delivery sytem. NSTI-Nanotech 2007;2:378–381.
[139] Li B, et al. Yeast glucan particles activate murine resident macrophages to secrete proinflammatory cytokines via MyD88- and Syk kinase-dependent pathways. Clin Immunol 2007;124(2):170–81.
[140] Yanase N, et al. OVA-bound nanoparticles induce OVA-specific IgG1, IgG2a, and IgG2b responses with low IgE synthesis. Vaccine 2014;32(45):5918–24.
[141] Lok AS, et al. Randomized phase II study of GS-4774 as a therapeutic vaccine in virally suppressed patients with chronic hepatitis B. J Hepatol 2016;65(3):509–16.
[142] Gaggar A, et al. Safety, tolerability and immunogenicity of GS-4774, a hepatitis B virus-specific therapeutic vaccine, in healthy subjects: a randomized study. Vaccine 2014;32(39):4925–31.
[143] King TH, et al. A whole recombinant yeast-based therapeutic vaccine elicits HBV X, S and Core specific T cells in mice and activates human T cells recognizing epitopes linked to viral clearance. PLoS One 2014;9(7):e101904.
[144] King TH, et al. Construction and Immunogenicity Testing of Whole Recombinant Yeast-Based T-Cell Vaccines. Methods Mol Biol 2016;1404:529–45.

Part III

Assessment of vaccine efficacy and its delivery

Chapter 9

Circadian rhythmicity and vaccination

María Maximina Bertha Moreno-Altamirano[a], Jacqueline Oliva-Ramírez[b], Francisco Javier Sánchez-García[a]

[a]*Laboratorio de Inmunorregulación, Departamento de Inmunología, Escuela Nacional de Ciencias Biológicas, Instituto Politécnico Nacional, Mexico City, Mexico,* [b]*Translational Molecular Pathology, MD Anderson Cancer Center, Houston, TX, United States*

9.1 Circadian cycles

Back in the 18th century, studies on phototropism in plants and animal behavior showed 24 h periodicity [1]. Daily physiological oscillations were later dubbed as "circadian" from the latin *circa* (about) and *diem* (a day) [2,3]. These daily oscillations include hormone secretion, brain activity, such as sleep-wake timing, body temperature, renal activity, blood pressure, and immune system responses [4–10]. Disruption of circadian rhythmicity has a negative impact on human health; as such, there is a higher risk to develop atherosclerosis and cardiovascular alterations, as well as cancer in shift workers (Fig. 9.1) [11,12,13]. A cohort of 78,562 nurses during a 10 years follow-up showed an increased risk of breast cancer, and circadian rhythm disruption might be more important than clinical family history [13].

The master regulatory circadian clock is the suprachiasmatic nucleus (SCN), located within the ventral hypothalamus, where several neurons are activated by external cues or zeitgebers (time-givers) (Fig. 9.2) [14]. The most common zeitgeber is day-light and the stimulation of the retinohypothalamic tract; light is received by the melanopsin-expressing retinal ganglion cells, also known as intrinsically photoreceptive retinal ganglion cells (ipRGCs) and transduced to the SCN neurons [15–17]. Experimental ablation of SNC in animals induced an arrhythmic behavior when under constant darkness, as compared to that in wild-type animals [18]. Furthermore, the rest/activity periods were delayed, as well as body temperature, indicating that the SNC dictates the length of the biological day/night switch [18,19]. In rodents, a lesion or ablation of the SNC disrupts the cyclic secretion of adrenal corticosterone [20] or impairs gonads development by an abnormal pituitary-gonadal axis [21,22]. Other studies indicate that transplantation of a healthy SNC to rats with damaged SNC recovers their circadian rhythmicity [23,24]. Retina-cells cultured in vitro show increased secretion of

System Vaccinology. https://doi.org/10.1016/B978-0-323-85941-7.00007-3

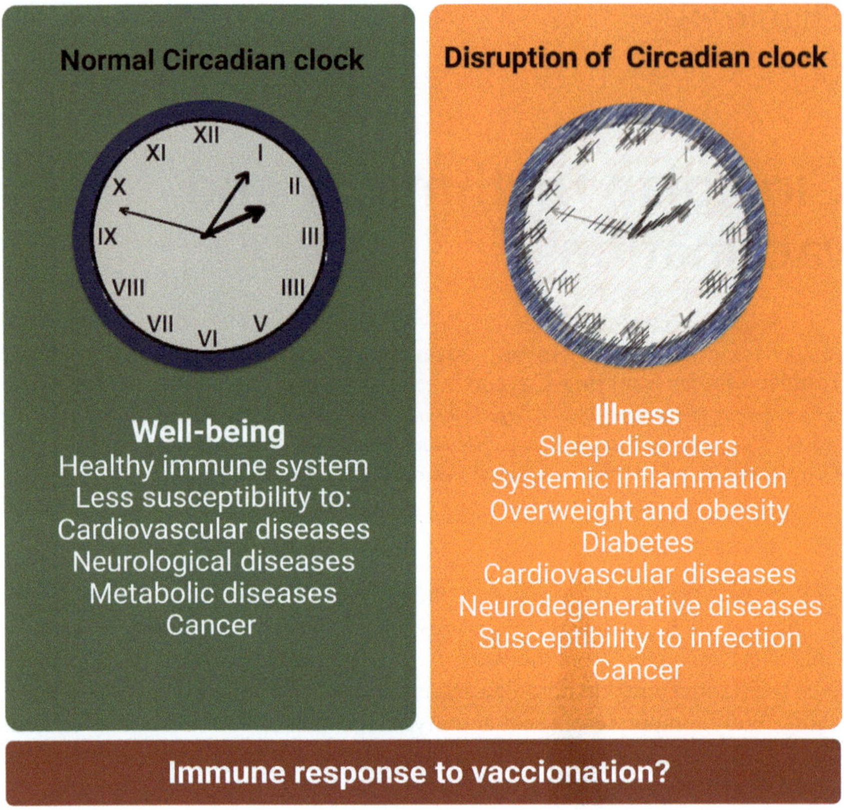

FIG. 9.1 Normal versus disrupted circadian clock.

melatonin [25], a hormone that in mammals is produced during the night by the pineal gland [26,27]. The main function of this *hormone of darkness* is to inhibit the SNC during the sleep period and to control the autonomous sympathetic nervous system [26,28]. Most of the physiological functions related to these brain functions are downregulated during the sleep period, such as urine production rate, body temperature, alertness, and blood pressure [29,30]. Rhythmicity in the levels of melatonin regulates sleep-wake behavior and inhibits the activity of the SNC at night-time [31]. Interestingly, in a small cohort of blind persons with no conscious perception of light, no loss in the ability to decrease plasma melatonin by bright light stimuli was observed, and still some individuals in this group retained a circadian response [32]. On the other hand, mice lacking retinal rods and cones photoreceptors showed no changes in their circadian behavior and responded normally to light, implying that the murine eye contains additional photoreceptors that regulate the circadian clock [33]. There are cues, other than light, also implicated in the control of rhythmic oscillations, notably, food intake and exercise [34–38]; moreover, environmental temperature can reset or synchronize the circadian cycle in homeothermic animals [39].

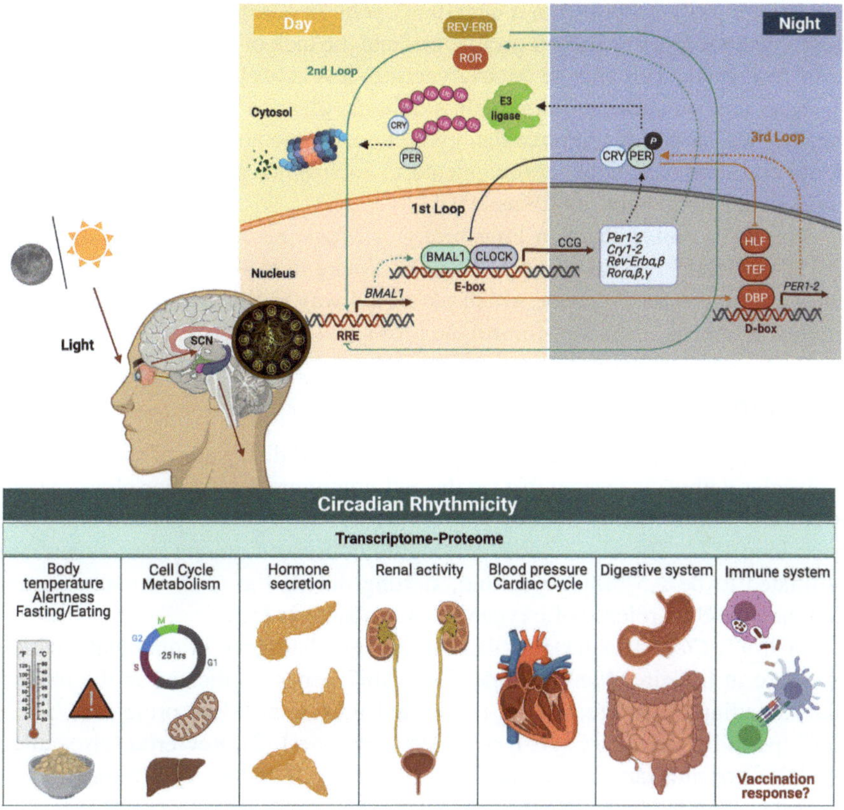

FIG. 9.2 The suprachiasmatic nucleus (*SCN*) is the master circadian clock.

General well-being is dependent on a fully functional circadian clock, disruption of circadian rhythmicity by genetic, physiological, environmental, or social factors compromise health.

SCN directs daily behavioral and physiological cycles including the immune response. Hence, circadian rhythmicity, or time of the day of vaccination, may have key roles in shaping the protective effect of vaccination.

It is estimated that ~10% of the whole transcriptome is controlled by the circadian cycle [40] and other physiological cycles such as the cardiac cycle [41,42] and the ovarian cycle [43] are better understood as circadian behaviors. In the murine oesophagus, the expression of cyclin A and DNA synthesis is higher during the night, thus implying that cell division follows a circadian cycle [44]. Furthermore, the DNA synthesis in the tongue, stomach, duodenum, jejunum, and rectum shows a delay of 6–8 h from tongue to rectum, suggesting that food intake-passage through the digestive system constitutes a circadian cue or zeitgeber [44,45]. The jejunum's metabolic enzymes, maltase, and sucrase [44], as well as insulin and 3-hydroxy-3-methylglutaryl coenzyme A reductase [46,47], and approximately 20% of the liver's secreted proteins [48] are differentially produced in a circadian cycle. In addition, 17% of the liver's lipidome undergoes circadian oscillations and the lack of clock genes regulation or of food intake can change the triglycerides levels [49].

Fatty acids oxidation, lipoprotein synthesis, glucose transporters, and some metabolites feedback the circadian cycle i.e., the metabolic pathways and the peripheral circadian cycle communicate to each other providing timed physiological harmony between tissues [50].

The 2017 Nobel Prize in Physiology or Medicine was awarded to Jeffrey C. Hall, Michael Rosbash, and Michael W. Young in recognition for their seminal work on circadian genes, which paved the way to the understanding of the molecular mechanisms that control the biological clocks.

9.2 Circadian clock

Over the past 20 years or so we have witnessed the discovery of the genes and molecular pathways responsible for the cell-autonomous circadian clock, which is currently described as a set of transcriptional factors autoregulated in a feedback loop [51]. The clock genes are highly conserved among species and are estimated to be 2.5 billion-year-old, starting during the great oxidation event and the circadian release of oxygen by cyanobacteria [52].

In 1997, *Clock* was the first discovered circadian gene in mammals, which is a core in the circadian network [53]. Other genes implicated in the molecular circadian clock are: *Bmal1* (brain and muscle arnt-like protein 1), *Per1*, *Per2* (period gene1, 2), *Cry1*, *Cry2* (Cryptochrome 1, 2), Rev-erbα (also called NR1D1/2 or nuclear receptor subfamily 1 group D) and *Rorα*/β (retinoic acid-related orphan receptor α/β) [54].

The circadian clock machinery is composed of three regulating loops (Fig. 9.2); the first one is formed by the transcriptional activator CLOCK dimerized with BMAL1, which binds to E-box elements and induces the gene expression of *Cry1*, *Cry2*, *Per1*, and *Per2*. The accumulated gene products repress CLOCK: BMAL1 transcription creating a negative feedback. This first loop takes around 24 h for PER and CRY to be ubiquitinated by E3 ubiquitin ligase complexes and degraded by proteasomes. The gradual proteolytic degradation during the day of CRY1, CRY2, and PER1 stops the repression of BMAL1-CLOCK to begin a new circadian cycle. In addition, CLOCK: BMAL1 dimer regulates other genes, such as *Nr1d1*, to produce REV-ERBα/β and form the second loop [55–57]. This product and the ROR (α/β/γ) receptors regulate the gene expression and transcription of BMAL1 and produce an antiphase *Per2* expression [58]. Finally, a third loop involves proline and acidic amino acid-rich basic leucine zipper proteins (PAR-bZip) family members: transcriptional activator albumin D-box binding protein (DBP), thyrotroph embryonic factor (TEF), and hepatic leukaemia factor (HLF). Likewise, DBP has been demonstrated to activate the *Per1* transcription through D-box gene regulation [56,59]. Interestingly, most of the proteins from the clock machinery are closely related or regulated by metabolic signals. The adenosine monophosphate-activated protein kinase (AMPK) phosphorylates and destabilizes CRY1 [55]. The poly ADP-ribose polymerase 1 (PARP-1) member of PARP family enzymes can poly ADP-ribosylate CLOCK and regulate the heterodimer activation with PER2 and CRYs [60]. In addition, post-translational modifications of clock proteins such as acetylation, methylation, phosphorylation, ubiquitination, and SUMOylation, also regulate the circadian clock; an example of this is that the dimerization of CLOCK/BMAL1 is enhanced, promoted, and stabilized by the phosphorylation of CLOCK and that the sub-nuclear relocation is caused by the SUMOylation of BMAL1 [61].

Several mutations in clock genes are associated with sleep disorders, such as in the familial advanced sleep phase disorder [62], schizophrenia [63], or depression [64]. A missense mutation in the casein kinase binding site of the *Per2* gene results in deficient phosphorylation, impairing degradation, and accumulation of its product within the nucleus; a missense mutation in the flavin binding domain of the *Cry2* gene, promotes the proteasomal degradation of its product. In the SCN, these clock genes are timely expressed following a circadian cycle [65].

Per1 and *Per2* mRNAs are rhythmically expressed outside the brain, in the liver, testis, heart, and skeletal muscle of BALB/C mice [66], and the peripheral expression of clock genes is conserved in different cell types. However, experimental jet-lag studies carried on *Per1*-luciferase transgenic rats showed that the SCN adapts faster to light-dark changes than peripheral tissues [67]. Moreover, when the time of feeding is changed during the light period, the SNC remains unaffected, but the liver is affected by this cue, and other studies report a synchronizing in peripheral organs [34,67]. Changes in the circadian cycles have a detrimental effect on human health; sleep-wake cycle under dim light and misalignment of fasting/feeding rhythmicity, are associated with a pre-diabetic condition characterized by high blood pressure, increased plasma insulin and glucose, decreased leptin levels [68] or impaired immunity [69].

Deletion of *Bmal1*, a master regulator of circadian cycle, can induce hypoglycemia [70], impaired glucose tolerance [71,72], cardiomyopathy [73], decrease fertility [74], obesity [75], and other pathologies.

9.3 Circadian rhythmicity and immunity

Circadian rhythmicity plays a key role in the regulation of human physiology [76], accordingly, its disruption leads to the loss of wellbeing, susceptibility to infection, and overt disease; these conditions include, sleep disorders, systemic inflammation, overweight and obesity, diabetes, cardiovascular and neuronal diseases, and cancer [71,77–83].

One of the first observations on the effect of time of the day fluctuations on immune responses was that peripheral blood leukocyte counts oscillated along the day, both in humans and mice [84,85], at a time when the molecular basis of circadian rhythmicity had not yet been unveiled. These early observations were

TABLE 9.1 Circadian rhythmicity and immunity.

Circadian rhythmicity	References
Peripheral blood leukocytes count	[84,85,86]
Leukocyte migration to peripheral organs	[93,94,95]
Expression of chemokine receptors	[89,91]
Expression of adhesion molecules	[91]
DCs migration to lymph nodes	[125]
Neutrophil infiltration into the liver	[88]
Monocytes infiltration into the heart	[90]
Macrophages gene expression	[96,110,111]
Monocytes/macrophages phagocytic and bactericidal activity and secretion of pro-inflammatory cytokines	[10,96,105, 106]
Expression of TLRs	[97]
TLRs-dependent cell response to ligands	[97]
Pro-inflammatory cytokines synthesis	[117]
NK cells cytotoxic activity	[104]
Lymphocyte counts in lymph nodes	[125]
T lymphocyte proliferation in response to TCR activation	[107]
T cell activation molecules and related signaling pathways	[144]
Granzyme and perforin levels	[104]
Th1 and Th17 cell differentiation	[101,109]
Aging neutrophils migration to bone marrow	[87]
Response to vaccination	[144,146–149]

followed by more detailed studies on the crosstalk between circadian rhythmicity and immunity, and the role of specific circadian clock proteins (Table 9.1). It is currently known that neutrophil blood counts oscillate in a circadian manner [86] and, very interestingly, that aging blood neutrophils ($CD62L^{low}$ $CXCR4^{high}$) migrate to the bone marrow at the end of the resting period in mice, where they are cleared by macrophages. The latter, in turn, triggers cholesterol-sensing nuclear receptors signaling that promote reductions in the size and function of the hematopoietic niche and the release of hematopoietic stem and progenitor cells. In this way, neutrophils regulate the homeostatic trafficking pattern of hematopoietic precursors and allow synchronization of immune and hematopoietic circadian rhythmicity [87]. Moreover, circadian rhythmic neutrophil infiltration into the liver modulates the expression of hepatic clock genes, such as hepatocyte *Bmal1*, through the secretion of neutrophil elastase; likewise, in vitro exposure of mouse hepatocytes to freshly isolated neutrophils but not to T or B lymphocytes, or macrophages, increases the hepatocyte expression of the clock genes *Bmal1* and *Clock* thus suggesting a neutrophil-hepatocyte communication that controls hepatocyte clock-gene expression [88].

Other immune cells like monocytes, also show maximal and minimal counts at the resting and active phases, respectively, due in part to the circadian expression of migratory factors [89]; the expression of the CCR2 receptor in circulating monocytes, for instance, is higher in the evening than in the morning, and correlates with higher infiltration of these cells into the heart [90].

As for neutrophils, these cells express differentially the adhesion molecules CD11a, ICAM-1, and L-selectin (CD62L), as well as the chemokine receptor, CXCR4, following a circadian pattern [91].

The homeostasis in the number of circulating immune cells may vary between cell subpopulations. In this regard, it has been shown that several days of sleep restriction increase the total numbers of circulating monocytes, neutrophils, and lymphocytes, and although the counts of monocytes and lymphocytes return to baseline levels after a single night of recovery sleep, neutrophil counts remain higher even 7 days after recovery sleep [92].

Deletion of the core clock gene *Bmal1*, in mice, results in the abolition of time of the day regulation in the number of circulating hematopoietic stem and progenitor cells and in leukocyte migration to peripheral organs [93–95]. In this regard, several immune cell types and lymphoid organs, tested to date, harbor functional circadian clocks [96,97].

As a whole, the numbers and cell types of circulating and tissue-resident cells (thymus, spleen, lymph node, liver, skin, gut, lung, and Peyer's patches) at a given time point depend on the highly tissue-specific temporal expression of adhesion molecules such as ICAM-1, ICAM-2, VCAM-1, and P-selectin, the initial points of contacts for leukocytes in the emigration process, as well as on the expression of chemokine receptors, such as CCR2, CCR7, CXCR4, and CXCR5, which vary among subsets, highlighting a unique rhythmic molecular signature for each cell lineage, as recently shown [89].

On the other hand, the retinoid acid receptor (RAR)-related orphan receptors RORα and RORγt are critical for the development of type 2 and type 3 innate lymphoid cells [98,99]. RORα promotes *Bmal1* transcription, and thus it maintains circadian rhythmicity [100] whereas the expression of RORγt is indirectly regulated by RORγ, a component of the transcriptional network of peripheral circadian clocks [101,102].

The response of NK cells to stimulating signals and their cytotoxic activity exhibits circadian rhythmicity, and disruption of *Per2* leads to the significant decrease of granzyme B and perforin levels [103,104].

The phagocytic and bactericidal activities of monocytes/macrophages as well as their capacity to secrete proinflammatory cytokines, such as TNF-α and IL-6, seem to follow a circadian rhythm pattern; however, differences among in vitro, ex vivo, and in vitro experimental conditions can be observed [10,96,105,106].

T lymphocytes proliferation in response to the engagement of their T cell receptor (TCR) shows a daily variation, which is dependent on the circadian rhythmic expression of the tyrosine kinase, ZAP70, a signaling protein immediately downstream of the TCR [107]. There is some controversy regarding the role of the clock protein, REV-ERBα, on Th17 cells. Yu et al. showed that *Nfil3* suppresses Th17 cell development by directly repressing RORγt transcription and REV-ERBα directly represses *Nfil3* transcription, even though that REV-ERBα is a positive regulator of TH17 cell differentiation [101]. Since REV-ERBα and its close homolog, REV-ERBβ, are components of the circadian clock circuitry by negatively regulating the circadian clock primary activators BMAL1 and CLOCK, these authors conclude that Th17 cell differentiation is regulated by the circadian clock [101]. On the other hand, Amir et al. showed that during naive CD4+ T cells differentiation into Th1, Th2, Th17, or inducible T regulatory cells (iTregs), REV-ERBα, but not REV-ERBβ, was upregulated at the mRNA level only in TH17 cells, acting as a negative regulator of pro-inflammatory Th17 cell development and autoimmunity, by competing with RORγt, thus, repressing RORγt-dependent genes, including Il17a [108]. More recently, Inokawa et al. using a chronic circadian misalignment-conditioned mouse model (non-adjustive light–dark shift condition, specifically a 8-h phase advance every 4 days), found that, in LN cells cultured under conditions favoring differentiation into either Th1, Th2, and Th17 cells, differentiation of IL-17A+ Th17 cells was elevated, and that IFNγ+ Th1 cells tended toward elevation, but not significantly, whereas IL-4+ Th2 cells remained unchanged, suggesting that chronic circadian misalignment accelerates T cell senescence and enrichment of Th17 and Th1 cells [109].

In addition to the circadian nature of immune cells tissue homing and cell effector functions, it is estimated that approximately 8% of the macrophage genes, among them a number of regulators of pathogen clearance [96] and at least 40% of protein-coding genes, in a tissue-specific manner, are expressed in a circadian fashion [110,111] many of which could regulate innate as well as adaptive immune responses.

9.4 Circadian rhythmicity and infection

Right at the beginning of Swann´s way, Remembrance of things past, volume one, Marcel Proust wrote:

> *"For a long time I used to go to bed early. Sometimes, when I had put out my candle, my eyes would close so quickly that I had not even time to say I'm going to sleep. And half an hour later the thought that it was time to go to sleep would awaken me [...] I would lay my cheeks gently against the comfortable cheeks of my pillow, as plump and blooming as the cheeks of babyhood. Or I would strike a match to look at my watch. Nearly midnight. The hour when an invalid, who has been obliged to start on a journey and to sleep in a strange hotel, awakens in a moment of illness and sees with glad relief a streak of daylight shewing under his*

bedroom door. Oh, joy of joys! it is morning. The servants will be about in a minute: he can ring, and some one will come to look after him. The thought of being made comfortable gives him strength to endure his pain. He is certain he heard footsteps: they come nearer, and then die away. The ray of light beneath his door is extinguished. It is midnight; some one has turned out the gas; the last servant has gone to bed, and he must lie all night in agony with no one to bring him any help" [112].

This lively literary account of life and illness resembles the fact of circadian clock misalignment as a result of infection.

Pathogen infection triggers an inflammatory response, characterized by the synthesis and release of pro-inflammatory cytokines [113,114]. The lipopolysaccharide (LPS), an endotoxin from gram-negative bacteria, has largely been used as a mice model of septic shock, a leading cause of death from infection [114,115]. Interestingly enough, the administration of LPS delays the phase of circadian rhythm in mice by -43+/-10 minutes during the early subjective night [116], and induces mortality, depending on the time of administration, partly due to the higher production of IL-1, IL-6, MCP-1, and MIP1 [117]. Moreover, the administration of LPS at the beginning of the active period in rats (night) induces more severe responses in temperature and cytokines than at resting time (morning), and this correlates with increased SCN basal neuronal activity, thus showing a direct influence of inflammation on the central master clock [118].

Three recent comprehensive reviews highlight the impact of infectious agents on circadian rhythmicity [119–121]. Of note, the course of experimental infection with bacteria, such as *Salmonella enterica* serovar Thyphimurium [119,120,122], *Listeria monocytogenes* [119,120,123], *Streptococcus pneumoniae* [119,120,124], *Helicobacter pylori* [119,120,125], and *Chlamydia spp.* [119,120,126], was always dependent on time of the day, in terms of bacterial colonization, proinflammatory response, effector immune cells recruitment, bacterial clearance, and incidence of histopathological signs. Ablation of clock genes, such as *Clock* in the study with *S. enterica* [122] or *Bmal1* in the study with *L. monocytogenes* [123] abolishes the time effect on infection, and there is a correlation between effector cell recruitment and bacterial colonization: a lower colonization of the spleen by *L. monocytogenes* correlates with maximal recruitment of inflammatory monocytes at ZT 8 [123], and *S. pneumoniae* burden is lower at ZT12, concurrent with the peak of neutrophils recruitment [124].

Viruses are obligate intracellular organisms and therefore unable to complete their life cycle without exploiting the machinery of a suitable host and they have evolved mechanisms to ensure replication and to avoid the immune system. One such mechanism is the subversion of circadian cycles and clock genes involved in antiviral defence.

Dengue virus (DENV), for instance, increases the amplitude of rhythmic movement in the *Aedes aegypti* mosquito, perhaps as a way to increase the vector's capacity to transmit the dengue virus to other humans [127]; about 70% of adults living with human immunodeficiency virus (HIV) do experience sleep difficulties, as compared to 30% prevalence of insomnia among U.S. adults [128] and, interestingly, mean levels of serum melatonin have been shown to be significantly lower in HIV-1-infected individuals as compared to healthy controls and, within the HIV-1 positive individuals, the lower the melatonin levels the more severe the clinical status [129]. Considering that the circadian rhythm of pineal melatonin is the best marker of internal time under low ambient light levels and that endogenous melatonin rhythm is closely associated with the endogenous circadian component of the sleep propensity rhythm [130], it follows that HIV-1 may disrupt circadian rhythmicity.

On the other hand, clock genes expression is subjected to seasonal changes and so Bmal1 expression reaches its lowest values in winter, contributing to the high occurrence of respiratory viral diseases [131]; likewise, deletion of the core clock gene, Bmal1, or environmental disruption of the circadian function by jet-lag exacerbate acute viral bronchiolitis caused by the Sendai virus (SeV) and the influenza A virus (IAV) in mice [132].

Murid Herpesvirus 4 replication is 10-fold higher in mice infected at the onset of the resting phase (ZT0; lights on) as compared to viral replication in mice infected just before their active phase (ZT10); this effect is dependent on a functional clock, since Bmal1–/– mice exhibited high levels of MuHV-4 infection when inoculated at either time of day. In addition, loss of Bmal1 also significantly augments Influenza A virus (IAV) replication [133]. Moreover, the time of day of IAV infection determines the outcome of influenza infection; being the worse outcome when mice are infected just prior to their active phase (ZT11), this correlates with increased cellularity in broncho-alveolar lavage, more severe lung injury and a distinct transcriptomic signature consistent with enhanced inflammation [134]. Edgar et al. analyzed IAV replication as a function of time of infection [133] whereas Sengupta et al. showed that the clock does not directly affect the pathogen burden, but the inflammatory process [134].

Some molecular clock proteins may exert a role on viral replication. In this regard, it has been shown that PER1 is a negative regulator that restricts HIV-1 replication in resting CD4+ T-cells in vitro and that *Per1* transcript levels in the peripheral blood mononuclear cells of HIV-1 positive patients inversely correlate with viral loads and positively correlate with CD4+ T-cells counts in rapid progressors, but not in long-term non-progressors, suggesting that PER1 plays a role in the control of HIV-1 infection and disease progression in rapid progressors [135].

The circadian components, BMAL1 and REV-ERBα, influence several steps in the hepatitis C virus (HCV) life cycle, including particle entry into hepatocytes and RNA genome replication. Likewise, REV-ERB regulates HCV, DENV, and Zika virus (ZIKV) RNA replication by repressing stearoyl-CoA-desaturase, leading to 60% reduction in total cellular phosphatidic acid concentration, which is likely to induce a profound effect on cellular membranes [136].

Future research will allow us to understand better how viruses interact with the molecular clockwork to improve treatments of viral infections.

9.5 Aging, immunosenescence, and circadian rhythmicity

With age comes the gradual decline of most physiological processes, including the immune response, hence the term of immunosenescence. Whether immunosenescence can be delayed, therapeutically treated or reverted, is currently a matter of intensive research [137,138]. Meanwhile, it is widely recognized that the aging process is associated with the increased production of pro-inflammatory cytokines, leading to a condition of chronic low-grade inflammation, currently known as inflamm-ageing, which also helps to explain other age-related conditions like neurodegenerative diseases, cognitive decline, reduction in metabolic function [137,138], as well as atherothrombosis and cardiovascular disease [139]. In regard to the latter two conditions, it has been shown that platelets hyper-reactivity and the formation of larger thrombi in aged-frail adults and in old mice is dependent on TNF-α, a key aging-associated pro-inflammatory cytokine. In addition, platelets from old mice exhibit significant mitochondrial changes, characterized by elevated mitochondrial mass and increased oxygen consumption, as well as age-dependent metabolic profiles that may poise platelets for activation [139].

TNF-α is able to modify circadian rhythmicity, by reducing the expression of PER2 and REV-ERBα and increasing the expression and association between BMAL1 and RORα in rheumatoid synovial cells [138], and mitochondria, which appear to coordinate the communication among circadian rhythmicity, metabolism and the immune system [140], contribute, when mitochondria have a decline in quality and activity, to cellular senescence, chronic inflammation and decline in stem cell activity, all being hallmarks of aging [141], closing the Aging—Immunosenescence—Circadian Rhythmicity circuitry.

Aging disrupts circadian rhythmicity, and disruption of circadian rhythmicity accelerates immunosenescence. Adler et al. have shown, by comparing the hippocampal proteomes of young and middle-aged mice across two circadian cycles, that 214 proteins display circadian rhythms in abundance in the hippocampus of young mice, while only 23 proteins were rhythmic in middle-aged mice [83], and Inokawa et al. have shown that chronic circadian misalignment in mice accelerates T cell senescence and enrichment of Th1 and Th17 cells, contributing to inflammation and autoimmunity [109]. An aging genomic signature, shared by women and men, was recently described by Márquez et al., this includes declines in T cell functions, and increase in NK cells, memory CD8+ T cells, and monocyte cell functions, consistent with the characteristic decline of adaptive immunity and increased systemic inflammation during the aging process. However, after the age of 65, men exhibit a higher innate and pro-inflammatory activity and lower adaptive activity than women of the same age [142].

9.6 Time of the day immunization/vaccination and immune response

Charles A. Janeway Jr. first proposed a role of innate immunity in the priming of adaptive immune responses and the need for pattern recognition receptors (PRRs) in antigen presenting cells (APCs) for their activation [143]. It is now recognized that expression of PRRs, such as Toll like-receptors (TLRs) in APCs, follow a circadian rhythmic pattern: in a recent study, for instance, Silver et al. analysed the expression of eight *Tlr* mRNAs (Tlr-1 to Tlr-8) throughout 24 h in the adherent population of mice spleen cells, primarily composed of B cells, dendritic cells (DCs), and macrophages, all APCs. Their results showed that except for *Tlr2* and *Tlr5*, all other *Tlr* exhibit a circadian rhythmic expression; even more, except for TLR8, the rest of TLRs undergo daily variations in their response to stimulation with their respective ligands [97]. Antigen-bearing DCs migration to lymph nodes (LNs), as well as lymphocyte counts in LNs, also follows a circadian rhythmic pattern, suggesting a time-of-day dependence for adaptive immune responses [125]. In this regard, Nobis et al. have shown that antigen-specific CD8 T cell proliferative response to OVA vaccination, using a model of DCs loaded with the $OVA_{257-264}$ peptide antigen (DC-OVA), is higher in animals vaccinated in the middle of the day as compared to other time points, which correlates with higher T cell activation markers and related signaling pathways such as the AKT and mTOR pathway [144]. These authors showed also a time-of-the-day effect of vaccination on the capacity of T cells to fight a bacterial infection (*L. monocytogenes*-OVA); the CD8 T cell clock is essential for these time of vaccination effects [144]. Mice immunized with 4-hydroxy-3-nitrophenyl acetyl (NP) hapten conjugated with chicken γ-globulin (NP-CGG), exhibited higher titres of NP-specific IgM and IgG1 antibodies when mice had been immunized at ZT17, a time when lymphocyte numbers in LNs are at their peak, as compared to ZT5 immunization [145]. Taken together, these findings highlight how circadian rhythmicity controls the sequential events leading to an efficient adaptive immune response, from APCs activation, migration of both APCs and lymphocytes to LNs and other immune organs, T lymphocyte activation, cell proliferation and, anti-microbial capacity. Although growing experimental evidence in mouse models strongly suggests that effective vaccination is time of the day dependent, human clinical trials of vaccination in a circadian rhythmicity setting are still scarce.

In an early study, published in 2003, two groups of healthy humans ($n = 19$) not previously infected with hepatitis A virus (HAV) were vaccinated with inactivated HAV in the morning (0900 h). On the day of vaccination, one group had regular sleep whereas the other stayed awake and did not sleep before 2100 h on the following day. Four weeks later, anti-HAV antibody titers were almost twofold higher in the regular sleep group than the group that stayed awake. The authors attributed the difference to the release of immune-stimulating hormones such as growth hormone, prolactin, and dopamine during sleep [146]. In a larger (n =125) and longer time-framed study, the clinical protection for hepatitis B, as assessed by anti-hepatitis B surface antigen IgG titers, was evaluated 6 months after the standard 3-dose hepatitis B vaccination series had been completed; regression analyses showed correlation between sleep duration during the course of the study and the IgG response, the shorter the sleep duration the lower the IgG titers [147]. Although these studies have evident experimental design differences and only indirectly analyzed the role of circadian clocks, both are indicative that circadian rhythmicity influences postvaccine protection.

In a randomized trial in humans, influenza vaccination elicited a higher titer of antibodies against H1N1A but not to H1N1B or H3N2A strains when the vaccine was administered in the morning rather than in the afternoon [148,149].

Münch et al. observed that enhancing daily light exposure increases the antibody response to influenza vaccination. In their study, a group of dementia patients with long-term brighter daytime light exposure (> 392.65 lux) showed significantly greater circadian interdaily stability and higher relative amplitude of circadian rest-activity cycles along with higher antibody production in response to the influenza A virus strain N3H2 (but not to influenza A virus strain H1N1 or influenza B virus) than the patient group with lower bright light exposure (< 392.65 lux). Nevertheless, seroconversion and seroprotection rates showed that both light exposure groups were well protected against the three strains of influenza virus contained in the trivalent vaccine Fluarix. These authors suggest that the improved immune response associated with brighter light exposure may not only be due to increasing circadian stability but also to the light-induced positive emotions including improved mood, greater alertness, and quality of life [150].

Another report analyzed the impact of immunization time and sample collection time in two different groups, an elderly group of people older than 65 years ($n = 80$) and a group of younger individuals, with ages within 30 and 40 years ($n = 59$). The participants were vaccinated with the inactivated influenza vaccine either *ante meridiem* (8–12 am) or *post meridiem* (12–5 pm) and blood samples were collected at days 0, 7, 14, and, in some cases, up to 28 days, also at 8–12 am or 12–5 pm. Results showed differences in antibody titers, including those at baseline, depending on the time of vaccination and sample collection in the aged, but not the younger group. Moreover, a significant increase in IgG and IgM titres at day 7 post-vaccination was observed in the older but not in the younger group when samples were collected in the afternoon. These authors caution that sample collection time can affect the interpretation of vaccination trial outcomes and suggest that both timing of vaccination and sample collection should be recorded carefully in future vaccine trials [151].

A more recent study showed that BCG vaccination in the morning elicits a strong trained immunity phenotype, characterized by the enhanced synthesis of interleukin 1β (IL-1β) and tumor necrosis factor α (TNF-α) following in vitro stimulation of peripheral blood monocytes with *S. aureus*, 2 weeks and/or 3 months after BCG vaccination; in contrast, no induction of trained immunity was observed in the evening-vaccinated individuals. Likewise, specific

Mycobacterium tuberculosis IFN-γ responses were significantly higher in morning-vaccinated as compared to evening-vaccinated individuals, 3 months after BCG vaccination [152]. Although induction of innate immune training suggests a better protection against tuberculosis (TB), long-term TB protection in morning-vaccinated vs. evening-vaccinated individuals should clarify this matter.

9.7 Challenges, outstanding questions, and future directions

Modern living styles, which involve prolonged light exposure, shift-working schedules, transcontinental travel, and social jet lag, lead to circadian disruption. The latter, together with a high-fat diet, alcohol use (and abuse), and sedentary habits, compromise, for a significant proportion of the world population, the promising advantage of discovering/knowing "the most effective time of the day for vaccination."

For instance, indoor illumination is enough to reset the circadian clock [153], making it difficult to calculate the best time for vaccination, as a general rule. In addition, it is estimated that 16% of workers in the United States worked, during 2019, a non-daytime schedule, including those that had a rotating shift, a split shift, an irregular schedule, or some other schedule [154], affecting their circadian rhythmicity. Obesity, being a major health concern and regarded as a continuous low-grade inflammatory pathology [155], is related to disruption of circadian rhythms [156,157]. According to the WHO, worldwide obesity has nearly tripled since 1975; in 2016, more than 1.9 billion adults and over 340 million children and adolescents aged 5 to 19 years were overweight or obese [158]. Moreover, in 2019, 38 million children under the age of 5 were overweight or obese [158,159]. As a whole, these figures and considering that the current world population is estimated to be around 7.8 billion [160], it is likely that more than 25% of the world population has somehow a disrupted circadian rhythmicity, due solely to overweight/obesity. Alcoholism is yet another important health concern that also modifies circadian rhythmicity [161]. Alcohol-consuming individuals have lower expression of several clock genes, including *Clock, Bmal1, Per1, Per2, Cry1,* and *Cry2*, in peripheral blood immune cells [161,162].

Other important variables to take into account when addressing the role of circadian rhythmicity in vaccination and in searching for the most effective time of the day for vaccination is age and gender. Circadian functions change with age [83,163] and with age comes adaptation or remodeling (not necessarily detrimental) of the immune system, which is mostly associated with a chronic, sterile, low-grade inflammation, now called inflamm-aging [164]. Both immunosenescence and inflammaging coexist in the elderly and the ways to intervene on the aging immune system are currently underway [164,165]. In addition, age-related epigenomic changes associated with the immune function have been described. Interestingly, these epigenomic changes that are first evident around the late-thirties show similar timing and magnitude between sexes. However, genomic differences between sexes increase after age 65 [142].

Most vaccines are delivered at an early age, but the question is as to when a clear day/night circadian rhythm arises. Sleep in newborn infants is distributed throughout the day and night and diurnal sleep rhythms only begin to emerge at around 10–12 weeks after birth, when infants increasingly sleep during the night. However, an important proportion of infants are reported to experience sleep problems in the first 6 months of life [166,167]. Whether this determines vaccination outcomes remains to be investigated.

Virus and bacteria reprogram host cell metabolism for their replication and evasion of host immune responses [168,169]; metabolic requirements are different for viral (influenza virus strain A/WSN/33) versus bacterial (*L. monocytogenes* strain 10403s) infections. Of note, whereas glucose utilization is required for survival in models of viral inflammation, it is lethal in models of bacterial inflammation [170]. Whether viral and bacterial vaccines induce metabolic reprograming in the vaccine recipients is to be further analyzed; however, some studies already point to that direction. High-resolution metabolomics analyses have shown that post-vaccination (hantavirus vaccine, hantavax) antibody responses are associated with higher serum concentrations of cholesteryl nitrolinoleate, octanoyl-carnitine, tyrosine, ubiquinone-9, and benzoate in high responders, whereas increased serum concentrations of chenodeoxycholic acid and methyl palmitate are found in non-responders and in low responders [171]. In the context of circadian rhythmicity and vaccination, it is necessary to take into account that a number of metabolites present in several biological samples, such as serum, urine, and breath, have consistently revealed that circadian rhythmicity is prevalent in almost every tissue and metabolic pathway [172,173]. Hence, the immune response elicited by vaccination may be determined not only by circadian rhythmicity but also by metabolism and perhaps other variables, such as the host-microbiome [140]; other important factor is night shift work [174].

While it is clear that more studies are needed to understand fully the role of circadian rhythmicity on vaccination and to define the best (theoretical) time of the day for vaccination, it is also clear that a significant part of the world population is out of the circadian phase relative to the "normal," as a result of living styles, age, metabolic disorders, et cetera. This invites us to posit yet another question: Is it possible to exert some control on circadian rhythm previously to vaccination? We leave this an open question.

Acknowledgments

The authors thank Bruno Alejandro Aguilar-López for critical reading of the manuscript. Current work in the *Laboratorio de Inmunorregulación* is being funded by *Consejo Nacional de Ciencia y Tecnología* (grant 284602); *Secretaria de Investigación y Posgrado-IPN* (grant 2020-1688); and by the Global Challenges Research Fund Networks in Vaccines Research and Development, VALIDATE Network, co-funded by the MRC and BBSRC (grant P020). Figures were created using Biorender.

References

[1] Roenneberg T, Merrow M. Circadian clocks - the fall and rise of physiology. Nat Rev Mol Cell Biol 2005;6(12):965–71.

[2] Fu L, Lee CC. The circadian clock: pacemaker and tumour suppressor. Nat Rev Cancer 2003;3(5):350–61.

[3] Bollinger T, Schibler U. Circadian rhythms - from genes to physiology and disease. Swiss Med Wkly 2014;144:w13984.

[4] Spies CM, et al. Circadian rhythms in rheumatology–a glucocorticoid perspective. Arthritis Res Ther 2014;16(Suppl 2):S3.

[5] Dijk DJ, Czeisler CA. Contribution of the circadian pacemaker and the sleep homeostat to sleep propensity, sleep structure, electroencephalographic slow waves, and sleep spindle activity in humans. J Neurosci 1995;15(5 Pt 1):3526–38.

[6] Waterhouse J, et al. The circadian rhythm of core temperature: origin and some implications for exercise performance. Chronobiol Int 2005;22(2):207–25.

[7] Firsov D, Tokonami N, Bonny O. Role of the renal circadian timing system in maintaining water and electrolytes homeostasis. Mol Cell Endocrinol 2012;349(1):51–5.

[8] Douma LG, Gumz ML. Circadian clock-mediated regulation of blood pressure. Free Radic Biol Med 2018;119:108–14.

[9] Scheiermann C, et al. Clocking in to immunity. Nat Rev Immunol 2018;18(7):423–37.

[10] Oliva-Ramirez J, et al. Crosstalk between circadian rhythmicity, mitochondrial dynamics and macrophage bactericidal activity. Immunology 2014;143(3):490–7.

[11] Morris CJ, et al. Circadian misalignment increases cardiovascular disease risk factors in humans. Proc Natl Acad Sci USA, 2016;113(10):E1402–11.

[12] Morris CJ, et al. Circadian misalignment increases C-reactive protein and blood pressure in chronic shift workers. J Biol Rhythms 2017;32(2):154–64.

[13] Schernhammer ES, et al. Rotating night shifts and risk of breast cancer in women participating in the nurses' health study. J Natl Cancer Inst 2001;93(20):1563–8.

[14] Gregson N, et al. Pricing medicines: theory and practice, challenges and opportunities. Nat Rev Drug Discov 2005;4(2):121–30.

[15] Berson DM, Dunn FA, Takao M. Phototransduction by retinal ganglion cells that set the circadian clock. Science 2002;295(5557):1070–3.

[16] Bellingham J, et al. Evolution of melanopsin photoreceptors: discovery and characterization of a new melanopsin in nonmammalian vertebrates. PLoS Biol 2006;4(8):e254.

[17] Do MT, Yau KW. Intrinsically photosensitive retinal ganglion cells. Physiol Rev 2010;90(4):1547–81.

[18] Ralph MR, et al. Transplanted suprachiasmatic nucleus determines circadian period. Science 1990;247(4945):975–8.

[19] Ruby NF, et al. Ablation of suprachiasmatic nucleus alters timing of hibernation in ground squirrels. Proc Natl Acad Sci USA, 1996;93(18):9864–8.

[20] Moore RY, Eichler VB. Loss of a circadian adrenal corticosterone rhythm following suprachiasmatic lesions in the rat. Brain Res 1972;42(1):201–6.

[21] Mosko S, Moore RY. Neonatal suprachiasmatic nucleus ablation: absence of functional and morphological plasticity. Proc Natl Acad Sci USA, 1978;75(12):6243–6.

[22] Mosko SS, Moore RY. Neonatal ablation of the suprachiasmatic nucleus. Effects on the development of the pituitary-gonadal axis in the female rat. Neuroendocrinology 1979;29(5): 350–61.

[23] Sujino M, et al. Suprachiasmatic nucleus grafts restore circadian behavioral rhythms of genetically arrhythmic mice. Curr Biol 2003;13(8):664–8.

[24] Aguilar-Roblero R, Morin LP, Moore RY. Morphological correlates of circadian rhythm restoration induced by transplantation of the suprachiasmatic nucleus in hamsters. Exp Neurol 1994;130(2):250–60.

[25] Tosini G, Menaker M. Circadian rhythms in cultured mammalian retina. Science 1996;272(5260):419–21.

[26] Robertson LM, Takahashi JS. Circadian clock in cell culture: I. Oscillation of melatonin release from dissociated chick pineal cells in flow-through microcarrier culture. J Neurosci 1988;8(1):12–21.

[27] Cahill GM. Circadian regulation of melatonin production in cultured zebrafish pineal and retina. Brain Res 1996;708(1-2):177–81.

[28] Amaral FGD, Cipolla-Neto J. A brief review about melatonin, a pineal hormone. Arch Endocrinol Metab 2018;62(4):472–9.

[29] Kalsbeek A, et al. Circadian rhythms in the hypothalamo-pituitary-adrenal (HPA) axis. Mol Cell Endocrinol 2012;349(1):20–9.

[30] Kalsbeek A, et al. Mammalian clock output mechanisms. Essays Biochem 2011;49(1):137–51.

[31] Pevet P, Challet E. Melatonin: both master clock output and internal time-giver in the circadian clocks network. J Physiol Paris 2011;105(4-6):170–82.

[32] Czeisler CA, et al. Suppression of melatonin secretion in some blind patients by exposure to bright light. N Engl J Med 1995;332(1):6–11.

[33] Freedman MS, et al. Regulation of mammalian circadian behavior by non-rod, non-cone, ocular photoreceptors. Science 1999;284(5413):502–4.

[34] Xie X, et al. Natural food intake patterns have little synchronizing effect on peripheral circadian clocks. BMC Biol 2020;18(1):160.

[35] Sasaki H, et al. Phase shifts in circadian peripheral clocks caused by exercise are dependent on the feeding schedule in PER2::LUC mice. Chronobiol Int 2016;33(7):849–62.

[36] Tahara Y, Aoyama S, Shibata S. The mammalian circadian clock and its entrainment by stress and exercise. J Physiol Sci 2017;67(1):1–10.

[37] Bruns DR, et al. The Peripheral Circadian Clock and Exercise: Lessons from Young and Old Mice. J Circadian Rhythms 2020;18:7.

[38] Vollmers C, et al. Time of feeding and the intrinsic circadian clock drive rhythms in hepatic gene expression. Proc Natl Acad Sci USA, 2009;106(50):21453–8.

[39] Buhr ED, Yoo SH, Takahashi JS. Temperature as a universal resetting cue for mammalian circadian oscillators. Science 2010;330(6002):379–85.

[40] Panda S. Circadian physiology of metabolism. Science 2016;354(6315):1008–15.

[41] Massin MM, et al. Circadian rhythm of heart rate and heart rate variability. Arch Dis Child 2000;83(2):179–82.

[42] Black N, et al. Circadian rhythm of cardiac electrophysiology, arrhythmogenesis, and the underlying mechanisms. Heart Rhythm 2019;16(2):298–307.

[43] Rahman SA, et al. Endogenous circadian regulation of female reproductive hormones. J Clin Endocrinol Metab 2019;104(12):6049–59.

[44] Scheving LA. Biological clocks and the digestive system. Gastroenterology 2000;119(2):536–49.

[45] Scheving LA, Russell WE. It's about time: clock genes unveiled in the gut. Gastroenterology 2007;133(4):1373–6.

[46] Brown MS, Goldstein JL, Dietschy JM. Active and inactive forms of 3-hydroxy-3-methylglutaryl coenzyme A reductase in the liver of the rat. Comparison with the rate of cholesterol synthesis in different physiological states. J Biol Chem 1979;254(12):5144–9.

[47] Rogers DH, et al. Circadian variation of 3-hydroxy-3-methylglutaryl coenzyme A reductase activity in swine liver and ileum. J Lipid Res 1981;22(5):811–9.
[48] Reddy AB, et al. Circadian orchestration of the hepatic proteome. Curr Biol 2006;16(11):1107–15.
[49] Adamovich Y, et al. Circadian clocks and feeding time regulate the oscillations and levels of hepatic triglycerides. Cell Metab 2014;19(2):319–30.
[50] Grimaldi B, et al. PER2 controls lipid metabolism by direct regulation of PPARgamma. Cell Metab 2010;12(5):509–20.
[51] Partch CL, Green CB, Takahashi JS. Molecular architecture of the mammalian circadian clock. Trends Cell Biol 2014;24(2):90–9.
[52] Sartor F, et al. Are there circadian clocks in mon-photosynthetic bacteria? Biology (Basel) 2019;8:41.
[53] King DP, et al. The mouse Clock mutation behaves as an antimorph and maps within the W19H deletion, distal of Kit. Genetics 1997;146(3):1049–60.
[54] Curtis AM, et al. Circadian clock proteins and immunity. Immunity 2014;40(2):178–86.
[55] Mohawk JA, Green CB, Takahashi JS. Central and peripheral circadian clocks in mammals. Annu Rev Neurosci 2012;35:445–62.
[56] Gachon F. Physiological function of PARbZip circadian clock-controlled transcription factors. Ann Med 2007;39(8):562–71.
[57] Lowrey PL, Takahashi JS. Mammalian circadian biology: elucidating genome-wide levels of temporal organization. Annu Rev Genomics Hum Genet 2004;5:407–41.
[58] Ueda HR, et al. Genome-wide transcriptional orchestration of circadian rhythms in Drosophila. J Biol Chem 2002;277(16):14048–52.
[59] Yamaguchi S, et al. Role of DBP in the circadian oscillatory mechanism. Mol Cell Biol 2000;20(13):4773–81.
[60] Asher G, et al. Poly(ADP-ribose) polymerase 1 participates in the phase entrainment of circadian clocks to feeding. Cell 2010;142(6):943–53.
[61] Lee Y, Kim K. Posttranslational and epigenetic regulation of the CLOCK/BMAL1 complex in the mammalian. Animal Cells Syst 2012;16(1):1–10.
[62] Toh KL, et al. An hPer2 phosphorylation site mutation in familial advanced sleep phase syndrome. Science 2001;291(5506):1040–3.
[63] Johansson AS, et al. Altered circadian clock gene expression in patients with schizophrenia. Schizophr Res 2016;174(1-3):17–23.
[64] Lavebratt C, et al. CRY2 is associated with depression. PLoS One 2010;5(2):e9407.
[65] Rijo-Ferreira F, Takahashi JS. Genomics of circadian rhythms in health and disease. Genome Med 2019;11(1):82.
[66] Zylka MJ, et al. Three period homologs in mammals: differential light responses in the suprachiasmatic circadian clock and oscillating transcripts outside of brain. Neuron 1998;20(6):1103–10.
[67] Yoo SH, et al. PERIOD2::LUCIFERASE real-time reporting of circadian dynamics reveals persistent circadian oscillations in mouse peripheral tissues. Proc Natl Acad Sci USA 2004;101(15):5339–46.
[68] Scheer FA, et al. Adverse metabolic and cardiovascular consequences of circadian misalignment. Proc Natl Acad Sci USA, 2009;106(11):4453–8.
[69] Castanon-Cervantes O, et al. Dysregulation of inflammatory responses by chronic circadian disruption. J Immunol 2010;185(10):5796–805.
[70] Lamia KA, Storch KF, Weitz CJ. Physiological significance of a peripheral tissue circadian clock. Proc Natl Acad Sci USA, 2008;105(39):15172–7.

[71] Marcheva B, et al. Disruption of the clock components CLOCK and BMAL1 leads to hypoinsulinaemia and diabetes. Nature 2010;466(7306):627–31.
[72] Perelis M, et al. Pancreatic beta cell enhancers regulate rhythmic transcription of genes controlling insulin secretion. Science 2015;350(6261):aac4250.
[73] Lefta M, et al. Development of dilated cardiomyopathy in Bmal1-deficient mice. Am J Physiol Heart Circ Physiol 2012;303(4):H475–85.
[74] Liu Y, et al. Loss of BMAL1 in ovarian steroidogenic cells results in implantation failure in female mice. Proc Natl Acad Sci USA, 2014;111(39):14295–300.
[75] Paschos GK, et al. Obesity in mice with adipocyte-specific deletion of clock component Arntl. Nat Med 2012;18(12):1768–77.
[76] Bass J, Lazar MA. Circadian time signatures of fitness and disease. Science 2016;354(6315):994–9.
[77] Kim JH, Duffy JF. Circadian Rhythm sleep-wake disorders in older adults. Sleep Med Clin 2018;13(1):39–50.
[78] Noh J. The effect of circadian and sleep disruptions on obesity risk. J Obes Metab Syndr 2018;27(2):78–83.
[79] Musiek ES, Holtzman DM. Mechanisms linking circadian clocks, sleep, and neurodegeneration. Science 2016;354(6315):1004–8.
[80] Muller JE, et al. Circadian variation in the frequency of onset of acute myocardial infarction. N Engl J Med 1985;313(21):1315–22.
[81] Papagiannakopoulos T, et al. Circadian Rhythm disruption promotes lung tumorigenesis. Cell Metab 2016;24(2):324–31.
[82] Thosar SS, Butler MP, Shea SA. Role of the circadian system in cardiovascular disease. J Clin Invest 2018;128(6):2157–67.
[83] Adler P, et al. Aging disrupts the circadian patterns of protein expression in the murine Hippocampus. Front Aging Neurosci 2019;11:368.
[84] Elmadjian F, Pincus G. A study of the diurnal variations in circulating lymphocytes in normal and psychotic subjects. J Clin Endocrinol Metab 1946;6:287–94.
[85] Brown HE, Dougherty TF. The diurnal variation of blood leucocytes in normal and adrenalectomized mice. Endocrinology 1956;58(3):365–75.
[86] Ella K, Csepanyi-Komi R, Kaldi K. Circadian regulation of human peripheral neutrophils. Brain Behav Immun 2016;57:209–21.
[87] Casanova-Acebes M, et al. Rhythmic modulation of the hematopoietic niche through neutrophil clearance. Cell 2013;153(5):1025–35.
[88] Crespo M, et al. Neutrophil infiltration regulates clock-gene expression to organize daily hepatic metabolism. Elife 2020;9:e59258.
[89] He W, et al. Circadian expression of migratory factors establishes lineage-specific signatures that guide the homing of leukocyte subsets to tissues. Immunity 2018;49(6):1175–90 e7.
[90] Schloss MJ, et al. Ly6C(high) Monocytes Oscillate in the heart during homeostasis and after myocardial infarction-brief report. Arterioscler Thromb Vasc Biol 2017;37(9):1640–5.
[91] Niehaus GD, et al. Circadian variation in cell-adhesion molecule expression by normal human leukocytes. Can J Physiol Pharmacol 2002;80(10):935–40.
[92] Lasselin J, et al. Effect of long-term sleep restriction and subsequent recovery sleep on the diurnal rhythms of white blood cell subpopulations. Brain Behav Immun 2015;47:93–9.
[93] Mendez-Ferrer S, et al. Haematopoietic stem cell release is regulated by circadian oscillations. Nature 2008;452(7186):442–7.
[94] Scheiermann C, et al. Adrenergic nerves govern circadian leukocyte recruitment to tissues. Immunity 2012;37(2):290–301.

[95] Pick R, et al. Time-of-day-dependent trafficking and function of leukocyte subsets. Trends Immunol 2019;40(6):524–37.
[96] Keller M, et al. A circadian clock in macrophages controls inflammatory immune responses. Proc Natl Acad Sci USA, 2009;106(50):21407–12.
[97] Silver AC, et al. Daily oscillations in expression and responsiveness of Toll-like receptors in splenic immune cells. Heliyon 2018;4(3):e00579.
[98] Wong SH, et al. Transcription factor RORalpha is critical for nuocyte development. Nat Immunol 2012;13(3):229–36.
[99] Eberl G, et al. An essential function for the nuclear receptor RORgamma(t) in the generation of fetal lymphoid tissue inducer cells. Nat Immunol 2004;5(1):64–73.
[100] Akashi M, Takumi T. The orphan nuclear receptor RORalpha regulates circadian transcription of the mammalian core-clock Bmal1. Nat Struct Mol Biol 2005;12(5):441–8.
[101] Yu X, et al. TH17 cell differentiation is regulated by the circadian clock. Science 2013;342(6159):727–30.
[102] Eberl G. RORgammat, a multitask nuclear receptor at mucosal surfaces. Mucosal Immunol 2017;10(1):27–34.
[103] Arjona A, Sarkar DK. The circadian gene mPer2 regulates the daily rhythm of IFN-gamma. J Interferon Cytokine Res 2006;26(9):645–9.
[104] Arjona A, Sarkar DK. Evidence supporting a circadian control of natural killer cell function. Brain Behav Immun 2006;20(5):469–76.
[105] Hayashi M, Shimba S, Tezuka M. Characterization of the molecular clock in mouse peritoneal macrophages. Biol Pharm Bull 2007;30(4):621–6.
[106] Geiger SS, et al. Daily variation in macrophage phagocytosis is clock-independent and dispensable for cytokine production. Immunology 2019;157(2):122–36.
[107] Fortier EE, et al. Circadian variation of the response of T cells to antigen. J Immunol 2011;187(12):6291–300.
[108] Amir M, et al. REV-ERBalpha Regulates TH17 Cell Development and Autoimmunity. Cell Rep 2018;25(13):3733–49 e8.
[109] Inokawa H, et al. Chronic circadian misalignment accelerates immune senescence and abbreviates lifespan in mice. Sci Rep 2020;10(1):2569.
[110] Zhang R, et al. A circadian gene expression atlas in mammals: implications for biology and medicine. Proc Natl Acad Sci USA, 2014;111(45):16219–24.
[111] Anafi RC, et al. CYCLOPS reveals human transcriptional rhythms in health and disease. Proc Natl Acad Sci USA 2017;114(20):5312–7.
[112] Proust, M, *Swann's Way*, in *Swann's Way: Remembranceof Things Past*. Neeland Media LLC, Kansas, US.
[113] Bosmann M, Ward PA. The inflammatory response in sepsis. Trends Immunol 2013;34(3):129–36.
[114] Mul Fedele ML, et al. Differential Thermoregulatory and Inflammatory Patterns in the Circadian Response to LPS-Induced Septic Shock. Front Cell Infect Microbiol 2020;10:100.
[115] Singer M, et al. The third international consensus definitions for sepsis and septic shock (Sepsis-3). JAMA 2016;315(8):801–10.
[116] Marpegan L, et al. Circadian responses to endotoxin treatment in mice. J Neuroimmunol 2005;160(1-2):102–9.
[117] Marpegan L, et al. Diurnal variation in endotoxin-induced mortality in mice: correlation with proinflammatory factors. Chronobiol Int 2009;26(7):1430–42.
[118] Guerrero-Vargas NN, et al. Reciprocal interaction between the suprachiasmatic nucleus and the immune system tunes down the inflammatory response to lipopolysaccharide. J Neuroimmunol 2014;273(1-2):22–30.

[119] Costantini C, et al. Microbes in the era of circadian medicine. Front Cell Infect Microbiol 2020;10:30.

[120] Diallo AB, et al. For whom the clock ticks: clinical chronobiology for infectious diseases. Front Immunol 2020;11:1457.

[121] Mazzoccoli G, et al. The circadian clock, the immune system, and viral infections: the intricate relationship between biological time and host-virus interaction. Pathogens 2020;9(2).

[122] Bellet MM, et al. Circadian clock regulates the host response to Salmonella. Proc Natl Acad Sci USA, 2013;110(24):9897–902.

[123] Nguyen KD, et al. Circadian gene Bmal1 regulates diurnal oscillations of Ly6C(hi) inflammatory monocytes. Science 2013;341(6153):1483–8.

[124] Gibbs J, et al. An epithelial circadian clock controls pulmonary inflammation and glucocorticoid action. Nat Med 2014;20(8):919–26.

[125] Druzd D, et al. Lymphocyte circadian clocks control lymph node trafficking and adaptive immune responses. Immunity 2017;46(1):120–32.

[126] Lundy SR, et al. Effect of time of day of infection on chlamydia infectivity and pathogenesis. Sci Rep 2019;9(1):11405.

[127] Lima-Camara TN, et al. Dengue infection increases the locomotor activity of Aedes aegypti females. PLoS One 2011;6(3):e17690.

[128] Taibi DM. Sleep disturbances in persons living with HIV. J Assoc Nurses AIDS Care 2013;24(1 Suppl):S72–85.

[129] Nunnari G, et al. Reduction of serum melatonin levels in HIV-1-infected individuals' parallel disease progression: correlation with serum interleukin-12 levels. Infection 2003;31(6):379–82.

[130] Cajochen C, Krauchi K, Wirz-Justice A. Role of melatonin in the regulation of human circadian rhythms and sleep. J Neuroendocrinol 2003;15(4):432–7.

[131] Dopico XC, et al. Widespread seasonal gene expression reveals annual differences in human immunity and physiology. Nat Commun 2015;6:7000.

[132] Ehlers A, et al. BMAL1 links the circadian clock to viral airway pathology and asthma phenotypes. Mucosal Immunol 2018;11(1):97–111.

[133] Edgar RS, et al. Cell autonomous regulation of herpes and influenza virus infection by the circadian clock. Proc Natl Acad Sci USA, 2016;113(36):10085–90.

[134] Sengupta S, et al. Circadian control of lung inflammation in influenza infection. Nat Commun 2019;10(1):4107.

[135] Zhao L, et al. The Per-1 Short Isoform Inhibits de novo HIV-1 Transcription in Resting CD4+ T-cells. Curr HIV Res 2018;16(6):384–95.

[136] Zhuang X, et al. The circadian clock components BMAL1 and REV-ERBalpha regulate flavivirus replication. Nat Commun 2019;10(1):377.

[137] Aiello A, et al. Immunosenescence and Its Hallmarks: How to Oppose Aging Strategically? A Review of Potential Options for Therapeutic Intervention. Front Immunol 2019;10:2247.

[138] de Souza Teixeira AA, Lira FS, Rosa-Neto JC. Aging with rhythmicity. Is it possible? Physical exercise as a pacemaker. Life Sci 2020;261:118453.

[139] Davizon-Castillo P, et al. TNF-alpha-driven inflammation and mitochondrial dysfunction define the platelet hyperreactivity of aging. Blood 2019;134(9):727–40.

[140] Aguilar-López BA, et al. Mitochondria: an integrative Hub coordinating circadian rhythms, metabolism, the microbiome, and immunity. Front Cell Dev Biol 2020;8:51.

[141] Sun N, Youle RJ, Finkel T. The mitochondrial basis of aging. Mol Cell 2016;61(5):654–66.

[142] Marquez EJ, et al. Sexual-dimorphism in human immune system aging. Nat Commun 2020;11(1):751.

[143] Janeway Jr CA. Approaching the asymptote? Evolution and revolution in immunology. Cold Spring Harb Symp Quant Biol 1989;54(Pt 1):1–13.

[144] Nobis CC, et al. The circadian clock of CD8 T cells modulates their early response to vaccination and the rhythmicity of related signaling pathways. Proc Natl Acad Sci USA, 2019;116(40):20077–86.

[145] Suzuki K, et al. Adrenergic control of the adaptive immune response by diurnal lymphocyte recirculation through lymph nodes. J Exp Med 2016;213(12):2567–74.

[146] Lange T, et al. Sleep enhances the human antibody response to hepatitis A vaccination. Psychosom Med 2003;65(5):831–5.

[147] Prather AA, et al. Sleep and antibody response to hepatitis B vaccination. Sleep 2012;35(8):1063–9.

[148] Long JE, et al. Morning vaccination enhances antibody response over afternoon vaccination: A cluster-randomised trial. Vaccine 2016;34(24):2679–85.

[149] Long JE, et al. Corrigendum to 'Morning vaccination enhances antibody response over afternoon vaccination: a cluster-randomised trial' [Vaccine 34 (2016) 2679-2685]. Vaccine 2016;34(40):4842.

[150] Munch M, et al. Bright light delights: effects of daily light exposure on emotions, restactivity cycles, sleep and melatonin secretion in severely demented patients. Curr Alzheimer Res 2017;14(10):1063–75.

[151] Kurupati RK, et al. The effect of timing of influenza vaccination and sample collection on antibody titers and responses in the aged. Vaccine 2017;35(30):3700–8.

[152] de Bree LCJ, et al. Circadian rhythm influences induction of trained immunity by BCG vaccination. J Clin Invest 2020;130(10):5603–17.

[153] Boivin DB, Czeisler CA. Resetting of circadian melatonin and cortisol rhythms in humans by ordinary room light. Neuroreport 1998;9(5):779–82.

[154] U. S. Bureau of Labor Statistics, Job flexibilities and work schedules in September 2019. www.bls.gov/news.release/flex2.nr0.htm (accessed January 2020).

[155] Rodriguez-Hernandez H, et al. Obesity and inflammation: epidemiology, risk factors, and markers of inflammation. Int J Endocrinol 2013;2013:678159.

[156] Obayashi K, et al. Exposure to light at night, nocturnal urinary melatonin excretion, and obesity/dyslipidemia in the elderly: a cross-sectional analysis of the HEIJO-KYO study. J Clin Endocrinol Metab 2013;98(1):337–44.

[157] Covassin N, Singh P, Somers VK. Keeping Up With the Clock: Circadian Disruption and Obesity Risk. Hypertension 2016;68(5):1081–90.

[158] WHO. 2020; www.who.int/news-room/fact-sheets/detail/obesity-and-overweight (accessed January 2020).

[159] Bluher M. Obesity: global epidemiology and pathogenesis. Nat Rev Endocrinol 2019;15(5):288–98.

[160] WorldoMeter. United Nations population division. https://www.worldometers.info/world-population (accessed January 2020).

[161] Voigt RM, Forsyth CB, Keshavarzian A. Circadian disruption: potential implications in inflammatory and metabolic diseases associated with alcohol. Alcohol Res 2013;35(1):87–96.

[162] Huang MC, et al. Reduced expression of circadian clock genes in male alcoholic patients. Alcohol Clin Exp Res 2010;34(11):1899–904.

[163] Chen CY, et al. Effects of aging on circadian patterns of gene expression in the human prefrontal cortex. Proc Natl Acad Sci USA 2016;113(1):206–11.

[164] Franceschi C, et al. Inflamm-aging. An evolutionary perspective on immunosenescence. Ann N Y Acad Sci 2000;908:244–54.

[165] Fulop T, et al. Immunosenescence and Inflamm-Aging As Two Sides of the Same Coin: Friends or Foes? Front Immunol 2017;8:1960.
[166] Armstrong KL, Quinn RA, Dadds MR. The sleep patterns of normal children. Med J Aust 1994;161(3):202–6.
[167] Iwata S, et al. Dependence of nighttime sleep duration in one-month-old infants on alterations in natural and artificial photoperiod. Sci Rep 2017;7:44749.
[168] Eisenreich W, et al. How viral and intracellular bacterial pathogens reprogram the metabolism of host cells to allow their intracellular replication. Front Cell Infect Microbiol 2019;9:42.
[169] Moreno-Altamirano MMB, Kolstoe SE, Sánchez-García FJ. Virus control of cell metabolism for replication and evasion of host immune responses. Front Cell Infect Microbiol 2019;9:95.
[170] Wang A, et al. Opposing effects of fasting metabolism on tissue tolerance in bacterial and viral inflammation. Cell 2016;166(6):1512–25 e12.
[171] Khan A, et al. A systems vaccinology approach reveals the mechanisms of immunogenic responses to Hantavax vaccination in humans. Sci Rep 2019;9(1):4760.
[172] Martinez-Lozano Sinues P, et al. Circadian variation of the human metabolome captured by real-time breath analysis. PLoS One 2014;9(12):e114422.
[173] Dyar KA, Eckel-Mahan KL. Circadian metabolomics in time and space. Front Neurosci 2017;11:369.
[174] Ruiz F, et al. Night shift work and immune response to the meningococcal conjugate vaccine in healthy workers: a proof of concept study. Sleep Med 2020;75:263–75.

Chapter 10

Controlled human infection modeling and vaccine development

Adrian Wildfire
Director, Scientific and Business, Strategy, hVIVO

10.1 Introduction

The history of vaccinology mirrors that of human challenge trials (HCTs) being founded upon the deliberate infection of human subjects with disease-causing materials and observations on subsequent protection from reinfection and disease. Edward Jenner (1749–1823) challenged individuals with live vaccinia virus to promote a protective immunological response to variola (1796). Jenner's novel smallpox vaccine became accepted practice prior to any knowledge of antigenic priming and pioneered the use of a challenge model in exploring induced immunity in infectious diseases. Jenner's theorem was however not unfamiliar even at that time and was likely an extrapolation of folkloric wisdom regarding variola immunization with live vaccinia preparations practiced both locally (Benjamin Jesty, 1774) and in mainland Europe from 1770 to 1791. The observation that direct or cross-protective immunity could be induced by the deliberate inoculation of infective matter from diseased individuals had been recognized since 1000 AD when the nasal inhalation of dried and powdered smallpox scabs (insufflation) was noted in Taoist culture. This practice was resurrected in China during the 15th Century, most likely following regional epidemics from 735 AD onwards in Asia Minor and Japan, evolving into the inoculation of pustular materials, scabs, or fluid, from mild cases of the disease into scarified skin (variolation). These early attempts at immunization, using whole pathogens, alive, dead and dried (fractionated), paved the way for later vaccines using attenuated strains of bacteria and viruses. The rabies virus vaccine of Louis Pasteur and Emile Roux (1885) and the *Mycobacterium bovis* "Bacilli of Calmet and Guerin" (BCG) for tuberculosis (1921) demonstrated the effectiveness of such an approach with polio and BCG preparations being adopted as essential elements of the first national immunization programs to be seen in the 20th century.

System Vaccinology. https://doi.org/10.1016/B978-0-323-85941-7.00002-4

Attenuated strains of viruses and bacteria have also been applied in clinical experiments to in healthy volunteers to study disease progression and as a discovery process to identify relevant markers of infection (e.g., T and B cell responses), pathogenesis, contagion (transmissibility), and recovery. Attenuated strains may be indicated where wild-type organisms offer an element of risk either incommensurate with study endpoints or outcomes or where attenuation ameliorates disease to an extent that measurements of drug or vaccine efficacy (VE) become indistinguishable from baseline or placebo. Typically challenge experiments in animals during preclinical investigations use pathogenic forms of the target organism or a surrogate where human pathogens are incapable of infection or disease in the animal model of choice. However, it has been well described that such preclinical data may frequently transcribe poorly into human field trials due to limiting factors associated with the pathogen, animal model, or extrinsic confounding factors such as high false discovery rates (FDR) in preclinical science. FDR translates as the proportion of genuine relationships available for discovery plus the Type 1 (false-positive) and Type 2 (false negative) error rates of experiments created to uncover them. Vaccine failure rates from preclinical to clinical testing may be as high as 76% with approximately only 19% of biological products proceeding from Phase 1 to approval and vaccines performing more poorly than other biologicals [1]. Where animal modeling is deemed inappropriate or poorly prognostic the early adoption of human modeling may be appropriate to bridge what has been referred to as a translational "valley of death" [2]. First-in-human (FIH) trials are routinely used in the development of biologicals as a proof of safety and to ensure that prognostic data from in vitro and non-human in vivo experimentation may be validated in small numbers of healthy, human volunteers. Such FIH studies are too small to provide irrefutable evidence of safety where a low incidence of adverse events may be extant, but it is an essential step in the translation of preclinical inferences into clinical practice. Likewise, measures of efficacy in animal models may be difficult to emulate in community trials where incidence of infection and disease is low. Seasonal infections, e.g., influenza, may be difficult to translate from animal modeling to the field as the gulf between deliberate infection and natural infection is only cost-effectively bridged where the prevalence of disease is high. The spectrum of disease may also confound studies where large numbers of subjects remain asymptomatic. This is especially true where populations are serially exposed to antigenically similar strains of the disease-causing agent. Malarial studies in Kenya at the coastal town of Kilifi and in the city of Nairobi, 500 km toward the interior, have demonstrated immunological responses to be radically different between the two populations upon deliberate sporozoite challenge, corresponding to prior exposure to *Plasmodium sp.* Kilifi residents frequently display a profound, pre-existing immunity to *Plasmodium falciparum* with complete suppression of growth observed in up to 40% of those challenged with direct venous inoculation (DVI) of GMP sporozoites (PfSPZ) (parasite densities meeting treatment criteria in only 39.5% of volunteers using qPCR) [3]. In malaria non-endemic regions, inoculation with the same dose (3.2 × 103 of PfSPZ) invariably leads to infection and in vivo parasite growth in 100% of volunteers.

10.2 The history of human challenge

Human challenge has been used as a therapy, an experimental investigational tool and to generate proof of concept (PoC) data in drug and efficacy trials. John Hunter infected both patients and, apocryphally, himself with both *Neisseria sp.* and *Treponema pallidum* containing material to study "syphilitic fever" through human experimentation from 1748 to 1761 [4]. During the First World War, Felix d'Herelle published an article in the proceedings of the French Academy of Sciences regarding "...an invisible microbe antagonistic to dysentery bacilli" and this work informed the use of bacteriophage challenge (ingestion) in treating enteric fevers. Also at this time the "Reading Bacillus" was cultured and used as a therapeutic inoculation in cases of intractable gangrene [5]. Malaria challenge was used as a treatment for neurosyphilis from the 1920s until the 1950s prior to the introduction of penicillin. Around this time (1936) the first human challenge experiment was trialed in Russia by a team led by A. A. Smorodintsev. An atomized, droplet suspension of two influenza A/H1N1 strains, previously passaged through mice, was used to inoculate 72 subjects. Data from such early trials was later used to inform the development of active immunization against influenza using live attenuated vaccines developed at the Smorodintsev Institute. With the standardization of the influenza challenge model came a realization that candidate drugs and vaccines could be trialed for efficacy prior to field studies thus potentially reducing both costs and lowering failure rates at late-phase development. Influenza has proven particularly intractable over the years with historically low VE estimates of 10%–60% over the past two decades, depending on the age of the cohort studied and strain targetted [6]. Clinical trials using human volunteers for Respiratory Syncytial Virus (RSV), human Rhinovirus (hRV) and even for *Neisseria gonococcus* were practiced at the Common Cold Research Unit in Salisbury and nearby Venereal Diseases Research Centre at Harnham Down. These centres were housed in ex-WWII barracks and recruited and consented volunteers to be inoculated with viral and bacterial pathogens to study new interventions to disease as well as to estimate the value of traditional remedies.

In contrast, unethical, illegal and unconsented episodes of deliberate infection have marred public perceptions of human challenge. The renowned bacteriologist Albert Neisser, who discovered *Neisseria gonococcus* in 1879 and was seminal in charting the course of syphilitic illness, injected cell-free serum recovered from syphilis patients into prostitutes and orphans in order to test VE. Although widely supported at the time by fellow medics and other leading researchers, public concern regarding Neisser's covert experimentation led first to a fine for misconduct and then, in 1900, to the issue of a directive from the

Minister for Religious, Educational, and Medical Affairs advising that medical interventions other than for "*diagnosis, healing, and immunisation*" were to be excluded under any and all circumstances if the subject "*was a minor or not competent for other reasons*" or if the physician had not obtained "*unambiguous consent*" in writing following explanation of possible sequelae relating to the procedure or treatment. This new emphasis on consent was further enshrined in German law by the Reich minister of the interior who issued "Guidelines for new therapy and human experimentation" in 1931 [7]. For the first time, ethical considerations considering the individual's right to freedom from clinical negligence and harm were clearly set out, with the essential differences and appended rights between therapeutic ("*new therapy*") and non-therapeutic research ("*human experimentation*") delineated.

Human challenge studies may be considered as having been potentiated by this regularisation of subjects' rights and certainly from 1900 studies into a wide range of pathogens were undertaken although many still transgressed the implicit understanding that written and informed consent was an essential element of such experimentation. Roestenberg et al. [8] estimated that some 23,000 volunteers were experimentally infected with different pathogens from 1900 to 2017 (PubMed listings). The heterogeneity of challenge agents is represented in the chart below (Fig. 10.1). The prevalence of some studies as compared to others may be a product of a range of disparate factors including availability of inoculum, priority to public health bodies, resistance to interruption of transmission or clinical failure of drugs and vaccines in reducing disease, frequency, or severity of sequelae, public health burden (e.g. as estimated from Disease Adjusted Life Years (DALYs)), age cohort of severe disease/mortality

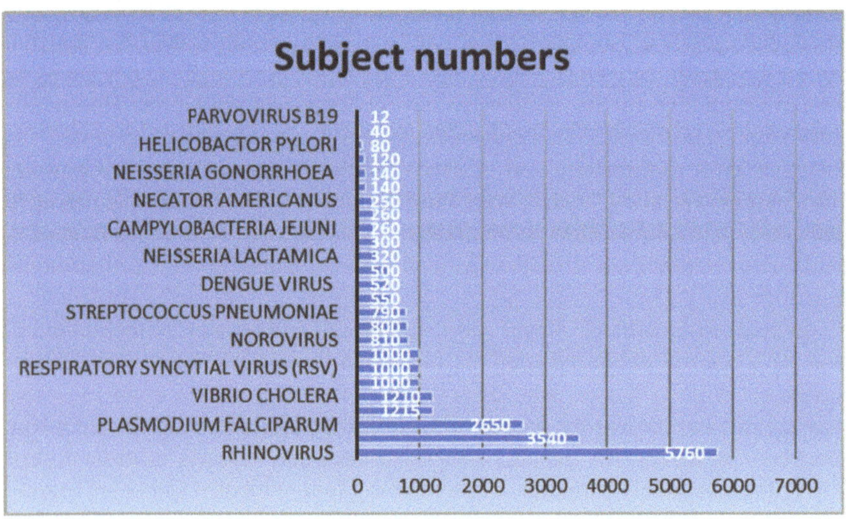

FIG. 10.1 Subjects challenged as part of an experimental, human challenge trial by agent and number.

and availability of predictive markers e.g. correlates of protection or disease. Any one or a combination of these elements may serve to make studies possible or impossible, ethical or unethical to perform in practice.

Scientific advancements in the collection and analysis of clinical samples with regard to disease initiation and progression are allowing novel insights into host and pathogen pathways. HCTs offer a perhaps unique opportunity to look at such interactions during the entire course of a disease, from inoculation to recovery. Early 'observation data' is increasingly being augmented and contextualized by findings at the cellular and even molecular level. It is this ability to link causality with outcomes that makes the longitudinal potential of challenge trials so appealing to fundamental, academic research as well as commercial drug and vaccine developers alike. What started out as individual observations regarding immunity has become an industry in itself and this industry may yet bring solutions to local, epidemic, or even pandemic threats of the future. Currently, the world's first SARS-CoV-2 challenge trial is in progress and the outcome of that may predicate the development of the second wave of vaccines aimed at disruption of transmission by reducing or eliminating viral shedding.

10.3 Principles of human challenge

Controlled human infection modeling (CHIM) modeling or HCTs serve to enshrine the twin principles that underpin traditional estimations of efficacy: 1. Statistically relevant subject numbers relating to infection and subsequent disease (n), and; 2. Statistically robust amplitude data (also referred to as magnitude or delta) correlating with the effect or effects of investigational drug or vaccine on the course of a disease (e.g. peak viral load, viral area under the curve (vAUC)). By controlling for elements that may obfuscate or confound such measurements e.g. low infection rates, coinfection, or comorbidities, within a controlled environment it is possible to decrease cohort sizes whilst preserving powering. Combining both vaccination and pathogen challenge into a single model negates the requirement for naturally high incidences of infection within the cohort and decreases the impact of chance elements, such as high levels of natural immunity to the challenge agent, by screening subjects against a panel of exclusion criteria prior to challenge.

The amalgamation of an investigatory, prophylactic intervention e.g. immunization, with deliberate, controlled infection presents both advantages and disadvantages. Although HCT modeling is designed to control for both incidence of infection and therefore prevalence of disease, the delta of symptoms associated with challenge agents may be restricted where homologous e.g. young and fit, cohorts are preselected for. Relative to this, measures associated with efficacy may provide restricted prognostic value for subjects with substantially different baseline characteristics e.g. the elderly, paediatric or the infirm. To augment challenge trial data, more broadly inclusive or pivotal trials may be performed within small Phase 2 field studies following initial proof of efficacy

(PoE) challenge studies. It has been noted that influenza challenge trials have similar proportions of asymptomatic, paucisymptomatic, and symptomatic individuals as compared to household infection (Fig. 10.2) [9].

Where such clinical homology to household infections is observed, this offers an element of justification to claims that challenge studies with wild-type organisms, able to recreate viral and host conditions as seen in the field, may act as surrogates in estimating VE. Typically, severe illness is absent in challenge cohorts and host markers of disease are primarily mild to moderate. Fever in influenza HCTs is markedly reduced for example. The drivers behind disease moderation are unknown but it has been suggested that they may be largely artifactual and a byproduct of inoculation titre, route of delivery, attenuation of the agent during manufacture or associated with covert mechanisms of host immunity e.g. pre-exposure; T cell activation [10]. The reduced spectrum of disease observed in challenge studies may be the product of a number of factors, including but not limited to infectious titre, route of inoculation, pre-existing immunity and cohort age and relative fitness (absence of cofactors).

Experimentation as early as 1966 by Robert H. Alford et al, Bethesda (NIAID) [11] demonstrated that extremely low titres of cell-culture derived influenza virus (A2/Bethesda/10/63) when administered orally (inhalation vs

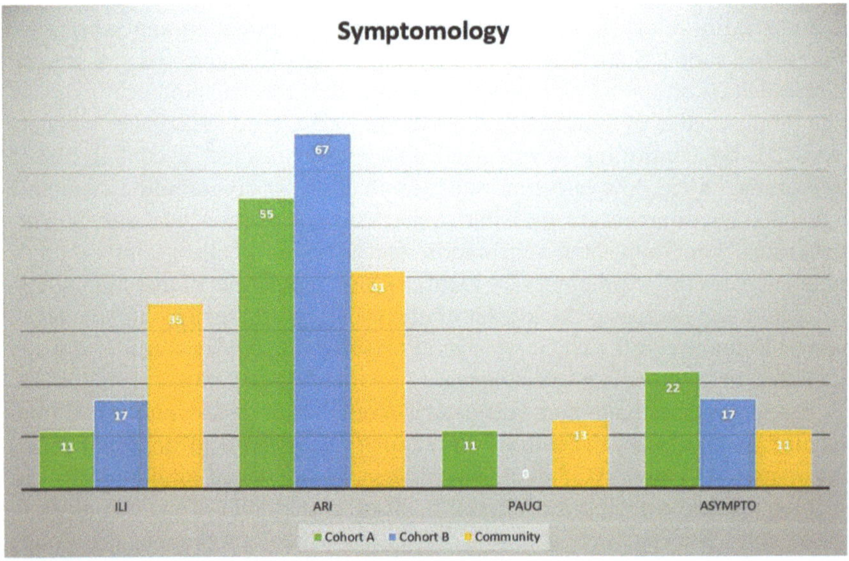

FIG. 10.2 Percentages of influenza like illness (*ILI*), acute respiratory illness (*ARI*), paucisymptomatic and asymptomatic disease in two cohorts from a viral challenge study relative to published data on community infections. (Cohort A: 11% ILI, 55% ARI, 11% pauci-symptomatic and 22% asymptomatic and Cohort B: 17%ILI, 67% ARI, 0% pauci-symptomatic and 17% asymptomatic vs observational data from a community study: 35% ILI, 41% ARI, 13% pauci-symptomatic and 11% asymptomatic). *Data from author study, presented WVC, 2017.*

Wild-type influenza virus challenge studies with nasal inoculation.

Reference	Virus type	Dose ($TCID_{50}$)	Exposed	Infected	Ill
Henle et al. (1946)	A (F-12)	10^{10a}	4	...[b]	1
	A (F-99)	$10^{8.5a}$	6	...[b]	0
Murphy et al. (1973)	A/Bethesda/88 (H3N2)	$10^{4.5}$	7	7	7[c]
Murphy et al. (1980)	A/Hong Kong/77 (H1N1)	$10^{4.2}$	6	6	5
	A/Udorn/72 (H3N2)	$10^{4.0}$	6	5	5
	A/Alaska/77 (H3N2)	$10^{4.2}$	8	8	4
Clements et al. (1983)	A/Alaska/6/77 (H3N2)	$10^{4.2}$	8	8	4
Clements et al. (1984b)	A/Washington/897/80 (H3N2)	$10^{6.0}$	24	23	11
Clements et al. (1984a)	A/Washington/897/80 (H3N2)[d]	$10^{6.0}$	24	23	11
Murphy et al. (1984)	A/California/10/78 (H1N1)	$10^{4.0}$	9	9	5
Murphy et al. (1985)	A/Washington/897/80 (H3N2)[d]	$10^{6.0}$	24	23	11
Clements et al. (1986)	A/Washington/897/80 (H3N2)[d]	$10^{6.0}$	24	23	11
Snyder et al. (1986)	A/California/10/78 (H1N1)	$10^{4.5}$	14	13	6
	A/Korea/1/82 (H3N2)	$10^{6.2}$	14	14	7
Sears et al. (1988)	A/Texas/1/85 (H1N1)	$10^{6.4}$	28	26	12
	A/Bethesda/1/85 (H3N2)	$10^{7.0}$	10	10	3
Youngner et al. (1994)	A/Kawasaki/9/86 (H1N1)	$10^{7.0}$	14	14	6

[a] Not tissue culture but ID_{50} in chick embryos.
[b] Not studied.
[c] Of these subjects, 6 had severe symptoms with fever, 1 had mild symptoms without fever.
[d] Same as Clements et al. (1984b).

Wild-type influenza virus challenge studies with aerosol inoculation.

Reference	Virus type	Dose ($TCID_{50}$)	Exposed	Infected	Ill
Henle et al. (1946)	A (F-12)	0.6×10^{10a}	4	...[b]	4
		0.6×10^{10a}	4	...[b]	4
		0.6×10^{9a}	4	...[b]	1
		0.6×10^{8a}	4	...[b]	1
	A (F-99)	$0.6 \times 10^{8.5a}$	6	...[b]	5
		$0.6 \times 10^{8.5a}$	4	...[b]	4
		$0.6 \times 10^{7.5a}$	6	...[b]	2
	A (PR-8)	$0.6 \times 10^{8.2a}$	33	...[b]	27
Jao et al. (1965)	A2 (Elisberg)	30	30	...[c]	12
Alford et al. (1966)	A2/Bethesda/10/63	126	3	0	0[d]
		78	3	0	0[d]
		59	3	1	0
		1	1	1	1
		2	4	1	0
		5	9	4	3

[a] Not tissue culture but ID_{50} in chick embryos.
[b] Not studied.
[c] Virus excretion and seroconversion studied but not reported.
[d] These subjects were presumably immune, as they had high antibody levels to the virus.

FIG. 10.3 Intranasal vs aerosolised virus inoculation (oral cavity) studies. Cohort numbers reflecting comparative infection and disease per $TCID_{50}$ dose of challenge agent [boxed, red]. *Source: Teunis, P., Brienen, N. and Kretzschmar, M. High infectivity and pathogenicity of influenza A virus via aerosol and droplet transmission. Epidemics (2010), 215–222.*

intranasal instillation of virus by droplets or atomizer) could induce significantly higher rates of symptomatic illness compared to nasopharyngeal inoculation of the same strain (inhaled 4 to 1000 $TCID_{50}$ illness severity was equal to that produced previously by IN administration of 80,000 to 180,000 $TCID_{50}$) with a mean maximum temperature of 38.8°C in the inhalation cohort [12].

Henle et al (1946) [13] in 1946 had also noted the difference in inoculation routes in inducing symptomatic disease: *"Febrile responses were observed in 58 of 65 subjects following inhalation of 0.4 to 0.8 cc. of finely atomized undiluted allantoic fluid; fluid diluted 1/10 or 1/100 was usually noninfective. When 1 cc. amounts of virus were instilled intra-nasally no fever occurred in 14 of 16 persons."* Following such early studies, inhaled virus studies declined and by the 1980s IN inoculation became the accepted practice owing to concerns regarding subject safety. With the preponderance of influenza challenge trial data now relating to mild to moderate influenza disease (MMID) care must be taken in translating challenge trial data directly into protective responses to severe disease Fig. 10.3.

10.4 Applications and limitations

The majority of experimental challenge studies are pivoted toward induction of mild symptomology by nature of the intelligent design. The selection of challenge agents is centered on the assumption of *primum non nocere* and, although it may justifiably be said that challenge trials induce 'harm' in the subject by intent, the duty of care is enshrined in the selection and screening of cohorts, by sustained and intensive clinical monitoring during the study and the choice and titre of agent employed. Challenge agent selection is based upon both the inherent properties of the pathogen e.g. self-limiting disease, and other criteria or thresholds that have been assessed during preclinical studies and early FIH characterization trials e.g. sufficient number and delta of symptoms; a defined and consistent shedding periodicity. Challenge studies may be said to represent a state of equipoise whereby the model recreates representative mild to moderate disease states within a controlled environment. This control extends to a marked reduction or elimination of severe disease and extremely elevated attack rates (ARs).

Where a challenge model is not able to fully able to recreate the natural course of the disease state to be studied due to elevated risk of, for example, severe adverse events (SAE), unacceptable sequelae, or irreversible changes in the subject's pathology then it is necessary to control the drivers of disease to reduce or eliminate said risk. Challenge agents may be amenable to chemotherapeutic intervention to halt the progression of disease. This is observed in malaria challenge trials where curative regimens (rescue therapy) are given as soon as the erythrocytic stage of the parasite reaches a set numerical threshold. Previously, *Plasmodium falciparum* trials have used primaquine (an anti-gametocytic drug) to eliminate the risk of onward transmission during a study and artemether and lumefantrine (Riamet®) as first-line rescue treatment of subjects at the conclusion of the trial. Where resistance to a first-line regimen is experienced a second-line regimen is frequently stipulated in the protocol to ensure patient safety e.g. atovaquone and proguanil hydrochloride (Malarone®). Such antimalarial cover is typical of malaria challenge trials and this practice may be observed in other intractable or refractile disease models such as *Salmonella typhi*, *Vibrio cholera* and similar enteric bacteria studies. Colonisation models e.g. *Neisseria lactamica* or *Streptococcus pneumoniae*, also have elimination therapies built into their design where natural elimination is unlikely or unexpected.

Typically human challenge modeling has been utilized to study intractable disease states or those with a strong epidemic or pandemic potential. Thus a self-limiting illness (usually an acute infection) with moderate to high states of morbidity, amenable to intervention, with a low potential for mortality or other severe sequelae in healthy adult cohorts would be expected as a passport to adoption. Such diseases predicate infection with a challenge strain that follows 'Type' or, in other words, is representative of the most commonly observed characteristics of the infective agent. Such agents should preferentially exemplify predominantly circulating or most frequently isolated strains, ideally accompanied by a global pattern of distribution (for worldwide relevance). Furthermore, such highly prevalent variants (relative to pathogen and locale) should be associated with both clinically and ethically acceptable levels of inducible disease. Ideally, any infection should also be readily induced with small numbers of the chosen pathogen, representative of natural infection. To achieve this paradigm there is an expectation that limited adaptive immunity should be observed within the community or that known correlates of protection (CoP) are amenable to allow for seroscreening for infection-permissive individuals. Recruitment of statistically significant numbers of immunonaive or serosusceptible subjects is frequently a barrier to performing challenge studies cost-effectively and has proven especially problematic for upper respiratory tract infections where yearly vaccination programs and seasonal exposure to circulating variants may excessively impact the incidence of serosuitable volunteers.

However, despite such barriers, challenge trials for RSV, influenza, and rhinovirus are performed with relevant cohort sizes by a number of research organizations.

The characteristics appending the choice of challenge agent to model such diseases may be said to follow some straightforward principles:

1. Known route and mode of transmission.
2. Self-limiting disease following inoculation.
3. Naturally inferred immunity.
4. Described disease state inducible in healthy adults.
5. Defined disease progression: host and pathogen, characteristic of type disease.
6. High AR achievable (>70%).
7. Effective therapeutic(s) available as rescue therapy.
8. Absent, minor, or preventable long-term sequelae.
9. Agent shows little attenuation or deviation from wild-type.

In the past, such criteria have limited challenge studies to infectious diseases that have been classified as mild, acute, self-limiting, or amenable to rescue medication. However, the potential for deliberate infection to study even previously taboo agents as hepatitis C virus (HCV) and dengue has recently been augmented by, for HCV, breakthrough curative regimens and for other agents, a lessening of the regulatory grip on human challenge through familiarization of the model and reliably safe clinical outcomes. As exemplars, despite the risk factors for Zika being well known and including the possibility to development a genetically-modified, attenuated strain of the virus, a bioethics panel convened by the National Institute of Allergy and Infectious Diseases and the Walter Reed Army Institute of Research rejected a Zika challenge model on grounds of safety and scientific value; to paraphrase:

(1) At the time, there was not enough was known about Zika transmission to eliminate potential risk to individuals outside of the study who had not given their consent to participate, and; (2) As existing studies were ongoing, the panel could not be confident that a Zika challenge model gave sufficient or critical data capable of accelerating the course of current vaccine development.

These findings highlighted a pertinent observation, i.e., where a live, infectious organism retained the potential to be disseminated outside of contained, clinically controlled environment, infection control measures should be deemed adequate, and proportional to knowledge regarding shedding and transmission of that organism. In the case of any "at risk" challenge model, a fundamental requirement would be the "known route and mode of transmission" element coupled to an estimation of infectious titre. Containment of the agent within a bounded structure alone may not be sufficient to prevent uncontrolled spread into vulnerable or broadly naïve populations. Where shedding of live organisms is sporadic, unpredictable or covert, it may persist beyond any set period of isolation. A recent discovery of an ebola outbreak linked to sequestered virus persisting in an infectious state for 5 years gives pause for thought [14]. To ensure the safety of bystanders it is necessary to perform characterization studies where a serosusceptible cohort is deliberately infected with rising titres of the challenge agent to observe, measure and define pertinent agent and host parameters during the course of the illness. Such titration or characterization trials are an essential step in challenge agent development and are a prerequisite to authorization of HCTs using a novel agent.

10.5 Challenge agents—selection and manufacture

The manufacture of a challenge agent, e.g., influenza virus, for use as a challenge agent in clinical trials is expected to conform cGMP according to both EMA and Food and Drug Administration (FDA) advisories. This expectation is predicated upon previous experience with EU/US clinical trials where both the dose-ranging and the POC studies are likely to be considered as a 'clinical study' and where the inoculating virus may be classified as an IND (hence following cGMP in the US) or IMP/NIMP in the European Union. Therefore to ensure a clinical trial utilizing a challenge agent is approved in the EU and reciprocally in the United States, the appropriate cGMP requirements should be applied during manufacture and reflected in the IMPD or IND item 7.

The manufacturing process for viruses may vary between species according to their target, host cells, or receptors. RSVs may be cultured only in cell lines (BEAS, HEp2, HELA, CAP, AMKC). However, influenza viruses may be grown both in embryonated eggs from specific pathogen-free flocks or in AGE1.CR or Madin-Darby canine kidney cell-lines. There are advantages and disadvantages to both approaches—embryonated egg-derived challenge virus may select for lower-lung epitopes owing to induced sialic-acid tropism (avian receptor α2,3-terminally-linked sialic acids (α2,3 SA)) and viral aspirates may contain high levels of antigenic ovalbumin, associated with atopic reactions. Cell lines, being highly permissive to extraneous, contaminating organisms, may also become infected with Mycoplasma or other adventitious agents and have been associated with low yields. Regulations governing cGMP, whether relative to cell-lines, growth media (plates or broths), or organic systems (eggs or animal or plants species) stipulate the same overall approach to production, with standards-based upon proofs of purity and of safety regarding the final product.

For viral and bacterial challenge agents, seed-stock may be acquired from community sampling, e.g., prevalence or other surveillance programs, or from institutes holding stocks for academic research or quality assurance schemes. Malaria challenge isolates have also been sourced from patients, e.g., NF-54 was initially obtained from a patient living near Schiphol Airport, Amsterdam, who had never left the Netherlands but it is posited that the parasite originated in Africa, but there is also the possibility to generate clones from source material (e.g., 7G8 – a Brazilian *P. falciparum*). Recently reverse-genetics has been employed to create viral challenge agents using intelligent design. This approach may allow for a reduced testing burden and the performance of such agents is being evaluated.

Community acquired agents have several advantages including known source of origin, documented patient characteristics, medical history including symptoms, and sequelae and the potential for follow-up samples; but approved, institutional stock may be well characterized through passage in cell lines, e.g., growth kinetics and dynamics relative to vaccine manufacture, and have antiserum available for use in adventitious agent testing. Live virus (i.e., cultures) are subject to rigorous Health and Safety restrictions relating to the transport and handling of dangerous goods and are subject to compliance with specific import and export licensure as well as shipping regulations, e.g., UN Recommendations on the Transport of Dangerous Goods; IATA-DGR (International Air Transport Association Dangerous Goods Regulations), prior to shipment across borders from the supplier to the client or manufacturer. Licensing may take several weeks to progress (e.g., USDA permits) and consideration should be given to including other products on the permit that may be required for future use to avoid delays, e.g., antiserum for target viruses. The source agent should be amplified to create seed stock under GMP conditions. This stock is the seeding agent for the manufacturing process and subject to its own purity testing program.

Once seed stock has been transferred to a manufacturing site there may be a requirement for pilot studies on limited numbers of eggs or in the target cell line to investigate infective titres and subsequent harvest counts according to the Technical Transfer protocol. Infectivity may vary widely between isolates and may be associated with attenuation, due to extended passage in vivo in communities or previous in vitro amplification and purification rounds, media formulation, the presence of defective infective particles or contamination with other organisms e.g. *Mycoplasma spp.*

Following identification of the optimal infective titre and completion of the Master Batch Records, the main manufacturing round may take place in a designated clean room. Challenge agents may be utilized for many years so it is important to generate sufficient volume for multiple trials. For an influenza agent, inoculation of up to 300 eggs may produce ~2.5 to 3.0 L of pooled harvest over 3–4 weeks. Up to 1.5 L may be used in adventitious and toxin testing as well as gene sequencing (to ensure homology to the original sample is maintained), therefore consideration should begiven to how much stock is remaindered after such analyses. The seed virus for inoculation is usually taken from the passage pool generated during the pilot studies. Harvest of the challenge stock (e.g., allantoic fluid; cell line culture medium) is followed by clarification using low speed centrifugation. Cell line harvests (e.g., two-stage bioreactor) may take place continuously or as a final extract at a specific period postinfection. In both cases, the final harvest should then be formulated (plaque-forming units (pfu), $TCID_{50}$, viral titre, haemagglutinin inhibition, or microneutralization test depending on the agent), filtered, aliquoted and flash frozen in liquid nitrogen for storage at ≤−70°C or −196°C prior to further analysis.

The detrimental effect of freeze-thaw cycles on viral challenge agent titres is well documented [15], therefore aliquots of the viral harvest should be created early to allow for distribution of samples to sites for adventitious testing without recourse to thawing the bulk product. Assessing the purity of the harvested agent is essential prior to use in healthy volunteers for both ethical and scientific reasons. Impure, contaminated or co-infected inoculum may produce adverse effects in subjects and may lead to unplanned illness and adversely affect the safety and PoC data. Adventitious testing should reflect risk, expressed as the likelihood of a specific pathogen having contaminated the seed stock or clinical sample and the types of organism that may be associated with the source subject or amplification medium. Testing may encompass a wide range of agents, from ubiquitous human pathogens (e.g., Human Parainfluenza Virus Types I and II) to organisms associated with the culture medium (e.g., Avian Sarcoma Leukosis Virus). Adventitious testing usually takes several months owing to complexity of the assays (co-culture, RT-PCT, product enhanced reverse transcriptase) and prolonged incubation periods (e.g., *Mycobacterium spp*.).

Once the concentration and purity of virus has been established as part of the Release Testing programme, the relative infectivity and pathogenicity of the challenge stock must be established in an animal model. For influenza, ferrets (*Mustela putorius furo*) have proven to express the best approximation to human disease; cotton rats (*Sigmodon hispidus*) are permissive to RSV with high respiratory tract titres of virus and translatable immunological markers for estimations of VE. Ferrets make good mammalian models owing to their small size, lung physiology, emulation of human symptomology following infection and the presence of $\alpha 2 \rightarrow 6$ sialylated glycan receptors in the respiratory tract. Preclinical studies in ferrets provide in vivo safety data for the challenge stock Investigators Brochure (IB), typically consisting of symptomology scores, viral load counts, cytokine analyses, and autopsy observations (tissue damage, compartmentalization of virus, immune-activation).

Although the a challenge stock may be approved for use by the relevant authority following review of the IB, IMPD/IND Chemistry and Manufacturing Controls (CMC) data, use of cGMP challenge stock should not be considered until a characterization study has been performed in healthy volunteers.

10.6 Characterization trials

The prognostic value of challenge modeling is derived from a comprehensive understanding of the disease-causing agent including the sequential elements of disease that follow-on from initiation of infection. Deviations from an expected course of occurrences relating to infection and illness (i.e., alterations in the presence, absence or sequence of events) or changes in their magnitude (the ɖ or delta) may provide information regarding the efficacy of experimental interventions, e.g., prophylactics and therapeutics, on the fitness of the agent studied or the immunological state of the host. To distinguish the likelihood of intervention related events being associated with chance observation and to better understand their relevance to events associated with natural or typical disease-related outcomes (such as changes in shedding, symptomologies and/or time-to-recovery for example) there must be a comprehensive understanding of the natural course of the disease and the measurable parameters associated with infection. Disease Emergent Adverse Events (EAEs, e.g., viral (VEAEs) and bacterial or parasitological AEs) must be distinguishable from Treatment Emergent Adverse Events if such events are to be contextualized and assigned the appropriate importance. Characterisation studies provide data relating not only to the drug emergent adverse events (DEAEs) but also the expected timing and delta of events. For viral challenge models typically the time to peak shedding, peak viral load, peak symptoms, number of symptoms, delta of symptoms, and time to recovery inclusive of cessation of shedding (genetic material and live virus) are key parameters.

Typically characterization studies comprise the inoculation of small cohorts of healthy, naïve individuals aged between 18 and 45 with escalating titres of challenge agent; similar to Phase 1 FIH Single-Ascending-Dose (SAD) studies. Depending on the anticipated pathogenicity of the agent, sentinel groups of 2–4 subjects may precede the inoculation of larger cohorts. Acceptable safety data from the low-dose subjects is considered a gateway to escalation. Minimum infectious dose (MID) may vary considerably according to characteristics intrinsic to the pathogen, e.g., inherent replicatory capacity (often described as multiplicity of infection or MOI, for viruses this is the number of genomes of a given virus species that infect individual host cells), strain variation (e.g., immune evasion mechanisms such as IFN downregulation), or growth medium, cell-line, or egg-adaptation during manufacture (see Gag-protein truncation of RSV strains grown on VERO) [16]; and to the host, e.g., age, health status, prior exposure to the challenge agent. The starting dose of the agent to be administered is frequently determined from prior experimentation; including cell culture infectivity assays where the presence of the infectious virus may be detected by its ability to cause cytopathic effects (CPEs) within a monolayer of cultured cells or in restricted regions of the monolayer (plaque formation). Viral titres are expressed either as the dilution of virus sufficient to CPE in 50% of the inoculated culture ($TCID_{50}$) or as plaque-forming units (pfu). For both viruses and bacteria, preclinical data from animal experimentation may provide data regarding MID. Suckling mice and infant rabbit models have been used to estimate MID for cholera but in general the human infective dose (HID_{50}) varies considerably depending on species, strain, route of inoculation, and experimental model. Animal modeling has limitations as the trophism and kinetics of the pathogen including accompanying symptomologies may differ markedly from that seen in humans. Typically, most influenza A and B strains, inoculated intranasally into BALB-c mice, do not result in an overt infection. Mouse adapted strains have been developed (two (2) A/H1N1 strains: A/Puerto Rico/8/1934 (PR/8) and A/WSN/1933 (WSN) and a single influenza B strain: B/Lee/1940) but these are now 80+ years old and may no longer be antigenically relevant to currently circulating virus. Upon infection with mouse-adapted influenza virus, mice display a marked weight loss (anorexia), huddling, hunching, and fur ruffling owing to cessation of grooming and dehydration as well as other signs of physical discomfort. Conversely, mice may become hypothermic upon infection, in contrast to a marked pyrexia noted in up to 70% of human influenza cases. Most notably, influenza in mice primarily manifests as a viral pneumonia, characterized by labored breathing and cyanosis and at postmortem by severe pulmonary histopathology. Increasing titres of virus or altered route of delivery in mice (e.g., intratracheal delivery) may manifest in earlier onset of systemic symptoms, a rapid onset of pneumonia, or an accelerated decline resulting in death. Challenge experiments with influenza in humans typically results in an acute and self-limiting upper respiratory tract illness characterized by fever, dry cough, pharyngitis, nasal congestion, and malaise. Timing of symptom onset is also clearly different for mice as compared to humans with peak symptoms in humans occurring at approximately day 3 (72 hours) but at day 4 to 5 in mice. Thus dosing studies in mice offers limited translatable information for HCTs. Ferret modeling of influenza offers more transferable data but may easily be confounded as the clinical severity of influenza infection via intranasal instillation is highly dependent on the volume of inoculum [17] even where titres remain equal.

Primary outcomes for titration or characterization studies of novel pathogens are usually premised upon shedding. The demonstration of dose-related responses in preclinical studies may guide the baseline titre but where such data is absent, inconsistent (e.g., non-correlative) or equivocal previous HCTs or community studies regarding MID may provide predictive data. The correlation between infectious dose and disease severity may vary between pathogens. There is some evidence that low dose challenge in influenza may promote an increase in both the number and seriousness of symptoms although ARs may be reduced [18]. Replication and shedding of the challenge agent must be balanced with measures of infectivity rates and subject safety. The aim of the majority of challenge models is to achieve an AR of >70% but <95% with a disease profile similar to that seen in community infections. Inoculum titres may also be manipulated so as to provide predictability in the course of a disease. For example, in the DVI model of malaria, an inoculum dose of 3,200 sporozoites ensures a predictable progression of stages with parasitaemia occurring consistently from d7 to d9 post-challenge. Similarly, 25-50 filariae provide a consistent infectivity and disease progression (time to patency or detection of eggs in faeces) for hookworm challenge models (e.g. *Necator americanus*). Such consistency reduces the risk of outliers e.g. prolonged incubation periods, and allows for improved patient management.

Secondary outcomes in characterization studies are primarily related to symptomology. Again, increasing titres must be balanced against patient safety. A threshold may be observed where low levels of innate immunity, neutralizing antibody, or adaptive T cell responses may be overcome by high inoculum titres.

10.7 Clinical aspects of performing human challenge trials

10.7.1 Trial population/cohort

PoC trials, including a challenge studies, have been safely conducted for many years for non-infectious diseases, for instance allergen challenge trials in mild asthma. For such trials, a subject should be susceptible or sensitive to the allergen employed. For asthma and chronic obstructory pulmonary disease (COPD), susceptibility is related to an underlying illness that may be both triggered and promulgated by the challenge agent. In essence, this is no different from a viral or bacterial challenge study, where the subjects should be capable of infection by the pathogen of choice. Where commonly circulating, e.g., seasonal, viral pathogens are prevalent in a population in which a viral challenge trial is to be conducted, the presence or absence of pre-existing immunity must first be established through testing. This is most commonly achieved via measuring neutralizing antibody. Identifying seronegative subjects, those without serological markers of pre-existing infection and immunity or those below a protective threshold, e.g., titre, decreases the risk of non-infection or confounding immunology and (lack of) symptoms following challenge; therefore increasing the power of the data derived per subject. Additional to this scientific rationale, there are valid considerations regarding the medical implications of pre-existing antibodies. Antibody-dependent enhancement (ADE) of infection may be a concern where non-specific antibodies predominate; such risks were highlighted for subunit and whole, inactivated viral vaccines during the SARS-CoV-2 pandemic based upon observations of ADE in animal vaccine models following the SARS and MERS outbreaks in 2002–2003 and 2013, respectively [18]. In ADE, the presence of non-neutralizing antibodies following infection may enhance viral entry into macrophages and monocytes via Fc binding. Enhanced antibody-dependent phagocytosis has the potential to upregulate innate cells into a highly inflammatory state, with an increased risk of immune-associated injury [19,20]. This rationale would equally apply when considering acceptable vaccination status. The simplest solution to achieving high ARs and large symptom deltas would be to only consider non-vaccinated subjects as suitable participants for a HCT, but this is not always feasible. Dependent on the product under development and disease being studied, this may not prove desirable either. In the instance of seasonal vaccination, the issue of prime and boost is important and the degree of benefit derived from vaccinating pre-exposed individuals may be explored using subsequent pathogen challenge only by selecting an antigen-experienced cohort. Enrolling preimmune or prevaccinated subjects for your challenge trial should always be considered in relation to the developmental program of the IMP and be aligned with implications for both safety and efficacy parameters of any individual study. For certain pathogens it may be acceptable to vaccinate pre-exposed individuals as this may decrease the prognosticated severity of disease; however, for others pre-exposure may increase risk via immune enhancement or downregulation.

10.7.2 Eligibility criteria and adverse events

Serological prescreening may be seen as a preliminary barrier to entry for any challenge study where a raised prevalence of the challenge agent is noted in the study population. Such data may be obtained through serosurveillance programs or observations on disease incidence. Where cohorts are ostensibly naïve, e.g., subjects from high-income countries in controlled human malaria infection (CHMI with *Plasmodium spp.*) or cholera studies, the relevance and thus value of prescreening is diminished. In such a case, succeeding investigations (true screening) should primarily focus on subject safety with eligibility criteria tailored to the disease and IMP under investigation. For respiratory pathogens, subjects with a healthy pulmonary system should be targeted to reduce the probability of a descending infection. For (parasite) pathogens with hepatic involvement during their life-cycle, normal baseline liver function tests (LFT) would be a prerequisite. Coinfection with chronic pathogens such as hepatitis or HIV may not only impact on a volunteer's immune system but also give rise to chronic, inflammatory states within a range of tissues leading to AEs or sequelae that may be incorrectly attributed to the challenge agent or otherwise more directly impact upon subject safety. A comprehensive viral and bacteriological screening panel may thus be appropriate to identify confounding agents alongside a haematological, biochemical, and physical work-up to baseline individuals prior to challenge with either IMP or pathogen. Certain immunological conditions may predispose subjects to worsened outcomes and should be excluded. A history of idiopathic anaphylaxis (an acute state of hypersensitivity of unknown origin) would preclude enrolment of a subject into any early development stage study. Other generic conditions or disorders which may be classed as PK influencers, such as a gastric bypass or known CYP polymorphism, would also be prohibited but should be identified during screening by conducting a thorough medical history. Equally, rare but potentially lethal postinfectious complications such as Guillain Barré syndrome or transverse myelitis (that may be attributable to prior infection or vaccination) or possibly permanent complications like Bell's palsy should be identified and such subjects equally excluded on grounds of subject safety [21,22].

With reference to the above, a careful consideration of confounding symptoms should also form part of the study's eligibility section, alongside those safety criteria as already discussed. In order to be able to differentiate DEAEs from concomitant illness, it may be beneficial to consider excluding certain pathologies. As an example, allergic rhinitis may confound symptoms from a challenge agent causing upper respiratory symptoms; equally irritable bowel syndrome could impact gastro-intestinal symptomatology and obesity could impact the subject's baseline liver function [23]. As ever, eligibility criteria should be tailored to allow for maximal scientific harvest while securing subject's safety, thus achieving equipoise relative to recruitment and enrolment.

10.7.3 Ethical considerations and study restrictions

The thought of deliberately infecting human volunteers may be perceived as bordering on unethical upon first reflection. There has been a history of covert, unconsented, experimental inoculation with a range of pathogenic organisms which, despite furthering the understanding of infectious diseases has infringed both human rights and the ethics embodied in *primum no nocere*. For the last 50 years, the moral imperative has been toward safe, consented, and regulated clinical studies, based upon agreements reached postconflict such as the Nuremburg Code (1947), the Universal Declaration of Human Rights (1948), and later the World Medical Association's 'Declaration of Helsinki' (1964) founding the ethical principles that underlie the International Conference for Harmonisation—Good Clinical Practice (ICH-GCP) (1996) regarding the individual rights to freedom of choice and freedom from harm: "It is the duty of the physician to promote and safeguard the health of the people. The physician's knowledge and conscience are dedicated to the fulfillment of this duty" (Declaration of Helsinki, General Principles [24]). In addition, there is substantial precedence of ethically acceptable CHIM studies operating by the mid-20th century with the Common Cold Research Unit (CCRU) performing intentional, experimental infections with cold viruses under the aegis of the Medical Research Council from 1946 until the early 1990s. The first coronaviridae were isolated at the CCRU during this period. Since the current coronaviridae COVID-pandemic was by declared the WHO in January 2020, (30 Jan 2020—"The Director-General (has) declared the novel coronavirus outbreak a public health emergency of international concern (PHEIC), WHO's highest level of alarm") [25], the debate about the functionality and use of challenge trials has gained momentum with the WHO publishing a manifest on how an acceptable (COVID) challenge trial should be structured [26]. In line with international guidelines, maximizing scientific benefit whilst minimizing individual participant risk, remain the main prerogatives in conducting a SARS-CoV-2 deliberate infection study. There are specific measurements, markers, and associated data that may only be observed within an HCT; such data may be difficult or even impossible to gain from a field trial, e.g., initiation or transmission events at the point of pathogen entry. Yet there exists an ethical bandwidth to the appropriateness of conducting such trials. The value of clinical trial data has to be proportional to individual risk versus societal gain. Covert restrictions on volunteer behavior may appear to contravene their basic human rights yet be essential to data integrity. Alongside protocol derived healthy volunteer restrictions (defined within the inclusion and exclusion criteria), maintaining a regularized diet to preserve baseline LFTs [27], there may be additional constraints in regard to pathogen containment and thus a necessity for subject isolation for an extended period of time (relative to shedding of live, infectious organisms). Constraints relative to infection control may even extend out to third parties, such as family members of participants, trial staff members and the wider society with secure containment and adequate disposal of medical waste, secretions, excretion and circulatory-fluids for blood-borne or faeco-oral challenge agents. Airborne bacteria or virus challenge studies typify the need for full containment by means of quarantine and various grade of personal protective equipment up to filtering facepiece 2/3 (FFP2/3) face masks or even Powered Air-Purifying Respirators to protect staff from infection and acting as an onward transmission vehicle and thus escape into potentially vulnerable populations [26,28].

10.8 Regulatory considerations

HCTs have been accepted as a useful model in discussions with regulators in obtaining estimations of efficacy. Challenge trial data presented within the Investigator's Brochure (IB) will be considered by both the US FDA and the European Medicines Agency (EMA). To date, regulators have accepted HCTs within the context of POC or dose finding studies. Most recently, a novel cholera vaccine (Vaxchora), aimed at preventing moderate to severe disease in travelers, received marketing authorization approval based upon a pivotal efficacy data from single, large scale HCT ($n = 201$). The challenge trial was supported by a large safety and immunogenicity trial ($n = 3235$). The rationale for both the FDA and the EMA agreeing to accept a challenge study as a pivotal efficacy trial for cholera was predicated on the extreme difficulty in performing a meaningful Phase III trial in such an indication resulting in conclusive, statistically relevant results, given that such "traveler" populations are transient and recruitment and retention is a primary concern.

Several regulators have published guidelines on the use of HCTs in drug and vaccine development. In 2016 the World Health Organization (WHO) published a guidance document titled: "Human challenge trials for vaccine development: regulatory considerations" [29]. Within the document there is specific text offering advice for regulators when considering data obtained from challenge studies: "whether the purpose of the study or studies is to provide supportive evidence for licensure or to help inform and design traditional efficacy studies or vaccine design, human challenge trials may contribute to the preponderance of evidence upon which regulators could take a clinical trial or licensure decision."

Additionally, in its "Guidelines on clinical evaluation of vaccines: regulatory expectations," [30] the WHO counsels that "If it is not feasible to perform VE trials and there is no immunological correlate of protection, it may be possible to obtain evidence in support of VE and/or to derive an immunological marker of protection from ...a human challenge trial" (relevant to that condition). The guidance also specifies that where such studies are performed, HCTs may be of particular use: "When there is no appropriate nonclinical model (e.g. when a candidate vaccine is intended to protect against an infectious disease that is confined to humans), when there is no known immune correlate of protection (ICP)" and/or "when VE trials are not feasible." As an example, there is to-date no known, definitive correlate, threshold or sliding-scale of protective marker relevant to SARS-CoV-2 infection or re-infection. COVID-19 field trials may prove increasingly difficult as populations become largely immune through vaccination and natural exposure or as seasonal prevalence may fluctuate. In such a case an HCT could prove an essential tool for obtaining efficacy data for second-generation vaccine candidates, that could not otherwise be obtained.

In further consideration of COVID-19 challenge trials, the WHO published a paper in 2020 termed: "Key criteria for the ethical acceptability of COVID-19 human challenge studies" [31] and the research and development blueprint: "Feasibility, potential value and limitations of establishing a closely monitored challenge model of experimental COVID-19 infection and illness in healthy young adult volunteers" [32] to discuss the ethical considerations of a COVID-19 HCT and the conditions under which such a trial could be performed. Several discussion points remain unresolved and should be considered with the applicable regulators and ethical bodies at a scientific advice meeting prior to any clinical trial application for a COVID-19 challenge study.

The regulatory requirements for viral (such as SARS-CoV-2) challenge studies in humans can be divided into two parts: firstly the requirements for the studies, and secondly, requirements for the supporting infrastructure, i.e., Phase I units where such studies may be performed. As a generalization, relatively little guidance exists around the development and performance of viral challenge/inoculation studies due to their novelty. There is no guidance on this subject provided by the EMA or any individual, European national authority. An FDA guideline on the development of influenza drugs only mentions this type of study briefly [33].

Following authorization for the use of any new viral challenge agent (dependent on a satisfactory review of the agents Investigator's Brochure (IB), including the CMC or manufacturing dossier, by the local regulatory agency) there is a requirement for a (virus) dose-finding study, often referred to as a characterization trial. In a characterization trial, healthy volunteers are inoculated with escalating titres of virus to establish a safe and effective dose of virus that has an infection or AR of $\geq$X% (for influenza an acceptable AR for a viral challenge agent is $\geq$75%). The optimal titre may thus be defined as the dose that has the appropriate safety and illness/infectivity profile inclusive of shedding and symptomologies representative of community infection. Challenge strains should retain homology to pathogens circulating within the community wherever possible. For vaccine trials, this is especially important if challenge data is to be prognostic to performance in the field. Where antigenic relevance is not achieved false positive or false negative data may result. For each challenge agent, only a single dose-finding study is required. Once characterized, the strain (at the designated optimal dose) may then be used in multiple challenge studies.

Whether or not a characterization trial can be considered a clinical study in the strictest sense remains an open question. The objectives of such a stand-alone experiment are not in line with the definition of a clinical study as described in Directive 2001/20/EC article 2 (a): "clinical trial": any investigation in human subjects intended to discover or verify the clinical, pharmacological and/or other pharmacodynamic effects of one or more investigational medicinal product(s) (IMPs), and/or to identify any adverse reactions to one or more IMP(s) and/or to study absorption, distribution, metabolism, and excretion of one or more IMP(s) with the object of ascertaining its (their) safety and/or efficacy [34].

In accordance with the Directive, a characterization trial may thus be regarded as an "experiment," only requiring approval from an ethics committee and not from health authorities per se. However, classifying characterization or challenge studies in general as experimentation should be the subject of careful consideration. Although the European directive may not consider challenge trials to be a clinical study in the strictest sense, individual national legislators take an alternative view and require conformity to ICH-GCP or Code of Federal Regulations Title 21 (FDA, CFR 21) in their execution. There is also a not insignificant risk that a dose-finding study may have to be repeated if it is performed without relevant health authority approval. This risk is elevated in a case where the CMC data of the virus is considered insufficient by the regulatory authority at the time of submission relative to an IMP, PoC study. PoC studies (in which the challenge agent and a vaccine or antiviral (the IMP) are both administered) fall under the definition of a clinical study according to Directive 2001/20/EC. Dose-finding studies are thus generally treated as per clinical studies to ensure acceptance across multiple jurisdictions. Somewhat paradoxically, challenge agents are not always considered to be an IMP as they do not fulfil the definition of an IMP as defined in both the Directive 2001/20/EC, Article 2 (d) [35] and the Guidance on IMPs and Non Investigational Medicinal Products (NIMPs) [33]. In the new European Clinical Trials Regulation (Regulation 536/2014) challenge agents will be considered Auxiliary Medicinal Products (AMP) [36].

To clarify further, if an inoculating virus is used to evaluate the efficacy of an investigational product, the inoculating virus is classified as a "condition" and not as an "intervention" (i.e., a disease or health issue worth studying in a clinical study, according to FDA classification [37]. According to Eudralex Volume 10, guidance on IMPs and NIMPs, revision March 1, 2011 [35]), the inoculating virus could be classified as NIMP in the European Union. In this case, the inoculating virus is a "challenge agent." A challenge agent, by definition, is a product, substance, or pathogen given to study subjects to produce a physiological response that is necessary before the pharmacological action of the IMP can be assessed. A challenge agent may be a substance without marketing authorization but may have a long tradition of clinical use.

Information regarding the quality of the inoculating agent should be provided in the non-investigational medicinal product dossier (NIMPD). There is no standard format available for presenting the information regarding such agents; however, guidelines on the requirements for quality documentation concerning biological IMPs in clinical studies, EMA/CHMP/BWP/534898/2008 [38] is frequently used as a reference. The quality information regarding an inoculating virus can be presented in Sections 2.1.S, 2.1.P, and 2.1.A of the NIMPD, similar to the quality documentation requirement for IMPs [38]. It is not necessary to provide extensive information, as per a biological drug used for marketing authorization; the NIMPD should mainly focus on the quality attributes related to safety aspects, considering the state of development or clinical phase. The quality part of the NIMPD should include information related to the quality, manufacture, and control of the NIMP. It is preferable to present data in tabular form accompanied by a brief narrative highlighting the main points. The information that should be provided includes source of origin, seed stock isolation, manufacturing process, control of materials, including growth medium e.g. master cell bank and working cell bank systems, control of seed stock (i.e., quantity, identity, and purity), analysis, and stability among others. In section 2.1.A.2 of the NIMPD (adventitious agents safety evaluation), information assessing the risk with respect to potential adventitious agents and other human pathogens contaminations should be provided (guideline on virus safety, EMEA/CHMP/BWP/398498/05) [39].

A number of important regulatory and operational aspects of running a human challenge study should also be considered. It is extremely important to avoid cross-infection between subjects infected with a pathogen as part of a clinical trial and the study staff performing duties within proximity of those subjects. Both proactive and reactive measures should be put in place to reduce the risk of harm for both parties. For example, study staff may be immunized against the challenge agent where possible (where such a vaccine a. exists and; b. is available), additionally a contingency plan to treat volunteers with rescue medication (e.g. antiviral, antibiotic, or antiparasitic) or other drugs (e.g., palliative) following challenge, where subjects may develop severe, prolonged, unusual (unexpected) or repeat/recrudescent disease, should be developed. Such measures apply equally for dose-finding studies as for challenge trials and should form part of the risk/benefit analysis and clinical study plan. Primarily, infection control is paramount where deliberate exposure is contemplated with the aim being to avoid the challenge agent from being released from either the containment facility or the subjects. Such measures also serve to ensure that secondary, natural agents are not accidentally introduced into the study.

Superinfection or coinfections may confound a study where symptomologies are a primary endpoint and prescreening for commonly occurring infectious diseases, prequarantine isolation, and on-going local, environmental disinfection may all lessen the risk of infected study staff or subjects transmitting infectious agents within study cohorts.

As challenge studies may frequently use agents that are transmissible by shedding, e.g., aerosols, fomite contamination, or droplet infection, once infected, the subjects are required to isolate within a quarantine unit and will be treated according to the principle of "reversed-barrier nursing." This method is comparable to barrier nursing used in an intensive care unit (ICU) setting, where the aim is to keep pathogens away from the ICU patients by creating a barrier between the outside world and the inside of a patient room by using personal protective equipment (gloves, masks, gowns) in addition to regular disinfection (hand-washing, surface treatments, fomite control). With reverse-barrier nursing, the aim is to not only keep the challenge agent confined within the facility but also to keep other, secondary agents out, using the same principles.

10.9 Summary

The history of deliberate infection has encompassed over 1000 years of usage. From origins in vaccination with attenuated or related strains of pathogen it has grown into a dedicated scientific model bridging the gap between animal testing and human field trials. HCTs have provided pivotal efficacy data for vaccine authorization and allowed for the rapid identification of superior vaccine candidates and formulations through the direct measurement of endpoints relating to markers and the observation of indirect effects such as symptoms or sequelae. Through controlling of the cohort for confounding factors and promoting high ARs, the negative predictive value of HCTs is high, i.e., if the drug or vaccine does not work in an optimized cohort then it is unlikely to be effective in a broadly heterologous population. Direct translation of positive HCT results into communities is less assured although work on the antiviral drug oseltamivir, demonstrating reductions in vAUC and symptoms scores has since been seen to be repeatable in the field [40]. Through the standardization of challenge trials, employing GMP agents and regularized IC/EC and schedules of assessments, data may increasing be compared between models and further explored via meta-analysis, offering assurances of both consistency and fidelity between studies.

Since 2000, a relative upsurge in challenge trials has occurred with expansions not only in the size of the cohorts and the variety of the models e.g. viral exacerbation of asthma, COPD, but also the range of pathogenic species shown to be amenable to such modeling.

With the emergence of novel, zoonotic diseases with pandemic potential and with some pre-existing pathogens showing substantial changes in both antigenicity (e.g., H3N2 influenza A) and susceptibility (e.g., *P. falciparum* and artemisinin-based therapies), an accelerated pipeline of new treatments is urgently needed. HCTs offer a route to early licensure for many drugs and may play a critical role in the selection of novel or effective repurposed candidates for further development as solutions to epidemic and pandemic agents.

References

[1] Struck M. Vaccine R&D success rates and development times. Nat Biotechnol 1996;14(5):591–3. doi:10.1038/nbt0596-591. PMID: 9630948 https://www.nature.com/articles/nbt0596-591.pdf?origin=ppub.

[2] Seyhan A. Lost in translation: the valley of death across preclinical and clinical divide—identification of problems and overcoming obstacles. Transl Med Commun 2019;4(18). doi:10.1186/s41231-019-0050-7.

[3] Kapulu M, Njuguna P, Hamaluba M, Kimani D, Ngoi J, Musembi J, Ngoto O, Otieno E, Billingsley P. Naturally acquired immunity among Kenyan adults suppresses the West African P. falciparum NF54 strain in controlled human malaria infection (CHMI) - CHMI-SIKA Study Team. medRxiv 2020:20172411. doi: https://doi.org/10.1101/2020.08.11.20172411.

[4] Wright, D John Hunter and venereal disease, Annals of the Royal College of Surgeons of England (1981) vol. 63. https://www.ncbi.nlm.nih.gov/pmc/articles/PMC2493930/ (accessed April 16, 2021).

[5] Robert Donaldson R. Character and properties of the "Reading" bacillus, on which a new method of treatment of wounds has been based. Jour Path and Bact 1919;22(2):129–51. https://doi.org/10.1002/path.1700220203.

[6] Centres for Disease Control and Prevention (CDC). (2020). [Statistical data on *Adjusted vaccine effectiveness estimates for influenza seasons from 2004-2018*]. *Past Seasons Vaccine Effectiveness Estimates*, https://www.cdc.gov/flu/vaccines-work/past-seasons-estimates.html (accessed April 16, 2021).

[7] Metzger W, Ehni H, Kremsner P, Mordmüller B. Experimental infections in humans—historical and ethical reflections. (2019). doi:10.1111/tmi.13320.

[8] Roestenberg M, Hoogerwerf M-A, Ferreira D, Mordmüller B, Yazdanbakhsh M. Experimental infection of human volunteers. Lancet Infect Dis 2018;18:e312–22.

[9] Ip D, Lincoln L, Leung N, Fang V, Kwok-Hung C, Chu D, Leung M, Peiris G, Uyeki T, Cowling B. Viral shedding and transmission potential of asymptomatic and paucisymptomatic influenza virus infections in the community. Clin Infect Dis 2017;64(6):736–42. doi:10.1093/cid/ciw841. Published online [2016] Dec 22. PMCID: PMC5967351, PMID: 28011603.

[10] Furuya-Kanamori L, Cox M, Milinovich G, Magalhaes R, Mackay I, Yakob L. Heterogeneous and dynamic prevalence of asymptomatic influenza virus infections. Emerg Infect Dis 2016;22(6):052–1056. https://dx.doi.org/10.3201/eid2206.151080.

[11] Alford R, Kasel J, Gerone P, Knight V. Human influenza resulting from aerosol inhalation. Proc Soc Exp Biol Med 1966;122(3):800–4. doi:10.3181/00379727-122-31255. PMID: 5918954. https://pubmed.ncbi.nlm.nih.gov/5918954/.

[12] Teunis P, Brienen N, Kretzschmar M. High infectivity and pathogenicity of influenza A virus via aerosol and droplet transmission. Epidemics 2010:215–22.

[13] Henle W, Henle G, Stokes J, Maris E. Experimental exposure of human subjects to viruses of influenza. J Immunol 1946;52(2):145–65.

[14] Kupferschmidt K. New Ebola outbreak likely sparked by a person infected 5 years ago. Science, Health 2021. doi:10.1126/science.abi4876. https://www.sciencemag.org/news/2021/03/new-ebola-outbreak-likely-sparked-person-infected-5-years-ago (accessed April 16, 2021).

[15] Greiff D, Blumenthal H, Chiga M, Pinkerton H. The effects on biological materials of freezing and drying by vacuum sublimation. II. Effect on influenza virus. J Exp Med 1954;100(1):89–101. doi:10.1084/jem.100.1.89.

[16] Kwilas S, Liesman R, Zhang L, Walsh E, Pickles R, Peeples M. Respiratory syncytial virus grown in vero cells contains a truncated attachment protein that alters its infectivity and dependence on glycosaminoglycans. J Virol 2009;83(20):10710–8. doi:10.1128/JVI.00986-09. PMCID: PMC2753119, PMID: 19656891.

[17] Bodewes R, Kreijtz J, van Amerongen G, Fouchier R, Osterhaus A, Rimmelzwaan G, et al. Pathogenesis of Influenza A/H5N1 virus infection in ferrets differs between intranasal and intratracheal routes of inoculation. Am J Pathol 2011;179:30–6. doi:10.1016/j.ajpath.2011.03.026.

[18] Song Y, Wang X, Zhang H, et al. Repeated low-dose influenza virus infection causes severe disease in mice: a model for vaccine evaluation. J Virol 2015;89(15):7841–51. doi:10.1128/JVI.00976-15.

[19] Tirado S, Yoon K. Antibody-dependent enhancement of virus infection and disease. Viral Immunol 2003;16(1):69–86. doi:10.1089/088282403763635465. PMID: 12725690.

[20] Vabret N, Britton G, Gruber C, Hegde S, Kim J, Kuksin M, Levantovsky R, Malle L, Moreira A, Park M, Pia L, Risson E, Saffern M, Salomé B, Selvan M, Spindler M, Tan J, van der Heide V, Gregory J, Alexandropoulos K. Sinai Immunology Review Project. Immunology of COVID-19: Current State of the Science. Immunity 2020(6):910–41. https://www.cell.com/immunity/fulltext/S1074-7613(20)30183-7?_returnURL=https%3A%2F%2Flinkinghub.elsevier.com%2Fretrieve%2Fpii%2FS1074761320301837%3Fshowall%3Dtrue.

[21] Rodríguez Y, Rojas M, Pacheco Y, Acosta-Ampudia Y, Ramírez-Santana C, Monsalve D, Gershwin M, Anaya J. Guillain-Barré syndrome, transverse myelitis and infectious diseases. Cellular Mol Immunol 2018;15(6):547–62. https://doi.org/10.1038/cmi.2017.142.

[22] Principi N, Esposito S. Do vaccines have a role as a cause of autoimmune neurological syndromes? Front Public Health 2020;8:361. doi:10.3389/fpubh.2020.00361 PMID: 32850592; PMCID: PMC7399175.

[23] Takyar V, Nath A, Beri A, Gharib A, Rotman Y. How healthy are the "Healthy volunteers"? Penetrance of NAFLD in the biomedical research volunteer pool. Hepatology 2017;66(3):825–33. https://doi.org/10.1002/hep.29247.

[24] World Medical Association (WMA). (Policy /Current Policies) (2018). *WMA Declaration of Helsinki—Ethical Principles for Medical Research Involving Human Subjects*. https://www.wma.net/policies-post/wma-declaration-of-helsinki-ethical-principles-for-medical-research-involving-human-subjects/ (accessed April 19, 2021).

[25] https://www.who.int/emergencies/diseases/novel-coronavirus-2019/interactive-timeline#! (accessed April 19, 2021).

[26] Jamrozik E, Littler K, Bull S, Emerson C, Kang G, Kapulu M, Rey E, Saenz C, Shah S, Smith P, Upshur R, Weijer C, Selgelid M. Key criteria for the ethical acceptability of COVID-19 human challenge studies: Report of a WHO Working Group. Vaccine 2021;39(4):633–40. ISSN 0264-410X. https://doi.org/10.1016/j.vaccine.2020.10.075.

[27] Purkins L, Love E, Eve M, Wooldridge C, Cowan C, Smart T, Johnson P, Rapeport W. The influence of diet upon liver function tests and serum lipids in healthy male volunteers resident in a Phase I unit. Br J Clin Pharmacol 2004;57(2):199–208. https://doi.org/10.1046/j.1365-2125.2003.01969.x.

[28] Verbeek J, Rajamaki B, Ijaz S, Tikka C, Ruotsalainen J, Edmond M, Sauni R, Kilinc Balci FS. Personal protective equipment for preventing highly infectious diseases due to exposure to contaminated body fluids in healthcare staff. Cochrane Database Syst Rev 2019;7(7):CD011621. https://doi.org/10.1002/14651858.CD011621.pub3.

[29] WHO. Human challenge trials for vaccine development: regulatory considerations. 2016. https://www.who.int/biologicals/expert_committee/Human_challenge_Trials_IK_final.pdf (accessed April 20, 2021).

[30] WHO. Guidelines on clinical evaluation of vaccines: regulatory expectations. Revision of WHO TRS 924, Annex 1. https://www.who.int/biologicals/BS2287_Clinical_guidelines_final_LINE_NOs_20_July_2016.pdf?ua=1 (accessed April 20, 2021).

[31] WHO. Key criteria for the ethical acceptability of COVID-19 human challenge studies. WHO Working Group for Guidance on Human Challenge Studies in COVID-19, 2020 https://www.who.int/ethics/publications/key-criteria-ethical-acceptabilityof-covid-19-human-challenge/en/ (accessed April 20, 2021).

[32] WHO. Feasibility, potential value and limitations of establishing a closely monitored challenge model of experimental COVID-19 infection and illness in healthy young adult volunteers. Report from the WHO Advisory Group on Human Challenge Studies: https://www.who.int/publications/m/item/feasibility-potential-value-and-limitations-of-establishing-a-closelymonitored-challenge-model-of-experimental-covid-19-infection-andillness-in-healthy-young-adult-volunteers (accessed April 20, 2021).

[33] FDA, Guidance for industry influenza: developing drugs for treatment and/or prophylaxis (Rockville, MD, 2011). https://www.fda.gov/regulatory-information/search-fda-guidance-documents/influenza-developing-drugs-treatment-andor-prophylaxis (accessed April 20, 2021).

[34] EC Directive 2001/20/EC, Approximation of the laws, regulations and administrative provisions of the Member States relating to the implementation of good clinical practice in the conduct of clinical trials on medicinal products for human use (Brussels, 2001). https://eur-lex.europa.eu/LexUriServ/LexUriServ.do?uri=OJ:L:2001:121:0034:0044:en:PDF (accessed April 20, 2021).

[35] EC, Guidance on Investigational Medicinal Products (IMPs) and Non-Investigational Medicinal Products (NIMP) (Brussels, 2011).

[36] Regulation (EU) No 536/2014 of the European Parliament and of the Council of 16 April 2014 on clinical trials on medicinal products for human use, and repealing Directive 2001/20/EC. https://ec.europa.eu/health/sites/default/files/files/eudralex/vol-1/reg_2014_536/reg_2014_536_en.pdf (accessed April 20, 2021).

[37] Final Rule for Clinical Trials Registration and Results Information Submission (42 CFR 11.10(a)). https://clinicaltrials.gov/ct2/manage-recs/fdaaa (accessed April 20, 2021).

[38] Guideline on the requirements for quality documentation concerning biological investigational medicinal products in clinical trials EMA/CHMP/BWP/534898/2008. https://www.ema.europa.eu/en/documents/scientific-guideline/guideline-requirements-quality-documentation-concerning-biological-investigational-medicinal_en-0.pdf (accessed April 20, 2021).

[39] EC, Guidance: virus safety evaluation of biotechnological investigational medicinal products (London 2008). https://www.ema.europa.eu/en/virus-safety-evaluation-biotechnological-investigational-medicinal-products (accessed April 20, 2021).

[40] Hayden F, Treanor J, Fritz R, et al. Use of the oral neuraminidase inhibitor oseltamivir in experimental human influenza: randomized controlled trials for prevention and treatment. JAMA 1999;282(13):1240–6. doi:10.1001/jama.282.13.1240.

Chapter 11

Preclinical testing of vaccine candidates in animal models

Katharine C. Carter[a], Derya T. Ata[a], Raphael T. Aruleba[b], Ramona Hurdayal[b]

[a]*Strathclyde Institute of Pharmacy and Biomedical Sciences, University of Strathclyde, Glasgow, United Kingdom,* [b]*Department of Molecular and Cell Biology, University of Cape Town, Cape Town, South Africa*

11.1 Introduction

The importance of vaccination in preventing diseases was exemplified by the eradication of smallpox following an international effort to ensure the transmission of this disease, which was responsible for 7 million deaths [1]. More recently the COVID19 pandemic, caused by infection with the virus with the SARS-COV-2, has shown how the vaccine can have a beneficial effect on human health and survival [2]. Successful vaccination is dependent on a clear understanding of the type of immune response required to protect against the particular infection or condition, and identification of the antigen(s) that can induce this response without inducing any adverse side effects. This type of information is based on years of studies on a particular pathogen of condition, but there are some general principles on the type of immune response required for different pathogens and/or conditions (Table 11.1).

The type of vaccine candidates that have been used over time can be divided into different categories, which may require the use of an adjuvant to boost the immune system to an adequate level to induce a sufficient level of immunity to protect against infection (Table 11.2).

Despite years of research there are very relatively few vaccines to protect against infection (<25). An up-to-date list of clinically approved vaccine available for different infectious diseases can be found be found on the World Health Organisations website (https://www.who.int/health-topics/vaccines-and-immunization#tab=tab_1, accessed 05/03/21). And different websites can be used to identify vaccines that are undergoing clinical trials (e.g. https://www.centerwatch.com/clinical-trials/, accessed 05/03/21). Development of therapeutic vaccines can use in silico methods to predict features such as B and T cells epitopes, antigenicity, allergenicity, toxicity, and protein-peptide docking [11].

System Vaccinology. https://doi.org/10.1016/B978-0-323-85941-7.00001-2

TABLE 11.1 The type of immune response required to protect against different type of infections/conditions.

Condition	Location	Example	Type of immune response involved	References
Viral	Intracellular	HIV	Cellular ($CD4^+$ and $CD8^+$ T cells)	Collins et al. (2020)
Bacteria	Intracellular	*Mycobacterium tuberculosis*	Cellular ($CD4^+$ T cells)	[3]
	Extracellular	*Staphylococcus aureus*	Humoral/Cellular (IgA,IgM,IgG/$CD4^+$ T cells)	[4]
Fungi	Intracellular	*Histoplasma Capsulatum*	Cellular ($CD4^+$and $CD8^+$ T cells)	[5]
	Extracellular	*Pneumocystis jirovecii*	Humoral (IgG,IgM)	[6]
Protozoan parasite	Intracellular	*Leishmania major*	Humoral/Cellular (IgG/ $CD4^+$ T cells)	[7]
	Extracellular	*Toxoplasma gondii*	Cellular ($CD4^+$ T cells)	[8]
Multicellular parasite	Intracellular	*Trichinella spiralis*	Humoral/Cellular (IgE,IgG/$CD4^+$ T cells)	[9]
Cancer	Intracellular	*Mycobacterium tuberculosis*	Cellular ($CD4^+$and $CD8^+$ T cells	[10]

However, in vivo models are required to demonstrate that a vaccine can protect against the particular pathogen or condition and its biological effect on whole organ living systems [12]. Preclinical animal testing in a variety of species and models is therefore paramount to evaluating efficacy, safety, and immunogenicity of a vaccine candidate. Granted, the success of these studies dictates progression of the candidate through further clinical trials. Thus, an important criterion to consider is the choice of animal species and model used to evaluate the vaccine candidate considering that animal models are different from humans in some respects, in terms of population genetics, disease manifestation, and immune response, amongst others. Naturally, vaccine testing in animal species that more closely resemble humans would be preferred, such as non-human primates [12], however financial, logistical, and ethical constraints often prevent routine use of these more complex models [13]. In this review, we will look at the role animal models have had in the development of vaccines against infectious diseases.

TABLE 11.2 Main type of vaccines used to protect against infections/conditions with examples of each vaccine type.

Type of vaccine	Nature of vaccine antigen	Adjuvant used	Type of immunity induced	Example (with reference)
Live, e.g., Dengue vaccine (Dengvaxia)	Whole organism	Not required	Humoral/ Cellular Immunity (IgG,IgM/$CD4^+$and $CD8^+$ T cells)	Guy et al. (2020)
Killed, e.g., Influenza virus (Formalin-Inactivated H1N1 whole virion vaccine)	Whole organism	Not required	Cellular Immunity ($CD8^+$ T cells)	Sabbaghi et al. (2019)
Attenuated organism, e.g., Yellow fever (17D)	Whole organism	Not required	Humoral/Cellular Immunity (IgG/$CD4^+$and $CD8^+$ T cells)	Collins et al. (2017) and Bovay et al. (2020)
Purified components, e.g., Dengue (Dengue virus serotype 1 (DENV-1))	Protein	Alum	Cellular Immunity ($CD4^+$and $CD8^+$ T cells)	Zutshi et al. (2019) and Friberg et al. (2020)
Recombinant protein, e.g., CO-VID-19 (NVX-CoV2373)	Protein	Matrix-M1	Humoral/ Cellular Immunity (IgG/$CD4^+$and $CD8^+$ T cells)	Pollet et al. (2021) and Keech et al. (2020)
Subunit vaccine, e.g., Tuberculosis (Bacillus Calmette-Guérin (BCG))	Protein	Glucopyranosyl Lipid	Cellular Immunity ($CD4^+$and $CD8^+$ T cells)	Bellini et al. (2020)
DNA vaccine, e.g., Influenza (H5 DNA vaccine)	Deoxyribonucleic acid oligonucleotides	Lipofectin	Humoral/Cellular Immunity (IgA/$CD4^+$and $CD8^+$ T cells)	Lee, et al. (2018) and Ghaemi et al. (2021)
RNA vaccine, e.g., COVID-19 (BNT162b2)	Deoxyribonucleic acid oligonucleotides	Not required	Cellular Immunity ($CD4^+$and $CD8^+$ T cells)	Cagigi et al. (2021) and Polack et al. (2020)

11.2 Types of animal models used in vaccine studies

The hallmark of vaccinology is the ability to induce immune protection and immunological memory against a particular pathogen. Accordingly, translation of vaccine research into efficient clinical therapies requires testing of the vaccine candidate in an appropriate model to determine how well it "works" [14]. Animal models are particularly useful for this purpose and encompass a wide variety including transgenic, cloned, and gene-deficient animals; outbred species; neonatal and aging animals to study age-specific effects; surgical models, to isolate certain immune compartments for analysis and "humanized" animals. They can be modeled to suit experimental needs to study single infections versus co-infections with pathogenic species, but they can also be used to model chronic diseases/conditions and autoimmune diseases [15]. Collectively, animal models are therefore used to assess how well a vaccine "works" by analyzing safety and toxicity, vaccine formulation, optimal dose, and delivery of the vaccine, induction of host protective immunity against challenge with the particular pathogen or condition, quality, quantity, onset, and duration of the host immune response induced and finally, reduction in disease pathology and/or disease transmission [12,15,16]. Not surprising, human studies are the gold standard for vaccine testing in comparison to unvaccinated groups. Realistically, however, vaccine studies in humans are complex requiring large numbers of participants and prone to ethical issues, which in turn may be compromised by geographic and demographic biases. Altogether this increases costs substantially. In contrast, animal models provide a cost-effective and faster alternative, and they are essential for preclinical safety testing. The type of animal model may be case-specific as the animal model must be permissive to infection, should mimic pathophysiology of disease by the pathogen to some extent, and exhibit immune responses that resemble human immune responses to determine protection from infection and/or disease transmission. In terms of logistics, the model should have immunological tools and reagents available for assessing the quality and quantity of the host immune response. Given these points, choosing an appropriate animal model is critical in vaccine research to make the translation from preclinical to clinical application. Caution should be noted however that no individual animal model provides all the resources and information necessary for passing a new vaccine through the preclinical stage [12]. Similarly, one should bear in mind that using animals for research also comes with ethical obligations to treat the animals in the most humane manner with appropriate ethical protocols in place, rigorously assessed by national and/or international experts [13].

11.2.1 Small and large animal models

A surfeit of animal models is available for use and can loosely be divided into two main types, small animal or large animal models (Fig. 11.1). Small animal models, such as mice, rats, hamsters, guinea pigs, and ferrets, are easy to procure, cost-effective to maintain, have consistent genetic backgrounds,

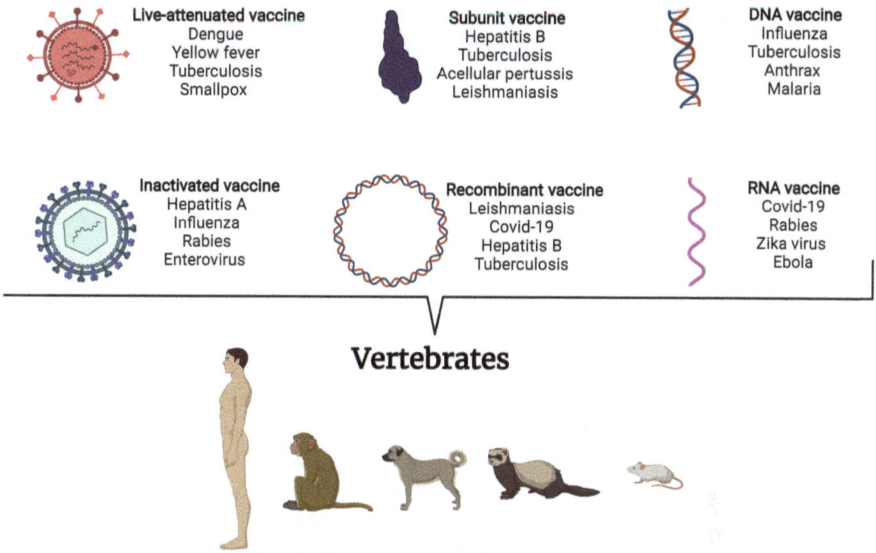

FIG. 11.1 Various vaccine platforms have been designed to provide immunity against different infectious agents affecting vertebrates, such as humans, dogs, ferrets, and rodents. Figure created in Biorender.com.

and have well-characterized immune systems to mimic essential aspects of mammalian immunity [15]. Small rodents have the added advantage of well-characterized inbred strains, so that differences in responses can be attributed to specific effects rather than genetic differences. Moreover, an abundance of reagents is available for in-depth mechanistic immunological analyses. In this regard, mice are a model species as advances in murine genetics have led to the generation of transgenic and gene-deficient models to study different genes and proteins in host immunity to infection and vaccination. Animals can be typed as "resistant" or "highly susceptible" to the pathogen so that it is possible to determine the influence of genotype on vaccine efficacy as people can have a range of immune responses to a vaccine. An example of strain-dependent susceptibility to an infection is the well-characterized mouse strains susceptibility to *Leishmania* infection [17]. Understanding the basis of this variability in susceptibility showed that a single gene, solute carrier family 11a (proton-coupled divalent metal ion transporters) member 1 or *Slc11a1*, controlled innate resistance to *Leishmania donovani* and led to the identification of similar genetic traits in humans [18].

Large animal models, such as pigs, cattle, goats, and non-human primates, are also used in preclinical vaccine studies. These models are not only physiologically closer to humans but often, are natural hosts to various human pathogens and can therefore mimic interactions between host and pathogen in an appropriate biological environment [19]. A further advantage is that larger animal models are outbred, thereby allowing greater insight into vaccine efficacy, and are useful for studies looking at the effect of scaling up a vaccine dose or collection of larger volumes for analysis. Altogether, these advantages could accelerate the development of a vaccine product from preclinical trials to human Phase I clinical trials [12]. Realistically, however, studies in large animal models are often limited by the range of immunological reagents available, a clear understanding of their immunological mechanisms in protection against infection, and their overall cost (reviewed by [12]).

11.2.2 Natural, surrogate, surgical, and experimental models

Generally, animal models can be grouped as natural, surrogate, surgical, and experimental models [15]. All these models encompass both small and large animals but there is a predominance of small animals in surrogate and experimental models. While each model differs in scope, cost, and practicality, each model can offer some assessment of immune responses, but no model is able to recapitulate the dynamics of human vaccine studies in its entirety (described in Table 11.3).

All four models can be used as single versus co-infection or co-condition models. Interestingly, natural animal models are preferred for studying co-infections and several have been well-established in large animals, e.g., combination of *Respiratory Bovine Coronaviruses* (RBCV)/*Pasteurella haemolytica* amongst others [15,20] Coinfections contribute substantially to the establishment of disease as well as progression to a severe or lethal outcome. Thus, co-infection can have a major impact on vaccine efficacy as different pathogens can stimulate polar changes in the host's immune responses (reviewed by [21]). For instance, people coinfected with influenza and SARS-CoV-2 are more than twice as likely to die as someone only infected with SARS-CoV-2 [22] hence a detailed understanding of how a vaccine against one pathogen can influence the immune response to a second pathogen is required. This type of study is currently being considered by the UK's Joint Committee on Vaccination and Immunisation and will be an issue for any country where they want integrate COVID vaccination into their normal influenza vaccine program [23]. In another study, co-infection with the helminth *Litomosoides sigmodontis* significantly reduced the efficacy of influenza vaccine in a murine model [24]. Coinfected vaccinated mice produced lower amounts of influenza-specific neutralizing IgG1, IgG2b, and IgG2c antibody ($P < 0.01$), lost more body weight over the course of infection ($P < 0.05$), and gave a lower amount of sterile immunity (31% vs 73%) compared to uninfected vaccinated mice challenged with the pathogenic Influenza A H1N1 A/HH/NY/1580/09 strain, which replicates in mice without further adaptation [24]. Interesting, vaccination had no significant effect on parasite burdens in the coinfected mice.

11.2.3 Humanized mice

The creation of humanized mice, which are generated by the transfer of human hematopoietic stem cells, peripheral blood mononuclear cells, or tissue

TABLE 11.3 Animal model groups for vaccine studies.

Type of model	Definition	Animal types	Important features
Natural model	Species that is a natural host for a pathogen	Pathogen specific host used, e.g., rodents, cats, dogs, pigs, cows	Allow influence of normal coinfections on vaccine efficacy, role of vertical transmission, on transfer of vaccine induced immunity, assessment of role of "responders" and "non-responders" on vaccine efficacy
Surrogate model	Species that can be only infected with pathogen under experimental conditions	Pathogen specific as species must be amenable to infection, e.g., mice, rats, cotton rats, Guinea pigs ferrets, pigs, monkeys	Allow influence of specific components of the immune response to a vaccine can be assessed using genetic "knockout" or "knock in host strains," animals can be "humanized" for vaccine screening studies
Surgical model	Allow administration of vaccine to a specific site within the body	Species used depends on intricacy of surgery involved—may favor larger species, e.g., pigs, cows	Allow influence of specific compartments on vaccine immunity to be defined
Experimental model	Used for preclinical testing—where regulatory authorities require two models	Defined by regulators: species include rodents, dogs, pigs, monkeys	Allow safety, efficacy, route of administration, and dosing regimen to be defined

transplants into immunodeficient animals, has potentially enhanced the success of surrogate models [15,25]. However, this system is still a work-in-progress as these mice do not fully mimic human immune responses yet [25]. Moreover, the popular NOD/Shi-scid-IL2Rγ^{null} (NOG) and NOD SCID γC (NSG) models will need further complex gene manipulations to study specific human immune responses and this is likely to require technological advances in gene manipulation [26,27]. Therefore, it may be a long while before humanized mice are able to accurately recapitulate essential components of the human immune system. To-date, no licensed vaccine has been validated in humanized mouse models for predicting efficacy and/or human immune responses [25].

11.3 Immunity to vaccines

Considering that effector immune responses are tailored to different microbes, an important aspect in vaccine development and design is identifying and targeting the relevant pathway of immune activation for host protection against a particular pathogen or condition [16]. Subsequent immunological evaluation of the vaccine candidate is one way of defining whether a vaccine "works" [14]. While many organizations and countries may advocate for the replacement of animal experiments for research purposes [28], an animal model is unquestionably critical in vaccine development to assess vaccine-induced immunity in a biological living system. Natural, surrogate, and experimental animal models are all applicable to assessing immunity and may include small (mice, rats, rabbits, ferrets, hamsters, and guinea pigs) or large animals (non-human primates, cattle, horses, and goats) [15]. Generally, the immune response to a vaccine follows the same trajectory as that of infection with a pathogen and involves a combination of innate immune compartments, such as antigen presenting cells (APC) and natural killer (NK) cells, and adaptive immune compartments namely $CD4^+$ and $CD8^+$ T and B cells.

11.3.1 $CD4^+$ T cell activation

Activation and differentiation of antigen-specific $CD4^+$ T cells requires three different signals. The first signal is the recognition of pathogens by antigen presenting cells (APCs). Upon immunization with a vaccine, diverse pattern-recognition receptors (PRRs) on professional APCs (DCs, macrophages and monocytes) recognize vaccine antigens via distinct pathogen-associated molecular patterns (PAMPs) on the antigen. This, in turn, activates NF-κB and inflammasome activation to promote phagocytosis of the vaccine antigen/s and secretion of immunomodulatory mediators (such as cytokines, chemokines, and killing-effector molecules). Following this, the activated DC processes the internalized antigens and loads peptide fragments in complex with MHC class II molecules. Peptide-loaded MHC Class II molecules are then transported to the surface of the APC for presentation to naïve $CD4^+$ T cells. This concludes signal one. The antigenic peptides are recognized by the naïve $CD4^+$ T cells via their unique T cell receptor (TCR)-CD3 complex. In addition, APC activation promotes costimulatory signals between CD80/CD86 on the APC with CD28 on the T cell that aids T cell activation. This constitutes signal two. Finally, immunomodulatory cytokines secreted by the activated APC enables the polarization of effector $CD4^+$ T cells into distinct subtypes such as Th1, Th2, Th17, or Tregs and memory T cells. The type of T response responses elicited by a vaccine will depend on local immune response and will be strongly influenced by ongoing innate immune responses [29] which will, in turn, be influenced by the route the antigen is introduced into the body [30]. However, long-term priming of innate immune responses can have a profound effect on immune responses to diverse infections, by a process named "trained immunity." Human studies suggest that live vaccines, e.g., measles vaccine, smallpox vaccine, oral polio vaccine had beneficial, non-specific protective effects against non-target diseases (reviewed by [31]). Therefore, the interaction between innate and specific immune cells is a multifactorial process and animal models should perhaps consider the role of vaccination on both target and non-target diseases.

11.3.2 CD8$^+$ T cell activation

The activation of CD8$^+$ T cells or cytotoxic T lymphocytes (CTLs) may occur via two routes. In the classical route, endogenous antigens are produced from pathogen replication within the APC. These antigens are cleaved within the proteasome of the cells for presentation to naïve CD8$^+$ T cells loaded onto MHC Class I molecules. In the non-classical route, DCs could present external antigens in the context of MHC class I molecules to CD8$^+$ T cells in a process termed "cross-presentation." As the name suggests, CTLs employ cytotoxicity to clear infected cells.

11.3.3 B-cell activation

Most vaccines in current use confer immune protection through humoral immunity [32]. This is mediated by high-affinity antibody-secreting plasma cells and memory B cells, which are products of B cell activation, and usually involve interaction with cognate CD4$^+$ T cells classically defined as T cell-dependent activation [33]. The opposite to this is T cell-independent activation, involving polysaccharide and/or lipopolysaccharide structures, whereby additional signals to activate the B cells come from binding of antigen to toll-like receptors (TLRs) or by extensive crosslinking of BCRs on the B cell, rather than from T cell stimulation (reviewed in [34]). Generally, T cell-independent activation results in the secretion of low-affinity IgM whilst T cell-dependent activation results in high-affinity IgG, the latter favored in vaccination ([33,34]) and hence will be our focus going forward. B-cell activation begins in secondary lymphoid organs (SLO) when the B cell recognizes and binds antigenic PAMPs via its BCR. As professional APCs, B cells can internalize the antigen, process it and present it on the B cell surface in complex with MHC-II molecules, to Th cells, specifically T follicular helper (T_{FH}), in the T cell zone of the SLO [33,35]. T_{FH} cells bind the peptide-MHC II complex via their TCR. This interaction is further stabilized by co-stimulatory signals between CD40 on B cells and CD40 ligand on CD4$^+$ T cells [35]. In addition, cytokines secreted by T_{FH} cells are bound by B cell cytokine receptors and promote B cell proliferation, differentiation, somatic hypermutation, and immunoglobulin class switching forming a germinal centre (GC) in the SLO. Somatic hypermutation directs affinity maturation whereby variable regions of the BCR undergo random mutations to generate a BCR with higher affinity for the antigen. B cells, with the newly generated BCR, then compete for survival signals from follicular dendritic cells in the GC [33,35]. B cells that manage to form a BCR with high enough affinity exit the GC as long-lived plasma cells and memory B cells. Vaccination is dependent on memory B cells that circulate throughout the body ready to quickly respond to the previously encountered antigen via their high-affinity BCR. Identification of a quantifiable "target" for a vaccine would allow rationale selection of an immunization schedule or help predict how long immunity can last after vaccination. This type of standardization is possible, for example, a hemagglutination inhibition titer of 1:40 is associated with 50% protection against influenza.

11.4 Predictors of vaccine-induced protective immunity in animal models

Immunogenicity to a vaccine candidate in animal models is often defined as a measure of innate and acquired immune responses, with the latter involving humoral and cell-mediated immunity regulated by distinct T cell subsets namely, Th1, Th2, Th17, T regulatory (Treg), T follicular helper (T_{FH}), and cytotoxic T (Tc) cells. In the simplest sense, cell-mediated immunity is particularly important in the clearance of intracellular pathogens whilst antibody-mediated humoral immunity protects against extracellular pathogens.

Since innate immune responses instructs the quality and quantity of adaptive immune responses, activation of innate immunity involving pathogen recognition, and uptake by activated phagocytes upon vaccination is a desirable outcome. To achieve this, vaccine formulations have incorporated adjuvants to stimulate innate signaling pathways thereby enhancing the induction of vaccine-specific T and B cell responses downstream, rather than by direct effects on the lymphocytes themselves (reviewed in [36]). This is especially relevant for non-living vaccine products (e.g., inactivated vaccines or recombinant protein vaccines) that are poorly immunogenic on their own [36]. In this respect, nearly all PRR families are potential adjuvant targets. Examples include NOD-like receptors (NLRs), C-type lectin receptors (CLRs), retinoid acid-inducible gene-I (RIG-I)-like receptors (RLRs) and TLRs [36]. TLRs are the most well-studied and the live attenuated yellow-fever vaccine 17D (YF-17D) is perhaps the earliest and most successful model to exemplify this [37] YF-17D elicits a strong pro-inflammatory response involving IL-12p40, IL-6, and IFN-α from activation of innate DC subsets via TLR2, TLR7, TLR8, and TLR9, which results in the activation and proliferation of antigen-specific $CD8^+$ T cells [38]. Comparatively, Leish-111f, a *Leishmania*-derived polyprotein composed of three antigens, is an efficacious vaccine candidate against all forms of leishmaniasis when combined with monophosphoryl lipid A (MPL), as MPL acts as a TLR4 agonist selectively inducing TLR4 activation and subsequent Th1-type immune responses [39]. Indeed, MPL and alum are now a licensed component of vaccines for HBV and papilloma due to its safety and effective polarization of Th1-responses [40]. Altogether, recognition of pathogen-associated ligands via PRRs directs the predominant pathway by which DCs become activated, mature, and provide signals to naïve T cells and B cells to tailor adaptive (humoral and cell-mediated) immune responses [41].

Cell-mediated immunity results from the activation of APCs and lymphocytes [16] and can be used to identify cell-mediated surrogates of protection, such as, lymphocyte activation and recruitment, T cell phenotype, cytokine, and chemokine secretion, cytotoxic killing, and proliferative capacity. To identify immune populations, chemokine expression and assess T and B cell phenotype and activation, flow cytometry is primarily used, and when combined with intracellular staining protocols, can be extended to cytokine and transcriptional factor analyses at the protein level. In addition, mass spectrometry, genomics, and proteomics (even at single-cell level) allow greater specificity in immune monitoring of vaccine candidates in animal models; however, the high cost of these methods restrict their routine use [25]. Other common assays include delayed-type hypersensitive (DTH) assays, cytotoxicity assays, and macrophage activation assays to determine effector function.

At the onset, to achieve cell-mediated immunity, the vaccine candidate must possess the ability to activate (or enter) target cells and activate specific T and B cells with high specificity and efficiency [42]. Most often, the activation and function of effector and memory T cells are assessed as correlates of protection to vaccination. For instance, in animal models of leishmaniasis, groups of dogs immunized with *Leishmania donovani* centrin-1 deleted ($LdCen^{-/-}$) parasites had a higher proliferation of B cells and $CD8^+$ T cells compared to vaccinated controls [43]. Moreover, $LdCen^{-/-}$ vaccination-induced type 1 immune responses, characterized by increased levels of TNF-α and IL-12/IL-23p40, one of the hallmarks associated with protective immunity to intracellular parasites (Table 11.2) [43]. Similarly, immunization of BALB/c mice with p27 gene-deficient Ld1S2D strain of *L. donovani* ($Ldp27^{-/-}$) induced significant secretion of *Leishmania* antigen-specific type 1 cytokines (IL-12p70, IFN-γ and TNF-α) postimmunization [44].

Humoral immunity is antibody/immunoglobulin (Ig)-mediated, and require affinity-matured plasma B cells to be produced, which requires T cell help [16]. Primary protection against several viruses, extracellular parasites, fungi and bacterial infections is mediated by humoral immunity [16], resulting in protection by a number of pathways such as neutralization of a pathogen by blocking its entry into cells, or antibody-dependent cytotoxicity by increasing activation of phagocytes or natural killer (NK) cells (Fig. 11.2). Indeed, vaccination may fail if the vaccine candidate is unable to activate humoral immunity under these infectious processes [32]. Routine serological assays such as neutralization and hemagglutination assays as well as enzyme-linked immunosorbent assay (ELISA) are often used to measure levels of serum antibody as correlates or surrogates of host protective humoral immunity to a proposed vaccine candidate (Fig. 11.3) [45]. For example, SARS-CoV2 requires the production of high avidity neutralizing IgG [46].Vaccination with the spike glycoprotein of SARS-CoV induced protective immunity in BALB/c mice and related to the presence

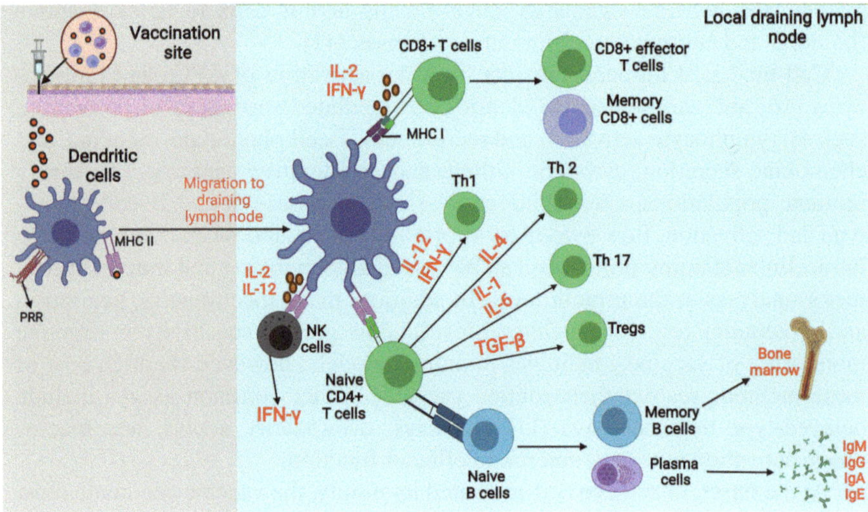

FIG. 11.2 Humoral or cellular immune responses or both, may be induced in a vertebrate after administration with a vaccine candidate. Antigen presenting cells (*APCs*) such as dendritic cells (*DCs*) recognize the vaccine candidate, or parts thereof, by their pathogen recognition receptors (*PRRs*), and process the signal following internalization. The activated DCs migrate to a secondary lymphoid organ (*SLO*) and present antigenic peptides on either MHC class I or MHC class II molecules, leading to specific T cell activation. Activated $CD4^+$ T cells proliferate and differentiate into various subpopulations in a process influenced by the cytokine milieu of the activated DC. Effector T cells in turn secrete cytokines that activate B cells or other cells that express the relevant cytokine receptors. Activated B cells undergo somatic hypermutation and class switching in the geminal center of the SLO and differentiate into plasma cells producing antibodies of different isotypes that bind to the specific pathogen at its site within the body. IgM is the first antibody produced, followed by IgG, which is a more efficient neutralizing antibody, and it binds to the surface of the pathogen and aids in opsonization. Other antibody classes, e.g., IgA, IgD, or IgE are produced by the plasma cells, their production depends on class of pathogen and the type of immune response stimulated. Some of the effector T and B cells differentiate into memory T and B cells so that an accelerated response can occur on second exposure to the pathogen/vaccine. Memory B cells move to the bone marrow where they live for a long time and function as APCs to T cells upon re-exposure to the same antigen. Furthermore, IL-2 and IL-12-derived DC production activates NK cells to produce IFN-γ. They present antigen to $CD8^+$ T cells via antigen expressed on MHC class I and stimulate the production of effector cytotoxic T cells (CTL). CTL can kill infected cells by inducing apoptosis or activate innate cytotoxicity via their IFN-γ production. Some CTL develops into memory cells that can be activated on second exposure to the pathogen. Figure created in Biorender.com.

of specific antibody (IgG) titres and the presence of strongly neutralizing antibodies (range 1:50 to 1:150 dilution) [47].

Cellular immunity may collaborate with humoral immunity to give an enhanced immunological response. For example, vaccination of mice with recombinant hydrophilic acylated surface protein B1 (HASPB1) induced a substantial IFN-γ response in $CD8^+$ T cells and IL-12p70 production by DCs with a concomitant (type 2) antibody response, altogether mediating host protection to VL in BALB/c mice [48]. In addition, studies have shown that protection induced by vaccination with Leishmune, Leish-Tec, or LBSap (60 μg

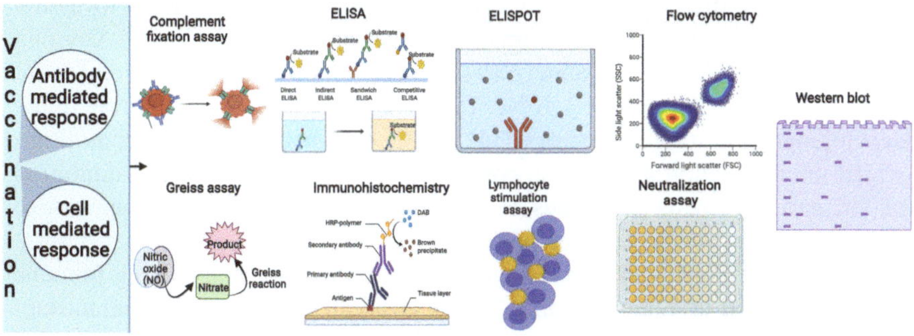

FIG. 11.3 Common immunological techniques used to identify vaccine specific immune responses. These assays use a blood samples obtain from vaccinated individuals and controls. The ability of antibodies to recognise a specific antigen is determined by carrying out an ELISA based assay, immunohistochemistry or Western blot studies, whereas the efficacy of the antibody responses to mediate in host immune responses can be determined using a neutralization assay. The ability of vaccination to induce specific cell-mediated immune responses is often determined using a lymphocyte proliferation assay or using flow cytometry to phenotype the cells present. The type of cell-mediated immune response can also be determined by assessing the products produced using assays such as an ELISPOT for cytokines or Greiss assay for the production of nitric oxide. An immunological assay can have multiple uses, for example an ELISA assay, flow cytometry or immunohistochemistry can also be used to determine the products produced by immune cell. Figure created in Biorender.com.

L. braziliensis antigen and 50 μg saponin/dose) was associated with increased levels of NK $CD3^{-}CD49^{+}$ cells and specific immunoglobulin is known to increase the activity of NK cells [49]. In this study, vaccination resulted in increased specific IgG1 and IgG2a levels [50] and a strong IgG1 response was unexpected in both studies [48,50] indicating that immunoglobulin subtype profiling is important when evaluating immune responses as the class produced is important in antibody mediate cytotoxicity for innate cells [63].

As reviewed by [45], another aspect of humoral and cell-mediated immunity is immunological memory. Importantly, direct protection is not provided by memory cells induced immediately after vaccination but is rather a vital second line of defense on re-exposure to the original pathogen. Much of our knowledge on memory T cells have been gleaned from animal models involving mice, again exemplifying the power of animal models. Upon antigen recognition, naïve T cells differentiate into central memory (T_{CM}) within lymphoid tissues and effector memory (T_{EM}) within peripheral tissues, both of which circulate in the blood [51]. T_{CM} and T_{EM} express effector functions like cytolytic activity (CD8 only) and cytokine production (both CD4 and CD8) but importantly, T_{CM} are more potent inducers of protective immunity [52] due to their high proliferative capacity. For instance, a novel vaccine against *Mycobacterium tuberculosis*, L91, was evaluated in mice in combination with BCG. Incorporation of L91 elicited greater expansion of T_{EM} and T_{CM} populations when compared to BCG alone [53]. Memory subsets are usually evaluated via flow cytometry however, a limitation is the differences in markers used in flow cytometry to assess memory subsets in preclinical animal models vs human clinical trials. Coming back to the yellow-fever vaccine, YF-17D vaccination induces upregulation of IRF7 and expression of type 1-IFNs. Type 1-IFN plays a significant role in the development and stabilization of $CD4^+$ and $CD8^+$ T cells with T_{CM} capabilities, whilst in conjunction with IL-12, contributes to T_{EM} production and inhibition of Th2 and Th17 cells [54]. Thus, the paramount success of YF-17D appears to tick all boxes of vaccine immunogenicity.

Regulatory T cells are immunosuppressors critical for maintaining immune homeostasis and immune tolerance [55]. Considering their role in immunosuppression, they could also suppress APC, T and B effector, and memory cells, thereby inhibiting protective immune responses to infection and vaccination, which is particularly important for viral infections. Several viruses support the expansion of Tregs at the expense of effector and memory T cells and allow their uncontrolled replication. This effect was confirmed in studies where depletion of Tregs led to beneficial outcomes in HSV-1, rotavirus, and influenza infection [56]. Therefore, it is important to carry out studies determining the phenotype of T cells induced as systematic monitoring of this population is overlooked when analyzing effector Th and CTL immune responses to vaccination [56]. Tregs have been shown to suppress vaccine-induced immune responses [55,56], for example, depletion of Tregs enhanced primary and memory CTL responses to HSV-1 DNA vaccine in mice, conferring greater protection upon viral challenge [57]. Based on these observations, recent studies now advocate that assays used to evaluate vaccine-induced effector T cells should also take antigen-specific Tregs into account. To this effect, flow cytometric analysis can be used focusing on markers associated with Tregs ($FoxP_3$) and activation markers such as CD25, OX40 (CD134), CD39, and IL-35, amongst others [55,56]. Overall, the immune response elicited after vaccination depends on various contributing factors, however, best protection if often associated with strong humoral and cell-mediated immune responses.

11.5 Examples of disease models used in development of preclinical vaccines in animal models

Probably the best way to understand and reflect on how different animal models have been used in preclinical vaccine studies to assess induction of host protective immunity to vaccine candidates is to review specific disease examples where these models have led to licensure of a vaccine. The following section discusses influenza, where preclinical vaccine studies translated into clinical therapies and licensure, and leishmaniasis, where preclinical vaccine studies were unsuccessful in translating into clinical therapies and hence, to-date, there is no licensed vaccine.

11.5.1 Influenza

Influenza is responsible for responsible for significant morbidity and mortality, where it can cause up to 650,000 deaths/year [58]. Currently, there are a number of clinical vaccines available and protective immunity can be correlated with an anti-hemagglutinin (HA) titre of >1:40, measured using an influenza hemagglutination inhibition assay [59] and the induction of $CD8^+$ T cells [60], often evaluated in small animal models. The development of a universal vaccine that protects against different strains of influenza may be possible if the immune response is directed against the conserved stalk domain of the HA rather than the variable globular head domain of the protein. One candidate vaccine in development is a chimeric HAs (cHA) protein, expressed in H1 HA stalk structures. Female BALB/c mice were immunized using a prime/boost protocol where animals were immunized in the left calf muscle with DNA encoding for the chimeric protein and then given a second immunization 3 weeks later intramuscularly or intranasally with 5 μg of the same protein with 5 μg poly(I•C) as adjuvant. Four weeks later, mice were infected with a lethal dose of different influenza viruses. The effect of vaccination on specific antibody titres, the ability to neutralize particles and mouse body weight were determined [61]. Vaccinated mice did not lose much weight after infection whereas control mice lost weight from day 3 postinfection and died by day 9. Vaccination was associated with the induction of humoral immunity, evidenced by stalk HA-specific IgG serum antibodies and IgA antibodies in nasal washes. Evidence suggested that the antibodies induced were protective as serum from vaccinated animals inhibited cell entry of the "pseudo viral particles" and protected mice against a lethal challenge in passive transfer experiments.

Another model that is often used in influenza studies is the ferret model, as ferrets are susceptible to human influenza strains, have a similar lung physiology to humans, and can have similar clinical symptoms, although these are usually milder [62]. The effect of immunization with Chimpanzee Adenovirus Oxford 1 (ChAdOx1) or modified vaccinia Ankara (MVA) virus, transfected to co-express cHA, an internal nucleoprotein (NP) and matrix 1 (M1) protein, was determined. Animals were primed with 5×10^8 infectious units (IU) of the ChAdOx1-cH14/3-NP + M1 and boosted 4 weeks later with 5×10^8 infectious units (IU) MVA-cH15/3-NP + M1. Six weeks later, vaccinated ferrets and controls were challenged intranasally (IN) with 10^6 PFU of A/Wyoming/03/2003 H3N2 virus and sacrificed on day 3 or day 4 postchallenge. The effect on vaccination on viral titres, cytokine production, and antibody levels were determined. Vaccination resulted in significantly lower nasal and oropharyngeal viral burdens compared to controls ($P < 0.01$), and vaccinated ferrets also had higher specific H3 anti-HA stalk, NP, and M1 IgG antibodies. Protection was also associated with an enhanced cell-mediated immune response as vaccinated ferrets had higher number or $CD8^+$ T cells in their nasal cavity at day 3 postchallenge compared to controls. Moreover, higher numbers of virus specific IFN-γ^+ T cells in the spleen and mesenteric lymph node cells were found on day 4 postchallenge ($P < 0.001$) [63], indicating that both humoral and cell-mediated immune responses were associated with protection. Recently a chimeric hemagglutinin-based vaccine was used in Phase I clinical trials to assess its safety and ability to elicit broadly cross-reactive antibodies against the hemagglutinin stalk domain. Individuals were primed on by giving live-attenuated influenza virus ($10^{7.5}$ 50% egg infectious dose), transfected with gene sequence for a H1 HA stalk protein (H8/1 HA) and a neuraminidase protein (N1 from pandemic H1N1 strain A/California/04/09). The vaccinees were given an intramuscular booster 84 later, using AS03-adjuvanted inactivated influenza virus vaccine expressing a different H1 HA stalk protein (cH5/1 HA) and the N1 NA on day 85. After priming the most common side effects reported were headache (33%), fatigue (21%), myalgia (18%), and nausea (18%), but all vaccine-related effects resolved within 4 days. The most common side effect after boosting was pain at the injection site (8%), headache (31%), and fatigue (23%). No IgA or IgG-specific anti-stalk protein antibodies were detected after priming but significant titres were detected after boosting, and inclusion of the adjuvant AS03 had a positive effect on antibody titres. Passive transfer studies in a BALB/c mouse model, using preimmunization (day 1) and postserum from patients (day 113 or day 420 serum) were carried out. Day 1 serum did not stop virally infected mice losing weight but mice given postboost serum lost less weight than infected controls. Determination of viral titres after challenge gave some evidence of lower viral titres in mice given day 113 serum. An area under the curve antistalk antibody titre above 1280 was an indicator to protection against infection with H1N1. In this study, 93.8% of vaccinees had thus level of specific antibody in this range, indicating that it is feasible to develop a universal anti-influenza vaccine, although it may require inclusion of more stalk protein entities to give better protection. This study show that animal models may still be relevant in preclinical studies, where they can be used to assess the ability of a component of the immune response, in this case, specific antibody, to protect against a live infection, as this would not be possible in a Phase I clinical study where safety rather than efficacy is the primary endpoint of the study.

11.5.2 Leishmaniasis

Leishmaniasis, a disease caused by infection with the protozoan parasite *Leishmania*, affects 350 million people worldwide. Female sandflies transmit infective metacyclic promastigotes to uninfected people when they take a blood meal. Clinical symptoms depend on the infecting species and host susceptibility but there are three main types; cutaneous leishmaniasis, where lesions are present on the skin, mucocutaneous leishmaniasis where lesions and found on the skin and mucosal membranes, and visceral leishmaniasis where parasites infect internal organs such as the spleen and liver. Species can only be infective to humans but other hosts, e.g., rodents and dogs can act as reservoirs that help maintain parasites in endemic areas [64]. Immunity to *Leishmania* mainly relies on cell-mediated immunity as the parasite resides within macrophages, a cell that normally helps protect against infection. Activation of humoral immunity is also noted, indicative of systemic infection. The type of immune response associated with protection against infection depends on the infecting species, activation of macrophage microbicidal effectors is required, usually by the production of IFN gamma by parasite-specific $CD4^+$ and/or $CD8^+$ T cells. Currently, there is no clinically approved vaccine for human use but there are vaccine products on the market to protect against canine leishmaniasis, e.g., CaniLeish and Leishmune [65]. A variety of approaches have been used in vaccine studies from live promastigote parasites to purified protein and DNA vaccines [66]. Most studies have shown using a single vaccine target as a recombinant protein [67] or DNA vaccine [68] can induce protection but does not induce sterile immunity, so production of an antileishmanial vaccine should be feasible but it is likely to require a combination approach e.g. polyproteins are present in the vaccine formulation. Live promastigotes vaccines are also being investigated, usually using genetically modified parasites which over express a vaccine candidate but cannot cause an infection in the host [69]. A whole range of different types of vaccines have been tested using both small and large animal models i.e. mice, hamsters, dogs and monkeys.

The murine model is one of the main models used in *Leishmania* research, as there are well-characterized parasite strains used for infection and the main responses associated with protective immunity are well known. In many cases, BALB/c mice are used as they are very susceptible to *Leishmania* infection. A study in 2004 showed that immunization with two doses of 0.5–3 μg poly protein Q, which contained five genetically fused antigenic determinants from *L. infantum*, gave a dose-dependent increase in specific IgG responses [70]. Inclusion of different adjuvants significantly increased the antibody titres compared to antigen given in PBS alone, but there was no significant difference in the IgG levels or IgG2a/IgG1 ratio between adjuvants. However, analysis of the antibody response against the individual antigens within the poly protein showed that the response varied between antigens and that specific adjuvants gave different effects. Thus, most of the antibody response was directed against LiP2a component and the presence of an adjuvant did not boost antibody levels to this antigen but did enhance the response to other antigens, with CpG (short single-stranded synthetic DNA molecules) or plasmid DNA resulting in higher IgG2a levels compared to IgG1. Therefore, it is important that antibody titres against individual antigens are determined in vaccine studies using polyproteins. Assessment of lymph node cell populations in mice immunized with the polyprotein and CpG or plasmid DNA showed that CpG enhanced the levels of dendritic cells based on higher number of $CD11c^+$ cells, but this did not occur for plasmid DNA. Challenge of poly protein Q and CpG immunized mice with *L. infantum*, resulted in a 99% reduction in splenic and liver parasite burdens ($P < 0.001$). This protection was associated with a Th1 response as significantly higher amount of IFN gamma were present in the serum ($P < 0.01$) and supernatants of spleen cells ($P < 0.01$), taken from vaccinated mice and incubated with poly protein Q, compared to controls. Taken together, vaccination with poly protein Q not only enhanced innate immunity, in the form of DC activation, but also adaptive immunity in terms of humoral and cell-mediated responses.

Hamsters are often used as a model of visceral leishmaniasis as they exhibit the type of clinical symptoms observed in human visceral leishmaniasis, whereas BALB/c mice, whilst highly susceptible, can tolerate a chronic infection [71]. Intradermal immunization of hamsters with 2μg of a *Lutzomyia longipalpis* salivary gland protein (LJM19) and boost vaccination with 2μg LJM19 and 10^7 stationary phase promastigotes, genetically engineered to be deficient in centrin (*LdCen*$^{-/-}$), and therefore cannot replicate, protected animals against challenge with virulent *L. donovani* compared to controls ($P < 0.05$) [72]. Protection was associated with significantly higher specific IgG2 response compared to controls ($P < 0.01$) and an elevated IgG_2/IgG_1 ratio ($P < 0.01$). This enhanced Th1 response correlated with significantly higher IFN-γ, iNOS in the lymph node and spleen ($P < 0.05$), and IL-12 in the lymph node ($P < 0.05$) of vaccinated hamsters compared to controls. This study indicated that the same immunological criteria can be used to predict protective immunity in rodent species.

Larger models using dogs are incorporated for human vaccine development in leishmaniasis for a number of reasons. They are important reservoir host for *L. infantum* and can be involved in the transmission of visceral leishmaniasis, they are companion animals and important veterinary market and their size allows scale-up of vaccine doses [73]. Like humans, dogs can exhibit asymptomatic infections and factors age, gender and proportion of time spent outdoors influence susceptibility to infection. Protective immunity does correlate with the induction of specific Th1 cells which of IFN-γ, IL-2 and TNF-α, but systemic and tissue-specific responses can vary greatly [74]. Currently, that are three vaccines available for canine leishmaniasis, CaniLeish, LetiFend, and Leish-Tec (reviewed by [75]). A meta-analysis of vaccine studies showed how dogs were challenged after vaccination, i.e., experimental challenge given by the intravenous or natural infection via the vector, do not give different results in vaccine efficacy studies, where vaccination with CaniLeish (25% protection) was found to be more effective than LetiFend (9% protection) in protecting against *L. infantum* infection. Both humoral and cellular immune responses are assessed after vaccination. Specific antibody levels are determined using a ELISA, where IgG titres are determined, usually using a crude soluble antigen prepared from lysed promastigote parasites [76]. Peripheral blood mononuclear cells are used in lymphocyte proliferation assay, and cytokine levels, e.g., IFN gamma are determined by ELISA. A recent study evaluated the efficacy of CaniLeish in a native heterogeneous population of dogs living in a *L. infantum* endemic region. Dogs were given the vaccine using three subcutaneous injections, three weeks apart, and the effect of vaccination was determined up to 12 months postvaccination. Vaccination was associated with the production of specific IgG but both vaccination and control animals had similar titres at 12 months postvaccination. Cells from vaccinated animals produced significantly higher levels of IFN gamma compared to control at one month after vaccination ($P < 0.001$), but by their cell produced similar levels at 12 months postvaccination. A year after vaccination, there was no significant difference in number or severity of active infections in the two groups whereas a previous study using beagle dogs a protection level of 92% was reported, based on the percentage of vaccinated animals which do not develop clinical signs [77]. Therefore, the breed of dog and the conditions used to carry out a vaccine study can have a profound effect. Some dogs have natural immunity to *L. infantum* and therefore need to be excluded from vaccine studies, so a phase III study of a canine leishmaniasis vaccine will require a large sample size, using dogs from different geographical areas.

There are relatively few studies using monkeys, which probably reflects difficulties associated with housing this model, reagents available for immunological analysis, and their relative cost compared to other animal models. However, this model is phylogenetically nearer to humans and therefore may give results that are more indicative of the outcome in human studies. Vervet monkeys (*Ceropithecus aethiops*), share~92% of their DNA with humans and their susceptibility to cutaneous leishmaniasis is similar to humans. Outbred vervet monkeys were vaccination intradermally with 100 or 200 μg recombinant *Leishmania* histone H1 protein fused to glutathione-S-transferase (rGST-H1) or a recombinant GST (rGST) alone mixed with the adjuvant Montanide ISA 720 (MISA720), using three doses given 3 weeks apart [78]. Animals were challenged 6 weeks after the last immunization by intradermal injection on the right eyebrow ridge with 5×10^6 virulent *L. major* promastigotes mixed with 20 μl of a *Phlebotomus duboscqi* salivary-gland lysate preparation. Both groups of animals produced a specific IgG response compared to control animals, which increased with the number of vaccine doses given. All vaccinated animals gave a positive delayed hypersensitivity response to an intradermal injection of 200 μg of respective vaccine protein, indicating that the vaccines induced a cell-mediated immune response. Assessment of lesion development after challenge infection showed that monkeys immunized with rGST-H1 developed smaller lesions compared to the other two groups, which had a nodular appearance rather classic wet, ulcerative lesions. Unfortunately, significant differences between treatments were not presented in this study, presumably because the sample size was too small. This study showed that the vaccines used did not induce sterile immunity. Previous studies by the same researchers using BALB/c mice also showed that a histone 1 based vaccine failed to induce sterile immunity against *L. major* [79], indicating that the murine model could be used to predict the outcome in vervet monkeys. Although non-human primates can be used in *Leishmania* studies [80] very few studies have been published in the past 10 years, which probably reflects a move away from using this type of model because of their cost and the experience of researchers in using these types of models.

11.6 Conclusion

One of the key criterium for any vaccine study is identifying a diagnostic test that can be used to predict successful vaccination. Ideally, using a sample collected from the vaccinee by a low invasive route, e.g., a saliva sample is desirable [81]. For example, detection of salivary IgA against SARS-CoV-2 can be used to monitor the effect vaccine program within a population [82]. In using animal models for vaccine efficacy, it must be noted however that in translational studies, animal models have had mixed success in predicting outcomes in human studies. For instance, [83] reported only partial concordance between animal models and humans of six interventions studied. The outcome of vaccination is a multifactorial process which is dependent on vaccine-specific factors, e.g., antigen(s) used, dose, presence of adjuvants, administration route, and vaccine-specific effects, e.g., genotype, influence of prior antigen exposures, co-infections, and what is required is an understanding of what effect priming has on both local innate and specific immune responses and the effect of components of the body that are not traditional associated with the immune system, e.g., non-immune cells and their products. We are often limited by the technology we have available to dissect the influence of different facets of the response to an antigenic challenge. However technical advances such as the use of technologies that allow single-cell analysis of immune responses [84–86] will help unravel some of the players involved in immunity and in situ imaging studies will allow monitoring of immune responses in real-time [87] if cell-specific products are available that give enough of a bioluminescent/fluorescent signal to track the movement of the cell type over time. At a more simplistic level, it would help if vaccine studies collected the same type of data so that comparisons can be made between studies. Often vaccine studies using the same commercial vaccine use different doses/protocols, etc., to make comparisons difficult. Although it is not possible to identify a single mechanism of immune protection for every disease to predict the outcome of vaccination, and hence, a range of immunological readouts appear to be required to determine humoral and cell-mediated protective immune responses induced in the host. That said, identification of an "International Standard Minimum Norm" as an immunological benchmark for all vaccine studies would be very beneficial, e.g., all studies to quote specific end point titres for IgG subtypes, amount of cytokine produced in lymphocyte proliferation studies using x μg/ml antigen, percentage of $CD4^+$ and $CD8^+$ cells present in FACs studies. As well as standard vaccination protocol, at least in animal models, to be included, e.g., two doses three weeks about with 50 μg/dose for recombinant protein antigens.

References

[1] Riedel S. Smallpox and biological warfare: a disease revisited. Baylor University Medical Center Proceedings.; 2005 Taylor & Francis.

[2] Calina D, et al. Towards effective COVID-19 vaccines: Updates, perspectives and challenges. Int J Mol Med 2020;46(1):3–16.

[3] Sheedy FJ, Divangahi M. Targeting immunometabolism in host defence against Mycobacterium tuberculosis. Immunology 2021;162(2):145–59.

[4] Armentrout EI, Liu GY, Martins GA. T cell immunity and the quest for protective vaccines against staphylococcus aureus infection. Microorganisms 2020;8(12):1936.

[5] Mittal J, et al. Histoplasma capsulatum: mechanisms for pathogenesis. In: Fungal Physiology and Immunopathogenesis; 2018, pp. 157–91.

[6] Tomás AL, et al. Detection of anti-Pneumocystis jirovecii antibodies in human serum using a recombinant synthetic multi-epitope kexin-based antigen. Eur J Clin Microbiol Infect Dis 2020;39(11):2205–9.

[7] Dubie T, Mohammed Y. Review on the role of host immune response in protection and immunopathogenesis during cutaneous leishmaniasis infection. J Immunol Res 2020;2020:1–12.

[8] Fisch D, Clough B, Frickel E-M. Human immunity to Toxoplasma gondii. PLoS Pathog 2019;15(12):e1008097.

[9] Ding J, et al. Trichinella spiralis: inflammation modulator. J Helminthol 2020;94:e193, 1–11.

[10] Cao S, et al. Mycobacterium tuberculosis antigens repress Th1 immune response suppression and promotes lung cancer metastasis through PD-1/PDl-1 signaling pathway. Cell Death Dis 2019;10(2):1–12.

[11] Kardani K, Bolhassani A, Namvar A. An overview of in silico vaccine design against different pathogens and cancer. Expert Rev Vaccines 2020;19(8):699–726.

[12] Gerdts V, et al. Large animal models for vaccine development and testing. ILAR J 2015;56(1):53–62.

[13] Kiros S, Vol 6. No 2 The principle of the presumption of innocence and its challenges in the Ethiopian criminal process. 2012.

[14] Herati RS, Wherry EJ. What is the predictive value of animal models for vaccine efficacy in humans? Consideration of strategies to improve the value of animal models. Cold Spring Harb Perspect Biol 2018;10(4):a031583.

[15] Kiros TG, et al. The importance of animal models in the development of vaccines. In: Innovation in Vaccinology; 2012, pp. 251–64.

[16] Griffin JFT. A strategic approach to vaccine development: animal models, monitoring vaccine efficacy, formulation and delivery. Adv Drug Deliv Rev 2002;54(6):851–61.

[17] Blackwell J, Plant J. Expression of the natural resistance gene (Lsh) in wild mice infected experimentally with Leishmania donovani or Salmonella typhimurium. In: The Wild Mouse in Immunology; 1986, pp. 323–30.

[18] Blackwell JM, Mohamed HS, Ibrahim ME. Genetics and visceral leishmaniasis in the Sudan: seeking a link. Trends Parasitol 2004;20(6):268–74.

[19] Gerdts V, et al. Oral DNA vaccination in utero induces mucosal immunity and immune memory in the neonate. J Immunol 2002;168(4):1877–85.

[20] Storz J, et al. Coronavirus and Pasteurella infections in bovine shipping fever pneumonia and Evans' criteria for causation. J Clin Microbiol 2000;38(9):3291–8.

[21] Driciru E, et al. Immunological considerations for Schistosoma vaccine development: transitioning to endemic settings. Front Immunol 2021;12:635985.

[22] Iacobucci G, Covid-19: risk of death more than doubled in people who also had flu, English data show. 2020.

[23] Robinson, E, Jones, A, Daly, M. International estimates of intended uptake and refusal of COVID-19 vaccines: A rapid systematic review and meta-analysis of large nationally representative samples. Vaccine 2020;39(15):2024–34.

[24] Hartmann W, et al. Helminth infections suppress the efficacy of vaccination against seasonal influenza. Cell Rep 2019;29(8):2243–56.e4.

[25] Koff WC, Gust ID, Plotkin SA. Toward a human vaccines project. Nat Immunol 2014;15(7):589–92.

[26] Jameson SC, Masopust D. Understanding subset diversity in T cell memory. Immunity 2018;48(2):214–26.
[27] Kametani Y, et al. Humanized mice as an effective evaluation system for peptide vaccines and immune checkpoint inhibitors. Int J Mol Sci 2019;20(24):6337.
[28] Wiles S, et al. Modelling infectious disease—time to think outside the box? Nat Rev Microbiol 2006;4(4):307–12.
[29] Jain A, Pasare C. Innate control of adaptive immunity: beyond the three-signal paradigm. J Immunol 2017;198(10):3791–800.
[30] Mohanan D, et al. Administration routes affect the quality of immune responses: a cross-sectional evaluation of particulate antigen-delivery systems. J Control Release 2010;147(3):342–9.
[31] Netea MG, et al. Defining trained immunity and its role in health and disease. Nat Rev Immunol 2020;20(6):375–88.
[32] Plotkin SA. Correlates of protection induced by vaccination. Clin Vaccine Immunol 2010;17(7):1055–65.
[33] Palm A-KE, Henry C. Remembrance of things past: long-term B cell memory after infection and vaccination. Front Immunol 2019;10:1787.
[34] Allman D, Wilmore JR, Gaudette BT. The continuing story of T-cell independent antibodies. Immunol Rev 2019;288(1):128–35.
[35] Parker JD, et al. Factorial validity of the 20-item Toronto Alexithymia Scale. Eur J Personality 1993;7(4):221–32.
[36] Coffman RL, Sher A, Seder RA. Vaccine adjuvants: putting innate immunity to work. Immunity 2010;33(4):492–503.
[37] Dowling JK, Mansell A. Toll-like receptors: the Swiss army knife of immunity and vaccine development. Clin Trans Immunol 2016;5(5):e85.
[38] Querec T, et al. Yellow fever vaccine YF-17D activates multiple dendritic cell subsets via TLR2, 7, 8, and 9 to stimulate polyvalent immunity. J Exp Med 2006;203(2):413–24.
[39] Coler RN, et al. Leish-111f, a recombinant polyprotein vaccine that protects against visceral Leishmaniasis by elicitation of CD4+ T cells. Infect Immun 2007;75(9):4648.
[40] Casella CR, Mitchell TC. Putting endotoxin to work for us: monophosphoryl lipid A as a safe and effective vaccine adjuvant. Cell Mol Life Sci 2008;65(20):3231–40.
[41] Duthie MS, et al. Heterologous immunization with defined RNA and subunit vaccines enhances T cell responses that protect against Leishmania donovani. Front Immunol 2018;9:2420.
[42] Bolhassani A, Zahedifard F. Therapeutic live vaccines as a potential anticancer strategy. Int J Cancer 2012;131(8):1733–43.
[43] Fiuza JA, et al. Induction of immunogenicity by live attenuated Leishmania donovani centrin deleted parasites in dogs. Vaccine 2013;31(14):1785–92.
[44] Dey R, et al. Live attenuated Leishmania donovani p27 gene knockout parasites are nonpathogenic and elicit long-term protective immunity in BALB/c mice. J Immunol 2013;190(5):2138–49.
[45] Amanna IJ, Slifka MK. Contributions of humoral and cellular immunity to vaccine-induced protection in humans. Virology 2011;411(2):206–15.
[46] Bauer G. The potential significance of high avidity immunoglobulin G (IgG) for protective immunity towards SARS-CoV-2. Int J Infect Dis 2021;106:61–4.
[47] Yang Z-y, et al. A DNA vaccine induces SARS coronavirus neutralization and protective immunity in mice. Nature 2004;428(6982):561–4.
[48] Stäger S, Smith DF, Kaye PM. Immunization with a recombinant stage-regulated surface protein from Leishmania donovani induces protection against visceral leishmaniasis. J Immunol 2000;165(12):7064–71.

[49] Murin CD. Considerations of antibody geometric constraints on NK cell antibody dependent cellular cytotoxicity. Front Immunol 2020;11:1635.

[50] de Mendonça LZ, et al. Multicomponent LBSap vaccine displays immunological and parasitological profiles similar to those of Leish-Tec® and Leishmune® vaccines against visceral leishmaniasis. Parasites Vectors 2016;9(1):1–12.

[51] Flaxman A, Ewer KJ. Methods for measuring T-Cell memory to vaccination: from mouse to man. Vaccines 2018;6(3):43.

[52] Wherry EJ, et al. Viral persistence alters CD8 T-cell immunodominance and tissue distribution and results in distinct stages of functional impairment. J Virol 2003;77(8):4911.

[53] Rai PK, et al. A lipidated peptide of Mycobacterium tuberculosis resuscitates the protective efficacy of BCG vaccine by evoking memory T cell immunity. J Transl Med 2017;15(1):1–14.

[54] Foulds KE, Shen H. Clonal competition inhibits the proliferation and differentiation of adoptively transferred TCR transgenic CD4 T cells in response to infection. J Immunol 2006;176(5):3037–43.

[55] Bayry J. Regulatory T cells as adjuvant target for enhancing the viral disease vaccine efficacy. Virusdisease 2014;25(1):18–25.

[56] Brezar V, et al. T-regulatory cells and vaccination "pay attention and do not neglect them": Lessons from HIV and cancer vaccine trials. Vaccines 2016;4(3):30.

[57] Toka FN, Suvas S, Rouse BT. CD4+ CD25+ T cells regulate vaccine-generated primary and memory CD8+ T-cell responses against herpes simplex virus type 1. J Virol 2004;78(23):13082–9.

[58] Lampejo T. Influenza and antiviral resistance: an overview. Eur J Clin Microbiol Infect Dis 2020;39(7):1201–8.

[59] Lopez CE, Legge KL. Influenza A virus vaccination: immunity, protection, and recent advances toward a universal vaccine. Vaccines 2020;8(3):434.

[60] Clemens EB, et al. Harnessing the power of T cells: the promising hope for a universal influenza vaccine. Vaccines 2018;6(2):18.

[61] Margine I, et al. Hemagglutinin stalk-based universal vaccine constructs protect against group 2 influenza A viruses. J Virol 2013;87(19):10435–46.

[62] Belser JA, Pulit-Penaloza JA, Maines TR. Ferreting out influenza virus pathogenicity and transmissibility: Past and future risk assessments in the ferret model. Cold Spring Harb Perspect Med 2020;10(7):a038323.

[63] McMahon M, et al. Vaccination with viral vectors expressing chimeric hemagglutinin, NP and M1 antigens protects ferrets against influenza virus challenge. Front Immunol 2019;10:2005.

[64] Hong A, et al. One health approach to leishmaniases: Understanding the disease dynamics through diagnostic tools. Pathogens 2020;9(10):809.

[65] Ikeogu NM, et al. Leishmania immunity: advancing immunotherapy and vaccine development. Microorganisms 2020;8(8):1201.

[66] Iborra S, et al. Vaccine candidates against leishmania under current research. Expert Rev Vaccines 2018;17(4):323–34.

[67] Henriquez F, et al. Vaccination with recombinant Leishmania donovani gamma-glutamylcysteine synthetase fusion protein protects against L. donovani infection. J Parasitol 2010;96(5):929–36.

[68] Carter K, et al. DNA vaccination against the parasite enzyme gamma-glutamylcysteine synthetase confers protection against Leishmania donovani infection. Vaccine 2007;25(22):4502–9.

[69] Pandey SC, Kumar A, Samant M. Genetically modified live attenuated vaccine: a potential strategy to combat visceral leishmaniasis. Parasite Immunol 2020;42(9):e12732.

[70] Parody N, et al. Adjuvant guided polarization of the immune humoral response against a protective multicomponent antigenic protein (Q) from Leishmania infantum. A CpG+ Q mix protects Balb/c mice from infection. Parasite Immunol 2004;26(6-7):283–93.
[71] Melby PC, et al. The hamster as a model of human visceral leishmaniasis: progressive disease and impaired generation of nitric oxide in the face of a prominent Th1-like cytokine response. J Immunol 2001;166(3):1912–20.
[72] Fiuza JA, et al. Intradermal immunization of Leishmania donovani centrin knock-out parasites in combination with salivary protein LJM19 from sand fly vector induces a durable protective immune response in hamsters. PLoS NeglTrop Dis 2016;10(1):e0004322.
[73] Ribeiro RR, et al. Canine leishmaniasis: an overview of the current status and strategies for control. Biomed Res Int 2018;2018.
[74] Hosein S, Blake DP, Solano-Gallego L. Insights on adaptive and innate immunity in canine leishmaniosis. Parasitology 2017;144(1):95–115.
[75] Calzetta L, et al. Immunoprophylaxis pharmacotherapy against canine leishmaniosis: a systematic review and meta-analysis on the efficacy of vaccines approved in European Union. Vaccine 2020:6695–703.
[76] Velez R, Gállego M. Commercially approved vaccines for canine leishmaniosis: a review of available data on their safety and efficacy. Tropical Med Int Health 2020;25(5):540–57.
[77] Oliva G, et al. A randomised, double-blind, controlled efficacy trial of the LiESP/QA-21 vaccine in naïve dogs exposed to two Leishmania infantum transmission seasons. PLoS Negl Trop Dis 2014;8(10):e3213.
[78] Masina S, et al. Protection against cutaneous leishmaniasis in outbred vervet monkeys, using a recombinant histone H1 antigen. J Infect Dis 2003;188(8):1250–7.
[79] Solioz N, et al. The protective capacities of histone H1 against experimental murine cutaneous leishmaniasis. Vaccine 1999;18(9-10):850–9.
[80] André S, et al. Non-human primates and Leishmania immunity. Cytokine: X 2020;2(4):100038.
[81] Yoshizawa M, Klosterman JK. Molecular architectures of multi-anthracene assemblies. Chem Soc Rev 2014;43(6):1885–98.
[82] Pisanic N, et al. COVID-19 serology at population scale: SARS-CoV-2-specific antibody responses in saliva. J Clin Microbiol 2020;59(1):e02204–e20.
[83] Perel P, et al. Comparison of treatment effects between animal experiments and clinical trials: systematic review. BMJ 2007;334(7586):197.
[84] Noé A, et al. The application of single-cell RNA sequencing in vaccinology. J Immunol Res 2020;2020.
[85] Khater IM, Nabi IR, Hamarneh G. A review of super-resolution single-molecule localization microscopy cluster Analysis and quantification methods. Patterns 2020;1(3):100038.
[86] Armingol E, Officer A, Harismendy O, Lewis NE, Deciphering cell–cell interactions and communication from gene expression. Nat Rev Genet 2021;22(2):71–88.
[87] McCarthy CE, et al. In vivo imaging technologies to monitor the immune system. Front Immunol 2020;11:1067.

Chapter 12

Vaccine human clinical trial

Bhawana Singh[a,#], Shyamali[b,#], Dharmendra Kumar Maurya[b,#], Rajiv Kumar[c,#], Shashi Bhushan Chauhan[a], Shyam Lal Mudavath[d], Ram Niwas Meena[e], Shyam Sundar[a], Om Prakash Singh[b,#]

[a]Department of Medicine, Institute of Medical Sciences, Banaras Hindu University, Varanasi, India, [b]Department of Biochemistry, Institute of Science, Banaras Hindu University, Varanasi, India, [c]Centre for Experimental Medicine and Surgery, Institute of Medical Sciences, Banaras Hindu University, Varanasi, India, [d]Infectious Disease Biology Laboratory, Institute of Nano Science & Technology, Mohali, Punjab, India, [e]Department of Surgery, Institute of Medical Sciences, Banaras Hindu University, Varanasi, India

#Joint First Author.

12.1 Introduction

Infectious diseases severely impact the indigenous and rural populations worldwide, accounting for enormous morbidity and mortality, and major costs to health care budgets. Vaccination is the simple and effective way to develop long-life protection against these diseases. So far vaccines have revolutionized the healthcare sector by saving millions of lives and improving the healthcare structure worldwide. The recent advances in the vaccination strategies and platforms have tried to provide better protection against the debilitating infectious diseases and brought the vaccination in reach of poorest communities at lower costs. Before the advent of vaccines, infectious diseases topped the list of killers for the world community. Vaccines have greatly accelerated the containment of many infectious diseases, especially in the developed countries. It is estimated that vaccines have prevented more than 100 million disease cases in the last century (in the United States alone) [1]. Variolation remains to be the most ancient forms of vaccination used against variola virus and it was used many centuries before Edward Jenner tested its utility against cowpox. Jenner's work laid the skeletal framework for modern vaccinology to induce adaptive immunity. Thus, vaccines work by priming the immune system, in other words, triggering and/or preparing the body to fight against particular invading pathogens, subvert disease pathology and prevent its spread in a population.

In the current era, emerging and re-emerging infectious diseases has continuously threatened mankind. Continuous modifications in the ecosystem, modernization, migration, etc., has greatly facilitated the exposure and spread

System Vaccinology. https://doi.org/10.1016/B978-0-323-85941-7.00019-X

of newer pathogens. In 1918, during Spanish flu, one of the dedliest pandemic in the history of mankind devoured millions and current emergence of the novel coronavirus disease (COVID-19) engulfed millions in the world. With more than 100 million people infected with SARS-Cov-2, it seems that the vaccination strategy has been the only hope to control the pandemic [2]. These reasons compelled the scientists and the policymakers for their immediate attention and redesign the vaccination strategies for managing the pandemic. To date, several vaccine candidates have arisen on the horizon however, vaccine designing, manufacturing, and dissemination remains a considerable challenging task. In the light of these facts, this chapter aims to gain an insight into the different stages of vaccine development, their complexities and recent innovative strategies that have accelerated the vaccine development in the pandemic era.

12.2 Vaccine development and complexities

Although vaccine development is quite intricate procedure starting from the selection of appropriate vaccine candidate, suitable adjuvant to development of stable formulation, pre-clinical studies, clinical trial, and finally licensing as well as manufacturing. Usually, the vaccines are derived from pathogenic gene products or synthetic analogues, that serves to trigger the immune system. A variety of immunization strategies using inactivated pathogens (heat-, chemical- or irradiation-based inactivation), attenuated pathogens (culture passage based attenuation or serologically related pathogens) have helped in the elimination/control of several diseases, including polio, smallpox, mumps, measles, rubella, tetanus, pertussis, and diphtheria [3]. Other formulation such as toxoid (inactivated version of toxin; e.g., tetanus), subunit vaccine (antigens of pathogens that stimulates immune responses), conjugate vaccine (pathogens that are poorly recognized by the immune system are conjugated with other biomolecules for their easy recognition), DNA/RNA vaccines (genetic material from pathogen) are also being used. Apart from the active antigenic component, vaccines also contain stabilizers (e.g., albumin, gelatin, sugar), preservatives (e.g., phenols or antibiotics), and adjuvants (alums, MPL-A, AS-04). Recent vaccine platforms and innovations have greatly revolutionized the vaccine research by facilitating the improvements in immunogenicity and vaccine efficacy.

An ideal vaccine is expected to be produced efficiently and delivered in acceptable format. It is well-known that entire process of vaccine development is exhaustive, time-consuming, and resource intensive task. Additionally, it remains quite arduous to determine rare safety issues for establishing the efficacy. Also, some pathogens which exhibit subtypes or formulations that include more than one component or possess difficulty in activating the immune system further adds to the complexity during vaccine development. The entire process is also strictly determined by the target population, for example, for healthy individuals, vaccines intend to prevent infection however in the case of healthy infants there remains a need of careful regulatory assessment during the development protocol. Likewise, lack of information regarding the infectious exposure of the target recipient population also creates a major setback in vaccine development pipeline as this prior exposure may result into rapid development of immune regulatory network which can influence the subsequent immunity [4]. Vaccines usually targets healthy population of all age groups for providing life-long immunity and therefore, there remains a need to establish vast safety database with safety profiles from thousands of subjects before a vaccine is licensed. Furthermore, most of the vaccines are available in an injectable form that requires trained personnel, appropriate storage, and transportation conditions which further affect the shelf-life of the vaccines. Additionally, improving the vaccine delivery modality to enhance the immunogenicity includes changing the route of administration, vaccination strategy (sequential, repeated, prime-boost, etc.), duration, or number of doses. These issues can further add to the complexity of the vaccination process. Also, different routes of administration can be the cause for unanticipated outcomes, such as altered antigen availability, different epitope recognition patterns [5,6].

Conversely, different vaccination strategy also plays important role in determining the immune responses, for example, sequential vaccination has been proven to be more efficacious (induces broadly neutralizing antibody responses) than repeated vaccination [7]. The type of vaccine also determines the outcome of vaccination, for example, subunit vaccine induces humoral responses while, cell-mediated immune responses are induced by attenuated viral and recombinant vectors-based vaccines [8,9]. Although great strides have been made over current decade to develop and commercialize effective vaccines for a variety of diseases, however, development of vaccine against difficult to treat diseases (such as HIV, Zika, tuberculosis, and malaria) remains grandiose task due to the inherent properties of the causative agent. High rates of antigenic shift in the pathogens forms the major cause of the emergence of new variants that requires identification, surveillance, and redesigning of the vaccine antigens or strains [10]. To add to the complexity, adjuvant selection remains one of important steps in determining immune responses and vaccine efficacy. Further, there are myriad of antigens to identify and carry forward for development with each type possessing its own safety and efficacy features [11]. The genetic diversity across different strains of pathogens also complicates the target selection process and therefore, remains the leading cause of geographical variability.

Another important reason that complicates the vaccine development is insufficient and inadequate preclinical testing models that also attribute to the failure of the clinical trials. This fact highlights the need for development of adequate animal model and need to increase the sample size (for clinical trial) for precisely determining the experimental success of the trial. Apart from the technicalities, high costs of the vaccine development remains to be the major cause for the premature termination of trials on potentially useful products. Also, it becomes leading cause for the inadequate vaccine supplies in the poorer parts of the globe. The long and rigorous research process (the exploratory phase) and preclinical assessment (animal testing and human trials) where target antigen is identified followed by years-long process of clinical testing before the vaccine is licensed, involves different phases (phases I–III) and the post licensure (phase IV) takes on an average ten to fifteen years (as discussed in next section).

Most importantly, it is noteworthy that many vaccines tested in disease-endemic regions have not performed as well as when tested in healthy volunteers during clinical trials. For example, the RTS,S/AS01 vaccine in children and infants affords 36% and 25% efficacy against clinical malaria, respectively [12], while a recent study showed that the efficacy of the same vaccine in healthy volunteers in controlled human malaria infections studies was 52% [13]. Similarly, BCG-mediated protection against pulmonary tuberculosis varies geographically and appears to be much less effective in areas with high incidence of the previous infection with *M. tuberculosis* or sensitization with environmental *Mycobacteria* [14].

12.3 Human clinical trial

Vaccine antigens are identified and developed in the laboratory where its safety and efficacy are tested on animals and non-human primates. After we have a vaccine that remains safe and promising in preventing infection in laboratory, we begin testing in humans. At this stage, we do not know whether or not this vaccine will work in human, therefore we began with very structure set up of study called clinical trials. These studies involve human healthy volunteers who are told in details about how and why this vaccine is being tested and about any potential harm. This process is called informed consent that goes on before entering the trial. There is continuous discussion between researchers and study volunteers, describing the study, informing the volunteers about any new information that occurs at any time during study, and answering all questions that volunteers have. The study researcher also confirms whether the volunteers meet all eligibility criteria to participate, which involves physical examinations and blood tests [15]. After completing inclusion and exclusion criteria, this newly developed vaccine usually undergoes through several phases of human clinical trials before it can be licensed for human use. Human vaccine trials are usually randomized, double blinded clinical trial meaning that after enrolment of healthy volunteers in the study, a computer randomly decides the vaccine and placebo group of volunteers. In this way neither the study researcher nor healthy volunteer knows about who is getting which type of injection. This prevents both researchers and volunteers from over or under-reporting symptoms.

Importantly, clinical trials usually go through three phases, each of which has specific purpose that determines the safety, immunogenicity, effectiveness, and its adverse events/side effects. All these information are recorded for assessment and final approval. An adverse event defined as any untoward medical occurrence (any unfavorable and unintended sign, symptom, or disease, including an abnormal laboratory finding) in temporal association with the use of the investigational vaccination and may or may not be causally related to it. This includes an exacerbation of pre-existing conditions or events, inter-current illnesses, or events, or the significant worsening of the disease under investigation that is not recorded elsewhere in the case report form under specific efficacy assessments. Anticipated day-to-day fluctuations of pre-existing conditions, (including the disease under study), that do not represent a clinically significant exacerbation or worsening of the condition, usually do not considered as adverse events.

12.3.1 Phase I clinical trial

This phase of trial which can last up to 2 years, is designed to test safety, tolerability and preliminary dosing into small group (20-80 participants) of human volunteers (Fig. 12.1). In this phase, researchers gather information related to the human immune response to the candidate vaccine to see whether is promising approach in preventing infection through stimulating both humoral and cellular antibody response.

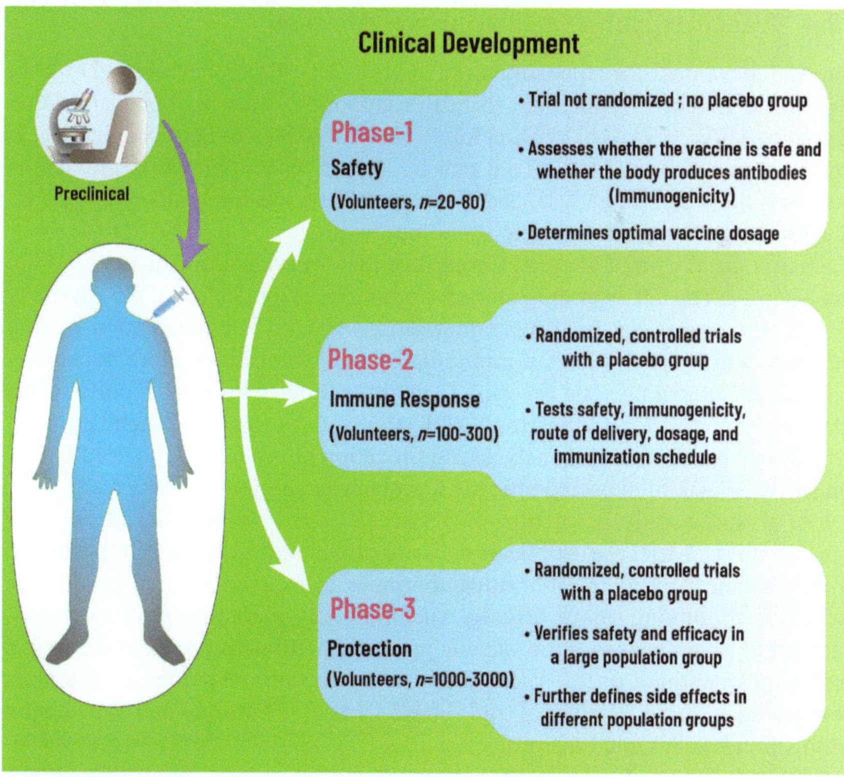

FIG. 12.1 Overview of human vaccine clinical trial phases.

12.3.2 Phase II clinical trial

After successful completion of Phase I trial, phase II trial which can last longer than 2 years, confirm the safety in larger group of volunteers (100–300 participants) and focus on the best dose level and the best timing of vaccination to generate strongest immune response (Fig. 12.1). Adverse effects are also evaluated to generate common recommendation. However, in some situation, candidate vaccine undergoes Phases I and II trial which is randomized, placebo-controlled, and multicentric to find more precise and effective doses.

12.3.3 Phase III clinical trial

Candidate vaccines that are safe and generate strong immune response in Phase-II trial move to Phase-III trial that is the largest clinical trials (>1000 participants) and compared the rate of infection in the vaccine and placebo group, while monitoring for the adverse effects at the optimal dose (Fig. 12.1). Results of this phase trial tell us whether the vaccine is able to prevent infection in all of the vaccinated volunteers or only in the specific subgroup.

12.4 Vaccine license and approval process

Vaccine developer or sponsor must submit Investigational New Drug or Biological License Application to health authorities such as Food and Drug Administration, USA [16] or Directorate General of Health Services, India [17] before making clinical trial. Trial can be started once approval is granted. It proceeds through Phases I, II, and III stages. There are few trials where phase II and phase III are combined to speed up the process, e.g., COVID vaccines. Each trial usually has a Steering Committee that overview the trial and report to the Sponsor. The Chair of the Steering Committee is a member of the Advisory Board who makes the final recommendations for the implementation of trial outcome and it usually have a minimum of five members or more depending on Country guideline. The Steering Committee after reviewing reports of the Data and Safety Monitoring Board (DSMB), and on the recommendations of DSMB can request interim analyses, modification of protocol if required (based on safety or lack of expected efficacy if an interim analysis is performed), etc.

After successful completion of Phase III trials, vaccine developer submits Biological License Application for approval and licensing. Importantly, these vaccine approving authorities continues to oversee vaccine production to ensure continuing safety. Usually, such monitoring continues till the manufacturer holds a license for the vaccine production. Sometimes, pharmaceutical companies continue to test vaccine for safety and efficacy after a vaccine is released as a Phase IV clinical trial. Phase IV trail is optional and depends on production batches and other potential uses. The whole process of the development of new vaccine to its license takes around 10 years or more (Fig. 12.2).

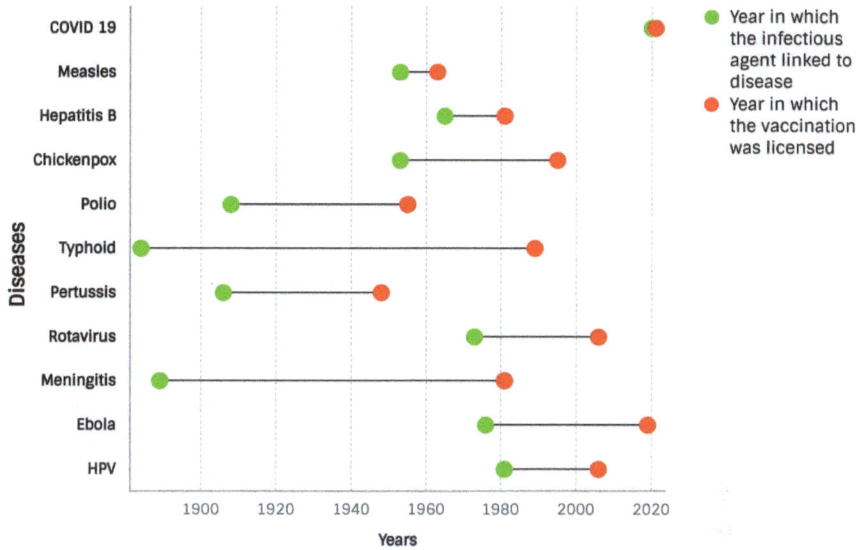

FIG. 12.2 History of human vaccine development for the infectious diseases.

However, in the COVID-19 pandemic, the vaccine development pathway is accelerated (Fig. 12.2).

12.5 Innovative strategy in vaccine development during times of pandemics

The current period is experiencing the best time of vaccine development era, when a larger number of vaccine products are flooding the market than ever. The incidence of vaccine-preventable diseases has dramatically reduced. Four vaccine-preventable diseases have been eliminated from the United States (polio, rubella, smallpox, and congenital rubella syndrome). Epidemiological surveys have suggested for the success of immunization programs in low-income countries by saving lives of 23.3 million people [18].

The biggest hurdle for vaccine development was the time constraint and availability of the stocks. Major breakthrough in the field of vaccine development came during the pandemic of H1N1 infection, when injectable monovalent vaccines emerged in October 2009. The virus yields from cell culture were lower than expected and the optimal quantity of hemagglutinin per dose, as well as the adjuvants, were also unknown. These factors instigated the manufacturers to work toward vaccine development and increase its reach to the resource poor countries of the world. The intramuscular formulation covered the largest part of H1N1 vaccine market. Conversely, intranasal formulation was another format that required suitable device for nasal administration, due to the requirement of low delivery volumes [19,20].

Newly emerging and re-emerging pathogens as influenza and SARS-CoV2-spreading by air-borne routes are amongst the most threatening pandemics. During the times of pandemics, rapid responses are needed in this context, passive antibody administration for infectious diseases have been the most trusted protocol for containing the viral spread. The Pandemic Prevention Platform program of the Defense Advanced Research Projects Agency (USA) has aimed to develop new version of passive antibody-based protection that slows viral epidemics until the vaccine becomes available. Newer technologies like reverse vaccinology have accelerated the vaccine development process and condensed the decade-long process of vaccine development. Experimental vaccines ready for phase I trial were developed in 20 months for SARS (in 2003) [21] and in approximately 3 months for Zika (in 2016) [22]. Likewise, in spite of the significant scientific and financial challenges, major breakthroughs in the form of development of COVID-19 vaccine have been one of the major milestones [23].

By the time COVID-19 was declared as a pandemic in March 2020, approximately 37 groups had already started the search for the vaccine candidates in different formats including the live attenuated, cell-based, viral-vector, inactivated, nanoparticle, spike protein based, DNA, mRNA-based vaccines [24]. COVID-19 research has made a remarkable mark from viral sequencing to analyses of vaccine efficacy with a well-designed pipeline within 300 days [25]. Many of these programs are collaborative projects between the biotechnology and pharmaceutical companies as well as the academia. These combined efforts led to the completion of COVID-19 efficacy trials in less than a year's time and gained authorization for human usage. Earlier approved vaccines employed the attenuated or killed viruses without gaining insight into the viral pathogenesis but current strategies do not follow the same track. Current strategies rely on innovative platforms for understating the host immune responses and host-pathogen interactions.

Accelerated vaccine development during the COVID-19 pandemic can also be attributed to the smart coordinated approach and previous knowledge from SARS-CoV-1 (severe acute respiratory syndrome) as well as MERS-CoV (Middle East Respiratory Syndrome) that resembled to greater extent with the SARS-CoV2 [21,26]. The previous works on MERS and SARS vaccines significantly reduced the overall duration required for preclinical assessment for the COVID-19 candidates. Approximately 2 months after viral sequencing, clinical trials began in March 2020. Overlapping the different phases of clinical was the need of the hour that led to beginning of the phase II while phase I trials were still ongoing. Likewise, for different candidates, phase III began before completion of phase II trials, an overlapping approach was proven to accelerate the overall agenda, without compromising the safety, dosage, and immunogenicity parameters [27,28]. Conversely, for another set of candidates, phase II and phase III were combined. By December 2020, several vaccine developers declared promising results on a large cohort of the population, bringing into the market the products from Pfizer (in collaboration with German firm BioNTech) and later Moderna vaccines. Overall, compressing different phases without compromising the safety and efficacy that required huge funding and planned manufacturing strategies along with international collaborations has severely shortened the time frame to approximately ten months. Thus, compressing and simultaneously operating different phases instead of proceeding with sequential testing has proven to be a boon for vaccine developers to fight against the COVID-19 pandemic. Also, the impact of vaccines to maximum extent can only be evaluated once the testing includes subjects from diverse geographical areas. Compressing different phases of trials can ensure better success rates if the trials are conducted in newer areas, i.e., diversifying the target population for inclusion in the study. This will allow broader vaccine coverage and eventually robust results for vaccine efficacy. The trials are thought to include the adolescents (less than 16 years of age) and also the subjects with chronic illnesses in order to gain additional safety and efficacy datasets. Although the trials are aimed to diversify the population, there will still be many variables that will eventually need to be addressed due to differing infection rates in different subjects.

Another aspect for an accelerated trials for vaccine includes recruiting a greater number of subjects in each trial phases to improve the trial accuracy. Larger sample sizes allow researchers to obtain better confidence scores however, there still remains the need to go for the in-depth vaccine efficacy studies. To increase the likelihood of obtaining an efficacious vaccine candidate, researchers can modify study site, sample size at that site, or utilizing a mobile trial structure that allows targeting the population at risk to be included in the study. Furthermore, the selection of controls for the randomized trials remains an important criterion for preventing the disease and making the differences between the controls and the cases more apparent easily and quickly [29]. An efficacious vaccine candidate is used as a positive control for evaluating other potential candidates and evaluate their efficacy and defining the beneficial criteria of the potential candidate.

Indeed, the global community received the COVID-19 vaccine quickly due to the years-long efforts directed toward understanding the related corona viruses. Also, sufficient funding opportunities, greatly facilitated the efforts for conducting several trials in parallel. These factors might be translated for other diseases for speeding up the vaccine efforts however, in a way scientists had considerable luck while working with SARS-CoV2 due to its low mutation rates and less efficient host evasion strategy.

12.6 COVID-19: reported clinical trials worldwide

Vaccines play vital role in inducing herd immunity, reducing disease burden and preventing disease severity against COVID-19. Serious global efforts aiming to normalize the pandemic threat led to the development of unprecedented number of vaccine candidates, with several under different phases of trials as discussed in the previous sections. Several trials have shown satisfactory efficacy and safety profiles. Many others are in preclinical phases including the DNA-based, RNA based, inactivated virus, replicating, and non-replicating viral vector based, virus like particle-based, cell-based, and protein subunit-based vaccine formulations. Vaccine approvals are based on randomized, blinded, controlled trials that evaluate the safety and efficacy for controlling the pandemic [2]. According the WHO, there are approximately 112 candidates in clinical development while 184 candidates are undergoing different phases of preclinical development. Although different strategies of vaccine development have been employed by different groups of researchers however, currently, protein subunit-based strategy has been the most explored by the majority of researchers as compared to other vaccination strategies known.

The scientific collaborations and hand-in-hand cooperation between the stakeholders, government, and researchers have significantly accelerated the pace of clinical trials for vaccine development. With the adequate financial support, vaccine development protocols can be accelerated smoothly with appropriate collaboration, for example, Moderna's mRNA vaccine entered phase I trial on March 16, after 10 weeks of the release of the entire genetic sequence. Later, several other nucleic acid-based vaccine candidates entered phase I trial, after regulatory approval. Conversely, for other potential candidates, clinical trial material for phase II was prepared and later trials required solid preparation in terms of scaling up manufacturing for commercial purposes. Manufacturing requirements, safety, and immunogenicity trials required huge investments and novel technological platforms for speeding up the manufacturing process. Thus, large manufacturing platforms have been developed for mass production of the potential candidate without compromising the safety and the efficacy parameters. As discussed earlier, plethora of clinical trials are underway, compiling up all the trials would be an exhaustive task thus, we have presented Table 12.1 here giving a comprehensive overview of currently ongoing different clinical trials (in phase IV) and the vaccine strategy employed in their development.

Overall, the combined well-developed system of financial support, large-scale manufacturing, procedure implementation and wise collaboration of researchers, policymakers and stakeholders allows fair allocation of resources and protects the economic losses in the pandemic situations.

12.7 Regulatory challenges

The study protocol for the trial is designed in accordance with the general ethical principles outlined in the Declaration of Helsinki, 2000 and ICH guidelines for Good Clinical Practice (International Committee for Harmonization). Trial protocol usually reviewed by Local-, National- and an International-independent ethics committee (IEC) before its implementation that is time taking and cumbersome process. As discussed in the previous section, there are more than hundreds of clinical trials that have been undertaken by academic and pharmaceutical companies however, there remains

TABLE 12.1 Overview of vaccine candidates in phase IV trial for COVID-19.

Vaccine strategy	Vaccine candidate	Route of adminis-tration	Developer	Number of doses required	Vaccination schedule (days)	Clinical trial registries
Inactivated virus	CoronaVac (vero cells)	Intramuscular (IM)	Sinovac R&D Co Ltd.	2	0+14	NCT04756830, NCT04747821, NCT04775069, NCT04789356, NCT04754698, NCT04801888, NCT04894227, NCT04892459, NCT04911790, NCT04953325, NCT04962308, NCT04993365
Inactivated virus	BBIBP- CoV (Vero cells)	IM	Sinopharm+ China National Biotec Group+ Beijing Institute of Biological products	2	0+21	NCT04560881, NCT04917523, NCT04510207, NCT04984408
Viral vector(non-replicating)	ChAdOx 1-S-(AZD-1222) Covishield Vaxzevria	IM Intranasal (IN)	AstraZeneca+University of Oxford University of Oxford	1-2 1-2	0+28 0+28	ISRCTN89951424, NCT04516746, NCT04540393, NCT04536051, EUCTR2020-005226-28-DE, NCT04864561
Viral vector	Ad 5-nCoV (Adenovirus type 5 vector)	IM	CanSino Biological Inc./Beijing Institute of Biotechnology	1	0	NCT04526990, NCT04540419
Viral vector	Ad 2. CoV2.S	IM	Janssen Pharmaceuticals	1-2	0 or 0+56	NCT04505722, NCT04614948, NCT04838795

(Continued)

TABLE 12.1 Overview of vaccine candidates in phase IV trial for COVID-19. *(Continued)*

Vaccine strategy	Vaccine candidate	Route of adminis-tration	Developer	Number of doses required	Vaccination schedule (days)	Clinical trial registries
RNA based	mRNA-1273	IM	Moderna+National Institute of Allergy and Infectious Diseases (NIAID)	2	0+28	NCT04470427, NCT04811664, NCT04805125, NCT04806113, NCT04860297
RNA based	BNT162b2(3 lipid nanoparticle-mRNA) also called Comirnaty	IM	Pfizer/BioNTech+Fosun Pharma	2	0+21	NCT04368728, NCT04713553, NCT04800133, NCT04805125, NCT04816669, NCT04951323
RNA based	mRNA 1273.351 LNP encapsulated mRNA based vaccine that encodes for S-protein of SARS-CoV2	IM	Moderna +NIAID	3	0, 0+28 or 56	EUCTR2021-000930-32, NCT04878211, NCT04869358

considerable financial, scientific and ethical issues that still needs attention. Several scientists, bioethicists and regulators have focused on gaining better insight into the long-term safety and efficacy data from different randomized control trials [30].

There are considerable challenges in determining the vaccine efficacy in higher risk subjects including the diabetics, older age, and obesity. Further, we still lag behind in understanding the extent of vaccine-induced protection in severe cases of COVID-19 and viral transmission abilities in vaccinated subjects [31]. The scientists, clinicians, and policymakers face considerable challenges in building confidence amongst general masses regarding the transparency adopted in releasing the safety and efficacies of the vaccines. Additionally, multiple candidates have been authorized for emergency usage in short span of time however, ensuring the continuous development of candidate, authorization, distribution, monitoring, and administration remains a big challenge. Vaccine trials and development protocols also experience major hurdles in monitoring safety, efficacy and transparency, manufacturing sufficient quantities for meeting global demands, maintaining supply chain and strong R&D incentives, running coordinated clinical trials, ensuring fair vaccine allocations, secure transport, encouraging general masses to get vaccinated, etc. [32–34].

Vaccine distribution remains another major area that possesses significant challenge in terms of storage; for example, some vaccines can be stored in normal refrigerator (AstraZaneca and University of Oxford vaccine), making their distribution feasible while others (Pfizer and BioNTech vaccine) require storage condition of −70° to −80°C before usage. Another controversial area of vaccine remains the prices, with wide variation in the vaccine prices affecting mainly the poorer countries of the world. The situation can be evaluated by the fact that Saudi Arabia and Africa pay more than five USD per dose for AstraZeneca vaccine while, European Commission pays only 3.5 USD per dose. These price differences exists for many other vaccines even in the scenario when the vaccines are hugely subsidized by local governments [35]. Newer financing R&D models have been emerging that tries to meet the needs of the purchaser and the manufacturer and eventually provide fair and sustainable prices for vaccines. This comes into picture in the scenario of booster dosing, for emerging newer variants and/or maintaining vaccine efficacy over longer duration as in the case of seasonal flu vaccines [36]. There also remains a pressing need to maintain enough stocks of the vaccines and crude products as a part of preparation for the future outbreak in case of antigenic shift and/or drift. Furthermore, the need for detecting viral mutations calls upon for global sharing of the genetic sequence, develop newer candidates, and/or repurposing the existing candidates to pathogens, if needed [36].

Although there remains issues and challenges however, global scientific partnership is thought to play an important role in effectively fighting against emerging pathogens and vaccine development and dissemination of vaccine.

12.8 Conclusion

Vaccine development remains the mainstay for combating infectious diseases however, stringent testing and regulatory norms makes it a tedious task for healthcare sector. The regulatory processes involved in the clinical evaluation are meant to safeguard healthy population but it requires time and resources from the authorities including the ethical committees, policymakers, and the manufacturers. Although vaccines are crucial tools for disease prevention, the entire process of clinical trial for a potential candidate can take up to ten to twelve years, highly expensive (>100 million USD), and require thousands of human volunteers to validate its success. Furthermore, the selection of adequate adjuvants and generation of robust memory responses also remains amongst the key ingredients for long-term vaccine success against infectious diseases. Considering all the safety parameters and clinical trials, COVID-19 vaccine was developed in a record time of 11 months. During the pandemic era, novel strategies of vaccine trials have outpaced the conventional vaccine development/trial protocols but still there remain several gaps that needs to be filled.

It is general assumption that the success of disease prevention program lies on the shoulders of the successful vaccination trials and/or campaign that directly relies on the long-term safety, immunological correlates, and efficacy parameters. Addressing other issues such as misinformation, vaccine hesitancy, political, and geographical divisions as well as deception remains the key challenge in the development of herd immunity. Despite all these barriers and obstacles, substantial progress has been made over the last two decades resulting in the development of vaccine for 17 deadly infectious diseases that have already saved millions of lives worldwide.

Funding

This study was funded and supported by the Science & Engineering Research Board (SERB) [Grant No. SRG/2020/002558], UGC-BSR Research start-up Grant, and Institute of Eminence (IoE) grant of Banaras Hindu University and SERB-DST (EEQ/2020/000563).

Acknowledgements

Authors would like to dedicate this article to all those COVID patients who have lost their lives during drug / vaccine trails in various part of the world.

References

[1] van Panhuis WG, Grefenstette J, Jung SY, Chok NS, Cross A, Eng H, Lee BY, Zadorozhny V, Brown S, Cummings D, et al. Contagious diseases in the United States from 1888 to the present. N Engl J Med 2013;369:2152–8.

[2] Excler JL, Saville M, Berkley S, Kim JH. Vaccine development for emerging infectious diseases. Nat Med 2021;27:591–600.

[3] Bonanni P, Picazo JJ, Remy V. The intangible benefits of vaccination—what is the true economic value of vaccination? J Mark Access Health Policy 2015;3(1). doi:10.3402/jmahp.v3.26964.

[4] Montes de Oca M, Good MF, McCarthy JS, Engwerda CR. The impact of established immunoregulatory networks on vaccine efficacy and the development of immunity to malaria. J Immunol 2016;197:4518–26.

[5] Nossal GJ. Current concepts: immunology. The basic components of the immune system. N Engl J Med 1987;316:1320–5.

[6] Arvin AM. Humoral and cellular immunity to varicella-zoster virus: an overview. J Infect Dis 2008;197(Suppl 2):S58–S60.

[7] Pantaleo G, Koup RA. Correlates of immune protection in HIV-1 infection: what we know, what we don't know, what we should know. Nat Med 2004;10:806–10.

[8] The Immune System and Infectious Diseases, 1989. National Research Council (US) Committee on Research Opportunities in Biology. https://www.ncbi.nlm.nih.gov/books/NBK217803/.

[9] Pulendran B, Ahmed R. Immunological mechanisms of vaccination. Nat Immunol 2011;12:509–17.

[10] Nachbagauer R, Feser J, Naficy A, Bernstein DI, Guptill J, Walter EB, Berlanda-Scorza F, Stadlbauer D, Wilson PC, Aydillo T, et al. A chimeric hemagglutinin-based universal influenza virus vaccine approach induces broad and long-lasting immunity in a randomized, placebo-controlled phase I trial. Nat Med 2021;27:106–14.

[11] Shah RR, Hassett KJ, Brito LA. Overview of vaccine adjuvants: introduction, history, and current status. Methods Mol Biol 2017;1494:1–13.

[12] Efficacy and safety of RTS, S/AS01 malaria vaccine with or without a booster dose in infants and children in Africa: final results of a phase 3, individually randomised, controlled trial. Lancet 2015;386:31–45.

[13] Ockenhouse CF, Regules J, Tosh D, Cowden J, Kathcart A, Cummings J, Paolino K, Moon J, Komisar J, Kamau E, et al. Ad35.CS.01-RTS,S/AS01 heterologous prime boost vaccine efficacy against sporozoite challenge in healthy malaria-naïve adults. PLoS One 2015;10:e0131571.

[14] Nguipdop-Djomo P, Heldal E, Rodrigues LC, Abubakar I, Mangtani P. Duration of BCG protection against tuberculosis and change in effectiveness with time since vaccination in Norway: a retrospective population-based cohort study. Lancet Infect Dis 2016;16:219–26.

[15] Mazraani M, Barbari A. Anti-Coronavirus Disease 2019 vaccines: need for informed consent. Exp Clin Transplant 2021;19:753–62.

[16] U.S. Food & Drug Administration. https://clinicaltrials.gov.

[17] Central Drugs Standard Control Organization, Directorate General of Health Services, Ministry of Health & Family Welfare, Government of India. https://cdsco.gov.in/opencms/opencms/en/Home/.

[18] Lee LA, Franzel L, Atwell J, Datta SD, Friberg IK, Goldie SJ, Reef SE, Schwalbe N, Simons E, Strebel PM, et al. The estimated mortality impact of vaccinations forecast to be administered during 2011–2020 in 73 countries supported by the GAVI Alliance. Vaccine 2013;31(Suppl 2):B61–72.

[19] Lambert LC, Fauci AS. Influenza vaccines for the future. N Engl J Med 2010;363:2036–44.

[20] Leung GM, Nicoll A. Reflections on pandemic (H1N1) 2009 and the international response. PLoS Medicine 2010;7(10):e1000346. doi:10.1371/journal.pmed.1000346.

[21] Li YD, Chi WY, Su JH, Ferrall L, Hung CF, Wu TC. Coronavirus vaccine development: from SARS and MERS to COVID-19. J Biomed Sci 2020;27:104.

[22] Shan C, Xie X, Shi PY. Zika virus vaccine: progress and challenges. Cell Host Microbe 2018;24:12–7.

[23] Pascual-Iglesias A, Canton J, Ortega-Prieto AM, Jimenez-Guardeño JM, Regla-Nava JA. An overview of vaccines against SARS-CoV-2 in the COVID-19 pandemic Era. Pathogens 2021;10(8):1030. doi:10.3390/pathogens10081030.

[24] Gerberding JL, Haynes BF. Vaccine innovations—past and future. N Engl J Med 2021;384:393–6.

[25] Ball P. The lightning-fast quest for COVID vaccines—and what it means for other diseases. Nature 2021;589:16–8.

[26] Schaefer GO, Tam CC, Savulescu J, Voo TC. COVID-19 vaccine development: time to consider SARS-CoV-2 challenge studies? Vaccine 2020;38:5085–8.

[27] Poland GA, Ovsyannikova IG, Kennedy RB. SARS-CoV-2 immunity: review and applications to phase 3 vaccine candidates. Lancet 2020;396:1595–606.

[28] Tu YF, Chien CS, Yarmishyn AA, Lin YY, Luo YH, Lin YT, Lai WY, Yang DM, Chou SJ, Yang YP, et al. A review of SARS-CoV-2 and the ongoing clinical trials. Int J Mol Sci 2020;21.

[29] Palacios R, Patino EG, de Oliveira Piorelli R, Conde M, Batista AP, Zeng G, Xin Q, Kallas EG, Flores J, Ockenhouse CF, et al. Double-blind, randomized, placebo-controlled Phase III clinical trial to evaluate the efficacy and safety of treating healthcare professionals with the adsorbed COVID-19 (Inactivated) vaccine manufactured by Sinovac - PROFIS-COV: a structured summary of a study protocol for a randomised controlled trial. Trials 2020;21:853.

[30] Forman R, Anderson M, Jit M, Mossialos E. Ensuring access and affordability through COVID-19 vaccine research and development investments: A proposal for the options market for vaccines. Vaccine 2020;38:6075–7.

[31] The COVID vaccine challenges that lie ahead. Nature 2020;587:522.

[32] Cohen J, Kupferschmidt K. Countries now scrambling for COVID-19 vaccines may soon have surpluses to donate. Science 2021. doi:10.1126/science.abh4476.

[33] Forman R, Atun R, McKee M, Mossialos E. 12 Lessons learned from the management of the coronavirus pandemic. Health Policy 2020;124:577–80.

[34] Irwin A, Nkengasong J. What it will take to vaccinate the world against COVID-19. Nature 2021;592:176–8.

[35] Check P: Nations pay wildly different prices for vaccines. Goats and Soda; p. 2021. https://www.npr.org/sections/goatsandsoda/2021/02/19/969529969/price-check-nations-pay-wildly-different-prices-for-vaccines.

[36] Brewer NT, Chapman GB, Rothman AJ, Leask J, Kempe A. Increasing vaccination: putting psychological science into action. Psychol Sci Public Interest 2017;18:149–207.

Chapter 13

Systems vaccinology for the design of rational vaccines against protozoan parasites

Mariela Luján Tomazic[a,*], Virginia Marugan-Hernandez[b], Anabel Elisa Rodriguez[c]

[a]*Instituto de Patobiología Veterinaria (IPVET), INTA-CONICET. Nicolás Repetto y De los Reseros s/n, Hurlingham, Argentina,* [b]*The Royal Veterinary College, University of London, Hawkshead Lane, United Kingdom,* [c]*Instituto de Patobiología (IP), IPVET, INTA-CONICET, Hurlingham, Argentina,* **Universidad de Buenos Aires, Facultad de Farmacia y Bioquímica, Cátedra de Biotecnología, Ciudad Autónoma de Buenos Aires, Argentina*

13.1 State-of-the-art of vaccines in protozoan parasites

Apicomplexan and Trypanosomatid parasites are a major cause of disease in humans and animals worldwide. Most of these pathogenic, unicellular microorganisms are zoonotic or cause an economic impact on farm animals, reason why they are in the focus of a large number of research groups. Examples of human diseases caused by Trypanosomatid parasites of the class Kinetoplastea and phylum Euglenozoa are leishmaniasis, which comes in four main forms visceral (VL), cutaneous (CL), cutaneous diffuse (DCL), and mucocutaneous (MCL), and Chagas disease; caused by *Leishmania* spp., and *Trypanosoma cruzi*, respectively. The most relevant human parasite, *Plasmodium* spp., belongs to the phylum Aplicomplexa and is the etiological agent of malaria in humans. Other zoonotic Apicomplexans are the cyst forming *Toxoplasma gondii* (model organism within the phylum) and *Cryptosporidium parvum*. Parasites of this phylum also encompass several species causing diseases with welfare and economic impact in livestock and poultry, as well as in wild animals and pets, some examples are babesiosis, eimeriosis (coccidiosis), neosporosis, besnoitiosis, and theileriosis among others, caused by species from the genera *Babesia, Eimeria, Neospora*, *Besnoitia* and *Theileria*, respectively.

For many decades, vaccines against parasites have been addressed by conventional methodologies based on the “Pasteurian principle of the 3Is” (isolate, inactivate and inject), this is to say isolation, inoculation of the parasites (live, live-attenuated, or inactivated), and testing the immunological response and protection against the infectious agent. Conventional vaccinology (also known as

System Vaccinology. https://doi.org/10.1016/B978-0-323-85941-7.00003-6

vaccinology 1.0) started in humans in 1798 with the smallpox vaccine [1], however, vaccines were not developed in the veterinary field until a century later, with the first animal vaccine against chicken cholera tested in 1879 and only a few years later against bovine babesiosis [2,3]. The first vaccines against avian coccidiosis were developed in the 1950s. However, the major contribution to the development of parasite vaccines came from efforts to combat malaria in the 1960s [4].

To date, a small number of vaccines against protozoan parasites of veterinary or human importance are available [5]. However, there are solid ongoing strategies and plans of action to improve the availability of veterinary vaccines against different pathogens (including protozoa parasites) addressed by the European Medicines Agency (EMA, europa.eu) and The Heads of Medicines Agencies (HMA). Together they have developed a joint high-level strategy for the network "EU Medicines Agencies Network Strategy" and a multiannual work plan (MAWP) for its implementation [6].

The limited number of vaccines against protozoan parasites, despite their importance for public health, contrasts markedly with the situation for vaccines against viral and bacterial diseases, for which a wide range of immunoprophylactic compounds are available both in human and veterinary medicine. The main barriers in protozoal vaccinology relate to their more complex and multifaceted lifecycles, presenting different stages and intricated interactions with the host, not yet well understood. Furthermore, in some cases, disease is caused by multiple species infections, e.g. coccidiosis, and the development of a universal vaccine that protects against heterologous species is not a simple goal to achieve. Fig. 13.1 shows the complex nature of the life cycle of these obligated intracellular protozoan parasites which are of utmost importance for systems-based analysis, as parasites display stage-dependent gene expression [7]. Overall, apicomplexan and trypanosomatids parasites develop their life cycle into one host (monoxenous), two hosts (dixenous), or several hosts (heteroxenous). The particular biology of each parasite will have impact in the discovery of a successful vaccine. For example, the ability of Apicomplexa parasites to reside in a parasitophorous vacuole (PV) to escape the host immune surveillance, or mechanisms such as the ability to form tissue cysts (e.g. *T. gondii and Neospora caninum*) as evasion mechanism to the host immune system, could hinder vaccine efficacy. Successful routes for transmission and long-term survival strategies can also compromise different measures of control against these parasitic diseases. In this way, *Eimeria* spp., *C. parvum* and *T. gondii* oocysts can survive for long periods in adverse environmental conditions, contaminating food, or water to facilitate further transmission [8,9]. Additionally, the limitations for *in vitro* cultivation for most of the life cycle stages in these parasites also hinder the advances in the field of vaccine development.

Effective—but limited—vaccines are available for some protozoal diseases in animals, and are detailed in Table 13.1, including the zoonotic disease leishmaniasis.

In comparison to human medicine, vaccine development for veterinary medicine has practical advantages such as the ability to perform experiments in the natural host, the possibility of making formulations with live parasites, and lower

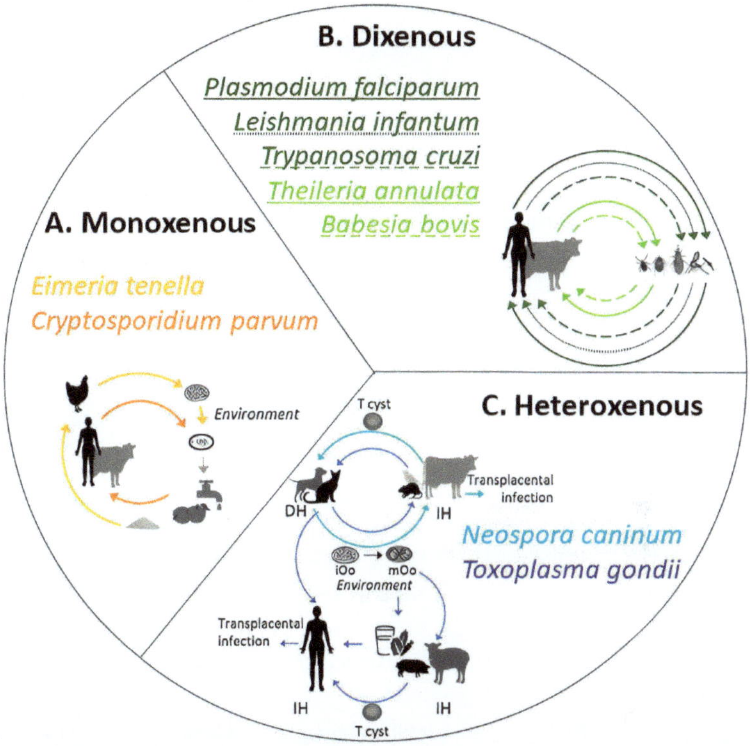

FIG. 13.1 Schematic life cycle examples of protozoan parasites. (A) The monoxenous apicomplexans species *C. parvum* (infects humans and cattle causing cryptosporidiosis; orange arrows) and avian *Eimeria* spp. (causing coccidiosis; yellow arrows) complete their entire cycle in a single host. Both parasitic genera develop asexual and sexual stages in a single organism. The vertebrate species affected depends on the parasite species involved. *Eimeria* oocysts sporulate in the environment, whereas *Cryptosporidium* oocysts are excreted sporulated. Oocysts are excreted with feces contaminating the food and water causing new rounds of infections. (B) Parasites exhibiting dixenous life cycle are the apicomplexans *P. falciparum* (causing human malaria; dark green solid arrows), the trypanosomatids *L. infantum* (causing leishmaniasis; dark green dotted arrows), *T. cruzi* (causing Chagas disease; dark green dashed arrows), *T. annulata* (causing theileriosis; light green solid arrows) and *B. bovis* (causing bovine babesiosis; light green dashed arrows). They complete their life cycle in two different organisms: vector and hosts. These diseases are transmitted by vectors such as female mosquitoes (for *P. falciparum*), sandflies (for *L. infantum*), ticks (for *T. annulata* and *B. bovis*) and triatomine bug (for *T. cruzi*), which are specific of each parasite genus. In the case of apicomplexans, sexual stages are developed in the vector and asexual stages in vertebrates causing disease. In trypanosomatids different asexual stages take place in vector and animal host, casing disease in the latter (C). The Apicomplexa *T. gondii* (causing toxoplasmosis; blue arrows) and *N. caninum* (causing neosporosis; light blue arrows) have a heteroxenous life cycle with felids or dogs, respectively, as definitive hosts (*DH*) and a wide range of species as intermediate hosts (*IH*). In DH the parasites reproduce by asexual and sexual multiplication in intestinal cells resulting in diploid oocysts (iOo) that are excreted with feces, contaminating the environment where sporulation (mOo) takes place. In IH the parasites reproduce asexually causing a systemic infection (usually asymptomatic), developing later to tissue cyst (T cyst) in specific organs (e.g., brain, skeletal muscle), stablishing a chronic infection. Horizontal transmission can occur through the environment by consuming vegetables or water contaminated with oocysts, or by consumption of uncooked food, containing tissue cysts. Additionally, vertical transmission can occur through transplacental infection of the offspring.

TABLE 13.1 Current licensed vaccines against protozoan parasites in veterinary medicine.

Parasite	Type of vaccine	Company	Target population	References
Babesia bovis, B. bigemina	Live attenuated	Local veterinary institutes[a]	Cattle	[10]
Babesia canis	Inactivated	Merial[b] and Intervet	Dog	[17]
Theileria annulata	Live attenuated	Local veterinary institutes	Cattle	[13]
Theileria parva	Live attenuated	CTTBD, Malawi	Cattle	[93]
Eimeria spp.	Live attenuated and unattenuated	MSD, Intervet Inc[c], Hipra, others[d]	Fowl	[11]
Eimeria maxima	Subunit	Novartis AH	Chicken	[20]
Neospora caninum	Inactivated	Intervet Inc.	Cattle	[16]
Toxoplasma gondii	Live attenuated	MSD Animal Health	Ovine	[14]
Leishmania donovani	Recombinant	Hertape Calier Saúde Animal; CEDIVEP[e]	Dog	[24]
Leishmania infantum	Li- ESP[f]	Virbac Santé Animale	Dog	[22]
Leishmania donovani	Recombinant	Laboratorios Leti	Dog	[23]

[a]*Reviewed by Florin-Christensen and collaborators [10].*
[b]*Now part of Boehringer Ingelhemim.*
[c]*Now part of MSD.*
[d]*Reviewed by Ahmad and collaborators [11].*
[e]*Reviewed by Solano Gallego and collaborators [178].*
[f]*Li-ESP, Purified excreted–secreted proteins of Leishmania infantum.*

safety requirements. Live attenuated vaccines are widely used, and most of them have been marketed for both bovine babesiosis and avian coccidiosis (reviewed by [10,11], respectively). They are composed of several species, as for example commercial vaccines for avian coccidiosis, containing between 3 (Livacox-T) to 8 (Paracox-8) infecting species or serotypes [11], they are produced in the natural host, i.e. in birds, which highly increase the production costs. Several live vaccines are also produced *in vitro*. This is the case for a babesiosis vaccine (currently in used in Argentina) that is produced in bovine erythrocytes [12]. Bovine tropical theileriosis vaccines are produced *in vitro* either in lymphoid or monocytic cells, and are manufactured by local veterinary institutes, mainly in government-sponsored laboratories [13] (Table 13.1). An attenuated vaccine prevents *T. gondii*-induced abortion in sheep [14] that has been continuously produced since 1988 and is currently marketed in New Zealand and some countries of Europe. A multivalent *Theileria parva* vaccine against East Coast fever (the Mugaga cocktail) is commercialized and distributed in Kenya, Tanzania, and Malawi [15].

Killed vaccines for *N. caninum* and *Babesia canis* are also commercialy available [16,17].

These first generation of vaccines, so called Vaccinology 1.0, can confer good levels of immunoprotection against protozoan parasites; nonetheless, they have drawbacks such as safety (potential to cause disease), short stability, high production cost, and often multiple doses are needed to induce an effective immunoprotective response. Vaccinology 2.0 or second-generation vaccines, consists of the administration of a fractionated microbial component (i.e., subunit), avoiding the safety issues (reversion to virulence is not possible). One example is the commercially available subunit vaccine for poultry is CoxAbic (licensed in some countries, Table 13.1). This is an oil emulsion vaccine that induces maternally derived antibodies aimed at protecting the broiler progeny [18,19]. This is the only available commercial cocidiosis vaccine based on the transmission of passive immunity through the yolk of hatching eggs to the progeny. The acquired immunity in the chicken is developed against purified gametocyte antigens 230kDa, 82kDa, and 56kDa from *E. maxima* that are the antigens present in the vaccine [20]. However, the production costs are still expensive since the antigens are purified from parasites previously produced in chickens. Another example of subuint vaccine is commercialized under the tradename CaniLeish (Virbac, France) and is composed of purified excreted–secreted proteins of *L. infantum* [22]. So far, there are two recombinant vaccines licenced for canine leishmaniasis [23,24] under the trade names Leish-Tec and LetiFend (Table 13.1).

Vaccinology has moved forward to third-generation along with the advances in many new technologies, opening a new era also known as Vaccinology 3.0. Third-generation vaccines or recombinant vaccines are based on recombinant DNA technologies, can use one or multiple antigens to induce immunological responses and immunoprotection, and are characterized by rational design and plan. The development of these new generation vaccines has been accompanied by the development of vaccine adjuvants, a growing area of research. Adjuvants are required to enhance immunological responses that otherwise would not be possible due to the low stimulatory properties of most recombinant antigen formulations.

Therefore, there is an urgent need for new cost-effective control strategies and third-generation vaccines offer a promising strategy. There are a wide variety of veterinary and human vaccines against protozoa parasites in research stage or in preclinical phase. Further phases before obtaining approval from the regulatory agencies involve controlled clinical trials in humans (involving phases 0, 1, 2, and 3) or field trials for animals. After being licensed, human vaccines undergo phase 4 (for further information related to vaccines information see the [25]). Veterinary and human vaccines in the most advanced phases are summarized in Table 13.2. Many efforts have been made to control human malaria disease, between 2010 and 2017, the incidence has only be reduced by 18% [26]. Despite its importance in public health and the progress achieved on malaria vaccines (for more information please refer to [27] and [29]), there is only one licensed vaccine against human malaria: Mosquirix (RTS, S)—GlaxoSmithKline.

Therefore, antimalarial vaccines are urgently needed. According to the national library of Medicine of the United States [28] there are at least 40 vaccines in differentes controlled trials, i.e., phases 1, 2, or 3, (antimalarial vaccines against the pre-erythrocytic stage were reviewed in [29]); from these, only the RTS,S vaccine has received a positive regulatory assessment. RTS,S is a relevant example of a third-generation vaccine, consisting of a recombinant fusion protein of *Plasmodium falciparum* NF54 strain, containing a tandem repeat region, and T cell epitopes of the circumsporozoite (CS) antigen that is co-expressed in yeast with hepatitis B surface antigen (HBsAg) and assembled with native HBsAg into virus-like particles [30]. The vaccine is formulated with AS01/AS02, a liposome-based adjuvant comprised of monophosphoryl lipid A.

In summary, despite the significant contribution that vaccines have done toward the control of these infectious diseases, many parasites of public health and veterinary importance are still not controlled by immunoprophylaxis; therefore, new affordable and sustainable vaccines based on recombinant or live-vectored antigens seems the way forward.

13.2 Host-immune response

Parasitic protozoa exhibit complex life cycles and have evolved to highly sophisticated strategies to evade host immune responses. Immune responses are often multifaceted and specific against different parasitic stages. Mechanisms that normally protect hosts from infection also can cause tissue injury, contributing to the pathology observed. There are important gaps in the knowledge of the immunological mechanisms that triggers protective responses that are essential to understand and predict the vaccine responses needed. The following section reviews some relevant finding of host-immune response against Apicomplexa and Tripanosomatid parasites.

13.2.1 Immunological response upon primary infection

13.2.1.1 Innate immunity

The innate response of the host is a non-specific first acting reaction that takes place after the parasitic infection and comprises physical and chemical barriers,

TABLE 13.2 Most advanced veterinarian and human vaccines against protozoan parasites under investigation.

Genus	Species	Antigen number	Vaccinology				Host Response	References/Vaccine name**
			1.0	2.0	3.0	Phase		
Cryptosporidium	*C. parvum*	2			D (2)	PC	Mouse	[25]
Babesia	*Bbo, Bbi, Bd*	13	LA (5) SPA (10)	S (6)	R (8)	F	Cattle	[93]
	B. canis	1	SPA (2)		R (1)	F	Dog	
	B. orientalis		SPA (1)			F	Buffalo	
	B. microti	2			R (2)	PC	Mouse	
Eimeria	*Ea, Et, Ema*	23	LA (1)	S (7)	R (18) D (11)	F	Chicken	[11]
Plasmodium[a]	*Pf*		LA (1)		R (1)	P3	Human	[28] RTS,S/AS01; RTS,S/AS02; BCG
				S	R	P1		[28] FMP010; FMP012; FMP1; FMP2.1/Ad35.CS.01
			LA		R	P2		PfSPZ; ChAd63/; Pfs25; MVA; PfCS; ME-TRAP; AMA-1; Rh5.1; MSP3; FP9; PEV3A

(Continued)

TABLE 13.2 (Cont'd)

Genus	Species	Antigen number	Vaccinology				Host Response	References/Vaccine name**
			1.0	2.0	3.0	Phase		
Leishmania	*VL*		K (1)			P1; P2/3	Human	[28] Leish-111f, LEISH -F2, LEISH-F3+ MPL-SE; Alum-ALM-BCG
	VL/PKDL				R (1)	P1; P2		[28] LEISH-F2;+ MPL-SE; ChAd63-KL
	CL				R (1)	P1/2		[28] Leish-111f+MPL-SE; Alum-ALM + BCG; LEISH-F2+ MPL-SE
Toxoplasma	*T. gondii*	11	M (3)	S (1)	R (2) D (9)	PC	Mouse	[25]
Neospora	*N. caninum*	9		S (6)	R (2) D (2)	PC	Mouse / Gerbil	[25]
Theileria	*T. annulata*	2		S (2)		F	Cattle	[25]
	T. parva	1		S (1)		F	Cattle	

Bbo- *B. bovis*; Bbi- *B. bigemina*; Bd.- *B. divergens*; Ea- *E. acervulina*; Et, *E. tenella*; Ema- *E. maxima*; LA, Live Attenuated; SPA, soluble parasite antigens; K, killed; T, Transgenic; S, Subunit; D, DNA vaccine; R, Recombinant; PC, Preclinical trials (animal models); F, Field trials (animal target population); P1/2 phases 1 and 2; P2: phase 2; P2/3: Phases 2 and 3; P3: phase 3. The number of vaccines is indicated in parentheses.

[a] *Antimalarial vaccine were reviewed by Zhen et al., 2019 [27] and vaccine candidates of pre-erythrocytic stages in clinical phase trials were recently review by Molina-Franky and collaborators 2020 [29].*

phagocytic cells, blood proteins and cytokines. This early response blocks the entry and eliminates or limits the growth of parasites. The initial sites for interaction between parasites and hosts are the skin or the gastrointestinal tract, depending on the specific parasite transmission route. The skin acts as the first line of defense against parasites like *P. falciparum,* after a female mosquito bite and inoculate sporozoites the initial infective stage. It has been shown that antibodies found in the skin tissues inhibit sporozoite motility in the dermis [31]. Other physical barriers for parasites transmitted by the oral route are the intestinal epithelial cells, that produces inflammation and biochemical factors, which can influence innate and stimulate adaptive immune cell function [32]. A recent study has identified the cytokine Interferon- λ3 (IFN-λ3), an IFN type III, as a key epithelial defense mechanism against *C. parvum* in a neonatal piglet model [33].

If protozoan parasites successfully trespass these barriers, they will encounter cells related to the innate immunity. Parasites contain substances that stimulate cells related to the innate immunity that are known as pathogen-associated molecular patterns (PAMPs). They are recognized by Pattern Recognition Receptors (PRRs, e.g., Toll-like receptors (TLRs) present in natural killers (NK), phagocytes (macrophages and neutrophils), and dendritic cells (DCs) and can induce their proliferation and cytokines production [34. Upon *Cryptosporidium* infection, TLR2 and TLR4 expressed in epithelial cells induce the production of human β-defensin 2 to help parasite clearence [35]. In murine models it has been shown that the innate recognition of *T. gondii* depends on the interaction of profilin with TLR11 and TLR12 (functionally absent in humans), and that monocytes and DCs drives Interleukine-12 (IL-12) response [36]. It has been also demonstrated that IL-12 induces the production of IFN-γ, activating T cell-mediated immunity, which controls intracellular parasites and cell-autonomous host defense [37].

Protozoan parasites can induce non-specific activation of different cell populations of the innate response [38–40]. Macrophages, produces nitric oxide, or toxic oxygen intermediates and cytokines which showed inhibition of growth of *T. gondii* [41], *N. caninum* [42] and *Eimeria* spp. [43]. During experimental *Leishmania* infection in mice, parasites infect macrophages where they replicated and survived. The parasite induced a decrease in toxic oxygen intermediates, and cytokines like Tumoral Necrosis Factor-alpha (TNF-α), and IL-12 (which are necessary for parasite clearance), together with an increase in IL-10, prostanglandin E2 (PGE2), and Transforming Growth Factor-beta (TGF-β) expression, demonstrating that *Leishmania* can manipulate the host immune response, which in turns determine to the persistent of the infections [44].

NK cytotoxicity is important for the clearance of intracellular parasites. After *T. cruzi* infection NK are involved in killing the parasite; however, the parasite is able to modulate their function [39]. NK are critical in early and continuous control of *Plasmodium* spp. infections in both mouse and humans models [45]. A recent work has shown how *Plasmodium* can activate NK cells, responding with natural cytotoxicity, and inhibiting the growth of parasites via antibody-dependent cellular cytotoxicity mechanisms [46]. The role of NK in cryptosporidiosis is also an active area of research [40]. The cytotoxic response of NK through the production of IFN-ɣ depending on IL-12 is well known; however, their role is not clear in some apicomplexans like *T. gondii* [47]. Furthermore, the effector functions of NK have been recently reconsidered [48] since innate lymphoid cells (ILC) derived from common lymphoid progenitor have been re-classified [49]. ILC is comprised of three groups that are important effector cells both in tissue homeostasis and disease. Additionally, ILCs are highly plastic, which is important for a successful response against infections and normal tissue integrity. Their involvement in apicomplexan infections has been investigated and recently reviewed by Ivanova and colleagues [48]. A recent study from Klose and colleagues in toxoplasmosis has shown that after oral infection with *T. gondii* high levels of IFN-ɣ and TNF-α were found in the small intestine mainly produced by ILC1s [49]. Another work carried out in deficient mice (Ahr-deficient) has indicated that ILC3s indirectly regulate immune responses to *T. gondii* infection [50]. Nontheless, the mechanism that activates ILCs is currently unknown.

13.2.1.2 Adaptive immunity

The adaptive immune response is specific and more effective than the innate response. The stimulation of immunological memory through the activation of memory lymphocytes will have effects during secondary infections against protozoan parasites [51], which is the goal of vaccination. The adaptive response is comprised of two types of responses: cell-mediated and humoral immunity.

There are functionally different subpopulations of lymphocytes that are distinguishable by their surface phenotypes: αβ T lymphocytes (comprising CD4+ helper, CD8+ cytotoxic T, and regulatory T cells), ɣδ T lymphocytes, and B lymphocytes. In addition to NK, NKT (a small population of T lymphocytes that are so named because they express a surface molecule typically found on NK cells) plays key roles in innate immunity.

Cell-mediated immune responses: Dendritic cells (DCs) are the link with the innate response and are critical for the initiation of the adaptive immune response. DCs are specialized antigen-presenting cells (APCs) that capture and present antigens through their mayor histocompatibility complexes (MHC) class II. These are recognized by the T cell receptor (TCR) of naive T helper (Th) lymphocytes (CD4+) for their stimulation and activation into effector T cells. Upon activation, CD4+ T cells differentiate to effector cells, usually Th1, or Th2 depending on the cytokines produced by APCs and by the T cells themselves. Th1 mediates classical macrophage activation and phagocytes intracellular parasites, whereas Th2 mediates differentiation of B cells to plasma cell with the consequent production of immunoglobulins, among other functions. Recognition of peptides presented by MHCs class I (present in all nucleated cells) by TCRs of cytotoxic T cells (CTL, CD8+) induces their activation and leads to three simultaneous strategies aiming to inactivate infected cells. Firstly, the release of granules containing perforins and granzymes, which respectively assemble in pore-like structures through the target's membrane, activate pro-caspases that initiate a cellular death cascade. Secondly, the expression of death ligands-such as FasL-that bind death receptors (FasR) on the target's surface. When one receptor is bound, it triggers the trimerization of the complete receptor around its ligand, and promotes the activation of pro-caspases. Finally, cytotoxic T cells express cytokines, among which TNF-α, promoting apoptosis through its death receptor TNFR1. Activated T cells may differentiate into memory cells, which survive for long periods and respond rapidly to a second antigen challenge.

MHC genes comprise the most polymorphic loci known in genetics, with over 10,000 alleles of classical class I and class II genes among the roughly 7.5 billion people currently on our planet. In comparison, very few alleles have been reliably described in farm animals [52]. The most polymorphic human MHC class I and class II proteins (human leukocyte antigens, HLAs) are each expressed from three gene regions (MHC class I: HLA-A, -B, -C; MHC class II: HLA-DR, -DP, -DQ). The counterpart in cattle is the bovine leukocyte antigen (BoLA) and are products of DRB and DQ genes [53]. The allelic variation mainly affects the nature and composition of the peptide-binding groove and thus modulates the peptide repertoire that is presented by MHC class I or MHC class II proteins to CD8+ or CD4+ T cell, respectively. Active invasion and formation of the parasitophorous vacuole (PV) in infected macrophages and dendritic cells seem critical for the priming CD4+ and CD8+ T cell responses [54]. Apicomplexa parasites remain sequestered within the PV and it is unclear how parasite-derived antigens access the MHC class I pathway for presentation to CD8 + T cells. Goldszmid and collegues [55], have demonstrated that recruitment of host endoplasmic reticulum (ER) to the PV in *T. gondii*–infected dendritic cells directly correlates with cross-priming of CD8 + T cells, indicating that pathogen-driven recruitment of the host ER as an important route of entry into MCH-I pathway. Additional line of evidence supporting several proteins from rhoptries or dense granules suppress antigen presentation by MHC-I to reduce CD8+ T cell recognition and consequent clearance of *T. gondii* infected host cells [56].

Humoral responses: Immunoglobulins (Igs) or antibodies (Abs) are secreted after activation and differentiation of B cells to plasma cells. The repertoire of B cell receptors is given by somatic recombination at the clonal level (variable, diversity and joining region (V(D)J) recombination), which is a late event along with isotype switching, affinity maturation, generation of memory B cells, and induction of long-lived plasma cell (for further insight see [57,58]). Different isotypes of Igs can be found, depending on the animal species [57]. The generic structure of receptors and Abs among vertebrates is very heterogeneous and redundant; therefore, each animal species has some particular properties that can impact on how they respond against different pathogens [57]. Effector functions, depending on the constant region, are the ability to opsonize, to fix complement protein (classical pathway), to cross the placenta, or to activate NK.

Both cell-mediated and humoral responses are involved in the control of parasitic infections and it is partially described for some of them such as bovine neosporosis [59], bovine cryptosporidiosis [40], toxoplasmosis, human malaria, [60], leishmaniasis, and Chagas disease [39]. For instance, after *Cryptosporidium* infection in calves, downregulation of Th1 cells has been observed consistent with the development of diarrhea and the progression of disease [61]. A mediated Th2 response was also demonstrated [62] with titers of parasite-specific IgG and IgA increased after infection. In particular, mucosal IgA avoids attachment of the infective stages to epithelial host cells [62]. However, antibodies are not enough to control and prevent *Cryptosporidium* infection. A local immune response against *C. parvum* [63] mediated by CD8+ was also shown [64]. Furthermore, it was suggested a role of Th17 in *C. parvum* infections but its role in protection is not well understood [65]. T cell responses were reported upon *Leishmania* infection. Whereas a Th1 mediated response is needed for clearance of *Leishmania* a Th2 response is associated with persistence and disease progression in mice [67]. A recent work additionally demonstrated a role of Th17 regulated by a prostaglandin (E2) produced by DCs in humans and mice [68].

Human antimalarial antibodies are important both in pre-erythrocytic and erythrocytic stages of *Plasmodium*. For example, Abs against free sporozoites and the circumsporozoite protein (CSP) prevent invasion of hepatocytes by neutralizing proteins required for cell traversal and invasion. This also activates complement fixation, phagocytosis, and lysis by cytotoxic NK and NKT cells (small population of T cells expressing markers that are found on NK cells; [60]). At the erythrocytic stage, human antibodies mediates cellular killing, blocks adhesion of infected red blood cells to endothelium and neutralizes parasite toxins among others effector functions [66]. Cell-mediated immunity in humans through CD8+ T cells, NK, and NKT is responsible of elimination of intrahepatic parasites (pre-erythrocytic stage). However, their role in the posterior stage is not well understood [60].

13.2.2 Immunological components involved in protection

Adaptive immunity is usually assumed to have rapid effects on the clearance of secondary infections [51] and, therefore, this is the type of response that vaccines aim to achieve. Vaccines pursue to trigger the adaptive immune response, activating cell and humoral-mediated immunity and generating antibodies and memory cells. For some pathogens, the immunologic responses that correlate to protection, either against natural infection or vaccines, are known and well-defined, but it is not the case for the vast majority of the protozoan parasites covered in this chapter, as a consequence significant research in this area is under way.

In *Eimeria*, the presence of T cells specifically reacting to the parasite antigens was demonstrated by an *in vitro* lymphoproliferation assay [69]. In addition, the abrogation of T cells function by using cyclosporin A [70], betamethasone or dexamethasone [71] affected the development of protective immunity against *Eimeria* reinfection, proposing an essential role for cell-mediated immunity in host protection. Recent studies have highlighted the role of other T cell subsets (distinct from the Th1/Th2 paradigm) involved in gut homeostasis after coccidian infection: CD4+ T helper 17 (Th17) and CD4+ CD25+ regulatory T cells (Treg) [72]. Interleukin-17, produced by Th17, can play both protective and pathological roles in protozoan infections. In coccidiosis, IL-17 has a proinflammatory role and is related to schizont maturation and migration of parasitized epithelial cells into the lamina propria [73]. Treg cells show suppression of activated immune cells by the production of high amounts of IL-10, which is considered to play an important role in host immune evasion. It has been suggested that *Eimeria* could stimulate Tregs to express IL-10 leading to the IFN-γ-related Th1 response, critical for the regulation of the protective immunity [72]. Also, Treg cells could reduce pathology caused by *Eimeria* infection by suppression of Th17 cells [72].

Regarding protection mediated by vaccination, in *P. falciparum* it has been shown that NF-κB may induce protection after antimalarial vaccination, in addition to IFN-γ [74]. It has been suggested that a greater complexity of interactions and cross-talk between adaptive and innate cells in protected subjects against malaria may exist [75]. Clinical trials in malaria using RTS,S vaccine have demonstrated that Abs against CSP and CD4+ T cell responses serve as good correlation for protection [76]. Moreover, CD8+ T cells are also implicated as effector cells in protection against the pre-erythrocytic stage of malaria [77]. Another work with *Plasmodium yoelii* model has demonstrated that NK cells are required for vaccine-induced protection in addition to CD8+ [78].

Studies in bovine cryptosporidiosis showed that passive transfer of immunoglobulins to calves, achieved by the feeding of the first milking colostrum, was able to protect them. The vaccination of pregnant cows with recombinant vaccines carrying the antigen P23 of *C. parvum* resulted in the production of a hyperimmune colostrum that was protective for *C. parvum*-challenged calves [79,80]. A Th1-like immune response involving IFN-γ in lymphocytes of the lamina propria, accompanied by IgG2 subclass fecal antibodies against *C. parvum* p23 was observed in gut mucosa of calves recovering from cryptosporidiosis, which was later confirmed in *in vitro* assays performed with T cells from calves that had recovered from *C. parvum* infection [81].

In canine visceral leishmaniasis was demonstrated that after vaccination with the recombinant vaccine Leish-Tec® the IgG2 subclass was found, indicating a protective role of IgG [82]. A recent transciptomics analysis were performed both in *Leishmania* amazonensis and human host, i.e. in lesions of infected patients [83]. The study has found that IgG4 isotype was produced by atypical B cells infiltrated in *L. amazonensis* biopsies and the absence of CD8+T cells and Th2 responses. Altogether the results provide further information regarding parasite transcriptome during difuse cutaneous leishmaniasis that would aid to fill the gaps regarding host immune response [83].

13.3 Antigen discovery

13.3.1 Classic approaches and their limitations

The scientific community agrees in the need for new affordable and sustainable vaccines based on recombinant or live-vectored well-defined parasite antigens to combat protozoa parasites. Back in the 1990s, the first promising results from small-scale experiments using recombinant antigens started to be reported [84]. However, despite numerous efforts, a fairly low number of antigens have been defined and tested as vaccines, typifying the general difficulties faced by scientists trying to identify effective vaccine antigens in complex pathogens. Antigen discovery in the past thirty years has mainly followed two principles:

a. A popular approach for antigen discovery has been the selection of antigens based in the presence of specific antibodies (humoral immune response) in the host against some of the stages of the life cycle.

b. Some of the proteins involved in relevant biological processes such as invasion or in host/parasite interactions are naturally exposed and they could be likely to bind receptors on the host cell and are therefore amenable targets for the host immune response. Some of these proteins were discovered without the intention of developing a vaccine but their specific function or localization makes them good vaccine targets.

Apicomplexa parasites contain an apical complex composed of the conoid and specialized secretory organelles that includes micronemes, rhoptries, and dense granules, which are involved in host cell attachment, invasion, and the establishment of an intracellular parasitophorous vacuole within the host cell. Proteins related to the invasion and early interaction with the host have been typical candidates in vaccine development. These include surface antigens (SAGs) and proteins secreted by organelles of the apical complex (micronemes—MICs, rhoptries—RON/ROPs) or form dense granules (GRAs). They have been very popular as antigens tested against *T. gondii* and *N. caninum* [85,86]. Most of the candidates has been from the tachyzoite stage with some vaccination trials done using bradyzoites surface antigens SRS9 and BSR4 [87,88]. In *Eimeria* microneme proteins MIC1 MIC2, MIC3, and AMA1 have been focus of most trials, together with the refractile body SO7 [89]. Most of the research in vaccine antigens against *Cryptosporidium* are based on the surface antigens CSL, Cp900, Cp23/27, Cp40/45, Cp15/17, Muc4, and Muc5 [90]. Antigens GST-12D3 and GST-11C5 derived from a crude extract of *B. bovis* have been also investigated for their protective potential [91] as well as the surface protein p67 against *T. parva* [92,93]. Interestingly, most advanced babesiosis vaccines are comprised of "soluble parasite antigens" (SPA), which are released into the culture medium containing actively growing *Babesia*-infected red blood cells [94]. The *B. canis* SPA vaccine demonstrated high protection against homologous challenges, but limited protection against heterologous challenges. SPA vaccines were subsequently tested against other *Babesia* spp. with promising outcomes (Table 13.2). However, the level of protection against heterologous challenges raising concerns about the development of an effective universal vaccine in endemic regions.

Popular candidates for *Plasmodium* have been CSP, TRAP (pre-erythrocyte stage), SP1, and AMA1 (asexual blood-stage) all related to the blocking of the host cell invasion for the respective stages [7]. Multiple antigens have been assayed against different species of *Leishmania* showing that gp36 and Hsp70 are some of the most promising results [95].

It is important to highlight that after more than 25 years of research in recombinant vaccine candidates, very few of these antigens has reached further than the preclinical stages of the vaccine development process (Table 13.2). A potential reason for this could be that few tested antigens have provided reproducible levels of parasite reduction and there is, in general, a lack of protection for most of the candidate antigens. Some antigens have been shown to have B cell epitopes (selected by the presence of antibodies as described above—"a"). Some other vaccine antigens were chosen by their roles in the biology of the parasite (as described above—"b"); therefore, they could affect the viability of the infection by alternative mechanisms to those that act in natural protection and would have subsequent limitations to improve their efficacy. In general, a primary infection triggers a natural immunological process leading to protection against further infections, however, most of the strategies for antigen discovery do not include an "immune screen" for antigen discovery. Furthermore, since it is generally agreed that a recombinant vaccine would require a pool of different antigens due to the complexity of these parasites, most advances have only focus on very few stages of the development (usually those amendable for cultivation but not always the most relevant in the pathogenicity). In addition, the outcomes of any of these studies vaccine candidates significantly relay in the delivery system and formulated adjuvant to achieve an optimal immune response and resulting protection. Adjuvants act at different levels after immunization starting for induction of dendritic cell maturation and migration and ending with the generation of a significantly enhanced long-lasting immune response [96], in consequence, the success of any of these vaccine candidates (and those identified by more sophisticated methods) will depend on the success of the adjuvant employed.

Therefore, the development of new approaches for antigen discovery to provide new or complementary alternatives that could enhance the levels of protection achieved by the current candidates is still necessary.

13.3.2 Multiomics and cutting-edge technologies

The discovery of novel antigens by classical approaches is slow and limited to very few antigens identified and analyzed in each study. High throughput approaches based on the expansion of the "omics", defined as the "characterization and quantification of pools of biological molecules" such DNA, RNA—, proteins, metabolites, and lipids denominated genomics, transcriptomics, proteomics, metabolomics, and lipidomics, respectively, has facilitated the functional annotation of the genome for many of these parasites, significantly improving the understanding of the parasite biology, interactions with the host, as well as providing novel targets for vaccine development.

In general, these protozoa parasites have large genomes with complex proteomes [97,98], where most of their proteins remain uncharacterized [99]. Recently, omics for Apicomplexa were reviewd by Tomazic et al., 2022 [100].

Recenlty, dual-transcriptomics performed on leishmaniasis has identify highly expressed parasite genes in cutaneous lesions and diffuse cutaneous leishmaniasis that would be novel targets for vaccine devolpement against *L. braziliensis* and *L. amazonensis*, respectively [101,83].

All this work in "multiomics" of protozoan parasites has supported the development of open access databases with comprehensive collections of curated nucleotide and amino acid sequences products. These databases together with advanced computational approaches that predict protein features and statistical models have allowed the prediction of novel antigens correlated with the induction of immunity. The quality and of these databases is essential to accurately retrieve sequences of interest. The "Eukaryotic Pathogen, Vector, and Host Informatics Resource" (VEuPathDB) is one of the "Bioinformatics Resource Center" (BRCs) that provides public access to diverse genomic and other large-scale datasets focused on eukaryotic pathogens and invertebrate vectors of diseases [102,103]. Projects from VEuPathDB include parasite Informatics Resources such as PlasmoDB for *Plasmodium* spp. [104]; ToxoDB for *T. gondii* and another coccidian such as and *Eimeria* spp. [105]; TriTrypDB for trypanosomatid parasites, including *Leishmania* and *Trypanosoma* [106]; CryptoDB for *Cryptosporidium* spp. [107]; PiroplasmaDB for *Babesia* spp. and *Theileria* spp. [108]; and VectorBase for invertebrate vector of human pathogens [109].

Furthermore, a comparative genomics and transcriptomics database for *Plasmodium* spp., *T. parva,* and *T. gondii* called Malaria.tools is available at [110]. This is a valuable tool for the identification of novel genes relevant to a biological process of interest since it has been developed based on gene co-expression networks that identify clusters of genes with similar expression profiles [111]. The use of Malaria.tools has allowed the identification of a gene that is co-expressed with another 91 genes related to erythrocyte invasion [111]. This powerful database would allow the identification of novel targets for therapy. Computational tools for the prediction of protein features or biological functions have been used to find alternative vaccine candidates to those discovered by classical approaches. Protein features that can make them accessible to the immune systems (e.g., surface location or secretion/excretion) can be predicted using bioinformatic tools including prediction of signal peptides (SignalP; signalBLAST) [112,113], transmembrane regions (TMHMM, Phobius) [114,115], excretory proteins from prediction of unconventional protein secretion (OutCyte) [116], or prediction of glycosylphosphatidylinositol anchor (PredGPI, NetGPI) [117,118], are some examples. There are several bioinformatic tools available for the prediction of protein signatures, biological functions, or orthology such as InterPro [119]; GeneOntology [120,121], and OrthoMCL [122], respectively.

Many novel tools are based on machine-learning algorithms built on experimental evidence, which allows the prediction of immune features that were not possible to identify by other methodologies. Prediction of T and B cell epitopes, also so-called immunoinformatics, is a key step in the vaccine design, providing additional information for the identification of peptides that can activate host T cells or binding to antibodies. Some popular predictors of B-epitopes either continous or discontinous are (1) ABCpred: [123], an algorithm that creates datasets of fixed length, using neural network [124], with applications for many pathogens, including parasites; (2) BCEpred [125], a server that predicts linear B cell epitopes based on physic-chemical properties of the BciPep database, which comprises 1029 B-cell epitopes, and 1029 non-epitopes obtained randomly from the Swiss-Prot database [126]; (3) BEPIpred-2.0 [127]; and (4) BEpro [128], for dicontinuos B-epitopes.

As was described above (see Section 13.2.1), MHCs (class I or II) present peptides to lymphocytes (CD4+/CD8+) after the proteins have been degraded intracellularly. The binding of peptides to MHC is a necessary step in the onset and effectiveness of an adaptive immune response and predicting the peptide-MHC binding can correlate positively with eliciting an immune response. Several tools are available for pattern recognition base on machine-learning and they are continuously updated based on new experimental evidence. As for example NetMHCII pan 4.0 [129] and NetMH pan 4.1 [130] allow predictions for a set of HLA (human), Bola (cattle), H-2 (mouse), Patr, Mamu, and Gogo (primates), SLA (swin), and Eqca (equine). Importantly, the latest version has been trained from an extensive experimental dataset (binding affinity and eluted ligand mass spectrometry), using a neural network algorithm (NNAlign, machine learning) [131,132]. The database and analysis resource Immune Epitope Database [133] provides a valuable dataset from experimental data on antibody and T cell epitopes studied in vertebrates in the context of infectious disease and autoimmunity. The IEDB also provides tools for the prediction and analysis of epitopes allowing the selection of different hosts (e.g., mammals, bird, or fish) [134].

The application of reverse vaccinology in human pathogens started two decades ago in humans pathogens [135], and today it has moved forward to a 2.0 version [136] thanks to the increasing amount of datasets, sequences available of B and T cell repertories and protective antigens. This approach explores the genome to find novel antigens, overcoming the lack of parasite culture or the different expression patterns in between the different life cycle stages and predicting immunological features of proteins. Examples of the use of reverse vaccinology applied to protozoan parasites are the prediction of the glycosylphosphatidylinositol (GPI) proteome of *Babesia* [137] and *C. parvum* [138,139]. GPI-anchored proteins are usually surface-expressed and are known to play a key role in parasites [137,140]. GPIs in *T. godii*, *T cruzi* and *P. falciparum,* among others [141–143] have shown to stimulate innate response through TLRs. Some proteins anchored to the surface by GPI have been demonstrated to be effective vaccinogens against *B. divergens* and *B. canis*, when expressed as recombinant GPI-anchored proteins [144,145]. Recently, a GPI-Anchored Surface Antigen-1 (GASA-1) was identified by a reverse approach from *B. bovis* GPI-anchored proteome. In vitro assays with the recombinant protein indicated that the novel protein carries neutralization-sensitive antibody epitopes as well as T cell epitopes [91].

Despite the general consensus that parasitic protein features like surface localization, excreted/secreted proteins (from micronemes, rhoptries, or dense granules), or relevant biological functions (e.g., proteases) are accessible to the host immune system and, as a consequence, are attractive vaccine candidates, a recent study provides additional characteristics to potentially identify novel vaccine candidates by reverse vaccinology. Goodswen et al. [146] have proposed a high-throughput *in silico* approach to predict positive selection sites, protein subcellular localization and sequence locations of medium to high T cell MHC class I binding peptides for *T. gondii*.

Another recent approach applied to *T. cruzi* consist of the synthesis of peptides to evaluate which of them can activate T cells [147] (which play a key role in the chronic stage of Chagas disease). This involves a combination of bioinformatics and synthetic combinatorial chemistry, previously applied in a "T cell driven" approach in the identification of peptides derived from highly immunogenic vaccinia proteins after smallpox vaccination [148]. The major finding of this work was the discovery of T cell activating peptides with a great potential for the development of new therapies. This innovative approach comprised a combination of *in silico* and in vitro assays to explore new insights into the immune systems, that finally described seven novel parasite-derived peptides that were recognized by CD4+ and CD8+ T cells (from which three of them were previously reported as class I epitopes) and which had the ability to activate CD4+ T cells [147]. This approach could be applied to study other related parasites, helping to achieve a deeper knowledge regarding the immune response of the host against these microorganisms.

There are many other computational biology techniques available such as molecular docking approach that can be used to model the interaction between a small molecule and a protein at the atomic level. There are online software available, such as GalaxyWeb [149]), which provides protein structure prediction, and refinement [150], and could allow the study of the binding of a peptide to an MHC molecule. Furthermore, predicted peptides or vaccine candidates derived from computational approaches will still requite require experimental validation in currently available animal models for the different diseases, evaluating vaccine-specific immune responses, immunoprotection, and safety.

Current advances in genetic manipulation of parasites with human or veterinary importance have allowed the generation of transgenic populations to experimentally validate the gene function predicted by the different approaches described above. There is a wide range of emerging tools applied now adapted to many of these parasites, allowing the discovery of antigens with potential interest as vaccine targets. Next-generation technologies of gene editing such as CRISPR (Clustered Regularly Interspaced Short Palindromic Repeats)/ Cas9 (CRISPR-associated protein 9) has contributed to this issue, moving forward gene functional studies, by knocking-out, repressing, activating, or tagging genes in species where it was not possible before by other methods. This has enhance and speed-up the understanding of the biology of these parasites, providing newly characterized genes as potential targets for vaccine development. CRISPR/ Cas9 was originally found in *Escherichia coli* as part of an RNA-based immune system against viruses. It has revolutioned parasitology research [151], being successfully applied to the Apicomplexa *P. falciparum* [152,153] in first placce, and then to many other tripanosomatid parasites like *Leishmania donovani, Leishmania mexicana, Leishmania major, Trypanosoma brucei,* and *T. cruzi* [154–156]) (for more information regarding CRISPR/Cas9 applied to Apicomplexa refer to [100]). For *T. cruzi* [157], and *Leishmania* spp. [155] step-by-step protocols have been published, becoming an invaluable resource for the research community. Interestly, Beneke et al. [156] have recently developed a CRISPR/ Cas9 toolkit for trypanosomatids based on a cloning free-method and a website (LeishGEdit.net), for the designing of primers required for sgRNAs and DNA repair templates, allowing a rapid tagging and gene knockout. Nevertheless, either predicted peptides or vaccine candidates derived from computational approaches or proteins with a validated a specific biological function by genetic manipulation approaches, will still requite require experimental validation in currently available animal models for the different diseases, evaluating vaccine-specific immune responses, immunoprotection, and safety. In summary, the implementation of omics and cutting-edge technologies, as reviewed in the current section, would lead to the identification of novel vaccine candidates of protozoan parasites (Fig. 13.2).

13.4 Systems biology applied to protozoan parasites

Systems biology is defined as an interdisciplinary approach within the area of biomedical research that combines big data derived from multiomic studies with computational and statistical analysis, aimed to understand interactions and dynamics from single to complex biological level [159]. This is an emerging approach that needs close collaborations with specialists from different disciplines such as biology, infectology, bioinformatics, mathematics, and immunology, necessary in the process of understanding the components and their interactions to generate knowledge on vaccine-induced immune responses. The use of data generated through high-through sequencing technologies combined with computational and experimental methods in the context of vaccination has raised the new field of "systems-vaccinology," aimed to predict the biological behaviour involved in vaccine-induced immunity as a holistic view [160]; that is, the system and their properties are analyzed as a whole and not just through single parts that make them up. Also, these approaches have been defined by Polland as vaccinomics "integration of immunogenetics and immunogenomics with systems biology and immune profiling" [161]. In addition, systems vaccinology analysis could provide useful surrogate markers or could assay vaccine efficacy without the need for a challenge [162]. However, well-established standard protocols are necessary for the assessment of vaccine efficacy in animal models for each disease to allow comparative evaluation, and these are not well unified at the moment for the evaluation of animal diseases [163]. In contrast, studies in malaria infections have adopted a standardized safety procedure, known as controlled human malaria infection (CHMI) that has been applied, among other purposes, to the fields of malaria vaccine and drug development, supporting immunology studies [164] and systems vaccinology approaches. Systems biology-based approaches have been applied in malaria research since the last decade. Tan & Crompton [165], and Smith & Styczynski [166] have reviewed and well-documented all the information regarding this issue. This section is focused on findings on leishmaniasis, coccidiosis, and toxoplasmosis-besides malaria-systems biology applied to vaccinology and immunology. Studies involve bioinformatics, mathematical and computational models and immunological analysis in addition to transcriptomics, and are summarised in Table 13.3.

Among studies carried out on malaria in systems vaccinology, it is interesting to mention that Vahey et al. [162] have found genes of the immunoproteasome pathway (related to the degradation of proteins for later presentation into MHCs) correlating with protection against *P. falciparum* infection after the third vaccination with RTS,S, suggesting a potential role in mediating protection in vaccinated people that may represent a useful surrogate marker. Other studies carried out by Van de Berg et al. [74], Kazmin et al. [167], and Tran et al. [75] have provided further insight into how vaccine-mediated protection, providing molecular signatures of protective immunity against malaria (Table 13.3). By analyzing longitudinal peripheral blood transcriptome and immunogenicity data from a clinical efficacy trial, in which healthy adults received three RTS,S doses four weeks, followed by CHMI two weeks later, Van de Berg and colleagues [74] have found that NF-κB and IFN-γ pathways may induce protection in RTS,S vaccination.

On the other hand, a previous study carried out by Kazmin et al. [167] has suggested that multiple mechanisms can induce protective immunity against *P. falciparum* given that specific antibody titers were associated with protection in the first vaccinated group but not in the second vaccinated group, where protection was associated with polyfunctional CD4+ T cell responses. It is interesting to highlight that in this study different vaccine protocols was used, where the first group of 21 volunteers received three consecutive immunizations of RTS,S/ AS01 (RRR regimen), whereas in the second group the 25 volunteers received two immunizations with RTS,S/ AS01 followed by immunization with Adenovirus serotype 35 expressing CSP (ARR regimen).

Further advances in systems vaccinology in visceral leishmaniasis was also achieved. Recently, a combination of methods that integrates immunoinformatics, modeling, simulation, and molecular docking has been applied to design a multi-epitope vaccine candidate against visceral leishmaniasis, providing functional and mechanistic knowledge of vaccines for the elicitation of the host immune responses [168] (Table 13.3). A similar approach was performed to *Eimeria* spp. for the design of a vaccine against coccidiosis. Retrieving data

TABLE 13.3 Systems biology approaches in the field of vaccinology and immunology applied to tripanosomatid and apicomplexan parasites (adapted of Tomazic et al., 2022) [194].

Field	Species	Target population/host	Disease[c]	Finding	Methods	References
Vaccinology	*L. infantum*, *L. donovani*	Human (*in silico*)	VL	Design of a multiepitope vaccine and *in silico* evaluation of its immunodynamics	Bioinformatics, modeling, simulation, molecular docking	[168]
	Eimeria spp.	Chicken (*in silico*)[d]	AC	Prediction of epitopes and disgn of multiepitope vaccine that induces immunity and boosts the host immune system	Immunoinformatics, molecular docking and simulation	[169]
	P. falciparum[a]	RTS,S vaccinated volunteers	HM	Up-regulation of genes associated with the efficient processing of MHC peptides that suggests a potential role in mediating protection in vaccinated people	Transcriptomics, gene set enrichment analysis, predictive modeling	[162]
		RTS, S vaccinated volunteers	HM	Pathways involved the protein complex NF-κB and the cytokine IFN-γ may induce protection in vaccinated population	Transcriptomics, gene set enrichment analysis, Predictive modeling	[74]
		CSP[b] vaccinated volunteers	HM	Differential expression of genes enriched in modules related to T cells, NK cells, protein synthesis, and mitochondrial processes were detected in fully protected individuals four weeks after the first immunization	Transcriptomics, network analysis	[75]

(*Continued*)

TABLE 13.3 (Cont'd)

Field	Species	Target population/host	Disease[c]	Finding	Methods	References
Immunology	*P. falciparum*[a]	Human	M	Immune signatures. Upregulation of Toll-like receptor signaling through NF-κB pathways, downregulation of genes involved in phagocytosis and inflammation (i.e. TNF-α, IFN-γ, and IL-1β). Modulation of other genes and induction of MHC class I and II expression. Differences in apoptosis genes between symptomatics and presymtomatics	Transcriptomics, computational approaches	[170]
				The proinflamatory immune response, and apoptosis pathways are upregulated at the time of acute illness in uncomplicated *P. falciparum* malaria	Transcriptomics, computational approaches	[171]
				Changes in the human innate immune, TLR2 and TICAM2 correlate with the severity. Genetic variation, calling single nucleotide polymorphisms tags, associated with severe malaria symptoms and with drug-resistance genes.	Transcriptomics, bioinformatics	[172]
	Plasmodium ashfordi	Birds, Mice	M	A large number of genes differentially expressed during both peaking and decreasing parasitemia stages, positive T-cell activation and lymphocyte differentiation were downregulated during decreasing parasitemia	Transcriptomics, gene set enrichment	[173]

Field	Species	Target population/host	Disease[c]	Finding	Methods	References
	T. gondii	Mice	T	Host genes associated with the immune response are more abundant during chronic infection than in acute	Dual-transcriptomics, ontological analysis	[174]
				Parasite actively regulates host genes related to the immune responses between acute and chronic infection	Transcriptomics and MiRNA–gene network analysis	[175]
	L. braziliensis	Human	CL	Differences in host immune responses correlates with active transcription of parasite genes. In lesions with parasite presence, infiltrated B cell, Igs and up-regulation of immune inhibitory molecules were found. In lesions without detection of parasite, absence of B cell activation, but increased expression of antimicrobial genes and genes encoding skin barrier function were found. Putative parasite virulence factors were highly expressed	Transcriptomics (RNA-seq), gene network analysis	[101]

[a] *Most recent studies, for further information refer to Tran & Crompton 2019 [75].*

[b] *CSP: immunization with live sporozoites.*

[c] *VL, visceral leishmaniasis; AC: avian coccidiosis; HM: human malaria; M: malaria; T: toxoplasmosis; CL: cutaneous leishmaniasis.*

[d] *In addition to chicken MHC human HLA alleles were also used.*

from databases, derived from omics, and using informatics and modeling tools, a multi-epitope vaccine was designed that included 7 cytotoxic T cell epitopes, 21 helper T cell epitopes, and 6 B cell epitopes fused to the cholera toxin subunit B. The designed vaccine showed immunogenicity and non-allergenicity [169].

Additionally, systems vaccinology has also been applied for the analyses of adjuvants [74,162,167], discerning new the mechanism of action that allows the amplification of immune responses. Hence, this would allow increasing the reduced number of adjuvants currently in use for human vaccine formulations.

Although systems vaccinology has been applied to a limited number of protozoan parasites (i.e. *P. falciparum, Eimeria* sp. and *Leishmania* sp.), systems biology studies have been extensively applied to elucidate of host-parasite interactions in some of them, recently reviewed by Swann et al. [99]. The analysis of transcriptomics data from both, parasite and host, has revealed some new aspects of parasite immunology, summarized in Table 13.3. Systems biology-based approaches applied to the study, analysis and understanding of the immune system are also known as "systems immunology." This has applied to identify immune signatures upon infection of *Plasmodium* sp. [170–173], *T. godii* [174,175] and *Leishmania* sp. [101] (Table 13.3).

A recent study carried out using blood from people with uncomplicated *P. falciparum* malaria indicated that the innate immune response, cytokines (IL-1β, IL-6, TNF-α, and IFN-ɣ), and apoptosis pathways were acutely upregulated in the group under study with concomitant downregulation of immune-modulatory and apoptosis inhibitory genes [171]. The results are in contrast with a previous report from Ockenhouse and colleagues [170] that showed that genes involved in phagocytosis and inflammation, including the cytokines TNF-α, IFN-γ, and IL-1β were downregulated. Hence, the results and the different interpretations that raise from the different datasets are affected by variations in the population under study, and clinical phenotype. Likewise, due to the high degree of heterogeneity between biological samples, high variability is expected. Additionally, immune responses are affected by other factors such as age, genetics, stress, comorbidity, that hinder the interpretation of the immune mechanisms. Therefore, the more data is collected the more hypothesis would arise and novel findings and biomarkers will be generated.

Yamagishi and collaborators have performed a transcriptomic analysis both in *P. falciparum* and humans to elucidate mechanism of host-interactions. This work has identified human and parasite genes and pathways that correlated with various clinical data (Table 13.3), providing novel targets for therapy. Furthermore, it has been identified genetic variations in anti-malaria drug resistance-related genes as well as associated with severe malaria symptoms [172].

Another transcriptomic analysis focused on avian malaria has revealed differences in the sets of RNA between infected and uninfected birds (*Eurasian siskins*), demonstrating shifts in response to malaria infection [173] (Table 13.3).

Global transcriptome analysis for both host and *T. gondii* during the establishment of chronic infection in mice was performed by Pittman and collaborators [174]. The results demonstrated the influence of parasite development on host gene transcription as well as the influence of the host environment on parasite gene transcription. Importantly, the host genes associated with the immune response were more abundant, during the chronic infection than in the acute phase. Conversely, parasite genes that are highly expressed in both acute and chronic infection were involved in transcription and translation, highlighting that both stages of the parasites can actively synthesizing proteins. A recent study has shown that microRNA (miRNA) expression in pigs is altered by *T. gondii*. In addition, genes related to immune responses are differently regulated when comparing to the splenocyte miRNA expression profiles during acute and chronic toxoplasmosis [175].

A study carry out by Christensen et al. [101] on cutaneous leishmaniasis has shown differences in immune response that correlated with active transcription of parasite genes. One of the major finding was that infiltrated B cell, Igs and upregulation of immune inhibitory molecules were found in cutaneus leishmania lesions where *Leishmania braziliensis* is detectable, whereas in lesions where the parasite was not detectable, absence of B cell activation, but increased expression of antimicrobial genes and genes encoding skin barrier function were found (Table 13.3).

Systems biology applied to vaccinology and immunology can improve the understanding of protective immune responses after vaccination as well as the molecular mechanisms behind host-parasite interactions, helping to fill the current gaps, and allowing the discovery of potential novel targets for chemoprophylaxis, vaccine development, and valuable surrogate markers.

13.5 Rational vaccine design: future and prospects

Third-generation vaccines or vaccinology 3.0 has emerged in protozoan parasites as the most suitable strategy for vaccines design and development. Several recombinant veterinary vaccines are commercially available for bacterial or viral pathogens [176] in contrast to the situation for protozoan parasites. The transition to vaccinology 3.0 has been possible thanks to several technological advancements such as reverse vaccinology, high-throughput omics, and other cutting-edge technologies, detailed in the present chapter. There is an increasing amount of open online software for the prediction of protein attributes as well as simulation and modeling that can significantly improve the prediction of the "desired properties" as well as immunological features for the prediction of novel vaccine candidates and their behaviour after administration into the host.

This chapter has covered the latest finding in the immunological responses against protozoan parasites as well as classical and novel approaches for antigen discovery and vaccine development in protozoa parasites, outlined in Fig. 13.2. The first step for vaccine development is the discovery of antigens with the potential to confer immunity, and this has undergone a significant improvement facilitated by the availability of bioinformatics for the prediction of desirable

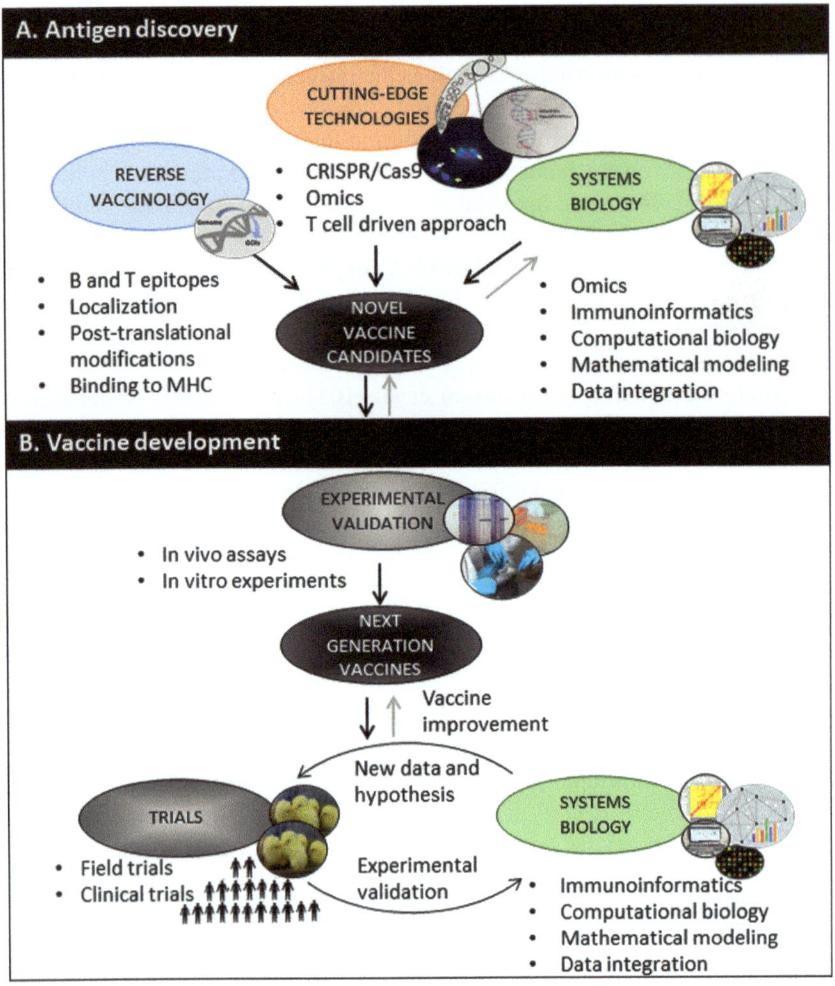

FIG. 13.2 Current approaches for antigen discovery and vaccine development applied to protozoan parasites. (A) Antigen discovery leading to novel candidates for development of novel vaccines. Reverse vaccinology is based on bioinformatics tools that support the selection of Genes Of Interest (*GOIs*) from annotated genomes. Following a designed pipeline, protein features, such as B cell epitopes, protein localization, post-translational modifications, and/or T cell epitopes binding MHC can be predicted, which require further experimental validation. Cutting-edge technologies such as comparative genomics or CRISPR/Cas9-based technologies allow functional characterization of genes with an hypothetical annotation. T cell-driven approach allows experimentally validation of MHC binding predictions through the synthesis of peptides that activate T- cells. Lately, systems biology approaches, by combining the use of data generated by molecular biology and high-throughput technologies with immunoinformatics, computational biology and mathematical modeling, have enabled the study of host immune responses and host-parasite interactions, leading to the discovery of novel potential vaccine antigens. This scheme is an iterative process (indicated with grey arrows) that allows the design, construction, and evaluation of vaccines, giving positive/negative dynamic feedback. (B) Vaccine development. Once the vaccine candidates are selected, they are evaluated under different formulations and regimens in animal/human models. Systems biology, in the context of controlled in vivo trials—i.e., field or clinical—will integrate immunological, experimental and 'omics' data, assessing vaccine efficacy in the specific target populations (animals or humans), support further improving approaches for next generation vaccines.

antigen features (T and B cells epitopes, protein localization, or posttranslational modifications), leading to the development and application of reverse vaccinology. Cutting-edge technologies such as comparative genomics, "T cell driven" approaches, and gene editing by CRISPR-Cas9 have also allowed the discovery and functional characterization of potential novel antigens. As further improvement, the expansion of systems biology to this field has allowed the study of the host-immune responses and host-parasite interactions in an integrative way, which can lead to the discovery of novel antigens based on integrated mechanisms of action. Once vaccine candidates are selected, and tested, efficacy and safety need to be evaluated within specific formulation (i.e. co-administration with an efficient adjuvant to improve efficacy and guarantee the absence of physical, chemical, or biological instability of the formulation). Systems based approaches can also provide relevant information before vaccine efficacy and safety is assessed in clinical or field trials, by predicting these features and behaviour (Fig. 13.2).

Nonetheless, achieving successful vaccines against protozoa parasites needs to overcome some limitations. For some of these parasites, the functional annotation of the genome is incomplete and the proteome coverage is very restricted [99]. Moreover, protocols to assess the vaccine efficacy are inconsistent and therefore not comparable. All these factors together hamper the development of vaccines for these species. In addition, most previous studies have focused on the evaluation of the individual parts of a biological system following traditional "reductionist" approaches. In this way, only few specific stages of the parasites are studied (usually that amendable for cell culture), or specific proteins of a particular biological mechanism (e.g., attachment and invasion) without considering the whole system; in consequence, the global immune components required for protection cannot be well characterized. Improvements on high throughput technologies or multiplex platforms (RNA-seq or gene microarrays, among others) has allowed the study of both parasites and hosts, providing relevant information on how they influence each other. Systems biology-based approach combines experimental data with mathematical models and computational tools, and offers the possibility to integrate the complex biology of protozoan parasites and their hosts, allowing a better understanding of the mechanisms used by the parasites to avoid host immune defenses and how hosts can balance these actions.

Newer technologies that are being developed on transcriptomics like single-cell RNA-seq platforms that overcome current limitations based on bulk measures that provides great heterogeinty and analytical variability [177], and the integration of other omics (such as proteomics, metagenomics of microbiota where parasites interacts, or metabolomics) would facilitate and increase the number of systems-based studies, generating new understandings on host-parasites interactions and on immunological responses. Therefore, systems biology could provide novel insights into mechanisms of action of vaccines and molecular signatures involved in protection, to improve their design and effectiveness. These integrative and interdisciplinary approaches have started to be incorporated into vaccine development of most relevant trypanosomatids and apicomplexan parasites, beyond malarial vaccines research, which was pioneering in the field about a decade ago (recently reviewed [165]).

The expansion of systems biology to other protozoa parasites beyond *T. gondii, Plasmodium* sp., *Eimeria* sp., and *Leishmania* sp. combined with subsequent evaluation of the novel vaccine candidates in animal models can significantly improve the rational design of vaccines against these parasites of zoonotic and economical relevance, opening a new era of vaccinology research that could lead to an expansion in licensed products after decades of significant but slow advances.

References

[1] Jenner E. An inquiry into the causes and effects of the variole vaccine, or cow-pox, 1798. On Vaccination Against Smallpox 1798.
[2] Pound J. Tick fever. Notes on the inoculation of bulls as a preventive against tick fever at Rathdowney and Rosedale. Queensl Agric J 1897:1471–7.
[3] Connaway J, Francis M. Texas fever. Experiments made by the Missouri experiment station and the Missouri state board of agriculture in cooperation with the Texas experiment station in immunizing northern breeding cattle against Texas fever for the southern trade Mo. Agric Exp Stn Bull 1899;48:1–64.
[4] Barriga OO. A review on vaccination against protozoa and arthropods of veterinary importance. Vet Parasitol 1994;55:29–55.
[5] Singh AK, Verma AK, Neha, et al. Trends and advances in vaccines against protozoan parasites of veterinary importance: A review. J Biol Sci 2014. doi:10.3923/jbs.2014.95.109. Epub ahead of print.
[6] Report on the operation of the Steering Group for the Joint EMA/HMA action plan on availability of veterinary vaccines European Medicines Agency EMA/565300/2017. https://www.ema.europa.eu/en/documents/report/report-operation-steering-group-joint-ema/hma-action-plan-availability-veterinary-vaccines-2016-2017_en.pdf.
[7] Hall N, Karras M, Raine JD, et al. A comprehensive survey of the Plasmodium life cycle by genomic, transcriptomic, and proteomic analyses. Science 2005. doi:10.1126/science.1103717. Epub ahead of print.
[8] Shapiro K, Bahia-Oliveira L, Dixon B, et al. Environmental transmission of Toxoplasma gondii: Oocysts in water, soil and food. Food Waterborne Parasitol 2019. doi:10.1016/j.fawpar.2019.e00049. Epub ahead of print.
[9] Sińskі E, Behnke JM. Apicomplexan parasites: Environmental contamination and transmission. Pol J Microbiol 2004;(53):67–73.
[10] Florin-Christensen M, Suarez CE, Rodriguez AE, et al. Vaccines against bovine babesiosis: where we are now and possible roads ahead. Parasitology 2014;141:1563–92.
[11] Ahmad TA, El-Sayed BA, El-Sayed LH. Development of immunization trials against Eimeria spp. Trials Vaccinol 2016. doi:10.1016/j.trivac.2016.02.001. Epub ahead of print.
[12] Mangold AJ, Vanzini VR, Echaide IE, et al. Viability after thawing and dilution of simultaneously cryopreserved vaccinal Babesia bovis and Babesia bigemina strains cultured in vitro. Vet Parasitol 1996. doi:10.1016/0304-4017(95)00839-X. Epub ahead of print.
[13] Pipano E, Shkap V. Vaccination against tropical theileriosis. Ann N Y Acad Sci 2000. doi:10.1111/j.1749-6632.2000.tb05328.x. Epub ahead of print 2000.
[14] Buxton D, Innes EA. A commercial vaccine for ovine toxoplasmosis. Parasitology 1995. doi:10.1017/S003118200000144X. Epub ahead of print.

[15] Patel EH, Lubembe DM, Gachanja J, et al. Molecular characterization of live Theileria parva sporozoite vaccine stabilates reveals extensive genotypic diversity. Vet Parasitol 2011. doi:10.1016/j.vetpar.2011.01.057. Epub ahead of print.

[16] Romero JJ, Pérez E, Frankena K. Effect of a killed whole Neospora caninum tachyzoite vaccine on the crude abortion rate of Costa Rican dairy cows under field conditions. Vet Parasitol 2004. doi:10.1016/j.vetpar.2004.06.016. Epub ahead of print.

[17] Vidor E, Bissuel G, Dubreuil N. Vaccination against canine babesiosis: an overview of field observations. Trans R Soc Trop Med Hyg 1989. doi:10.1016/0035-9203(89)90611-1. Epub ahead of print.

[18] Ziomko I, Karamon J, Cencek T, et al. Prevention of broiler chick coccidiosis using the inactivated subunit vaccine Coxabic®. Bull Vet Inst Pulawy 2005;49(3):299–302.

[19] Titilincu A, Fit N, Salagean M, et al. Maternal transfer and evolution of humoral immune effectors in chickens from breeders vaccinated with coxabic (ABIC, Israel). Bull Univ Agric Sci Vet Med Vol 2005;62:593–599.

[20] Wallach MG, Ashash U, Michael A, et al. Field application of a subunit vaccine against an enteric protozoan disease. PLoS One 2008;3:1–7.

[21] Wallach M, Halabi A, Pillemer G, et al. Maternal Immunization with Gametocyte Antigens as a Means of Providing Protective Immunity against Eimeria maxima in Chickens. Inf and Imm 1992;60(5):2036–9.

[22] Moreno J, Vouldoukis I, Martin V, et al. Use of a liesp/qa-21 vaccine (canileish) stimulates an appropriate th1-dominated cell-mediated immune response in dogs. PLoS Negl Trop Dis 2012. doi:10.1371/journal.pntd.0001683. Epub ahead of print.

[23] Carcelén J, Iniesta V, Fernández-Cotrina J, et al. The chimerical multi-component Q protein from Leishmania in the absence of adjuvant protects dogs against an experimental Leishmania infantum infection. Vaccine 2009. doi:10.1016/j.vaccine.2009.07.069. Epub ahead of print.

[24] Regina-Silva S, Feres A, França-Silva JC, et al. Field randomized trial to evaluate the efficacy of the Leish-Tec® vaccine against canine visceral leishmaniasis in an endemic area of Brazil. Vaccine 2016;34:2233–9.

[25] Vaccine investigation and online information network (VIOLIN) http://www.violinet.org/ [Accessed 2021 Feb 26].

[26] World Health Organization. The World malaria report 2018.

[27] Zheng J, Pan H, Gu Y, et al. Prospects for malaria vaccines: pre-erythrocytic stages, blood stages, and transmission-blocking stages. Biomed Res Int 2019. doi:10.1155/2019/9751471. Epub ahead of print.

[28] NIH U.S. National Library of Medicine. https://www.clinicaltrials.gov. [Accessed 18 Jan 2021].

[29] Molina-Franky J, Cuy-Chaparro L, Camargo A, et al. Plasmodium falciparum pre-erythrocytic stage vaccine development. Malar J 2020;19:1–18.

[30] Gordon DM, Mc Govern TW, Krzych U, et al. Safety, immunogenicity, and efficacy of a recombinantly produced plasmodium falciparum circumsporozoite protein-hepatitis b surface antigen subunit vaccine. J Infect Dis 1995. doi:10.1093/infdis/171.6.1576. Epub ahead of print.

[31] Rénia L, Goh YS. Malaria parasites: the great escape. Front Immunol 2016. doi:10.3389/fimmu.2016.00463. Epub ahead of print.

[32] Petry F, Jakobi V, Tessema TS. Host immune response to Cryptosporidium parvum infection. Exp Parasitol 2010;126:304–9.

[33] Ferguson SH, Foster DM, Sherry B, et al. Interferon-λ3 promotes epithelial defense and barrier function against cryptosporidium parvum infection. Cell Mol Gastroenterol Hepatol 2019;8:1–20.

[34] Brownlie R, Allan B. Avian toll-like receptors. Cell Tissue Res 2011. doi:10.1007/s00441-010-1026-0. Epub ahead of print.

[35] Chen X-M, O'Hara SP, Nelson JB, et al. Multiple TLRs Are Expressed in Human Cholangiocytes and Mediate Host Epithelial Defense Responses to Cryptosporidium parvum via Activation of NF-κB. J Immunol 2005. doi:10.4049/jimmunol.175.11.7447. Epub ahead of print.

[36] Tosh KW, Mittereder L, Bonne-Annee S, et al. The IL-12 Response of Primary Human Dendritic Cells and Monocytes to Toxoplasma gondii Is Stimulated by Phagocytosis of Live Parasites Rather Than Host Cell Invasion. J Immunol 2016. doi:10.4049/jimmunol.1501558. Epub ahead of print.

[37] Sasai M, Pradipta A, Yamamoto M. Host immune responses to Toxoplasma gondii. Int Immunol 2018;30:113–9.

[38] Goodswen SJ, Kennedy PJ, Ellis JT. Discovering a vaccine against neosporosis using computers: Is it feasible? Trends Parasitol 2014;30:401–11.

[39] Acevedo GR, Girard MC, Gómez KA. The unsolved jigsaw puzzle of the immune response in Chagas disease. Front Immunol 2018;9:1929.

[40] Lemieux MW, Sonzogni-Desautels K, Ndao M. Lessons learned from protective immune responses to optimize vaccines against cryptosporidiosis. Pathogens 2018;7:1–20.

[41] Zhao Y, Wilson D, Matthews S, et al. Rapid elimination of Toxoplasma gondii by gamma interferon-primed mouse macrophages is independent of CD40 signaling. Infect Immun 2007. doi:10.1128/IAI.00738-07. Epub ahead of print.

[42] Yamane I, Kitani H, Kokuho T, et al. The inhibitory effect of interferon gamma and tumor necrosis factor alpha on intracellular multiplication of neospora caninum in primary bovine brain cells. J Vet Med Sci 2000. doi:10.1292/jvms.62.347. Epub ahead of print.

[43] Hériveau C, Dimier-Poisson I, Lowenthal J, et al. Inhibition of Eimeria tenella replication after recombinant IFN-γ activation in chicken macrophages, fibroblasts and epithelial cells. Vet Parasitol 2000. doi:10.1016/S0304-4017(00)00275-2. Epub ahead of print.

[44] Gupta G, Oghumu S, Satoskar AR. Mechanisms of Immune Evasion in Leishmaniasis. Adv Appl Microbiol 2013. doi:10.1016/B978-0-12-407679-2.00005-3. Epub ahead of print 2013.

[45] Wolf AS, Sherratt S, Riley EM. NK cells: Uncertain allies against malaria. Front Immunol 2017. doi:10.3389/fimmu.2017.00212. Epub ahead of print.

[46] Arora G, Hart GT, Manzella-Lapeira J, et al. NK cells inhibit plasmodium falciparum growth in red blood cells via antibody-dependent cellular cytotoxicity. Elife 2018. doi:10.7554/eLife.36806. Epub ahead of print.

[47] Gigley JP. The diverse role of NK cells in Immunity to Toxoplasma gondii Infection. PLoS Pathog 2016. doi:10.1371/journal.ppat.1005396. Epub ahead of print.

[48] Ivanova DL, Denton SL, Fettel KD, et al. Innate lymphoid cells in protection, pathology, and adaptive immunity during apicomplexan infection. Front Immunol 2019;10:1–15.

[49] Klose CSN, Flach M, Möhle L, et al. Differentiation of type 1 ILCs from a common progenitor to all helper-like innate lymphoid cell lineages. Cell 2014. doi:10.1016/j.cell.2014.03.030. Epub ahead of print.

[50] Wagage S, Pritchard GH, Dawson L, et al. The group 3 innate lymphoid cell defect in aryl hydrocarbon receptor deficient mice is associated with T cell hyperactivation during intestinal infection. PLoS One 2015. doi:10.1371/journal.pone.0128335. Epub ahead of print.

[51] Florin-Christensen M, Schnittger L. *Parasitic protozoa of farm animals and pets*. 2018. Epub ahead of print 2018. doi:10.1007/978-3-319-70132-5.

[52] Potts ND, Bichet C, Merat L, et al. Development and optimization of a hybridization technique to type the classical class I and class II B genes of the chicken MHC. Immunogenetics 2019. doi:10.1007/s00251-019-01149-2. Epub ahead of print.

[53] Glass EJ, Oliver RA, Russell GC. Duplicated DQ Haplotypes Increase the Complexity of Restriction Element Usage in Cattle. J Immunol 2000. doi:10.4049/jimmunol.165.1.134. Epub ahead of print.

[54] Dupont CD, Christian DA, Selleck EM, et al. Parasite fate and involvement of infected cells in the induction of CD4+ and CD8+ T cell responses to Toxoplasma gondii. PLoS Pathog 2014. doi:10.1371/journal.ppat.1004047. Epub ahead of print.

[55] Goldszmid RS, Coppens I, Lev A, et al. Host ER-parasitophorous vacuole interaction provides a route of entry for antigen cross-presentation in Toxoplasma gondii- I nfected dendritic cells. J Exp Med 2009. doi:10.1084/jem.20082108. Epub ahead of print.

[56] Rommereim LM, Fox BA, Butler KL, et al. Rhoptry and dense granule secreted effectors regulate CD8+ T cell recognition of Toxoplasma gondii infected host cells. Front Immunol 2019. doi:10.3389/fimmu.2019.02104. Epub ahead of print.

[57] Sun Y, Huang T, Hammarström L, Zhao Y. The Immunoglobulins: new insights, implications, and applications. Annu Rev Anim Biosci. 2020;8:145–169. doi: 10.1146/annurev-animal-021419-083720. Epub 2019 Dec 17.

[58] Litman G, Rast J, SD F. The origins of vertebrate adaptive immunity. Alergol Immunol 2010;10:543–53.

[59] Goodswen SJ, Kennedy PJ, Ellis JT. A review of the infection, genetics, and evolution of Neospora caninum: from the past to the present. Infect Genet Evol 2013;13:133–50.

[60] Belachew EB. Immune response and evasion mechanisms of plasmodium falciparum parasites. J Immunol Res 2018. doi:10.1155/2018/6529681. Epub ahead of print 2018.

[61] Wyatt CR, Riggs MW, Fayer R. Cryptosporidiosis in Neonatal Calves. Vet Clin North Am—Food Anim Pract 2010;26:89–103.

[62] Petry F, Jakobi V, Tessema TS. Host immune response to Cryptosporidium parvum infection. Exp Parasitol 2010;126:304–9.

[63] Wyatt CR, Brackett EJ, Perryman LE, et al. Activation of intestinal intraepithelial T lymphocytes in calves infected with Cryptosporidium parvum. Infect Immun 1997;65:185–90.

[64] Abrahamsen M, Lancto C, Walcheck B, et al. Localization of a/b and g/d T Lymphocytes in Cryptosporidium parvum-infected tissues in naive and immune calves. Infect Immun 1997;65:2428–33.

[65] Zhao GH, Fang YQ, Ryan U, et al. Dynamics of Th17 associating cytokines in Cryptosporidium parvum-infected mice. Parasitol Res 2016. doi:10.1007/s00436-015-4831-2. Epub ahead of print.

[66] Gomes PS, Bhardwaj J, Rivera-Correa J, et al. Immune escape strategies of malaria parasites. Front Microbiol 2016. doi:10.3389/fmicb.2016.01617. Epub ahead of print.

[67] Locksley RM, Scott P. Helper T-cell subsets in mouse leishmaniasis: induction, expansion and effector function. Immunol Today 1991. doi:10.1016/S0167-5699(05)80017-9. Epub ahead of print.

[68] Boniface K, Bak-Jensen KS, Li Y, et al. Prostaglandin E2 regulates Th17 cell differentiation and function through cyclic AMP and EP2/EP4 receptor signaling. J Exp Med 2009. doi:10.1084/jem.20082293. Epub ahead of print.

[69] Rose ME, Hesketh P. Infection with Eimeria tenella: modulation of lymphocyte blastogenesis by specific antigen, and evidence for immunodepression. J Protozool 1984. doi:10.1111/j.1550-7408.1984.tb05500.x. Epub ahead of print.

[70] Lillehoj HS. Effects of immunosuppression on avian coccidiosis: Cyclosporin A but not hormonal bursectomy abrogates host protective immunity. Infect Immun 1987. doi:10.1128/iai.55.7.1616-1621.1987. Epub ahead of print.

[71] Isobe T, Lillehoj HS. Dexamethasone suppresses T cell-mediated immunity and enhances disease susceptibility to Eimeria mivati infection. Vet Immunol Immunopathol 1993. doi:10.1016/0165-2427(93)90073-D. Epub ahead of print.

[72] Kim WH, Chaudhari AA, Lillehoj HS. Involvement of T Cell Immunity in Avian Coccidiosis. Front Immunol 2019. doi:10.3389/fimmu.2019.02732. Epub ahead of print.

[73] Del Cacho E, Gallego M, Lillehoj HS, et al. IL-17A regulates Eimeria tenella schizont maturation and migration in avian coccidiosis. Vet Res 2014;45:1–9.

[74] van den Berg RA, Coccia M, Ballou WR, et al. Predicting RTS,S vaccine-mediated protection from transcriptomes in a malaria-challenge clinical trial. Front Immunol 2017;8:1–13.

[75] Tran TM, Bijker EM, Haks MC, et al. Whole-blood transcriptomic signatures induced during immunization by chloroquine prophylaxis and Plasmodium falciparum sporozoites. Sci Rep 2019. doi:10.1038/s41598-019-44924-7. Epub ahead of print.

[76] White MT, Bejon P, Olotu A, et al. The relationship between RTS,S vaccine-induced antibodies, CD4+ T cell responses and protection against plasmodium falciparum infection. PLoS One 2013. doi:10.1371/journal.pone.0061395. Epub ahead of print.

[77] Crompton PD, Moebius J, Portugal S, et al. Malaria immunity in man and mosquito: insights into unsolved mysteries of a deadly infectious disease. Annu Rev Immunol 2014. doi:10.1146/annurev-immunol-032713-120220. Epub ahead of print.

[78] Doolan DL, Hoffman SL. IL-12 and NK cells are required for antigen-specific adaptive immunity against malaria initiated by CD8+ T cells in the Plasmodium yoelii model. J Immunol 1999;163(2):884–892.

[79] Perryman LE, Kapil SJ, Jones ML, et al. Protection of calves against cryptosporidiosis with immune bovine colostrum induced by a Cryptosporidium parvum recombinant protein. Vaccine 1999;17:2142–9.

[80] Askari N, Shayan P, Mokhber-Dezfouli MR, et al. Evaluation of recombinant P23 protein as a vaccine for passive immunization of newborn calves against Cryptosporidium parvum. Parasite Immunol 2016;38:282–9.

[81] Wyatt CR, Lindahl S, Austin K, et al. Response of T lymphocytes from previously infected calves to recombinant Cryptosporidium parvum P23 vaccine antigen. J Parasitol 2005;91:1239–42.

[82] Testasicca MC de S, dos Santos MS, Machado LM, et al. Antibody responses induced by Leish-Tec®, an A2-based vaccine for visceral leishmaniasis, in a heterogeneous canine population. Vet Parasitol 2014;204:169–76.

[83] Christensen SM, Belew AT, El-Sayed NM, et al. Host and parasite responses in human diffuse cutaneous leishmaniasis caused by L. amazonensis. PLoS Negl Trop Dis 2018;13:1–23.

[84] Vermeulen AN. Progress in recombinant vaccine development against coccidiosis. A review and prospects into the next millennium. Int J Parasitol 1998. doi:10.1016/S0020-7519(98)00080-0. Epub ahead of print 1998.

[85] Zhang NZ, Chen J, Wang M, et al. Vaccines against Toxoplasma gondii: New developments and perspectives. Expert Rev Vaccines 2013. doi:10.1586/14760584.2013.844652. Epub ahead of print.

[86] Horcajo P, Regidor-Cerrillo J, Aguado-Martínez A, et al. Vaccines for bovine neosporosis: current status and key aspects for development. Parasite Immunol 2016. doi:10.1111/pim.12342. Epub ahead of print.

[87] Jiménez-Ruiz E, Álvarez-García G, Aguado-Martínez A, et al. Low efficacy of NcGRA7, NcSAG4, NcBSR4 and NcSRS9 formulated in poly-e{open}-caprolactone against Neospora caninum infection in mice. Vaccine 2012. doi:10.1016/j.vaccine.2012.05.033. Epub ahead of print.

[88] Sun X, Mei M, Zhang X, et al. The extracellular matrix protein mindin as a novel adjuvant elicits stronger immune responses for rBAG1, rSRS4 and rSRS9 antigens of Toxoplasma gondii in BALB/c mice. BMC Infect Dis 2014. doi:10.1186/1471-2334-14-429. Epub ahead of print.

[89] Blake DP, Pastor-Fernández I, Nolan MJ, et al. Recombinant anticoccidial vaccines—a cup half full? Infect Genet Evol 2017;55:358–65.

[90] Mead JR. Prospects for immunotherapy and vaccines against Cryptosporidium. Human Vaccines Immunotherapeutics 2014. doi:10.4161/hv.28485. Epub ahead of print.

[91] Flores DA, Rodriguez AE, Tomazic ML, et al. Characterization of GASA-1, a new vaccine candidate antigen of Babesia bovis. Vet Parasitol 2020;287. doi:10.1016/j.vetpar.2020.109275. Epub ahead of print.

[92] Uilenberg G. Immunization against diseases caused by Theileria parva: A review. Tropical Medicine and International Health 1999;4(9):12–20. doi:10.1046/j.1365-3156.1999.00446.x. Epub ahead of print.

[93] Boulter N, Hall R. Immunity and vaccine development in the bovine theilerioses. Adv Parasitol 1999. doi:10.1016/s0065-308x(08)60230-4. Epub ahead of print.

[94] Rathinasamy V, Poole WA, Bastos RG, et al. Babesiosis vaccines: lessons learned, challenges ahead, and future glimpses. Trends Parasitol 2019;35:622–35.

[95] Zutshi S, Kumar S, Chauhan P, et al. Anti-leishmanial vaccines: Assumptions, approaches, and annulments. Vaccines 2019. doi:10.3390/vaccines7040156. Epub ahead of print.

[96] Awate S, Babiuk LA, Mutwiri G. Mechanisms of action of adjuvants. Front Immunol 2013. doi:10.3389/fimmu.2013.00114. Epub ahead of print.

[97] El-Sayed NM, Myler PJ, Bartholomeu DC, et al. The genome sequence of Trypanosoma cruzi, etiologic agent of chagas disease. Science (80-) 2005. doi:10.1126/science.1112631. Epub ahead of print.

[98] Gardner MJ, Hall N, Fung E, et al. Genome sequence of the human malaria parasite Plasmodium falciparum. Nature 2002. doi:10.1038/nature01097. Epub ahead of print.

[99] Swann J, Jamshidi N, Lewis NE, et al. Systems analysis of host-parasite interactions. Wiley Interdiscip Rev Syst Biol Med 2015;7:381–400.

[100] Tomazic ML, Marugan-Hernandez V, Rodriguez AE. Next-Generation Technologies and Systems Biology for the Design of Novel Vaccines Against Apicomplexan Parasites. Front Vet Sci 2022;8(800361). doi:10.3389/fvets.2021.800361.

[101] Christensen SM, Dillon LAL, Carvalho LP, et al. Meta-transcriptome profiling of the human-leishmania braziliensis cutaneous lesion. PLoS Negl Trop Dis 2016;10:1–17.

[102] Bioinformatics Resource Center' (BRCs). https://veupathdb.org/veupathdb/app/. [Accessed 2022 Jan 13].

[103] Warrenfeltz S, Basenko EY, Crouch K, et al. EuPathDB: the Eukaryotic pathogen genomics database resource. Methods Mol Biol 2018;1757:69–113.

[104] PlasmoDB for Plasmodium spp. https://plasmodb.org/plasmo/app. [Accessed 2022 Jan 13].

[105] ToxoDB. https://toxodb.org/toxo/app/. [Accessed 2022 Jan 13].

[106] TriTrypDB. https://tritrypdb.org/tritrypdb/app. [Accessed 2022 Jan 13].

[107] CryptoDB. https://cryptodb.org/cryptodb/app/. [Accessed 2022 Jan 13].

[108] PiroplasmaDB. https://piroplasmadb.org/piro/app/. [Accessed 2022 Jan 13].

[109] VectorBase. https://vectorbase.org/vectorbase/app. [Accessed 2022 Jan 13].

[110] Malaria.tools. https://malaria.sbs.ntu.edu.sg. [Accessed 2022 Jan 13].
[111] Tan QW, Mutwil M. Malaria.tools-comparative genomic and transcriptomic database for Plasmodium species. Nucleic Acids Res 2020;48:D768–75.
[112] Almagro Armenteros JJ, Tsirigos KD, Sønderby CK, et al. SignalP 5.0 improves signal peptide predictions using deep neural networks. Nat Biotechnol 2019. doi:10.1038/s41587-019-0036-z Epub ahead of print.
[113] Frank K, Sippl MJ. High-performance signal peptide prediction based on sequence alignment techniques. Bioinformatics 2008. doi:10.1093/bioinformatics/btn422 Epub ahead of print.
[114] Krogh A, Larsson B, Von Heijne G, et al. Predicting transmembrane protein topology with a hidden Markov model: application to complete genomes. J Mol Biol 2001. doi:10.1006/jmbi.2000.4315 Epub ahead of print.
[115] Käll L, Krogh A, Sonnhammer ELL. A combined transmembrane topology and signal peptide prediction method. J Mol Biol 2004. doi:10.1016/j.jmb.2004.03.016 Epub ahead of print.
[116] Zhao L, Poschmann G, Waldera-Lupa D, et al. OutCyte: a novel tool for predicting unconventional protein secretion. Sci Rep 2019;9:19448.
[117] Gíslason MH, Nielsen H, Almagro Armenteros JJ, et al. Prediction of GPI-anchored proteins with pointer neural networks. Curr Res Biotechnol 2021. doi:10.1016/j.crbiot.2021.01.001 Epub ahead of print.
[118] Pierleoni A, Martelli PL, Casadio R. PredGPI: a GPI-anchor predictor. BMC Bioinformatics 2008;9:392.
[119] Jones P, Binns D, Chang H-Y, et al. InterProScan 5: genome-scale protein function classification. Bioinformatics 2014;30:1236–40.
[120] The gene ontology resource: enriching a GOld mine. Nucleic Acids Res 2021. doi:10.1093/nar/gkaa1113 Epub ahead of print.
[121] Ashburner M, Ball CA, Blake JA, et al. Gene ontology: tool for the unification of biology. The Gene Ontology Consortium. Nat Genet 2000;25(1):25–9. doi:10.1038/75556.
[122] Chen F, Mackey AJ, Stoeckert CJ, et al. OrthoMCL-DB: querying a comprehensive multi-species collection of ortholog groups. Nucleic Acids Res 2006;34:D363–8.
[123] ABCpred: *https://webs.iiitd.edu.in/raghava/abcpred/ABC_submission.html.*
[124] Saha S, Raghava GPS. Prediction of continuous B-cell epitopes in an antigen using recurrent neural network. Proteins 2006;65:40–8.
[125] BCEpred. https://webs.iiitd.edu.in/raghava/bcepred/bcepred_submission.htmle. [Accessed 2022 Jan 13].
[126] Saha S, Raghava GPS. BcePred: prediction of continuous B-cell epitopes in antigenic sequences using physico-chemical properties. Lect Notes Comput Sci (including Subser Lect Notes Artif Intell Lect Notes Bioinformatics) 2004. doi:10.1007/978-3-540-30220-9_16 Epub ahead of print.
[127] BEPIpred. http://www.cbs.dtu.dk/services/BepiPred/. [Accessed 2022 Jan 13].
[128] BEPro. http://pepito.proteomics.ics.uci.edu/. [Accessed 2022 Jan 13].
[129] NetMHCII pan 4.0. http://www.cbs.dtu.dk/services/NetMHCIIpan/. [Accessed 2022 Jan 13].
[130] NetMH pan 4.1. http://www.cbs.dtu.dk/services/NetMHCpan/abstract.php. [Accessed 2022 Jan 13].
[131] Reynisson B, Barra C, Kaabinejadian S, et al. Improved prediction of MHC II antigen presentation through integration and motif deconvolution of mass spectrometry MHC Eluted Ligand Data. J Proteome Res 2020. doi:10.1021/acs.jproteome.9b00874 Epub ahead of print.

[132] Reynisson B, Alvarez B, Paul S, et al. NetMHCpan-4.1 and NetMHCIIpan-4.0: improved predictions of MHC antigen presentation by concurrent motif deconvolution and integration of MS MHC eluted ligand data. Nucleic Acids Res 2020. doi:10.1093/nar/gkaa379 Epub ahead of print.

[133] Immune Epitope Database (IEDB, www.iedb.org/). [Accessed 2022 Jan 13].

[134] Vita R, Mahajan S, Overton JA, et al. The Immune Epitope Database (IEDB): 2018 update. Nucleic Acids Res 2019. doi:10.1093/nar/gky1006 Epub ahead of print.

[135] Rappuoli R. Reverse vaccinology. Curr Opin Microbiol 2000;3:445–50.

[136] Rappuoli R, Bottomley MJ, D'Oro U, et al. Reverse vaccinology 2.0: Human immunology instructs vaccine antigen design. J Exp Med 2016;213:469–81.

[137] Rodriguez AE, Florin-Christensen M, Flores DA, et al. The glycosylphosphatidylinositol-anchored protein repertoire of Babesia bovis and its significance for erythrocyte invasion. Ticks Tick Borne Dis 2014. doi:10.1016/j.ttbdis.2013.12.011 Epub ahead of print.

[138] Tomazic ML, Rodriguez AE, Lombardelli J, et al. Identification of novel vaccine candidates against cryptosporidiosis of neonatal bovines by reverse vaccinology. Vet Parasitol 2018;264:74–8.

[139] Manque PA, Tenjo F, Woehlbier U, et al. Identification and immunological characterization of three potential vaccinogens against Cryptosporidium species. Clin Vaccine Immunol 2011;18:1796–802.

[140] Rodríguez AE, Couto A, Echaide I, et al. Babesia bovis contains an abundant parasite-specific protein-free glycerophosphatidylinositol and the genes predicted for its assembly. Vet Parasitol 2010;167. doi:10.1016/j.vetpar.2009.09.024 Epub ahead of print.

[141] Zhu J, Krishnegowda G, Gowda DC. Induction of proinflammatory responses in macrophages by the glycosylphosphatidylinositols of Plasmodium falciparum: The requirement of extracellular signal-regulated kinase, p38, c-Jun N-terminal kinase and NF-κB pathways for the expression of proinflamm. J Biol Chem 2005. doi:10.1074/jbc.M413539200 Epub ahead of print.

[142] Oliveira A-C, Peixoto JR, de Arruda LB, et al. Expression of Functional TLR4 Confers Proinflammatory Responsiveness to Trypanosoma cruzi Glycoinositolphospholipids and Higher Resistance to Infection with T. cruzi. J Immunol 2004. doi:10.4049/jimmunol.173.9.5688 Epub ahead of print.

[143] Denkers EY. Toll-like receptor initiated host defense against toxoplasma gondii. J Biomed Biotechnol 2010. doi:10.1155/2010/737125 Epub ahead of print 2010.

[144] Hadj-Kaddour K, Carcy B, Vallet A, et al. Recombinant protein Bd37 protected gerbils against heterologous challenges with isolates of Babesia divergens polymorphic for the bd37 gene. Parasitology 2007. doi:10.1017/S0031182006001399 Epub ahead of print.

[145] Moubri K, Kleuskens J, Van de Crommert J, et al. Discovery of a recombinant Babesia canis supernatant antigen that protects dogs against virulent challenge infection. Vet Parasitol 2018. doi:10.1016/j.vetpar.2017.11.002 Epub ahead of print.

[146] Goodswen SJ, Kennedy PJ, Ellis JT. A gene-based positive selection detection approach to identify vaccine candidates using Toxoplasma gondii as a test case protozoan pathogen. Front Genet 2018;9:1–16.

[147] Acevedo GR, Juiz NA, Ziblat A, et al. Silico Guided Discovery of Novel Class I and II Trypanosoma cruzi Epitopes Recognized by T Cells from Chagas' Disease Patients. J Immunol 2020;204:1571–81.

[148] Judkowski V, Bunying A, Ge F, et al. GM-CSF production allows the identification of immunoprevalent antigens recognized by human CD4+ T cells following smallpox vaccination. PLoS One 2011;6. doi:10.1371/journal.pone.0024091 Epub ahead of print.

[149] GalaxyWeb. http://galaxy.seoklab.org/index.html. [Accessed 2022 Jan 13].
[150] Ko J, Park H, Heo L, et al. GalaxyWEB server for protein structure prediction and refinement. Nucleic Acids Res 2012;40:W294–7.
[151] Bryant JM, Baumgarten S, Glover L, et al. CRISPR in Parasitology: Not Exactly Cut and Dried!. Trends Parasitol 2019;35:409–22.
[152] Wagner JC, Platt RJ, Goldfless SJ, et al. Efficient CRISPR-Cas9-mediated genome editing in Plasmodium falciparum. Nat Methods 2014;11:915–8.
[153] Ghorbal M, Gorman M, MacPherson CR, et al. Genome editing in the human malaria parasite Plasmodium falciparum using the CRISPR-Cas9 system. Nat Biotechnol 2014;32:819–21.
[154] Zhang WW, Matlashewski G. CRISPR-Cas9-mediated genome editing in Leishmania donovani. MBio 2015;6:1–14.
[155] Zhang W-W, Lypaczewski P, Matlashewski G. Application of CRISPR/Cas9-Mediated Genome Editing in Leishmania. In: Michels PA, Ginger ML, Zilberstein D, editors. Trypanosomatids. Methods in Molecular Biology. New York, NY: Springer Protocols; 2020. pp. 199–225.
[156] Beneke T, Madden R, Makin L, et al. A CRISPR Cas9 high-throughput genome editing toolkit for kinetoplastids. R Soc Open Sci 2017. doi:10.1098/rsos.170095 Epub ahead of print.
[157] Lander N, Chiurillo MA, Docampo R. CRISPR/Cas9 Technology Applied to the Study of Proteins Involved in Calcium Signaling in Trypanosoma cruzi. Methods Mol Biol 2020;2116:177–97.
[158] Sateriale A, Pawlowic M, Vinayak S, et al. Genetic Manipulation of Cryptosporidium parvum with CRISPR/Cas9. In: Mead JR, Arrowood MJ (eds) *Cryptosporidium: Methods and Protocols*. New York, NY: Springer, pp. 219–228.
[159] Tavassoly I, Goldfarb J, Iyengar R. Systems biology primer: The basic methods and approaches. Essays Biochem 2018. doi:10.1042/EBC20180003 Epub ahead of print.
[160] Hagan T, Pulendran B. Will systems biology deliver its promise and contribute to the development of new or improved vaccines?: From data to understanding through systems biology. Cold Spring Harb Perspect Biol 2018;10. doi:10.1101/cshperspect.a028894 Epub ahead of print.
[161] Poland GA, Ovsyannikova IG, Kennedy RB, Haralambieva IH, Jacobson RM. Vaccinomics and a New Paradigm for the Development of Preventive Vaccines Against Viral Infections. OMICS 2011;15(9):625–36. doi:10.1089/omi.2011.0032 Epub 2011 Jul 6.
[162] Vahey MT, Wang Z, Kester KE, et al. Expression of genes associated with immunoproteasome processing of major histocompatibility complex peptides is indicative of protection with adjuvanted RTS,S malaria vaccine. J Infect Dis 2010. doi:10.1086/650310 Epub ahead of print.
[163] Soutter F, Werling D, Tomley FM, et al. Poultry Coccidiosis: Design and Interpretation of Vaccine Studies. Front Vet Sci 2020;7:1–12.
[164] Stanisic DI, McCarthy JS, Good MF. Controlled human malaria infection: Applications, advances, and challenges. Infect Immun 2018. doi:10.1128/IAI.00479-17 Epub ahead of print.
[165] Tran TM, Crompton PD. Decoding the complexities of human malaria through systems immunology. Immunol Rev 2020;293:144–62.
[166] Smith ML, Styczynski MP. Systems Biology-based Investigation of Host-Plasmodium Interactions. Trends Parasitol 2018;34(7):617–32. doi:10.1016/j.pt.2018.04.003.
[167] Kazmin D, Nakaya HI, Lee EK, et al. Systems analysis of protective immune responses to RTS,S malaria vaccination in humans. Proc Natl Acad Sci USA 2017. doi:10.1073/pnas.1621489114 Epub ahead of print.

[168] Ojha R, Pandey RK, Prajapati VK. Vaccinomics strategy to concoct a promising subunit vaccine for visceral leishmaniasis targeting sandfly and leishmania antigens. Int J Biol Macromol 2020. doi:10.1016/j.ijbiomac.2020.04.097 Epub ahead of print.

[169] Madlala T, Adeleke VT, Fatoba AJ, Okpeku M, Adeniyi AA, Adeleke MA. Designing multiepitope-based vaccine against Eimeria from immune mapped protein 1 (IMP-1) antigen using immunoinformatic approach. Sci Rep 2021;11(1):18295. doi:10.1038/s41598-021-97880-6.

[170] Ockenhouse CF, Hu WC, Kester KE, et al. Common and divergent immune response signaling pathways discovered in peripheral blood mononuclear cell gene expression patterns in presymptomatic and clinically apparent malaria. Infect Immun 2006. doi:10.1128/IAI.00408-06 Epub ahead of print.

[171] Colborn JM, Ylöstalo JH, Koita OA, et al. Human Gene Expression in Uncomplicated *Plasmodium falciparum* Malaria. J Immunol Res 2015;2015:162639.

[172] Yamagishi J, Natori A, Tolba MEM, et al. Interactive transcriptome analysis of malaria patients and infecting Plasmodium falciparum. Genome Res 2014;24:1433–44.

[173] Videvall E, Cornwallis CK, Palinauskas V, et al. The Avian Transcriptome Response to Malaria Infection. Mol Biol Evol 2015;32:1255–67.

[174] Pittman KJ, Aliota MT, Knoll LJ. Dual transcriptional profiling of mice and Toxoplasma gondii during acute and chronic infection. BMC Genomics 2014;15:1–19.

[175] Hou Z, Liu D, Su S, et al. Comparison of splenocyte microRNA expression profiles of pigs during acute and chronic toxoplasmosis. BMC Genomics 2019;20:97.

[176] Jorge S, Dellagostin OA. The development of veterinary vaccines: a review of traditional methods and modern biotechnology approaches. Biotechnol Res Innov 2017;1:6–13.

[177] Papalexi E, Satija R. Single-cell RNA sequencing to explore immune cell heterogeneity. Nat Rev Immunol 2018. doi:10.1038/nri.2017.76 Epub ahead of print.

[178] Dantas-Torres F, Miró G, Baneth G, et al. Canine leishmaniasis control in the context of one health. Emerg Infect Dis 2019. doi:10.3201/eid2512.190164 Epub ahead of print.

Chapter 14

Cancer vaccine's multiverse and the future ahead

Víctor Chavarria[a], Rubén Figueroa[a], Aleli Salazar[a], Verónica Pérez de la Cruz[b], Benjamín Pineda[a]

[a]*Neuroimmunology and Neuro-Oncology Unit, Instituto Nacional de Neurología y Neurocirugía (INNN), Mexico City, Mexico,* [b]*Neurobiochemistry and Behaviour Laboratory, Instituto Nacional de Neurología y Neurocirugía (INNN), Mexico City, Mexico*

14.1 Introduction

Cancer is considered one of the most harmful chronic diseases and a major public health problem; almost two million new cancer cases were reported in 2020, causing 600,000 cancer-related deaths in the United States [1]. Although in the last years, the treatment has become quite successful, even with the use of chemo and radiotherapy, the survival after the diagnosis remains dismal.

The failure of this modality of treatment has forced the search of new alternatives to deal with this disease, to increase both, quality life and survival. Currently, there are very promising therapeutics that could be used either as an adjuvant therapy altogether in the current first line treatment or as a monotherapy. In this sense, vaccines could be considered as a new therapeutic tool with the potential to increase the survival rate of cancer patients, awakening the immune system by supporting and directing the immune response to attack tumor cells (TCs).

14.2 Cancer vaccines

The earliest literature recording the use of foreign material inoculation to induce protection dates from the mid-16th century, where the Indians and Chinese describe a method called variolation, which was able to provide some protection against smallpox. Variolation consisted of either inoculation of smallpox scab material into a lesion inflicted on the skin of a healthy person, or inhalation of such material. Although effective, this technique had a high mortality rate among inoculated individuals [2].

The term "vaccine" comes from the Latin word "*vacca*" or cow, an allusion to the first man-made vaccine. It was in 1796 when Edward Jenner, an English

System Vaccinology. https://doi.org/10.1016/B978-0-323-85941-7.00010-3

physician, provided the basis for vaccination. He extracted the pustule liquid of a milkmaid infected with cowpox to inoculate an 8-year-old-boy with this fluid. Later, when the boy was exposed to smallpox, he did not develop the disease. This procedure resulted to be less dangerous and just as effective as variolation [3,4]. It was not until 1881 that, thanks to Louis Pasteur's observations, the deliberate effort to generate immunity through the inoculation of microorganisms processed by the principles of attenuation and inactivation began, paving the way for the production of standardized vaccines [5]. Currently, vaccines have been used as a prophylactic treatment in several diseases, decreasing the rates of measles [6], poliomyelitis [7], diphtheria [8] and even, eradicating diseases, such as the smallpox [9].

The seminal concept of vaccine, which involved the ability to prevent infectious diseases through the generation of a new specific immune response in naïve patients, has been shaped over time. The current concept involves the modeling of the immune system to build response phenotypes for each type of antigen allowing a therapeutic approach and offering the possibility of improving the response to infections, autoimmune diseases, autoinflammatory diseases, and cancer [10].

Due to the wild success of vaccines in infectious diseases, the idea of finding a vaccine against cancer sounded plausible. The idea arose due to the findings made by Coley in 1890. Coley observed that advanced cancer patients presented a spontaneous tumor regression after being treated with the now known "Coley's toxin" an admixture of heat-killed S. pyogenes and Serratia marcescens. Later, it was clear that the combination of Gram-positive and Gram-negative bacteria induced a strong innate immune response, leading to tumor regression [11,12]; however, these findings were flashed by the novel use of the radiotherapy, which showed a better response for the treatment of cancer.

Nowadays, Coley's principle has been the baseline of immunotherapy, and particularly, the bedrock of cancer vaccines, which main goal is to stimulate and direct the immune system to recognize and induce cytotoxicity against cancer cells [13]. Additionally, cancer vaccines can also be used to reduce the growth of advanced tumors or to inhibit tumors that are refractory to the conventional cancer treatment [14].

However, most clinical trials focused on the therapeutic activity of cancer vaccines have shown dismal results, having mild efficacy at best. Among the reasons why tumor vaccination has not been successful is the development of immune tolerance since most of these vaccines used autoantigens that are normally expressed in cells and tissues of the body; but also, the tumor-driven immunosuppressive and tolerogenic microenvironment contributes to an ineffective antitumor response.

The new research approaches are directed to the use of mutated self-antigens (neoantigens), which are molecules predominantly expressed by virus-infected cells and tumoral cells, thus not induced immune tolerance and could allow the development of an enhanced and effective targeted inflammatory response [15].

14.3 Targeted antigens

Initially, vaccines were defined by their use as preventive measures, now a shift is taking place in the field of vaccine development, as vaccines have also acquired a therapeutic focus aimed at the integrated management of diseases involving the immune response, becoming a new reality and a tool of great interest.

During the vaccine development process, one of the first steps to consider is the target antigen of interest against which the immune response will be directed. An antigen is defined as any substance that is able to elicit a specific immune response. Classically, there are several factors that determine the ability of an antigen to initiate the immune response; factors such as size and foreignness of the molecule, heterogeneity of chemical composition, and susceptibility to antigenic processing and presentation have been highlighted [16].

However, the changing nature of TCs during carcinogenesis caused by their high mutation rate due to genomic instability and by their ability to adaptively modify their functions, leads to continuous changes in the antigens presented by TCs, making it very difficult to identify a specific antigen that could be exploited for therapeutic purposes [15,17].

In this regard, tumoral antigens can be classified into three groups, depending on their origin and differential expression:

a. Tumor associated antigens (TAA): defined as antigens that can be found in both healthy and tumoral tissues. This type of antigens could be generated during any stage of protein synthesis, from gene transcription to protein degradation, through mRNA translation and post-translational modifications. However, these steps are carried out aberrantly, so that the expressed proteins may exhibit or hide epitopes involved in their recognition [18].

The National Cancer Institute proposed the classification of the 75 most representative TAA used in the development of cancer vaccines, with the purpose of emphasizing the ideal antigens most likely to have therapeutic efficacy (Fig. 14.1). This classification is based on TAA's reported therapeutic function, immunogenicity, role of the antigen in oncogenicity, specificity, level of expression and percentage of positive cells, expression in stem cells, number of patients with antigen-positive tumor, number of epitopes, and cellular localization. Although none of the evaluated antigens met all the criteria for ideal antigen, it was possible to identify some TAAs with therapeutic potential, including antigens as Wilms' Tumor 1 Protein (WT1), mucin 1 (MUC1), Human Papillomavirus E6/E7 (HPV E6/E7), Epidermal growth factor receptor variant III (EGFRvIII), Human Epidermal Growth Factor Receptor-2 (HER2/neu), Melanoma-Associated Antigen A3 (MAGE-A3), non-mutant Tumour Protein 53 (p53), Carcinoembryonic Antigen (CEA), Melanoma Antigen Recognized by T cells 1 (MART1), mutant RAS, glycoprotein 100 (gp100), survivin, prostate-specific antigen (PSA), Human Telomerase Reverse Transcriptase (hTERT), and prostatic acid phosphatase

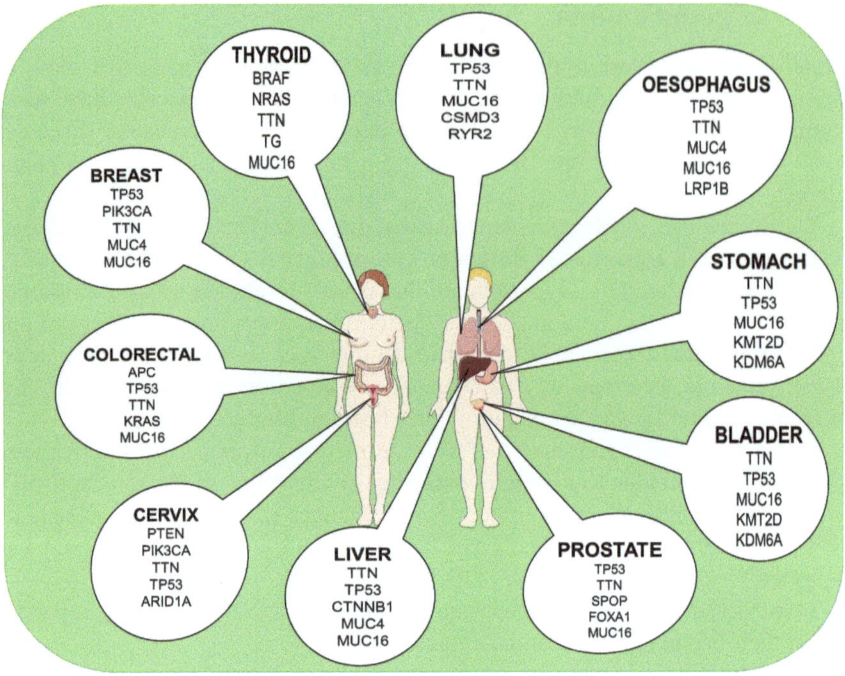

FIG. 14.1 TAAs expressed in different types of Cancer. Illustration shows the main TAAs expressed in the 10 most common types of Cancer according to National Cancer Institute (USA, 2021).

(PAP) [15]. At the same time, these TAAs can be subclassified into overexpressed antigens, differentiation antigens, and germline antigens.

Overexpressed antigens are the most common antigens associated with tumors, leading to their use in the development of the first wave of modern cancer vaccines [19]. These proteins are aberrantly expressed at higher levels within tumoral cells when compared to normal cells and tissues of the body, they are generally characterized by low immunogenicity, since there is a low number of T lymphocytes able to recognize these antigens due to negative selection in the thymus [20]. Thus, overexpressed antigens are capable of inducing an antitumor immune response only if their expression level is high enough to reach the recognition threshold of T lymphocytes to overcome immune tolerance [21]. However, the major disadvantage in the use of TAAs as an anticancer target is the potential induction of autoimmunity against normal tissues that also express them [22]. Overexpressed antigens that had been tested in vaccine development are MUC-1, CEA, HER2, p53, hTERC, survivin, among others. While overexpressed antigens have been widely used as therapeutic targets in the development of anticancer vaccines, lack of specificity still poses an obstacle to overcome.

Differentiation antigens are a class of TAAs derived from proteins that are expressed selectively according to the differentiation stage of the tissues, showing a highly restricted distribution, especially for the tumor, and the normal tissue of origin. This feature of TAAs allows for avoidance to a greater extent of the nonspecific effects of targeted therapy that do occur with overexpressed antigens. As these antigens are normally expressed by the tissue of origin and are subject to thymic expression for T lymphocyte selection, they could be considered as antigens with low immunogenicity [23]. The differentiation antigens that have been tested in clinical trials are mesothelin, gp100, PAP, PSA, and MART1.

Nevertheless, an FDA-approved vaccine, Sipuleucel-T, consists of PAP-loaded dendritic cells fused with the granulocyte-macrophage colony stimulating factor (GM-CSF) to overcome tolerance, has been developed for the treatment of minimally symptomatic/asymptomatic patients with metastatic castrate-resistant prostate cancer [24].

Germline Antigens are proteins whose expression is restricted to testicular and placental tissue as well as tumors with different histologic origin, lacking expression by somatic cells [25]. The most representative characteristic of germline antigens is that they are antigens expressed in tissues that have been considered as "immunoprivileged." It should be noted that germline antigens are also expressed in the thymus during the maturation process of T lymphocytes, however, current evidence points to the lack of tolerance development against these antigens; therefore, their immunogenic capacity could be exploited in favor of immunotherapy.

Some of the most studied antigens currently under investigation are MAGE-A3 for the management of melanoma and New York Esophageal Squamous Cell Carcinoma 1 (NY-ESO-1), with about 50 clinical studies focused on this last antigen.

Germline antigens are often associated with critical roles in tumor progression [25] and they could be used as cancer diagnostic biomarkers [26]. Interestingly, the expression of germline antigens may occur predominantly on carcinogenic stem cells, which have been linked to chemotherapeutic resistance and recurrence in some solid tumors. Because of their involvement in carcinogenesis and their important role in the performance of various cellular functions, the focus of immunotherapy has been redirected in a promising way toward the creation of vaccines against carcinogenic stem cells [27].

b. Neoantigens: also called tumor-specific antigens, neoantigens are proteins characterized by an expression restricted to tumoral cells. The emergence of neoantigens is closely related to the mutational burden and genomic instability of TCs; these alterations include non-synonymous somatic mutations, insertions, deletions, frameshift mutations, single nucleotide variations, and fusion genes, which allow the de novo synthesis of proteins exclusively expressed by TCs carrying such a mutation [28].

Importantly, neoantigens represent novel proteins that have not generated prior immunological tolerance and therefore have great immunogenic potential [29] in relation to their presentation on Major Histocompatibility Complex (MHC) class-I molecules and their increased binding affinity to T lymphocyte receptors (TCR), having thus demonstrated efficacy in eliciting T lymphocyte-dependent antitumor response [30].

During the development of personalized cancer vaccines in the context of neoantigens, the application of bioinformatics analysis has allowed the prediction of immunogenicity, processing, and expression in MHC class-I molecules as well as recognition by TCR, improving the ability to identify and prioritize neoantigens. However, findings from clinical studies with neoantigens still pose a challenge in clinical translation [31].

The greatest limitation involved in neoantigen-dependent vaccines is that they are strictly individual, i.e., TCs from one individual are likely to have a different mutational burden than those from another individual with the same type of cancer; and their identification depends on sequencing analyses that are difficult to apply on a large scale. Likewise, the same mutational rate of TCs could alter the expression of these neoantigens in an individual with whom they were previously identified [32].

c. Oncogenic viral antigens: about 15% of the worldwide incidence of cancer has been linked to viral infection, with specific mechanisms of carcinogenesis for each type of virus. Oncogenic viral antigens are a set of proteins and peptides of viral origin expressed by infected cells, tumoral or not [33].

To date, several viruses with carcinogenic potential have been identified, such as the human papillomavirus (HPV) and its relationship with cervical, vulvar, anal, penile, oropharyngeal carcinoma, among others; alongside the related E6 and E7 oncoproteins [34]. A relationship has also been found between hepatitis B/C virus (HBV/HCV) with hepatocellular carcinoma, the human T-lymphotropic virus-1 (HTLV-1) with T-cell lymphoblastic leukemia, the human herpesvirus 8 (HHV-8) with Kaposi's sarcoma, and the Epstein-Barr virus (EVB) mainly with lymphoma [35,36].

Despite the contagious spread of oncogenic viruses, the identification of oncogenic viral antigens has led to the development of preventive cancer vaccines being one of the greatest advances in modern public health. Due to the high immunogenicity of viral elements and the expression of conserved viral peptides among individuals, it has been possible to generate highly effective vaccines for cancer prevention [37].

The therapeutic efficacy of a vaccine, in addition to the proper selection of the antigen, depends to a large extent on the delivery method and the use of adjuvants that enhance the immune response.

14.4 Delivery platforms

The intensity of the immune response triggered by immunization is largely determined by the antigen integrity when it is administrated, so multiple platforms have been developed to deliver antigens that retain their integrity [38].

These platform technologies are based on the construction or coupling of antigens with the aim to generate the best possible immune response. To date, multiple types of platforms have been developed, including those based on peptides/proteins, nucleic acids, whole TCs, dendritic cells, viral vectors, extracellular vesicles, and nanoparticles (Fig. 14.2) [39].

a. Protein/peptide-based vaccine: This cancer vaccine platform relies on protein fragments or whole proteins as a source of antigens present in TCs [14].

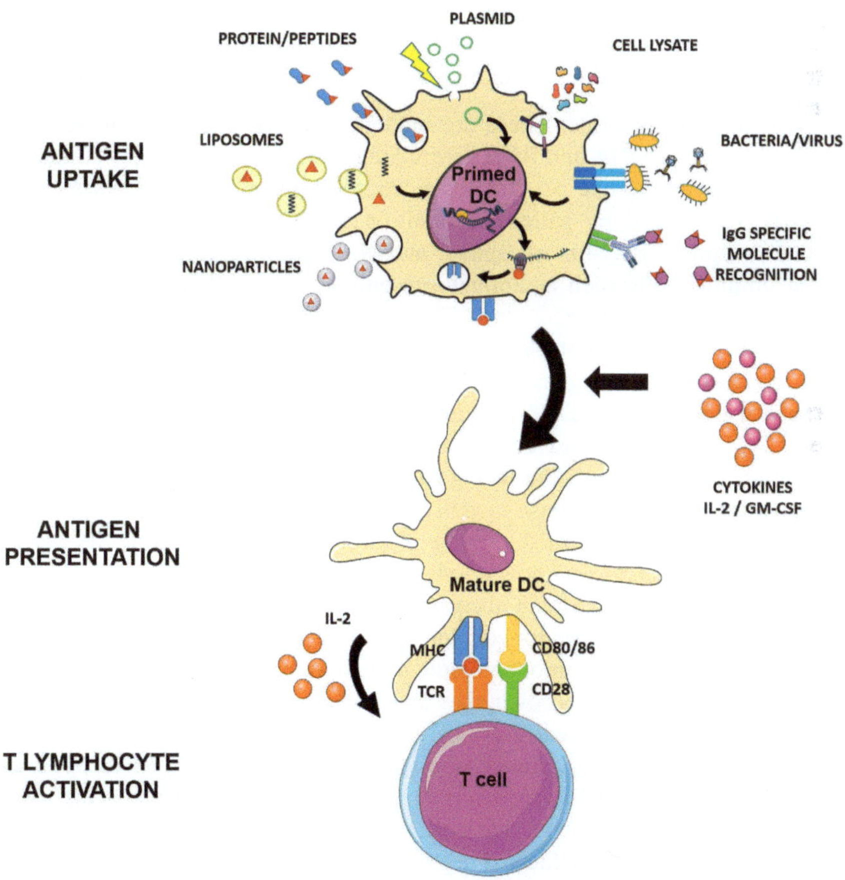

FIG. 14.2 Antigen platforms and adjuvants. The combination of the different antigen platforms and adjuvants available to date enable to shape the intensity and type of immune response.

Peptide-based vaccines are based on protein subunits, which show ease of *de novo* design and synthesis, biocompatibility, and degradability; peptides are useful in the selection and use of specific antigenic sequences [40], which can be a TAA, a neoantigen, or an oncogenic virus antigen. Peptide vaccines are usually obtained by chemical synthesis, which is cost-effective and rapid [41]. Peptides with low binding affinity to MHC molecules are less immunogenic and the immune response is usually transient or ineffective. Although it is possible to synthesize them on a large scale and direct the response to highly specific epitopes. Peptide vaccines immunogenic threshold is usually not reached unless coupled to an adjuvant substance [42,43].

Protein-based vaccines are selected proteins that are expressed by TCs, which retain their three-dimensional structure and are thus able to induce a cellular and humoral immune response [44]. These proteins offer exposure to a greater number of epitopes, providing a polyclonal activation of the immune response, with a higher probability of being a successful immunization. This formulation with multiple epitopes has allowed overcoming the problems related to the loss or modification of tumor antigens [45].

b. Genetic-based vaccine: These are nucleic acid-dependent vaccines, comprising mainly DNA and RNA formulations, which are relatively simple to synthesize, but unlike peptide-dependent vaccines, nucleic acids are prone to be recognized by pattern recognition receptors (PRRs) such as Toll-like receptors, RIG-like receptors, and Nod-like receptors present mainly on immune cells such as antigen-presenting cells (APCs), enhancing the inflammatory response.

The basis of gene-based vaccines is the induction of the synthesis of tumor-associated antigens or tumor-specific antigens in the host cells. The most widely used are DNA plasmids and messenger RNA.

DNA-based vaccines emerged in the 1990s, early reports termed this platform as "gene guns," inducing an effective cellular and humoral immune response in in vivo disease models. The methods surrounding DNA-based vaccines have been refined over the past few decades to become the cancer vaccine platform as we know it today [46].

The DNA plasmid method consists of the transfection of host cells with a plasmid expression vector coupled with a target genetic sequence, specific for the synthesis of a tumor antigenic protein, or a sequence characterized as an epitope [47]. On their own, they are immunogenic due to the presence of unmethylated CpG repeat sites [48].

RNA-based vaccines started when the messenger RNA (mRNA) application in vivo was initially carried out by Wolff and colleagues, proving to be effective in inducing protein-antigen synthesis as DNA plasmid-based constructs [49]. Few years later, it began to be explored as a therapeutic device in cancer, effectively inducing protective immunity in melanoma models [50]. One of the main advantages over DNA plasmids is that transfection of host cells is carried out more efficiently and does not require passage into the nucleus to induce synthesis of the antigens encoded by the administered sequence [51].

Recently, the therapeutic potential of mRNA vaccines has been brought to public attention by the high efficiency of mRNA SARS-CoV-2 vaccines [52]. Notably, the mRNA platforms have shown tangible goals, especially when used in combination with immune checkpoint inhibitors.

Both DNA-based and RNA-based platforms require that the delivery method retains its stability and guarantees its entry into the host cells. These methods include the use of gene guns, microneedle injection, cell membrane electroporation, liposomes, intracellular delivery nanoparticles, and direct delivery to autologous dendritic cells [53,54].

c. Dendritic cell-based vaccine: Dendritic cells (DC) are considered as a natural platform and adjuvant; thus, they have become a major target in the development of cancer vaccines. DC mechanistic is based on the intrinsic ability to capture, process and present antigens by coupling them to the MHC molecules on their surface, with the capacity to elicit the T lymphocyte-dependent immune response, thus generating a specialized vehicle for antigenic presentation [55]. The potential of DCs to initiate a protective antitumor immune response derives from the interaction with specific T lymphocytes and their activation with costimulatory molecules.

DC vaccination consists of the extraction and isolation of autologous DCs, pulsed with tumor antigens, and matured with the co-administration of immunostimulatory adjuvants such as cytokines and PRR ligands and revaccination of DC to the patient [56].

Despite the pivotal role played by DCs in the development of the antitumor immune response, most of the results obtained from clinical studies are still unfavorable, which is why the use of combination therapy with immune checkpoint inhibitors has been implemented, finding more encouraging results [57,58]. The development of DC vaccines still needs to be standardized and evaluated on a larger scale, allowing to discern between patterns of immune response and individual variations among each cancer patient [59].

d. TC-based vaccine: They derive from the use of whole TCs from the autologous or allogeneic origin, as a source of multiple antigens, resulting in polyclonal activation of the immune response [60].

Autologous TCs are derived from the primary culture of surgically resected TCs from each patient. This type of platform offers the use of cells with the same genetic background and mutational burden as the cells of origin, so there will be a theoretical matching of antigens expressed by remaining TCs. The use of autologous cells is considered to be an individualized therapy, so their development is expensive and difficult to perform on a large scale [61,62].

Allogeneic TCs are derived from established human cell lines with defined mutation and gene expression patterns, making it straightforward to identify associated antigens and tumor-specific antigens. Availability and ease of production make them desirable platforms in the construction of cancer vaccines [63].

TC-based vaccines can also be classified depending on the presentation or fragment obtained, dividing them into apoptotic cells, cell lysates, and extracellular microvesicles [60].

Apoptotic cells are obtained from ultraviolet irradiation of TCs. Apoptotic bodies generated during the progression of apoptosis express phosphatidylserine (PS) on the outer membrane surface, which allows recognition by PS receptors on DCs, enhancing their phagocytosis for the retrieval and processing of tumor antigens [64–66]. A major drawback arises from the anti-inflammatory nature of apoptosis, although it increases phagocytosis of apoptotic bodies and antigen processing, it also stimulates the secretion of IL-10 and TGF-β from APCs, cytokines known to be potent regulators of the inflammatory response [67].

Cell lysates are obtained from cell stress caused by freeze/thaw cycles, repeated irradiation, and heating. Based on obtaining a mixture of cell fragments and components resulting from necrosis, with the exposure of damage-associated molecular patterns (DAMP's), which are associated with the initiation of an inflammatory response and DC maturation [68]. Whole TC lysates can be administered without the need of a carrier; however, they can be associated with immunostimulatory adjuvants in order to induce effective and long-lasting immune responses [60].

Extracellular microvesicles are rounded organelles, with diameters ranging from 50 to 1000 nm, enclosed by a phospholipid bilayer, including exosomes. Extracellular microvesicles are actively secreted through exocytosis, both under normal and pathological conditions. Despite being an outstanding source of tumor antigens, the biological activity of microvesicles has been related to immune evasion by inducing suppressor phenotypes in myeloid cells and inducing apoptosis of T lymphocytes [69–71]. In contrast, the immunogenicity of microvesicles can be enhanced by exposing TCs to stressful stimuli, such as heat shock and even radiation, generating an effective antitumor immune response [72,73]. Although the use of microvesicles has great potential in immunotherapy, it requires an optimization process to overcome their immunosuppressive properties.

Unfortunately, these platforms are unstable and, at times, unpredictable; findings show that antigenic uptake by DCs may be low and cross-presentation of tumor antigens is insufficient to produce a sustained antitumor response.

e. Microorganism-based vaccine: This type of vaccine platform takes advantage of the intrinsic immunogenicity of microorganisms to elicit an inflammatory response through stimulation of various PRR's on immune cells. The two main variants used in the development of cancer vaccines are virus-based vaccines and bacterial-based vaccines.

Virus-based vaccines use genetic engineering techniques to modify viruses so that they lose their infectivity but express one or more target tumor antigens acting as a vector. The high immunogenicity of this type of platform generates a neutralizing immune response to the viral particles, which hinders the administration of repeated doses of the same vector. In addition, there is a risk of obtaining a suboptimal immunization due to the induction of the large number of viral particles elimination before an effective response against the tumor antigen has been triggered [74,75]. These challenges can be overcome as long as an adequate immunization regimen is established, considering heterologous immunization, with different viral vectors at each step of vaccination, as recently applied in the formulation of a vaccine against COVID-19 [76]. The most commonly exploited viruses as a vaccine platform are adenoviruses, along with alphaviruses and poxviruses [77].

Bacterial-based vaccines employ the high immunogenicity of attenuated bacteria to polarize the immune response toward an inflammatory phenotype and induce the synthesis of TNF-α, IFN-γ, IL-12, and other inflammatory mediators associated with a better antitumor response. Bacteria can also be transfected to express tumor antigens. Vaccines with live attenuated bacteria are currently being developed with application in cancer, including Salmonella, Listeria monocytogenes, and Lactococcus lactis strains [78]. The main advantages associated with their use derive from their high immunogenicity, low production cost, biosafety, and easy management of infectious complications [79].

f. Nanoparticle-based vaccine: Recently, research has been directed to the use of nanoscale elements (<1 μm) as delivery platforms with potential adjuvant effect. The use of nanoparticles is related to the maintenance of antigenic structural stability and controlled antigen release, thus maintaining constant and prolonged exposure to the immune system. The uptake of nanoparticle vaccines by APCs depends on factors such as size, shape, and composition, which are related to the nanoparticle ability to diffuse across the membrane, to be endocytosed and phagocytosed leads to specific antigen processing, thus enhancing the T-lymphocyte-dependent response. Among these are liposomes, inorganic nanoparticles, and organic nanopolymers [38,80].

These platforms can be combined with each other to enhance and direct the immune response against the tumor antigens of interest. In addition, their intrinsic conformation allows them to function as both platform and adjuvant.

14.5 Adjuvants

While the identification of tumor antigens has allowed the development of cancer vaccines, most formulations have low immunogenicity, which is reflected as poor clinical efficiency. This challenge can be faced through the selection and coupling of the vaccine to the ideal adjuvant that extends the antigen availability and potentiates the associated immune response, with the aim of generating a protective antitumor immunity [81]. A great advantage is that several of the platforms used in the development of vaccines have adjuvant activity that depends on their conformation and origin, regulating the release of the antigen and promoting immune activation, which can be aimed at obtaining the ideal response [82]. The action mechanism of adjuvants varies in relation to their nature, but in general, they are understood to play an important synergistic role in the initiation and maintenance of the immune response [83].

Classification according to their main function allows us to identify adjuvants as immunostimulatory molecules and depot delivery systems, although they may possess both characteristics (Fig. 14.2).

a. Immunostimulatory molecules: They are one of the most promising tools as an antitumor response enhancer. Their use should be strictly followed since they have the capacity to shape the immune response, producing local inflammation, activation of dendritic cells, synthesis of cytokines, and development of an adaptive response by T lymphocytes [84].

However, it should be considered that an inadequate formulation of immunostimulants is related to sequestration, anergy, and elimination of T lymphocytes, completely limiting the generation of an effective immune response [85].

Cytokines are the effector molecules par excellence of the immune response. They act through the activation of intracellular signaling cascades that determine the functional phenotype of the cells of the organism, with the potential to develop cellular and humoral immunity [86]. The most commonly used cytokine is GM-CSF, widely demanded in the development of vaccines in the clinical phase due to the biological effects attributed to this cytokine, involved in haematopoiesis, inflammatory response, maturation of myeloid cells, and induction of cellular immunity [87].

Toll-like receptor ligands are adjuvants whose molecular structure is recognized through PRRs. These ligands have the ability to activate cells on contact, promoting the synthesis, and secretion of proinflammatory cytokines and chemokines, the recruitment and activation of new immune cells, and the increased expression of costimulatory molecules on APCs necessary to establish a T-lymphocyte immune response [88]. To date, the only FDA-approved TLR-ligands for cancer vaccines are Bacillus Calmette-Guerin (TLR2/TLR4 ligand), monophosphoryl lipid A (TLR4 ligand), and imiquimod (TLR7 ligand). However, there are other ligands under study that have demonstrated efficacy in inducing an antitumor immune response, among them poly-I:C (TLR3 ligand), flagellin (TLR5 ligand), and CpG oligodeoxynucleotide (TLR9 ligand) [89].

Saponins are chemical compounds with great immunological activation capacity, initially originated from the extraction of the bark of the *Quillaja saponaria* tree. The most representative adjuvant agent is QS-21, the combination of two isomeric saponins whose activity stimulates a balanced Th1/Th2 response and adequate generation of specific cytotoxic T lymphocytes [90]. Several action mechanisms attributed to the saponins have been proposed, including NLRP3 inflammasome activation and caspase-1-dependent IL-1β production [91], and the costimulatory function by direct binding to the amino-terminal region of the TCR [92]; however, the mechanism of action involved in the immunogenicity generated by the saponins is still unknown.

Stimulator of interferon genes agonists are molecules designed to bind and stimulate STING, endoplasmic reticulum-coupled proteins, highly responsive to cytoplasmic DNA-cGAS signaling, whose activity culminates in the activation of the type I interferon response [93]. The purpose of this adjuvant is the differentiation of myeloid cells into dendritic cells more suitable for initiating a cellular immune response. The downside of the use of STING agonists is that they are able of inducing lymphocyte apoptosis if doses are inadequate, so their delivery should ideally be directed to cells of myeloid lineage [94].

Biomolecules-based targeting is a set of techniques based on the synthesis of fusion proteins, where one fragment corresponds to a conformational antigen classically recognized by its own IgG, and the other fragment is a tumor-associated antigen or tumor-specific antigen. They rely on the generation of immune-complexes with IgG, whose Fc fragment will subsequently be recognized by the Fc gamma receptor (FcγR) expressed by APCs, acting as an immunostimulant by facilitating antigenic uptake. There is only a few research using this approach, and most have focused on an antigenic fragment of tetanus toxoid and its coupling to tumor antigens. The main challenge is the high cost of production of these therapies, which is even higher when using antibodies [95–97].

b. Depot-delivery systems: Depot adjuvants mainly act by stabilization of antigens, protection against degradation, and enhancing their uptake and processing by dendritic cells.

Mineral salts are characterized by enabling a depot effect and a slow antigen release, with low production cost and low toxicity. The most common mineral salt used in human vaccines is Alum [98]. Alum agents essentially result in a sustained Th2-lymphocyte response eliciting antibody production, but generally fail to mount a strong Th1 and cytotoxic response, so an effective antitumor activity is not completely achieved [99,100]. By modifying the presentation of aluminum toward the generation of nanoparticles, it has been possible to increase the antigen loading and delivery capacity and enhance the response of dendritic cells [101,102].

Emulsions are commonly based in water-in-oil or oil-in-water formulation and act by the controlled delivery of antigens in the injection site. Complete Freund's adjuvant was the first-in-class emulsion to be developed in 1930, although its use in humans is not allowed due to the intense inflammatory reaction generates by having heat-killed mycobacteria. On the other hand, incomplete Freund's adjuvant, water-in-oil only, has proven to induce a sufficient cellular and humoral response; for human usage, a water-in-oil emulsion named Montanide ISA-51 was developed and widely used in vaccine development and research at present [103].

Liposomes are lipid bilayer constructs that encapsulate an aqueous core. In 1974, Gregoriadis and Allison first reported the value of liposomes as adjuvants [104]. Since then, the versatility that characterizes liposomes has been exploited to shape them and target their performance. Currently, cationic liposomes have emerged as the main candidate, by generating greater dendritic cell uptake, hence greater antigenic uptake [105]. A series of characteristics have been listed that make liposomes one of the most promising adjuvants/platforms in the development of vaccines, including high loading capacity, antigenic stability, biocompatibility, and easy handling [106].

Virosomes are considered a specialized variant of liposomes, where the phospholipid bilayer has been fused to the viral envelope, preserving the viral glycoproteins on its surface. The antigens of interest can be included within the lumen of the virosome or attached to the lipid surface. Virosomes allow antigen processing and expression on both MHC class-I molecules by recognition as a viral particle, and MHC class-II molecules by being phagocytosed by dendritic cells, thus eliciting an effective immune response [107]. Virosomes have been successfully used in the generation of preventive vaccines against HPV subtypes 16 and 18, exhibiting effectiveness in the prevention of HPV-associated premalignant and malignant lesions [108,109].

Nanoparticles are formulations where a substance acquires unique properties by forming structures on the nanoscale. Nanocarriers are prone to target APCs by a wide range of mechanisms [110]. Currently, the most commonly used nanoparticles as adjuvants are metallic nanoparticles, carbon nanotubes, and polymeric particles. Nanoparticles are easily modified to promote stronger immune responses when combined with diverse platforms and adjuvants. In addition, their nanometric size allows them to be more effectively transported to lymphatic tissues, where they can be taken up readily by APCs [111].

In cancer, the most commonly used adjuvants are GM-CSF, Montanide ISA-51 (water-in-oil emulsion), poly-I:C, cationic liposomes, IL-2, tetanus/diphtheria toxoid, heat shock protein, imiquimod and CD40L [81].

14.6 Current clinical trials

We performed research through the ClinicalTrial.gov database and the European Union Clinical Trials Register available by June 2021, introducing the keywords: cancer + vaccine; plus, the specific filters: completed study + with results + study phase I/II/III/IV; obtaining a total of 263 and 39 clinical trials to date, respectively. Only trials with a statistical analysis comparing overall survival against a control group were included in Table 14.1.

Most trials reporting survival analysis were predominantly peptide and whole TC-based vaccines, and 70% were in trial phases I and II. Nearly 30% of the registered clinical trials evaluated the preventive effect of different HPV vaccinations on the development of cervical, anal, perineal, penile, and head squamous cell carcinoma on diverse populations.

Of the clinical trial results, only three showed a statistically significant increase in overall survival compared to the control group, including HSPPC-96, Provenge, and Tecemotide. It should be noted that these results are to be expected as long as they are used under the specified conditions.

Non-serious adverse events reported in more than 10% of patients included in the clinical trials present in Table 14.1 were fever, chills, fatigue, asthenia, anemia, thrombocytopenia, leukopenia, headache, insomnia, dizziness, peripheral neuropathy, tachycardia, hypotension, hypertension, cough, dyspnea, abdominal pain, nausea, vomiting, diarrhea, constipation, hyporexia, lumbago, myalgia, arthralgia, application site reaction, pruritus, and alopecia.

Additionally, these clinical trials have also reported serious adverse events associated with vaccination, highlighting chills, fever, fatigue, weakness, hypertension, hypokalemia, pneumonia, dyspnea, pancytopenia, thromboembolic events, seizures, and metastasis, among others. In vaccines effective at improving overall survival [24,112,113], these serious adverse events have shown a cumulative incidence higher than 20%.

14.7 Perspectives and limitations

Cancer vaccines continue to be a developing arm of immunotherapy. The importance of integrating the most pertinent characteristics of each antigen, delivery platform, and adjuvant lies in the formulation of an effective vaccine; highlighting the critical understanding of how the vaccine components interact with each other to elicit a desired immune response.

To date, only a few therapeutic vaccines in clinical trials have shown a statistically significant improvement in overall survival, and some of them have even been demonstrated to be deleterious.

The search for specific antigens in cancer should be done, if possible, on a case-by-case basis; this could be achieved through the application of individualized medicine. Currently, the realization of this type of individualized therapeutics is expensive and involves exhaustive multidisciplinary work. At the same time, reaching a consensus on the use of shared antigens in each cancer is a subject of intense debate.

TABLE 14.1 Cancer vaccines in current clinical trials, showing type of vaccine platform, specifications, combination therapy, delivery route, cancer indications, phase of trial, statistical analysis of overall survival, and registration number.

Name	Specifications	Therapy	Delivery	Cancer	Phase	Results	Registration	References
DCVAC/OvCa *Type*: Peptide-loaded DC	SK-OV-3 and OV-90 cell line's antigens-loaded dendritic cells	CARB + GEM	SC	Ovarian cancer (Relapse)	II	OS 24.1 months vs 21.7 (control); HR 0.63, CI 95% (0.26–1.54), $P = 0.3028$	NCT02107950	[114]
CVAC *Type*: Peptide-loaded DC	MUC1 antigen-specific dendritic cells	None	ID	Ovarian cancer (Remission)	II	OS >42 mo vs 26 (control); HR 0.17, CI 95% (0.02–1.44), $P = 0.07$	NCT01068509	[115]
HSPPC-96 *Type*: Peptide	Autologous tumor-derived Hsp peptide complex-96	TMZ + XRT	ID	Glioblastoma	II	OS 18 mo (PD-L1 high) vs 47 (PD-L1 low); HR 3.3, CI 95% (1.4–8.6), $P = 0.007$	NCT00905060	[112]
GVAX pancreas vaccine *Type*: Whole cell	Irradiated GM-CSF-transfected allogeneic pancreatic tumor cells.	CRS-207 + CP	ID	Pancreatic adenocarcinoma (Advanced or metastatic)	IIb	OS 3.7 mo vs 4.6 (control); HR 1.17, CI 95% (0.84–1.64), $P = 0.1499$	NCT02004262	[116]

Name	Specifications	Therapy	Delivery	Cancer	Phase	Results	Registration	References
KLH+OPT-821 *Type:* Peptide	Polyvalent antigen (Globo-H, GM2, MUC1-TN,TF)-KLH conjugate with adjuvant OBI-821	None	SC	Ocarian cancer (Remission)	II	OS 47 mo vs 46 (control); HR 0.83, CI 95% (0.55–1.24), $P = 0.18$	NCT00857545	[117]
GVAX pancreas vaccine *Type:* Whole cell	Irradiated GM-CSF-transfected allogeneic pancreatic tumor cells	Ipilimumab	ID	Pancreatic adenocarcinoma (Advanced or metastatic)	II	OS 9.38 mo vs 14.7 (control); HR 1.75, CI 95% (1.09–2.79), $P = 0.019$	NCT01896869	[118]
Provenge *Type:* Peptide-loaded DC	PAP/GM-CSF loaded dendritic cells	None	IV	Prostate cancer (Metastatic hormone-refractory)	III	OS 25.8 mo vs 21.7 (control); HR 0.78, CI 95% (0.61–0.98), $P = 0.03$	NCT00065442	[24]
210M *Type:* Peptide	Modified gp100 melanoma peptide	IL-2	IV	Melanoma (stage III-IV, HLA-A0201 positive)	III	OS 17.8 mo; CI 95% (11.9–25.8) vs 11.1 mo (control); CI 95% (8.7–16.3), $P = 0.06$	NCT00019682	[119]

(Continued)

TABLE 14.1 Cancer vaccines in current clinical trials, showing type of vaccine platform, specifications, combination therapy, delivery route, cancer indications, phase of trial, statistical analysis of overall survival, and registration number.

Name	Specifications	Therapy	Delivery	Cancer	Phase	Results	Registration	References
Tecemotide *Type:* Peptide	Liposomal-based synthetic lipopeptide from MUC1	CP + XRT	SC	Non-small cell lung cancer (Unresectable stage III)	III	OS 29.4 mo vs 20.8 (control); HR 0.81, CI 95% (0.68–0.98), $P = 0.026$	NCT00409188	[113]
IMA901 *Type:* Peptide	Multiple tumor associated peptides	Sunitinib + GM-CSF + CP	ID	Renal cell carcinoma (Advanced or metastatic)	III	OS 33.17 mo vs 33.67 (control); HR 1.34, CI 95% (0.96–1.86), $P = 0.087$	NCT01265901	[120]
Rindopepimut *Type:* Peptide	EGFRvIII-specific peptide conjugated to KLH	TMZ	ID	Glioblastoma (EGFRvIII-positive)	III	MRD population: OS 20.1 mo vs 20 (control); HR 1.01, CI 95% (0.79–1.30), p=0.93; SDR population: OS 14.8 mo vs 14.1 (control); HR 0.79, CI 95% (0.61–1.02), $P = 0.066$	NCT01480479	[121]

Name	Specifications	Therapy	Delivery	Cancer	Phase	Results	Registration	References
PROSTVAC-V/F *Type:* Viral vector	Viral vector vaccinia/fowl-pox virus-PSA-TRICOM	GM-CSF	SC	Prostate cancer (Metastatic hormone-refractory)	III	OS 33.2 mo vs 34.3 (control); HR 1.02, CI 95% (0.86–1.22), $P = 0.59$	NCT01322490	[122]
DCVAC/PCa *Type:* WCL-loaded DC	Whole prostate tumor cell lysate loaded dendritic cells	DTX + PDN	SC	Prostate cancer (Metastatic hormone-refractory)	III	OS 29.7 mo vs 26.7.8 (control); HR 0.908, CI 95% (0.74–1.1), $P = 0.335$	NCT02111577	[123]

CARB, carboplatin; CI, confidence interval; CP, cyclophosphamide; CRS-207, live attenuated mesothelin-expressing Listeria monocytogenes; DTX, docetaxel; EGFRvIII, Epidermal Growth Factor Receptor Variant III; GEM, gemcitabine; Globo-H, globo-H hexasaccharide; GM-CSF, granulocyte-macrophage colony stimulating factor; GM2, ganglioside GM2; Hsp, heat shock protein; HR, hazard ratio; ID, intradermal; IL-2, interleukin-2; IV intravenous; KLH, keyhole limpet hemocyanin; mo, months; MRD, minimal residual disease; MUC1, mucine 1; MUC1-Tn, glycosylated mucine 1; OS, overall survival; PAP, prostatic acid phosphatase; PD-L1, programmed cell death-ligand 1; PDN, prednisone; PSA, prostatic-specific antigen; SC, subcutaneous; SRD, significant residual disease; TF, Thompson Friedrich antigen; TMZ, temozolomide; TRICOM, Three costimulatory molecules for T cells (B7.1, leukocyte function-associated antigen-3, and intercellular adhesion molecule-1); vs, versus; XRT, radiotherapy.

14.8 Concluding remarks

The identification of highly immunogenic antigens specific against TCs, the development of appropriate delivery strategies, and the use of suitable adjuvants with combination therapies will enable the optimal development of effective vaccines that will have a significant impact on clinical outcomes in cancer patients.

The hope for the future is to find optimal antigens for cancer vaccine formulation that works for most people and to properly discern who will require a personalized vaccine, considering combination with other immunotherapy arms to optimize the antitumor immune response and overcome the immunosuppressive profile of cancer.

References

[1] Siegel RL, Miller KD, Fuchs HE, Jemal A. Cancer Statistics, 2021. CA Cancer J Clin 2021;71(1):7–33.

[2] Boylston A. The origins of inoculation. J R Soc Med 2012;105(7):309–13.

[3] Barquet N, Domingo P. Smallpox: the triumph over the most terrible of the ministers of death. Ann Intern Med 1997;127(8 Pt 1):635–42.

[4] Lombard M, Pastoret PP, Moulin AM. A brief history of vaccines and vaccination. Rev Sci Tech 2007;26(1):29–48.

[5] Plotkin SA. Vaccines: past, present and future. Nat Med 2005;11(4 Suppl):S5–S11.

[6] Xu J, Doyon-Plourde P, Tunis M, Quach C. Effect of early measles vaccination on long-term protection: A systematic review. Vaccine 2021;39(22):2929–37.

[7] Falleiros-Arlant LH, Ayala SEG, Domingues C, Brea J, Colsa-Ranero A. Current status of poliomyelitis in Latin America. Rev Chilena Infectol 2020;37(6):701–9 Estado actual de la poliomielitis en Latinoamerica.

[8] Meng Q, et al. The maternal antibody against diphtheria, tetanus and pertussis showed distinct regional difference in China. BMC Pediatr 2019;19(1):480.

[9] Heymann DL, Wilder-Smith A. Successful smallpox eradication: what can we learn to control COVID-19? J Travel Med 2020;27(4).

[10] Saxena M, van der Burg SH, Melief CJM, Bhardwaj N. Therapeutic cancer vaccines. Nat Rev Cancer 2021;21(6):360–78.

[11] Decker WK, Safdar A. Bioimmunoadjuvants for the treatment of neoplastic and infectious disease: Coley's legacy revisited. Cytokine Growth Factor Rev 2009;20(4):271–81.

[12] Wang J, Mamuti M, Wang H. Therapeutic vaccines for cancer immunotherapy. ACS Biomater Sci Eng 2020;6(11):6036–52.

[13] Tran T, Blanc C, Granier C, Saldmann A, Tanchot C, Tartour E. Therapeutic cancer vaccine: building the future from lessons of the past. Semin Immunopathol 2019;41(1):69–85.

[14] Guo C, Manjili MH, Subjeck JR, Sarkar D, Fisher PB, Wang XY. Therapeutic cancer vaccines: past, present, and future. Adv Cancer Res 2013;119:421–75.

[15] Cheever MA, et al. The prioritization of cancer antigens: a national cancer institute pilot project for the acceleration of translational research. Clin Cancer Res 2009;15(17):5323–37.

[16] Broker M, Berti F, Costantino P. Factors contributing to the immunogenicity of meningococcal conjugate vaccines. Hum Vaccin Immunother 2016;12(7):1808–24.

[17] Zhou G, Lu Z, McCadden JD, Levitsky HI, Marson AL. Reciprocal changes in tumor antigenicity and antigen-specific T cell function during tumor progression. J Exp Med 2004;200(12):1581–92.

[18] Haen SP, Loffler MW, Rammensee HG, Brossart P. Towards new horizons: characterization, classification and implications of the tumour antigenic repertoire. Nat Rev Clin Oncol 2020;17(10):595–610.

[19] Bright RK, Bright JD, Byrne JA. Overexpressed oncogenic tumor-self antigens. Hum Vaccin Immunother 2014;10(11):3297–305.

[20] Strasser A, Puthalakath H, O'Reilly LA, Bouillet P. What do we know about the mechanisms of elimination of autoreactive T and B cells and what challenges remain. Immunol Cell Biol 2008;86(1):57–66.

[21] Buonaguro L, Petrizzo A, Tornesello ML, Buonaguro FM. Translating tumor antigens into cancer vaccines. Clin Vaccine Immunol 2011;18(1):23–34.

[22] Dudley ME, et al. Cancer regression and autoimmunity in patients after clonal repopulation with antitumor lymphocytes. Science 2002;298(5594):850–4.

[23] Gotter J, Brors B, Hergenhahn M, Kyewski B. Medullary epithelial cells of the human thymus express a highly diverse selection of tissue-specific genes colocalized in chromosomal clusters. J Exp Med 2004;199(2):155–66.

[24] Kantoff PW, et al. Sipuleucel-T immunotherapy for castration-resistant prostate cancer. N Engl J Med 2010;363(5):411–22.

[25] Fratta E, et al. The biology of cancer testis antigens: putative function, regulation and therapeutic potential. Mol Oncol 2011;5(2):164–82.

[26] Grizzi F, Franceschini B, Hamrick C, Frezza EE, Cobos E, Chiriva-Internati M. Usefulness of cancer-testis antigens as biomarkers for the diagnosis and treatment of hepatocellular carcinoma. J Transl Med 2007;5:3.

[27] Gordeeva O. Cancer-testis antigens: unique cancer stem cell biomarkers and targets for cancer therapy. Semin Cancer Biol 2018;53:75–89.

[28] Lurquin C, et al. Structure of the gene of tum- transplantation antigen P91A: the mutated exon encodes a peptide recognized with Ld by cytolytic T cells. Cell 1989;58(2):293–303.

[29] De Plaen E, et al. Immunogenic (tum-) variants of mouse tumor P815: cloning of the gene of tum- antigen P91A and identification of the tum- mutation. Proc Natl Acad Sci U S A 1988;85(7):2274–8.

[30] Lennerz V, et al. The response of autologous T cells to a human melanoma is dominated by mutated neoantigens. Proc Natl Acad Sci USA 2005;102(44):16013–8.

[31] Chen I, Chen MY, Goedegebuure SP, Gillanders WE. Challenges targeting cancer neoantigens in 2021: a systematic literature review. Expert Rev Vaccines. 2021;20(7):827–37.

[32] Buonaguro L, Tagliamonte M. Selecting target antigens for cancer vaccine development. Vaccines (Basel) 2020;8(4).

[33] zur Hausen H. Viruses in human cancers. Science 1991;254(5035):1167–73.

[34] Vonsky M, et al. Carcinogenesis associated with human papillomavirus infection. Mechanisms and Potential for Immunotherapy. Biochemistry (Mosc) 2019;84(7):782–99.

[35] Ringelhan M, McKeating JA, Protzer U. Viral hepatitis and liver cancer. Philos Trans R Soc Lond B Biol Sci 2017;372(1732).

[36] Tagaya Y, Gallo RC. The exceptional oncogenicity of HTLV-1. Front Microbiol2017;8:1425.

[37] Finn OJ. The dawn of vaccines for cancer prevention. Nat Rev Immunol 2018;18(3):183–94.

[38] Gregory AE, Titball R, Williamson D. Vaccine delivery using nanoparticles. Front Cell Infect Microbiol 2013;3:13.

[39] Gatti-Mays ME, Redman JM, Collins JM, Bilusic M. Cancer vaccines: enhanced immunogenic modulation through therapeutic combinations. Hum Vaccin Immunother 2017;13(11):2561–74.

[40] O'Neill CL, Shrimali PC, Clapacs ZP, Files MA, Rudra JS. Peptide-based supramolecular vaccine systems(-). Acta Biomater 2021;133:153–67.

[41] Li W, Joshi MD, Singhania S, Ramsey KH, Murthy AK. Peptide vaccine: progress and challenges. Vaccines (Basel) 2014;2(3):515–36.

[42] Slingluff Jr. CL. The present and future of peptide vaccines for cancer: single or multiple, long or short, alone or in combination? Cancer J 2011;17(5):343–50.

[43] Peres Lde P, et al. Peptide vaccines in breast cancer: The immunological basis for clinical response. Biotechnol Adv 2015;33(8):1868–77.

[44] Saylor K, Gillam F, Lohneis T, Zhang C. Designs of antigen structure and composition for improved protein-based vaccine efficacy. Front Immunol 2020;11:283.

[45] Aldous AR, Dong JZ. Personalized neoantigen vaccines: a new approach to cancer immunotherapy. Bioorg Med Chem 2018;26(10):2842–9.

[46] Kutzler MA, Weiner DB. DNA vaccines: ready for prime time? Nat Rev Genet 2008;9(10):776–88.

[47] Yang B, Jeang J, Yang A, Wu TC, Hung CF. DNA vaccine for cancer immunotherapy. Hum Vaccin Immunother 2014;10(11):3153–64.

[48] Klinman DM, Ishii KJ, Verthelyi D. CpG DNA augments the immunogenicity of plasmid DNA vaccines. Curr Top Microbiol Immunol 2000;247:131–42.

[49] Wolff JA, et al. Direct gene transfer into mouse muscle in vivo. Science 1990;247(no. 4949 Pt 1):1465–8.

[50] Zhou WZ, et al. RNA melanoma vaccine: induction of antitumor immunity by human glycoprotein 100 mRNA immunization. Hum Gene Ther 1999;10(16):2719–24.

[51] Bettinger T, Carlisle RC, Read ML, Ogris M, Seymour LW. Peptide-mediated RNA delivery: a novel approach for enhanced transfection of primary and post-mitotic cells. Nucleic Acids Res 2001;29(18):3882–91.

[52] Jackson LA, et al. An mRNA Vaccine against SARS-CoV-2 - Preliminary Report. N Engl J Med 2020;383(20):1920–31.

[53] Broos K, et al. Particle-mediated intravenous delivery of antigen mRNA results in strong antigen-specific T-cell responses despite the induction of Type I interferon. Mol Ther Nucleic Acids 2016;5(6):e326.

[54] Esprit A, de Mey W, Bahadur Shahi R, Thielemans K, Franceschini L, Breckpot K. Neoantigen mRNA vaccines. Vaccines (Basel) 2020;8(4):776.

[55] Palucka K, Banchereau J. Cancer immunotherapy via dendritic cells. Nat Rev Cancer 2012;12(4):265–77.

[56] Matsuo K, Yoshie O, Kitahata K, Kamei M, Hara Y, Nakayama T. Recent progress in dendritic cell-based cancer immunotherapy. Cancers (Basel) 2021;13(10).

[57] Wculek SK, Amores-Iniesta J, Conde-Garrosa R, Khouili SC, Melero I, Sancho D. Effective cancer immunotherapy by natural mouse conventional type-1 dendritic cells bearing dead tumor antigen. J Immunother Cancer 2019;7(1):100.

[58] Anguille S, Smits EL, Lion E, van Tendeloo VF, Berneman ZN. Clinical use of dendritic cells for cancer therapy. Lancet Oncol 2014;15(7):e257–67.

[59] Figdor CG, de Vries IJ, Lesterhuis WJ, Melief CJ. Dendritic cell immunotherapy: mapping the way. Nat Med 2004;10(5):475–80.

[60] Chiang CL, Benencia F, Coukos G. Whole tumor antigen vaccines. Semin Immunol 2010;22(3):132–43.

[61] Chiang CL, Coukos G, Kandalaft LE. Whole tumor antigen vaccines: where are we? Vaccines (Basel) 2015;3(2):344–72.

[62] Sondak VK, et al. Adjuvant immunotherapy of resected, intermediate-thickness, node-negative melanoma with an allogeneic tumor vaccine: overall results of a randomized trial of the Southwest Oncology Group. J Clin Oncol 2002;20(8):2058–66.

[63] Srivatsan S, et al. Allogeneic tumor cell vaccines: the promise and limitations in clinical trials. Hum Vaccin Immunother 2014;10(1):52–63.

[64] Deacon DH, et al. The use of gamma-irradiation and ultraviolet-irradiation in the preparation of human melanoma cells for use in autologous whole-cell vaccines. BMC Cancer 2008;8:360.

[65] Luo L, Lv M, Zhuang X, Zhang Q, Qiao T. Irradiation increases the immunogenicity of lung cancer cells and irradiation-based tumor cell vaccine elicits tumor-specific T cell responses in vivo. Onco Targets Ther 2019;12:3805–15.

[66] Larsson M, Fonteneau JF, Bhardwaj N. Dendritic cells resurrect antigens from dead cells. Trends Immunol 2001;22(3):141–8.

[67] Szondy Z, Sarang Z, Kiss B, Garabuczi E, Koroskenyi K. Anti-inflammatory mechanisms triggered by apoptotic cells during their clearance. Front Immunol 2017;8:909.

[68] Sauter B, Albert ML, Francisco L, Larsson M, Somersan S, Bhardwaj N. Consequences of cell death: exposure to necrotic tumor cells, but not primary tissue cells or apoptotic cells, induces the maturation of immunostimulatory dendritic cells. J Exp Med 2000;191(3):423–34.

[69] Valenti R, et al. Human tumor-released microvesicles promote the differentiation of myeloid cells with transforming growth factor-beta-mediated suppressive activity on T lymphocytes. Cancer Res 2006;66(18):9290–8.

[70] Andreola G, et al. Induction of lymphocyte apoptosis by tumor cell secretion of FasL-bearing microvesicles. J Exp Med 2002;195(10):1303–16.

[71] Huber V, et al. Human colorectal cancer cells induce T-cell death through release of proapoptotic microvesicles: role in immune escape. Gastroenterology 2005;128(7):1796–804.

[72] Gastpar R, et al. Heat shock protein 70 surface-positive tumor exosomes stimulate migratory and cytolytic activity of natural killer cells. Cancer Res 2005;65(12):5238–47.

[73] Pineda B, et al. Malignant Glioma Therapy by Vaccination with Irradiated C6 Cell-Derived Microvesicles Promotes an Antitumoral Immune Response. Mol Ther 2019;27(9):1612–20.

[74] Ong HK, Tan WS, Ho KL. Virus like particles as a platform for cancer vaccine development. PeerJ 2017;5:e4053.

[75] Caldeira JC, Perrine M, Pericle F, Cavallo F. Virus-like particles as an immunogenic platform for cancer vaccines. Viruses 2020;12(5).

[76] Logunov DY, et al. Safety and immunogenicity of an rAd26 and rAd5 vector-based heterologous prime-boost COVID-19 vaccine in two formulations: two open, non-randomised phase 1/2 studies from Russia. Lancet 2020;396(10255):887–97.

[77] Choi Y, Chang J. Viral vectors for vaccine applications. Clin Exp Vaccine Res 2013;2(2):97–105.

[78] Flickinger Jr. JC, Rodeck U, Snook AE. Listeria monocytogenes as a vector for cancer immunotherapy: current understanding and progress. Vaccines (Basel) 2018;6(3).

[79] Bolhassani A, Zahedifard F. Therapeutic live vaccines as a potential anticancer strategy. Int J Cancer 2012;131(8):1733–43.

[80] Gutierro I, Hernandez RM, Igartua M, Gascon AR, Pedraz JL. Size dependent immune response after subcutaneous, oral and intranasal administration of BSA loaded nanospheres. Vaccine 2002;21(1-2):67–77.

[81] Cuzzubbo S, Mangsbo S, Nagarajan D, Habra K, Pockley AG, McArdle SEB. Cancer vaccines: adjuvant potency, importance of age, lifestyle, and treatments. Front Immunol 2020;11:615240.

[82] McKee AS, Munks MW, Marrack P. How do adjuvants work? Important considerations for new generation adjuvants. Immunity 2007;27(5):687–90.

[83] O'Hagan DT, Lodaya RN, Lofano G. The continued advance of vaccine adjuvants—'we can work it out'. Semin Immunol 2020;50:101426.

[84] Hollingsworth RE, Jansen K. Turning the corner on therapeutic cancer vaccines. NPJ Vaccines 2019;4:7.
[85] Hailemichael Y, et al. Persistent antigen at vaccination sites induces tumor-specific CD8(+) T cell sequestration, dysfunction and deletion. Nat Med 2013;19(4):465–72.
[86] Commins SP, Borish L, Steinke JW. Immunologic messenger molecules: cytokines, interferons, and chemokines. J Allergy Clin Immunol 2010;125(no. 2 Suppl 2):S53–72.
[87] Clive KS, et al. Use of GM-CSF as an adjuvant with cancer vaccines: beneficial or detrimental? Expert Rev Vaccines 2010;9(5):519–25.
[88] Steinhagen F, Kinjo T, Bode C, Klinman DM. TLR-based immune adjuvants. Vaccine 2011;29(17):3341–55.
[89] Urban-Wojciuk Z, et al. The Role of TLRs in Anti-cancer Immunity and Tumor Rejection. Front Immunol 2019;10:2388.
[90] Wang P. Natural and Synthetic Saponins as Vaccine Adjuvants. Vaccines (Basel) 2021;9(3).
[91] Marty-Roix R, et al. Identification of QS-21 as an inflammasome-activating molecular component of saponin adjuvants. J Biol Chem 2016;291(3):1123–36.
[92] Rhodes J. Covalent chemical events in immune induction: fundamental and therapeutic aspects. Immunol Today 1996;17(9):436–41.
[93] Zhu Y, An X, Zhang X, Qiao Y, Zheng T, Li X. STING: a master regulator in the cancer-immunity cycle. Mol Cancer 2019;18(1):152.
[94] Gulen MF, et al. Signalling strength determines proapoptotic functions of STING. Nat Commun 2017;8(1):427.
[95] Mangsbo SM, et al. Linking T cell epitopes to a common linear B cell epitope: a targeting and adjuvant strategy to improve T cell responses. Mol Immunol 2018;93:115–24.
[96] Patel PM, et al. Targeting gp100 and TRP-2 with a DNA vaccine: Incorporating T cell epitopes with a human IgG1 antibody induces potent T cell responses that are associated with favourable clinical outcome in a phase I/II trial. Oncoimmunology 2018;7(6):e1433516.
[97] Fletcher EAK, et al. Formation of immune complexes with a Tetanus-Derived B cell epitope boosts human T cell responses to covalently linked peptides in an ex vivo blood loop system. J Immunol 2018;201(1):87–97.
[98] Gupta RK. Aluminum compounds as vaccine adjuvants. Adv Drug Deliv Rev 1998;32(3):155–72.
[99] Kool M, Fierens K, Lambrecht BN. Alum adjuvant: some of the tricks of the oldest adjuvant. J Med Microbiol 2012;61(Pt 7):927–34.
[100] Oleszycka E, Lavelle EC. Immunomodulatory properties of the vaccine adjuvant alum. Curr Opin Immunol 2014;28:1–5.
[101] Zhong X, et al. An aluminum adjuvant-integrated nano-MOF as antigen delivery system to induce strong humoral and cellular immune responses. J Control Release 2019;300:81–92.
[102] Sun B, et al. Engineering an effective immune adjuvant by designed control of shape and crystallinity of aluminum oxyhydroxide nanoparticles. ACS Nano 2013;7(12):10834–49.
[103] van Doorn E, Liu H, Huckriede A, Hak E. Safety and tolerability evaluation of the use of Montanide ISA51 as vaccine adjuvant: A systematic review. Hum Vaccin Immunother 2016;12(1):159–69.
[104] Allison AG, Gregoriadis G. Liposomes as immunological adjuvants. Nature 1974;252(5480):252.
[105] Watson DS, Endsley AN, Huang L. Design considerations for liposomal vaccines: influence of formulation parameters on antibody and cell-mediated immune responses to liposome associated antigens. Vaccine 2012;30(13):2256–72.

[106] Wang N, Chen M, Wang T. Liposomes used as a vaccine adjuvant-delivery system: from basics to clinical immunization. J Control Release 2019;303:130–50.

[107] Kannan R, Madden K, Andrews S. Primer on immuno-oncology and immune response. Clin J Oncol Nurs 2014;18(3):311–7 326.

[108] Enokida T, Moreira A, Bhardwaj N. Vaccines for immunoprevention of cancer. J Clin Invest 2021;131(9).

[109] Harper DM, et al. Sustained efficacy up to 4.5 years of a bivalent L1 virus-like particle vaccine against human papillomavirus types 16 and 18: follow-up from a randomised control trial. Lancet 2006;367(9518):1247–55.

[110] Wen R, Umeano AC, Kou Y, Xu J, Farooqi AA. Nanoparticle systems for cancer vaccine. Nanomedicine (Lond) 2019;14(5):627–48.

[111] Silva JM, Videira M, Gaspar R, Preat V, Florindo HF. Immune system targeting by biodegradable nanoparticles for cancer vaccines. J Control Release 2013;168(2):179–99.

[112] Bloch O, et al. Autologous heat shock protein peptide vaccination for newly diagnosed glioblastoma: impact of peripheral PD-L1 expression on response to therapy. Clin Cancer Res 2017;23(14):3575–84.

[113] Mitchell P, et al. Tecemotide in unresectable stage III non-small-cell lung cancer in the phase III START study: updated overall survival and biomarker analyses. Ann Oncol 2015;26(6):1134–42.

[114] Rob L, et al. Autologous dendritic cell vaccination (DCVAC/OvCa) added to standard of care therapy in three open-label randomized phase 2 studies in women with advanced stage ovarian cancer. (OC) 2014;32(15):3134.

[115] Gray HJ, et al. Progression-free and overall survival in ovarian cancer patients treated with CVac, a mucin 1 dendritic cell therapy in a randomized phase 2 trial 2016;4(1):34.

[116] Le DT, et al. Results from a Phase IIb, randomized, multicenter study of GVAX pancreas and CRS-207 compared with chemotherapy in adults with previously treated metastatic pancreatic adenocarcinoma (ECLIPSE. Study) 2019;25(18):5493–502.

[117] O'Cearbhaill RE, et al. A phase II randomized, double-blind trial of a polyvalent Vaccine-KLH conjugate (NSC 748933 IND# 14384) + OPT-821 versus OPT-821 in patients with epithelial ovarian, fallopian tube, or peritoneal cancer who are in second or third complete remission: An NRG Oncology/GOG study. Gynecol Oncol 2019;155(3):393–9.

[118] Wu AA, et al. A Phase II Study of Allogeneic GM-CSF-transfected pancreatic tumor vaccine (GVAX) with ipilimumab as maintenance treatment for metastatic pancreatic cancer. Clin Cancer Res 2020;26(19):5129–39.

[119] Schwartzentruber DJ, et al. gp100 peptide vaccine and interleukin-2 in patients with advanced melanoma. N Engl J Med 2011;364(22):2119–27.

[120] Rini BI, et al. IMA901, a multipeptide cancer vaccine, plus sunitinib versus sunitinib alone, as first-line therapy for advanced or metastatic renal cell carcinoma (IMPRINT): a multicentre, open-label, randomised, controlled, phase 3 trial. Lancet Oncol 2016;17(11):1599–611.

[121] Weller M, et al. Rindopepimut with temozolomide for patients with newly diagnosed, EGFRvIII-expressing glioblastoma (ACT IV): a randomised, double-blind, international phase 3 trial. Lancet Oncol 2017;18(10):1373–85.

[122] Gulley JL, et al. Phase III Trial of PROSTVAC in asymptomatic or minimally symptomatic metastatic castration-resistant prostate cancer. J Clin Oncol 2019;37(13):1051–61.

[123] Vogelzang NJ, et al. Autologous dendritic cell vaccination (DCVAC/PCa) added to docetaxel chemotherapy in a double-blind, randomized phase III trial (VIABLE) in men with advanced (mCRPC) prostate. cancer 2015;33(15):5070.

Chapter 15

Emerging trends in vaccine delivery systems

Varsha Gautam[a], Pawan Kumar Maurya[b]
[a]*Amity Institute of Advanced Research and Studies (M&D), Amity University, Noida, Uttar Pradesh, India,* [b]*Department of Biochemistry, Central University of Haryana, India*

15.1 Introduction

Vaccines have been proven to save human lives in the past, saving millions of lives from different outbreaks [1]. Patients are administered vaccinations to promote immune responses that generate antibodies (humoral) or cell-mediated responses to avoid infection. According to the World Health Organization (WHO), effective immunization avoids approximately 2.5 million child deaths each year. Weak immunogenicity and sub-unit immunization, as well as poor patient compliance with booster doses that should improve prime doses, are only a few of the issues that drove the development of innovative preventative and therapeutic vaccines. Many of these compounds are adjuvants, and some of them are toxic and unfit for human consumption. As a result, alum compounds are employed in vaccines as a major adjuvant, either in combination with other chemicals or alone [2,4]. However, studies show that they are ineffective against influenza, Ebola, tuberculosis, malaria, HIV, and other diseases that need more stringent immunological responses, such as activation of CD8+ and CD4+ T cell-controlled immunity [3]. To elicit an immune response, traditional vaccinations employ either the whole pathogen or its traces [2]. Due to the lack of effective vaccines against common pathogens such as HIV, mycobacterium tuberculosis, and hepatitis C via traditional vaccinations, vaccine developers have shifted their focus to developing vaccines using recombinant proteins, nucleic acids, or using short peptidyl sequences that prioritize safety over efficiency and may need adjuvants or stimulating agents. The traditional vaccination technique depended on metallic salts called alum compounds, which work on the concept of precipitation, allowing the antigen to be released for a long time. Immunomodulators can potentially play the function of vaccine delivery mechanisms in rare cases by increasing immunogenicity via activating Th1/Th2 pathway [5]. However, some drawbacks such as acute and chronic tissue toxicity have been linked to these delivery methods, necessitating the development of

System Vaccinology. https://doi.org/10.1016/B978-0-323-85941-7.00020-6

immunologically neutral, and biocompatible vaccine delivery vehicles. Vaccine carriers are important for successful immunization because they control the geographical and temporal presentation of antigens to the immune system, aid in vaccine delivery, and assist overcome the constraints of a standard vaccination schedule. As a result, smaller doses of these non-immunogenic formulations can be employed to generate immunological responses, obviating the need for prime and booster doses in the standard vaccination schedule.

Nanoparticles (NPs) have found their way into vaccine delivery systems result of improved technology, and they can effectively act as antigen carriers. NPs-based drug delivery methods have proven to be excellent alternatives to conventional vaccinations [6]. These NPs have the capacity to encapsulate and preserve the desired quantity of antigen against in vivo destruction. Antigens combined with NPs function similarly to pathogens in traditional vaccinations. Antigen-presenting cells (APCs) may easily ingest these NPs via direct phagocytosis or receptor-mediated endocytosis since they are nanosized. Furthermore, APCs digested these antigens and presented them as peptides, causing Th cells to become activated. Th cells then stimulate additional Th and Tc cells, as well as B cells, to produce antigen-specific antibodies. A number of vaccine delivery adjuvants based on NPs are currently being investigated and developed. Liposomes, microspheres, and nanoparticles, as well as dendrimers, micellar systems, ISCOMs, and plant viruses, are all examples of these [7]. Virosomes and bacteriophage, which function as modern-day adjuvants for vaccine administration, are also used in several sophisticated delivery methods [8,9]. To induce an immune response against the disease, many ways can be utilized to deliver antigen encapsulated with a vaccine delivery system. In comparison to traditional delivery approaches, advanced delivery systems perform well in vivo due to their advantages of being biocompatible, nanosized, nontoxic, and executing targeted delivery. As a result, they improve the quality and effectiveness of the vaccine while also providing long-term immunity. Three advanced vaccine delivery methods namely polymers, liposomal, and bacteriophage, are discussed in this chapter.

15.2 Advantages of using advanced nanomaterials based vaccine delivery systems

In order to be immunogenic, a NPs vaccine must interact with a diverse range of cells. APCs, B cells, and macrophages are among the cells that process antigen-associated vaccines. Dimensions, shape, in vitro durability, and antigen copy adherence in living tissue are all variables that may be adjusted. Using a variety of NPs, researchers have attempted to increase the immunogenicity of an antigen by prolonging its persistence in the targeted region [10]. In a study conducted by researchers, shows that vaccination can be improved by interbilayer-crosslinked multilamellar vesicles that contain surface-conjugated

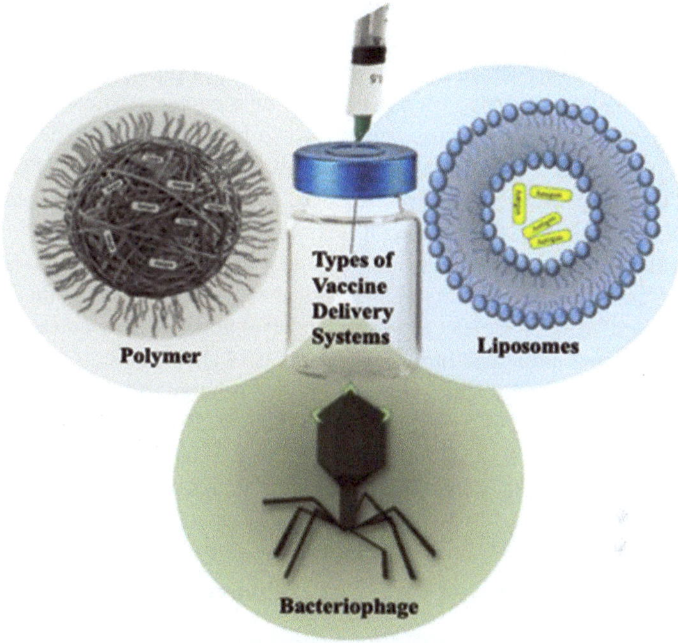

Graphical Abstract- Vaccine delivery systems

and encapsulated malarial antigens [11]. This is owing to the soluble antigen's long-term persistence in the draining lymph nodes. For robust cellular immune responses, APCs must efficiently ingest, process, and distribute antigens following cross-presentation of the antigen that is required for an efficient CD8+ T cell response. NPs that are sensitive to the endolysosomal route have been explored as a means of achieving this [12]. While free antigen does not accurately mimic some viral infections, this nanotechnological approach results in higher CD8+ T cell responses than free antigen delivery. The size of the NPs has a big role in how effectively they drain to the lymph nodes. The physical properties of NPs such as charge, shape, and flexibility have an influence on lymphatic drainage. As a result, NPs smaller than 100 nm tend to drain to lymph nodes [13]. Because mucus being a porous network of mucin glycopolymers, size, and surface characteristics affect whether NPs may flow through or adhere to it [14,15]. Cationic nanoparticle adhesion permits them to engage with immune cells for extended lengths of time in mucus. Hydrophilic polymers namely poly-ethylene glycol (PEG) [16–18] and the cationic polymer chitosan [19,20] derived from crustaceans shells, are being used to transport vaccinations to the mucosal delivery of vaccines against TB. Because of its phagocytic nature, macrophages swallow NPs; nevertheless, researchers have attempted to direct NPs absorption to certain sub-types of APC. The size, charge, and shape of NPs can be adjusted to promote macrophage absorption or to boost uptake by APCs. There have been findings that macrophages prefer cationic nanoparticles to ingest [21–23]. Also, dendritic cells endocytose particles as small as 20–200 nm, whereas macrophages phagocytose particles as large as 500–5000 nm [24]. As a result of regulating adjuvant release near or inside APCs, nanomaterials can help lower the overall dosage. In comparison with soluble antigen/MPLA vaccination, nanomaterial vaccines have the potential to improve adjuvant effectiveness while lowering unwanted local or systemic consequences such as inflammation or toxicity [25–27]. It was found in a study that multilamellar "stapled" lipid vesicles carrying a malarial antigen allowed for a 10-fold dose reduction and enhanced humoral responses [11]. As a result, even without TLR ligands or other adjuvants, some NPs have inherent adjuvating properties that might be the result of possible pathways such as complement activation, inflammasome signaling, and activation of B cell [13]. Because they reduce inflammation and toxicity caused by other adjuvants, these intrinsic adjuvating NPs may be beneficial.

15.3 Types of advanced vaccines delivery systems

15.3.1 Polymeric nanoparticles based vaccine delivery systems

These are important aspects of modern vaccines that are made of polymeric components or macromolecular complexes designed to improve the potency of vaccine and perdurance of immune responses. Despite of being non-immunogenic these non-viral vectors have high compatibility with biosystems and large surface area. Therefore, these polymeric NPs have been shown to be more efficient in delivering antigens and various antigens and adjuvants may be effectively encapsulated in these particles. The increased immunogenicity by using these NPs for delivering antigens is attributed to improved cellular responses as well as immune responses (Th1/Th2), increasing cytokine secretions, and antigen-specific antibodies, being able to be administered through various routes, having prolonged stay in the body, and single-dose formulations. The mechanism of action of polymeric particles as antigen delivery vehicles is shown in Fig. 15.1. A huge family of biodegradable and synthetic thermoplastic polymers has been investigated widely as vaccine carriers and potential adjuvants, as shown in Fig. 15.2 [28,29]. Synthetic polyesters are known to have great safety profiles and biocompatibility and they are also approved by the "European Medicines Agency" and US FDA for biomedical use cases [30].

Polyesters such as polyglycolide (PGA), polycaprolactone (PCL), polylactic-co-glycolic acid (PLGA), polylactides, polyanhydrides, and polyphosphazene are all being frequently utilized as vaccine delivery agents. The activation of the classical complement system occurs when PGA is hydrolyzed to glycolide, resulting in a powerful inflammatory response. Aliphatic polyesters

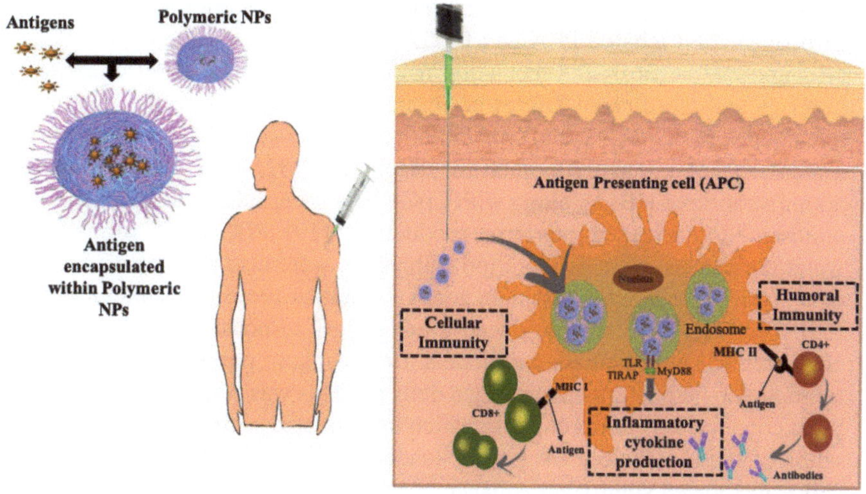

FIG. 15.1 Mechanism of action of polymeric particle for antigen delivery to cellular levels.

such as PLGA, PLA, and PCL, and their related copolymers, are often used biodegradable synthetic polymers in biomedical applications. One of the best examples of biodegradable polymer is PLGA as it is known to have superior degradability and biocompatibility and is used widely in microcapsules, microspheres, pellets, nanoparticles, film preparation, and implants. The use of PLGA and PLA NPs for pulmonary administration of hepatitis B vaccination has been widely studied. In comparison to hydrophilic NPs with a size of less than 500 nm, hydrophobic NPs with a size larger than 500 nm evoked a more

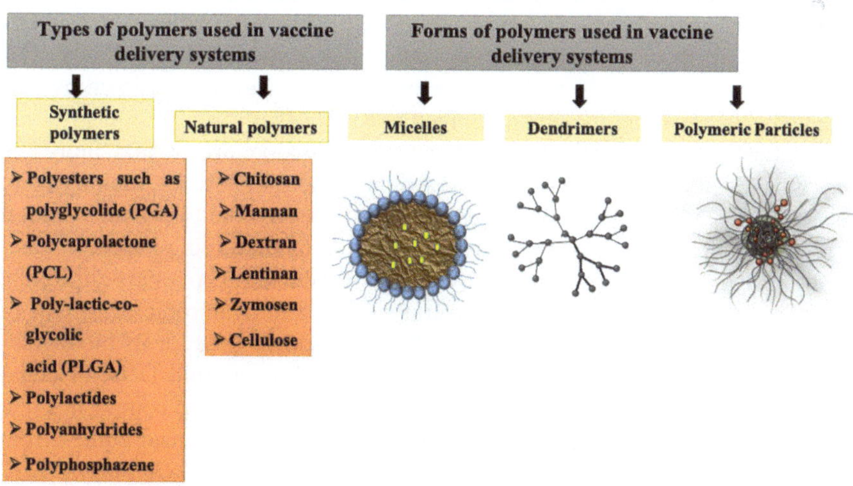

FIG. 15.2 Types and forms of polymers used for vaccine delivery.

substantial rise in the levels of IgA, interleukin-2, and interferon. The produced aerosolized and inhaled PLA and PLGA hepatitis B surface antigen (HBsAg) NPs improve hepatitis B vaccination responses (humoral, mucosal, and cytokine) [31]. According to Diwan et al., delivering CpG synthetic oligodeoxynucleotides (CpG/ODN) and toxoid antigens in biodegradable nanospheres is a more effective delivery method for vaccination [32]. In another study, nasal administration of HBsAg along with CpG/ODN encapsulated in alginate-coated chitosan NPs increased interferon production [119]. PLGA NPs formed using water/oil/water solvent evaporation techniques were also used for the delivery of a stable immunogenic domain four of Bacillus protective antigen (PAD4) [33]. The PAD4 systems produced a mixed IgG response (IgG1 and IgG2a), compared to controlled animal models. Besides these polymers, lipid-polymer hybrids also help in effective antigen delivery. This was confirmed in an experiment conducted by Lima et al., in which mice treated with live Mycobacterium with glycolipid trehalose dimycolate loaded Poly-DL-lactide-coglycolide outer cell wall showed significant enhancement in the inflammatory response in the lungs [34]. Polyphosphazene, a biodegradable macromolecular polymer with superior antigen delivery characteristics, is made up of phosphorus and nitrogen that are linearly connected by alternating single and double bonds [35].

In a research mucosal adjuvant properties of Poly-di[sodiumcarboxylatoethylphenoxy] phosphozene) (PCEP) were tested through coupling it with a variety of antigens, including, pneumococcal surface protein A, pertussis toxin, HIV-1 LAI, formalin-inactivated PR8 influenza virus, and trivalent influenza virus [36,120]. When F protein antigen for respiratory syncytial virus along with CpG/ODN and immunomodulatory innate defense regulator peptide were encapsulated in PCEP microparticles, their immunogenicity was increased [37]. Another category of biopolymers named as "polyanhydrides" are biopolymers with a high surface erodibility that have been studied as adjuvants or for antigen administration. Carboxylic acids are polyanhydride's metabolites. The USFDA has approved them as biocompatible and non-mutagenic [38]. Unlike PLGA polymers, which degrade by bulk erosion, polyanhydrides breakdown by surface erosion, ensuring maximum antigen release [39].

Natural polymers decompose into carbon dioxide, water, and inorganic compounds, and they may be derived from a variety of sources, making them eco-friendly. With several functional groups, it is possible to produce natural polymers with chemical and physical methods, or by modifying it as new material with nanotechnology. Some of the widely-used natural polymers are starch, chitosan, cellulose, alginate, chondroitin sulfate, and hyaluronic acid. Out of these natural polymers, alginate and chitosan is widely used for its biodegradability and biocompatibility. They can easily bind to plasmid DNA or negatively charged protein with electrostatic interaction to develop composites that can secure the DNA and protein from degrading [40]. Alginate comes from marine plants like "*Rhodophyceae,*" "*Cyanophyceae,*" and "*Chlorophyceae*" [41,42] as a natural polysaccharide. Calcium alginate, sodium alginate, and ammonium alginate are the widely used products made of alginate [43]. Alginate–poly(ethylenimine) (PEI) is a bio-reducible polymer material that self-assembles into a nanogel formulation for antigen loading and delivery, greatly improving vaccine-induced humoral and cellular immune responses [44]. In a research study, cholesterol-bearing hydrophobized pullulan and the protein that is a part of a family of cancer/testis antigens (NY-ESO-1) was studied as an immunogenic molecule in cancer patients [45]. Stimulation studies for CD8 and CD4 T cells from peripheral blood mononuclear cells was also conducted. The findings were highly encouraging in terms of developing a polyvalent cancer vaccine. In mice and guinea pigs, Saad et al. demonstrated that the Advax adjuvant can increase the immunogenicity of hepatitis B surface antigens [46]. In another research study coupling of a hyper-branched multifunctionalized polyglycerol with the combination of both T-cell epitope P2 from tetanus toxoid with tumor associated glycopeptide (MUC1) via "click chemistry" was done [47]. This resulted in an elicit immune response and increased IgG antibodies in mice models and human breast cancer cells. The researchers demonstrated that the polypeptide cationic micellar formulations poly(ethylene glycol)-b-poly(L-lysine)-b-poly(L-leucine) (PEG-PLL-PLLeu) significantly increased vaccine-induced antibody production by 70–90 times [48]. Zhang et al. link two different kinds of alginate to create alginate nanoparticles using $CaCl_2$ [49]. The mannose functionalized alginate nanoparticles were used to specifically target dendritic cells. The researchers also utilized ovalbumin (OVA) as a model antigen, conjugating it to alginates via the pH-sensitive Schiff base bond method. The impact of toll-like receptor (TLR) ligands on blood dendritic cells can be controlled using an alginate-coated chitosan nanogel [50]. Another natural biopolymer that is being used in vaccine delivery systems is mannan.

"Mannan" is a naturally occurring mannose biopolymer comprising of 1,4-linkage and have high affinity to binds with mannan-binding lectins (MBL). MBL has a role in phagocytosis, complement activation, and other immune responses requiring opsonization. According to recent studies [51], MBL interactions have been related to dendritic cell trafficking and the activation of both humoral as well as cellular responses. Inflammatory cytokines (Interleukines-1, TNF, and Interferons) and Th1/Th2 cytokines, are shown to be stimulated by mannan derivatives. When given intranasally to mice models, oxidized mannan coupled with recombinant protein antigens evoked a more stronger immune response than cholera toxin [52]. Dextran is another hydrophilic polymer generated by *Leuconostoc mesenteroides*. Dextran has been studied since the 1970s for its role as an adjuvant for influenza vaccines(H5 inactivated) [53]. DEAE-dextran and whole-cell cholera antigen have been demonstrated to boost immune responses through promoting and polarising Th2 response for antibody production, even though its mechanism of action is unclear [54]. In order to produce acetylated dextran (Ac-DEX), the hydroxyl groups of dextran are modified with acetal moiety [55]. Antigen presentation through MHC I/MHC II pathways can be altered by altering the characteristics of Ac-DEX-based particles [56]. p24, and HIV-1 capsid protein antigens have been shown to be effectively delivered with the help of dextran and chitosan-based polyelectrolyte complexes [57].

Anti-cancer effects of "Lentinan" (β-glu6) another natural compound have been well documented. Lentinan has been found to improve resistance to malignant transformation by stimulating the growth of blood mononuclear cells such as lymphocyte and macrophages. When DNA vaccines are administered with Lentinan, there has been an increase in the immune response [58]. Lentinan is an effective adjuvant when combined with DNA vaccines that encode HBV core antigen [(HBcAg) pB144] as demonstrated with experiments on mice models. In addition to boosting T cell population size, lentinan enhanced APC recruitment and maturation, as well as T cell (CD8+/CD4+) activation. Adjuvanted HBsAg vaccination enhanced both humoral and cell immunological responses in BALB/c mice, according to a study [59], by boosting APC maturation and antigen presentation, as well as activating CD4+T cells thereby generating interleukins and anti-HBV antibodies. *Saccharomyces cerevisiae* cell wall preparation, "Zymosan" is able to activate APCs via TLR-2 and Dectin-1, a phagocyte receptor expressed on dendritic cells and macrophage cells [60]. Through an alternate route that increased the recruitment of APCs, HIV-1 DNA vaccination in combination to zymosan improved the humoral as well as cellular immune responses in BALB/c mice [61]. Zymosan combined with double-stranded RNA polyriboinocinic polyribocytidylic acid in influenza vaccines may become more effective as an adjuvant by boosting the production of cytokines by dendritic cells [62].

15.3.2 Liposomes-based vaccine delivery systems

Liposomes were first utilized as vaccine delivery vehicles in 1974 and two vaccines based on liposomes, Epaxal, and Inflexal V, against hepatitis A and influenza, respectively, have already been licensed for human use [63,64]. Liposomes are spherical hollow structures consisting phospholipid bilayers able to entrap hydrophilic and hydrophobic moieties inside the aqueous compartment and the lipid bilayers, with cholesterol giving rigidity to the bilayers. They are useful in delivering DNA vaccines because the positive charge on liposomes is neutralized by the negative charge on DNA [65]. It is necessary to entrap and target virus particles, proteins, and glycoproteins in order to elicit immune responses at the subcellular and cellular levels. Liposomes are effective vaccine adjuvants that can easily cross these cellular barriers due to their particle structure and ability to interact with lipid receptors present on cell surface such as CD1a after complement activation [7]. The phospholipid bilayer combines with the cell wall, causing it to be quickly integrated into the system. Researchers have also synthesized polymer-lipid hybrid carriers and tested their effectiveness as vaccine carriers. Mucosal vaccination may potentially benefit from the creation of polymerized liposomes, as they have shown improved stability within the gastrointestinal system [66]. These polymerized liposomes can bind to particular cell surface receptors in mucosal tissues. Hydrophilic surfaces are present on stealth liposomes or sterically stabilized liposomes owing to the coating of liposomes with PEG, which covalently bonds with the polyethylene found in the lipid bilayer and prevent serum protein binding reducing opsonization. To combat *Campylobacter jejuni* infection, researchers encapsulated a nucleic acids encoding a protein from basal body part in liposomes combining with adjuvants and that it resulted in an immunogenic response against the infection [67]. Therefore, as a result of their physicochemical characteristics, liposomes provide a wide range of possibilities for vaccine administration. It was found that liposomes prepared using phosphophatidyl serine (PS) were less efficient in generating an immune response following transdermal administration than that made from phosphophatidyl glycerol (PG) or phosphatidylethanolamine (PE) [68,69]. DPPC/DMPE liposomes demonstrated substantially greater antibody titers than DPPC/DPPE and DPPC/PS liposomes when administered orally. The choice of fatty acids has a major impact on the immune response pathway. In a study, Ovalbumin bound to liposomes via saturated fatty acids activated CD4+ T cell, whereas liposomes containing unsaturated fatty acids activated both CD4+ as well as CD8+ T cells via cross-presentation and successfully produced a response from cytotoxic T lymphocytes in another [70].

The addition of cholesterol to liposomes changes the stiffness and fluidity of the bilayer, making them more stable and less prone to breakdown in the circulation. Following vaccination, there was a decrease in uptake of macrophages as well as cellular responses, which was confirmed by the reduction in interferon-gamma levels. The presence of cholesterol, on the other hand, had no effect on antigen biodistribution patterns or the total systemic immunoglobulin response (IgG) [71]. According to a study, the IgG response was significantly reduced in the ovalbumin conjugated liposomes that were given extra cholesterol concentration as compared to the control group that received liposomes without cholesterol. Therefore, cholesterol has a significant influence on the development of humoral immunity when coupled with cationic phospholipids. The cationic liposomes produced from DPPC/DC-cholesterol at a 1:1 molar ratio elicited more immunological responses than those prepared at a 9:1 molar ratio [72,73]. The immune response was related to liposome cholesterol concentration despite equal particle size, surface charge, and antigen loading, underlining the necessity of regulating the cholesterol content of liposome-based vaccines. Furthermore, there is no consistent relationship between the phospholipid/cholesterol ratio and immunogenicity [74].

As a result, liposome loading efficiency is influenced by the bilayer's physicochemical properties that include antigen polarity, partition coefficient (log P) values, and liposomal production processes [75]. After adding the lipid mixture, antigen can be added during the hydration phase. Antigens can be chemically bonded or adsorbed to the liposomal surface via covalent bonding or can be encapsulated within the lipid bilayer membrane or the inner aqueous core of the liposome [76].

Antigen processing along with antigen presentation may be influenced by the position of antigens in liposomes. Antigens on the liposome surface were shown to be more immunogenic than those that were encapsulated as protein antigens bind to cationic liposome surfaces via hydrophobic bonds, van der Waals forces, electrostatic interactions and are responsible for the adsorption. Liposomes can display antigens on their surface by covalently attaching them to phospholipids. Liposomes with hemagglutinin (HA) adsorbed to their surface were shown to be more immunogenic than liposomes with HA that was enclosed within the liposome. While B cells may readily detect surface-associated antigens, antigen-encapsulated liposomes must be phagocytosed before they can be identified by the immune system [77].

For a comprehensive range of immunological responses, liposomes can contain several copies of structurally different epitopes such as when cytotoxic T lymphocytes as well as the T-helper epitopes were conjugated on to the surface of liposomes, they induced strong antitumor immunity, according to the study's findings [78]. Using a single liposome vesicle, researchers were able to transmit two distinct epitopes that are a B cell and a universal Th epitope attached to the phospholipid surface and coupled to Pam3-cystinylalanyl-glycine, respectively [79,80]. The process of delivery two epitopes was found to generate a robust humoral response along with long-term memory against the antigens. In addition to peptide antigens, liposomes can contain exogenous immunostimulatory substances in the same vesicles.

When it comes to a liposome-based vaccination, factors such as the size of the liposomes, their ability to form lamellar hexagonal bilayers, and the inclusion of immunostimulatory lipids can have an impact on the vaccine's function and potential use. Liposomal vaccine vesicles should undergo stability tests in a variety of environments to ensure they do not change over time. Liposomes can be stabilized via a variety of methods (such as spray drying, sterilization, cryoprotection, and PEGylation) [81]. These approaches avoid unwanted changes in vesicle form, which might have a detrimental influence on the vaccine's immunological response [82]. The surface charge of liposomes should be taken into account while developing vaccinations. Antigen loading in vaccination might be altered by lipid adsorption or antigen interaction which is mainly dependent on charge [83].

15.3.2.1 Types of liposomes

There are several types of liposomes that are currently being used in vaccine delivery (Fig. 15.3). Double-bagged" or multivesicular vesicles are typical *vesosomes*, a liposome derivative that is very recent vesicles require two distinct formulas [84]. Ethanol is used to create a thin coating of lipid sheets that surround the liposomes within. An important advantage of utilizing vesosomes is that the outer liposome provides protection. Thus, liposomes imprisoned in the liposomes slowly release, increasing the circulation duration of the payload medication or antigen. Aside from that, vesosomes may be easily modified to

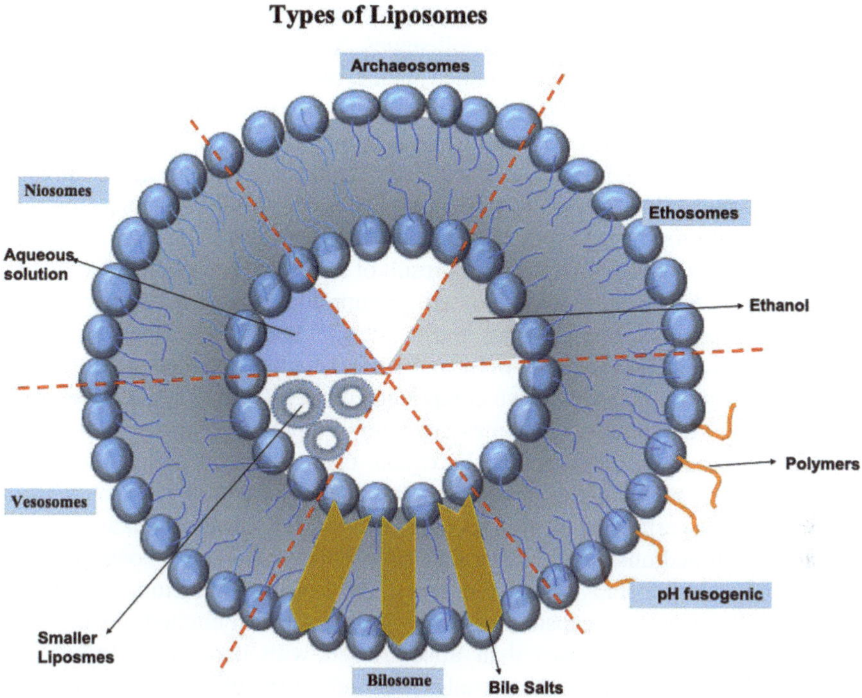

FIG. 15.3 Types of liposomes used for vaccine delivery.

suit different delivery methods. In contrast to normal liposomes, *niosomes* have a non-ionic surfactant in their formulation, which makes them different from liposomes [85]. Alkyl esters, ethers, and amides are the most widely utilized surfactants. These vesicles have a diameter of 10 to 100 nanometers. It was Brewer et al. that discovered niosomes were more effective than Freud's adjuvant at triggering an immune response in mice immunized with bovine serum albumin. Toutefois, these antibody titers lasted just one month following inoculation [86]. A *bilosome* is a liposome that contains bile salts as part of it. Bilayer instability and lysis are prevented by adding bile to liposomes, which allows the antigen to remain in place until the liposomes reach their target [87]. Because to their high gastrointestinal tract stability, they are mostly employed in oral vaccine/drug administration. To test the effectiveness of mucosal vaccine delivery methods, Jain et al. compared niosomes and two types of bilosomes that are glucomannan modified as well as bilosomes without any modifications [88]. After being encapsulated in thin films, Tetanus toxoid antigen was characterized by its physical and chemical characteristics.

Under certain acidic circumstances, *pH fusogenic liposomes* undergo a phase shift. This means they're stable at normal pH and can be taken up by the cells via the endocytosis [89]. Their instability occurs when they are maintained in endosomes after internalization [90]. As vaccine carriers, pH fusogenes were investigated by Watarai and colleagues. Mice were intraperitoneally vaccinated using ovalbumin encapsulated within two types of modified pH fusogenic polymer, the one modification comprised of succinylated poly(glycidol) and the unmodified liposome. IgG1, IgG2a, and IgG3 antibody titers in both cases were much higher in the mice [91]. Liposomes having significant levels of alcohol (20%–45%) are known as *Ethosomes* [92]. The interdigitation effect was thought to prevent ethanol and lipid vesicles from coexisting in a single delivery system for years. As a result of a study, it was shown that including alcohol in lipid vesicles increased stratum corneum penetration, that can be helpful for delivering vaccines into the dermal layers [93]. Because of their softness and malleability, they offer numerous benefits over liposomes, including the ability to transport active compounds more effectively. As derived from the archaean domain, archeosomes are a novel liposome type. *Archaeosomes* are often produced from archaeal extracts or synthesized archeal fats [94]. Archaea possess branching phytanyl chains linked by ether bonds to the glycerol backbone carbons at locations sn-2,3 in contrast to bacteria, eukarya, which include saturated/unsaturated fatty acyl chains attached via ester bonds at sn-1,2 [95,96]. In another study, it was found that animals vaccinated intraperitoneally using archaeosomes encapsulating bovin serum albumin elicited much greater humoral immune responses than mice treated with liposomal formulations in one of the early vaccination trials. Antibody titers elicited using archaeosomes were equivalent to those elicited by antigen prepared using a powerful, traditional Cholera toxin adjuvant [97]. *Proteoliposomes* vesicles structurally include the bacterial primary outer membrane proteins, lipopolysaccharides, and phospholipids [98]. When adjuvanting capabilities of proteoliposomes were discovered in the late 1980s, vaccine research began employing them. As part of this, for treating infection from *Neisseria meningitidis*, proteoliposome was used to create the most well-known Finlay adjuvant platform [99].

15.3.2.2 Methods involved in the preparations for liposomes

There are many liposome preparation methods, but the thin-film approach is perhaps the most used. An inner flask wall is coated with an ultrathin layer of lipids. The resulting film is then hydrated with either water or a buffer solution to complete the process [100]. In order to facilitate the formation of the bilayer, it is critical that the lipid film and water/buffer solution be warmed above the lipids transitional temperature (Tm). If this is done in conjunction with strong shaking and a possible ultrasound bath, the film can tear off the flask and create liposomes. As a result, the liposomes are multilamellar vesicles of various sizes. For lipophilic substances, the encapsulating material can be added along with lipids before the thin film is formed or along with water/buffer solution if they are hydrophilic in nature. Even when working with little amounts of chemicals, this technique is very reproducible, although it has a poor encapsulation efficiency. Encapsulation of lipophilic components in lower amounts is a particular advantage of this method. Another way to obtain liposomes is proliposomal technique. Comparatively, it has poor repeatability when producing smaller amounts of liposomes, but it achieves considerably greater encapsulation efficiency than thin-film technique. Dissolving lipids in water with alcohol, stirring at 60°C for 10 minutes, and resulting in a smooth paste is the basic technique. Following this, water/buffer is added dropwise together with stirring the lipids. As MLVs develop, the suspension is hydrated for 1 hour. Liposomal production with this technique is very beneficial for bigger batches, notably for TBARS tests. All of these methods involve injecting a lipid suspension for hydrophobic or hydrophilic organic solvents into water. Aside from being simple to prepare, these methods allow for a large amount of liposomes to be produced, but they do require significant quantities of often costly chemicals. Ethanol Injection is a technique utilized to create liposomes ranging in size from 30 to 170 nm, which are commonly employed to prepare Small unilamellar vesicles. As far as size is concerned, it is determined by the lipid content and injection speed. During stirring, lipids dissolved in ethanol, are injected into the aqueous phase, and the solvent is discarded to produce liposomes. The solution is then left to hydrate for another 15 minutes while stirring. A silica gel column or rotary evaporation can be used to remove the ethanol from the liposome suspension. The Ether Injection Method and the Ethanol Injection Method are quite similar, with the significant distinction that the lipid solvent employed in this case, ether, is kept away from water. Ether's ability to dissolve more fats than ethanol, as well as the fact that it does not interfere with liposome production, make it possible to produce liposomes in greater quantities. In the same way as ethanol, ether is eliminated from the solution after injection into the solution. Other disadvantages of this approach include the necessity for ether and water needs different temperatures during injection, ether's ability to alter the encapsulation of certain chemicals, and liposomes that are produced have very variable forms. Like injection techniques, emulsification involves dissolving lipids and mixing them with organic solvents. The water phase is delivered to the organic phase (i.e., at an inverted organic/water phase ratio). There is also no immediate removal of the organic phase, but rather a water-inorganic phase emulsion. After the lipids create a monolayer over the water droplets, they are evaporated, leaving behind the organic solvent. Liposomes are produced around water particles as the organic solvent evaporates. Emulsification has the advantage of better encapsulation efficiency than injection techniques. Also, reverse-phase evaporation is one of the most fundamental emulsification methods.

15.3.3 Bacteriophage-based vaccine delivery systems

Due to the advent of phage display technology 30 years ago, its usage has been immense in the areas of drug delivery, gene therapy as well as biosensors but the fact that antigen-antibody interactions can be improved by phage display, results in more effective vaccinations has been studies for some 10 years now.

This phage display usage as vaccines delivery systems relies on engineering bacteriophages to display antigens on their surface. It has been known for some time that phage display vaccines may be used to prevent or cure a wide range of diseases that includes tumor, viral, fungal, and parasitic infections. Anti-drug vaccines employ phages particles with antibodies that inhibit the toxicity of various substances (cocaine), in order to prevent drug misuse. Gene-engineered random proteins and peptides can be used in the early phases of vaccine creation to identify new antigens, allowing for the selection of the antigen that is best in regard to target binding. These viruses (Bacteriophages) infect and reproduce in bacteria and archaea, but are not capable of infecting eukaryotes. Genetic material, such as DNA or RNA, is used to create these viral particles, which are then packed in simple/complex structures of proteins known as capsids. Phage display implement the creation of peptides or proteins that have a high affinity to the phage's surface proteins.

15.3.3.1 Types of bacteriophage used in vaccines delivery system

Filamentous phages category of non-lytic viruses has single-stranded circular DNA due to this particles of this type can be formed in large concentrations in the presence of the reduced amount of bacterial contamination [101,102]. Structurally it is cylindrical in shape and is made up of five coat proteins (pIII, pVI, pVII, pVIII, and pIX) [103]. For vaccine development, this protein's immunogenic peptide content has been extensively utilized. The display level of the peptide is dependent on its length and sequence. Many copies of the protein pVIII can be successfully fused with short peptides (8 amino acids or less). For vaccine applications, phages have been used in for antigen display as they are stable in the face of extremes in pH and temperature [104]. Protein copies per virus particle are directly related to the immunological response they elicit, thus vaccine developers have relied heavily on protein pVIII's concentration of immunogenic peptides [106]. For vaccine applications, phages have been used in for antigen display as they are stable under harsh conditions such as pH and temperature [105]. While filamentous phages can show larger proteins at high copy numbers more effectively, capsid proteins found in T4 phages, Hoc and Soc can display larger proteins. Immune responses in humans and mice have been shown to be enhanced by the T4 phage capsid. To show heterologous peptides in antigen display methods, the carboxyl-terminus of phage T7 protein has been modified. The phage has been proposed as a substitute for filamentous phages, which are the most often employed vectors in antigen presentation [107]. The λ-phages have been shown to be capable of displaying appropriately folded antigenic peptides and two-three times larger fusion proteins in comparison to filamentous phages, making them a viable choice for complex antigen presentation [103,108]. When β-galactosidase, a 400 kDa protein, is shown appropriately on the phage surface, it has no effect on the survivability or shape of the phage [109]. There is more evidence that peptide display employing λ phage produces particles with greater antigen concentrations than peptide display using filamentous phages.

15.3.3.2 Types of bacteriophage-based vaccines delivery system

In 1988, the first study offering the role of phage particles as immunogenic delivery vehicles was published [110]. Currently, there are three primary forms of phage-based vaccinations: (1) phage display vaccines and (2) bacteriophage DNA vaccines (3) the hybrid phage vaccine, has emerged from the merging of these two procedures (Fig. 15.4).

Phage display vaccines—To generate viral particles (phage display vaccines) with particular immunogenic activity, antigens bound to phage surface proteins must be expressed properly [111,114]. A variety of populations of potential phages with varying antigens are generated by cloning various variants of natural as well as random cDNA sequence within the phage genome to express them on phage surface. Phages that have higher affinity for the required target (antibody for antigen identification) are chosen from these libraries, with the identification of DNA sequences that encode for a better affinity for the target antigen in these phage libraries. The reports of great efficiency and low expenses for the phage display technology for antigen identification have been beneficial. There have been reports of antigens such as Epidermal Growth Factor Receptor and the Melanoma Antigen Gene being studied for knowing the best antigen for cancer vaccines based on phages [111]. A single dosage of M13 and T4 phages containing 1 × 1011 plaque-forming units (pfu) administered subcutaneously to mice tumor models, resulted in elimination of tumor-associated macrophages [112]. According to a study, anti-tumor phages drive neutrophilic granulocyte infiltration, which leads to metastatic activity, which damages tumor tissue and reduces viable tumor cells. As a result of the great ability of phage particles to generate immunogenicity, phage-based vaccines for cancer immunotherapy are being developed [113].

Bacteriophage-based DNA vaccines delivery system—A bacteriophage DNA vaccine consists of an expression cassette that encodes an antigen and

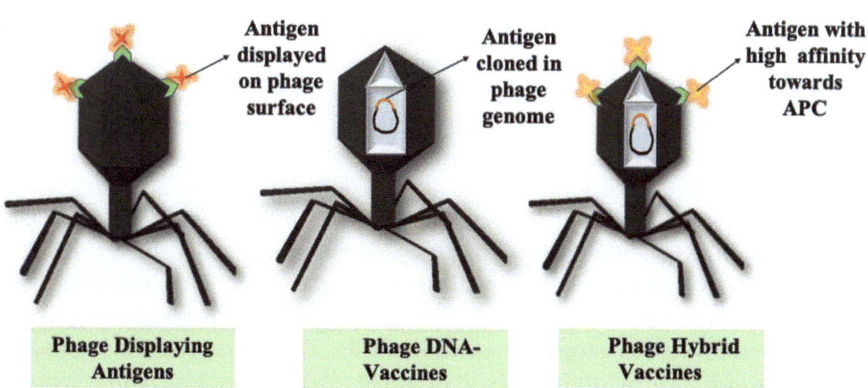

FIG. 15.4 Types of bacteriophage-based vaccine delivery modes.

is controlled by target-specific promoters found inside the bacteriophage [109,114]. Regulatory sequences must be present in the antigen's expression cassette to ensure proper gene expression and protein folding [116,117]. This method consists of phage particles serving as passive carriers and enabling the DNA-encoded antigen to be transmitted to eukaryotic cells where it will be expressed. It is believed that phage-DNA vaccines are preferable to regular DNA vaccinations due to the fact that phage-DNA vaccines have more stability when they are stored, transported, and orally delivered [116]. Phage is most commonly used for DNA vaccination, although other types of phages have also been tried, including filamentous phage. For filamentous phage-DNA vaccines, the ability of phagemid vectors to effectively transport multiple gene copies, allowing immunization with several epitopes or antigens with a single delivery vector, is essential. It has also been reported that these vaccines are more efficient in comparison to naked-DNA vaccinations [115]. Using a lambda-DNA vaccine, for example, elicited greater immune responses than a naked-plasmid vaccination, even at lower dosages. When utilizing DNA vaccines, Clark and co-workers have observed better immune responses than when using Engerix B, which uses recombinant protein along with HBsAg [117]. Protein folding, higher compatibility with post-translational modifications, their adjuvant effect, lipopolysaccharides presence including lipid incorporation during the time of protein secretion are all factors that contributed to the improved performance of the DNA vaccine [115]. In particular, phage DNA vaccines have shown to be more successful when given in several doses. Because the immunological response of the host is focused on phage coat proteins, which limit a portion of the DNA-carrying phages, this result has been linked to inadequate DNA expression in the initial vaccination. The fabrication of phage DNA vaccines is easy and inexpensive compared to other vaccine systems, the phage genome is ideal for the insertion of long DNA antigen sequences, i.e., up to 20 kb in lambda vectors, absence antibiotic resistance genes, and the phage genome is quite stable compared to standard DNA vaccines. Furthermore, because the bacteriophage cannot multiply in eukaryotic cells, phage DNA vaccines are much safer as compared to DNA vaccines utilizing adenovirus vectors.

Bacteriophage Vaccines with antigen display and DNA containing antigen specific sequences—Phage display and phage DNA vaccines are combined to create hybrid bacteriophage vaccinations. Recent advancements in phage-based vaccinations have focused on increasing the immune response by enhancing the contact and internalization of phage particles by APC. This approach relies on bacteriophages displaying high-affinity proteins or peptides for APCs or the antigen itself, while also carrying a eukaryotic expression cassette that encodes for specific antigen on their genome, with the goal of combining both effects to increase the immune response. Antigenic genes can be delivered by phages to immune response activators such dendritic cells. The process by which phages transport DNA has yet to be fully understood. There are evidence that recommended this method as an effective tool for the creation of anti-tumor vaccines after an increase in the CTL response has been noticed following the injection of hybrid phages [118].

15.4 Conclusion

The chapter summarizes various vaccine delivery vehicles that are based on polymers, liposomes, and phages. Biodegradable materials are less toxic and biocompatible, making them safe and efficient for therapeutic purposes. Polymers specially muco-adhesive polymers with inherent potential to enhance cross-presentation of antigens are known to have great improvement over traditional alum-based vaccines. They are known to promote clinical usage of new vaccines against tumor, HIV, TB, and Hepatitis. However, further research is needed about physicochemical properties of biomaterials like shape, size, and charge, and mechanisms to build immunity for developing more effective vaccines. Liposomes on the other hand have been known for efficient delivery of vaccine cargo because of their excellent safety and large loading capacity. Liposomes can be used as a flexible vaccine delivery vehicle when combined with functional molecules such as TLR ligands and adjuvanticity-bearing compounds. Many liposomes based vaccines have already been commercialized and many are in phase trials. As far as phage based delivery of vaccines is concerned they have immense potential in delivery DNA vaccines. The first clinical trial using phage treatment in humans has already received approval from the USFDA in which a bacteriophage-based vaccine formulation is used in a treatment study for resistant *Staphylococcus aureus* infection. Furthermore, the broad variety of phage-based vaccines may aid in the development of combinatorial vaccination techniques that might overcome the limitations of existing vaccination strategies.

References

[1] VanCott T. Vaccine adjuvants: preparation methods and research protocols edited by Derek O'Hagan, humana press. Trends Biotechnol 2000;18:511. https://doi.org/10.1016/s0167-7799(00)01508-0.

[2] Reed SG, Bertholet S, Coler RN, Friede M. New horizons in adjuvants for vaccine development. Trends Immunol 2009;30:23–32. https://doi.org/10.1016/j.it.2008.09.006.

[3] Sahdev P, Ochyl LJ, Moon JJ. Biomaterials for nanoparticle vaccine delivery systems. Pharm Res 2014;31:2563–82. https://doi.org/10.1007/s11095-014-1419-y.

[4] O'Hagan DT, De Gregorio E. The path to a successful vaccine adjuvant – "The long and winding road,". Drug Discov Today 2009;14:541–51. https://doi.org/10.1016/j.drudis.2009.02.009.

[5] Ryan EJ, Daly LM, Mills KHG. Immunomodulators and delivery systems for vaccination by mucosal routes. Trends Biotechnol 2001;19:293–304. https://doi.org/10.1016/s0167-7799(01)01670-5.

[6] Gregory AE, Titball R, Williamson D. Vaccine delivery using nanoparticles. Front Cellular Infection Microbiol 2013;3. doi:10.3389/fcimb.2013.00013.

[7] Lakshmi P, Bhaskaran S, Saroja C. Recent trends in vaccine delivery systems: A review. Int J Pharmaceutical Invest 2011;1:64. https://doi.org/10.4103/2230-973x.82384.

[8] González-Mora A, Hernández-Pérez J, Iqbal HMN, Rito-Palomares M, Benavides J. Bacteriophage-based vaccines: a potent approach for antigen delivery. Vaccines 2020;8. doi:10.3390/vaccines8030504.
[9] Asadi K, Gholami A. Virosome-based nanovaccines; a promising bioinspiration and biomimetic approach for preventing viral diseases: a review. Int J Biol Macromol 2021;182:648–58. https://doi.org/10.1016/j.ijbiomac.2021.04.005.
[10] Moon JJ, Suh H, Li AV, Ockenhouse CF, Yadava A, Irvine DJ. Enhancing humoral responses to a malaria antigen with nanoparticle vaccines that expand Tfh cells and promote germinal center induction. Proc Natl Acad Sci 2012;109:1080–5. https://doi.org/10.1073/pnas.1112648109.
[11] Swartz MA, Hirosue S, Hubbell JA. Engineering approaches to immunotherapy. Sci Transl Med 2012;4:148rv9. https://doi.org/10.1126/scitranslmed.3003763.
[12] Kaminskas LM, Porter CJH. Targeting the lymphatics using dendritic polymers (dendrimers). Adv Drug Deliv Rev 2011;63:890–900. https://doi.org/10.1016/j.addr.2011.05.016.
[13] Fries CN, Curvino EJ, Chen J-L, Permar SR, Fouda GG, Collier JH. Advances in nanomaterial vaccine strategies to address infectious diseases impacting global health. Nat Nanotechnol 2020;16:1–14. https://doi.org/10.1038/s41565-020-0739-9.
[14] Lai SK, Wang Y-Y, Wirtz D, Hanes J. Micro- and macrorheology of mucus. Adv Drug Deliv Rev 2009;61:86–100. https://doi.org/10.1016/j.addr.2008.09.012.
[15] Lai SK, Wang Y-Y, Hanes J. Mucus-penetrating nanoparticles for drug and gene delivery to mucosal tissues. Adv Drug Deliv Rev 2009;61:158–71. https://doi.org/10.1016/j.addr.2008.11.002.
[16] Leleux J, Atalis A, Roy K. Engineering immunity: Modulating dendritic cell subsets and lymph node response to direct immune-polarization and vaccine efficacy. J Control Release 2015;219:610–21. https://doi.org/10.1016/j.jconrel.2015.09.063.
[17] Kim Y-M, Pan JY-J, Korbel GA, Peperzak V, Boes M, Ploegh HL. Monovalent ligation of the B cell receptor induces receptor activation but fails to promote antigen presentation. Proc Natl Acad Sci 2006;103:3327–32. https://doi.org/10.1073/pnas.0511315103.
[18] Smirnov D, Schmidt JJ, Capecchi JT, Wightman PD. Vaccine adjuvant activity of 3M-052: an imidazoquinoline designed for local activity without systemic cytokine induction. Vaccine 2011;29:5434–42. https://doi.org/10.1016/j.vaccine.2011.05.061.
[19] Singh B, Maharjan S, Cho K-H, Cui L, Park I-K, Choi Y-J, Cho C-S. Chitosan-based particulate systems for the delivery of mucosal vaccines against infectious diseases. Int J Biol Macromol 2018;110:54–64. https://doi.org/10.1016/j.ijbiomac.2017.10.101.
[20] Bivas-Benita M, van Meijgaarden KE, Franken KLMC, Junginger HE, Borchard G, Ottenhoff THM, Geluk A. Pulmonary delivery of chitosan-DNA nanoparticles enhances the immunogenicity of a DNA vaccine encoding HLA-A*0201-restricted T-cell epitopes of Mycobacterium tuberculosis. Vaccine 2004;22:1609–15. https://doi.org/10.1016/j.vaccine.2003.09.044.
[21] Champion JA, Mitragotri S. Role of target geometry in phagocytosis. Proc Natl Acad Sci 2006;103:4930–4. https://doi.org/10.1073/pnas.0600997103.
[22] Yu S, Lau T, Jerome D, Giorgio T, Hubbell M. Size- and charge-dependent non-specific uptake of PEGylated nanoparticles by macrophages. Int J Nanomed 2012:799. doi:10.2147/ijn.s28531.
[23] Fröhlich E. The role of surface charge in cellular uptake and cytotoxicity of medical nanoparticles. Int J Nanomed 2012;5577. https://doi.org/10.2147/ijn.s36111.
[24] Xiang SD, Scholzen A, Minigo G, David C, Apostolopoulos V, Mottram PL, Plebanski M. Pathogen recognition and development of particulate vaccines: does size matter? Methods 2006;40:1–9. https://doi.org/10.1016/j.ymeth.2006.05.016.

[25] Smirnov D, Schmidt JJ, Capecchi JT, Wightman PD. Vaccine adjuvant activity of 3M-052: an imidazoquinoline designed for local activity without systemic cytokine induction. Vaccine 2011;29:5434–42. https://doi.org/10.1016/j.vaccine.2011.05.061.

[26] Ilyinskii PO, Roy CJ, O'Neil CP, Browning EA, Pittet LA, Altreuter DH, Alexis F, Tonti E, Shi J, Basto PA, Iannacone M, Radovic-Moreno AF, Langer RS, Farokhzad OC, von Andrian UH, Johnston LPM, Kishimoto TK. Adjuvant-carrying synthetic vaccine particles augment the immune response to encapsulated antigen and exhibit strong local immune activation without inducing systemic cytokine release. Vaccine 2014;32:2882–95. https://doi.org/10.1016/j.vaccine.2014.02.027.

[27] Hanson MC, Crespo MP, Abraham W, Moynihan KD, Szeto GL, Chen SH, Melo MB, Mueller S, Irvine DJ. Nanoparticulate STING agonists are potent lymph node–targeted vaccine adjuvants. J Clin Invest 2015;125:2532–46. https://doi.org/10.1172/jci79915.

[28] Fei Liu X, Lin Guan Y, Zhi Yang D, Li Z, De Yao K. Antibacterial action of chitosan and carboxymethylated chitosan. J Appl Polym Sci 2000;79:1324–35. https://doi.org/10.1002/1097-4628(20010214)79:7<1324::aid-app210>3.0.co;2-l.

[29] Morán JI, Vázquez A, Cyras VP. Bio-nanocomposites based on derivatized potato starch and cellulose, preparation and characterization. J Mater Sci 2013;48:7196–203. https://doi.org/10.1007/s10853-013-7536-x.

[30] Civalleri D, Scopinaro G, Balletto N, Claudiani F, Decian F, Camerini G, Depaoli M, Bonalumi U. Changes in vascularity of liver tumours after hepatic arterial embolization with degradable starch microspheres. Br J Surg 1989;76:699–703. https://doi.org/10.1002/bjs.1800760716.

[31] Thomas C, Rawat A, Hope-Weeks L, Ahsan F. Aerosolized PLA and PLGA nanoparticles enhance humoral, mucosal and cytokine responses to Hepatitis B vaccine. Mol Pharm 2011;8:405–15. https://doi.org/10.1021/mp100255c.

[32] Diwan M. Enhancement of immune responses by co-delivery of a CpG oligodeoxynucleotide and tetanus toxoid in biodegradable nanospheres. J Control Release 2002;85:247–62. https://doi.org/10.1016/s0168-3659(02)00275-4.

[33] Manish M, Rahi A, Kaur M, Bhatnagar R, Singh S. A Single-Dose PLGA encapsulated protective antigen Domain 4 nanoformulation protects mice against bacillus anthracis spore challenge. PLoS One 2013;8:e61885. https://doi.org/10.1371/journal.pone.0061885.

[34] Lima VMF, Bonato VLD, Lima KM, Dos Santos SA, Dos Santos RR, Gonçalves EDC, Faccioli LH, Brandão IT, Rodrigues-Junior JM, Silva CL. Role of trehalose Dimycolate in recruitment of cells and modulation of production of cytokines and NO in tuberculosis. Infect Immun 2001;69:5305–12. https://doi.org/10.1128/iai.69.9.5305-5312.2001.

[35] Teasdale I, Brüggemann O. Polyphosphazenes: multifunctional, biodegradable vehicles for drug and gene delivery. Polymers 2013;5:161–87. https://doi.org/10.3390/polym5010161.

[36] Payne LG, Jenkins SA, Woods AL, Grund EM, Geribo WE, Loebelenz JR, Andrianov AK, Roberts BE. Poly[di(carboxylatophenoxy)phosphazene] (PCPP) is a potent immunoadjuvant for an influenza vaccine. Vaccine 1998;16:92–8. https://doi.org/10.1016/s0264-410x(97)00149-7.

[37] Garlapati S, Garg R, Brownlie R, Latimer L, Simko E, Hancock REW, Babiuk LA, Gerdts V, Potter A, van Drunen S, Littel-van den H. Enhanced immune responses and protection by vaccination with respiratory syncytial virus fusion protein formulated with CpG oligodeoxynucleotide and innate defense regulator peptide in polyphosphazene microparticles. Vaccine 2012;30:5206–14. https://doi.org/10.1016/j.vaccine.2012.06.011.

[38] Wilson-Welder JH, Torres MP, Kipper MJ, Mallapragada SK, Wannemuehler MJ, Narasimhan B. Vaccine adjuvants: current challenges and future approaches. J Pharm Sci 2009;98:1278–316. https://doi.org/10.1002/jps.21523.

[39] Torres MP, Wilson-Welder JH, Lopac SK, Phanse Y, Carrillo-Conde B, Ramer-Tait AE, Bellaire BH, Wannemuehler MJ, Narasimhan B. Polyanhydride microparticles enhance dendritic cell antigen presentation and activation. Acta Biomater 2011;7:2857–64. https://doi.org/10.1016/j.actbio.2011.03.023.

[40] Won R. Properties and biomedical applications of chitosan. J Chitin Chitosan 2018;23:143–51. https://doi.org/10.17642/jcc.23.3.1.

[41] Parkes J. A clinical in-market evaluation of an alginate fibre dressing. Br J Nurs 2015;24:S28–35. https://doi.org/10.12968/bjon.2015.24.sup15.s28.

[42] Rowley JA, Madlambayan G, Mooney DJ. Alginate hydrogels as synthetic extracellular matrix materials. Biomaterials 1999;20:45–53. https://doi.org/10.1016/s0142-9612(98)00107-0.

[43] Jeon O, Alt DS, Ahmed SM, Alsberg E. The effect of oxidation on the degradation of photocrosslinkable alginate hydrogels. Biomaterials 2012;33:3503–14. https://doi.org/10.1016/j.biomaterials.2012.01.041.

[44] Li P, Luo Z, Liu P, Gao N, Zhang Y, Pan H, Liu L, Wang C, Cai L, Ma Y. Bioreducible alginate-poly(ethylenimine) nanogels as an antigen-delivery system robustly enhance vaccine-elicited humoral and cellular immune responses. J Control Release 2013;168:271–9. https://doi.org/10.1016/j.jconrel.2013.03.025.

[45] Hasegawa K. In vitro stimulation of CD8 and CD4 T cells by dendritic cells loaded with a complex of cholesterol-bearing hydrophobized pullulan and NY-ESO-1 Protein: identification of a New HLA-DR15-Binding CD4 T-Cell epitope. Clin Cancer Res 2006;12:1921–7. https://doi.org/10.1158/1078-0432.ccr-05-1900.

[46] Saade F, Honda-Okubo Y, Trec S, Petrovsky N. A novel hepatitis B vaccine containing Advax™, a polysaccharide adjuvant derived from delta inulin, induces robust humoral and cellular immunity with minimal reactogenicity in preclinical testing. Vaccine 2013;31:1999–2007. https://doi.org/10.1016/j.vaccine.2012.12.077.

[47] Glaffig M, Palitzsch B, Hartmann S, Schüll C, Nuhn L, Gerlitzki B, Schmitt E, Frey H, Kunz H. A fully synthetic glycopeptide antitumor vaccine based on multiple antigen presentation on a hyperbranched polymer. Chem Eur J 2014;20:4232–6. https://doi.org/10.1002/chem.201400256.

[48] Luo Z, Li P, Deng J, Gao N, Zhang Y, Pan H, Liu L, Wang C, Cai L, Ma Y. Cationic polypeptide micelle-based antigen delivery system: a simple and robust adjuvant to improve vaccine efficacy. J Control Release 2013;170:259–67. https://doi.org/10.1016/j.jconrel.2013.05.027.

[49] Zhang C, Shi G, Zhang J, Song H, Niu J, Shi S, Huang P, Wang Y, Wang W, Li C, Kong D. Targeted antigen delivery to dendritic cell via functionalized alginate nanoparticles for cancer immunotherapy. J Control Release 2017;256:170–81. https://doi.org/10.1016/j.jconrel.2017.04.020.

[50] Démoulins T, Bassi I, Thomann-Harwood L, Jandus C, Kaeuper P, Simon H-U, von Gunten S, McCullough KC. Alginate-coated chitosan nanogel capacity to modulate the effect of TLR ligands on blood dendritic cells. Nanomed Nanotechnol Biol Med 2013;9:806–17. https://doi.org/10.1016/j.nano.2013.01.002.

[51] Apostolopoulos V, Thalhammer T, Tzakos AG, Stojanovska L. Targeting antigens to dendritic cell receptors for vaccine development. J Drug Del 2013;2013:1–22. https://doi.org/10.1155/2013/869718.

[52] Stambas J, Pietersz G, McKenzie I, Cheers C. Oxidised mannan as a novel adjuvant inducing mucosal IgA production. Vaccine 2002;20:1068–78. https://doi.org/10.1016/s0264-410x(01)00456-x.

[53] Joye IJ, McClements DJ. Biopolymer-based nanoparticles and microparticles: fabrication, characterization, and application. Curr Opin Colloid Interface Sci 2014;19:417–27. https://doi.org/10.1016/j.cocis.2014.07.002.

[54] Houston WE, Crabbs CL, Kremer RJ, Springer JW. Adjuvant effects of diethylaminoethyl-dextran. Infect Immun 1976;13:1559–62. https://doi.org/10.1128/iai.13.6.1559-1562.1976.

[55] Bachelder EM, Beaudette TT, Broaders KE, Dashe J, Fréchet JMJ. Acetal-derivatized dextran: an acid-responsive biodegradable material for therapeutic applications. J Am Chem Soc 2008;130:10494–5. https://doi.org/10.1021/ja803947s.

[56] Broaders KE, Cohen JA, Beaudette TT, Bachelder EM, Frechet JMJ. Acetalated dextran is a chemically and biologically tunable material for particulate immunotherapy. Proc Natl Acad Sci 2009;106:5497–502. https://doi.org/10.1073/pnas.0901592106.

[57] Drogoz A, Munier S, Verrier B, David L, Domard A, Delair T. Towards biocompatible vaccine delivery systems: interactions of colloidal PECs based on polysaccharides with HIV-1 p24 antigen. Biomacromolecules 2008;9:583–91. https://doi.org/10.1021/bm701154h.

[58] Lemieszek M, Rzeski W. Anticancer properties of polysaccharides isolated from fungi of the Basidiomycetes class. Współczesna Onkologia 2012;4:285–9. https://doi.org/10.5114/wo.2012.30055.

[59] Dong S-F, Chen J-M, Zhang W, Sun S-H, Wang J, Gu J-X, Boraschi D, Qu D. Specific immune response to HBsAg is enhanced by β-glucan oligosaccharide containing an α-(1→3)-linked bond and biased towards M2/Th2. Int Immunopharmacol 2007;7:725–33. https://doi.org/10.1016/j.intimp.2007.01.004.

[60] Dillon S. Yeast zymosan, a stimulus for TLR2 and dectin-1, induces regulatory antigen-presenting cells and immunological tolerance. J Clin Invest 2006;116:916–28. https://doi.org/10.1172/jci27203.

[61] Ara Y, Saito T, Takagi T, Hagiwara E, Miyagi Y, Sugiyama M, Kawamoto S, Ishii N, Yoshida T, Hanashi D, Koshino T, Okada H, Okuda K. Zymosan enhances the immune response to DNA vaccine for human immunodeficiency virus type-1 through the activation of complement system. Immunology 2001;103:98–105. https://doi.org/10.1046/j.1365-2567.2001.01201.x.

[62] Ainai A, Ichinohe T, Tamura S, Kurata T, Sata T, Tashiro M, Hasegawa H. Zymosan enhances the mucosal adjuvant activity of poly(I:C) in a nasal influenza vaccine. J Med Virol 2010;82:476–84. https://doi.org/10.1002/jmv.21694.

[63] Yeh M-K, Chang H-I, Cheng M-Y. Clinical development of liposome based drugs: formulation, characterization, and therapeutic efficacy. Int J Nanomed 2011:49. doi:10.2147/ijn.s26766.

[64] Allison AG, Gregoriadis G. Liposomes as immunological adjuvants. Nature 1974;252:252. https://doi.org/10.1038/252252a0.

[65] Zhang X-X, McIntosh TJ, Grinstaff MW. Functional lipids and lipoplexes for improved gene delivery. Biochimie 2012;94:42–58. https://doi.org/10.1016/j.biochi.2011.05.005.

[66] Bernasconi V, Norling K, Bally M, Höök F, Lycke NY. Mucosal vaccine development based on liposome technology. J Immunol Res 2016;2016:1–16. https://doi.org/10.1155/2016/5482087.

[67] Kobierecka PA, Wyszyńska AK, Gubernator J, Kuczkowski M, Wiśniewski O, Maruszewska M, Wojtania A, Derlatka KE, Adamska I, Godlewska R. Chicken anti-Campylobacter vaccine–comparison of various carriers and routes of immunization. Front Microbiol 2016;7:740.

[68] Phillips N. Influence of phospholipid composition on antibody responses to liposome encapsulated protein and peptide antigens. Vaccine 1996;14:898–904. https://doi.org/10.1016/0264-410x(96)82949-5.

[69] Phillips NC, Gagné L. Modulation of murine macrophage nitric oxide synthesis by liposomal phospholipids: correlation with liposome immune adjuvant activity. J Drug Target 1995;3:137–47. https://doi.org/10.3109/10611869509059213.

[70] Taneichi M, Ishida H, Kajino K, Ogasawara K, Tanaka Y, Kasai M, Mori M, Nishida M, Yamamura H, Mizuguchi J, Uchida T. Antigen chemically coupled to the surface of liposomes are cross-presented to CD8+ T cells and induce potent antitumor immunity. J Immunol 2006;177:2324–30. https://doi.org/10.4049/jimmunol.177.4.2324.

[71] Kaur R, Henriksen-Lacey M, Wilkhu J, Devitt A, Christensen D, Perrie Y. Effect of incorporating cholesterol into DDA:TDB liposomal adjuvants on bilayer properties, biodistribution, and immune responses. Mol Pharm 2013;11:197–207. https://doi.org/10.1021/mp400372j.

[72] Nakano Y, Mori M, Yamamura H, Naito S, Kato H, Taneichi M, Tanaka Y, Komuro K, Uchida T. Cholesterol inclusion in liposomes affects induction of antigen-specific IgG and IgE antibody production in mice by a surface-linked liposomal antigen. Bioconjug Chem 2002;13:744–9. https://doi.org/10.1021/bc0155667.

[73] Barnier Quer C, Elsharkawy A, Romeijn S, Kros A, Jiskoot W. Cationic liposomes as adjuvants for influenza hemagglutinin: more than charge alone. Eur J Pharm Biopharm 2012;81:294–302. https://doi.org/10.1016/j.ejpb.2012.03.013.

[74] Barnier-Quer C, Elsharkawy A, Romeijn S, Kros A, Jiskoot W. Adjuvant effect of cationic liposomes for subunit influenza vaccine: influence of antigen loading method, cholesterol and immune modulators. Pharmaceutics 2013;5:392–410. https://doi.org/10.3390/pharmaceutics5030392.

[75] Bozzuto G, Molinari A. Liposomes as nanomedical devices. Int J Nanomed 2015;10:975. https://doi.org/10.2147/ijn.s68861.

[76] Wagner A, Vorauer-Uhl K. Liposome technology for industrial purposes. J Drug Del 2011;2011:1–9. https://doi.org/10.1155/2011/591325.

[77] Hamborg M, Rose F, Jorgensen L, Bjorklund K, Pedersen HB, Christensen D, Foged C. Elucidating the mechanisms of protein antigen adsorption to the CAF/NAF liposomal vaccine adjuvant systems: effect of charge, fluidity and antigen-to-lipid ratio. Biochimica et Biophysica Acta (BBA) - Biomembranes 2014;1838:2001–10. https://doi.org/10.1016/j.bbamem.2014.04.013.

[78] Boeckler C, Dautel D, Schelté P, Frisch B, Wachsmann D, Klein J-P, Schuber F. Design of highly immunogenic liposomal constructs combining structurally independent B cell and T helper cell peptide epitopes. Eur J Immunol 1999;29:2297–308. https://doi.org/10.1002/(sici)1521-4141(199907)29:07<2297::aid-immu2297>3.0.co;2-5.

[79] Roth A, Rohrbach F, Weth R, Frisch B, Schuber F, Wels WS. Induction of effective and antigen-specific antitumour immunity by a liposomal ErbB2/HER2 peptide-based vaccination construct. Br J Cancer 2005;92:1421–9. https://doi.org/10.1038/sj.bjc.6602526.

[80] Jalali SA, Sankian M, Tavakkol-Afshari J, Jaafari MR. Induction of tumor-specific immunity by multi-epitope rat HER2/neu-derived peptides encapsulated in LPD Nanoparticles. Nanomed Nanotechnol Biol Med 2012;8:692–701. https://doi.org/10.1016/j.nano.2011.09.010.

[81] Gamvrellis A, Leong D, Hanley JC, Xiang SD, Mottram P, Plebanski M. Vaccines that facilitate antigen entry into dendritic cells. Immunol Cell Biol 2004;82:506–16. https://doi.org/10.1111/j.0818-9641.2004.01271.x.

[82] Badiee A, Khamesipour A, Samiei A, Soroush D, Shargh VH, Kheiri MT, Barkhordari F, Mc Master WR, Mahboudi F, Jaafari MR. The role of liposome size on the type of immune response induced in BALB/c mice against leishmaniasis: rgp63 as a model antigen. Exp Parasitol 2012;132:403–9. https://doi.org/10.1016/j.exppara.2012.09.001.

[83] Christensen D, Korsholm KS, Andersen P, Agger EM. Cationic liposomes as vaccine adjuvants. Expert Rev Vaccines 2011;10:513–21. https://doi.org/10.1586/erv.11.17.

[84] Boyer C, Zasadzinski JA. Multiple lipid compartments slow vesicle contents release in lipases and serum. ACS Nano 2007;1:176–82. https://doi.org/10.1021/nn7002025.

[85] Baillie AJ, Florence AT, Hume LR, Muirhead GT, Rogerson A. The preparation and properties of niosomes-non-ionic surfactant vesicles. J Pharm Pharmacol 1985;37:863–8. https://doi.org/10.1111/j.2042-7158.1985.tb04990.x.

[86] Brewer JM, Alexander J. Studies on the adjuvant activity of non-ionic surfactant vesicles: adjuvant-driven IgG2a production independent of MHC control. Vaccine 1994;12:613–9. https://doi.org/10.1016/0264-410x(94)90265-8.

[87] Wilkhu JS, McNeil SE, Anderson DE, Perrie Y. Characterization and optimization of bilosomes for oral vaccine delivery. J Drug Target 2013;21:291–9. https://doi.org/10.3109/1061186x.2012.747528.

[88] Jain S, Harde H, Indulkar A, Agrawal AK. Improved stability and immunological potential of tetanus toxoid containing surface engineered bilosomes following oral administration. Nanomed Nanotechnol Biol Med 2014;10:431–40. https://doi.org/10.1016/j.nano.2013.08.012.

[89] Straubinger RM, Düzgünes N, Papahadjopoulos D. pH-sensitive liposomes mediate cytoplasmic delivery of encapsulated macromolecules. FEBS Lett 1985;179:148–54. https://doi.org/10.1016/0014-5793(85)80210-6.

[90] Simões S. On the formulation of pH-sensitive liposomes with long circulation times. Adv Drug Deliv Rev 2004;56:947–65. https://doi.org/10.1016/j.addr.2003.10.038.

[91] Watarai S, Iwase T, Tajima T, Yuba E, Kono K. Efficiency of pH-Sensitive Fusogenic polymer-modified liposomes as a vaccine carrier. Scientific World J 2013;2013:1–7. https://doi.org/10.1155/2013/903234.

[92] Mishra D, Mishra PK, Dubey V, Nahar M, Dabadghao S, Jain NK. Systemic and mucosal immune response induced by transcutaneous immunization using Hepatitis B surface antigen-loaded modified liposomes. Eur J Pharm Sci 2008;33:424–33. https://doi.org/10.1016/j.ejps.2008.01.015.

[93] Touitou E, Dayan N, Bergelson L, Godin B, Eliaz M. Ethosomes—novel vesicular carriers for enhanced delivery: characterization and skin penetration properties. J Control Release 2000;65:403–18. https://doi.org/10.1016/s0168-3659(99)00222-9.

[94] Barbeau J, Cammas-Marion S, Auvray P, Benvegnu T. Preparation and characterization of stealth archaeosomes based on a synthetic PEGylated archaeal tetraether lipid. J Drug Del 2011;2011:1–11. https://doi.org/10.1155/2011/396068.

[95] Jacquemet A, Barbeau J, Lemiègre L, Benvegnu T. Archaeal tetraether bipolar lipids: structures, functions and applications. Biochimie 2009;91:711–7. https://doi.org/10.1016/j.biochi.2009.01.006.

[96] van de Vossenberg JLCM, Driessen AJM, Konings WN. The essence of being extremophilic: the role of the unique archaeal membrane lipids. Extremophiles 1998;2:163–70. https://doi.org/10.1007/s007920050056.

[97] Sprott G. Archaeosomes as novel antigen delivery systems. FEMS Microbiol Lett 1997;154:17–22. https://doi.org/10.1016/s0378-1097(97)00294-2.

[98] Tamargo B, Márquez Y, Ramírez W, Cedré B, Fresno M, Sierra G. New proteoliposome vaccine formulation from N. meningitidis serogroup B, without aluminum hydroxide, retains its antimeningococcal protectogenic potential as well as Th-1 adjuvant capacity. BMC Immunol 2013;14. https://doi.org/10.1186/1471-2172-14-s1-s12.

[99] Findlow J, Bayliss CD, Beernink PT, Borrow R, Liberator P, Balmer P. Broad vaccine protection against Neisseria meningitidis using factor H binding protein. Vaccine 2020. doi:10.1016/j.vaccine.2020.08.031.

[100] Chacra NAB. Liposomes: methods and protocols. Brazilian J Pharmaceutical Sci 2010;46:821. https://doi.org/10.1590/s1984-82502010000400029.

[101] Samoylova TI, Norris MD, Samoylov AM, Cochran AM, Wolfe KG, Petrenko VA, Cox NR. Infective and inactivated filamentous phage as carriers for immunogenic peptides. J Virol Methods 2012;183:63–8. https://doi.org/10.1016/j.jviromet.2012.03.032.

[102] van Houten NE, Henry KA, Smith GP, Scott JK. Engineering filamentous phage carriers to improve focusing of antibody responses against peptides. Vaccine 2010;28:2174–85. https://doi.org/10.1016/j.vaccine.2009.12.059.

[103] Nicastro J, Sheldon K, Slavcev RA. Bacteriophage lambda display systems: developments and applications. Appl Microbiol Biotechnol 2014;98:2853–66. https://doi.org/10.1007/s00253-014-5521-1.

[104] Pande J, Szewczyk MM, Grover AK. Phage display: Concept, innovations, applications and future. Biotechnol Adv 2010;28:849–58. https://doi.org/10.1016/j.biotechadv.2010.07.004.

[105] Hashemi H, Bamdad T, Jamali A, Pouyanfard S, Mohammadi MG. Evaluation of humoral and cellular immune responses against HSV-1 using genetic immunization by filamentous phage particles: A comparative approach to conventional DNA vaccine. J Virol Methods 2010;163:440–4. https://doi.org/10.1016/j.jviromet.2009.11.008.

[106] Hess GT, Cragnolini JJ, Popp MW, Allen MA, Dougan SK, Spooner E, Ploegh HL, Belcher AM, Guimaraes CP. M13 Bacteriophage display framework that allows sortase-mediated modification of surface-accessible phage proteins. Bioconjug Chem 2012;23:1478–87. https://doi.org/10.1021/bc300130z.

[107] Ghaemi A, Soleimanjahi H, Gill P, Hassan Z, Jahromi SRM, Roohvand F. Recombinant λ-phage nanobioparticles for tumor therapy in mice models. Genetic Vaccines Therapy 2010;8. doi:10.1186/1479-0556-8-3.

[108] Iwagami Y, Casulli S, Nagaoka K, Kim M, Carlson RI, Ogawa K, Lebowitz MS, Fuller S, Biswas B, Stewart S, Dong X, Ghanbari H, Wands JR. Lambda phage-based vaccine induces antitumor immunity in hepatocellular carcinoma. Heliyon 2017;3. https://doi.org/10.1016/j.heliyon.2017.e00407.

[109] Thomas BS, Nishikawa S, Ito K, Chopra P, Sharma N, Evans DH, Tyrrell DLJ, Bathe OF, Rancourt DE. Peptide vaccination is superior to genetic vaccination using a recombineered bacteriophage λ subunit vaccine. Vaccine 2012;30:998–1008. https://doi.org/10.1016/j.vaccine.2011.12.070.

[110] de la Cruz VF, Lal AA, McCutchan TF. Immunogenicity and epitope mapping of foreign sequences via genetically engineered filamentous phage. J Biol Chem 1988;263:4318–22. https://doi.org/10.1016/s0021-9258(18)68927-6.

[111] Ren S, Ren Z, Zhao M, Wang X, Zuo S, Yu F. Antitumor activity of endogenous mFlt4 displayed on a T4 phage nanoparticle surface. Acta Pharmacol Sin 2009;30:637–45. https://doi.org/10.1038/aps.2009.44.

[112] Dabrowska K, Opolski A, Wietrzyk J, Switala-Jelen K, Godlewska J, Boratynski J, Syper D, Weber-Dabrowska B, Gorski A, Anticancer activity of bacteriophage T4 and its mutant HAP1 in mouse experimental tumour models., 24(6):3991-5. (2004).

[113] Eriksson F, Tsagozis P, Lundberg K, Parsa R, Mangsbo SM, Persson MAA, Harris RA, Pisa P. Tumor-specific bacteriophages induce tumor destruction through activation of tumor-associated macrophages. J Immunol 2009;182:3105–11. https://doi.org/10.4049/jimmunol.0800224.

[114] Bazan J, Całkosiński I, Gamian A. Phage display—a powerful technique for immunotherapy. Hum Vaccin Immunother 2012;8:1829–35. https://doi.org/10.4161/hv.21704.

[115] Adhya S, Merril CR, Biswas B. Therapeutic and prophylactic applications of bacteriophage components in modern medicine. Cold Spring Harb Perspect Med 2014;4:a012518. https://doi.org/10.1101/cshperspect.a012518.

[116] March JB, Clark JR, Jepson CD. Genetic immunisation against hepatitis B using whole bacteriophage λ particles. Vaccine 2004;22:1666–71. https://doi.org/10.1016/j.vaccine.2003.10.047.

[117] Clark JR, Bartley K, Jepson CD, Craik V, March JB. Comparison of a bacteriophage-delivered DNA vaccine and a commercially available recombinant protein vaccine against hepatitis B. FEMS Immunol Med Microbiol 2011;61:197–204. https://doi.org/10.1111/j.1574-695x.2010.00763.x.

[118] Sartorius R, Pisu P, D'Apice L, Pizzella L, Romano C, Cortese G, Giorgini A, Santoni A, Velotti F, De Berardinis P. The use of filamentous bacteriophage fd to deliver MAGE-A10 or MAGE-A3 HLA-A2-restricted peptides and to induce strong antitumor CTL responses. J Immunol 2008;180:3719–28. https://doi.org/10.4049/jimmunol.180.6.3719.

[119] Zhao K, Chen G, Shi X, Gao T, Li W, Zhao Y, Zhang F, Wu J, Cui X, Wang Y-F. Preparation and efficacy of a live newcastle disease virus vaccine encapsulated in chitosan nanoparticles. PLoS One 2012;7:e53314. https://doi.org/10.1371/journal.pone.0053314.

[120] Bose RJ, Kim M, Chang JH, Paulmurugan R, Moon JJ, Koh W-G, Lee S-H, Park H. Biodegradable polymers for modern vaccine development. J Ind Eng Chem 2019;77:12–24. https://doi.org/10.1016/j.jiec.2019.04.044.

Part IV

Vaccine future and ethics

Chapter 16

Vaccine regulation and ethics

Hemant Arya, Tarun Kumar Bhatt
Department of Biotechnology, Central University of Rajasthan, Bandarsindri, Ajmer, Rajasthan, India

16.1 Introduction

The most significant and successful achievement of science and public health is a vaccine [1,2]. The vaccine is one of the safe and cost-effective medical interventions that protect human health from many infectious diseases [3]. It is an inactivated or weak form of a microorganism that is injected into a healthy human that improves immunity by triggering an immune response against the targeted deadly microorganism/pathogen [1,4]. In addition, it will generate and keep memories to eradicate the actual pathogen infection in the future. As per WHO, "Vaccine helps to trigger the body's immune system to recognize and fight against the pathogen infection and keep the human population safe from the diseases" (https://www.who.int/topics/vaccines/en/).

16.2 Role of vaccine in human health

Human health is one of the key factors that influence any country's economic growth and social security [5]. A vaccine is an important gift from science that has prevented millions of premature illnesses and deaths worldwide. According to Centers for Disease Control and Prevention (CDC), vaccines are available for deadly diseases such as Chickenpox, Rotavirus, Rubella, Hepatitis A and B, Diphtheria, Influenza, Pneumococcal, Human Papillomavirus, Measles, Meningococcal, Whooping Cough, Mumps, Polio, Smallpox, Tuberculosis, Shingles, Tetanus, Haemophilus influenzae type b, Adenovirus, Anthrax, Cholera, Japanese Encephalitis (JE), Yellow Fever Rabies, Typhoid Fever, and Gastroenteritis [5–8]. Millions of lives have been prevented by vaccines from deadly diseases. According to needs, the vaccines are being given to infants, children, teens, and adults. The vaccine prevents approximately 3 million deaths/year worldwide [7].

System Vaccinology. https://doi.org/10.1016/B978-0-323-85941-7.00016-4

16.3 Vaccination

In vaccination or immunization, vaccines are administered to healthy people, protecting them from deadly pathogen infections [3]. After getting vaccinated, humans develop immunity to that disease and therefore do not get ill due to that disease. Vaccination is essential because, from birth onwards, we are constantly exposed to different bacteria, many viruses, microbes, and pathogens [9]. Among them, many are beneficial and not harmful, but few of them may cause disease. Therefore, vaccination is important for a happy and healthy life.

Few reasons to get vaccinated for the betterment of human life [3,9,10]:

1. Low risk of getting an infection.
2. Vaccine promotes a healthy body for long life.
3. It can mean the difference between life and death.
4. Vaccines are safe and highly effective.
5. Save lives and costs.

16.4 Vaccine development and regulation

Vaccine development is an important process that includes the selection of a potential antigen through a complex research process [4,11–13]. Once the component is identified, developing it into a final vaccine construct also involves many critical steps such as selecting adjuvant and route of administration, etc [14]. The vaccine is made up of several components, and each of them is serving a specific purpose [9,15–17]. The components are antigens, adjuvant/s, preservatives, stabilizers, surfactants, residuals, and diluents. Each ingredient is tested for its safety during the manufacturing process. The vaccine development process is initiated with basic research, which includes identifying and purifying a potential antigen, appropriate cloning, creating a new vector system, and careful immunologic evaluation for a subunit vaccine. Different types of vaccines have different protocols and strategies to follow. Generally, the primary research is conducted at academics/research laboratories that are funded by government agencies [2,18,19]. Based on the promising outcomes of the basic and preclinical research, the decision to take the vaccine into clinical trials evaluation is determined (clinical phases1–4) (Table 16.1 and Fig. 16.1) [18,20–22].

Before licensing the vaccine, the developmental process is extensively tested, regulated, and reviewed for its safety, antigenicity, and efficacy (in the laboratory, on animals, and during clinical trials) [12,22]. Post-marketing surveillance, licensing, and vaccine use come under the vaccine regulation, and it is carried out after the use of the vaccine for human use has been granted [3,13].

For an effective vaccine regulatory system, six essential functions were identified by the WHO [23]:

1. A published set of precise requirements for licensing.
2. Surveillance of vaccine safety and efficacy.
3. System of lot release.

TABLE 16.1 Clinical phases during the vaccine development program.

Phase	Sample size	Purpose	Vaccination
I	10–100	Safety and immunogenicity analysis. Confirm immune response generation. Dose determination.	Healthy adult volunteers
II	100–1000	Expand safety and immunogenicity analysis. Monitor potential side effects and dose optimization.	Multiple trials on the various age groups
III	1K–10,000	Assess long-term safety and clinical efficacy. Monitor potential side effects.	Multiple countries and multiple sites
IV	10K–1M	Assess safety and effectiveness. Licensing and post-marketing surveillance.	Multiple countries and multiple sites

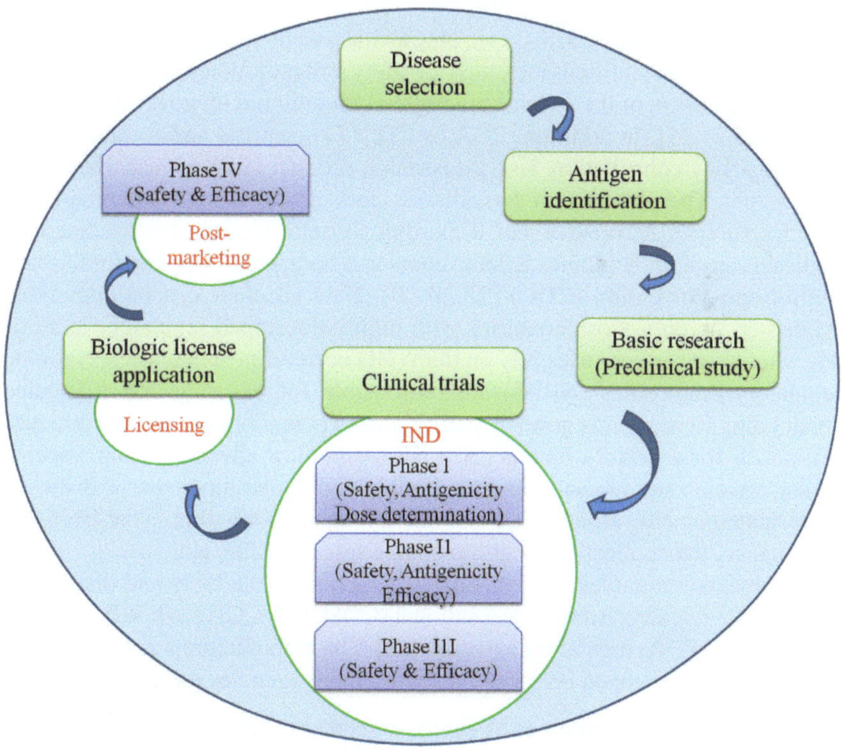

FIG. 16.1 Vaccine development and regulation process overview. A sequence of vaccine development events such as preclinical studies, an investigational new drug (IND) application, licensing phase, and post-marketing approval.

4. Use of laboratory when needed.
5. Regular inspections of manufacturers for good manufacturing practices (GMP) compliance.
6. Evaluation of clinical performance through authorized clinical trials.

16.5 Vaccine approval process

After the successful preclinical and clinical trials, the vaccine product should be approved by approval agencies such as The U.S. Food and Drug Administration's Center for Biologics Evaluation and Research in the United States, Central Drugs and Standards Control Organization (CDSCO) in India, Therapeutic Goods Administration (TGA) in Australia, MEDSAFE in New Zealand, Health Sciences Authority (HSA) in Singapore, Health Canada in Canada, etc. The pictorial representation explains the vaccine approval process of CDSCO (Fig. 16.2) and FDA (Fig. 16.3) [11–13,20,24–26].

16.6 Role of national and international agencies on vaccine regulation and distribution

The FDA, CDSCO, TGA, HSA, etc., play a vital role in the regulatory evaluation of vaccines. The scientific issues such as safety, efficacy, potency, effectiveness, and adverse effects of the vaccine are regularly monitored by government agencies [12,22,24,25]. In addition, FDA or CDSCO scientists and technical team evaluate policy contribution, risk assessment, product labeling, vaccine safety, efficacy, etc. The government surveillance team closely observes the marketed vaccines such as Adverse Event Reporting System, Centres for Medicare & Medicaid Services, Biologics Effectiveness and Safety, and Centres for Disease Control and Prevention (CDC) [25,27–29]. New vaccines can be authorized or licensed by only those countries with highly developed regulatory authorities, whereas other countries rely on the WHO or developed countries. National Regulatory Authorities (NRAs) are responsible for ensuring that a vaccine which going to be used is good in quality, shows potential efficacy and potency, and is safe for a healthy human [30]. NRAs monitor adverse events, vaccine quality, vaccine storage and handling, vaccine administration, sharps disposal, waste management, registration and marketing authorization, post-licensure surveillance, data collection, analysis update safety profile, etc.

Vaccines are manufactured in batches which are called lots and distributed through a lot release system by the national (CDSCO/DCGI) [29]; R.B. [31] and international (FDA) regulatory agencies [27]. The manufacturers need to submit the lot data as mentioned below to the government agencies for approval:

1. Protocol: vaccine developed as per the agreement (agreed-upon procedures).
2. Result: manufacturer testing results (emphasis on purity, potency, and sterility)
3. Samples: samples from the lot must be submitted to FDA for seeking permission.

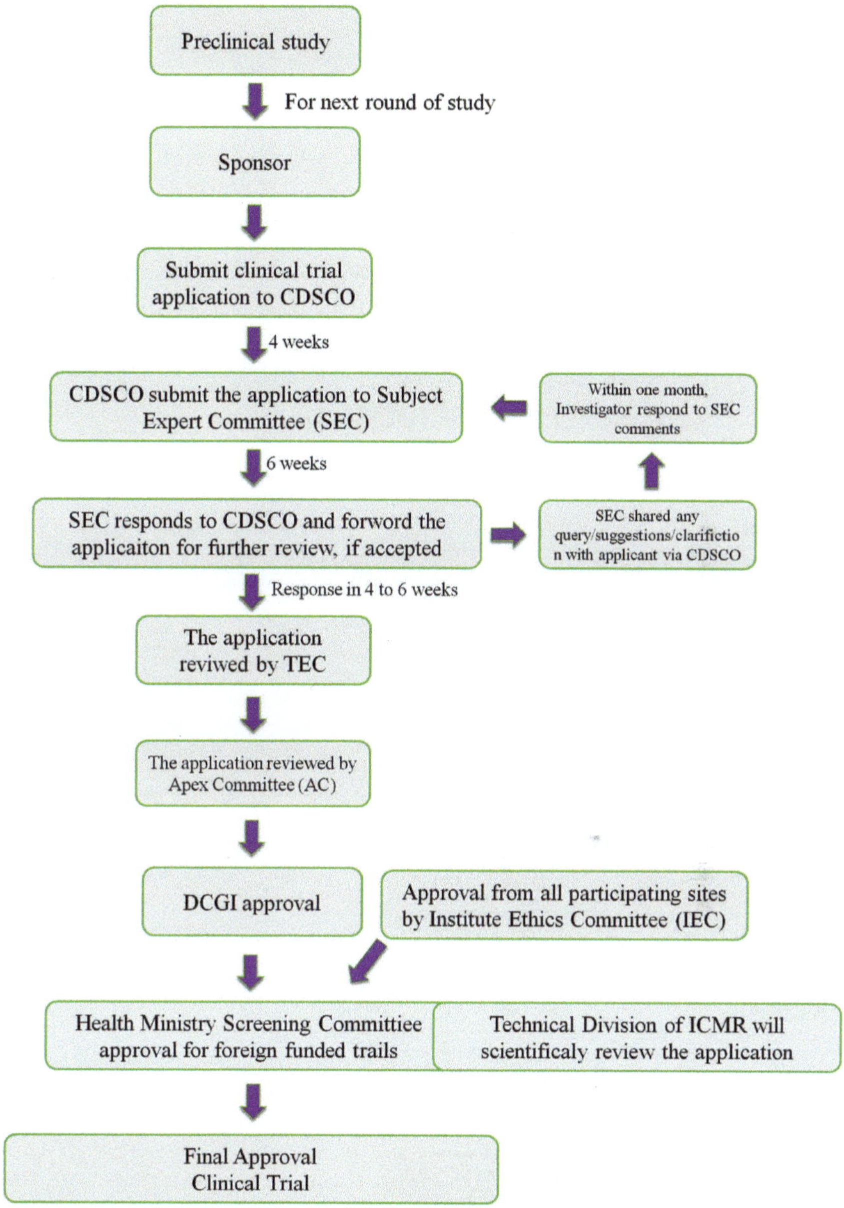

FIG. 16.2 A step-by-step process of vaccine regulatory approval by DCGI, CDSCO in India.

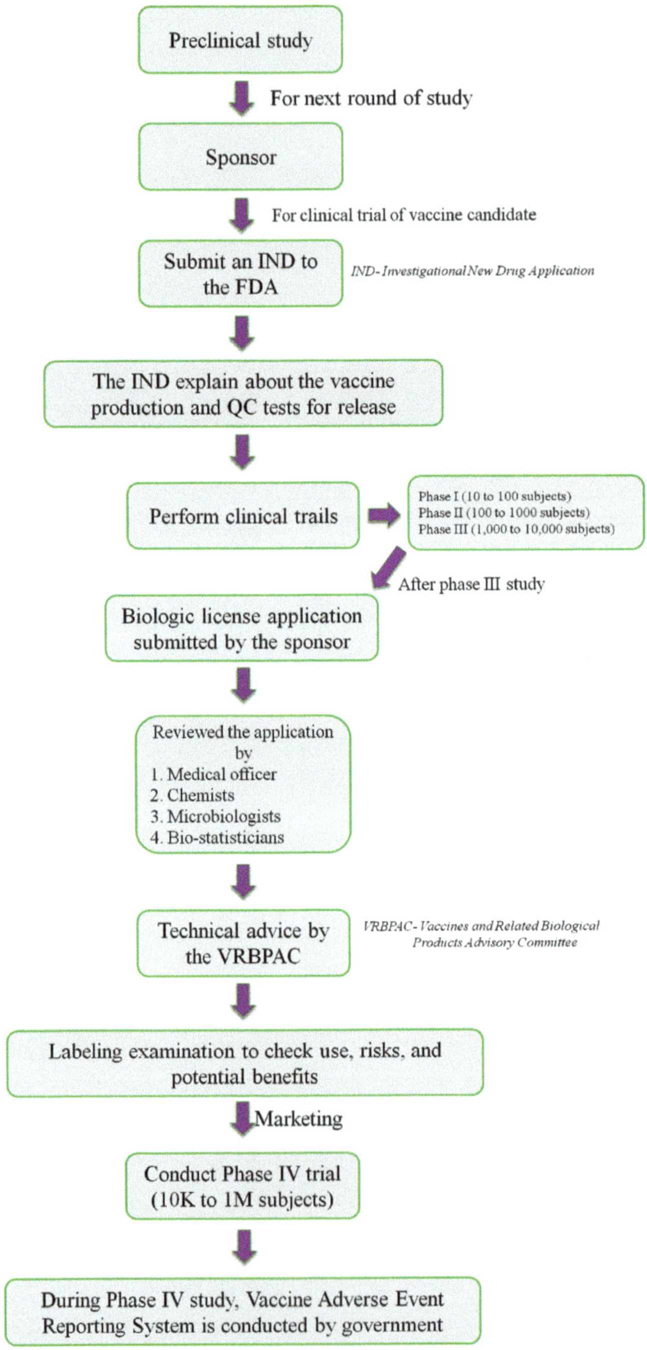

FIG. 16.3 Vaccine regulatory approval process by FDA in the United States.

Without FDA approval, the manufacturer is not authorized to distribute a specific lot of vaccines [32]. Distribution and supply of the product (vaccine) is in the control of national agencies (NRA). NRA releases the vaccine lot, and National Immunization Programme (NIP) takes responsibility from its appropriate storage to vaccine administration to the target people. An important part of the vaccine supply is maintaining a robust, reliable, and routinely monitored cold-chain, the system between manufacturer and end-user. Fig. 16.4 depicts the standard way of supplying vaccines in India and other countries. Individuals have a moral responsibility to get vaccinated, at least against certain infectious diseases in pandemic circumstances.

16.7 Vaccination ethics and issues

A vaccine is an effective tool to protect human health from infection [14]. It is an individual's moral duty to get vaccinated against certain infectious diseases to save others' lives. If 90%–95% of the population of any country/world gets immunized against a specific disease, it might stop the spreading of the disease and prevent the pandemic from making havoc. It also leads to "herd immunity" generation and keeps the checks on a pathogen to survive. Vaccination is the most successful medical approach that is capable of eliminating disease effectively [1,2]. Vaccination should be performed effectively,

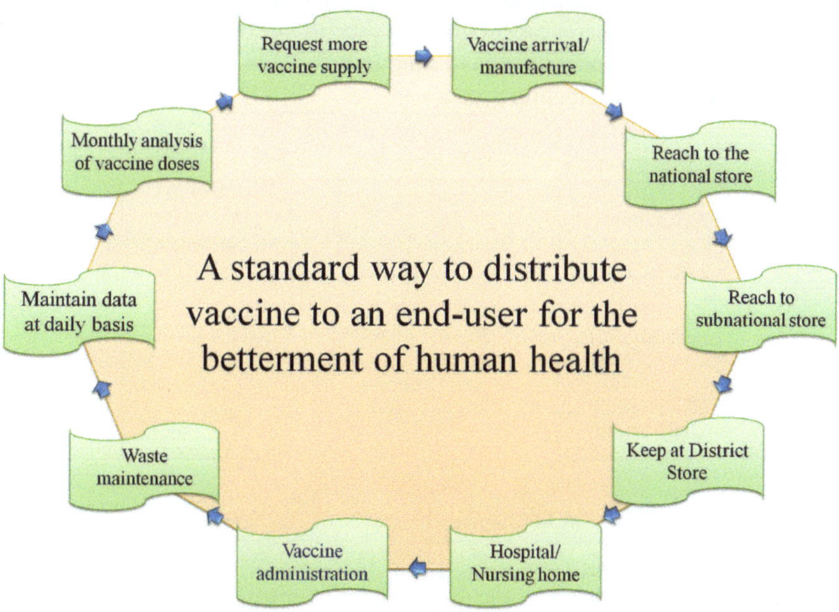

FIG. 16.4 An overview of standard vaccine supply from manufacturer to the end-user, followed by most national and international agencies.

efficiently, and with NRAs guidelines [10,33,34]. A few criteria's for effective global vaccination are;

1. The vaccine should be approved by the WHO or its authorized regulatory agencies.
2. Production of the vaccine should be on a large scale.
3. Prices must be affordable by common people, or government should provide the vaccine freely.
4. Proper infrastructure and efficient distribution of the vaccine at health centers.
5. Public must be aware of the benefits and harms of the vaccine.
6. Vaccine should be available wherever is required.
7. Reduce morbidity and mortality.
8. No political and individual influence in the vaccine use.
9. The vaccine should be available globally.

But the government policies, socio-economic consequences, myths, rumors, political influences, lack of public awareness, IPR issues, and many other reasons evoke specific ethical issues in the use and distribution of vaccines [9,10,33,35,36]. To minimize the conflicts in any vaccination program, the ethical principles (Fig. 16.5) need to be followed as:

1. Review and evaluate the vaccination by health jurisdiction.
2. Use of non-compulsory vaccination approach.
3. Vaccine safety concerns and benefits need to be discussed in public.
4. Conduct public awareness program of vaccine-preventable disease risks.
5. Make the public understand herd immunity.
6. Fairness in the vaccination process.

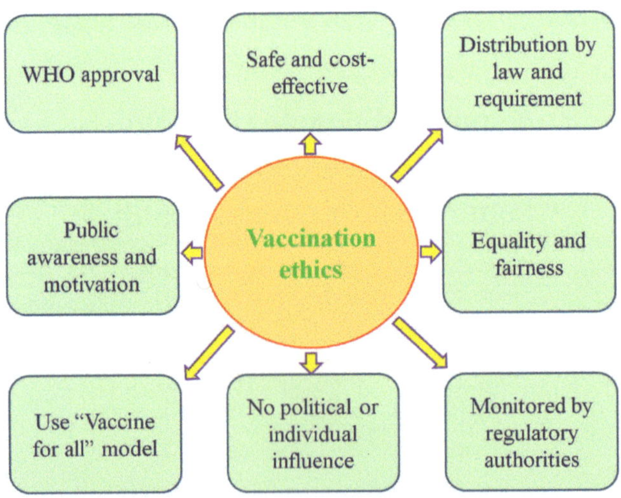

FIG. 16.5 A schematic representation of ideal vaccination ethics.

7. Distribute vaccines as per the requirement.
8. Autonomy-Patients should be informed about the benefits and risks of the vaccine.
9. The vaccination process does not harm the patients.
10. People need to be treated equally and fairly.
11. During pandemics and emergencies, the vaccine should be given to Health care personnel first and later to essential services personnel, a person with high-risk medical conditions, elderly individuals, and others.
12. Research and regular testing by the manufacturer as well as regulatory authorities.
13. The main aim of any vaccination program is to achieve herd immunity.
14. Vaccination should be performed as per the WHO guidelines.
15. Vaccine for all.

16.8 Vaccine for animal health

Vaccination is an effective way to overcome the disease burden in animals and pets [37,38]. Vaccinating animals is the easiest way to protect and provide a healthy life. Several vaccines such as West Nile virus (horse), avian influenza virus (birds), Apex-IHN (salmon), Ovastem (ewes), Suvaxyn PCV2 (pigs), feline leukemia virus (cat), etc., are available for animals [38–40]. World Small Animal Veterinary Association, The National Office of Animal Health (British), National Animal Disease Control Programme of The Department of Animal Husbandry and Dairying (India), Animal and Plant Health Inspection Service (USA), etc., are regulating the vaccine development program worldwide [41–43].

Vaccines have become an essential part of our life to keep us healthy. Vaccination makes a disease-free nation and also helps in the overall development of the country. The regulatory agencies play a vital role in vaccine development, vaccine regulations, vaccine distribution, and post-marketing analysis. Therefore, a robust vaccine regulatory system with considerate ethical issues is the key to a healthier and happy life in society.

Acknowledgment

Hemant Arya thanks the Indian Council of Medical Research (ICMR), Government of India, for the Research Associate Fellowship (Project ID: 2019-6285; File No. ISRM/11(35)/2019).

References

[1] Bartlett BL, Pellicane AJ, Tyring SK. Vaccine immunology. Dermatol Ther 2009;22(2):104–9. doi:10.1111/j.1529-8019.2009.01223.x.

[2] Plotkin SA. Vaccines: past, present and future. Nat Med 2005;11(S4):S5–S11. https://doi.org/10.1038/nm1209.

[3] Akan H, Bruns T, Pletz MW. Vaccine-Preventable Diseases. In: Cornely OA, Hoenigl M (eds) Infection Management in Hematology. Hematologic Malignancies. Springer, Cham. 2021:57–75. https://doi.org/10.1007/978-3-030-57317-1_6.

[4] Pollard AJ, Bijker EM. A guide to vaccinology: from basic principles to new developments. Nat Rev Immunol 2021;21(2):83–100. https://doi.org/10.1038/s41577-020-00479-7.
[5] Kumar P, Sharma P. Role of vaccines on human health—a review. SSR Inst Int J Life Sci 2019;5(1):2122–5. https://doi.org/10.21276/SSR-IIJLS.2019.5.1.1.
[6] Abath FGC, Montenegro SML, Gomes YM. Vaccines against human parasitic diseases: an overview. Acta Trop 1998;71(3):237–54. https://doi.org/10.1016/S0001-706X(98)00066-7.
[7] Doherty M, Buchy P, Standaert B, Giaquinto C, Prado-Cohrs D. Vaccine impact: benefits for human health. Vaccine 2016;34(52):6707–14. https://doi.org/10.1016/j.vaccine.2016.10.025.
[8] Oliveira LVN, Wang R, Specht CA, Levitz SM. Vaccines for human fungal diseases: close but still a long way to go. Npj Vaccines 2021;6(1):33. https://doi.org/10.1038/s41541-021-00294-8.
[9] Greenwood B. The contribution of vaccination to global health: past, present and future. Philosophical Trans Royal Society B: Biol Sci 2014;369(1645):20130433. https://doi.org/10.1098/rstb.2013.0433.
[10] Largeron N, Lévy P, Wasem J, Bresse X. Role of vaccination in the sustainability of healthcare systems. J Market Access Health Pol 2015;3(1):27043. https://doi.org/10.3402/jmahp.v3.27043.
[11] Gruber M, Marshall V. Regulation and testing of vaccines. In: Plotkin S, Orenstein W, Offit P, et al., (eds) Plotkin's Vaccines, Elsevier, Philadelphia, PA; 2017. pp. 1547–1565. https://doi.org/10.1016/B978-0-323-35761-6.00079-1.
[12] Marshall V, Baylor NW. Food and drug administration regulation and evaluation of vaccines. Pediatrics 2011;127(Supplement):S23–30. https://doi.org/10.1542/peds.2010-1722E.
[13] Singh K, Mehta S. The clinical development process for a novel preventive vaccine: An overview. J Postgrad Med 2016;62(1):4. https://doi.org/10.4103/0022-3859.173187.
[14] Ada GL. The ideal vaccine. World J Microbiol Biotechnol 1991;7(2):105–9. https://doi.org/10.1007/BF00328978.
[15] Clem A. Fundamentals of vaccine immunology. J Global Infectious Dis 2011;3(1):73. https://doi.org/10.4103/0974-777X.77299.
[16] Patronov A, Doytchinova I. T-cell epitope vaccine design by immunoinformatics. FEBS Open Bio 2013;3(1):120139. https://doi.org/10.1098/rsob.120139.
[17] Prugnola A. Vaccine design. Trends Biotechnol 1994;12(6):251. https://doi.org/10.1016/0167-7799(94)90132-5.
[18] Huang Z, Wang X, Liu Q. Vaccine development. In: The Norovirus, Academic Press; 2017: 187–206. https://doi.org/10.1016/B978-0-12-804177-2.00013-0.
[19] Leroux-Roels G, Bonanni P, Tantawichien T, Zepp F. Vaccine development. Perspectives Vaccinol 2011;1(1):115–50. https://doi.org/10.1016/j.pervac.2011.05.005.
[20] Gogtay NJ, Dhingra MS, Yadav A, Chandwani H. Vaccine policy, regulations and safety in India. Int J Risk Safety Med 2009;21(1–2):23–30. https://doi.org/10.3233/JRS-2009-0457.
[21] Singh K, Mehta S. The clinical development process for a novel preventive vaccine: An overview. Postgrad Med 2016;62(1):4. https://doi.org/10.4103/0022-3859.173187.
[22] Nafian F, Nafian S, Kamali Doust Azad B. Regulatory and biosafety challenges for vaccines. Iran J Med Microbiol 2020;14(1):17–29. https://doi.org/10.30699/ijmm.14.1.17.
[23] World Health Organization. Regulation of vaccines: building on existing drug regulatory authorities. Geneva, Switzerland: World Health Organization; 1999.
[24] Ruffin MT, Hausman BL. Vaccine refusals and regulations. Fam Med 2019;51(9):785. https://doi.org/10.22454/FamMed.2019.959213.
[25] Sathyanarayana SD, Fernandes SD, Castelino LJ, Vadakkepushpakath AN, Shriram RG. Vaccines in the United States: a systematic review on history of evolution, regulations, licensing, and future challenges. Clin Exp Vaccine Res 2020;9(2):69. https://doi.org/10.7774/cevr.2020.9.2.69.

[26] Sivanandan S, Jain K, Plakkal N, Bahl M, Sahoo T, Mukherjee S, Gupta YK, Agarwal R. Issues, challenges, and the way forward in conducting clinical trials among neonates: investigators' perspective. J Perinatol 2019;39(S1):20–30. https://doi.org/10.1038/s41372-019-0469-8.

[27] Anderson S. An FDA-CBER Update on Surveillance, epidemiology and risk management approaches for biologics. DIA PV and Risk Management Strategies Conference; 2020:1–25.

[28] CQ Press. Centers for Medicare and Medicaid Services. In: Federal Regulatory Guide CQ Press; 2020, pp. 728–33. https://doi.org/10.4135/9781544377230.n80.

[29] Lang J, Cluff L, Payne J, Matson-Koffman D, Hampton J. The Centers for Disease Control and Prevention. J Occupat Environ Med 2017;59(7):631–41. https://doi.org/10.1097/JOM.0000000000001045.

[30] Salman O, Topf K, Chandler R, Conklin L. Progress in Immunization Safety Monitoring—Worldwide, 2010–2019. MMWR. Morbidity and Mortality Weekly Report, 2021;70(15), 547–551. https://doi.org/10.15585/mmwr.mm7015a2

[31] Singh RB. A comparision of US, Europe, Japan and India Biosimilar regulations. Int J Drug Develop Res 2013;5(2):35–9.

[32] WHO. Guideline on the international packaging and shipping of vaccines. *World Health Organization*, 2005;30. http://whqlibdoc.who.int/hq/2005/WHO_IVB_05.23_eng.pdf.

[33] Giubilini A. Vaccination ethics. Br Med Bull 2021;137(1):4–12. https://doi.org/10.1093/bmb/ldaa036.

[34] Schwartz JL, Caplan AL. Ethics of vaccination programs. Curr Opin Virol 2011;1(4):263–7. https://doi.org/10.1016/j.coviro.2011.05.009.

[35] Quilici S, Smith R, Signorelli C. Role of vaccination in economic growth. J Market Access Health Policy 2015;3(1):27044. https://doi.org/10.3402/jmahp.v3.27044.

[36] Wouters OJ, Shadlen KC, Salcher-Konrad M, Pollard AJ, Larson HJ, Teerawattananon Y, Jit M. Challenges in ensuring global access to COVID-19 vaccines: production, affordability, allocation, and deployment. Lancet North Am Ed 2021;397(10278):1023–34. https://doi.org/10.1016/S0140-6736(21)00306-8.

[37] Francis MJ. A veterinary vaccine development process map to assist in the development of new vaccines. Vaccine 2020;38(29):4512–5. https://doi.org/10.1016/j.vaccine.2020.05.007.

[38] McVey S, Shi J. Vaccines in Veterinary Medicine: A Brief Review of History and Technology. Veterinary Clinics North America: Small Animal Practice 2010;40(3):381–92. https://doi.org/10.1016/j.cvsm.2010.02.001.

[39] Crisci E, Bárcena J, Montoya M. Virus-like particles: the new frontier of vaccines for animal viral infections. Vet Immunol Immunopathol 2012;148(3–4):211–25. https://doi.org/10.1016/j.vetimm.2012.04.026.

[40] Yang D-K, Kim H-H, Lee K-W, Song J-Y. The present and future of rabies vaccine in animals. Clinical Exp Vaccine Res 2013;2(1):19. https://doi.org/10.7774/cevr.2013.2.1.19.

[41] CQ Press. Animal and Plant Health Inspection Service. In: Federal Regulatory Guide CQ Press; 2020, pp. 593–8. https://doi.org/10.4135/9781544377230.n44.

[42] Dent N, Visanji R. National Office of Animal Health. In: Veterinary Clinical Trials From Concept to Completion CRC Press; 2001, pp. 333–6. https://doi.org/10.1201/9781482294170-35.

[43] Niemiec B, Gawor J, Nemec A, Clarke D, McLeod K, Tutt C, Gioso M, Steagall PV, Chandler M, Morgenegg G, Jouppi R. World small animal veterinary association global dental guidelines. J Small Anim Pract 2020;61(7). doi:10.1111/jsap.13132.

Chapter 17

Future of system vaccinology

Dhaneswar Prusty
Department of Biochemistry, School of Life, Sciences, Central University of Rajasthan, Ajmer, India

17.1 Introduction

Human civilization has been challenged with major pandemics, including cholera, plague, dengue, and influenza. We have experienced the loss of human life, millions of working hours, and economic growth throughout the last decade due to disease outbreaks and pandemics created by viruses including Zika, Ebola, H7N9, and SARS. The deadliest pandemic of Spanish flu of 1918 infected one-third of the world population and took 50 million lives [1]. The first known cases of SARS CoV-2 occurred in Dec 2019 in Wuhan, China. In just a few months, the virus made its way throughout the globe, even though the mode of viral transmission was well known. As of Sep. 14, 2021, the viral pandemic claimed 226,844,344 cases and 4,666,334 deaths worldwide, reported to WHO. There was no proper medication for the disease; however, the global effort at finding an effective vaccine happened at a pandemic speed. The advanced knowledge of system vaccinology, nucleic acid vaccine platform, viral vectors, and licensed adjuvants allowed many effective vaccine candidates to be developed in an unprecedented time limit [2]. As per the WHO report, 5,634,533,040 vaccine doses were administered until Sep. 14, 2021, resulting in a significant death rates decline.

Similarly, vaccines have been proven to bring a "paradigm shift" in diminishing mortality and morbidity of many infectious diseases in world history. In the view of the dynamic relationships between host-pathogen leads to host switching, the emergence of new life-threatening infectious agents and their rapid spread remains a potential threat to human civilization. The development and production of the vaccine, the best pharmaceutical product to counter emerging infections, are costly and time-consuming processes. Hence, the central agenda of now and in the future is to develop effective, safe, and new generation vaccines quickly. In recent years, the design of new generation vaccines has been revolutionized by the system vaccinology. This chapter has discussed how system vaccinology can guide every step of vaccine development, beginning from

System Vaccinology. https://doi.org/10.1016/B978-0-323-85941-7.00013-9

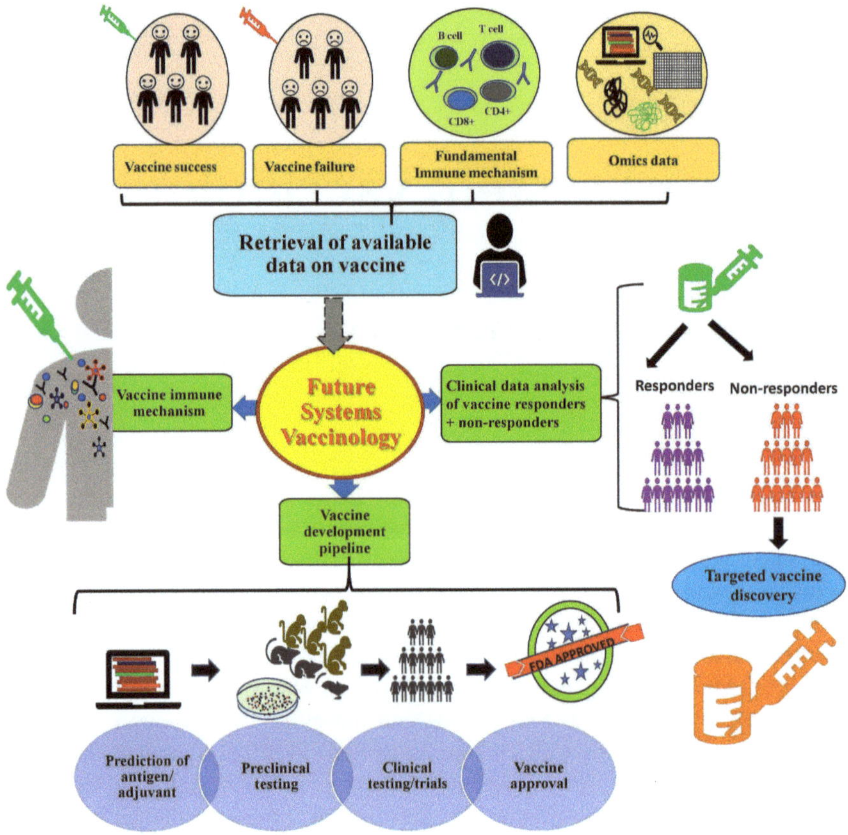

FIG. 17.1 Future aspects of system vaccinology in diverse field of vaccine research.

antigen prediction to the final stage of clinical trials, for faster development of new generation vaccines. Furthermore, the application of system vaccinology will reveal the molecular mechanism of clinical success and failures of different vaccines to fine-tune future vaccine development (Fig. 17.1).

17.2 System vaccinology: a rational approach to reduce time and cost of vaccine development

In the current decade, emerging and re-emerging viral diseases resulting from dynamic interplays of host-parasite interactions demand faster vaccine development to control and prevent the diseases. Developing a new vaccine is a resource-intensive and lengthy process of about 10 years [3]. Divergence regulatory requirements in different countries for clinical trials and approvals are complex issues that significantly delay developing novel vaccines. A systemic analysis of the cost of vaccine development from preclinical trials to phase 2a, assuming no risk of failure, for a single infectious disease indicated a cost of US$31-68 million [4]. In addition to that, as clinical trials are conducted in healthy individuals, safety issues are a significant concern. The timing of vaccine availability to combat a pandemic has been incredibly realized in the era of COVID-19. The danger of allergenic reactions is associated with traditional techniques such as inactivated or live-attenuated vaccines [5].

The recent advancements in proteomics, transcriptomics, bioinformatics, structural biology, immunogenomics, and immunoinformatics allow system vaccinology, over traditional vaccinology, to offer a computational speed in vaccine development through various rational designing methods. Vast numbers of servers and software tools are now available to study several antigenic and physiological properties of vaccine candidate proteins of dangerous microorganisms. In order to reduce the time and cost of vaccine development, the best vaccine candidates obtained from system biology studies can be tested for their immunogenicity and safety by employing various in vitro and in vivo assays [6]. An excellent example of how system vaccinology can revolutionize vaccine developments is the H7N9 influenza vaccine. In the influenza pandemics series of H2N2 (1957), H3N2 (1968), and H1N1 (2009), every time new vaccine development missed the timing to challenge the pandemic at its peak. In 2013, when WHO declared the outbreak of the H7N9 influenza virus, a team of scientists of the J. Craig Venter Institute in San Diego, California, could do cell-free synthesis of two vaccine candidates genes such as neuraminidase and hemagglutinin by accessing sequencing data published by the Chinese Center for Disease Control and Prevention [7]. Later these synthetic genes were transferred to scientists of Novartis Vaccines, Massachusetts, which resulted in the development of synthetic RNA vaccine in a record time of one week [8].

During the COVID-19 pandemic, the SARS-CoV-2 genome sequence was posted by scientists from Fudan University and their collaborators in January 2020. The availability of genomic sequence information of the virus translated to the development of around 200 vaccines in a short time. The remarkable advances in reverse vaccinology together with structural vaccinology, synthetic biology, and vaccine adjuvants, allowed the development of several vaccines at a pandemic speed [9]. Thus system vaccinology retains the potential to make significant value additions in terms of quality and speed required for vaccine development to respond to any future pandemics.

17.3 System vaccinology: a guide in the vaccine development chain

Vaccine development usually is a complicated process that is accomplished in five standard phases such as (1) exploratory, (2) preclinical, (3) clinical development, (4) approval, and (5) pharmacovigilance. The application of system vaccinology can enhance the accuracy and qualities of most vaccine development phases to avoid any possible late-stage failure.

Exploratory is the first and research-intensive stage intended to find natural or synthetic antigens that can trigger an immune response capable of preventing or treating a disease. System vaccinology does the comprehensive qualitative, and quantitative analysis of vaccine composition, including antigen and adjuvant based on data sets obtained through cell-mediated responses, transcriptomics, proteomics, and metabolomics. At present, there are various alternative system vaccinology websites and downloadable software available for selecting the best antigen(s) based on different antigenic and physiochemical properties. It is important to mention that system vaccinology primarily identifies protein antigenic molecules. Host cells related to the immune system recognize and interact with proteins present on the surface of pathogens; thus, the proteins present on the pathogen's plasma membrane can be better antigens to generate protective responses [10]. In addition to various software tools such as ANTIGENpro and AllerTop that use amino acid sequence information, protein databases such as eSLDB, LocDB, and LOCATE provide useful information to find out membrane-localized proteins. Adhesin properties have also been considered as an important criterion for some vaccine candidates, so vaccine target prediction programs predict the adhesin probability of proteins [11]. The expression and purification of proteins with more than one transmembrane are complex [12]; thus, proteins with a low transmembrane helix are filtered for vaccine designing. The similarity between the amino acid sequence of the antigen under study and with the host and other etiological agents have different effects. The high degree similarity with the host is undesirable as it may induce an autoimmune response, whereas the high degree of similarity with other etiological agents is preferred as it can develop cross-protection. The pathogen-induced immune response is of two kinds: cellular or humoral, depending on different pathogens. The knowledge obtained through the insightful analysis of pathogen-induced response enables system vaccinology to identify biomarkers and mechanisms required for the infection's natural clearance.

Further, this information is quite helpful to examine the desired vaccine-induced response such as cellular response for tuberculosis or Leishmaniasis vaccine [13,14] and humoral response for influenza or HIV [15,16]. In order to identify vaccine candidates for induction of cellular response, software including TEpredict, ProPred-I, MAPPP, GPS-MBA, PREDIVA identify antigens that can be presented by major histocompatibility complex (MHC) of T cells. Similarly, software including BCEP, IgPred, PEPITO, BCPREDS, and BEpro predict sequential epitope for B cells, and Websites including DiscoTope, SEPPA, and CEP, search conformational epitopes for B cells. Furthermore, based on the similarity of amino sequence and physiochemical properties with known antigens with higher in vivo and in vitro immune responses, the antigenicity of proteins can be independently evaluated [17]. There is a constant need for adjuvants to combine with protein subunit vaccines to elicit the expected vaccine-induced immune response. The molecular markers, pathways, and immune cell subset activities induced by the use of adjuvants have been studied by different proteomic [18] and transcriptomic [19] approaches. In the first system-based studies on the adjuvant-induced response of MF59, a-GalCer, CpG ODN, and alum, it has been demonstrated that CpG showed a profound, systematic immune response as compared to alum and MF59 [20]. With reference to the vaccine-induced molecular signatures in animal models, system vaccinology has also been applied to compare the potency of adjuvatted vaccine and simple antigen alone [21].

System vaccinology can assist the evaluation of the vaccine-induced immune response, referring to the molecular and cellular signatures of the effective infection-induced immunity. For example, the molecular signature of B. pertussis infection, such as induction of T helper type 17 (Th17) cells and mucosal IgA responses and activation of the innate immune system marked by the pulmonary recruitment of Th17 cells and CCR6+ B-cells are used for comparative network analysis [22]. It has been demonstrated that the Outer Membrane Vesicle Pertussis vaccine (omvPV) caused similar immune responses but with different kinetics and intensity [23]. This comparative network analysis worked as an evaluator for concluding the better protection power of omvPV than the cutaneous vaccine. Furthermore, immune responses such as polyfunctional CD8+ T cells and neutralizing antibodies are the molecular signatures of many vaccines. Thus system vaccinology can utilize such predictive signatures of protective immunity to develop vaccine chips for rapid screening of vaccines [24].

System vaccinology would be of great value in different phases of clinical trials by providing predictive markers to assess safety and efficacy rapidly. A system-based gene expression profile analysis of human blood of over 500 studies was curated to identify universal signatures of antibody and cellular mediated immune response of different vaccines. In that study, the 334 Blood Transcription Module (BTMs) analysis indicated that inactivated vaccines induce an antibody response associated with plasmablast differentiation. In contrast, live-attenuated vaccines have been shown to induce antibody response mediated by innate immunity and type-1 interferon [25]. Further, a database "MSigDB" was created to provide information related to immunologic signatures specifying a wide range of activation and suppression of genes of the immune system cells [26]. Regulatory bodies study the adverse reactions caused by vaccines before approval. Any severe adverse reactions are not acceptable. System vaccinology can assist study vaccines' safety by identifying clinical and genetic markers related to adverse reactions. For instance, Immunological characterization of immune response of yellow fever vaccination demonstrated that 1 in 250,000 cases had a fatal viscerotropic disease caused by the 200-fold elevation of CD14+CD16+ inflammatory monocytes [27]. Similarly, the investigation on incidences of narcolepsy arisen in response to the swine influenza A (H1N1) vaccination campaign with Pandemrix showed an association of genetic marker HLA-DQB1*06:02 genotype with the Pandemrix-induced narcolepsy [28]. These findings led to the belief that system vaccinology studies of such predictive clinical and genetic markers are essential for assessing any possible severe adverse reactions of a vaccine. Considering the practical applicability of system vaccinology for studying the reactogenicity and efficacy of vaccines, a unique public-private partnership project entitled "BIOVACSAFE" was initiated in 2011. This project will identify biomarkers for clinical evaluation of reactogenicity related to post-immunization and natural infection [29].

The early correlation of reactogenicity of a new vaccine with the reactogenicity molecular signatures of approved vaccines obtained from post-marketing surveillance studies will be valuable for predicting the further clinical development of a vaccine. System vaccinology is yet to define the molecular signatures induced during early vaccination to predict the future adaptive immune response. However, some pioneering studies have shown that the gene expression profiles of blood within the first week of vaccination could predict the antibody titers and antigen-specific CD8+ T-cell levels of post-60-days of immunization [30–32]. In a clinical phase study of two seasonal influenza vaccine formulations such as MF59-adjuvanted TIV (ATIV) and trivalent inactivated influenza vaccine (TIV), it has been shown that the antibody titers of post-one-month immunization can be predicted from the analysis of specific immune signatures related to plasmablasts and innate immunity [33,34].

17.4 System vaccinology: a tool to reveal the mechanism of vaccine action

How the immune system senses empirically designed successful vaccine remains elusive [35,36]. In addition, wide variations remain in the vaccine efficacy among people of a given region [37], which is sometimes up to 100-fold [38]. Vaccine immunogenicity also varies among different regions of the world. For example, immunity obtained by vaccines designed for malaria, yellow fever, rotavirus, and poliomyelitis provides better protection to people of the United States and Europe than people of Asia and Africa [39–42]. Similarly, the BCG vaccine has been reported to be more effective in Europe than in Africa [43,44]. In this scenario, system vaccinology can do a meaningful analysis of a sea of data obtained by vaccinologists, immunologists, clinicians, and systems biologists to reveal the possible immunological mechanisms underlying the efficacy of successful vaccines and variations in vaccine efficacy. Vaccine immunity is determined by the complex interplay of genetics, metabolic state, and an individual's microbiota. Several new insights into the mechanism of vaccine-induced immune response have been made by finding the set of genes differentially regulated upon vaccination with different vaccines. Therefore, to facilitate the immunogenomics studies, the Immunological Genome Project was established in 2008 [45]. A gene transcriptional profile analysis of peripheral blood mononuclear cells (PBMCs) of yellow fever vaccine (YF-17D) vaccinated individuals identified several immune genes, including signal transducer and activator of transcription 1 (STAT1), transcription factors that regulate the expression of type I IFNs, IRF7, and innate sensing receptors (i.e., TLR7, RIG-I) involved in antiviral immunity [46,47]. Moreover, in the same study, a group of transcription factors was recognized that regulate the early immune response to the YF-17D vaccine. Later ETS2 was found to be upregulated in activated and proliferating T cells for induction of IL-5 (Th2) and IL-12 p40 (Th1) gene expression [48,49]. The genes required for differentiation and maturation of macrophages NK cells, T cells, and B cells were also identified [47]. Further investigation revealed that YF-17D vaccine-induced amplification of antibody titers and antigen-specific CD8+ T-cell responses had a strong correlation with the expression profile of two genes—eukaryotic translation initiation factor 2 α kinase 4 (EIF2AK4) and solute carrier family 2, member 6 (SLC2A6) [46]. Subsequent animal model studies have demonstrated that the activation of EIF2AK4, also identified as the general control nonderepressible 2 kinase (GCN2) plays an important role in enhanced CD8+ T cells and programming of dendrtitic cells to intiate autophagy [57]. System-level approaches have also been used to understand genetic signatures induced by virus-like particle (VLP)-based HIV vaccines in monocyte-derived DCs (MDDCs) and PBMCs. Several regulatory genes involved in antiviral immunity such as transcription factors for the expression of IRF1, STAT2, and type I IFNs and innate sensing of viruses, including TLR2 (innate sensing receptor), were reported to be upregulated [50–52]. Genetic polymorphisms can adversely affect the immune system and alter host-pathogen interactions and molecular signaling [53]. The effect of TLRs' single nucleotide polymorphisms (SNPs) on immune response to measles vaccination has been well studied. The SNP in the 3' UTR of TLR3 was found to be associated with low cellular and humoral to the vaccine [54]. It has also been reported that allele variants of MyD88, intracellular adapter involved in signaling TLRs, caused by SNPs influenced lower antibody response to the vaccine [54]. A similar study was also conducted to investigate the effect of polymorphism in intronic regions and promoter regions of TLR4 and TLR3 on vaccine immunity of the rubella vaccine. Two SNPs of TLR3 gene were found to alter the secretion of IFN-γ [55]. Interestingly, those SNPs also reported to cause low lymphoproliferative responses to measles vaccine [54]. The association of antibody response to pertussis (PT) vaccine and SNPs of TLR4 gene's promoter and its signaling cascade gene's has been well studied [56,57]. Furthermore, the effects of SNPs in the TOLLIP gene on PT vaccine-induced antibody response found to be linked with its biological role. TOLLIP, a small protein, coordinates optimal signaling through IL-1 receptor type I (IL-1RI) and TLR4 by binding with the activated TLR2, TLR4, and IL-1RI complexes [58,59]. Similarly, the SNPs of the TLR signaling pathway's modulator proteins such as TIRAP and TICAM1 as well as SNPs of the Toll and IL-1R family member proteins such as IRAK4 and IRAK3 have been observed to influence the immune response to PT vaccine [56,57]. All these studies are strongly indicating that genetic polymorphisms in the TLR signaling pathway remain important factors underlying the heterogeneous immune response to vaccines. Hence, such comprehensive system-level analysis will address the cause of eventual failures of vaccines at different trial levels and assist the formulation of suitable antigens and antigen-adjuvant mixture to deal with people having genetic variants in immune signaling pathways.

The robust connectivity between the metabolism and the immune response has been well established [60,61]. Emerging shreds of evidence emphasize the role of metabolic disorders such as obesity [62,63] and undernutrition [64–66] in eliciting defects in immune responses. It has been found that the sensors such as heme-regulated inhibitor kinase, GCN2, and R-like endoplasmic reticulum kinase are shared for both environmental stress and pathogen-induced stress [25,67]. As metabolic disorders, including obesity, are rising worldwide, systems vaccinology can play a critical role in delineating the poorly understood effects of metabolic disorders on vaccine-induced protective immunity.

Through immunological stimuli, many diverse microbial communities, settled in all the epithelial cell surfaces, including skin, lung, and gut, potentially impact the host immune system to develop immunological imprints from a very early stage of life. The local and distal impacts of microbiota on host immune response and their influences on vaccine-induced immune protection are recently reviewed elsewhere [68]. An increasing number of studies indicate that microbiota modulates immunity to a vaccine [69]. The gut microbiome profoundly interacts with live-attenuated microorganisms of oral vaccines and thereby potentially influences the immune responsiveness of the vaccines [70]. Evidence for the role of a particular species of gut bacteria in vaccine responses has been obtained from studies in Bangladesh, Pakistan, and Ghana. There were differences in immune responses to oral rotavirus vaccination due to microbiota composition between non-responders and responders among Pakistani and Ghanian infants [71,72]. Furthermore, the dominant effect of Bifidobacterium colonization in early infancy was reflected in the immune response to the oral route-based polio vaccine, tetanus toxoid, BCG vaccine, and hepatitis B virus vaccine [73,74]. However, the extent to which the lung microbiota impacts the response to a live-attenuated vaccine, such as influenza vaccine, administered through the intranasal route remains to be seen.

The identification of microbiota-induced specific immune signals for determining vaccine efficacy in humans has been a difficult task. However, shreds of evidence for the role of microbiota in response to different vaccines in the animal models provide the cues to identify similar immune mechanisms in humans. In an oral immunization model study, Belkaid and colleagues have demonstrated a reduction in Th1 and Th17 responses to mutant *Escherichia coli* heat-labile toxin, LT(R192G/L211A due to depletion of gut microbiota [75,76]. Similar studies have shown that antigen-specific immunoglobulin G (IgG) production in response to a potent adjuvant, cholera toxin, after internasal immunization is critically regulated by microbiota [77]. The reduction of IgG and IgM antibody responses to the seasonal influenza vaccine in germ-free mice and restoration of the impaired response by the oral constitution by a flagellated strain of *E.coli* further support the robust association of microbiota and vaccine response in animal models [78].

Interestingly, the induction of TLR5, a pattern recognition receptor for flagellin, was observed in PBMCs in response to the seasonal influenza vaccine [38], and vaccine-induced antibody response was impaired in TLR5 knockout mice [78]. The comparative immune response analysis between adjuvanted YF-17D, Tdap, the recombinant hepatitis B, and HIV Env vaccine and non-adjuvanted inactivated polio vaccine indicated that microbiota only enhances the vaccine-induced immune response of non-adjuvanted vaccine [38]. These studies altogether suggest the possible role of microbiota-derived flagellin as a natural adjuvant.

The animal model study has recently shown the detrimental impact of antibiotic-driven dysregulation of the gut microbiota on adjuvanted and live vaccines routinely administered to infants [79]. Further, human cohort system vaccinology studies demonstrated that antibiotics-driven microbiota dysbiosis could cause impairment of seasonal influenza vaccine-induced immune response in individuals without pre-existing immunity [69]. The antibiotics-induced microbiota dysbiosis modulates pro-inflammatory state by inducing AP-1 and NR4A signature in response to seasonal influenza vaccination [69]. The importance of gut microbiota in the production of secondary bile acids from primary bile has been well recognized [80]. Later a significant correlation was noticed between the reduction of secondary bile acid and enhanced NLRP3 and AP-1 signature-based inflammatory activation [68]. Thus, it seems that microbiota affects immune function by direct interactions with immune cells and regulates immune mechanisms by modulation of critical secondary metabolites. The abovementioned system biology approaches to delineate the role of different factors in vaccine function further strengthen the notion that system vaccinology can be an essential tool in exploring the mechanism of successful vaccines and differential vaccine-induced immune protection.

17.5 Conclusion

Besides the increasing demand for effective, safe, and timely vaccines in recent years, there still exists a cascade of challenges starting from vaccine designing to vaccine approval in front of the scientific community and pharma industry. The inaccuracy of vaccines may create public mistrust, leading to a massive hindrance in the public health care system. Rapid improvement in system vaccinology allows rational vaccine (antigen/adjuvant) design, validation of immune response to the vaccine in the experimental/animal model, analytical tools for clinical data analysis, and logistic support for vaccine approval. Publicly available systems vaccinology's servers and analytical tools have further assisted in understanding the immune mechanism of successful vaccines, diverse immune responses to the vaccine of responders and non-responders, vaccine responsiveness of infants, elderly persons, immune-deficient individuals, and healthy individuals. System vaccinology can be significant in proposing a rational vaccine as a starting model for testing at a computational speed by predicting immune response beforehand.

Over the past two decades, researchers have shown the transformative role of system vaccinology in investigating many vaccines designed against infectious diseases caused by *M. tuberculosis* [81], *Plasmodium* spp [82], HIV [83], Ebola virus [84], and other diseases [85]. Such accumulating evidence will undoubtedly generate renewed interest for subsequent application of system vaccinology to develop safe, effective, and timely vaccines for the current and possible health issues.

References

[1] Beach B, Clay K, Saavedra M. The 1918 influenza pandemic and its lessons for COVID-19. J Econ Lit 2022 Mar;60(1):41–84.

[2] Rappuoli R, De Gregorio E, Del Giudice G, Phogat S, Pecetta S, Pizza M, et al. Vaccinology in the post– COVID-19 era. Proc Natl Acad Sci 2021 Jan 19;118(3):1–7.

[3] Rauch S, Jasny E, Schmidt KE, Petsch B. New vaccine technologies to combat outbreak situations. Frontiers in immunology 2018 sep 19;9:1–24.

[4] Gouglas D, Le TT, Henderson K, Kaloudis A, Danielsen T, Hammersland NC, et al. Estimating the cost of vaccine development against epidemic infectious diseases: a cost minimisation study. The Lancet Global Health 2018;6(12):e1386–96.

[5] Khalili S, Jahangiri A, Borna H, Ahmadi Zanoos K, Amani J. Computational vaccinology and epitope vaccine design by immunoinformatics. Acta Microbiol Immunol Hung 2014;61(3):285–307.

[6] Rappuoli R. Reverse vaccinology. Curr Opin Microbiol 2000;3(5):445–50.

[7] Dormitzer PR, Suphaphiphat P, Gibson DG, Wentworth DE, Stockwell TB, Algire MA, et al. Synthetic generation of influenza vaccine viruses for rapid response to pandemics. Sci Transl Med 2013;5(185):185ra168.

[8] Hekele A, Bertholet S, Archer J, Gibson DG, Palladino G, Brito LA, et al. Rapidly produced SAM® vaccine against H7N9 influenza is immunogenic in mice. Emerging Microbes Infections 2013;2(1):1–7.

[9] Rappuoli R, De GE, Del Giudice G, Phogat S, Pecetta S, Pizza M, et al. Vaccinology in the post—COVID-19 era. Proc Natl Acad Sci 2021;118(3):1–7.

[10] Chaudhuri R, Kulshreshtha D, Raghunandanan MV, Ramachandran S. Integrative immunoinformatics for Mycobacterial diseases in R platform. Systems Synthetic Biol 2014;8(1):27–39.

[11] He Y, Xiang Z. Databases and in silico tools for vaccine design. In: Silico Models for Drug Discovery, 993. Springer; 2013:115–27.

[12] Pizza M, Scarlato V, Masignani V, Giuliani MM, Arico B, Comanducci M, et al. Identification of vaccine candidates against serogroup B meningococcus by whole-genome sequencing. Science 2000;287(5459):1816–20.

[13] Pandey K, Sharma M, Saarav I, Singh S, Dutta P, Bhardwaj A, et al. Analysis of the DosR regulon genes to select cytotoxic T lymphocyte epitope specific vaccine candidates using a reverse vaccinology approach. Int J Mycobacteriol 2016;5(1):34–43.

[14] Seyed N, Taheri T, Rafati S. Post-genomics and vaccine improvement for Leishmania. Front Microbiol 2016;7:467.

[15] Rappuoli R, Bottomley MJ, D'Oro U, Finco O, De Gregorio E. Reverse vaccinology 2.0: human immunology instructs vaccine antigen design. J Exp Med 2016;213(4):469–81.
[16] Van Regenmortel MH. An outdated notion of antibody specificity is one of the major detrimental assumptions of the structure-based reverse vaccinology paradigm, which prevented it from helping to develop an effective HIV-1 vaccine. In: HIV/AIDS: Immunochemistry, Reductionism and Vaccine Design, 5. Springer; 2019:205–16.
[17] Doytchinova IA, Flower DR. VaxiJen: a server for prediction of protective antigens, tumour antigens and subunit vaccines. BMC Bioinformat 2007;8(1):1–7.
[18] Kooijman S, Brummelman J, van Els CA, Marino F, Heck AJ, Mommen GP, et al. Novel identified aluminum hydroxide-induced pathways prove monocyte activation and pro-inflammatory preparedness. J Proteomics 2018;175:144–55.
[19] Hancock DG, Shklovskaya E, Guy TV, Falsafi R, Fjell CD, Ritchie W, et al. A systems biology approach to the analysis of subset-specific responses to lipopolysaccharide in dendritic cells. PLoS One 2014;9(6):e100613.
[20] Mosca F, Tritto E, Muzzi A, Monaci E, Bagnoli F, Iavarone C, et al. Molecular and cellular signatures of human vaccine adjuvants. Proc Natl Acad Sci 2008;105(30):10501–6.
[21] Olafsdottir TA, Lindqvist M, Nookaew I, Andersen P, Maertzdorf J, Persson J, et al. Comparative systems analyses reveal molecular signatures of clinically tested vaccine adjuvants. Sci Rep 2016;6(1):1–14.
[22] Raeven RH, Brummelman J, van der Maas L, Tilstra W, Pennings JL, Han WG, et al. Immunological signatures after Bordetella pertussis infection demonstrate importance of pulmonary innate immune cells. PLoS One 2016;11(10):e0164027.
[23] Raeven RH, Brummelman J, Pennings JL, Van Der Maas L, Helm K, Tilstra W, et al. Molecular and cellular signatures underlying superior immunity against Bordetella pertussis upon pulmonary vaccination. Mucosal Immunol 2018;11(3):979–93.
[24] Pulendran B, Li S, Nakaya HI. Systems vaccinology. Immunity 2010;33(4):516–29.
[25] Systems vaccinology: probing humanity's diverse immune systems with vaccines. 2014; 111(34):12300–12306.
[26] Liberzon A, Subramanian A, Pinchback R, Thorvaldsdóttir H, Tamayo P, Mesirov JP. Molecular signatures database (MSigDB) 3.0. Bioinformatics 2011;27(12):1739–40.
[27] Pulendran B, Miller J, Querec TD, Akondy R, Moseley N, Laur O, et al. Case of yellow fever vaccine-associated viscerotropic disease with prolonged viremia, robust adaptive immune responses, and polymorphisms in CCR5 and RANTES genes. J Infect Dis 2008;198(4):500–7.
[28] Hallberg P, Smedje H, Eriksson N, Kohnke H, Daniilidou M, Öhman I, et al. Pandemrix-induced narcolepsy is associated with genes related to immunity and neuronal survival. EBioMed 2019;40:595–604.
[29] Lewis DJ, Lythgoe MP. Application of "systems vaccinology" to evaluate inflammation and reactogenicity of adjuvanted preventative vaccines. Journal of immunology research 2015;2015:1–11.
[30] Nakaya HI, Wrammert J, Lee EK, Racioppi L, Marie-Kunze S, Haining WN, et al. Systems biology of vaccination for seasonal influenza in humans. Nat Immunol 2011; 12(8):786–95.
[31] Querec TD, Akondy RS, Lee EK, Cao W, Nakaya HI, Teuwen D, et al. Systems biology approach predicts immunogenicity of the yellow fever vaccine in humans. Nat Immunol 2009;10(1):116–25.
[32] Gaucher D, Therrien R, Kettaf N, Angermann BR, Boucher G, Filali-Mouhim A, et al. Yellow fever vaccine induces integrated multilineage and polyfunctional immune responses. J Exp Med 2008;205(13):3119–31.

[33] Nakaya HI, Clutterbuck E, Kazmin D, Wang L, Cortese M, Bosinger SE, et al. Systems biology of immunity to MF59-adjuvanted versus nonadjuvanted trivalent seasonal influenza vaccines in early childhood. Proc Natl Acad Sci 2016;113(7):1853–8.
[34] Nakaya HI, Hagan T, Duraisingham SS, Lee EK, Kwissa M, Rouphael N, et al. Systems analysis of immunity to influenza vaccination across multiple years and in diverse populations reveals shared molecular signatures. Immunity 2015;43(6):1186–98.
[35] Plotkin SA. Vaccines: past, present and future. Nat Med 2005;11(4):S5–S11.
[36] Rappuoli R. From Pasteur to genomics: progress and challenges in infectious diseases. Nat Med 2004;10(11):1177–85.
[37] Praharaj I, John SM, Bandyopadhyay R, GJPTotRSBBS K. Probiotics, Antibiotics Immune Responses Vaccines 2015;370(1671):20140144.
[38] Nakaya HI, Hagan T, Duraisingham SS, Lee EK, Kwissa M, Rouphael N, et al. Systems analysis of immunity to influenza vaccination across multiple years and in diverse populations reveals shared molecular signatures. 2015;43(6):1186–1198.
[39] Hanlon P, Marsh V, Shenton F, Jobe O, Hayes R, Whittle H, et al. Trial of an attenuated bovine rotavirus vaccine (RIT 4237) in Gambian infants. 1987;329(8546):1342–1345.
[40] Muyanja E, Ssemaganda A, Ngauv P, Cubas R, Perrin H, Srinivasan D, et al. Immune activation alters cellular and humoral responses to yellow fever 17D vaccine. 2014;124(7):3147–3158.
[41] Sissoko MS, Healy SA, Katile A, Omaswa F, Zaidi I, Gabriel EE, et al. Safety and efficacy of PfSPZ Vaccine against Plasmodium falciparum via direct venous inoculation in healthy malaria-exposed adults in Mali: a randomised, double-blind phase 1 trial. 2017;17(5):498–509.
[42] Tate JE, Burton AH, Boschi-Pinto C, Steele AD, Duque J, Parashar U. 2008 estimate of worldwide rotavirus-associated mortality in children younger than 5 years before the introduction of universal rotavirus vaccination programmes: a systematic review and meta-analysis. 2012;12(2):136–141.
[43] Fine P Variation in protection by BCG: implications of and for heterologous immunity. 1995;346(8986):1339–1345.
[44] Hur Y-G, Gorak-Stolinska P, Lalor MK, Mvula H, Floyd S, Raynes J, et al. Factors affecting immunogenicity of BCG in infants, a study in Malawi, The Gambia and the UK. 2014;14(1):1–10.
[45] Heng TS, Painter MW, Elpek K, Lukacs-Kornek V, Mauermann N, Turley SJ, et al. The Immunological Genome Project: networks of gene expression in immune cells. Nat Immunol 2008;9(10):1091–4.
[46] Querec TD, Akondy RS, Lee EK, Cao W, Nakaya HI, Teuwen D, et al. Systems biology approach predicts immunogenicity of the yellow fever vaccine in humans. 2009;10(1):116–125.
[47] Gaucher D, Therrien R, Kettaf N, Angermann BR, Boucher G, Filali-Mouhim A, et al. Yellow fever vaccine induces integrated multilineage and polyfunctional immune responses. 2008;205(13):3119–3131.
[48] Sun H-J, Xu X, Wang X-L, Wei L, Li F, Lu J, et al. Transcription factors Ets2 and Sp1 act synergistically with histone acetyltransferase p300 in activating human interleukin-12 p40 promoter. 2006;38(3):194–200.
[49] Blumenthal SG, Aichele G, Wirth T, Czernilofsky AP, Nordheim A, D JrJJoBC. Regulation of the human interleukin-5 promoter by Ets transcription factors: Ets1 and Ets2, but not Elf-1, cooperate with GATA3 and HTLV-I Tax1. 1999;274(18):12910–12916.
[50] Aricò E, Wang E, Tornesello ML, Tagliamonte M, Lewis GK, Marincola FM, et al. Immature monocyte derived dendritic cells gene expression profile in response to Virus-Like Particles stimulation. 2005;3(1):1–14.

[51] Monaco A, Marincola FM, Sabatino M, Pos Z, Tornesello ML, Stroncek DF, et al. Molecular immune signatures of HIV-1 vaccines in human PBMCs. 2009;583(18):3004–3008.

[52] Buonaguro L, Monaco A, Aricò E, Wang E, Tornesello ML, Lewis GK, et al. Gene expression profile of peripheral blood mononuclear cells in response to HIV-VLPs stimulation. 2008;9(2):1–7.

[53] Georgel P, Macquin C, Bahram S. The heterogeneous allelic repertoire of human toll-like receptor (TLR) genes. PLoS One 2009;4(11):e7803.

[54] Dhiman N, Ovsyannikova IG, Vierkant RA, Ryan JE, Pankratz VS, Jacobson RM, et al. Associations between SNPs in toll-like receptors and related intracellular signaling molecules and immune responses to measles vaccine: preliminary results. 2008;26(14):1731–1736.

[55] Ovsyannikova IG, Dhiman N, Haralambieva IH, Vierkant RA, O'Byrne MM, Jacobson RM, et al. Rubella vaccine-induced cellular immunity: evidence of associations with polymorphisms in the Toll-like, vitamin A and D receptors, and innate immune response genes. 2010;127(2):207–221.

[56] Banus S, Bottema RW, Siezen CL, Vandebriel RJ, Reimerink J, Mommers M, et al. Toll-like receptor 4 polymorphism associated with the response to whole-cell pertussis vaccination in children from the KOALA study. 2007;14(10):1377–1380.

[57] Kimman TG, Banus S, Reijmerink N, Reimerink J, Stelma FF, Koppelman GH, et al. Association of interacting genes in the toll-like receptor signaling pathway and the antibody response to pertussis vaccination. 2008;3(11):e3665.

[58] Didierlaurent A, Brissoni B, Velin D, Aebi N, Tardivel A, Käslin E, et al. Tollip regulates proinflammatory responses to interleukin-1 and lipopolysaccharide. 2006;26(3):735–742.

[59] Bulut Y, Faure E, Thomas L, Equils O, A MJTJoI. Cooperation of Toll-like receptor 2 and 6 for cellular activation by soluble tuberculosis factor and Borrelia burgdorferi outer surface protein A lipoprotein: role of Toll-interacting protein and IL-1 receptor signaling molecules in Toll-like receptor 2 signaling. 2001;167(2):987–994.

[60] Hotamisligil G Inflammation and metabolic disorders. 2006;444(7121):860–867.

[61] Ouchi N, Parker JL, Lugus JJ, W KJNri. Adipokines in inflammation and metabolic disease. 2011;11(2):85–97.

[62] Lamas O, Marti A, M JAJEjocn. Obesity and immunocompetence. 2002;56(3):S42–S45.

[63] Bandaru P, Rajkumar H, Nappanveettil G The impact of obesity on immune response to infection and vaccine: an insight into plausible mechanisms. 2013;2(2):1000113–1000122.

[64] Savy M, Edmond K, Fine PE, Hall A, Hennig BJ, Moore SE, et al. Landscape analysis of interactions between nutrition and vaccine responses in children. 2009;139(11):2154S–2218S.

[65] Haque R, Snider C, Liu Y, Ma JZ, Liu L, Nayak U, et al. Oral polio vaccine response in breast fed infants with malnutrition and diarrhea. 2014;32(4):478–482.

[66] Qadri F, Bhuiyan TR, Sack DA, Svennerholm A-MJV. Immune responses and protection in children in developing countries induced by oral vaccines. 2013;31(3):452–460.

[67] Anderson P, Kedersha N. 壽 Visibly stressed: the role of eIF2, TIA-1, and stress granules in protein translation. Cell Stress Chaperones 2002 Apr;7(2):213.

[68] de Jong SE, Olin A, Pulendran B. The impact of the microbiome on immunity to vaccination in humans. Cell Host Microbe 2020;28(2):169–79.

[69] Hagan T, Cortese M, Rouphael N, Boudreau C, Linde C, Maddur MS, Das J, Wang H, Guthmiller J, Zheng NY, Huang M. Antibiotics-driven gut microbiome perturbation alters immunity to vaccines in humans. Cell 2019 Sep 5;178(6):1313–28.

[70] Olin A, Henckel E, Chen Y, Lakshmikanth T, Pou C, Mikes J, Gustafsson A, Bernhardsson AK, Zhang C, Bohlin K, Brodin P. Stereotypic immune system development in newborn children. Cell 2018 Aug 23;174(5):1277–92.

[71] Harris VC, Armah G, Fuentes S, Korpela KE, Parashar U, Victor JC, Tate J, de Weerth C, Giaquinto C, Wiersinga WJ, Lewis KD. Significant correlation between the infant gut microbiome and rotavirus vaccine response in rural Ghana. J Infect Dis 2017 Jan 1;215(1):34–41.

[72] Harris V, Ali A, Fuentes S, Korpela K, Kazi M, Tate J, Parashar U, Wiersinga WJ, Giaquinto C, de Weerth C, de Vos WM. Rotavirus vaccine response correlates with the infant gut microbiota composition in Pakistan. Gut Microbes 2018 Mar 4;9(2):93–101.

[73] Huda MN, Ahmad SM, Alam MJ, Khanam A, Kalanetra KM, Taft DH, Raqib R, Underwood MA, Mills DA, Stephensen CB. Bifidobacterium abundance in early infancy and vaccine response at 2 years of age. Pediatrics 2019 Feb 1;143(2).

[74] Huda MN, Lewis Z, Kalanetra KM, Rashid M, Ahmad SM, Raqib R, Qadri F, Underwood MA, Mills DA, Stephensen CB. Stool microbiota and vaccine responses of infants. Pediatrics 2014 Aug 1;134(2):e362–72.

[75] Hall JA, Bouladoux N, Sun CM, Wohlfert EA, Blank RB, Zhu Q, Grigg ME, Berzofsky JA, Belkaid Y. Commensal DNA limits regulatory T cell conversion and is a natural adjuvant of intestinal immune responses. Immunity 2008 Oct 17;29(4):637–49.

[76] Norton EB, Lawson LB, Freytag LC, Clements JD. Characterization of a mutant Escherichia coli heat-labile toxin, LT (R192G/L211A), as a safe and effective oral adjuvant. Clinical and Vaccine Immunology 2011 Apr;18(4):546–51.

[77] Kim D, Kim YG, Seo SU, Kim DJ, Kamada N, Prescott D, et al. Nod2-mediated recognition of the microbiota is critical for mucosal adjuvant activity of cholera toxin. Nat Med 2016 May;22(5):524–30.

[78] Oh JZ, Ravindran R, Chassaing B, Carvalho FA, Maddur MS, Bower M, Hakimpour P, Gill KP, Nakaya HI, Yarovinsky F, Sartor RB. TLR5-mediated sensing of gut microbiota is necessary for antibody responses to seasonal influenza vaccination. Immunity 2014 Sep 18;41(3):478–92.

[79] Lynn MA, Tumes DJ, Choo JM, Sribnaia A, Blake SJ, Leong LE, et al. Early-life antibiotic-driven dysbiosis leads to dysregulated vaccine immune responses in mice. Cell host & microbe 2018;23(5):653–60.

[80] Ridlon JM, Kang DJ, Hylemon PB. Bajaj JS Bile acids and the gut microbiome. Curr Opin Gastroenterol 2014 May;30(3):332.

[81] Van Den Berg RA, De Mot L, Leroux-Roels G, Bechtold V, Clement F, Coccia M, Jongert E, Evans TG, Gillard P, van der Most RG. Adjuvant-associated peripheral blood mRNA profiles and kinetics induced by the adjuvanted recombinant protein candidate tuberculosis vaccine M72/AS01 in bacillus Calmette–Guérin-vaccinated adults. Front Immunol 2018 Mar 26;9:564.

[82] Kazmin D, Nakaya HI, Lee EK, Johnson MJ, Van Der Most R, Van Den Berg RA, et al. Systems analysis of protective immune responses to RTS, S malaria vaccination in humans. Proc Natl Acad Sci 2017;114(9):2425–30.

[83] Anderson J, Olafsdottir TA, Kratochvil S, McKay PF, Östensson M, Persson J, Shattock RJ, Harandi AM. Molecular signatures of a TLR4 agonist-adjuvanted HIV-1 vaccine candidate in humans. Front Immunol 2018 Feb 26;9:301.

[84] Rechtien A, Richert L, Lorenzo H, Martrus G, Hejblum B, Dahlke C, Kasonta R, Zinser M, Stubbe H, Matschl U, Lohse A. Systems vaccinology identifies an early innate immune signature as a correlate of antibody responses to the Ebola vaccine rVSV-ZEBOV. Cell Rep 2017 Aug 29;20(9):2251–61.

[85] de Bree LCJ, Koeken VA, Joosten LA, Aaby P, Benn CS, van Crevel R, et al. Non-specific effects of vaccines: current evidence and potential implications. In: Seminars in immunology. Amsterdam, Netherlands: Elsevier; 2018;35–43.

Index

Page numbers followed by "*f*" and "*t*" indicate, figures and tables respectively.

Q

R

S

T

COLD SPRAY TECHNOLOGY

COLD SPRAY TECHNOLOGY

Professor Anatolii Papyrin
Professor Vladimir Kosarev
Dr. Sergey Klinkov
Professor Anatolii Alkimov
Professor Vasily Fomin

Khristianovich Institute of Theoretical and Applied Mechanics of Russian Academy of Science in Novosibirsk, Russia

ELSEVIER

Amsterdam • Boston • Heidelberg • London • New York • Oxford
Paris • San Diego • San Francisco • Singapore • Sydney • Tokyo

Elsevier
The Boulevard, Langford Lane, Kidlington, Oxford OX5 1GB, UK
Radarweg 29, PO Box 211, 1000 AE Amsterdam, The Netherlands

First edition 2007

British Library Cataloguing in Publication Data
A catalogue record for this book is available from the British Library

Library of Congress Cataloging-in-Publication Data
A catalog record for this book is available from the Library of Congress

ISBN-13: 978-0-08-045155-8
ISBN-10: 0-08-045155-1

For information on all Elsevier publications visit our website at books.elsevier.com

Typeset by Integra Software Services Pvt. Ltd, Pondicherry, India.
Printed and bound by CPI Antony Rowe, Eastbourne

Contents

Preface

Cold gas-dynamic spray (or simply cold spray) is a process of applying coatings by exposing a metallic or dielectric substrate to a high velocity (300–1200 m/s) jet of small (1–50 μm) particles accelerated by a supersonic jet of compressed gas. This process is based on the selection of the combination of particle temperature, velocity, and size that allows spraying at the lowest temperature possible. In the cold spray process, powder particles are accelerated by the supersonic gas jet at a temperature that is always lower than the melting point of the material, resulting in coating formation from particles in the solid state. As a consequence, the deleterious effects of high-temperature oxidation, evaporation, melting, crystallization, residual stresses, debonding, gas release, and other common problems for traditional thermal spray methods are minimized or eliminated. Eliminating the deleterious effects of high temperature on coatings and substrates offers significant advantages and new possibilities and makes cold spray promising for many industrial applications.

The cold spray process was originally developed in the mid-1980s at the Institute of Theoretical and Applied Mechanics of the Russian Academy of Sciences in Novosibirsk by Dr. Anatolii Papyrin and his colleagues. They successfully deposited a wide range of pure metals, metal alloys, and composites onto a variety of substrate materials, and demonstrated the feasibility of the cold spray process for various applications. A US patent was issued in 1994, and the European patent in 1995.

Outside of Russia, the cold spray process was presented first in the United States by Dr. Papyrin in 1994. In 1994–95 Dr. Papyrin, with a consortium formed under the auspices of the National Center for Manufacturing Sciences (NCMS) of Ann Arbor, MI, conducted the first research in the United States on cold spray. The membership included major US companies such as Ford Motor Company, General Motors, General Electric – Aircraft Engines, and Pratt & Whitney Division of United Technologies. This consortium established the first US cold spray capability, and the group published property measurements for several cold-sprayed materials.

At the present time, a wide spectrum of research is being conducted at several research centers and companies around the world, including the Institute of Theoretical and Applied Mechanics of the Russian Academy of Sciences; Sandia National Laboratories; the Pennsylvania State University; ASB Industries Inc., Ford Motor Company, Pratt & Whitney, Dartmouth College, Rutgers University, Army Research Laboratory,

Delphi Research Laboratory, (United States); the University of the Federal Armed Forces, European Aeronautic Defense and Space Company, Cold Gas Technology, Linde AG, Siemens (Germany); Cambridge University, University of Nottingham, University of Liverpool, Yasaki Europe, BOC Gases (England); Shinshu University, Plasma Gigen (Japan); National Research Council, University of Windsor (Canada); CRISO (Australia); Mahle Metal Leve (Brazil); companies in South Korea, China, India, and many other countries. The cold spray process propagates around the world so fast that it is difficult to mention all the companies and institutions involved in this activity. There has been a great surge in publications on the cold spray process. Many high level studies have been conducted at these centers and many very interesting and important results for further developments and improvements of cold spray have been obtained.

This book includes the results of more than twenty years of original studies (1984–2005) conducted at the Institute of Theoretical and Applied Mechanics of Siberian Branch of the Russian Academy of Sciences, as well as the results of studies conducted at many of the research centers around the world.

The authors' goal has been to explain the basic principles and advantages of the cold spray process, to give some practical information on technologies and equipment as well as to present the current state of research and development in this field.

Chapter 1 describes the experiments that resulted in the discovery of the cold spray process and established the basic physical principals of the process. Two aspects of the cold spray process are important for better understanding and improving the process. The first one is the physics of high speed particle impact (to explain bonding mechanism), and the second one is the gas-dynamics (to optimize spray parameters and provide as high particle velocity as possible). For this reason the authors paid close attention in the book to these topics (Chapters 2 and 3). Chapter 4 describes the equipment and some specific technologies, while Chapter 5 presents an overview of studies at different research centers around the world.

It should be noted that the portion of the book related to specific technologies and coating characterization (sections in Chapters 4 and 5) is not the strongest part of the book. The authors came to the cold spray process from gas-dynamics and do not have much experience in materials characterization. However, we believe that even brief and simple enough information on coatings and technologies and corresponding references can be useful for readers. We also believe that more detailed overview and analysis in this field will be made by material specialists in the nearest future.

The book is a research monograph, intended for specialists working in the field of surface technologies, in particular, applying coatings with thermal and cold spray processes. The book can be useful for the broad reading public, in particular, for engineers, scientists, undergraduate and postgraduate students who are interested in studies of advanced technologies, gas-dynamics of supersonic gas flows and physics of high speed interaction of the particles with the target.

We would like to thank all the scientists, engineers, and technicians of ITAM SB RAS (Russia), who assisted us in the development of the cold spray process and who participated in various cold spray projects, including Prof. A. Tushinskii, Dr. A. Gulidov, Dr. I. Shabalin, Dr. I. Golovnev, Dr. A. Bolesta, Mr. V. Lavrushin, Mr. P. Spesivcev, and others.

We would also like to thank Dr. M.Smith (Sandia National Laboratories, USA), Mr. A. Kay (ASB Industries, Inc., USA), Mr. R. Blose (Ktech Corp., USA), Dr. R. McCune (Ford Motor Company, USA), Prof. M. Amateeu (PennState University, USA), Prof. H. Kreye (University of the Federal Armed Forces, Germany), Mr. P. Richter (Cold Gas Technology, Germany), Mr. P. Heinrich (Linde AG, Germany) for their cooperation, support of cold spray activity, and useful discussions.

We express our appreciation to Mr. P. Richter (Cold Gas Technology, Germany), Mr. R. Blose (Ktech Corp.,USA), Dr. R. Maev and Dr. V. Leshchynsky (University of Windsor, Canada) for their contribution to the equipment description (Chapter 4).

We would like to thank Dr. N. Nesterovich, posthumously, for contribution in gas-dynamics research and Academics of RAN, M. Zhukov and N. Yanenko, for encouragement and support of cold spray activity in Russia. Finally, we would like to express our gratitude to Mrs. Meg Szulinski for her assistance in the editing and preparation of this book.

Anatolii N. Papyrin
Professor, Dr.Sc., Ph.D
President, Cold Spray Technology.

CHAPTER 1

Discovery of the Cold Spray Phenomenon and its Basic Features

As mentioned in the introduction, the phenomenon of cold gas-dynamic spraying (cold spray) was discovered in the early 1980s at the Institute of Theoretical and Applied Mechanics of the Siberian Branch of the Russian Academy of Sciences (ITAM of RAS) while studying models subjected to a supersonic two-phase flow (gas + solid particles) in a wind tunnel [1].

The issues associated with a two-phase flow and its interaction with the surface of the immersed body became urgent because of a large number of scientific and applied problems in various fields of research, including aviation, cosmonautics, coating-application technologies, and processing and development of new materials, etc. The presence of particles in the flow can significantly alter the flow field of the gas, as compared with the pure flow, and change the state of the body surface, flow parameters near the body, and its aerodynamic characteristics (drag, temperature field, heat flux, etc.).

The theoretical [2–9] and experimental [10–13] works known at that time (1980s) and related to the studies of a two-phase flow were mainly limited to determining the integral parameters: drag, heat flux, etc. In this aspect, one of the main problems was to formulate experiments that would allow one to study the microstructure of the processes responsible for the flow character with the use of laser diagnostics with high spatial and temporal resolution available at that time. Based on such diagnostics, a wide spectrum of studies in the field of gas-dynamics of two-phase flows was conducted in ITAM of RAS (see for example [14]).

Below, we would like to present results of wind tunnel studies that led to the discovery of cold spray process. These results are important for describing and understanding the cold spray process.

1.1. Supersonic Two-phase Flow around Bodies and Discovery of the Cold Spray Phenomenon

1.1.1. Experimental setup and research techniques

The layout of the experimental setup is shown in Fig. 1.1. A supersonic gas flow was generated by a plane-contoured nozzle. The gas in the pre-chamber had the following parameters: pressure $p_0 = 0.85\,\text{MPa}$, temperature $T_0 = 260–280\,\text{K}$, and Mach number at the nozzle exit $M^* = 3$. The models to be tested were mounted in the vicinity of the nozzle exit. There were windows designed for optical measurements. A wide range of particles with disparate sizes d_p and density ρ_p were used in experiments: bronze particles $100\,\mu\text{m}$, $8.6\,\text{g/cm}^3$; Plexiglas particles $200\,\mu\text{m}$, $1.2\,\text{g/cm}^3$; aluminum particles $15\,\mu\text{m}$, $2.7\,\text{g/cm}^3$; lycopodium particles $25\,\mu\text{m}$, $0.5\,\text{g/cm}^3$. The particles were injected into the gas flow at a distance of 300 mm upstream of the throat section.

Several laser-based techniques were used to diagnose the process. The particle velocity was measured by laser Doppler velocimetry (LDV) with a direct spectral method for the registration of the Doppler frequency shift. Pulsed shadowgraphy was used to register the microstructure of the density field. A ruby laser operating in the mode with a modulated Q-factor and pulse duration of 30 ns was used as a source of light. The displacement of

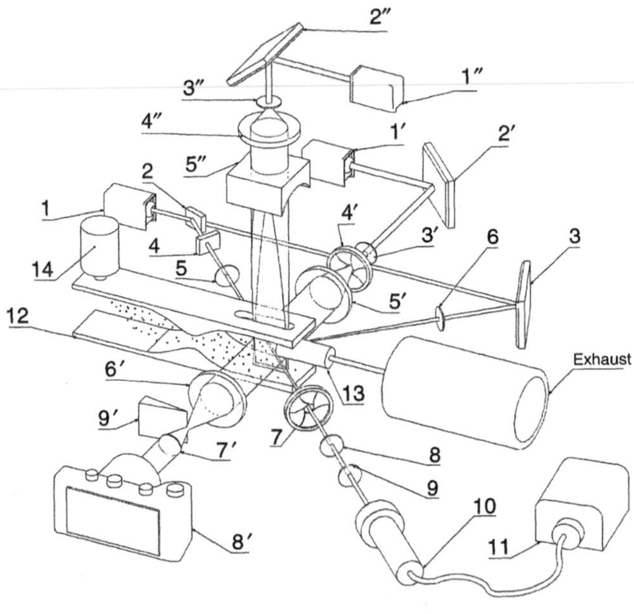

Fig. 1.1. Schematic of the setup and diagnostic equipment. LDV scheme: 1 – single-frequency laser; 2–9 – optical elements; 10 – confocal interferometer; 11 – recorder. Setup elements: 12 – plane supersonic nozzle; 13 – model under study; 14 – powder feeder. Scheme of mutli-frame Schlieren technique: 1′ – ruby laser with a modulator; 2′–7′ – optical elements; 8′ – camera, 9′ – sheet. Laser sheet technique: 1″ – ruby laser; 2″–5″ – optical elements.

particles during the exposure time was less than their diameter. Schlieren pictures were obtained with the use of a visualization diaphragm.

The time evolution of the wave structure was studied by the multi-frame Schlieren technique based on the use of a laser generating a series of pulses with a prescribed time interval between them (laser stroboscope).

The trajectories of particle motion were observed by the method of laser visualization in scattered light (laser sheet). The ruby laser operated in the "peak" generation mode. The duration of emission of a pulse series was $\sim 10^{-3}$ s.

1.1.2. Structure of disturbances induced by reflected particles

To study the global pattern of the two-phase flow around bodies and to clarify the main physical features of this process, the first experiments involved flow visualization with bodies of simple geometry (wedge, cylinder, and sphere) and injection of particles that differed in size and material.

Photographs obtained by flow visualization in scattered and transient laser radiation are shown in Figs 1.2 and 1.3. The photographs in scattered light (laser sheet technique) illustrate the particle trajectories. Reflected particles are clearly seen. Some of them have a reflection angle close to the incidence angle. After reflection and subsequent deceleration by the oppositely directed flow, these particles change their direction to the opposite one and, being accelerated toward the body, hit the body again. The presence of particles that can collide with the body many times with a gradual decrease in the rebound distance leads to their accumulation near the frontal part of the body. A zone with an elevated concentration of the disperse phase with intense interaction of incident and reflected particles is formed.

Figure 1.3 shows typical shadowgraphs illustrating the disturbance of the wave structure near the body owing to the presence of the disperse phase in the flow. One can clearly see local shock waves formed by a supersonic flow around the particles and the character of changes in the bow-shock structure, which is associated with the presence of particles. Photographs of each body in a "pure" airflow are also presented for comparison.

An analysis of a large amount of experimental data revealed that the following features related to the influence of particles on the structure of the bow-shock front. The character of variation of the wave structure around the body and, hence, its basic characteristics significantly depend on the body shape (blunted or sharp forebody) and on particle parameters. In the flow around bodies with a blunted forebody (sphere or stream-wise aligned cylinder) and injection of fine aluminum ($d_p = 1$–$40\,\mu$m) and lycopodium ($d_p =$ 25–28 μm) particles into the flow, the influence of the disperse phase on the bow-shock structure starts to manifest itself when the volume concentration of particles reaches $\varphi_p \geq (0.5$–$1)\%$. In the shadowgraphs (see, e.g., Fig. 1.3, frame 4), this phenomenon is manifested as a change in the distance between the shock-wave front and the body and as a deformation of the shock-wave front shape. In the flow around blunted bodies by a gas with coarser particles of Plexiglas ($d_p = 200\,\mu$m) and bronze ($d_p = 100\,\mu$m), the changes in the wave structure acquire a different character. Strong disturbances of the bow-shock

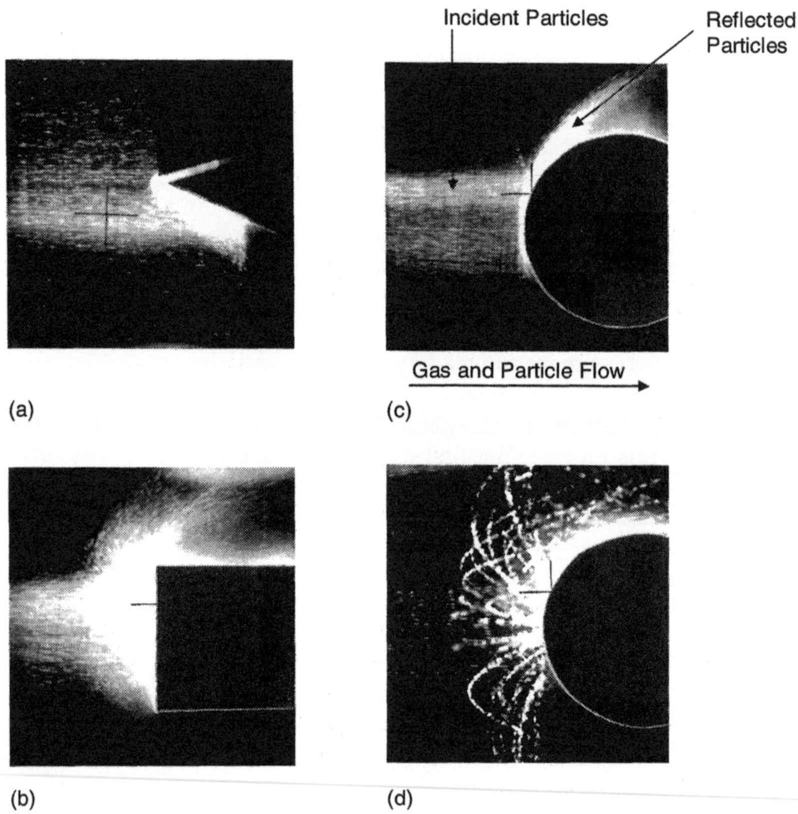

Fig. 1.2. Laser sheet visualization of a body in a supersonic two-phase flow illustrating particles trajectories. The body diameters are $D_b = 8\,\text{mm}$, $M_\infty = 3.0$. (a) wedge (Al particles); (b) cylinder (Al particles) (c) and (d) sphere (Al and Plexiglas particles).

structure is observed even in the case of a low concentration of particles $\varphi_p << 1\%$. These disturbances are manifested in the form of conical shock waves (Fig. 1.3a, frame 3; Fig. 1.3b, frames 3 and 4) with large apex angles and particles located at the apices. This is most clearly seen in the flow around a stream-wise mounted cylinder.

In the flow around sharp bodies (wedge, cone), the character of variation of the wave structure does not change significantly by injection of all particles, both fine and coarse. In this case, the effects of bow-shock disturbances are similar to those observed in the flow around blunted bodies in the presence of fine particles (aluminum and lycopodium) in the flow. For $\varphi_p > 1\%$, a change in the shape and position of the bow-shock front is observed; as in the case of blunted bodies, this can be explained by the effect of "concentration", i.e., changes in gas parameters upon its interaction with particles. In particular, for a wedge, the effects associated with the influence of particles on the gas were considered in, [e.g. 2], and a significant effect of the volume content of particles on the shock-wave front structure and on the character of pressure variation on the body surface was demonstrated.

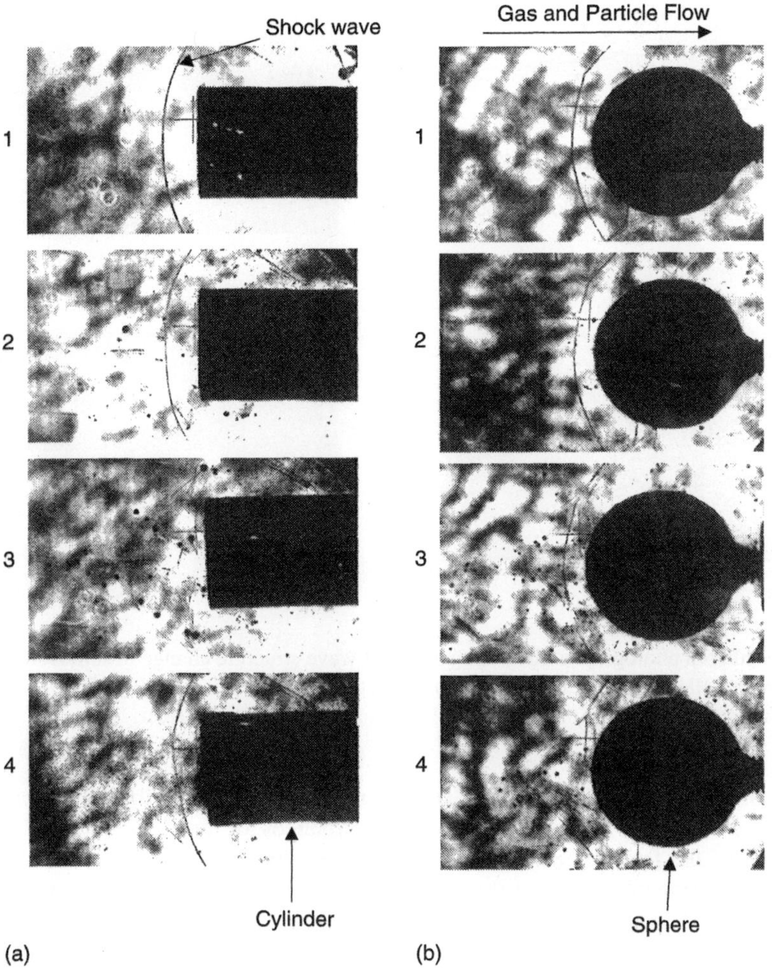

Fig. 1.3. Schlieren photographs illustrating effect of wave structure change in supersonic two-phase flow around (a) a cylinder and (b) a sphere. The body diameters are $D_b = 8\,\text{mm}$, $M_\infty = 3.0$, $t_{ex} = 30\,\text{ns}$. (a) 1 – without particles; 2, 3 – Plexiglas particles 50–200 μm; 4 – lycopodium particles. (b) 1 – without particles; 2 – Al particles; 3, 4 – Plexiglas particles.

In contrast to blunted bodies, the effect of the strong disturbance of the bow-shock wave in the presence of coarse particles for bodies with a sharp nose was not observed. This made it possible to assume that reflected particles moving away from the body, intersecting the bow-shock front, and entering the supersonic zone play some special role. To support this hypothesis, multi-exposure shadowgraphs were obtained, and additional experiments on the two-phase flow around a hollow cylinder were performed.

Figure 1.4 shows the shadowgraphs obtained for a two-phase flow with Plexiglas particles around a hollow cylinder. In this case, the probability of particle reflection is very low, and the main role belongs to interaction of incident particles with the shock wave. The

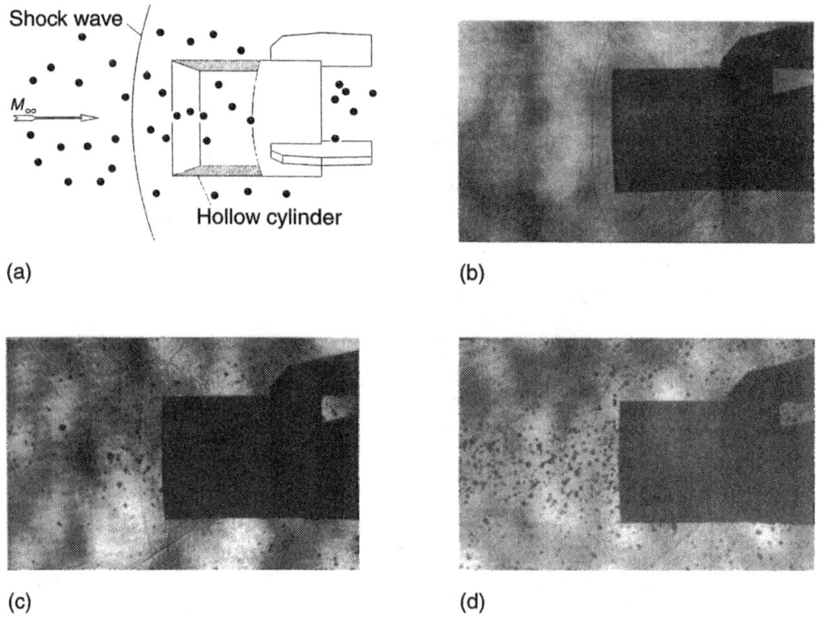

Fig. 1.4. Schlieren photographs illustrating effect of wave structure change in supersonic two-phase flow around a hollow cylinder (a). The body diameter is $D_b = 8\,\text{mm}$, $M_\infty = 3.0$, $t_{ex} = 30\,\text{ns}$. (b) – gas flow without particles; (c) and (d) with Plexiglas particles 50–200 μm.

character of bow-shock disturbance is significantly different from the flow around a solid cylinder and involves formation of local disturbances of the bow-shock front due to intersection of the front by incident particles. The typical size of these disturbances has the order of the transonic zone of the shock layer formed near the particles in a supersonic flow. Even if the concentration is high (Fig. 1.4, frame 3), the shape of the bow-shock wave typical of this body can be distinguished. No disturbances in the form of oblique shock waves with a large angle, which were registered in the flow around blunted bodies, are observed. Note also that the character of the disturbance formed as a single incident particle crosses the bow-shock wave is clearly seen in Fig. 1.3a, frame 2.

A simplified scheme of disturbances of the wave structure in the vicinity of the body, which is formed by the reflected particle, can be presented as follows (Fig. 1.5) [14]. As it follows from the Schlieren picture (Fig. 1.5b), the character of the disturbance introduced by such a particle involves formation of a shock wave with a close-to-conical shape propagating upstream together with the reflected particle. The cone angle is much greater than the corresponding Mach angle.

The experimental facts described above confirm the important role of the particle reflected from the body and entering the supersonic flow region through the bow-shock front. Because of the importance of this effect in science and potential applications, the structure of the flow ahead of a blunted body, formed by single particles moving from the frontal surface of the body upward the supersonic flow, was studied in detail.

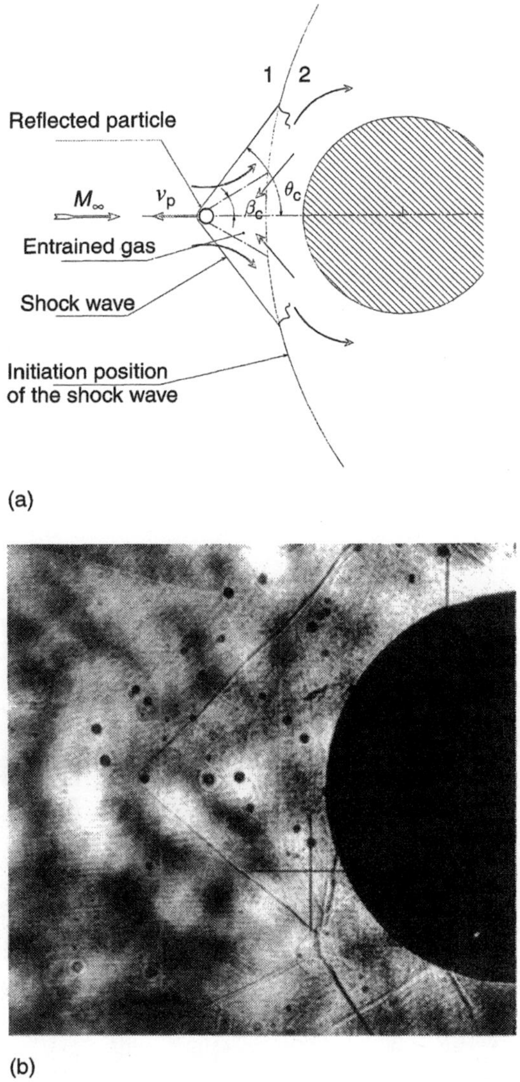

Fig. 1.5. Formation of a disturbed flow by a reflected particle. The body diameter is $D_b = 8\,\text{mm}$, $M_\infty = 3.0$, $t_{ex} = 30\,\text{ns}$. (a) schematic (b) Schlieren picture of the process.

The flight of a single particle was examined with the help of shadowgraphy and interferometry, which made it possible to explain the main features of the time evolution of the resultant flow. The experiments showed that as the particle passes through the shock wave, an elevated pressure region is formed behind the latter, and the apex of this zone together with the particle moves upstream. The shape of this zone and the shock wave is close to conical. Depending on the distance between the reflected particle and the body (rebound distance), we can distinguish two typical modes:

1. regime without separation of the elevated pressure region from the particle;
2. regime with separation of the elevated pressure region from the particle.

The first mode is converted to the second one as the rebound distance exceeds a certain critical value.

The first mode observed if the rebound distance is smaller than the critical value is characterized by the absence of flow reconstruction (i.e., breakdown of the elevated pressure region) over the entire range of particle motion from the body surface to the point where it stops and returns, and the particle is "rigidly" connected to the apex of the gas cone. The initial shape of the bow-shock wave upstream of the body is reconstructed when the particle returns to the subsonic region. The second mode is observed if the maximum rebound distance is greater than the critical value at which flow reconstruction leading to recovery of a supersonic flow ahead of the cylinder begins. Figure 1.6 shows typical photographs illustrating these two modes.

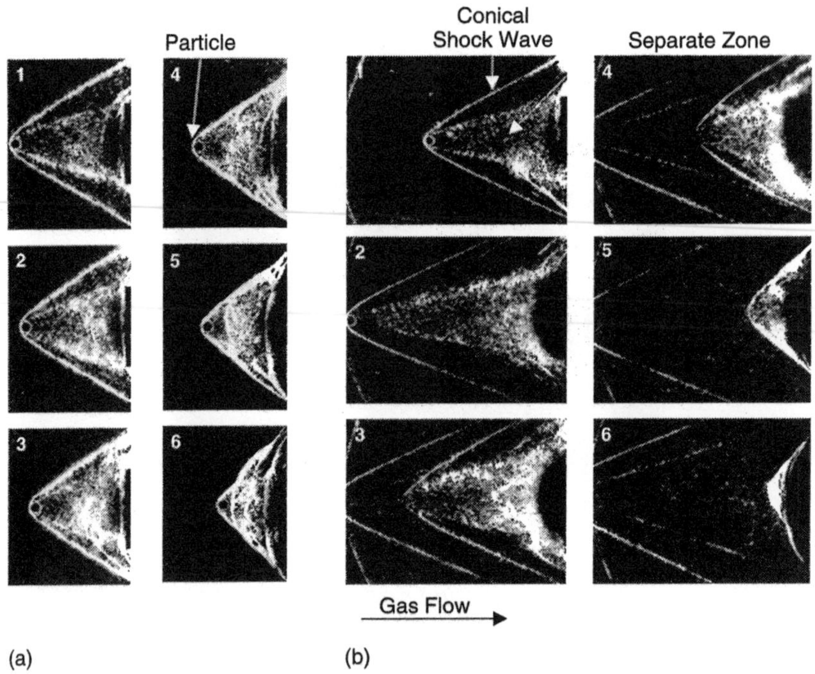

Fig. 1.6. Multiframe schlieren pictures illustrating the development of the disturbance ahead of the cylinder under escape of "particle" towards flow. The cylinder diameter is $D_b = 11\,\text{mm}$, and the "particle" diameter is $d_p = 1.5\,\text{mm}$, $M_\infty = 3.0$, $Re_D = 7.8 \times 10^5$, $t_{ex} = 30\,\text{ns}$. (a) regime without flow reconstruction (the particle returns to the body), the initial flight velocity is $v_{st} = 20\,\text{m/s}$. The interval between two neighboring frames is $\Delta t = 100\,\mu\text{s}$ and (b) regime with flow reconstruction, the initial flight velocity is $v_{st} = 30\,\text{m/s}$. The interval between two neighboring frames is $\Delta t = 30\,\mu\text{s}$.

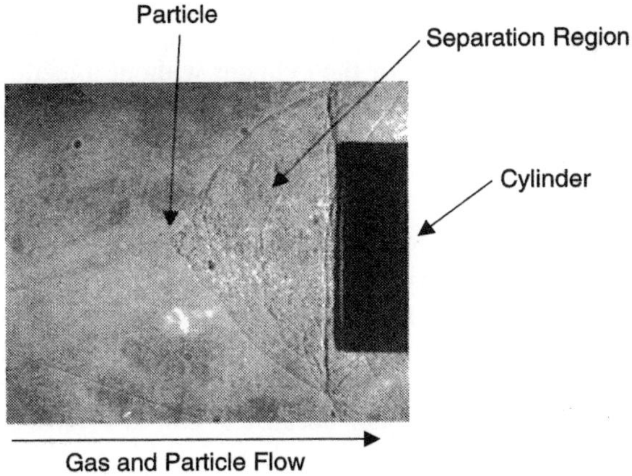

Fig. 1.7. Schlieren picture illustrating the formation of a separation region in front of the cylinder in supersonic two-phase flow by a particle with $d_p \leq 10\,\mu m$. $D_b = 11\,mm$, $M_\infty = 3.0$, $Re_D = 7.8 \times 10^5$, $\Delta p_{bl} = 1.4\,MPa$, $t_{ex} = 30\,ns$.

The Schlieren picture in Fig. 1.7 shows the disturbance of the bow-shock wave by the particle with $d_p \approx 10\,\mu m$. A single zone of elevated pressure between the particle and the cylinder is clearly visible; as it follows from this figure, the critical rebound distance is greater than 0.8 of the cylinder diameter.

Experiments were also performed which showed that a flux of particles exhausting from the frontal part of a blunted body upstream to a supersonic flow can substantially reduce the drag force of the body in a supersonic gas flow. Figure 1.8 shows the behavior

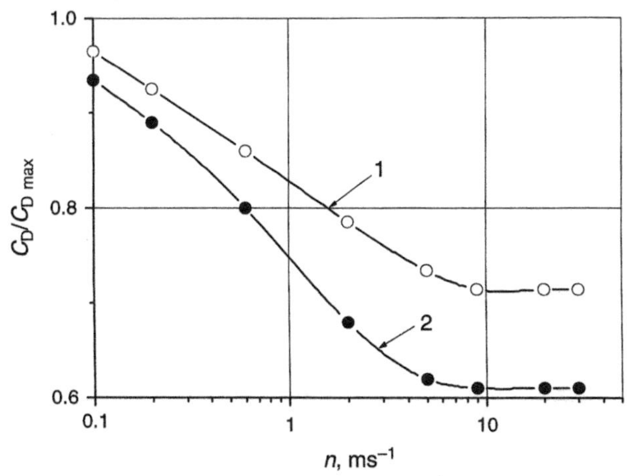

Fig. 1.8. Drag coefficient of a cylinder versus the number of the particles, which are taking off from a body in unit of time. Points 1 and 2 refer to $\Delta p_{bl} = 0.6\,MPa$ and $\Delta p_{bl} = 1.2\,MPa$, respectively.

of the drag coefficient of the cylinder $C_D{}^* = C_D/C_{D0}$ as a function of the number of the particles which are taking off from a body in time unit $\dot{n}_p$ for two values of the injection parameter (C_{D0} is the drag coefficient of the cylinder without injection of particles). The fact that C_D/C_{D0} differs from unity for $\dot{n}_p = 0$ is caused by the influence of the "pure" gas jet. Thus, there is a certain analogy between a spike mounted ahead of the body for decreasing its drag and a single particle located at a certain distance upstream of the body.

The study performed made it possible to offer a first explanation to the mechanism of formation and time evolution of disturbances ahead of blunted bodies with a flux of fine particles reflected or exhausted from them, and to submit an application and patent the method for drag reduction for such bodies in a supersonic gas flow [15]. It should be noted that the effect of the change of shock wave structure by reflected particles in front of the body was described in detail because it can also have an influence on the gas-dynamics of the cold spray process.

1.1.3. Interaction of a supersonic two-phase flow with the surface. Effect of coating formation

Results of investigations of the flow around bodies by a supersonic two-phase flow with a low content of the disperse phase described above reveal the specific features of formation of elevated pressure regions by single particles reflected (or exhausted) from the body at a distance greater than the thickness of the compressed layer. It was shown that the presence of such particles changes the character of the flow and can lead to a significant decrease in the force action of the gas flow on the body. Results of the study of shock interaction of particles with the surface of bodies exposed to a supersonic two-phase flow (gas + solid particles) with high flow rates of the disperse phase are presented below.

Pictures taken with the laser sheet technique in experiments with a supersonic two-phase flow are shown in Figs 1.2, 1.9, and 1.10. It is clear from these pictures that high mass flow rates of the disperse phase lead to formation of a buffer zone ahead of the body, where the concentration of particles is much higher than in the remaining free-stream region. The parameters of this zone (shape and typical size, concentration of particles, etc.) and its effect on the body largely depend on the body geometry and on particle properties.

The pictures show that the rebound distance for Plexiglas particles (~6 mm) is significantly greater than for aluminum particles (~1 mm). As it follows from Figs 1.9 and 1.10, the process of particle reflection from the surface is one of the main factors determining the character of formation of the buffer zone and its parameters, in particular the growth rate of concentration of the disperse phase as compared to the incoming flow.

It is much simpler to obtain single reflection in the flow around bodies with a rounded forebody and with the use of particles with a large rebound distance. For instance, in the photographs shown in Fig. 1.9a, illustrating the trajectories of Plexiglas particles interacting with the surface of a cross flow-mounted cylinder, it is clearly seen that the major part of these particles after one collision do not return to the body except for particles in the region of the critical point. In passing to bodies with a flat forebody and injection of aluminum particles, the situation becomes substantially different for the same

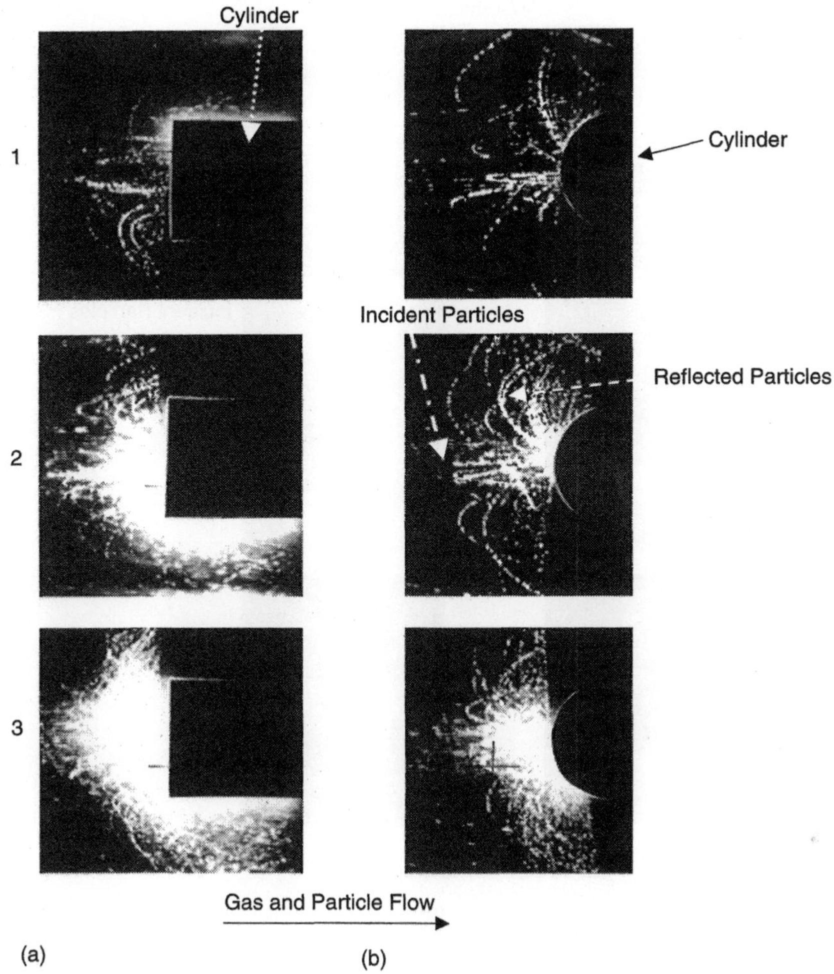

Fig. 1.9. Laser sheet photographs illustrating trajectories of particles under flow around a cylinder mounted (a) along and (b) across the flow with Plexiglas particles with mass flow rates of $1-0.1\text{g/s cm}^2$, $2-0.5\text{g/s cm}^2$, and $3-3\,\text{g/s cm}^2$. $M_\infty=3.0$, $Re_\text{D}=4\times10^5$.

mass flow rates. Figure 1.10b shows the results of optical observations for a streamwise-mounted cylinder, which display some principally new effects in the character of formation of the buffer zone. Thus, the photographs taken with the laser sheet technique (Fig. 1.10b) show that the thickness of the buffer zone after a certain time of the flow action increases with increasing flow rate of particles G_p in contrast to the flow around a sphere or a cross flow-mounted cylinder.

An analysis of the body surface after its treatment by a flow of aluminum particles showed that a continuous solid coating is formed from the particle material on the frontal surface of the cylinder (Fig. 1.11).

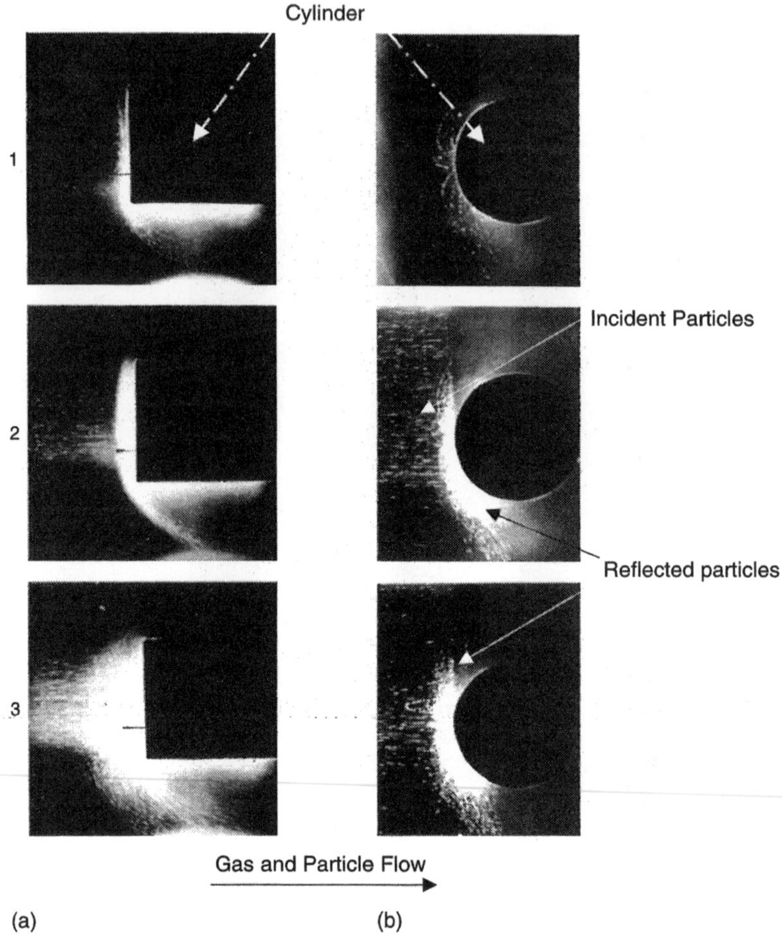

Fig. 1.10. Laser sheet photographs illustrating trajectories of particles under flow around a cylinder mounted (a) along and (b) across the flow with aluminum particles and mass flow rates of 1 – 0.3 g/s cm^2, 2 – 2 g/s cm^2, and 3 – 6 g/s cm^2, $M_\infty = 3.0$, $Re_D = 4 \times 10^5$.

These effects were not observed in the flow with Plexiglas or bronze around a streamwise-mounted cylinder, though the maximum flow rate of these particles (30 g/s cm^2) was greater than the corresponding value of G_p for aluminum (15 g/s cm^2). Bombardment of the target by bronze particles led to the "reverse" phenomenon: significant erosion of the steel-target material responsible for changes in the forebody shape.

Thus, the experiments performed showed that the process of formation of the buffer zone and its parameters in the case of high flow rates of the disperse phase are largely determined by the character of particle collisions with the target and by collisions of particles with each other. In addition, formation of a dense aluminum coating on the frontal surface was experimentally registered in the flow containing finely dispersed aluminum particles around the body.

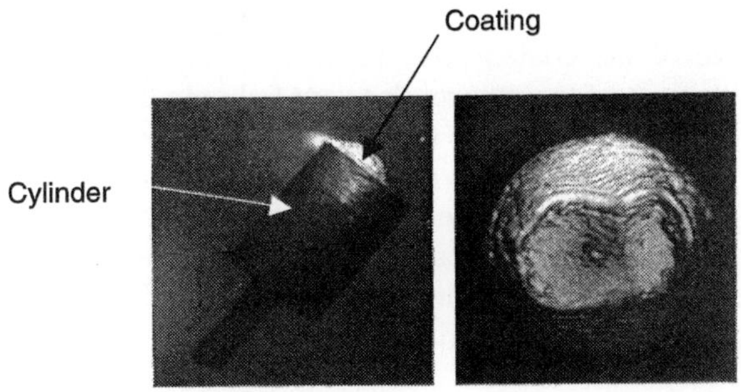

Fig. 1.11. Photographs of the coating formed from aluminum particles on a cylinder, $M_\infty = 3.0$, $T_0 = 300\,\mathrm{K}$, $d_{pm} = 20\,\mu\mathrm{m}$, $G_p = 15\,\mathrm{g/s\,cm^2}$.

The microphotographs of the sprayed layer showed that the coating consists of strongly deformed and densely packed particles uniformly covering the surface. The coating has a scaly structure with dense packing without noticeable pores and voids. Based on the microscope data, the mean strain of particles in the layer is ε_p in the range 0.6–0.8.

It is important to emphasize that the flow stagnation temperature was approximately 280 K. Thus, it follows from the results presented that the effect of coating formation on the frontal surface of the body in a "cold" ($T_0 = 280\,\mathrm{K}$), supersonic, two-phase flow with aluminum-particle velocity of 400–450 m/s was obtained for the first time, and it was supposed that the principal role in coating formation belongs to particle velocity. These experiments initiated the studies of a new low-temperature method for applying coatings: cold spray.

The scientific and practical importance of the above-noted effect of formation of a coating from solid particles at low temperatures (close to room temperature) of the gas and particles, stimulated experiments for a more detailed study of the phenomenon observed.

1.2. Spraying with a Jet Incoming onto a Target

The results described above and obtained in a wind tunnel with an external supersonic two-phase flow demonstrated that it is possible to obtain coatings from solid particles at room stagnation temperature of the flow. It should be noted that it was commonly accepted at this time (mid-1980s) that particles should be heated to high temperatures ensuring their melting in the gas flow to obtain a coating. For instance, it was argued in [16] that it is impossible to obtain a coating by spraying particles in the solid state.

Due to the importance of the effect observed, it was decided to perform additional studies. The objective of these studies was to find the main features of interaction of solid particles with a target at high impact velocities.

The effect of cold gas-dynamic spraying was registered in an external two-phase flow around bodies. Obviously, such a method is unsuitable for widely used applications. First, in the case of spraying in a wind tunnel, the fraction of particles hitting the body is rather low because the size of the coated body is considerably smaller than the nozzle-exit section, and the main mass of the powder does not fall onto the body surface. Second, the size of the coated body is restricted by the test-section size. It is important to emphasize that an increase in the test-section size does not allow a significant increase in the body size because the effect of particle deceleration ahead of the body becomes relevant, which can worsen the coating quality or prevent coating formation altogether. For these reasons, the cold spray method was implemented in the regime of a two-phase jet + moving target, which is typical of thermal coating techniques.

It is well known [17] that the target material is subjected to erosion in the case of low velocities ($v_p = 10–100\,\mathrm{m/s}$) of collisions of solid particles with the target at room temperature. Therefore, it was obvious that the observed effect of coating formation under conditions of an external flow is caused by the high velocity of particles (for aluminum particles, the velocity was $v_p = 400–450\,\mathrm{m/s}$). Therefore, the main problem at the first stage was to perform experiments on interaction of solid particles with a target in a wide range of velocities $v_p = 100–1000\,\mathrm{m/s}$ to register the transition from erosion of the substrate material to coating formation. It should be noted that there was no reliable data on collision of solid particles with the target in this range of velocities at that time. The main data was only available for low velocities ($v_p \leq 100\,\mathrm{m/s}$) because of the erosion problem and for high velocities ($\geq$1 km/s) due to military and space problems. The results of investigations in the field of thermal spraying methods were mainly obtained for interaction of particles in the melted state [16, 18].

The majority of experiments were performed with aluminum particles for the following reasons:

- It was with aluminum particles that the effect of coating formation in an external flow was detected. Therefore, it was important to continue investigations with the same particles to compare the results.
- Possibility of obtaining high particle velocities ($v_p \approx 1000\,\mathrm{m/s}$) because of the low density of aluminum particles being accelerated in a gas flow.
- High probability of observation of a possible effect of particle-material melting at the moment of the particle–substrate collision because of a comparatively low melting point of aluminum (670 °C).

1.2.1. Acceleration of particles in cold spray

Investigations performed already at the early stage of studying the cold spray process unambiguously showed that the velocity of the particle impact on the substrate surface plays the most important role in the application of coatings by this method. Therefore, before performing experiments in this aspect, it was necessary to work out the technique for velocity control and measurement. The particle velocity was controlled by deliberate changes in the test-gas composition (the test gas was a mixture of air and helium) and was determined numerically. Numerical results were first verified by experimental methods. Figure 1.12 shows the calculated velocity of aluminum particles of several different sizes

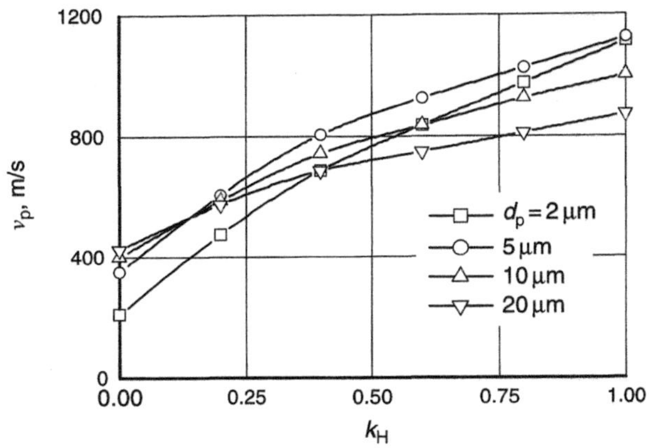

Fig. 1.12. Calculated aluminum-particle velocity near the substrate surface versus helium concentration in the mixture air-helium.

for their acceleration in a rectangular nozzle with a throat size 3 mm × 3 mm and exit size of 3 mm × 10 mm.

By changing the content of helium in the mixture, it is possible to change the particle velocity within the range $v_p = 200–1200\,\mathrm{m/s}$.

1.2.1.1. Diagnostic methods

The measurements were performed on a setup equipped by various laser-diagnostic tools (Fig. 1.13) including LDV, shadowgraphy and Schlieren methods as well as laser sheet technique [19]. The particle velocity was measured by two methods: LDV with a direct spectral method of registration of the Doppler shift of frequency [20] and the tracking technique [21]. The particle velocity was also evaluated on the basis of a one-dimensional model in the single-particle approximation. Thus, the measured and calculated data made it possible to determine the particle velocity, which could be varied in a wide range $v_p = 200–1200\,\mathrm{m/s}$.

One method of particle-velocity measurement was LDV with a direct spectral method of registration of the Doppler shift of frequency. Its detailed description and methodical features can be found in [22, 23]. LDV with a direct spectral analysis is most effective in studying high-velocity flows ($v_p \geq 10^2\,\mathrm{m/s}$). In addition, these schemes allow determining both the value of velocity and its direction. This is important for simultaneous registration of particle fluxes moving in the opposite directions, for example incident particles and particles reflected from the substrate. Velocities of copper and aluminum particles of different sizes were measured by the LDV technique. Figure 1.14 shows a typical signal obtained in measuring the velocity of aluminum particles accelerated by an air jet. In this case, LDV was calibrated so that the distance between these peaks (free-dispersion range) corresponded to 1500 m/s. The signal in the center is the signal from the flux of aluminum particles.

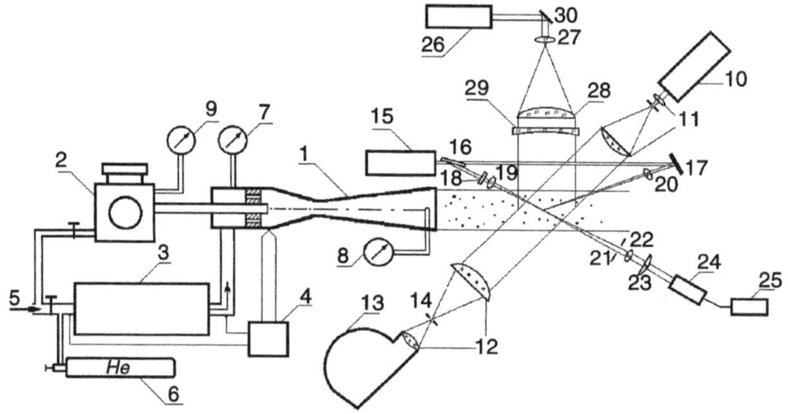

Fig. 1.13. Schematic of the experimental setup; 1 – plane supersonic nozzle; 2 – powder feeder; 3 – gas heater; 4 – system for controlling gas temperature; 5 – compressed air; 6 – compressed helium; 7–9 – pressure gauges in the pre-chamber, at the nozzle exit, and in the powder feeder; 10 – ruby laser operating in the regime with a modulated Q-factor and with pulse duration $t \approx 30 \times 10^{-9}$ s; 11 – telescopic system; 12 – detecting optical system; 13 – chamber; 14 – visualization element; 15 – LG-159-type single-frequency helium–neon laser; 16 – transparent dividing plate; 17 – rotating 100% mirror; 18 – polarizer used to adjust the reference-beam intensity; 19, 20 – focusing lenses; 21 – aperture diaphragm of the detecting optical system; 22 – collecting lens; 23 – matching objective; 24 – multibeam confocal interferometer with a photomultiplier at the exit; 25 – recorder.

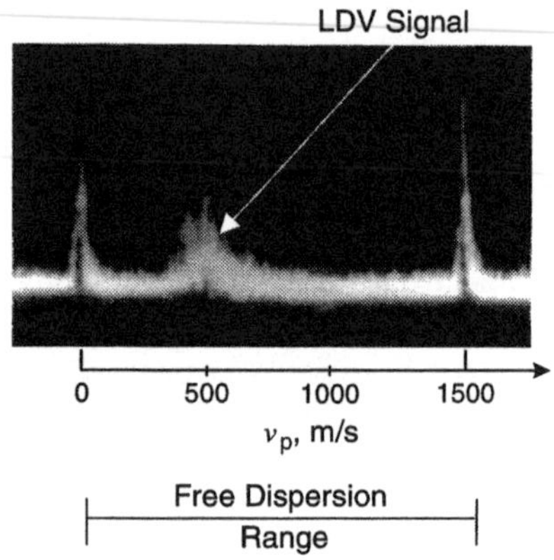

Fig. 1.14. Typical LDV signal. Aluminum particles, $d_{pm} = 20\,\mu m$, $v_{pm} \approx 500\,m/s$.

The other method used for velocity measurements was the tracking technique [19] shown schematically in Fig. 1.13. The basic elements of the scheme are a ruby laser operating in the free-generation mode, a telescopic system, an optical system forming the laser sheet, and a photo-recorder producing a continuous time sweep of moving particles. The images of particles from the peripheral regions of the jet were cut off by a screen; thus, the velocity of particles moving in the jet core was measured. With a stationary

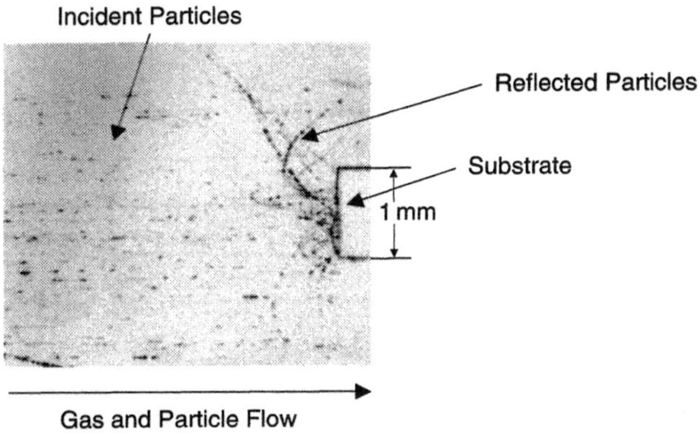

Fig. 1.15. Laser sheet photographs illustrating trajectories of incident and reflected Cu particles. $d_p = 30\text{–}60\,\mu\text{m}$, $v_{pm} \approx 150\,\text{m/s}$.

photo-recorder, it was possible to obtain the trajectories of particles incident onto the surface and particles reflected from the surface. As an example, Fig. 1.15 shows the photographs of particles in the jet and the particle reflected from the target.

The tracking technique allows reliable measurements of velocity of particles with $d_p \geq 5\,\mu\text{m}$ in the range of velocities $v_p = 200\text{–}1200\,\text{m/s}$. The use of this method was conditioned by its simplicity and certain advantages over LDV:

- This method allows measurements with extremely low concentrations of particles where they obviously have no influence on the carrier gas parameters.
- By processing one sweep, it is possible to obtain data on particle velocity at different distances from the nozzle exit simultaneously.
- It is rather simple to obtain the value of the mean velocity of particles and also their velocity distribution induced by their size distribution, and it is also possible to measure the velocity of single particles, whereas scanning LDV measurements require a certain minimum concentration of particles in the flow.

A necessary condition of applicability of this method is the absence of scattering of particles moving in the jet core toward the corners. An analysis of photographs similar to those in Fig. 1.15 showed that particles in the flow core move without any significant scatter toward the corners. As an example, Fig. 1.16 shows a sweep for moving aluminum particles.

Processing of such photographic records on a microscope by measuring the slopes of trajectories of moving particles to the film axis made it possible to determine the velocity of each individual particle at different distances from the nozzle exit within 0–10*h*, where *h* is the least size of the nozzle-exit cross section. The particle velocity was calculated by the formula

$$v_p = \frac{1}{k} v_{sc} \operatorname{tg} \alpha_{tr}, \tag{1.1}$$

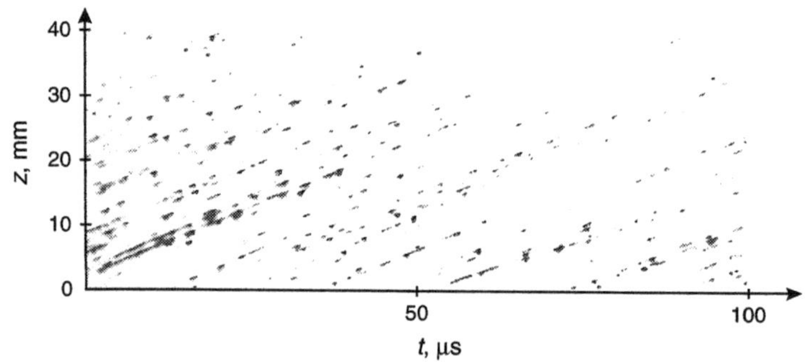

Fig. 1.16. Typical photographic sweep of moving aluminum particles. $d_{pm} = 30.2\,\mu m$; $v_{pm} = 394\,m/s$.

where k is the magnification of the optical system, v_{sc} is the linear velocity of the sweep of the image recorded on the film, which is set by the photo-recorder, and α_{tr} is the angle of inclination of the particle track on the film to the film axis.

An analysis of the accuracy of particle-velocity measurement by this method shows that the relative error is determined by the expression

$$\frac{\Delta v_p}{v_p} = \frac{\Delta k}{k} + \frac{\Delta v_{sc}}{v_{sc}} + \frac{2\Delta\alpha_{tr}}{\sin 2\alpha_{tr}} \tag{1.2}$$

where Δk is the accuracy of determining the optical system magnification, Δv_{sc} is the accuracy of setting the velocity of the image in the film, and $\Delta\alpha_{tr}$ is the accuracy of determining the slope of the trajectory on the film, which is induced by the accuracy of the measurement instrument and by scattering of particles in the jet toward the corners.

By choosing the image velocity such that $\alpha_{tr} \approx \pi/4$ and applying appropriate registration tools, the particle velocity could be measured within 10%.

1.2.1.2. Experimental measurement of particle velocity

The measurements performed showed that the velocity of particles under consideration remained practically unchanged in the examined region of the jet core, i.e., from the nozzle exit to the compressed layer. Measuring the velocity of a large number of particles on one photographic sweep, we plotted the particle-distribution functions in terms of their velocities, which were conditioned by the particle-size distribution and by random factors, such as turbulent fluctuations of velocity, density, etc. The mean velocity of particles $v_{pm} = \frac{1}{N}\sum_{i=1}^{N} v_p^i$ and the standard deviation $\sigma_v = \frac{1}{N-1}\sum_{i=1}^{N}\left(v_p^i - v_{pm}\right)^2$ were determined by processing the measured results.

We measured the velocity-distribution functions for various fractions of aluminum and copper particles accelerated by air and helium jets with isobaric exhaustion of the jet from the nozzle. Figure 1.17 shows the size-distribution functions for three fractions of

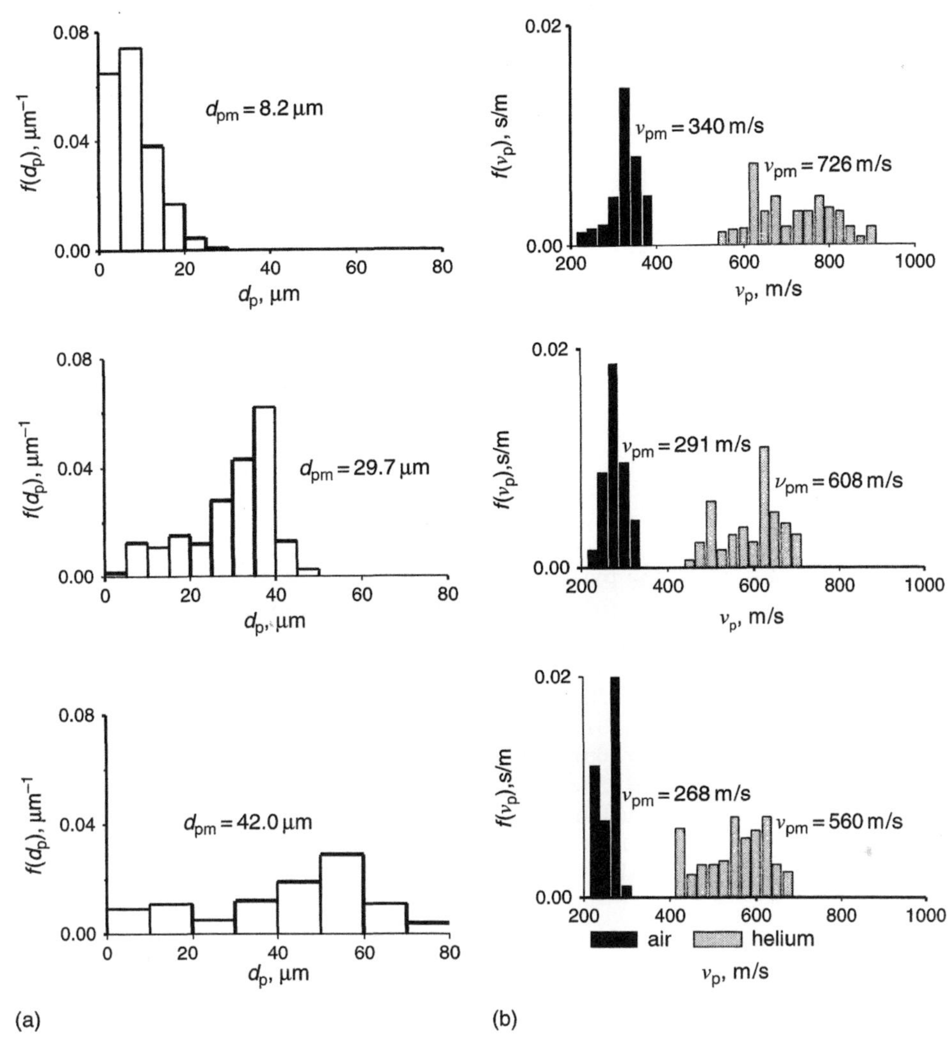

Fig. 1.17. (a) Particle size-distribution functions and (b) corresponding particle velocity-distribution functions near the jet centerline for three fractions of copper accelerated by air and helium jets.

copper and the corresponding velocity distributions for particle acceleration by pure air and helium.

These results clearly illustrate the influence of the particle size and the type of the accelerating gas. For all particle sizes, the mean velocity of particles accelerated by helium is approximately twice the mean velocity of particle accelerated by air; the scatter of particle velocities is also noticeably greater.

The experimentally measured values of particle velocity at the nozzle exit were compared with predicted values (the numerical technique is described in Chapter 3); plotted in

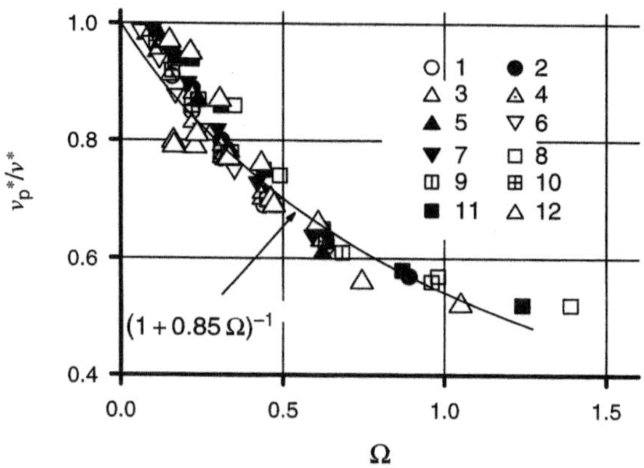

Fig. 1.18. Generalized dependence of the relative velocity of particles at the exit of a plane supersonic nozzle.

1. $L = 50\,\text{mm}$, $p_0 = 3.0\,\text{MPa}$
2. $L = 50\,\text{mm}$, $p_0 = 1.5\,\text{MPa}$
3. $L = 100\,\text{mm}$, $p_0 = 3.0\,\text{MPa}$
4. $L = 100\,\text{mm}$, $p_0 = 1.5\,\text{MPa}$
5. $L = 100\,\text{mm}$, $p_0 = 2.0\,\text{MPa}$
6. $L = 150\,\text{mm}$, $p_0 = 3.0\,\text{MPa}$
7. $L = 150\,\text{mm}$, $p_0 = 1.0\,\text{MPa}$

(1–7: $T_0 = 300\,\text{K}$)

8. $L = 50\,\text{mm}$, $p_0 = 1.0\,\text{MPa}$
9. $L = 100\,\text{mm}$, $p_0 = 2.0\,\text{MPa}$
10. $L = 150\,\text{mm}$, $p_0 = 3.0\,\text{MPa}$
11. $L = 100\,\text{mm}$, $p_0 = 3\,\text{MPa}$

(8–11: $T_0 = 500\,\text{K}$)

12. Experiment

1–7 – Al *8–11* – Cu

Fig. 1.18 is the ratio of particle velocity to the gas velocity versus the dimensionless quantity $\Omega = \sqrt{\frac{d_p}{L} \times \frac{\rho_p v^{*2}}{p_0}}$. The predicted values are shown by points *1–11*.

Figure 1.18 also shows the results of an experiment on determining the particle velocity (point *12*), which were obtained under test conditions used in the computations. The predicted and experimental values are in agreement and admit simple approximation convenient for rapid evaluation of the particle velocity at the nozzle exit:

$$\frac{v_p^*}{v^*} = (1+0.85\Omega)^{-1} = \left(1+0.85\sqrt{\frac{d_p}{L} \times \frac{\rho_p v^{*2}}{p_0}}\right)^{-1} \tag{1.3}$$

Another comparison of numerical results with the experimentally determined velocity of various particles at the nozzle exit is shown in Fig. 1.19 in the form of the particle velocity versus the particle size. The solid curves with squares show the numerically calculated velocity of particles at the nozzle exit, accelerated by air and helium jets. The figure also illustrates the test results on determining the velocity of these particles, which were obtained under conditions used in the computations. The good agreement of

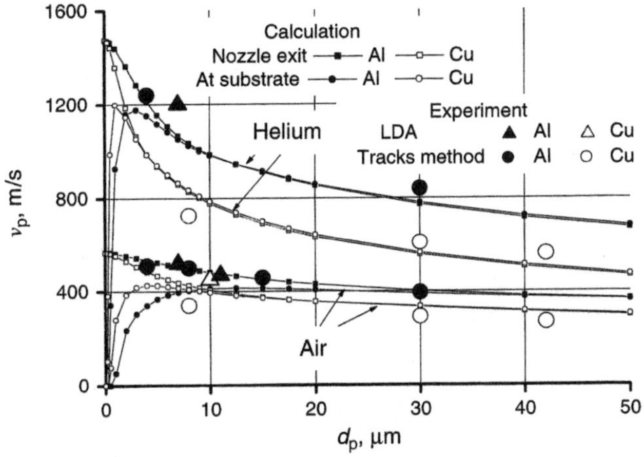

Fig. 1.19. Computed velocities of aluminum and copper particles at the nozzle exit and at the substrate surface versus the particle size as compared with experimental results. $L = 100\,\text{mm}$, $p_0 = 2.0\,\text{MPa}$.

numerical and experimental data allows us to consider these data to be reliable and to use computations in further evaluations of the particle velocity during spraying.

Figure 1.19 also shows the computed velocities of aluminum and copper particle at the substrate surface (dashed curves with circles). Small particles noticeably lose their velocity in the frozen gas region immediately ahead of the substrate. Copper particles are less inert and have a lower velocity at the nozzle exit, but they become less decelerated behind the shock wave. As a result, both copper and aluminum particles with a size of $(5\text{–}20) \times 10^{-6}\,\text{m}$, being accelerated by an air jet, have approximately identical velocities ($\sim 400\,\text{m/s}$) when they hit the substrate. In a helium jet, the influence of particle inertia on their final velocity has a more pronounced effect on their final velocity.

Based on these results, to obtain a sufficiently high particle velocity on the substrate, one has to not only choose a nozzle with a length sufficient for particle acceleration to a high velocity but also reduce the adverse decelerating action of the compressed gas immediately ahead of the substrate.

Thus, the experiments and numerical calculations allowed for an accurate determination of particle velocity as a function of various parameters of the spraying process. This allowed for starting the experiments on studying the main features of the cold spray process, first of all, its dependence on particle velocity.

1.2.2. Description of the setup

The experiments were performed in the regime of jet impact on a target [24] normally used for coating application by gas–thermal methods. The layout of this setup is shown in Fig. 1.20. Main elements are: pre-chamber and supersonic nozzle, gas heater, powder

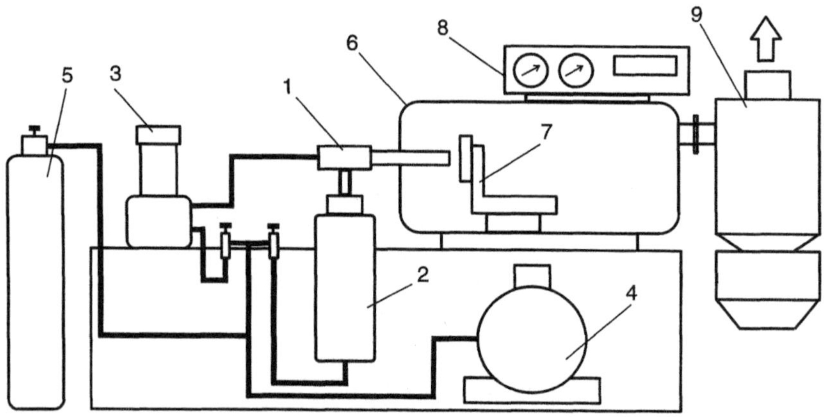

Fig. 1.20. Schematic of the Cold Spray setup. Its basic elements are 1 – the spraying unit consisting of a pre-chamber and a plane supersonic nozzle, 2 – the gas heater, 3 – the particle feeder, 4 – the source of compressed air, 5 – the source of helium, 6 – the spraying chamber, 7 – the traversing gear for moving the coated substrate, 8 – the panel for controlling and monitoring the process parameters (gas pressure in the pre-chamber and particle dispenser, gas temperature in the pre-chamber), and 9 – the particle separator.

feeder, compressed air and helium, spray chamber with motion system for substrate, and exhaust system for collecting powder. The setup ensured the possibility of accelerating particles $d_p = 1\text{–}50\,\mu\text{m}$ in supersonic nozzle up to velocities $v_p = 200\text{–}1200\,\text{m/s}$ for different concentrations of particles.

1.2.3. Interaction of individual particles with the surface

The first task was to study the process of interaction of individual particles with the substrate in a wide range of particle velocities in order to demonstrate the effect of transition from rebound to adhesion of "cold" particles to the "cold" substrate with an increase in particle velocity. The character of this interaction was considered with the use of a moving polished substrate; the concentration of particles in the jet and the substrate velocity were chosen such that it was possible to observe individual craters and attached particles on the substrate. Aluminum particles with a mean diameter $d_{pm} = 30.2\,\mu\text{m}$ were used; they are shown in the photograph in Fig. 1.21.

The particle velocity was controlled by forming different compositions of air–helium mixtures. A typical microphotograph of the substrate surface after its interaction with aluminum particles with $d_{pm} = 30.2\,\mu\text{m}$ and the mean particle velocity $v_{pm} = 730\,\text{m/s}$ is shown in Fig. 1.22a. There are only some individual craters formed by particle impact on the substrate, and there are no attached particles. With the increase in particle velocity the situation is changed. Particles start adhering to the substrate and the probability of particle attachment increases with the increase in particle velocity (Fig. 1.22b,c)

Thus, we can see that there are two characteristic processes in the course of interaction of "cold" particles with a "cold" substrate, which are separated by a certain critical

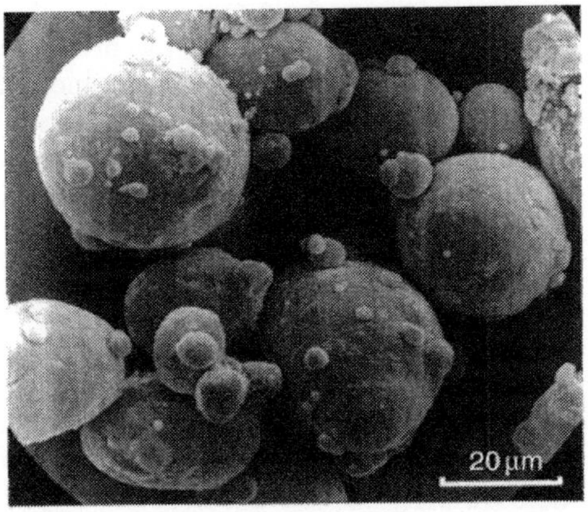

Fig. 1.21. Appearance of aluminum particles.

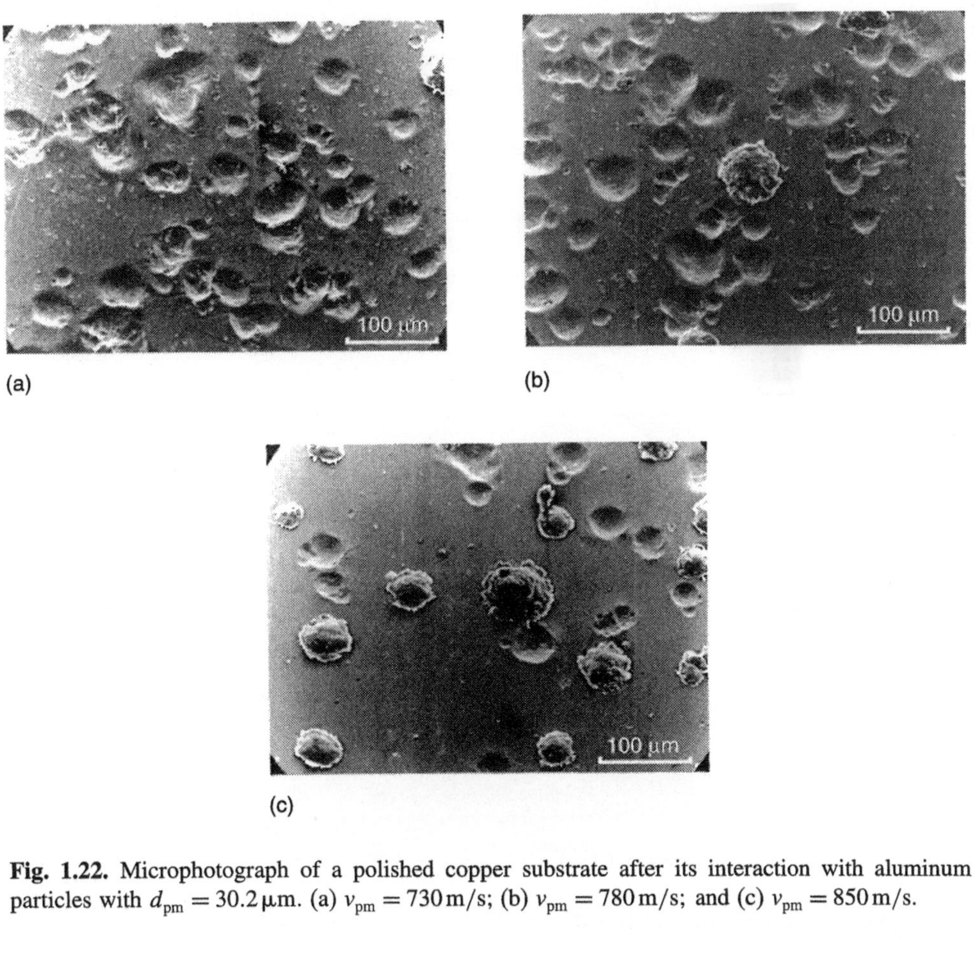

Fig. 1.22. Microphotograph of a polished copper substrate after its interaction with aluminum particles with $d_{pm} = 30.2\,\mu m$. (a) $v_{pm} = 730\,m/s$; (b) $v_{pm} = 780\,m/s$; and (c) $v_{pm} = 850\,m/s$.

velocity. If the particle velocity is low, particle rebound from the substrate occurs. With the particle velocity increasing to the critical value, the process of particle adhesion to the surface begins, and the particle-attachment probability increases with an increase in particle velocity. The experiments performed showed that the critical value of particle velocity depends on many factors, including particle and substrate materials, particle temperature and size, substrate-surface state, etc. For example, Fig. 1.23 shows that the critical velocity increases in the case of preliminary treatment of the substrate, and the probability of particle attachment increases almost to 100% for a particle velocity of 850 m/s.

Results of these experiments were of principal importance. They showed that in terms of coating formation by "cold" particles, a transition from the process of substrate erosion (due to particle rebound) to the process of coating formation (due to particle adhesion) with an increase in particle velocity should occur. To verify this idea, the following experiments were conducted in the regime of coating formation.

1.2.4. Transition from erosion to coating formation process. Critical velocity

The next step in the understanding of "cold" spraying phenomena was to observe the process of coating formation by "cold" particles. For this purpose, several metals were sprayed on a copper substrate with different particle velocities.

The measured deposition efficiency $k_d = \frac{\Delta m_s}{M_p}$ (Δm_s – change of weight of a substrate, M_p – weight of all particles interacting with a substrate) of various metallic particles accelerated by an air-helium mixture is shown in Fig. 1.24.

Figure 1.24 illustrates the fundamental concept of cold spray, namely, that the coating is formed by a high-velocity flow of "cold" particles on a "cold" substrate. The following results were obtained in investigations.

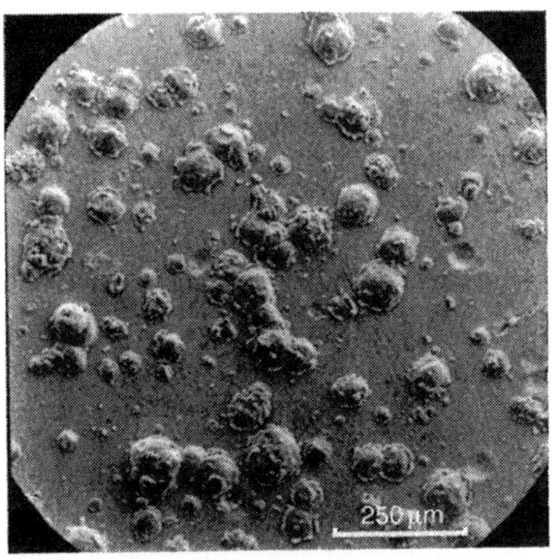

Fig. 1.23. Aluminum particles attached to the preliminary treated copper substrate, $v_{pm} = 850\,\mathrm{m/s}$.

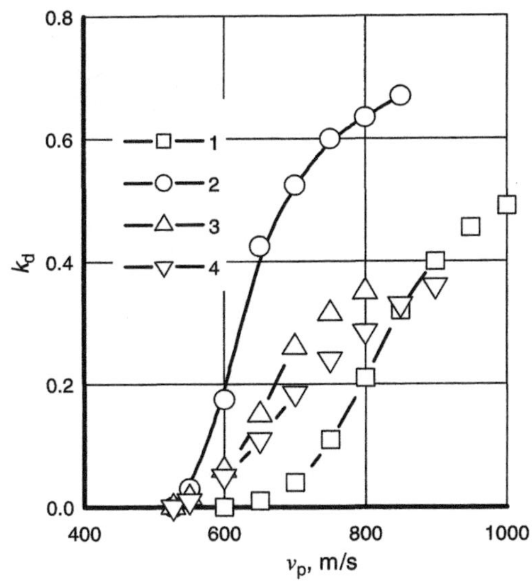

Fig. 1.24. Deposition efficiency versus particle velocity for of 1 – aluminum, 2 – copper, 3 – nickel, and 4 – zinc powders accelerated by an air-helium mixture at room stagnation temperature.

Two characteristic regions separated by the critical velocity v_{cr1} were found. The first region ($v_p < v_{cr1}$) corresponds to a well-known process of substrate erosion, which is undesirable in our case. However, as the particle velocity exceeds the critical value v_{cr1}, the coating process begins. The deposition efficiency rapidly increases to 50–70% as the particle velocity significantly exceeds the critical value.

The transition from erosion to coating formation process is illustrated by the photographs of the trajectories of incident aluminum particles and aluminum particles reflected from the substrate in Fig. 1.25. The processing of such photographs together with studying the substrate surface showed that all single particles with $v_p \le v_{cr1}$ ($v_p \approx 250\,\mathrm{m/s}$, Fig. 1.25a) are reflected. As the velocity increases within the range $v_p \ge v_{cr1}$, the character of particle–substrate interaction is drastically changed: a rapidly growing coating is formed on the substrate surface ($v_p \approx 900\,\mathrm{m/s}$, Fig. 1.25b).

It is seen from Fig. 1.24 that typical values of v_{cr1} for various metals (Al, Cu, Ni, and Zn) are within 500–700 m/s. Various metals and alloys can be sprayed by a jet with room stagnation temperature (without any heating) if the particles reach a necessary velocity. This transition from substrate erosion to formation of "viable" coatings by a flow of "cold" solid particles was the physical basis for the development of the cold spray method.

1.2.5. Effect of jet temperature on the deposition efficiency

As stated earlier, the test results plotted in Fig. 1.24 were obtained with the use of an air–helium mixture. Obviously, from a practical viewpoint, the use of expensive helium is not always justified.

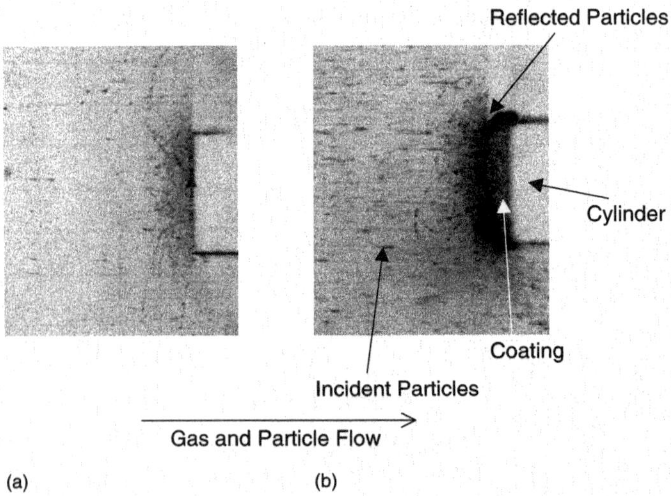

Fig. 1.25. Trajectories of incident and reflected aluminum particles; (a) $v_{pm} = 250\,m/s$ and (b) $v_{pm} = 900\,m/s$.

The use of a pure air jet at room temperature does not ensure formation of coatings for most materials. Therefore, investigations were performed with a slightly heated air jet with an objective to increase the gas velocity and, hence, the particle velocity. It is important to emphasize that the particle temperature under such heating was always much lower than the melting point of the particle material, providing coating formation from particles in the solid state.

Figure 1.26 shows the results of measurement of the deposition efficiency for various metallic powders (aluminum, copper, and nickel) as a function of stagnation temperature of the jet.

Curves 4–6 in Fig. 1.27 show the data of Fig. 1.26 for the materials mentioned, but the data is plotted versus the particle velocity used in the computations (with the corresponding temperatures of air heating). By comparing these dependences with those obtained with the use of an air–helium mixture as a driver gas at $T_0 = 300\,K$ (curves 1–3), we can conclude that the particle and substrate temperatures have also a significant effect on the spraying process; otherwise these two families of curves would coincide. As the air temperature in the pre-chamber increases, both the particle velocity and the particle and substrate temperatures increase. Therefore, the drastic increase observed for the deposition efficiency can be attributed to the growth of both the velocity of sprayed particles (which increases the pressure and temperature in the contact at the impact moment) and the temperatures of the sprayed particles and the substrate (which can lead to changes in their properties, increase in temperature in the particle–substrate contact, and hence, displacement toward lower values of the critical velocity v_{cr1}).

Thus, we can see that slight preheating of the jet allowed us to decrease the critical velocity and, as a consequence, to extend the range of sprayed materials with an air jet.

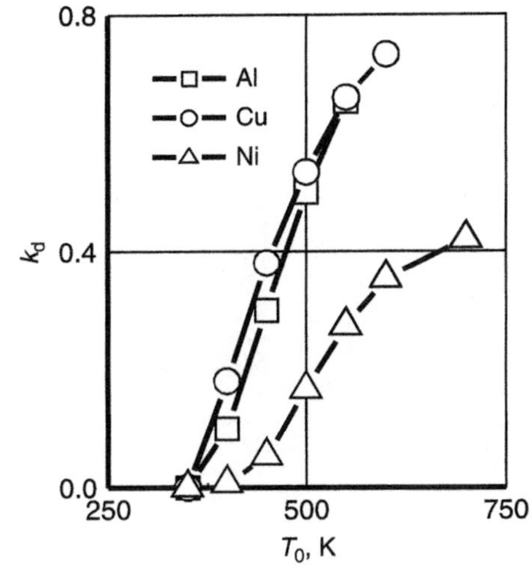

Fig. 1.26. Deposition efficiency of aluminum, copper, and nickel powders sprayed on copper substrates versus the air jet stagnation temperature.

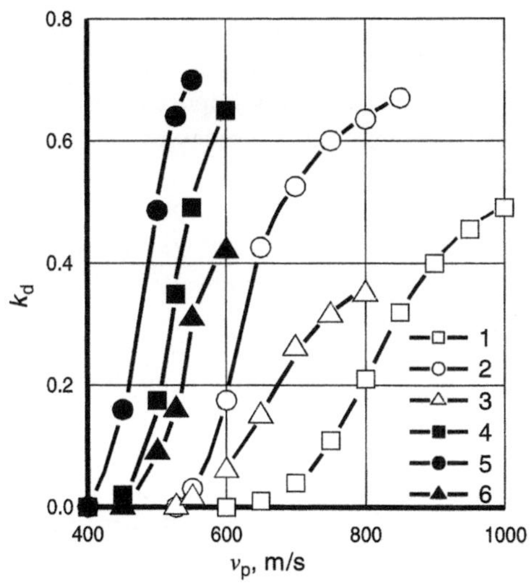

Fig. 1.27. Deposition efficiency for aluminum, copper, and nickel powders accelerated by an air-helium mixture (1–3) and by heated air (4–6) versus particle velocity. The curves refer to Al (1, 4), Cu (2, 5), and Ni (3, 6).

Thus, the results presented show that the use of a supersonic jet of air (nitrogen) mixture with helium and having a stagnation temperature of $\sim$300 K and the use of a slightly preheated ($\Delta T \leq$ 500–600 K) supersonic (M = 2.0–3.0) air (nitrogen) jet allowed us to obtain coatings from most metals and many alloys (Al, Cu, Ni, Zn, Pb, Sn, V, Co, Fe,

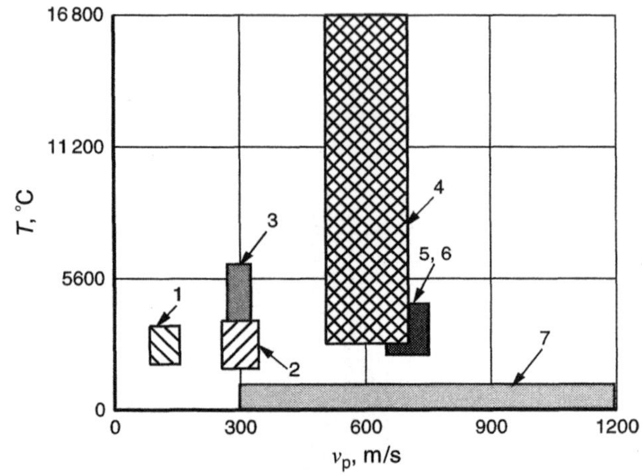

Fig. 1.28. Diagram of jet temperatures (T) and particle velocities (v_p) used in different spraying methods. 1 – low-velocity gas-plasma; 2 – high-velocity gas-plasma; 3 – electric-arc, 4 – plasma; 5, 6 – detonation and high-velocity oxygen-fuel; and 7 – cold spray.

Ti, bronze, brass, etc.) with particles of the size $d_p < 50\,\mu m$ onto various metallic and dielectric substances (in particular, glass, ceramics, etc.). The deposition efficiency of the powders reaches 0.5–0.8, which is extremely important from a practical point of view in the development of particular technological processes.

A comparison of the basic parameters of the two-phase flow for cold spray with parameters typical of traditional spraying methods shows that they are significantly different (Fig. 1.28). The characteristic features of the cold spray process are much lower temperature and higher velocity of particles.

It is important to emphasize that the key difference between cold spraying and conventional thermal spraying methods (Fig. 1.28) from the physical viewpoint is that the coating is formed from particles in the solid state. That is why the term "cold" was introduced into the name of the process despite some jet heating. As was mentioned above, according to the concept commonly accepted in mid-1980s [16], for the coating to be formed, the incident particles should be in the melted or almost-melted state. The presented results demonstrated that a high temperature of the jet is not a necessary condition for all sprayed materials, and many coatings can be obtained from particles whose temperature is substantially lower than their melting point.

Eliminating the harmful effects of high temperature on coatings and substrates offered significant advantages and new possibilities. These include

- *avoiding* oxidation and undesirable phases;
- *retaining* properties of initial particle materials;

- *inducing* low residual stresses;
- *conducting* heat and electricity easily through the coatings;
- *providing* high density, high hardness, cold-worked microstructure;
- *spraying* thermally-sensitive materials;
- *spraying* powders with a particle size <5–$10\,\mu m$;
- *working* with highly dissimilar materials;
- *preparing* the substrate minimally with surface preparation/masking, short standoff distance;
- *feeding* powder at a high rate, resulting in high productivity;
- *depositing* many materials at high deposition rates and efficiencies;
- *collecting and re-using* particles (powder utilization up to 100% with recycling);
- *heating* the substrate minimally;
- *increasing* operational safety because of the absence of high-temperature gas jets, radiation, and explosive gases.

The above-listed advantages make cold spray promising for producing and repairing a wide range of industrial parts. Examples include turbine blades, pistons, cylinders, valves, rings; and bearing components, pump elements, sleeves, shafts, and seals for many industries. Various coatings may add strengthening, hardening, wear resistance, corrosion resistance, electro-magnetic conductivity, thermal conductivity, and other properties. The process is also suitable for production of compact powder materials and for direct fabrication of parts.

Thus, the results presented allow us to state that a new concept, a new approach to spraying coatings, has been developed. This offers wide possibilities for developing new technologies and new equipment for spraying.

It should be noted that understanding the possibilities of this method in solving various problems associated with spraying coatings for specific powder and substrate materials requires detailed comprehensive investigations of physical processes accompanying particle–target interaction and also the main properties of coatings formed thereby. Results of these studies are presented in the following chapters.

Symbol List

p_0 Pressure in the pre-chamber (stagnation pressure)
T_0 Temperature in the pre-chamber (stagnation temperature)
M Mach number
M^* Mach number at the nozzle exit
M_∞ Mach number of the incident flow

d_p	Particle size
d_{pm}	Mean particle size
ρ_p	Density of the particle material
φ_p	Volume concentration of the particles
D_b	The air-flow body diameter (cylinder)
v_{st}	The initial velocity of the particle start
t_{ex}	Exposure time
Δt	Interval between two neighboring frames
$Re_D = \frac{\rho v D_b}{\mu}$	Reynolds's number of a air-flow body
ρ	Gas density
V	Gas velocity
μ	Gas viscosity
Δp_{bl}	Blowing pressure
$\dot{n}_p$	Number of the particles, which are taking off from a body in unit of time
$C_D^* = C_D/C_{D0}$	Drag coefficient of the cylinder
C_{D0}	Drag coefficient of the cylinder without injection of the particles
G_p	Particles flow rate
ε_p	Strain of the particle
v_p	Particle velocity
$v_{pm} = \frac{1}{N}\sum_{i=1}^{N} v_p^i$	Mean particle velocity
K	Magnification of the optical system
α_{tr}	Angle of inclination of the particle track on the film to the film axis
v_{sc}	Linear velocity of the sweep of the image recorded on the film
Δk	Accuracy of determining the optical system magnification
$\Delta\alpha_{tr}$	Accuracy of determining the slope of the trajectory on the film
Δv_{sc}	Accuracy of setting the velocity of the image in the film
H	Least size of the nozzle-exit cross section
$\sigma_v = \frac{1}{N-1}\sum_{i=1}^{N}\left(v_p^i - v_{pm}\right)^2$	Standard deviation of velocity distribution
$\Omega = \sqrt{\frac{d_p}{L} \times \frac{\rho_p v^{*2}}{p_0}}$	Dimensionless quantity
v_p*	Particle velocity at the nozzle exit
$V*$	Gas velocity at the nozzle exit
L	Length of a supersonic part of the nozzle
v_{cr1}	First critical velocity
ΔT_0	Heating of gas in pre-chamber
k_{He}	Helium concentration
$k_d = \frac{\Delta m_s}{M_p}$	Deposition efficiency
Δm_s	Change of weight of a substrate
M_p	Weight of all particles interacting with a substrate

References

[1] A.P. Alkhimov, V.F. Kosarev, and A.N. Papyrin, *Dokl. Akad. Nauk SSSR*, Vol. 315, 1990, pp. 1062–1065.

[2] A.G. Saltanov, *Supersonic Two-Phase Flows* [in Russian], Vysshaya Shkola, Minsk, 1972.

[3] J.H. Spurk and N. Gerber, *AIAA J.*, Vol. 10, No. 6, 1972, pp. 755–761.

[4] R.F. Probstein and F. Fassio, *AIAA J.*, Vol. 9, No. 4, 1971, pp. 772–779.

[5] J.D. Waldman and W.J. Reinecke, *AIAA J.*, Vol. 9, No. 6, 1971, pp. 60–67.

[6] W.A. Laitone, *J. Aircraft,* Vol. 16, No. 12, 1979, pp. 809–814.

[7] S.K. Matveev and L.P. Seyukova, Calculation of a gas–suspension flow around a disk and a flat end face of a cylinder, in *Gas Dynamics and Heat Transfer*, No. 6, Viscous and Inviscid Gas Flows, Izd. Leningr. Gos. Univ., Leningrad, 1981, pp. 3–12.

[8] A.P. Trunev and V.M. Fomin, *J. Appl. Mech. Tech. Phys.*, Vol. 25, No. 4, 1984, pp. 583–590.

[9] A.P. Trunev and V.M. Fomin, *J. Appl. Mech. Tech. Phys.*, Vol. 25, No. 5, 1984, pp. 732–734.

[10] B.A. Balanin and V.V. Zlobin, *Mekh. Zhidk. Gaza,* No. 3, 1979, pp. 159–162.

[11] A.J. Laderman, C.H. Lewis, and S.R. Byron, *AIAA J.*, Vol. 8, No. 10, 1970, pp. 1831–1839.

[12] D.T. Hove and A.A. Smit, *AIAA J.*, Vol. 13, No. 7, 1975, pp. 947–948.

[13] L.E. Dunbar, J.F. Courtney, and L.D. Memillen, *AIAA J.*, Vol. 13, No. 7, 1975, pp. 908–912.

[14] A.P. Alkhimov, N.N. Yanenko, N.I. Nesterovich, A.N. Papyrin, and V.M. Fomin, *Dokl. Akad. Nauk SSSR*, Vol. 260, No. 4, 1981, pp. 821–825.

[15] A.P. Alkhimov, V.F. Kosarev, N.I. Nesterovich, and A.N. Papyrin, Method of a Drag Reduction of a blunt-nosed body. Patent of Russian Federation No. 1228579 [in Russian], 1986.

[16] S.S. Bartenev, Y.P. Fedleo, and A.I. Grigirov, Detonation coatings in machine building [in Russian], Mashinostroenie, Leningrad branch,1982.

[17] C. Preece, (ed.), *Erosion*, Academic Press, New York, 1979.

[18] V.V. Kudinov, P.Yu. Pekshev, V.E. Belashchenko, O.P. Solonenko, and V.A. Safiulin, *Plasma-Induced Application of Coatings* [in Russian], Nauka, Moscow, 1990, p. 408

[19] A.P. Alkhimov, S.V. Klinkov, V.F. Kosarev, and A.N. Papyrin, *J. Appl. Mech. Tech. Phys.*, Vol. 38, No. 2, 1997, pp. 324–330.

[20] A.P. Alkhimov, V.M. Boiko, and A.N. Papyrin, *Avtometriya*, No. 3, 1982, pp. 38–45.

[21] A.P. Alkhimov and V.F. Kosarev, Laser diagnostics of supersonic two-phase jets, 8th Intern. Conf. on the Methods of Aerophysical Research, Sept. 1996, Proceedings, Part 2, Novosibirsk, 1996, pp. 3–8.

[22] A.P. Alkhimov, V.A. Arbuzov, A.N. Papyrin, R.I. Soloukhin, and M.S. Stein, *Comb. Expl. Shock Waves*, No. 4, 1973, pp. 507–514.

[23] A.P. Alkhimov, A.N. Papyrin, A.L. Predein, and R.I. Soloukhin, *J. Appl. Mech. Tech. Phys.*, Vol. 18, No. 4, 1977, pp. 496–502.

[24] A.P. Alkhimov, V.F. Kosarev, and A.N. Papyrin, *J. Appl. Mech. Tech. Phys.*, Vol. 39, No. 2, 1998, pp. 318–324.

CHAPTER 2

High-velocity Interaction of Particles with the Substrate. Experiment and Modeling

Cold Spray process has much in common with other methods of powder spraying (detonation, plasma, etc.); at the same time, there are some specific features, namely the particles are in solid state before their interaction with the substrate. The cold spray method can be used for coating application at room temperature. This circumstance allows one to track the effect of particle velocity (in pure form) on the deposition process and to eliminate temperature from consideration, which is impossible in gas-thermal methods. Using this unique property of cold spray method, we experimentally studied the high-velocity interaction of microparticles with the surface at low temperatures [1]. The calculations show that the impact temperature of particles accelerated by a supersonic gas flow with room stagnation temperature is 150–200 K, i.e., the particles incident onto the surface are in the "frozen" state. Another specific feature of the study performed is the neglect of collective effects, i.e., the main attention was paid to the so-called interaction of "single particles" with the mean distance between the particles in the jet and on the substrate surface being much greater than the particle size. This regime allows one to study physical laws of the phenomenon of particle-surface adhesion, which are common for all methods of powder deposition and have not been adequately addressed yet.

2.1. Deformation of Microparticles in a High-velocity Impact

Investigation of conditions of particle adhesion to the surface is a key problem whose solution could ensure understanding the mechanisms of coating formation. An important aspect of this problem, especially for the cold spray method, is the interaction of solid metallic microparticles with the substrate for impact velocities $v_p = 400$–$1200\,\mathrm{m/s}$, leading to particle deformation and attachment on the substrate surface [2].

A dimensional analysis of the problem of particle deformation in the case of a normal impact on the surface allows to conclude that possible parameters of the problem are $\rho_p v_p^2/H_p$, ρ_p/ρ_s, and H_p/H_s [3–5], where ρ_p, ρ_s, H_p, and H_s are the densities and dynamic hardness of the particle and the substrate, respectively. Deformation of spherical particles is independent of the particle size in the first approximation.

Deformation of particles made of a material with hardness lower than that of the substrate material was considered. The hardness of the substrate material was varied by means of thermal treatment and appropriate choice of particular materials. Thus, the role of the three parameters mentioned above was elucidated in the course of the experiment.

2.1.1. Experimental setup and materials

The setup included the gas heater, the feeder, and the nozzle unit. If the driver gas was helium, a standard gas holder with helium was connected to the setup. In all experiments, we used a supersonic nozzle with a rectangular cross section, the throat dimensions of 3 mm × 3 mm, exit-section dimensions of 3 mm × 10 mm, and supersonic-section length of 100 mm. Theoretically, this nozzle was designed for a Mach number $M_{id} = 2.75$, but the real Mach number at the jet centerline at the nozzle exit was $M^* = 2.5$ because of a fairly thick boundary layer on the nozzle walls. Thus, the pressure in the pre-chamber was equal to 1.7 MPa ensuring exhaustion of an isobaric jet.

After leaving the nozzle, the two-phase jet was directed onto the substrate at an angle of 90°. The substrate was an annular magazine with fixed specimens made of different materials; the specimens were cylinders with one butt-end face polished. The magazine was set into motion with an angular velocity of 5–10 rps. By varying the velocity of motion of the specimens, we could obtain different numbers of particles attached to the surface. The distance from the nozzle exit to the substrate surface was chosen within 15–20 mm. The materials used for the specimens were copper and unhardened or hardened steel. The experiments were performed with aluminum-powder particles shown in Fig. 2.1.

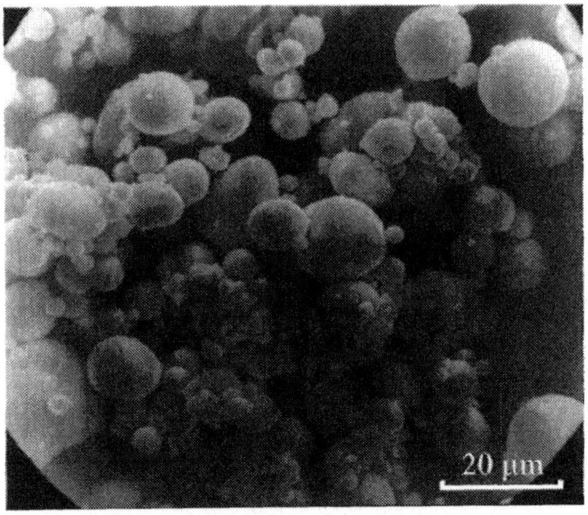

Fig. 2.1. Configuration of aluminum particles.

The shape of the particles was close to spherical, which allowed their acceleration to be calculated more precisely and facilitated simulation of the particle impact onto the substrate and the study of their deformation because the number of criteria was reduced. The mean particle size was 19.4 μm with a narrow range of scattering around this value.

The parameters varied in the experiments were the gas temperature in the pre-chamber and the type of the gas (helium or air), which allowed obtaining different impact velocities.

2.1.2. Measurement technique

Figure 2.2 shows the aluminum particles attached to the polished surface of the copper substrate. The particle in Fig. 2.2b became attached at $v_p \approx 1100\,\mathrm{m/s}$. Peripheral outbursts

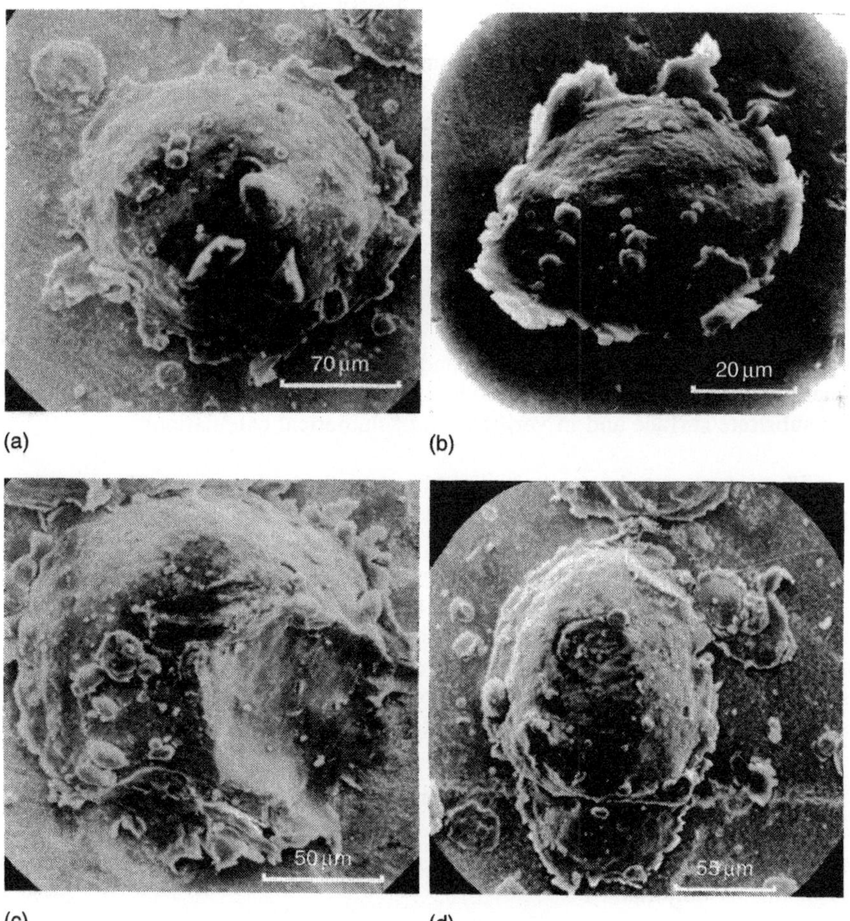

Fig. 2.2. Typical deformation of aluminum particles with different impact velocities on a polished copper substrate.

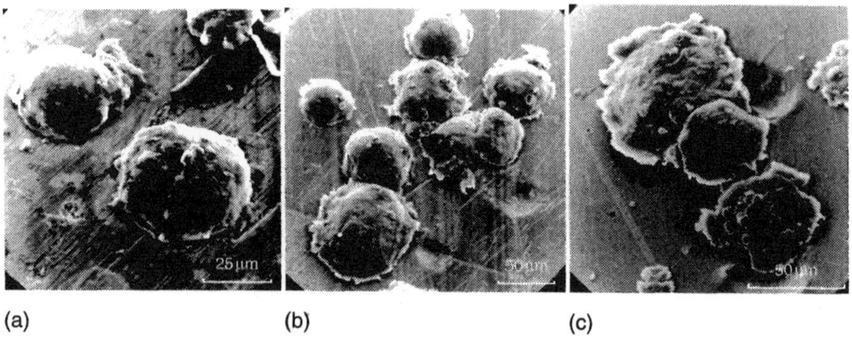

Fig. 2.3. Deformation of aluminum particles with different impact velocities on a polished copper substrate. Particle velocity $a = 625\,\mathrm{m/s}$, $b = 730\,\mathrm{m/s}$, and $c = 850\,\mathrm{m/s}$.

of metal are clearly visible. In Fig. 2.2c, the attached particle experienced an impact of the next particle, which did not get attached to the surface. In Fig. 2.2d, the next particle became attached due to its impact onto a previously attached particle.

Figure 2.3 shows the microphotographs of attached aluminum particles, which illustrate the character of particle deformation depending on the impact velocity. The photographs in Fig. 2.3a,b were obtained on a mechanically activated surface. For $v_{\mathrm{pm}} = 730\,\mathrm{m/s}$, a thin layer of crown-shaped outbursts appears over the periphery of attached particles, which is more noticeable at $v_{\mathrm{pm}} = 850\,\mathrm{m/s}$ and absent at $v_{\mathrm{pm}} = 625\,\mathrm{m/s}$. Inspection of a large number of photographs of particles of different sizes attached on the surface at different velocities allowed better understanding of the basic features of this process and subsequent use of this knowledge in modeling the adhesion interaction of microparticles with the substrate surface and in verification of numerical calculations.

The size of attached particles was measured by an optical microscope. The measurements were performed on individual particles whose planform shape was close to a circle with diameter D_{p}. The height of particles above the surface was measured on the basis of the effect of low depth resolution for short-focus microscope objectives ($\approx 1\,\mu\mathrm{m}$ for the objective used). Thus, the height h_{p} of the attached particle above the surface was determined from the difference between the objective positions with a clearly visible specimen surface and a clearly visible upper part of the particle. Based on these two values and on the assumption that the attached particle is a paraboloid of revolution, we reconstructed the particle volume and then its initial diameter:

$$d_{\mathrm{p}} = \left(\frac{3}{4} h_{\mathrm{p}} D_{\mathrm{p}}^2\right)^{1/3}.$$

Figure 2.4 shows a microphotograph of the attached particle profile, which confirms the validity of this assumption.

A comparison of the distribution function of attached particles based on the thus-reconstructed diameters with the initial distribution function shows that the representation of attached particles in the form of a paraboloid is fairly valid with a probability of 95%.

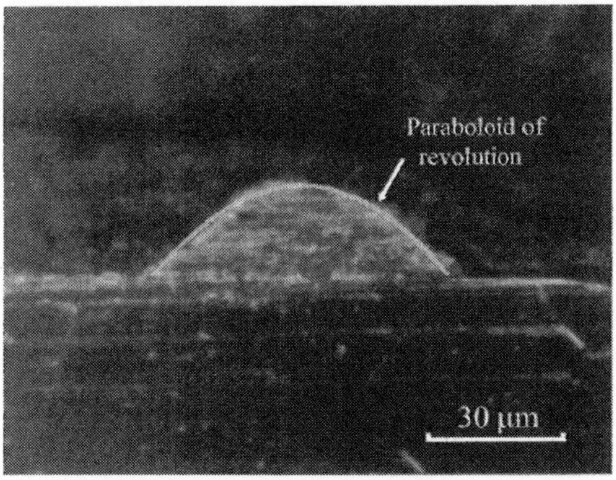

Fig. 2.4. Microphotograph of the attached particle profile.

From the reconstructed values of the initial particle diameter, we found the impact-induced strain by the formula

$$\varepsilon_p = 1 - \frac{h_p}{d_p},$$

2.1.3. *Statistical processing*

Due to the measurement errors and scattering of particles in terms of shape, size, velocity, etc., the realistic value of particle strain can be obtained on the basis of a large number of measurements and statistical processing of the results. The number of experiments for different specimen varied from 50 to 120, which ensures a standard deviation within 3.0%. The standard procedure includes finding the mean value and the root-mean-square deviation

$$\varepsilon_{pm} = \frac{1}{N}\sum_{1}^{N}\varepsilon_i,$$

$$\mathrm{sd} = \left(\frac{1}{N-1}\sum_{1}^{N}\left(\varepsilon_{pm} - \varepsilon_i\right)^2\right)^{0.5},$$

$$s = \frac{\mathrm{sd}}{\sqrt{N}}.$$

We can say that the true value of strain is located in the interval $\varepsilon_p = \varepsilon_{pm} \pm s$ with a probability of 68.3% and in the interval $\varepsilon_p = \varepsilon_{pm} \pm 2s$ with a probability of 95.5%.

In addition, it is important to know whether the two mean values found in processing different specimens are significantly different or if their difference can be neglected. For this purpose, the following procedure is used. Let similar values of strain be obtained in processing two different specimens with, e.g., different hardness: $\varepsilon_{pm1} \pm s_1$, $\varepsilon_{pm2} \pm s_2$. We have to determine whether the value of hardness affects the value of strain. We find $s_{12} = \sqrt{s_1^2 + s_2^2}$, $\Delta\varepsilon_{pm} = |\varepsilon_{pm1} - \varepsilon_{pm2}|$. If $\Delta\varepsilon_{pm} > 2.576 s_{12}$, then these values are different with a probability of 99%, i.e., it is possible to track the influence of the specimen hardness on the particle strain; if $\Delta\varepsilon_{pm} < 1.96 s_{12}$, the difference is insignificant with a probability of 95%, and the effect of hardness can be neglected. In the intermediate case, additional data have to be used.

To find strain as a function of the particle size on the basis of experimental data, one can use linear regression with the least squares technique, which is valid in the case of a narrow range of particle sizes.

2.1.4. Results of microscopic studies

The processing of the measured results for a large number of particles attached on one specimen included finding the initial diameter of all sampled particles and their strain. After that, we found the mean particle size and their strain for a given specimen and a prescribed root-mean-square deviation. All these data are summarized in Table 2.1.

In addition, linear regression by the least squares technique was performed. In identical acceleration modes, there is a weak but yet noticeable tendency of the particle strain to decrease with increasing particle diameter. A probable reason for this is the lower velocity of particles of greater diameters. The expected strain for particles 10 and 30 μm in diameter was found on the basis of the approximation curve. These values are compared with mean strains in Table 2.2.

To verify that microscopic measurements do not experience any subjective factors, the experiments were performed at two different times with the same specimen. The mean values and the root-mean-square deviations turned out to be similar. For instance, for

Table 2.1. Experimental data on particle strain under particle impact

Specimen number	d_{pm}, μm	$sd(d_{pm})$	$s(d_{pm})$	ε_{pm}	$sd(\varepsilon_{pm})$	$s(\varepsilon_{pm})$
1	19.8	4.4	0.62	0.37	0.083	0.012
2	18.6	3.2	0.46	0.35	0.152	0.022
3	18.3	5.2	0.48	0.43	0.085	0.008
4	16.3	5.7	0.53	0.44	0.096	0.009
5	21.1	4.4	0.70	0.48	0.082	0.013
6	20.5	5.0	0.85	0.47	0.078	0.013
7	19.6	4.7	0.73	0.52	0.103	0.016
8	18.7	5.4	0.62	0.63	0.065	0.008
9	17.8	4.6	0.58	0.63	0.077	0.010
10	19.6	4.6	0.44	0.72	0.069	0.006

Specimen material: unhardened steel (1, 3, 5, and 8), hardened steel (4, 7, 9, and 10), and copper (2 and 6).

Table 2.2. Mean strain for different particle sizes

Specimen number	1	2	3	4	5	6	7	8	9	10
$\varepsilon(30\,\mu m)$	0.29	0.25	0.39	0.41	0.44	0.45	0.44	0.63	0.64	0.66
$\varepsilon(d_{pm})$	0.37	0.35	0.43	0.44	0.48	0.47	0.52	0.63	0.63	0.72
$\varepsilon(10\,\mu m)$	0.44	0.42	0.45	0.46	0.53	0.48	0.60	0.64	0.63	0.77

specimen No. 4, we obtained $\varepsilon_{p1} = 0.45424 \pm 0.01045$ and $\varepsilon_{p2} = 0.44216 \pm 0.00878$, hence $\Delta\varepsilon_{pm} = 0.012 < 1.96 s_{12}$, i.e., these two samples indeed belong to one parent population. Thus, the chosen measurement procedure can be assumed to be correct and to ensure a high level of data reproducibility.

Observation of the surface with attached particles allows us to note that particles are often attached as clusters (see Fig. 2.3b), i.e., several particles are attached close to each other, and it is difficult to find the boundary between them. This possibly occurs because of the high activity of surface sections adjacent to the previously attached particle. Thus, a single attached particle plays the role of a nucleus triggering the growth of a continuous coating over the specimen surface. By comparing steel and copper specimens, we can note that a greater number of particles are attached on the copper specimen in all acceleration modes.

2.1.5. Dependence of strain on impact velocity

Based on the data of Tables 2.1 and 2.2 and using the calculated particle velocities, we find particle strain as a function of particle velocity. According to the dimensional analysis, the strain should depend on the dimensionless parameter $\rho_p v_p^2/H_p$ and on the ratios ρ_p/ρ_s and H_p/H_s. It is seen from the results presented above that the dependence on the first parameter dominates, and the dependence on the last two parameters can be neglected. Figure 2.5 shows the experimental results in the coordinates ε_p, $\rho_p v_p^2/H_p$. We use the value of 560 MPa as H_p [5]. The same plot shows the points obtained for particles 10 and 30 μm in diameter by the linear regression technique. It is seen from Fig. 2.5 that

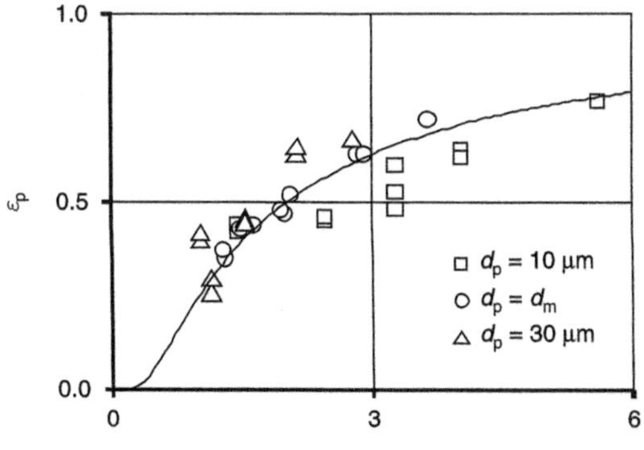

Fig. 2.5. Generic dependence of particle strain on impact velocity.

if we take into account the dependence of particle velocity on particle size, we find that the strain of fine particles is lower than the strain of coarse particles with an identical velocity, i.e., fine particles have better hardness properties (H_p) than coarse particles. This confirms the presence of scaling in the range of velocities and particle diameters considered, which is well known in the range of hypersonic impact [6, 7].

The solid curve is the approximation constructed on the basis of results obtained for the mean particle size. The experimental points for d_{pm} admit approximation by one curve. Note that the analytical expression for the approximation function

$$\varepsilon_p = \exp\left(-1.4\frac{H_p}{\rho_p v_p^2}\right) \tag{2.1}$$

has correct asymptotic curves, because $\varepsilon_p \to 1$ as $v_p \to \infty$ and $\varepsilon_p \to 0$ as $v_p \to 0$.

The experimental studies of high-velocity (400–1200 m/s) interaction of spherical aluminum particles with the surface, including microscopic inspection of the particle shape and methods of statistical processing of a large amount of data, allowed obtaining results on the particle strain as a function of the impact velocity. In the examined range of ρ_p/ρ_s and H_p/H_s, these parameters do not exert any substantial effect on particle strain, and the governing parameter is $\rho_p v_p^2/H_p$. The experimental results described in this section are indispensable in verification of particle-strain calculations, modeling of heat release under an impact, and adhesion interaction of the particle with the substrate.

2.2. Spraying of the Initial Layer and its Influence on the Coating Formation Process

Except for very thin coatings, the spray process can be considered as a process that consists of two stages: the spraying of the first layer of particles on a substrate and the buildup of the coating. During the first stage, the particles interact with the substrate, and this process determines the quality of the interface and coating adhesion. To improve adhesion, sand blasting is commonly used under thermal spraying. However, this method has certain disadvantages including the effect of interface contamination due to penetration of sand blasting particles into the substrate, especially for soft substrate materials. Sand blasting is undesirable in many applications, for example, in spraying on parts with thin walls, parts already coated, parts made of brittle materials, etc. In the cold spray process, the sprayed particles are in the solid state, and in some cases they can be used for preliminary treatment and preparation of the substrate, in particular, when the use of sand blasting is unacceptable.

The first stage of coating spraying turns out to be more complicated, because it depends on particle and substrate parameters (e.g., roughness, hardness, temperature, etc.) and on the state of the surface, which is obviously changed as the number of particle impacts increases. This change, in turn, leads to changes in conditions of particle–substrate interaction and, consequently, to unsteady growth of the coating.

This section presents some results of study of spraying of the first layer and its influence on the coating formation process.

2.2.1. Activation of the surface by the particles. Induction time.

The results of experiments on interaction of individual aluminum particles with a moving polished copper substrate at the initial stage of spraying are shown in Figs 2.6 and 2.7 Aluminum particles with a mean diameter of 30.2 μm were accelerated by a mixture of air and helium. The particle velocity was changed by varying the content of helium in the mixture. The objective of these experiments was to observe individual particles attached to the surface as well as craters from reflected particles for different particle velocities. Figure 2.6 shows a typical experimental dependence of the induction time as a function of the particle-impact velocity and an approximation curve of the form $t_i = a\left(\frac{1}{\sqrt{v_p - v_{cr1}}} - \frac{1}{\sqrt{v_{cr2} - v_{cr1}}}\right)$ with the values $a = 365$ s, $v_{cr1} = 550$ m/s, and $v_{cr2} = 850$ m/s.

The *induction* or *delay time* is the time between the beginning of surface treatment by the flow of particles and the beginning of particle attachment to the surface. The main results of these experiments are as follows. There are three characteristic regions of particle–substrate interaction, divided by two values of particle velocity: v_{cr1} and v_{cr2} (Fig. 2.6). In region 1, with v_p higher than v_{cr2} (850 m/s), particles adhere to the initial surface without any delay. As the particle velocity decreases, the situation is changed. In region 2, located between v_{cr1} and v_{cr2}, particles cannot adhere to the initial (original) surface. They start to adhere to the surface only after some delay, when the surface state is changed because of its treatment by the first impinging particles. In this region, the first particles rebound, thus, preparing the surface, and only after that does the coating start to form.

Figure 2.7 shows a typical photograph of the substrate surface in this regime after the surface treatment during 25 s by a flow of particles with a velocity of 600 m/s. The entire surface is covered by craters from reflected particles, and only very few particles adhered to the surface.

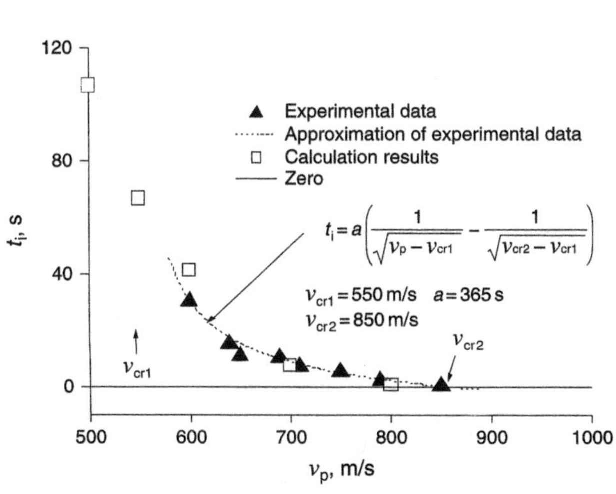

Fig. 2.6. Induction (deposition delay) time versus the mean impact velocity of aluminum particles on a polished copper substrate; $d_{pm} = 30.2\,\mu m$, $\varphi_p = 10^{-8}$ (the mass flow of particles per unit area is 0.06 kg/m^2 s).

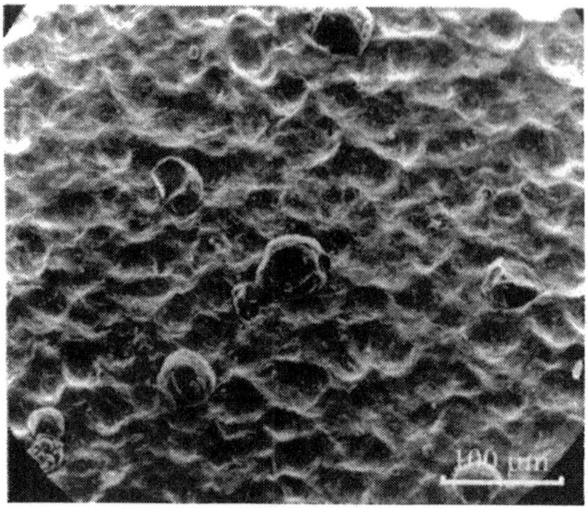

Fig. 2.7. Microphotograph showing the influence of surface activation by impacted particles on the process of particle attachment to the substrate.

Thus, it is clear that the surface was exposed to a large number of particle impacts before particles start to adhere to the surface. The first impinging particles increase the chemical activity of the surface owing to creation of an elevated concentration of dislocations in the superficial layer. In addition, particles may leave on the surface a certain amount of attached particle material, which obviously makes activation energy approach a value intrinsic for the particle. As a result, the activation energy of the particle–substrate interaction decreases. Intensive bombardment by the first particles results in cleaning and activation of the surface and preparing favorable conditions for adhesion of the following particles. It should be noted that adhesion of the first particles leads to a rapid increase in the number of attached particles and to formation of a continuous coating (avalanche-type process). With a decrease in particle velocity, the induction time increases (Fig. 2.6) because more intense treatment and activation of the surface are required.

In region 3, with an impact velocity lower than v_{cr1} (550 m/s), particles do not adhere to the surface regardless of the time of treatment; only the process of particle rebounding and, as a consequence, surface erosion are observed. This value of velocity was determined as a critical one for transition from erosion to coating formation in the experiments described in Chapter 1.

It is clear that the spraying induction time is related to the concentration of particles in the flow. To find this relation, we assume that the particle size is not much different from the mean size, i.e., we consider the motion of a monodisperse powder. Note that in the case of motion of a polydisperse powder, which is more typical in practice, two rather narrow ranges with characteristic mean particle size can be conventionally distinguished. In this case, considering each fraction separately, we can draw conclusions for the powder as a whole. The quantity measured in the experiment is normally the volume or mass flow rate of the powder. The relation between the volume $\dot{V}_p$ and numerical $\dot{N}_p$ flow rates of the powder is determined by formula (2.2), and the relation between the mass and numerical flow rates is found from formula (2.3):

$$\dot{V}_p = \frac{1}{k_p}\frac{\pi d_p^3}{6}\dot{N}_p, \tag{2.2}$$

where k_p is the packing factor of the powder (normally, about 0.5),

$$\dot{m}_p = \rho_p \frac{\pi d_p^3}{6}\dot{N}_p. \tag{2.3}$$

Knowing the total flow rate of particles from the powder feeder, we can estimate the flux of particles per unit area of the surface. For this purpose, we assume that the particles are uniformly distributed over the area of the exposed substrate surface, i.e., the average number of impacts at an arbitrary point of the exposed surface is identical. Note, this can be hardly achieved in the experiment, because the concentration of particles at the jet edges is usually lower, and it is difficult to predict the non-uniformity of particle distribution over the area in the case of a developed shock-wave structure induced by non-isobaric exhaustion of jets. Therefore, the density of the particle flux in the vicinity of a given point of the surface should be determined in the general case by some additional methods with additional assumptions. Assuming further that the area of the exposed surface coincides with the cross-sectional area of the jet and, moreover, with the nozzle-exit area S_{ex}, we can readily estimate the flux of particles per unit surface as $\dot{n}_p = \dot{N}_p/S_{ex}$. Obviously, this surface point experiences the impact of only those particles whose centers are located in a circle of diameter D_p around this point. Here, D_p is the diameter of the contact zone between the particle and the surface, which is determined via the particle diameter and its strain due to the impact by formula (2.4) derived, e.g., in [8–10]:

$$D_p = \frac{2d_p}{\sqrt{3(1-\varepsilon_p)}} \tag{2.4}$$

Assuming that the number of impacts obeys Poisson's ratio, we use formulas (2.5) borrowed from [11] to determine the probability of exactly m particles impacting a given point of the surface during the time t:

$$P_m = \frac{(\dot{n}_{im} t)^m}{m!}e^{-\dot{n}_{im} t}, \; \alpha = \dot{N}_p \frac{\pi D_p^2}{4 S_{ex}} = \dot{N}_p \frac{S_c}{S_{ex}} = \dot{N}_p s_c. \tag{2.5}$$

Here, $\dot{n}_{im}$ is the mean number of impacts at a given point of the surface per unit time, i.e., the mean frequency of impacts, $S_c = \pi D_p^2/4$ is the particle–substrate contact area, and $S_c = \dfrac{S_c}{S_{ex}}$ is the normalized particle–substrate contact area.

Poisson's ratio can be approximated by the Gaussian distribution if the expected number of impacts during the exposure time $\dot{n}_{im} t_{ex}$ is rather large. The variance (i.e., the squared root-mean-square deviation) should be set equal to the mean value. Knowing the mean frequency of impacts at the point, the mean number of impacts during the induction time is determined by the formula

$$\langle N_{im} \rangle_i = \dot{n}_{im} t_i. \tag{2.6}$$

As the number of impacts at a given point of the surface should remain approximately identical because it characterizes activation processes, it follows from formulas (2.5) and (2.6) that the spraying induction time is inversely proportional to the powder flow rate.

It should be noted that the experiments were performed with volume concentrations of the disperse phase $\varphi_p \approx 10^{-8}$. Clearly, for different particle concentrations in the jet, the induction time in the first approximation is determined as

$$t_i\left(v_p, \varphi_p\right) = t_i\left(v_p, 10^{-8}\right)\frac{10^{-8}}{\varphi_p}. \tag{2.7}$$

At such concentrations of particles, the effect of substrate heating by heat released in particle impacts onto the substrate and the effect of interaction of particles with each other are negligibly small. For instance, even with neglected heat exchange with the jet, a 10 g copper substrate is heated by one degree only during the time of $\approx$40 s. The probability of interaction of an incident particle with another particle contacting the substrate can be evaluated as $P \approx 6\varepsilon_p\varphi_p$, where ε_p is the particle strain. For our test conditions, we have $P \approx 3 \times 10^{-8}$.

The critical velocities v_{cr1} and v_{cr2}, as well as the induction time, depend on numerous interaction parameters: particle and substrate materials, particle size, initial state of the particle and substrate surfaces, etc.

The induction time t_i can be expressed via the parameters of the two-phase jet and the necessary (depending on the particle velocity) number of preliminary impacts $N_{pi}(v_p)$ at each point of the surface:

$$t_i\left(v_p, \varphi_p\right) = \frac{2}{3}\frac{d_p}{\varphi_p v_p}\left\langle N_{im}\left(v_p\right)\right\rangle_i. \tag{2.8}$$

Correspondingly, we obtain

$$\left\langle N_{im}\left(v_p\right)\right\rangle_i = \frac{3}{2}\frac{\varphi_p v_p}{d_p} t_i\left(v_p, \varphi_p\right), \tag{2.9}$$

which, after substitution of numerical values ($\varphi_p \approx 10^{-8}$; $v_p = 600$–$800\,\mathrm{m/s}$; $d_p = 30 \times 10^{-6}\,\mathrm{m}$), yields $\left\langle N_{im}\left(v_p\right)\right\rangle_i = (2 \div 4)\, t_i\left(v_p, 10^{-8}\right)$ (the values of all parameters are given in the SI measurement system), where $t_i(v_p, 10^{-8})$ can be found from Fig. 2.6. For example, for $v_p = 600\,\mathrm{m/s}$, we have $t(v_p, 10^{-8}) \approx 30\,\mathrm{s}$; correspondingly, $\langle N_{im}(600\,\mathrm{m/s})\rangle_i \approx 50$.

Thus, the results presented show that the sprayed particles in the cold spray process can play an important role in the preparation and activation of the substrate surface, and this effect can be used in applications when utilization of sand blasting is unacceptable or undesirable. In this case, however, additional effects associated with a delay of spraying of the first layer should be taken into account in the coating formation process analysis. Some results of such an analysis are presented further in this section.

2.2.2. Critical parameters

It should be noted that there exist a critical concentration of particles in the jet with a velocity of particles $v_{cr1} < v_p < v_{cr2}$ incident onto the substrate moving with a velocity v_w; below this critical concentration, no coating is formed on the substrate during one pass of the nozzle. Correspondingly, for a particular concentration of particles in the jet, there exists a maximum substrate velocity above which no coating is formed:

$$v_{w\,max} \approx \frac{h}{3t_i\left(v_p, \varphi_p\right)}. \tag{2.10}$$

The reason is that each point of the moving surface is activated by particles from the jet periphery and then arrives in the jet core, where the deposition proceeds (see Fig. 2.8).

We can estimate the minimum concentration of particles in the jet, necessary for each point of the surface to experience a necessary particle-velocity-dependent number of impacts before entering the jet core. We assume that the thickness of the peripheral region to be equal to one-third of the jet thickness. After some transformations, we obtain

$$\varphi_{p\,min} = 2\frac{d_p}{h}\frac{v_w}{v_p}\left\langle N_{im}\left(v_p\right)\right\rangle_i, \tag{2.11}$$

where v_w is the substrate velocity.

It follows from the relations presented that in the case of deposition onto a moving substrate in the regime with $v_{cr1} < v_p < v_{cr2}$, the critical concentration of particles is inversely proportional to the jet thickness h and depends linearly on the substrate velocity and, which is particularly important, on the diameter of sprayed particles.

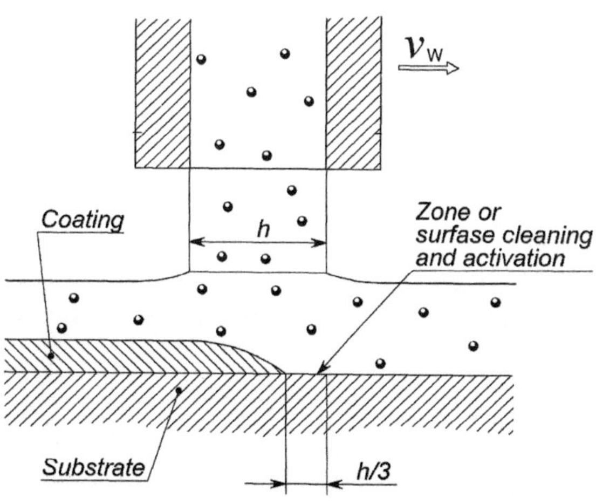

Fig. 2.8. Activation of the substrate by peripheral particles.

2.2.3. Determination of the mass of the first coating layer

To determine the mass of the first coating layer (coating layer at the time when there is no free surface left on the substrate), we use the following considerations. Let the exposed surface S_{ex} have a certain free surface S_{fr} (not occupied by particles) at a certain time. We introduce the normalized free surface $s_{fr} = S_{fr}/S_{ex}$. Further, suppose a small number of particles dN_p falls onto the exposed surface. Among these particles, $s_{fr}dN_p$ particles are incident onto the free surface. Among the latter number of particles, $P_1 s_{fr} dN_p$ particles adhere to the surface (P_1 is the probability of attachment on the free surface). The decrease in free surface is determined as

$$ds_{fr} = -P_1 s_c s_{fr} dN_p \tag{2.12}$$

On the other hand, $P_2(1 - s_{fr})dN_p$ particles adhere to the already covered surface (P_2 is the probability of particle attachment on the already covered surface). Hence, the total number of attached particles is

$$dN_c = [P_1 s_{fr} + P_2(1 - s_{fr})]dN_p \tag{2.13}$$

To estimate the mass of the first layer, we further simplify the model. We assume that the probability of particle attachment on the free surface P_1 equals zero at $t \le t_i$. As the coating grows, we assume that the probability of particle attachment on the free surface P_1 remains unchanged during the time of formation of the first layer. This allows us to obtain an analytical solution for Eqs (2.14) and (2.15) for the free surface and the mass of deposited particles m_c:

$$s_{fr} = \begin{cases} 1 & t < t_i \\ \exp\left[-P_1 \dot{n}_{pm}(t - t_i)\right] & t \ge t_i, \end{cases} \tag{2.14}$$

$$m_c = \begin{cases} 0 & t < t_i \\ P_2 \dot{m}_p (t - t_i) + \dfrac{P_1 - P_2}{P_1}\dfrac{\dot{m}_p}{\dot{n}_{pm}}\left[1 - \exp\left[-P_1 \dot{n}_{pm}(t - t_i)\right]\right] & t \ge t_i, \end{cases} \tag{2.15}$$

When condition (2.16) is satisfied, formation of the first layer is practically completed; as it follows from formula (2.15), further growth of the coating is almost linear, i.e., $dm_c/dt = \text{Const}$:

$$t_0 - t_i \approx 3\frac{1}{P_1 \dot{n}_{pm}} \tag{2.16}$$

Substituting the value of t_0 from formula (2.16) to formula (2.15), we obtain Eq. (2.17) for the mass of particles contained in the first layer of the coating m_{c0}:

$$m_{c0} = \frac{\dot{m}_p}{\dot{n}_{pm}}\left(1 + 2\frac{P_2}{P_1}\right) = S_{ex}\frac{\rho_p d_p}{2}(1 - \varepsilon_p)\left(1 + 2\frac{P_2}{P_1}\right) \tag{2.17}$$

It is worth noting that the number of particles in the first layer and its mass depend on probabilities and, hence, on the properties of the substrate and particle materials. This clearly affects the first layer roughness: the greater the first layer mass, the greater the roughness. The least roughness is obtained for the minimum value of m_{c0}, i.e., under the condition $P_2 \ll P_1$, which implies that adhesion of particles to each other is much weaker than adhesion of particles to the surface.

If the probabilities are commensurable in value (in the case of identical substrate and particle materials, the probabilities should be identically equal), the mass of particles in the first layer can be estimated by the expression

$$\frac{m_{c0}}{S_{ex}} \approx 3\frac{\rho_p d_p}{2}\left(1-\varepsilon_p\right) \tag{2.18}$$

The approach proposed here also allows us to estimate the characteristic value of surface roughness. Assuming that the stage of formation of the first layer is completed, and the coating growth is determined by the probability of particle attachment on the surface formed by particles themselves, P_2. We also assume that the number of attached particles at a given point obeys Poisson's ratio with a frequency $P_2\dot{N}_pS_c/S_{ex}$. To estimate the mean thickness and the coating and its roughness, the mean number of attached particles and its root-mean-square deviation found from Poisson's distribution should be multiplied by the characteristic height of the particle after its deformation h_p. After some simple transformations, we can obtain the following expression for normalized roughness:

$$\frac{\delta h_c}{h_c} = \sqrt{\frac{d_p\left(1-\varepsilon_p\right)}{h_c}}. \tag{2.19}$$

Hence, we can conclude that it is desirable to use a fine powder and high velocities to obtain a uniform coating, because $\varepsilon_p \to 1$ as $v_p \to \infty$.

2.2.4. *Steady stage of coating formation*

After the first layer is formed, we assume that the curve of the further increase in coating mass should have a constant slope, because the particles interact with the surface consisting of particles themselves. A decrease or an increase in the growth rate would indicate some changes in the particle–surface interaction conditions. We also assume that the first layer of the coating of mass m_{c0} is formed on the substrate surface at the time $t = t_0$. Then, the further increase in coating mass (or in the number of attached particles) is described by the linear dependence

$$m_c = m_{c0} + k_{d0}\dot{m}_p\left(t-t_0\right) = m_{c0} + k_{d0}\left(m_p - m_{p0}\right), t > t_0. \tag{2.20}$$

On the other hand, assuming that the exponent in Eq. (2.5) is negligibly small as compared to unity, we obtain the expression

$$m_c = P_2\dot{m}_p\left(t-t_0\right) + \frac{P_1 - P_2}{P_1}\frac{\dot{m}_p}{\dot{n}_{pm}} \text{ for } t > t_0 \tag{2.21}$$

Equation (2.21) is brought to the form of (2.20) if equalities (2.22) and (2.23) are satisfied:

$$P_2 = k_{d0}, \tag{2.22}$$

$$P_1 = \frac{3m_{c0}}{m_{p0} - m_{pi}} - 2k_{d0}, \tag{2.23}$$

2.2.5. *Kinetics of coating-mass growth*

To have an idea about the changes in mass of the sprayed layer, depending on the mass of the powder used (or on the time if the flow rate of the powder from the feeder is uniform), we consider Fig. 2.9. The x axis shows the mass of the powder used and the y axis shows the mass of the coating formed.

It is assumed in Fig. 2.9a,b that the probability of attachment of particles to each other (i.e., at the steady stage of coating formation) is identical and equal to 0.5. We consider the cases of better attachment to the substrate surface (case 1), worse attachment to the surface (case 2), and identical attachment to the surface (case 3), as compared to attachment to the surface formed by particles themselves. The straight line emanating from the origin describes the limiting case with zero induction time $t_i = 0$ (or $m_{pi} = 0$) and identical probabilities $P_1 = P_2 = 0.5$, i.e., identical surface and particle materials. Curves

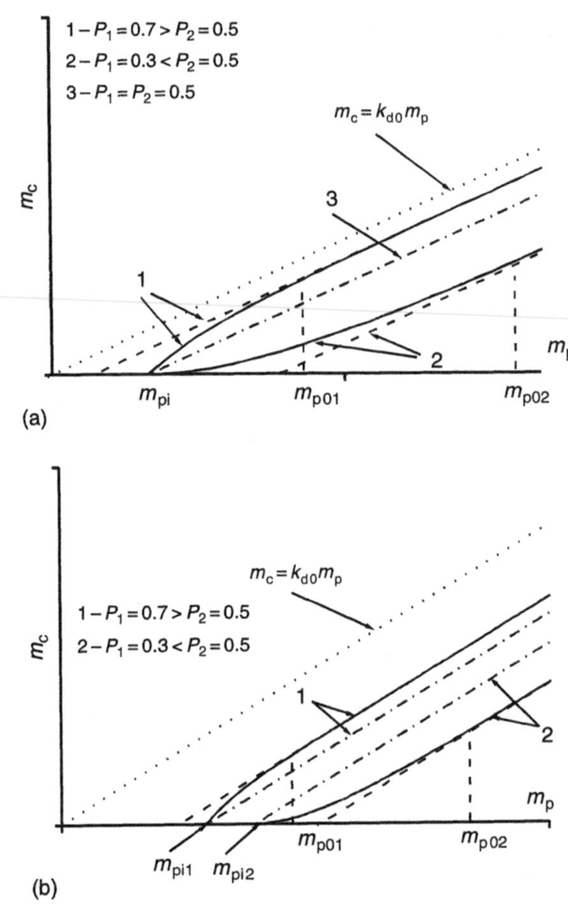

Fig. 2.9. Mass of the coating versus the mass of the powder used for identical induction times (a) and different induction times (b).

1 refer to case 1 ($P_1 > P_2$), and curves 2 refer to case 2 ($P_1 < P_2$). The induction times in Fig. 2.9a are identical. Figure 2.9b shows the case with different induction times $t_{i1} < t_{i2}$ (or $m_{pi1} < m_{pi2}$). The solid curves are constructed by formula (2.15) for cases 1 and 2, respectively. It is seen that the coating mass is zero as m_p changes from 0 to m_{pi}, increases in accordance with formula (2.15), and approaches the approximation curve determined by Eq. (2.21) for $m_p > m_{p0}$. The dot-and-dashed curves 3 refer to case 3 ($P_1 = P_2 = 0.5$).

Obviously, coating growth proceeds faster in case 1 in which the particle attachment to the surface is better than the attachment of particles themselves.

If the particle attachment to the surface is worse, it seems logical to expect a longer induction time. This variant is shown in Fig. 2.9b. Clearly, the coating growth is even slower in this case.

2.2.6. Deposition efficiency

We determine the deposition efficiency k_d as the ratio of the coating mass to the mass of the powder incident onto the substrate. We designate the derivative d_{mc}/d_{mp} at the steady stage of coating formation as k_{d0} and call it the theoretical deposition efficiency.

Let us track the changes in the deposition efficiency with time (with changes in mass of the powder used). From formula (2.15) one can produce formula (2.24)

$$k_d = P_2\left(1-\frac{m_{pi}}{m_p}\right)+P_2\frac{m_{pi}^*}{m_p}\left\{1-\exp\left[-\frac{P_1-P_2}{P_2}\frac{m_p}{m_{pi}^*}\left(1-\frac{m_{pi}}{m_p}\right)\right]\right\}, \tag{2.24}$$

where $m_{pi}^* = \dfrac{P_1-P_2}{P_1P_2}\dfrac{\rho_p d_p(1-\varepsilon_p)}{2}$ is the critical mass of fallen particles during induction time.

At $m_{pi} \ll m_{pi}^*$, which corresponds to small induction time, Eq. (2.24) can be simplified down to fashion (2.25)

$$k_d = P_2 + P_2\frac{m_{pi}^*}{m_p}\left\{1-\exp\left[-\frac{P_1-P_2}{P_2}\frac{m_p}{m_{pi}^*}\right]\right\} \tag{2.25}$$

At $m_{pi} \gg m_{pi}^*$ or at $P_1 = P_2$ (the materials of the deposited particles and the substrate are identical), second term in expression (2.24) can be neglected and then formula (2.24) can be simplified to formula (2.26)

$$k_d = \frac{m_c}{m_p} = \begin{cases} 0 & m_p < m_{pi} \\ k_{d0}\left(1-\frac{m_{pi}}{m_p}\right) & m_p \geq m_{pi} \end{cases}. \tag{2.26}$$

Estimates show that for typical values $P_1 = 0.7, P_2 = 0.5, \rho_p = 2700\,\text{kg/m}^3, d_p = 10^{-5}\,\text{m}, \varepsilon_p \approx 0.5$ critical value $m_{pi}^* \approx 3\times10^{-3}\,\text{kg/m}^2$. For induction time at typical for cold spray powder flow rate $\dot{m}_p \approx 30\,\text{kg/m}^2\text{s}$ $t_i^* \approx 10^{-4}\,\text{s}$ this time is significantly smaller than the characteristic time of the process (~1 s) and is comparable to the mean time between impacts of particles onto the selected point of surface $t_{\text{im}} = \frac{1}{\dot{n}_{\text{pm}}} = \frac{\rho_{\text{p}} d_{\text{p}}(1-\varepsilon_{\text{p}})}{2\dot{m}_{\text{p}}}$. It is obvious that even if for preparation of the surface only 1% of the common number of impacts of particles is consumed ($N_{\text{im}} \approx 5 \times 10^3$) then the value m_{pi} will be much greater than value m^*_{pi} $\left(\frac{m_{\text{pi}}}{m^*_{\text{pi}}} \approx 50\right)$. Thus, it is obvious that practically always $t_{\text{i}} \gg t^*_{\text{i}}$ and with a high accuracy for estimate of deposition efficiency one can use formula (2.25).

In Fig. 2.10, curves 1 and 2 show dependences of deposition efficiency upon mass of consumed powder. These curves were constructed using formula (2.24) in accordance with cases 1 and 2 at different induction times considered above. Curves 3 and 4 are constructed using formula (2.25) and correspond to cases 1 and 2. From comparison of curves 1 and 3 and also 2 and 4 it is followed that they have approximately equal type of shape.

For an arbitrary fixed number of particles leaving the feeder, there is always a certain error in determining the deposition efficiency. The greater the mass of the powder used (or the deposition time), the smaller the normalized error of the experimentally measured deposition efficiency:

$$\frac{|k_{\text{d}} - k_{\text{d0}}|}{k_{\text{d0}}} = \frac{m_{\text{pi}}}{m_{\text{p}}} \tag{2.27}$$

As is seen from formula (2.27), the experimental value can tend to zero not because there is actually no particle attachment but because the number of particles used approaches the number of particles necessary for surface activation. Thus, one has to know the induction time to describe the spraying phenomenon correctly.

In measuring deposition efficiency, the substrate normally moves with a constant velocity under the jet. The number of passes over one point on the surface can be greater than one. In practice, the substrate velocity and the number of passes is chosen such that a

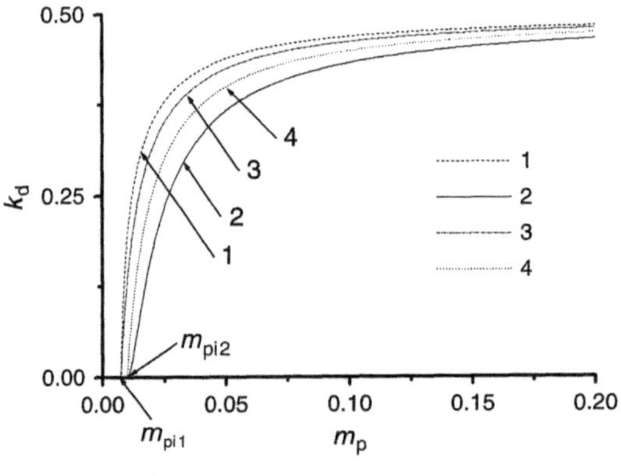

Fig. 2.10. Deposition efficiency as a function of mass of the powder used (deposition time in the case of a uniform flow rate of the powder).

sufficient coating mass necessary for accurate measurements is formed on the substrate surface. The flow rate of powder from the feeder is also constant in time.

Let us consider an elementary area $dxdy$. Moving under the jet in the x direction, it experiences particle impacts during the time $h(y)/v_w$. Thus, $(\dot{n}_p h(y)/v_w)\,dxdy$ particles are incident onto this area. If the number of incident particles is greater than the number of particles necessary for surface activation $n_{pi}dxdy$, then $n_c dxdy = P_2(\dot{n}_p h(y)/v_w - n_{pi})\,dxdy$ particles adhere to the elementary area $dxdy$. Thus, the total number of particles used is determined by the integral

$$N_p = \int_0^{L_c} dx \int_{-H/2}^{H/2} \frac{\dot{n}_p h(y)}{v_w} dy. \tag{2.28}$$

Note, expression (2.28) describes the simple fact that $N_p = \dot{N}_p L_c/v_w$ particles are used during the feeder-operation time L_c/v_w, where L_c is the length of the deposition band with allowance for the number of passes. Therefore, integration is not necessary in view of the simplicity of the physical interpretation.

The total number of attached particles is determined by the expression

$$N_c = \int_0^{L_c} dx \int_{-y_m}^{y_m} P_2\left(\frac{\dot{n}_p h(y)}{v_w} - n_{pi}\right) dy. \tag{2.29}$$

Here, the half-width of the deposition band y_m is found from the condition $n_{pi} = \dot{n}_p h(y_m)/v_w$ or $t_i = h(y_m)/v_w$.

The deposition efficiency measured in the experiment is determined by the ratio of the quantities described by Eq. (2.29) and Eq. (2.28). In the case of a plane nozzle, these relations are readily integrated, because the exposure time of the elementary area of the surface is independent of the coordinate y. We obtain the following expression for deposition efficiency:

$$k_d = k_{d0}\left(1 - \frac{m_{pi} v_w}{\dot{m}_p h}\right) = k_{d0}\left(1 - \frac{t_i v_w}{h}\right). \tag{2.30}$$

In the case of a conical nozzle, the expression becomes more difficult, because the variable h changes in accordance with the formula

$$h(y) = 2\sqrt{\left(\frac{D_j}{2}\right)^2 - y^2}. \tag{2.31}$$

Here, D_j is the jet diameter and y is the coordinate perpendicular to the substrate-motion direction and counted from the coating-band centerline.

In this case, the deposition efficiency is determined by the formula

$$k_d = k_{d0}\frac{2}{\pi}\left(\arcsin\sqrt{1-\beta_i^2} - \beta_i\sqrt{1-\beta_i^2}\right), \quad \beta_i = \frac{t_i v_w}{D_j}. \tag{2.32}$$

With accuracy sufficient for practical applications, the function in the right-hand part of formula (2.32) can be replaced by a simpler approximate expression$(1-\beta_i)^{1.35}$. Thus, the deposition efficiency can be generalized in the form of Eq. 2.33, where ω equals 1 or 1.35 for rectangular and circular nozzle cross sections, respectively:

$$k_d = k_{d0}\left(1-\frac{m_{pi}v_w}{\dot{m}_p h}\right)^{\omega} = k_{d0}\left(1-\frac{t_i v_w}{h}\right)^{\omega} \tag{2.33}$$

In the case of a circular nozzle, the nozzle-exit diameter should be used as h. Since the quantity in brackets is smaller than unity, the deposition efficiency k_d of the nozzle with a rectangular cross section is closer to the theoretical value k_{d0}.

2.2.7. Correction to the deposition efficiency

Using the data in Fig. 2.6, we can estimate the mass of the powder used for surface activation and the first layer formation. In experiments with deposition efficiency measurements, the weight dose was 100 mg, which yields a specific mass of $\sim$3.3 kg/m^2. Substituting the resultant values into formula (2.26), we find the correction factor for estimating the theoretical deposition efficiency on the basis of data obtained in the experiment [12]. Figure 2.11 shows the experimental data and the data calculated by the method described above.

It is seen that the weight dose of 100 mg is sufficient for obtaining reliable experimental data.

Nevertheless, if the weight dose is much smaller than 100 mg (as an example, Fig. 2.11 also shows the data that would be obtained with a dose of 17 mg), the differences would be fairly noticeable, for instance, the critical velocity would be 700 m/s rather than the real value 600 m/s.

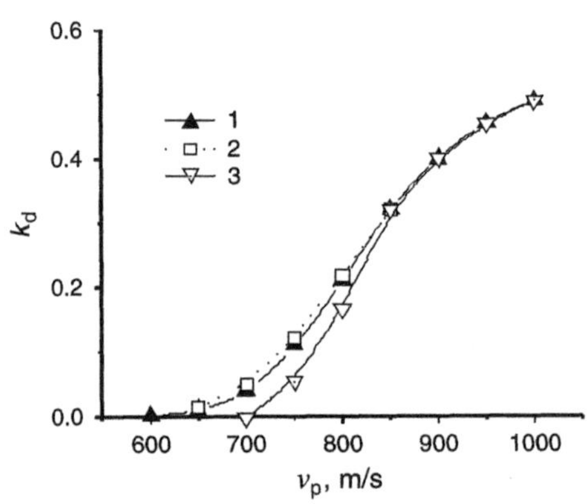

Fig. 2.11. Deposition efficiency measured in the experiment and the corrected value: 1 – experimental values, 2 – corrected values and the values that would be obtained in an experiment with a weight dose of 17 mg.

Thus, as we can see from results presented in this section, the effect of the first layer on the coating formation process and its characteristics can play an important role in the cold spray process, and it should be taken into account especially under spraying thin (a few monolayers of particles) coatings.

2.3. Modeling of Interaction of Single Particles with the Substrate within the Framework of Mechanics of Continuous Media

Experimental investigation of the dynamics of high-velocity ($v_p = 200$–$1200\,\mathrm{m/s}$) interaction of microparticles ($d_p = 1$–$50\,\mu\mathrm{m}$) with the substrate (especially its dynamics) is very complicated (at the moment, almost impossible). The reason for this is that the characteristic sizes and times in this problem are 1–50 μm and 10^{-7}–10^{-9} s, respectively. Therefore, the main tool for such investigations is mathematical modeling.

The quantitative description of the impact phenomenon is a complicated problem; and there is an associated field of research under intense recent development. The impact of bodies is accompanied by versatile processes whose relative role depends on the shape and physical parameters of the object and, which is more important, on the relative impact velocity. In addition, the impact often involves penetration of one body into the other. During the high-velocity impact, one or both colliding bodies can disintegrate, spread, or sprayed, which is accompanied by dissipation of significant amounts of energy.

Until a certain stage of development of computational equipment, the impact processes were mainly described by engineering and one-dimensional approaches. Though these approaches offered explanations to some qualitative and quantitative laws, the high-velocity impact processes can be considered in detail only by numerical methods in two-dimensional and three-dimensional formulations. Application of analytical methods for solving this class of problems (especially in the three-dimensional case) remains an extremely difficult problem.

The problem of the impact of a spherical deformable particle on a solid substrate was solved within the framework of the mathematical model and numerical algorithm described in [13–15]. The behavior of materials was described by the model of an ideal elastoplastic Prandtl–Reuss medium with a variable dynamic yield stress, which gained wide application after the famous Wilkins' publication [16] later on generalized in monobook [17]. Numerical solutions were obtained for some particular problems, which are of individual significance in addition to justification of the proposed approach to studying the impact of deformable bodies in the range of velocities up to 2–3 km/s. The method of solution is based on the Lagrangian approach of description of continuous deformable media [13].

The main attention was paid to studying the integral characteristics of the process. The process of microparticle adhesion to the substrate depends not only on the particle size and impact velocity but also on the contact time. Therefore, the dependence of the particle–substrate contact time on the impact velocity, particle size, and particle properties was primarily examined. It should be noted that we are not aware of any publications with the data on experimental investigations of a single act of microparticle–substrate interaction because of the small particle size and a very short interaction time. The theoretical analysis of this phenomenon is often reduced to estimates obtained from the one-dimensional theory. Mathematical simulations for a symmetrical axis case allow for obtaining more detailed information about this process. Another important parameter of the impact, which substantially affects the process of adhesion interaction of the microparticle and the substrate under an impact, is their contact area.

In the calculations, the particle size and velocity were chosen to take values typical for conditions of cold spray. Methodical calculations showed that the calculated results of the impact interaction of the particle and the substrate are strongly affected by the substrate size and propagation of elastic–plastic waves, generated as a result of an impact. The effect of the substrate size is no longer important as its mass becomes greater than the particle mass by a factor of 200–300. For particles with a diameter $d_p = 10\,\mu m$, the substrate radius and the substrate thickness were chosen to be 40 and $50\,\mu m$, respectively. As the diameter d_p increased, the substrate dimensions were increased accordingly. The conditions of zero displacements were imposed on the side and bottom boundaries of the substrate that corresponds to full damping of plastic waves, and amplitude of elastic waves is considered to be low.

2.3.1. Impact of a spherical particle on a rigid substrate

We considered the problem of a normal impact of a spherical particle with the initial velocity v_p varied from 5 to 800 m/s on an absolutely rigid substrate. The particle size was chosen to correspond to the microparticle size in the cold spray process: $d_p = 10$–$50\,\mu m$. The basic parameters of aluminum, copper, and iron materials used in the calculations are listed in Table 2.3 (K is the volume compression modulus, μ_{sh} is the shear modulus, E is Young's modulus, ν_P is Poisson's ratio, and Y_0 is the dynamic yield stress).

2.3.1.1. Impact of elastic particles

Kil'chevskii [18] derived an analytical expression for the contact time of two colliding elastic spheres on the basis of Hertz's theory:

$$t_c = 2.9432\left[\frac{25\pi^2}{8}\frac{(1-\nu_P)^4}{(1-2\nu_P)^2}\right]^{0.2}\frac{d_p}{2v_p^{0.2}c_{II}^{0.8}}, \tag{2.34}$$

Table 2.3. Mechanical properties of materials

Material	ρ_0, kg/m	K, GPa	μ_{sh}, GPa	E, GPa	ν_P	Y_0, GPa
Al	2.70	72	26.8	66	0.347	0.3
Cu	8.90	139	46.0	124	0.351	0.3
Fe	7.87	170	80.0	207	0.297	0.7

where $c_{II} = \sqrt{\frac{E(1-\nu_p)}{(1+\nu_p)(1-2\nu_p)\rho_p}}$ is the velocity of longitudinal waves in the medium. To obtain a solution in the approximation of the elastic behavior of the medium, the dynamic yield stress was given such a value that the plasticity condition was obviously unsatisfied in the range of impact velocities under consideration. The results of these calculations by formula (2.34) for copper and aluminum particles with a diameter $d_p = 10\,\mu m$ are plotted in Figs 2.12 and 2.13, respectively, as the contact time versus the initial impact velocity v_p. Determination of contact time at numerical modeling is described in details in [13, 18].

The calculated curves are lower than the theoretical data, and the approximation formulas obtained by the least squares technique have factors slightly different from 0.2. In our opinion, this difference is associated with the neglect of the wave processes in the sphere in formula (2.34).

2.3.1.2. *Elastoplastic impact*

A typical curve of the contact time as a function of the initial impact velocity in the case of the elastoplastic behavior of the particle material is plotted in Fig. 2.14. This figure shows the results of the calculation of the process of the impact of an aluminum particle with $d_p = 20\,\mu m$ and $Y_0 = 0.3\,GPa$ on obstacle. For low velocities of impact, the effect is plasticity is small, and the contact time decreases as that in the elastic case. The effect of plasticity increases with increasing velocity, and the rate of variation of the contact time decreases, reaches a minimum, and starts increasing again, because the influence of plasticity starts to prevail. The influence of the yield stress of the material on the contact time versus velocity is illustrated in Fig. 2.15.

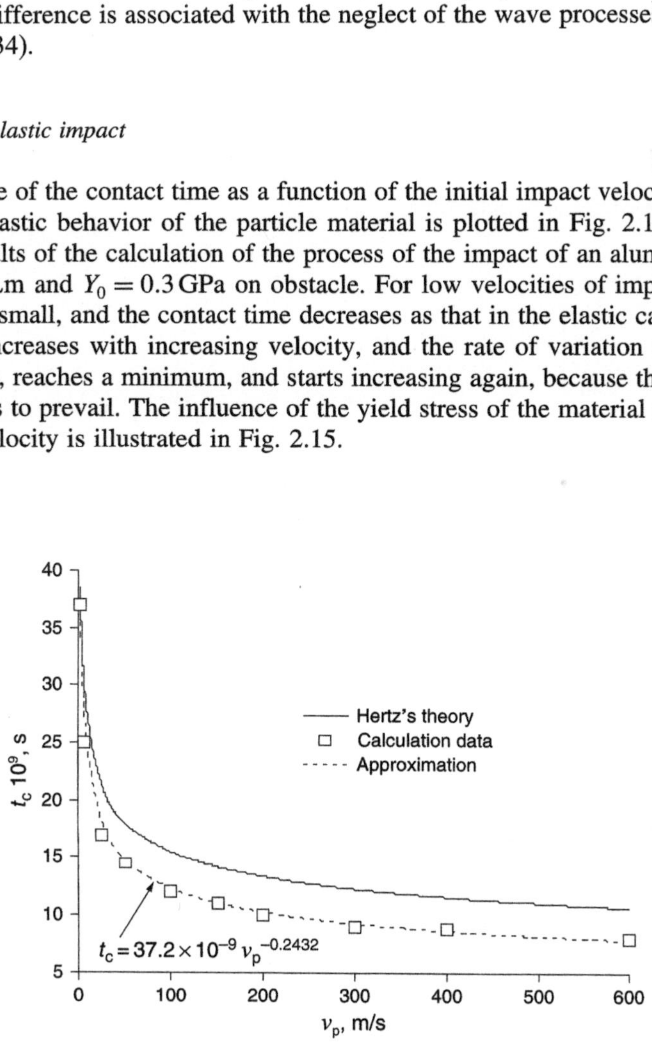

Fig. 2.12. Contact time versus the impact velocity of a copper particle on a rigid wall.

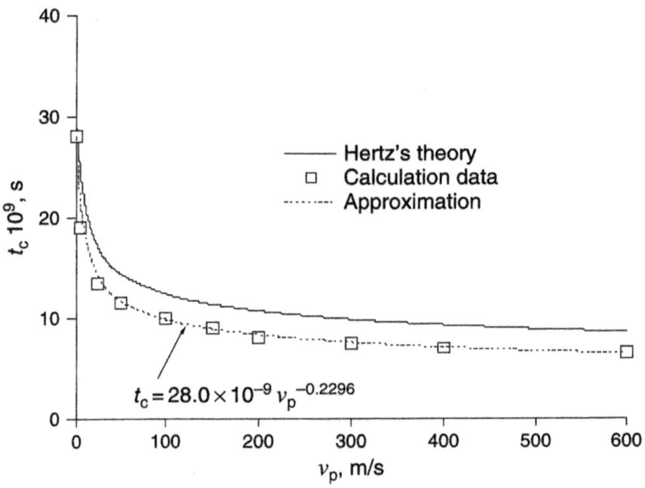

Fig. 2.13. Comparison of the theoretical and numerical solutions for the contact time for different initial impact velocities on a rigid wall.

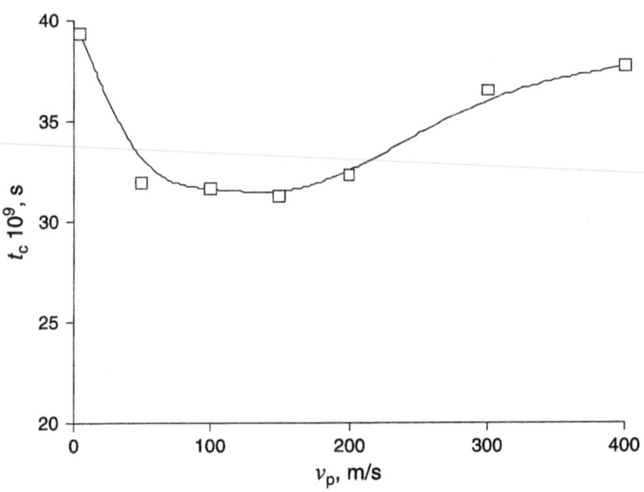

Fig. 2.14. Contact time for an elastoplastic aluminum particle. $d_p = 20\,\mu m$, $Y_0 = 0.3\,GPa$.

As the yield stress increases, the contact time decreases, and the minimum is reached at large values of Y_0. Thus, if the yield stress increases, then

1. the minimum point is shifted to the right;
2. the contact time decreases;
3. the growth of the contact time versus the impact velocity is slower.

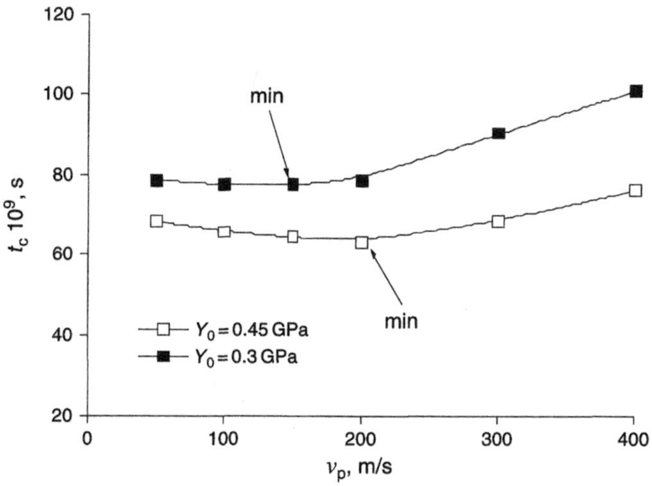

Fig. 2.15. Effect of the yield stress on the contact time with a rigid wall.

All mentioned conclusions are easy to explain by the wave character of process of interaction, see [18, 19].

This behavior of the contact time differs from the case of a rod impact on a substrate [19, 20], where the contact time remains constant until a certain impact velocity different for each particular material is reached and then increases. In the case of a spherical particle, the contact area with the substrate surface changes in the course of interaction and depends both on the impact velocity and on the strength parameters of the particle material. This is the governing factor in the behavior of the contact time for different impact velocities. Figure 2.16 shows deformation of a spherical aluminum particle with $d_p = 10\,\mu\text{m}$ and initial velocity of 200 m/s at different times.

Figure 2.17 shows deformation of the same particle at time $t = 18\,\text{ns}$ close to the end of the contact interaction for different initial velocities.

As it follows from formula (2.34), the contact time of an elastic spherical particle depends linearly on the particle radius. It is of interest that this is also true for an elastoplastic particle. Figure 2.18 shows contact time as a function of impact velocity for different diameters of the aluminum particle in the dimensionless variables $t'_c = t_{cp}/t_{ce}$ and $v' = \rho_p v_p^2/Y_0$, where t_{ce} and t_{cp} are the calculated contact times of the "elastic" and "elastoplastic" particles, respectively.

These curves almost coincide, which confirms the fact of the linear dependence of the contact time on the particle radius in the case the particle material manifests plastic properties. A similar situation is observed for particles of other materials. On the other hand, the contact time does not possess this property in the case of a constant impact velocity and different yield stress. Figure 2.19 shows the data calculated for an aluminum particle with $d_p = 10\,\mu\text{m}$ and different yield stress for impact velocities $v_p = 200\,\text{m/s}$ and $v_p = 400\,\text{m/s}$.

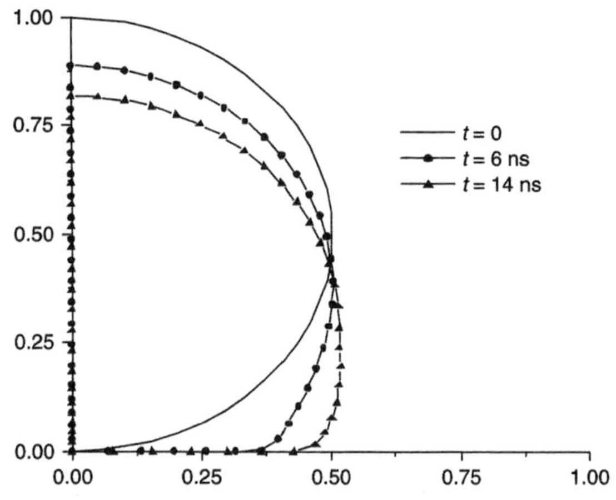

Fig. 2.16. Time evolution of the aluminum particle profile, $v_p = 200\,\mathrm{m/s}$.

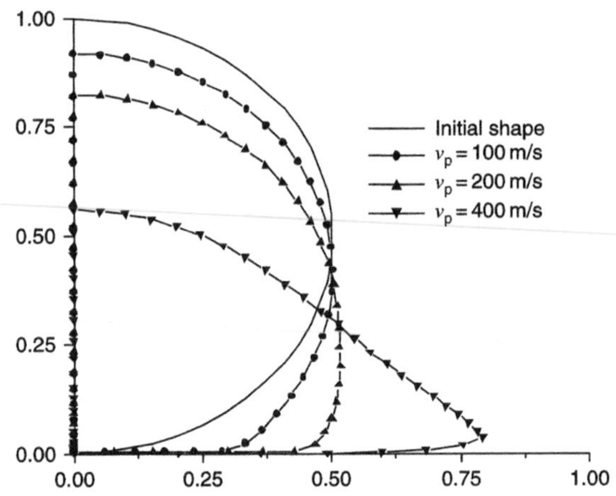

Fig. 2.17. Effect of the initial velocity of the particle on its shape at the end of the contact process, $t = 18\,\mathrm{ns}$.

A typical behavior of the force f_c acting at the aluminum particle–substrate interface versus time is shown in Fig. 2.20. Curve 1 refers to an "elastic" particle, and curve 2 corresponds to an inelastic particle with the yield stress $Y_0 = 0.3\,\mathrm{GPa}$. In both cases, the diameter is $d_p = 10\,\mu\mathrm{m}$ and the impact velocity is $v_p = 100\,\mathrm{m/s}$. The influence of plasticity decreases the force magnitude and increases the contact time.

Thus, it is shown that the phenomenon of rebounding of spherical particles from a solid substrate and the particle–substrate contact time are significantly different in the cases of elastic and elastoplastic behavior of the material.

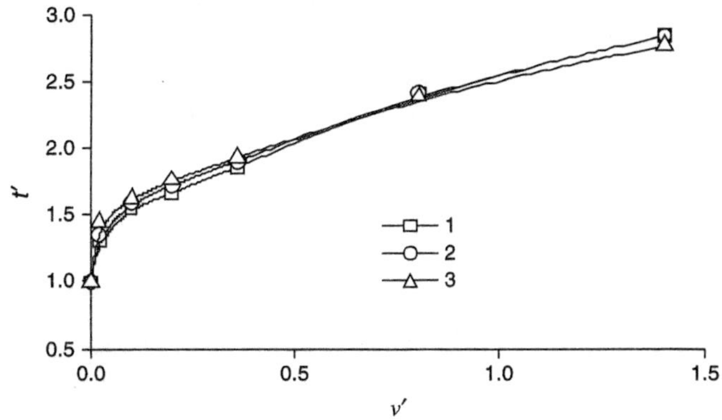

Fig. 2.18. Contact time versus the parameter $v' = \rho_p v_p^2 / Y_0$. Aluminum particles on a rigid wall. $Y_0 = 0.3\,\text{GPa}$, $1 - d_p = 50\,\mu\text{m}$, $1 - d_p = 20\,\mu\text{m}$, $1 - d_p = 10\,\mu\text{m}$.

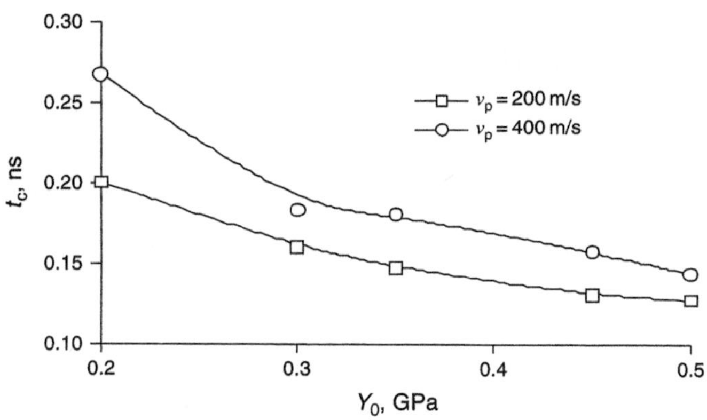

Fig. 2.19. Effect of the yield stress on the contact time.

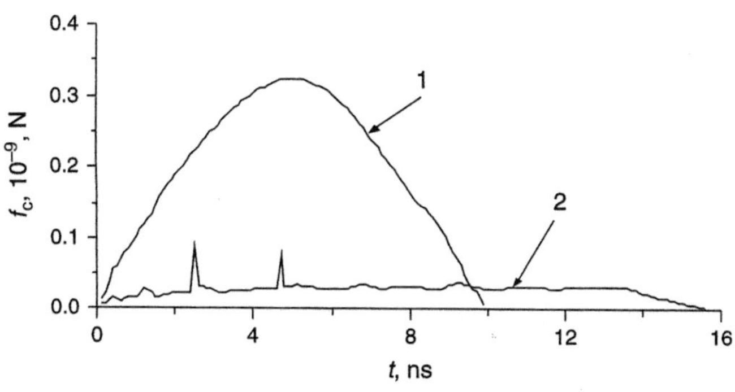

Fig. 2.20. Behavior of the force at the interface for 1 – elastic and 2 – plastic impact modes.

2.3.2. *Impact of microparticles on deformable substrates*

In real cold spray processes, the hardness of particles is often commensurable with the substrate hardness. Therefore, we calculated the impact of microparticles on a deformable substrate. In the variant considered, an aluminum particle impacted on an aluminum substrate along the normal. The following mechanical properties of aluminum were used:

$$\rho_p = 2700\,\mathrm{kg/m^3},\ K = 0.69\times10^5\,\mathrm{MPa},\ \mu_{sh} = 0.248\times10^5\,\mathrm{MPa},$$

$$Y_0 = 0.0045\times10^5\,\mathrm{MPa},\ Y = Y_0\left(1 - e/e_m\right),\ e_m = 5451\,\mathrm{MJ/kg},$$

where e is the specific internal energy and e_m is the specific internal energy at the melting point. The particle diameters were 10, 25, and 100 μm, and the range of impact velocities was from 300 to 1000 m/s.

Table 2.4 contains the integral characteristics obtained in some calculation variants. The numbers of the variants are listed in the first column. The contact time t_c was determined

Table 2.4. Results of calculation of particle impact parameters

Variant number	v_p, m/s	d_p, μm	t_c, ns	v_{pr}, m/s	$s'_{c\,max}$	e_r
1	300	10	15	39.6548	0.85512	0.01747
2	500	10	14	34.9222	1.44924	0.00488
3	600	10	13	55.8707	1.81546	0.00867
4	800	10	14	68.7954	2.13639	0.0074
5	300	25	36	37.6128	0.91253	0.01572
6	500	25	34	32.8245	1.59441	0.00431
7	600	25	33	41.4816	1.89548	0.00478
8	800	25	34	69.0858	2.42275	0.00746
9	300	10	15	33.0492	0.96103	0.01214
10	500	10	15	27.1565	1.50921	0.00295
11	600	10	15	30.4139	1.98021	0.00257
12	800	10	15	49.9595	3.00204	0.00390
13	300	25	36	33.0997	0.88056	0.01217
14	500	25	36	28.7338	1.65502	0.00330
15	600	25	36	31.3158	1.91590	0.00272
16	800	25	36	54.2441	2.56511	0.00460
17	300	100	143	33.3274	0.88460	0.01234
18	500	100	141	28.1185	1.62627	0.00316
19	600	100	141	31.6660	1.96176	0.00279
20	800	100	142	55.2212	2.68879	0.00476

as the time interval between the moment the particle touches the substrate and the moment when all boundary points of the particle depart from the substrate boundary. The dimensionless contact area s'_c and the coefficient of recovery of kinetic energy of the rebounded particle e_r were calculated by the formulas

$$s'_c = \frac{s_{c\,max}}{s_m}, \quad s_m = \frac{\pi d_p^2}{4}, \quad e_r = \left(\frac{v_{pr}}{v_p}\right)^2$$

where $s_{c\,max}$ is the contact area of the particle surface with the substrate at the time preceding the rebounding moment. The dynamic yield stress was constant in variants 1–8 and variable in the remaining variants (in this case, it was calculated by the formula given above).

It is seen from Table 2.4 that the contact time depends weakly on the impact velocity and almost linearly increases with increasing particle diameter. The behavior of other integral parameters is shown in Figs 2.21–2.24.

Figure 2.21 shows the particle contours ($d_p = 10\,\mu m$) at the time of rebounding and substrate fragments for different impact velocities. In Figs. 2.21–2.24, a and b refer to a constant yield stress and to a variable yield stress, respectively. For velocities v_p lower than 500 m/s, the interaction leads to particle flattening without its deep penetration into the substrate. For high velocities, a decrease in particle height is accompanied by an increase in penetration depth. It is of interest to note that the critical velocity in the cold spray method is approximately 600 m/s for aluminum powder, which was found in experiments in Chapter 1 [21].

Figures 2.22a,b show the particle–substrate contact time versus the impact velocity. The maximum differences in the velocity range considered are within 12%. The numbers 1, 2, and 3 in the figures indicate the dependences corresponding to initial particle diameters of 10, 25, and 100 μm.

Figure 2.23 illustrates the behavior of the dimensionless area of the contact surface as a function of the initial velocity v_p. The behavior of this function is close to linear and depends little on the initial particle diameter. For s'_c, we can use the formula

$$s'_c = \alpha v_p + \beta,$$

where α and β obtained by processing the calculated results are $\alpha = 2.5 \times 10^{-3}$ and $\beta = 0.25$ for variant *a* and $\alpha = 3.5 \times 10^{-3}$ and $\beta = -0.22$ for variant *b*.

Figure 2.22 shows the dependence of e_r on the impact velocity. For velocities up to 500 m/s, this parameter decreases, and then starts to increase insignificantly.

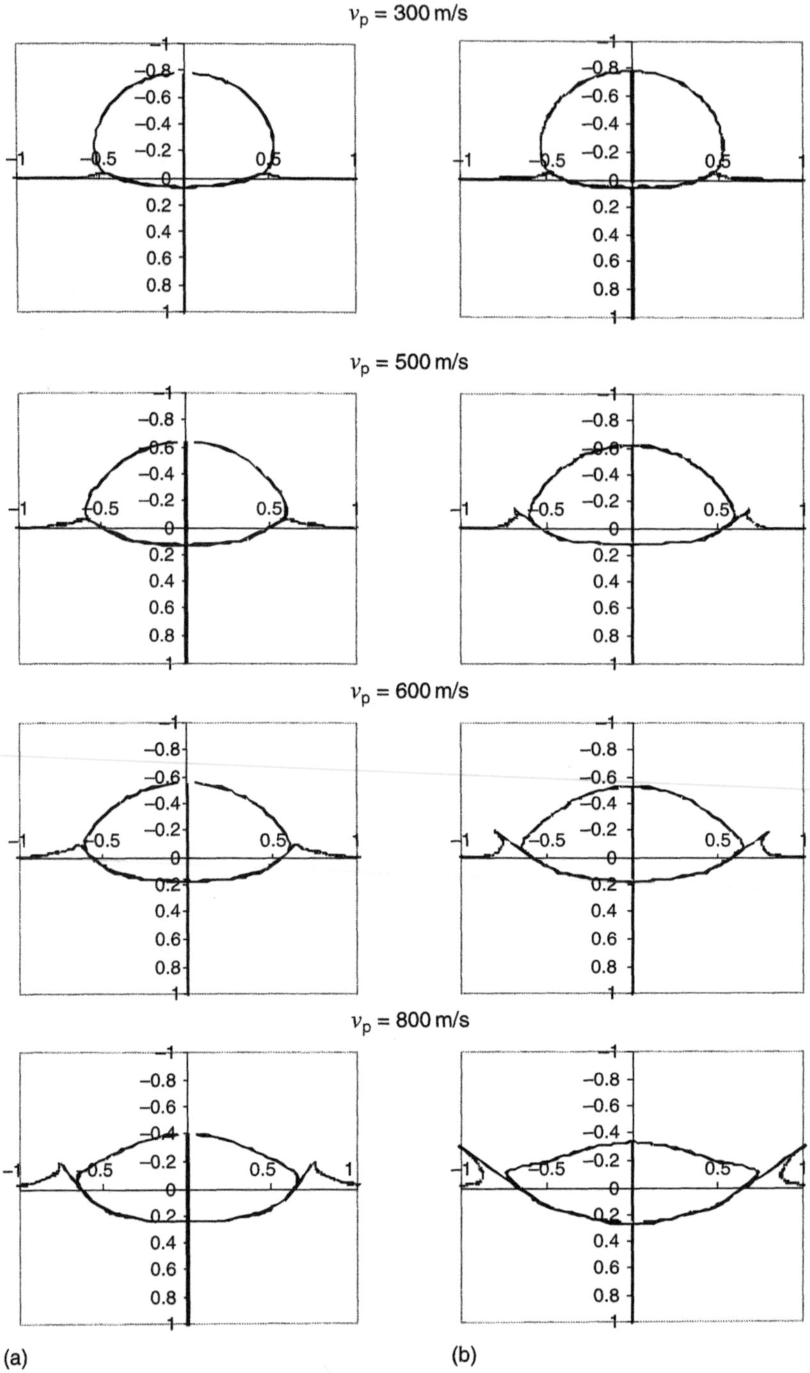

Fig. 2.21. Particle contours at the rebounding moment. (a) constant yield stress and (b) variable yield stress.

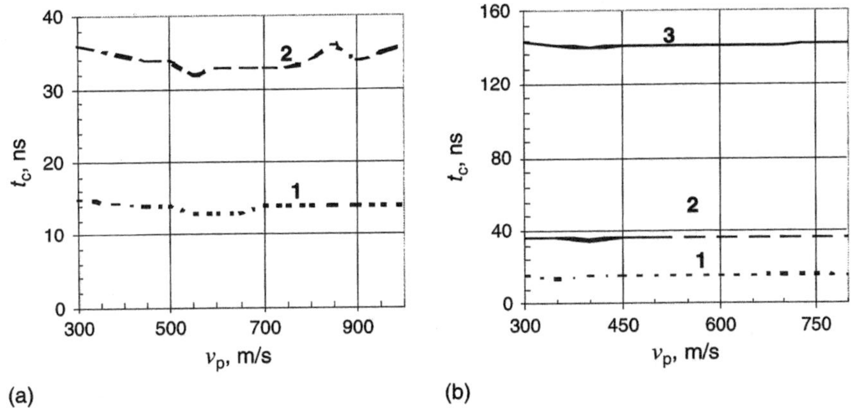

Fig. 2.22. Contact time versus the initial impact velocity. (a) constant yield stress and (b) variable yield stress.

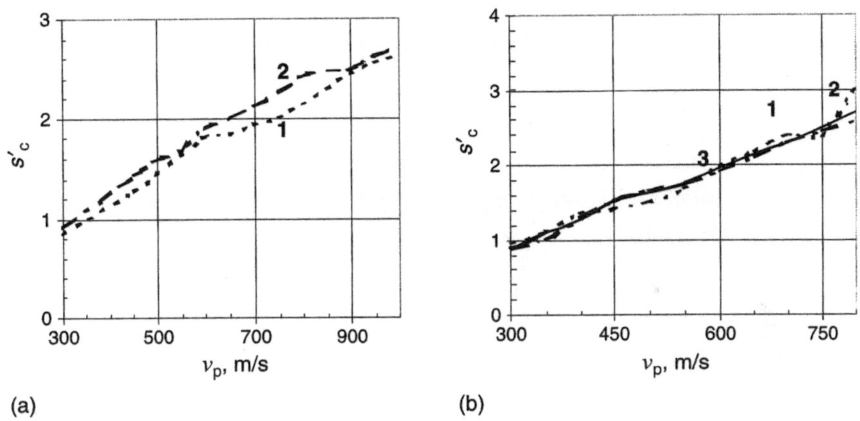

Fig. 2.23. Increase in the contact area with increasing impact velocity. (a) constant yield stress and (b) variable yield stress.

The calculated impact interaction of microparticles with the substrate allows to understand the dependence of the basic parameters of the impact (contact time and area, particle–substrate interaction force) on the particle size and velocity and on the basic mechanical properties of the particle and the substrate. These parameters can be further used as criteria in constructing the model of particle adhesion to the substrate.

2.4. Formation of a Layer of a High-velocity Flow in the Vicinity of the Microparticle–Solid Substrate Contact Plane

In this section, we consider an important issue of formation of a thin layer of a high-velocity flow in the vicinity of the contact area of an individual microparticle incident

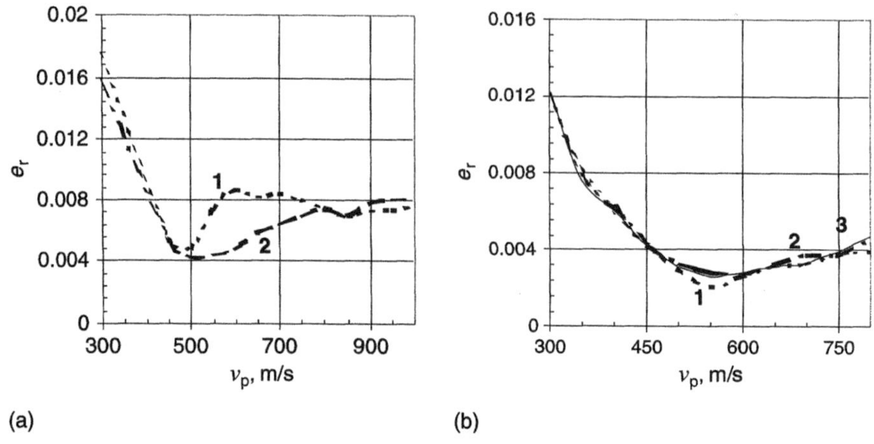

Fig. 2.24. Behavior of kinetic energy of the rebounded particle. (a) constant yield stress and (b) variable yield stress.

onto a solid substrate on the basis of experimental data and numerical simulation results (Section 2.3) [21].

2.4.1. Background

An electron and optical microscope analysis of particles attached on a polished substrate after an impact revealed some typical features of particle deformation (Figs 2.2 and 2.3). Crown-shaped outbursts of metal are formed at the contact periphery at the final stage of plastic deformation (Fig. 2.2b). The most probable reason for their emergence is the formation of a high-velocity radial metal jet near the wall, which resembles a shaped-charge jet. The main role here belongs to the processes in the vicinity of the contact area, where intense deformation and conversion of mechanical energy to thermal energy occur. Under these conditions, the impact may form a thin melted layer of metal near the wall. Formation of this layer depends on the balance of heat generation and removal.

Simulations (some results are described in the previous section) also reveal the presence of a high-velocity near-wall flow of metal in the radial direction (see, e.g., Figs 2.25 and 2.26, which show the results computed with a zero-friction boundary condition).

Figure 2.25 shows the distribution of the radial component of velocity u over the particle height at the time $t = 20 \times 10^{-9}$ s in three radial cross sections (a) and the particle contour at $t = 0$ and 20 ns (b). Naturally, the highest velocity is observed at a point with the greatest distance along the radius. In addition, in each cross section, velocity increases as the particle approaches the substrate and reaches the maximum values in the layer adjacent to the substrate (the thickness of this layer is approximately $0.05d_p$).

Figure 2.26 shows the distributions of the radial velocity over the radius for different times in the near-wall cells. At the early stage of the impact, the radius of the contact surface is smaller than $d_p/2$ (at $t = 10 \times 10^{-9}$ s, it becomes equal to $d_p/2$), and the

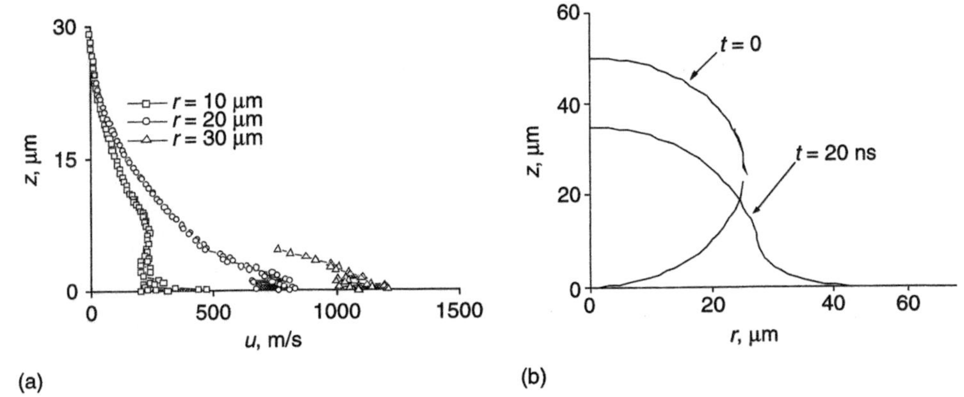

Fig. 2.25. Distribution of the radial component of velocity over the (a) particle height at $t = 20 \times 10^{-9}$ s and (b) particle contour at $t = 0$ and $t = 20$ ns.

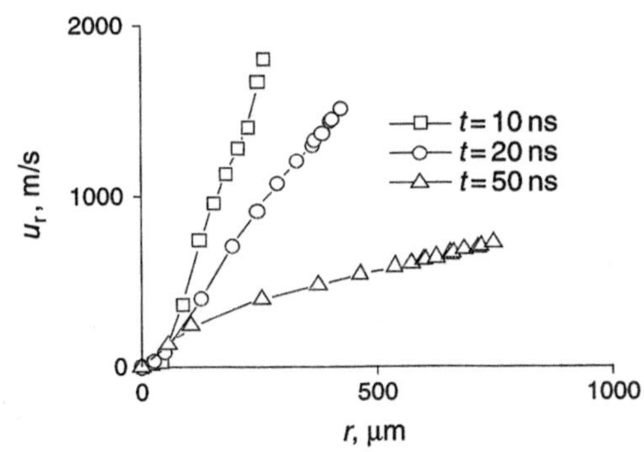

Fig. 2.26. Distribution of the radial component of velocity along the interface.

maximum velocity is approximately two times higher than the impact velocity v_p. In what follows, the radius of the contact surface increases because of the spreading of the particle material over the substrate; as a consequence, the extreme point of this surface is decelerated owing to radial expansion and resistance of the material to shear strains.

We also calculated the distribution of specific internal energy in cells of the different grid in a layer 1 μm thick adjacent to the substrate. The increase in internal energy equals the work of shear stresses on the corresponding plastic deformations. Further, we estimated the temperature in the particle material under the assumption that the relation $e = c_V T$ ($c_V = \text{const}$) is valid. The increase in temperature near the wall is $\Delta \approx 600$ K, as compared to the initial value.

Thus, numerical simulations confirmed the assumption about the presence of a high-velocity near-wall flow of metal in the radial direction (see Fig. 2.25). At certain times (under the condition of ideal slipping on the wall), the velocity at certain points of the near-wall flow is approximately twice the impact velocity. This flow is induced by the propagation of a wave of unloading of the pulsed pressure after the shock wave in the particle leaves the contact area. This flow can lead to outbursts of thin films of the particle material over the contact periphery, which is seen in Fig. 2.2b.

2.4.2. Modeling of the high-velocity flow layer

As the problem considered is rather complicated, we chose an approximate scheme of formation and self-sustaining of the melted metal layer, based on the classical laws of friction and heat transfer with the use of integral methods for the boundary layer.

Let us consider the balance of near-wall heat generation and removal with allowance for results obtained on particle deformation as a whole. Note, in the general case of a near-wall melted metal flow, the thickness of the temperature layer δ_T is greater than the thickness of the viscous boundary layer because the Prandtl number Pr is low. In our case, the thickness of the melted layer δ_m can be greater than or equal to the thickness of the viscous layer δ_μ. Let us determine conditions for each of these cases.

If $\delta_m > \delta_\mu$ for all r, then the viscous boundary layer is developed as that in the case of an incompressible viscous fluid in the vicinity of the stagnation point of a symmetrical-axis flow onto the wall, because the flow velocity at $z = 0$ in our problem has a linear dependence on the radius (see Fig. 2.26):

$$u_r = ar.$$

Here, u_r is the velocity at the layer edge (equal to the velocity on the wall obtained in numerical simulations of deformation of the entire particle); r is the distance from the axis of symmetry of the spherical particle; the constant a, as is seen from Fig. 2.26, is time-dependent, but this dependence can be neglected (by imposing quasi-steady boundary conditions) for approximate estimates to use the exact solution of the Navier–Stokes equations for a similar problem [22]. The exact solution yields

$$\delta_\mu = 2\sqrt{\frac{\mu}{\rho_p a}}, \tag{2.35}$$

where μ is the dynamic viscosity and ρ_p is the density.

In what follows, we estimate the parameter a as

$$a = \frac{2u_R}{d_p}, \tag{2.36}$$

where u_R is the velocity at the layer edge for $r = d_p/2$.

Viscosity of liquid metals near the melting point is approximated by the formula $\mu = (T_m/T) \times 2.75 \times 10^{-3}$ Pa s. It is further shown that T_m/T is slightly smaller than unity; hence, we assume that $\mu \approx 2.5 \times 10^{-3}$ Pa s.

The characteristic value of velocity u_R based on the calculated deformation of the particle with $d_p = 50\,\mu m$ for $v_p = 800\,m/s$ is $u_R \approx 1500\,m/s$. From Eqs (2.35) and (2.36), we obtain

$$\frac{\delta_\mu}{d_p} = \sqrt{\frac{2}{Re_d}} \tag{2.37}$$

where $Re_d = \dfrac{d_p u_R \rho_p}{\mu}$ is the Reynolds number.

Substituting the parameters for the aluminum particle into this formula, we obtain $Re_d = 0.91 \times 10^5$ and, correspondingly, $\delta_\mu / d_p = 0.43 \times 10^{-2}$. Thus, we validate the assumption of a small thickness δ_μ and the possibility of separating the problems for the external flow and the boundary layer.

To estimate the melted layer thickness δ_m in the case $\delta_m > \delta_\mu$, we consider the heat balance in the near-wall region in the integral approximation (see Fig. 2.27):

$$d \int_0^{\delta_m} 2\pi r u \rho_p b H_m dz \approx 2\pi r dr \int_0^{\delta_\mu} \mu \left(\frac{\partial u}{\partial z}\right)^2 dz \tag{2.38}$$

After some transformations, we obtain

$$\frac{d}{dr}\left[r \int_0^{\delta_m} u dz\right] \approx \frac{\mu}{\rho_p H_m} r dr \int_0^{\delta_\mu} \left(\frac{\partial u}{\partial z}\right)^2 dz. \tag{2.39}$$

Here, H_m is the specific melting heat ($\approx 400 \times 10^3$ J/kg for aluminum) and $\mu\,(\partial u/\partial z)^2$ is the volume source of heat due to viscous friction. The left-hand side of Eq. (2.39) is

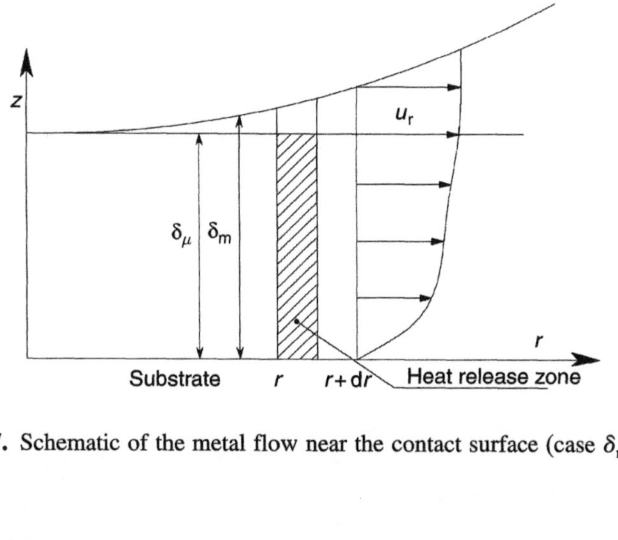

Fig. 2.27. Schematic of the metal flow near the contact surface (case $\delta_m > \delta_\mu$).

the increment of the heat flux through the cylindrical surface of radius r, entrained by melted metal in the form of latent melting heat.

Equation (2.39) is an approximate estimate because it does not contain additional heating of metal after melting and heat transfer outward the top and bottom boundaries of the layer δ_m.

We assume that the velocity profile in the viscous boundary layer corresponds to the distribution in a laminar flow. Then, we obtain

$$d\int_0^{\delta_m} 2\pi r u \rho_p H_m dz \approx 1.5\delta_m \pi r u_r \rho_p H_m,$$

$$2\pi r dr \int_0^{\delta_\mu} \mu \left(\frac{\partial u}{\partial z}\right)^2 dz \approx 1.5\delta_\mu \mu \left(\frac{u_r}{\delta_\mu}\right)^2 2\pi r dr.$$

With allowance for approximations used, simple transformations yield

$$r\frac{d\delta_m}{dr} = \frac{\delta_\mu u_r^2}{4H_m} - 2\delta_m. \tag{2.40}$$

Taking into account that δ_μ is independent of r in the case considered (Eq. 2.35), we write the resultant equation in the form

$$r\frac{d\left(\frac{\delta_m}{\delta_\mu}\right)}{dr} = \frac{u_r^2}{4H_m} - 2\frac{\delta_m}{\delta_\mu} \tag{2.41}$$

Let us consider the sign of the derivative at the point where $\delta_m = \delta_\mu$. If the derivative is positive ($u_r^2 \geq 8H_m$), the thickness of the melted layer increases along r faster than the thickness of the viscous layer. For aluminum, $H_m = 400 \times 10^3$ J/kg and $u_r \geq 1800$ m/s, which corresponds to $v_p \geq 1000$ m/s.

Now we consider the case $v_p \leq 1000$ m/s with $\delta_m = \delta_\mu = \delta$. We assume that the velocity profile in the boundary layer is linear. The integral balance of generated and entrained heat has the following form:

$$d\left(0.5\delta 2\pi r u_r \rho_p H_m\right) \approx \delta\mu\left(\frac{u_r}{\delta}\right)^2 2\pi r dr \tag{2.42}$$

After appropriate transformations, we obtain

$$\frac{1}{2}\frac{\delta}{r}\frac{d\delta}{dr} + \left(\frac{\delta}{r}\right)^2 = \frac{2u_R^2}{Re_d H_m}. \tag{2.43}$$

This equation has the solution

$$\frac{\delta}{r} = \frac{2}{\sqrt{3}}\frac{u_R}{\sqrt{Re_d H_m}}. \tag{2.44}$$

For $\delta_{\rm m} = \delta_\mu = \delta$, the boundary-layer thickness δ increases in proportion to r. In our case, $(\delta/r)_{r=R} \approx 0.96 \times 10^{-2}$. For $r = d_{\rm p}/2$, we obtain $\delta \approx 0.24\,\mu$m.

Let us evaluate the temperature in the boundary layer. The heat flux entrained by melted metal from a control volume bounded by the cylindrical surface of radius r is calculated by the formula

$$Q = 0.5\delta u_\delta \times 2\pi r\rho_{\rm p}H_{\rm m} = \frac{u_{\rm R}^2\rho_{\rm p}H_{\rm m}}{\sqrt{Re_{\rm d}H_{\rm m}}}\frac{2\pi r^3}{d_{\rm p}}. \tag{2.45}$$

If the wall is thermally insulated, the heat flux to the top boundary of the layer where the melting occurs is determined as

$$q = \frac{{\rm d}Q}{{\rm d}S} \approx \lambda\frac{\Delta T}{\delta/2}, \tag{2.46}$$

where $S = \pi r^2$, $\lambda = \mu c_{\rm p}/Pr$ is the thermal conductivity, $c_{\rm p}$ is the heat capacity, Pr is the Prandtl number, and $\Delta T = T - T_{\rm m}$ (T is the averaged temperature in the boundary layer). From Eqs (2.45) and (2.46), we obtain

$$\Delta T \approx \frac{1}{2}\frac{u_{\rm R}^2}{c_{\rm p}}Pr\left(\frac{2r}{d_{\rm p}}\right)^2. \tag{2.47}$$

For $r = d_{\rm p}/2$, the estimate for liquid aluminum ($c_{\rm p} = 1084\,{\rm J/kg}\,K$; $Pr = 0.037$) yields $\Delta T = 38\,{\rm K}$. This result confirms the validity of using the assumption of an insignificant overheating of metal in the boundary layer.

The allowance for heat transfer from the boundary layer into the wall, metal overheating in the layer, and metal heating to the melting point outside the layer yields even smaller values of the thickness δ. Thus, the data obtained can be regarded as the upper estimates.

The present analysis shows that because of the impact of a small metallic particle on a solid non-deformable substrate, a very thin ($\delta < 0.015d_{\rm p}$) surface layer of melted metal can be formed and sustained by heat release in the viscous boundary layer, the temperature of this thin layer being close to the melting point of the particle metal. Formation of such a layer can be responsible for the high adhesion of particles with the substrate in the course of cold spray.

2.5. Particle–Substrate Adhesive Interaction under an Impact

Coating formation by a "cold" high-velocity two-phase flow incident onto a substrate finds more and more various applications [23–27]. Nevertheless, the nature of adhesion of metallic particles with velocities $v_{\rm p} \sim 400$–$1200\,{\rm m/s}$ and temperatures much lower than the melting point of the particle material to the substrate is not clear. The factors that complicate the study of this phenomenon are the small size of particles ($d_{\rm p} \sim 10^{-5}\,{\rm m}$), the short time of interaction ($t_c \sim 10^{-8}$ s), the uncertainty of the phase state of interacting objects in micro-volumes near the contact boundaries, etc.

The process of adhesive particle–substrate interaction during cold spray can be considered within the framework of the approach widely used in gas-thermal spraying analysis [28–30]. It should be noted, however, that cold spray involves a much greater (than in gas-thermal methods) effect on kinetic energy of particles, leading to significant differences in interaction of cold particles and melted particles typical of gas-thermal deposition techniques. Thus, the temperature at the particle–substrate contact in the case of cold particles depends on heat release in the zone of high plastic strains, which is not important in the interaction of melted particles with the substrate. In addition, as is shown below, heat-transfer processes during the contact are essential for particles with $d_p \leq 50\,\mu\text{m}$, and the condition of process adiabaticity normally accepted in constructing the mathematical model of shock-induced deformation [31] becomes invalid.

2.5.1. *Estimates of the contact time and particle strain in a high-velocity impact*

Let us simulate deformation of a plastic particle with a velocity of 500–1500 m/s impacting a non-deformable substrate (e.g., an impact of an aluminum particle on a steel substrate).

We assume that the velocity of the backward point of the particle uniformly decreases from v_p at $\tau = 0$ to 0 at $\tau = 1$: $v(\tau) = v_p(1-\tau)$. In this case, the particle strain at an arbitrary time is determined via the velocity-dependent final strain $\varepsilon_p = (d_p - h_p)/h_p$ by the expression $\varepsilon(v_p, \tau) = \varepsilon_p \tau(2-\tau)$, where h_p is the final height of the deformed particle and $\tau = t/t_c$ is the normalized time. Under these assumptions, the contact time is

$$t_c = 2\varepsilon_p d_p / v_p, \tag{2.48}$$

where the final strain of the particle ε_p was determined by Eq. (2.1).

An analysis of the cross-sectional view of attached particles (see Fig. 2.4) shows that it can be rather accurately approximated by a paraboloid of revolution. Therefore, the particle shape at an arbitrary time $0 < \tau < 1$ can be represented in the form of a combination of a paraboloid of revolution and a spherical segment at $0 < \varepsilon(v_p, \tau) < 1 - 1/\sqrt{3}$ and in the form of a paraboloid of revolution at $1 - 1/\sqrt{3} < \varepsilon(v_p, \tau) < 1$. In this case, with allowance for the conservation of particle mass, the normalized current radius of the contact area $\zeta = r/d_p$ and the strain are related as

$$\zeta^2(v_p, \tau) = \begin{cases} \varepsilon(v_p, \tau)\left[1 - \varepsilon(v_p, \tau)\right] + \left\{\frac{\varepsilon^2(v_p, \tau)\left[3 - 2\varepsilon(v_p, \tau)\right]}{2}\right\}^{2/3} & \varepsilon(v_p, \tau) \leq 1 - \frac{1}{\sqrt{3}} \\ \zeta^2(v_p, \tau) = \frac{1}{3\left[1 - \varepsilon(v_p, \tau)\right]} & 1 - \frac{1}{\sqrt{3}} \leq \varepsilon(v_p, \tau) \leq 1 \end{cases} \tag{2.49}$$

Figure 2.28 shows the ratio of the current radius to the final radius versus the normalized time. The same figure shows the curves $y = \tau^{1/2}$ and $y = \tau^{1/3}$, which are adequate approximations for these dependences ($y = \tau^{1/3}$ for $v_p = 500\text{–}1000\,\text{m/s}$ and $y = \tau^{1/2}$ for $v_p = 1000\text{–}1500\,\text{m/s}$). Therefore, these curves are used in further estimates instead of rather complicated Eq. (2.49).

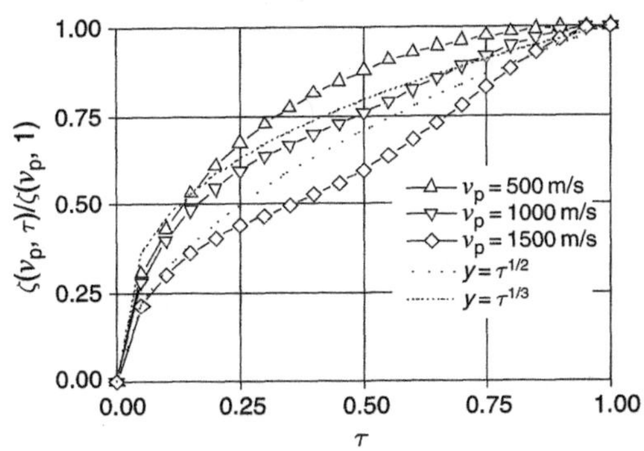

Fig. 2.28. Ratio of the radius of the contact area of the deformed particle to the final radius of the contact area versus normalized time for different impact velocities: $\upsilon_p = 300$, 500, 1000, and 1500 m/s.

2.5.2. *Temperature of the particle–substrate contact area in a high-velocity impact*

2.5.2.1. *Analytical modeling*

We define the temperature $T_c(\eta, \tau)$ of the particle–substrate contact area as the sum $T_c^0(\eta, \tau) + T_v(\eta, \tau)$($T_c^0$ is the temperature at the contact of two heated bodies with different temperatures and $T_v(\eta, \tau)$ is the temperature of additional heating of the contact area by heat released during the impact) [32]. In the first approximation, $T_c^0(\eta, \tau)$ can be estimated as the contact temperature of two semi-infinite bodies

$$T_c^0(\eta, \tau) = T_c^0 = \frac{T_s + K_p T_p}{1 + K_p}, \tag{2.50}$$

where $K_p = \sqrt{\frac{\lambda_p c_p \rho_p}{\lambda_s c_s \rho_s}}$ is the criterion of thermal activity of the particle relative to the substrate, T_s and T_p are the substrate and particle temperatures before the impact, and $\rho_s, \rho_p, \lambda_s, \lambda_p, c_s$, and c_p are the substrate and particle densities, thermal conductivities, and heat capacities.

The estimate of the particle–substrate contact temperature as the contact temperature of two semi-infinite bodies is fairly accurate if the condition $z^*/2\sqrt{\chi t} > 2$ is satisfied (where z^* is the characteristic size in the direction perpendicular to the contact plane and χ is the thermal diffusivity of the particle) because the particle temperature in the one-dimensional approximation can be determined by the formula

$$T_p(z, t) = T_p + \frac{T_s - T_p}{1 + K_p}\left[1 - \Phi\left(\frac{z}{2\sqrt{\chi t}}\right)\right]. \tag{2.51}$$

For $(z/2\sqrt{\chi t}) > 2$, we have the function $\Phi(z/2\sqrt{\chi t}) \approx 1$ and $T_p(z, t) = T_p$. Hence, the heat from the interface is removed in the same manner as it occurs in a semi-infinite body.

In our problem, we can assume that $z^* \approx d_p(1-\varepsilon_p)$ is the final height of the attached particle, $t = t_c$. Finally, we see that the condition $(z/2\sqrt{\chi t}) > 2$ is satisfied for particles of size

$$d_p > \frac{32\varepsilon_p \chi}{v_p\left(1-\varepsilon_p\right)^2}. \tag{2.52}$$

For finer particles, the estimate Eq. (2.50) is the bottom estimate of the contact temperature, i.e., $T_c^0(\zeta, \tau) \geq T_c^0$. For $d_p \geq 5\,\mu$m and velocities of interest, however, the difference between $T_c^0(\zeta, \tau)$ and T_c^0 is fairly small.

First, let us consider the increment of the contact temperature $T_v(\tau)$ due to heat release during the impact analytically, in the one-dimensional approximation with allowance for heat transfer during the contact.

We assume that the heat is released during the entire contact time t_c in the layer $h_H = \beta(1-\varepsilon_p)d_p$ (β is a coefficient that takes into account deformation localization in the particle, $0 \leq \beta \leq 1$) and propagates to both sides of the contact plane in an infinite medium with prescribed identical values of λ, c, and ρ (Fig. 2.29). The particle and substrate can be modeled by a semi-infinite medium if the temperatures of the backward sides of these objects remain unchanged during the contact time (as is shown below, this condition is satisfied rather accurately) and, hence, the heat from the heat-release zone propagates in a manner it propagates in semi-infinite media.

In this case, the temperature $T_v(\eta, \tau)$ at the point with the coordinate $\eta = z/d_p$ at the time $\tau \leq 1$ can be determined from the expression [33]

$$T_v(\eta, \tau) = \frac{d_p}{2c\rho}\sqrt{\frac{t_c}{\pi\chi}} \int_0^{\tau} \frac{d\tau'}{\sqrt{\tau-\tau'}} \int_0^{\beta(1-\varepsilon_p)} d\eta' A(\eta', \tau') \exp\left[-\frac{d_p^2(\eta-\eta')^2}{4\chi t_c(\tau-\tau')}\right] \tag{2.53}$$

where $0 \leq \eta' \leq \beta(1-\varepsilon_p)$ is the heat-release zone at the time τ' and $A(\eta', \tau')$ is the amount of heat released per unit volume per unit time. For $\tau > 1$, we can also use Eq. (2.53) with the upper limit of integration in time set to unity.

The specific heat release $A(\eta', \tau')$ is determined from the condition of conservation of energy by defining its functional dependence on η' and τ'. We find the total amount of

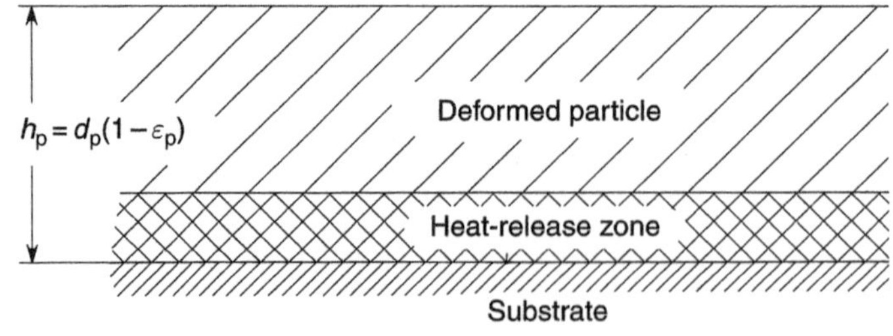

Fig. 2.29. One-dimensional approximation of heat release in the deformed particle.

heat released per unit contact area (taking into account that almost all kinetic energy is converted to heat at high impact velocities)

$$Q_{s1} = \rho \frac{v_p^2}{2} \frac{(1-\varepsilon_p) d_p}{2}. \tag{2.54}$$

with the limiting value $Q_{s1} \to 0.35 H_p d_p$ as $v_p \to \infty$.

The total amount of heat released per unit contact area increases with increasing particle diameter and velocity. On the other hand,

$$Q_{s1} = t_c d_p \int_0^1 d\tau' \int_0^{\beta(1-\varepsilon_p)} A(\eta', \tau') \, d\eta'. \tag{2.55}$$

Equating these two expressions, we can find the value of $A(\eta', \tau')$ for its particular form.

Let us consider the case of a uniform space–time distribution of heat-release intensity $A(\eta', \tau') = A_0$ in the layer $0 \le \eta' \le \beta(1-\varepsilon_p)$. In this case, from Eq. (2.54) we obtain $Q_{s1} = A_0 t_p d_p \beta(1-\varepsilon_p)$ and, finally,

$$A(\eta', \tau') = A_0 = \frac{\rho v_p^3}{8 \varepsilon_p d_p \beta}. \tag{2.56}$$

Expression (2.53) for temperature is rewritten as

$$T_v(\eta, \tau) = \frac{v_p^3}{16 c \varepsilon_p \beta} \sqrt{\frac{t_c}{\pi \chi}} \int_0^\tau \frac{d\tau'}{\sqrt{\tau - \tau'}} \int_0^{\beta(1-\varepsilon_p)} d\eta' \exp\left[-\frac{d_p^2 (\eta - \eta')^2}{4 \chi t_c (\tau - \tau')} \right]. \tag{2.57}$$

Integrating this expression with respect to η', we obtain

$$T_v(\eta, \tau) = \frac{v_p^3}{8 c \beta} \int_0^\tau d\tau' \left\{ \Phi\left[\frac{d_p \eta}{\sqrt{4 \chi t_c (\tau - \tau')}} \right] - \Phi\left[\frac{d_p (\eta - \beta(1-\varepsilon_p))}{\sqrt{4 \chi t_c (\tau - \tau')}} \right] \right\}. \tag{2.58}$$

For the contact plane $\eta = 0$, hence, we have

$$T_v(0, \tau) = \frac{v_p^3}{8 c \beta} \int_0^\tau d\tau' \Phi\left[\frac{d_p \beta (1-\varepsilon_p)}{\sqrt{4 \chi t_c (\tau - \tau')}} \right]. \tag{2.59}$$

For $\beta = 0$, we obtain

$$T_v(\eta, \tau) = \frac{v_p^3 (1-\varepsilon_p)}{16 c \varepsilon_p} \sqrt{\frac{t_c}{\pi \chi}} \int_0^\tau \frac{d\tau'}{\sqrt{\tau - \tau'}} \exp\left[-\frac{d_p^2 \eta^2}{4 \chi t_c (\tau - \tau')} \right] \tag{2.60}$$

$$T_v(0, \tau) = \frac{v_p^{5/2} d_p^{1/2} (1-\varepsilon_p)}{c \sqrt{32 \pi \chi \varepsilon_p}} \tau^{1/2}. \tag{2.61}$$

Thus, we see that the temperatures are always finite, even in the case of heat release in an infinitely thin layer at the interface.

2.5.2.2. Results

Let us analyze the contact temperature as a function of velocity for particles of different sizes at the final time. For coarse particles, the contact temperature is higher and increases approximately as $\sqrt{v_p}$ with increasing velocity (Fig. 2.30).

Let us analyze the temperature distribution in the region of the particle–substrate contact at the final time. Figure 2.31 shows the effect of the heat-release zone thickness β and the particle size on the temperature distribution. The final height of the particle deformed with an impact velocity of 1000 m/s is ≈0.25. The temperature of the backward side of the particle remains almost unchanged; hence, this method can be used to analyze the contact temperature.

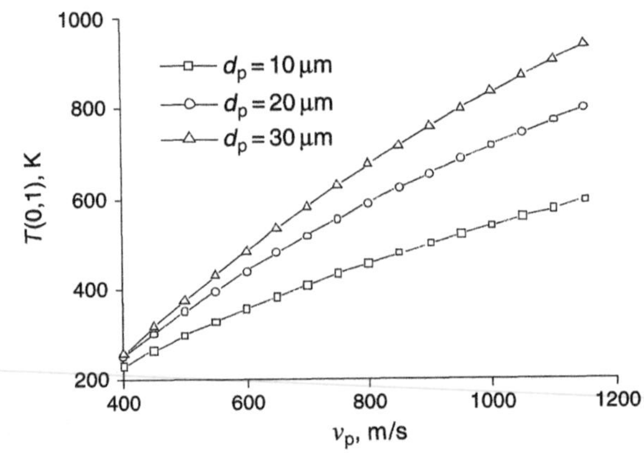

Fig. 2.30. Contact temperature at $t = t_c$ versus the particle velocity.

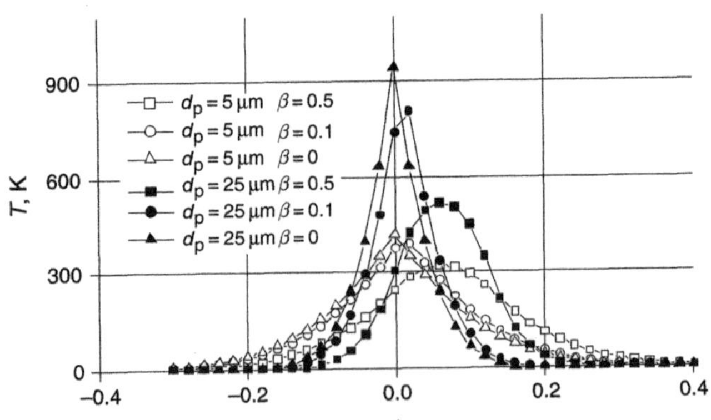

Fig. 2.31. Temperature distribution in the contact zone for $v_p = 1000\,\mathrm{m/s}$, $d_p = 5$ and $25\,\mu\mathrm{m}$, and $\beta = 0.5$, 0.1, and 0.

For small values of $0 \leq \beta \leq 0.1$ (the calculations of [21] show that the most intense plastic strains and, hence, the most intense heat release are observed in a thin layer near the interface corresponding to $\beta \approx 0.1$), the distributions almost coincide. This fact substantially simplifies the problem of modeling heat release due to particle impact because it allows the use (especially for the contact temperature) of simpler expressions obtained for a zero thickness of the heat-release zone.

Figure 2.31 also illustrates a significant effect of the particle size on the temperature distribution: the temperature peak decreases with decreasing particle size, and the width of the temperature distribution increases, i.e., the influence of heat transfer on the final temperature distribution is more profoundly manifested for fine particles, though the contact time for fine particles is shorter. Indeed, the space–time temperature distribution in the first approximation is determined by the parameter $z^{*^2}/4\chi t^*$, where z^* and t^* are the characteristic scale and time of the problem under consideration. In our case, $z^* = d_p$, $t^* = t_c = 2\varepsilon_p d_p/v_p$; hence, we have $z^{*2}/4\chi t^* \sim d_p$. Therefore, the smaller the particle, the smaller the value of $z^{*2}/4\chi t^*$ and the stronger the influence of heat transfer in the course of the impact.

The impact velocity affects the temperature in the contact zone; at a certain velocity depending on the particle size and heat-release zone thickness, the peak temperature exceeds the melting point, and the results obtained become incorrect because the model does not include melting. The velocity at which the melting point is reached at some point versus the particle diameter is plotted in Fig. 2.32 (curve $1 - T_p = T_s = 300\,\text{K}, \beta = 0.1$; curve $2 - T_p = T_s = 500\,\text{K}, \beta = 0.1$; curve $3 - T_p = T_s = 300\,\text{K}, \beta = 0$). The same figure shows the velocity of particles accelerated in a nozzle commonly used in cold spray by air (4, 5) and helium (6, 7) with stagnation temperatures $T_0 = 300\,\text{K}$ (4, 6) and $T_0 = 500\,\text{K}$ (5, 7).

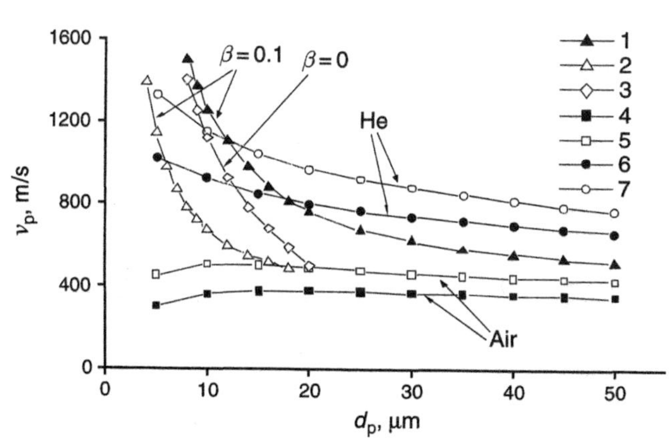

Fig. 2.32. Critical velocity at which the particle temperature reaches the melting point versus the particle diameter. $1 - T_p = T_s = 300\,\text{K}, \beta = 0.1$; $2 - T_p = T_s = 500\,\text{K}, \beta = 0.1$; $3 - T_p = T_s = 300\,\text{K}, \beta = 0$; $4, 6 - T_0 = 300\,\text{K}$; $5, 7 - T_0 = 500\,\text{K}$; acceleration by air (4, 5) and helium (6, 7).

As is seen from Fig. 2.32, the velocity at which the melting temperature is reached at a certain point of the particle in the particle-size range of interest depends on the particle diameter, initial temperatures of the particle and the substrate, and heat-release zone thickness. For $T_p = T_s = T_0 = 300\,K$ and $\beta = 0.1$, which is a realistic value, this can occur in the case of particle acceleration by helium for $d_p \geq 18\,\mu m$ and can never occur in the case of particle acceleration by air. For $d_p \leq 12\,\mu m$, the melting point is not reached even for a zero thickness of the heat-release zone (see intersection of curves 3 and 6). Heating of accelerating air slightly increases the particle velocity (curves 5 and 7), and the velocity necessary to reach the melting point decreases (curve 2) because of the higher initial temperatures of the particle and the substrate. At a certain temperature of jet heating, curves 2 and 5 intersect. This means that it is possible to reach the melting point in the case of acceleration by a heated air jet. As is seen from Fig. 2.32, this occurs for $d_p \geq 18\,\mu m$.

2.5.2.3. *Numerical estimates*

These estimates were obtained for identical thermo-physical properties of the substrate and the particle. The temperature distribution for different thermo-physical properties is somewhat different. The problem was solved numerically taking into account the finiteness of the particle and substrate size in the direction perpendicular to the contact plane and the difference in thermo-physical properties of the substrate and the particle.

A substrate of thickness δ_s made of a material with certain values of ρ_s, λ_s, and c_s is set at the time $t = 0$ into contact with a plate of thickness $\delta_p = d_p(1 - \varepsilon_p(v_p))$ modeling the particle. During the period $0 \leq t \leq t_c = 2\varepsilon_p(v_p)d_p/v_p$, a certain amount of heat determined by Eq. (2.56) is released in the plate in the region $0 \leq y \leq \delta_H = \beta d_p(1 - \varepsilon_p(v_p))$. Heat exchange with the ambient medium on the surfaces δ_s and δ_p was ignored (for $\alpha \leq 5 \times 10^4$ corresponding to heat transfer in the jet impacting on the substrate, its effect is insignificant). The initial temperature of the substrate was assumed to be equal to the stagnation temperature of the jet, and the particle temperature was set equal to the calculated value (depending on the particle size).

Figure 2.33 shows the temperature distribution in the aluminum particle–substrate system for different substrate materials with different thermo-physical properties. The particle was accelerated by a gas with a stagnation temperature $T_0 = 300\,K$ up to 800 m/s; therefore, the initial temperature of the substrate was assumed to be $T_s = 300\,K$, and the initial particle temperature was $T_p = 200\,K$ (the particle is cooled during its motion in a supersonic flow); the particle diameter was $d_p = 25\,\mu m$.

It is seen that interaction with a substrate made of a less-heat-conducting material significantly increases the temperature in the contact layer (from ~630 K in the Al–Cu system to ~970 K in the Al–Al_2O_3 system).

2.5.3. *Specific features of adhesive interaction of a non-melted particle with the substrate*

This section presents an attempt to construct a simple statistical model of adhesive interaction of particles with the substrate that allows receiving some qualitative data

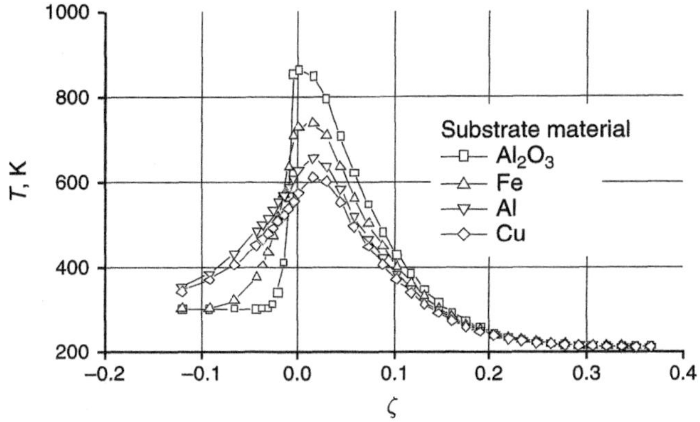

Fig. 2.33. Temperature distribution in the contact region for $v_p = 800\,m/s$, $d_p = 25\,\mu m$, and $\beta = 0.1$.

related to the cold spray process. All presented results are related to interaction of an aluminum particle with a steel substrate.

The model proposed is based on the following approach. The impact of a cold (non-melted) particle on the surface involves, on one hand, formation of bonds between the contacting surface atoms of the particle and substrate materials and, on the other hand, accumulation of elastic energy in the entire volume of the particle. During unloading, the accumulated elastic energy tends to get free in the form of the kinetic energy of particle rebounding. If the accumulated elastic energy is greater than the total adhesion energy, the particle rebounds from the surface. Otherwise, it remains attached to the surface (cold spray phenomenon [12]).

In constructing this statistical model, we faced the fact that the experience gained in studying this phenomenon is mainly qualitative. Many quantities necessary for constructing the model have not been adequately examined, and we had to make assumptions on their magnitude and character of distribution. The model proposed [9] focuses attention on these quantities, which should stimulate a more detailed study of the phenomenon. Nevertheless, the model proposed allows qualitative tracking of the influence of the governing parameters of spraying (first of all, the velocity and size of the deposited particles) on the process of particle attachment onto the substrate surface. Under certain assumptions on the constants used in the model and with the values of some quantities being chosen to ensure the best fit with the experiment, quantitative estimates can also be made.

2.5.3.1. Governing equation for the number of bonds formed

Let us consider the process of formation of bonds between the particle and the substrate due to the impact as a topochemical reaction (reaction at the interface of contacting bodies). This approach is very common for thermal spray [30, 34, 35].

The rate of bond formation at an arbitrary point of the particle–substrate contact can be written as

$$\frac{dN}{dt} = \nu (N_{\sigma 0} - N_{\sigma}) \exp\left(-\frac{E_a}{kT_c}\right). \tag{2.62}$$

From this equation, we can obtain the integral expression for the relative number of bonds formed by the contact

$$\frac{N_\sigma}{N_{\sigma 0}} = 1 - \exp\left[-\nu \int_{t_c(r)}^{t_c} \exp\left(-\frac{E_a}{kT_c}\right) dt\right], \tag{2.63}$$

where $t_c(r)$ is the time of the particle–substrate contact at a distance r from the center of the contact, $t_0(0) = 0$, the value of ν is assumed to be $10^{13}\,s^{-1}$, and $k = 1.38 \times 10^{-23}$ J/K is the Boltzmann constant. In the general case, the temperature at the contact point T_c is a function of the distance r and the time t.

The number of bonds averaged over the contact area is

$$\left\langle \frac{N_\sigma}{N_{\sigma 0}} \right\rangle = 1 - \int_0^{r_c} \frac{2r dr}{r_c^2} \exp\left[-\nu \int_{t_c(r)}^{t_c} \exp\left(-\frac{E_a}{kT_c}\right) dt\right]. \tag{2.64}$$

Passing to the normalized time $\tau = t/t_c$ and distance $\zeta = r/r_c$, we obtain the formula convenient for numerical simulations:

$$\left\langle \frac{N_\sigma}{N_{\sigma 0}} \right\rangle = 1 - \int_0^{1} \frac{2\zeta d\zeta}{\zeta_c^2} \exp\left[-\nu t_c \int_{\tau_c(r)}^{1} \exp\left(-\frac{E_a}{kT_c}\right) d\tau\right]. \tag{2.65}$$

Our next task is to determine the dependence of the number of bonds on the particle velocity and size. Mathematically, we have to pass from two independent variables t_c and T_c to two different independent variables, namely, v_p and d_p. For this purpose, we have to determine how the contact time and temperature depend on the particle velocity and size. These tasks are rather complicated, and we will use approximate models.

We estimate the contact time by Eq. (2.48), which is convenient because the final strain is directly measured in the experiment; hence, we can expect that this estimate of the contact time is fairly precise for impact velocities of 400–120 m/s (range of velocities where the value of ε_p was determined experimentally). The dependence of the final strain on the impact velocity for aluminum particles is known: it is expressed by formula (2.1) obtained by approximating experimental data.

It is currently impossible to measure the contact temperature and determine its dependence on the primary parameters, the particle velocity and size. Therefore, this can be done only by means of calculation. The most correct calculation is the numerical computation of the high-velocity impact of the particle onto the substrate with allowance for heat transfer during the contact. At the first stage of solving this problem, however, it was calculated on the basis of rather simple physical considerations and approximations to demonstrate how the contact temperature depends on the governing parameters of interaction (particle velocity and size, etc.). The procedure is described below.

2.5.3.2. Heated volume

During the contact time, the temperature front propagates inward the particle to a depth that can be determined by the following formula in the first approximation:

$$z = \sqrt{\chi_p t_c}. \tag{2.66}$$

Approximating the shape of the deformed particle by a paraboloid of revolution [2], we can readily estimate the particle volume subjected to heating during the contact time:

$$V_z = 1 - \left(1 - \frac{z}{h_p}\right)^2. \tag{2.67}$$

This estimate is valid for $z < h_p$. For $z \geq h_p$, the entire volume of the particle is heated, i.e., $V_z = 1$.

2.5.3.3. Critical velocities

Applying the law of conservation of energy, we can easily estimate the particle impact velocity for the moment the melting point is reached in the heated volume. For this purpose, we need to solve the equation

$$\eta \frac{v_p^2}{2} = c_p \left(T_m - T_p\right) V_z. \tag{2.68}$$

In this equation, η is a coefficient that accounts for the fraction of kinetic energy of the particle, which is spent on particle-material heating. It follows from the calculations described in Section 2.5.2.3 that η varies from 0.6 for a copper substrate to 0.9 for a ceramic substrate; its values for steel and aluminum substrates are approximately 0.75 and 0.65, respectively. Allowance for heat release in the substrate (it is important for substrates whose hardness is commensurable with that of aluminum, namely, aluminum or copper) slightly reduces this coefficient again, and the latter approaches the critical value of 0.5. We denote the value of particle velocity obtained from this equation by v_{p1} and the part of the heated volume by V_{z1}. Note that v_{p1} is a function of the particle size. The results calculated for $\eta = 0.5$ are shown by curve 1 in Fig. 2.34a and for $\eta = 0.75$ in Fig. 2.34b.

For higher values of kinetic energy of the particle, there arises a possibility of material melting in the heated volume. Using the law of conservation of energy, we estimate the impact velocity that ensures not only heating to the melting point but also particle-material melting itself. For this purpose, we have to solve the equation

$$\eta \frac{v_p^2}{2} = \left[c_p \left(T_m - T_p\right) + H_m\right] V_z. \tag{2.69}$$

We denote the particle velocity obtained from this equation by v_{p2} and the fraction of the melted volume by V_{z2}. The velocity v_{p2} is also a function of the particle diameter. This case is described by curve 2 in Fig. 2.34a,b.

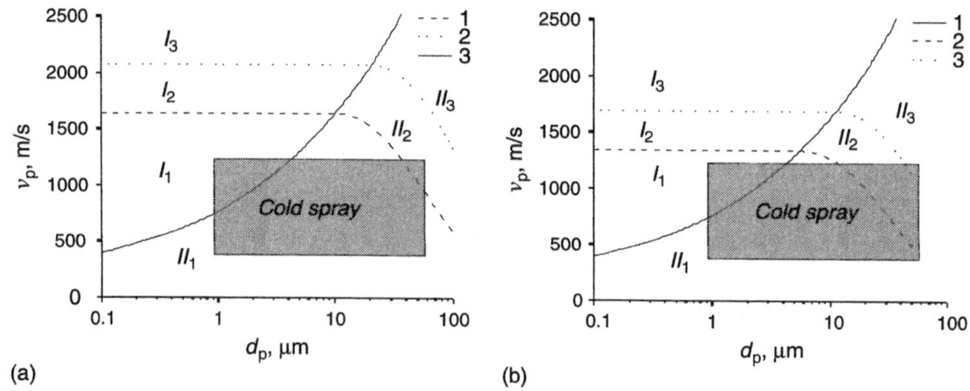

Fig. 2.34. Domains of complete and incomplete heating of the particle during the impact in terms of particle velocities and sizes for (a) $\eta = 0.5$, and (b) $\eta = 0.75$.

The condition that the heat extends over the entire particle during the contact time defines the third velocity. It is found by solving the equation

$$z = h_p. \tag{2.70}$$

This case is described by curve 3 in Fig. 2.34a,b. This curve separates the domains of complete (uniform) heating of particles during the impact (domain *I*) and incomplete (non-uniform) heating (domain *II*).

2.5.3.4. Diagram of thermal states

Let us consider domain *I* in more detail using Fig. 2.34a,b. This domain can be conventionally called the domain of small sizes and high velocities. Curves 1 and 2 divide this domain into three sub-domains I_1, I_2, and I_3. In sub-domain I_1, the particle energy during the impact is insufficient for reaching the melting point. Curve 1 refers to particle parameters that ensure a possibility of particle heating to the melting point. Curve 2 corresponds to particle melting due to the impact. Thus, the sub-domain I_2 between curves 1 and 2 corresponds to formation of a layer of the melted material whose fraction increases with increasing impact velocity. The sub-domain I_3 consists of completely melted particles.

Let us now consider the domain *II* located below curve 3 and corresponding to incomplete heating of particles during the impact. The sub-domain II_1 (it can be conventionally called the domain of low velocities) corresponds to particle heating to temperatures below the melting point. It can also be called the sub-domain of insignificantly non-uniform heating. Significantly non-uniform heating occurs in the sub-domain II_2 when the impact generates a melted sub-layer whose thickness increases with increasing particle velocity and size. The sub-domain II_3 corresponds to melting of the fraction of the particle, which is heated during the impact. It is in this range (range of macrobodies) that most experimental and theoretical investigations of the impact are performed.

Note that the high-velocity impact within this domain can be simulated with neglected temperature effects because the fraction of the heated and melted material rapidly decreases with increasing body size and becomes of little importance. The greater part of the particle volume is not subjected to significant heating. The ratio z/h_p for a fixed velocity decreases in proportion to $d_p^{-0.5}$ with increasing particle diameter. Expansion of expression (2.67) into a Tailor series with respect to the small parameter (which is valid in the sub-domain II_3 far from curve 2) yields the same law $\sim d_p^{-0.5}$. Nevertheless, simulations inside the sub-domain II_2 and in its neighborhood should be performed with allowance for the thermal characteristics of the materials. The domain of particle parameters where the cold spray phenomenon is observed adjoins curve 1 from the left and from below. Thus, to explain the cold spray nature, consideration of the thermal problem in addition to the dynamic problem is mandatory. It should be emphasized that the cold spray domain marked in Fig. 2.34a,b is the currently known domain.

2.5.3.5. Volume of the material at the melting point

For further consideration, we have to estimate the particle-material volume whose temperature is approximately equal to the melting temperature. We denote this volume by V_m. For the sub-domains I_1 and II_1, we have $V_m = 0$. In the sub-domains I_2 and II_2, the value of V_m is found by the relation

$$H_m V_m = \eta \frac{v_p^2}{2} - c_p (T_m - T_p) V_z. \tag{2.71}$$

In the sub-domains I_3 and II_3, we have the simple equality $V_m = V_z$. These cases are generalized by the relation

$$V_m = \begin{cases} 0 & v_p < v_{p1} \\ \dfrac{1}{H_m}\left(\eta \dfrac{v_p^2}{2} - c_p (T_m - T_p) V_z\right) & v_{p1} < v_p < v_{p2} \\ V_z & v_p > v_{p2} \end{cases}. \tag{2.72}$$

2.5.3.6. Contact temperature

To determine the contact temperature, we use simple estimates. In the sub-domains I_1 and II_1, we can write expression (2.73) and the boundary condition Eq. (2.74) valid on curve 1 (see Fig. 2.34a,b). Taking their ratio, we can readily obtain the temperature

$$\eta \frac{v_p^2}{2} = c_p (T_c - T_p) V_z, \tag{2.73}$$

$$\eta \frac{v_{p1}^2}{2} = c_p (T_m - T_p) V_{z1}. \tag{2.74}$$

In the sub-domains I_3 and II_3, we use relations (2.75) and (2.76) in the same manner:

$$\eta \frac{v_p^2}{2} = [c_p (T_c - T_p) + \mathrm{H_m}] V_z, \tag{2.75}$$

$$\eta \frac{v_{p2}^2}{2} = [c_p (T_m - T_p) + \mathrm{H_m}] V_{z2}. \tag{2.76}$$

In the sub-domains I_2 and II_2, the contact temperature can be simply assumed to be equal to the melting point because the melted material sub-layer should be expected to arise primarily at the interface. Let us unify the expressions for the contact temperature:

$$T_c = \begin{cases} T_p + (T_m - T_p)\dfrac{(v_p/v_{p1})^2}{V_z/V_{z1}} & v_p < v_{p1} \\ T_m & v_{p1} < v_p < v_{p2} \\ T_p + (T_m - T_p)\left[\dfrac{(v_p/v_{p2})^2}{V_z/V_{z2}}\left(1+\dfrac{H_m}{c_p(T_m-T_p)}\right) - \dfrac{H_m}{c_p(T_m-T_p)}\right] & v_p > v_{p2} \end{cases}. \quad (2.77)$$

Note that the solution to the problem in the entire volume (with allowance for the spherical shape of the particle and for the changes in material properties as functions of temperature and pressure) remains complicated from both the computational and the physical viewpoints.

The resultant temperature is in best agreement with the value at the central point of the particle–substrate contact. In view of the high-velocity radial flow of the particle material along the surface [21], however, we can assume that the contact temperature at the most remote radial points is close to the temperature at the central point. Thus, we assume that the points shifted to the periphery have the same temperature at the moment of the contact beginning at the central point at the same time. At later times, these temperatures are also identical. To determine the relative number of bonds, we assume that the temperature distribution over the contact surface is uniform. This allows us to substantially simplify the adhesion-energy calculation:

$$q = \left\langle \frac{N_\sigma}{N_{\sigma 0}} \right\rangle = 1 - \exp\left[-\nu t_c \exp\left(-\frac{E_a}{kT_c}\right)\right]. \quad (2.78)$$

2.5.3.7. Activation energy

In addition to the contact time and temperature considered above, expressions (2.34–2.37) contain one more parameter: adhesive activation energy E_a. Generally speaking, the value of the activation energy characterizes adhesive interaction of material pairs and should be determined in experiments. Nevertheless, based on an analogy between adhesive interaction and creep, diffusion, etc. in solids, we can draw some conclusions about the magnitude and the behavior of adhesive activation energy in a high-velocity impact.

It is known [36] that the activation energy of creep and diffusion in solids substantially decreases with increasing applied stresses. It can go down to values of approximately $0.5–1.5 \times 10^{-19}$ J, depending on the material (Fig. 2.35). Apparently, the same behavior should be expected for the activation energy of high-velocity adhesion. The theoretical calculated activation energies borrowed from [36] are summarized in Table 2.5.

Note that the metals listed in Table 2.5 are qualitatively distributed in the same order in terms of deposition difficulty. The deposition difficulty is understood as the necessity of increasing the flow temperature and velocity, and also as a reduction of deposition efficiency in identical deposition modes.

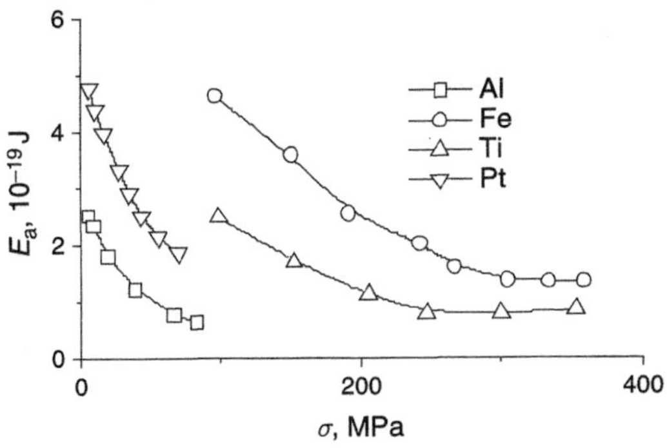

Fig. 2.35. Creep activation energy versus stress.

Table 2.5. Theoretical data on activation energies for some materials

Metal	Zn	Al	Ti	Cu	Fe	Ni	Cr
$E_a \times 10^{19}$, J	0.42	0.50	0.81	1.07	1.55	1.57	2.16

For aluminum, the limiting value of activation energy is reached already at stresses above 100 MPa. The mean dynamic pressure on the particle-contact area can be estimated as $\rho_p v_p^2/2$, and the pressure becomes significantly higher than 100 MPa for particle velocities of 400 m/s and higher. By analogy, for iron, limiting value of activation energy is reached at velocity of an aluminum particle near 470 m/s. This means that most of the bonds are formed during the time of action of dynamic pressure. This is the particle–substrate contact time mentioned above. Therefore, we assumed that it is possible to estimate the upper limit of integration in expressions (2.63) and (2.64) as t_c in accordance with formula (2.48). The activation energy was assumed to have the value 1.55×10^{-19} J (from Table 2.5 for Fe), as big from pair materials participating in interaction and $\eta = 0.75$ at a stage of a primary layer formation, further $E_a = 0.5 \times 10^{-19}$ J and $\eta = 0.65$.

Thus, using the above-adopted simplifications, we can find the dependence of the number of bonds averaged over the particle-contact area on the particle velocity and diameter in accordance with Eq. (2.78).

2.5.3.8. Adhesion energy

To determine the adhesion energy, we take into account that $E_{ad}/E_{ad}^0 = N_\sigma/N_{\sigma 0}$, where the maximum possible energy of adhesion of a given particle to the substrate E_{ad}^0 can be expressed as $E_{ad}^0 = S_c N_{\sigma 0} E_1$. $N_{\sigma 0}$is the maximum number of bonds per unit contact area, equal to the number of atoms in the contact plane, which can be evaluated in terms of the crystal lattice parameter a ($N_{\sigma 0} \approx 2/a^2$ for a face-centered lattice and $N_{\sigma 0} \approx 1/a^2$ for a volume-centered lattice).E_1 is and the energy of bonding of two atoms estimated by sublimation energy. For aluminum (a face-centered crystal lattice), we can assume [37] that $a \approx 4.05 \times 10^{-10}$ m ($N_{\sigma 0} \approx 12 \times 10^{18}$) and $E_1 \approx 0.52 \times 10^{-18}$ J; the corresponding values for iron (bulk-centered lattice) are $a \approx 2.87 \times 10^{-10}$ m($N_{\sigma 0} \approx 12 \times 10^{18}$) and $E_1 \approx 0.68 \times 10^{-18}$ J. Hence, the value $N_{\sigma 0}E_1 \approx 7.0\,\mathrm{J/m^2}$ was used in what follows. Expressing the contact area via the particle diameter and its strain, we can estimate the maximum adhesion energy:

$$E_{\mathrm{ad}}^{0} \approx \frac{\pi d_{\mathrm{p}}^{2} N_{\sigma 0} E_1}{3\left(1-\varepsilon_{\mathrm{p}}\right)} \sim d_{\mathrm{p}}^{2}. \tag{2.79}$$

The dependence of adhesion energy on the particle velocity and its size was calculated by Eq. (2.78).

2.5.3.9. *Elastic energy*

Analyzing expressions (2.78) and (2.48), we could have assumed that coarser particles should be used for more efficient deposition. Yet, this is not the case in reality. The reason is that coarser particles have a higher rebounding probability. The rebounding probability increases with increasing elastic energy stored in the particle U released in the form of the kinetic energy of rebounding when the dynamic impact pressure ceases to act. This energy is a parameter competing with the adhesion energy. In particular, in an impact of macrobodies (sub-domain II_3 in Fig. 2.34a,b), the major part of the particle volume is not subjected to significant heating; hence, it has a large amount of accumulated elastic energy, which is a powerful factor preventing attachment of coarse particles.

The rebound energy should be expressed by the difference between the accumulated elastic energy and adhesion energy in accordance with the equation

$$R = U_{\mathrm{e}} - E_{\mathrm{ad}}. \tag{2.80}$$

If the accumulated energy is sufficiently high to overcome the work of bonding forces with the substrate surface, the particle rebounds.

There are no data for the rebound energy for the examined range of parameters in the literature, and we will use an approximate estimate. It is known that the rebound energy is well approximated by the following relation in the range of low velocities (up to 100 m/s) [38]:

$$R = e_{\mathrm{r}}^{2} m_{\mathrm{p}} \frac{v_{\mathrm{p}}^{2}}{2} = \frac{p_{\mathrm{d}}^{2}}{E^{*}} V_{\mathrm{p}} f(\Omega), \quad \Omega = \frac{\rho_{\mathrm{p}} v_{\mathrm{p}}^{2}}{p_{\mathrm{d}}}. \tag{2.81}$$

Here $p_{\mathrm{d}} \approx 3\sigma_{\mathrm{s}}$ is the stress at the boundary at the rebounding moment (we chose the value of the yield stress of aluminum equal to 20 MPa [39]), E^* is the normalized elasticity modulus (for the aluminum particle–iron substrate pair, $E^* \approx 57$ GPa), and $f(\Omega) = 1.5\Omega^{3/4}$.

Adhesion of particles in an impact with velocities lower than 100 m/s is close to zero, and the accumulated elastic energy can be assumed to be completely converted to kinetic energy of rebounding.

We find the estimate for the accumulated elastic energy by Eq. (2.81), replacing the total volume of the particle by its portion that does not experience significant heating. As this part of the volume is determined by the difference between the initial particle volume and the volume that experiences significant heating (the latter is understood as the characteristic temperature reaching the melting point), we introduce the value of the rebound energy (elastic energy) U_{100} at a velocity of 100 m/s calculated by Eq. (2.81) and obtain the expression

$$\frac{U_e}{U_{100}} = \left(\frac{v_p}{100}\right)^{3/2} (1 - V_m). \qquad (2.82)$$

In what follows, it is more convenient to consider the value of elastic energy normalized to the maximum adhesion energy. Denoting this quantity by g, we obtain the expression

$$\frac{U_e}{U_{100}} = (1 - V_m)\left(\frac{v_p}{100}\right)^{3/2} (1 - \varepsilon_p)\, d_p C_0, \qquad (2.83)$$

where

$$C_0 = 0.75\frac{p_d^2}{E^*}\left(\frac{10^4 \rho_p}{p_d}\right)^{3/4} \frac{1}{E_1 N_{\sigma 0}}.$$

2.5.3.10. *Comparison of energies*

Let us analyze the dependence of the relation between elastic energy and adhesion energy on the particle velocity and size. Figure 2.36 shows the curves corresponding to the impact of particles of different sizes.

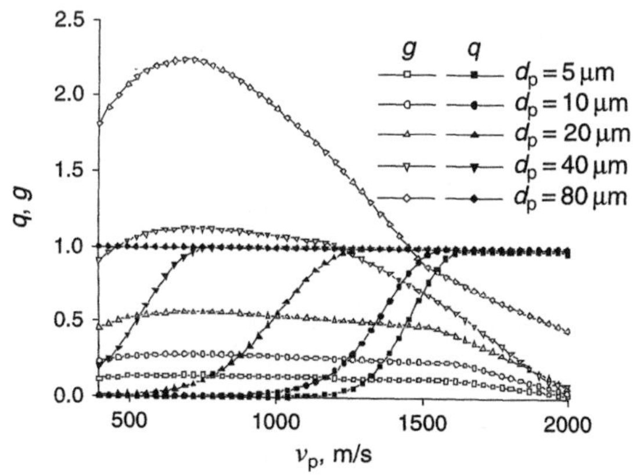

Fig. 2.36. Surface density of adhesion energy q and elastic energy g versus the impact velocity and particle size.

Taking into account that elastic energy is proportional to the particle volume $\sim d_p^3$ (see Eq. (2.81)), and adhesion energy is proportional to $\sim d_p^2$ (see Eq. (2.79)), we find that the ratio U_e/E_{ad}^0 increases in proportion to the particle size. Hence, we can conclude that the process of interaction of the solid particle with the substrate during cold spray significantly depends on the particle size. Regardless of the particle velocity, it rebounds from the substrate if its size is sufficiently large, even if the maximum number of bonds is formed during the contact time. Therefore, it is desirable to use fine particles to reduce the effect of elastic rebounding.

As is seen from Fig. 2.36, the adhesion energy becomes significantly lower than the elastic energy already for particles approximately 80 μm in diameter with a typical range of velocities of 400–200 m/s, and this difference increases with a further increase in particle diameter.

However, when the particle size decreases, the contact time of the particle-substrate to a substrate decreases (see Eq. (2.48)), and also the temperature in the contact area of the particle–substrate decreases (see Eq. (2.61) and Fig. 2.31), that results in reduction of adhesion. Therefore, at the chosen temperatures of a substrate and a particle, there is optimum size of a particle for fastening on a substrate (see Section 2.5.3.12).

2.5.3.11. Adhesion probability

By virtue of its statistical nature (it is known that the breakdown and formation of bonds is a clearly expressed statistical process), even for a rigorously prescribed activation energy and particle size and velocity, the number of bonds formed should be presented as a distribution function. In addition, as the particle size is commensurable with the typical size of the substrate-surface roughness and the grain structure of most materials, it should be expected that this should also contribute to the scatter of the values of adhesion energy and accumulated elastic energy.

The distribution function has the above-obtained mean value N_σ and the dispersion (peak half-width) σ. Because of the influence of a large number of factors, we believe that the use of normal distribution is fairly justified.

Note that a precise idea about the character of the distribution function of adhesion energy of particles and coatings as a whole could be obtained by processing a large number of adhesion tests of coatings deposited under identical conditions. These tests, however, are rather complicated; hence, only a few tests are performed, which offer a general idea about a certain mean typical level of coating adhesion but do not allow estimating the dispersion.

We introduce the number of broken bonds N_r proportional to the accumulated elastic energy. If the number of broken bonds N_r is greater than or equal to the number of formed bonds, the particle detaches from the surface. In the opposite case, the particle becomes attached; hence, the condition of particle attachment on the surface can be written as $x > N_r$, where x is a random quantity corresponding to the number of bonds formed in a particular sampling. The normal distribution function of the random variable x is given by the expression

$$\Phi\left(\frac{x-N_\sigma}{\sigma}\right)=\frac{1}{\sigma\sqrt{2\pi}}\int_{-\infty}^{x}\exp\left(\frac{(x-N_\sigma)^2}{2\sigma^2}\right)\mathrm{d}x. \tag{2.84}$$

The probability of hitting the interval $x > N_r$ is determined by the increment of the distribution function and can be described by the relation

$$P=1-\Phi\left(\frac{N_r-N_\sigma}{\sigma}\right)\equiv\Phi\left(\frac{N_\sigma-N_r}{\sigma}\right). \tag{2.85}$$

Substituting the value of dispersion, e.g. $\sigma \sim 0.3N_\sigma$, we can easily see that the probability of particle attachment is estimated by the function

$$P=\Phi\left(3\left(1-\frac{N_r}{N_\sigma}\right)\right)=\Phi\left(3\left(1-\frac{U_e}{E_{ad}}\right)\right). \tag{2.86}$$

Note that if the elastic and adhesion energies (i.e., the number of formed and broken bonds) are identical, the probability of particle attachment is 0.5, i.e., one half of all particles incident onto the surface remains there, and the other half of particles rebound from the surface.

Figure 2.37 shows the probability of particle attachment (deposition efficiency) as a function of the particle velocity and size.

The curves in Fig. 2.37 confirm the ideas put forward above. In addition, we can note that fine particle (about 5 c and smaller) and coarse particles (about 80 μm and larger) have higher impact velocities necessary for particle attachment than medium-sized particles (20–40 μm).

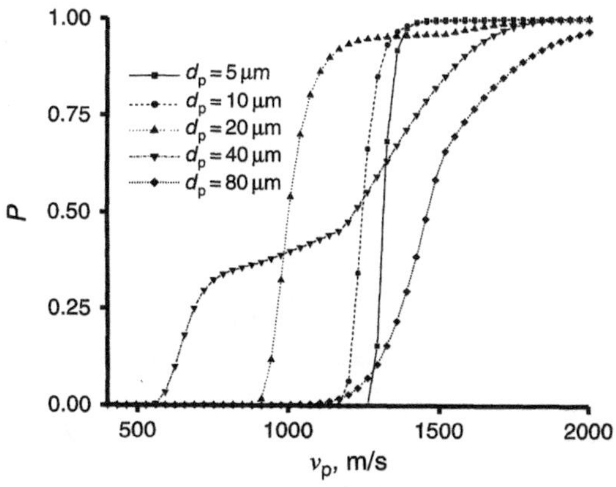

Fig. 2.37. Deposition efficiency versus the particle velocity and size.

2.5.3.12. Optimization problem

As it follows from Fig. 2.37, there is a certain particle size with a minimum impact velocity necessary for particle attachment with a certain prescribed probability. The mathematical formulation of the problem involves solving Eq. (2.86) with respect to v_p, where P is a prescribed probability of particle attachment. Figure 2.38 shows the results calculated for probabilities equal to 0.1, 0.5, and 0.9. The impact velocity and the particle diameter are plotted along the ordinate and abscissa, respectively. The curves have a clearly expressed minimum determining the most efficient parameters of particles for reaching a given value of the adhesion probability.

In practice, the choice of optimal parameters is affected by the structural features of the setup. Thus, if the structure allows acceleration of particles approximately 30 μm to velocities up to 800 m/s, the probability equal to 0.5 can be reached. The most efficient parameters for reaching the particle-adhesion probability of 0.9 are the impact velocities of approximately 1200 m/s for particle 20 μm in diameter, as is seen from Fig. 2.38.

The calculations show [40] that a nozzle of particular geometry is most efficient only in a certain range of particle sizes; hence, in solving optimization problems, one has to take into account the particle-size and particle-velocity distributions in addition to the particle-adhesion probability, because the former factors determine the use of a particular nozzle.

2.5.3.13. Polydispersity

It is rather difficult to produce a monodisperse fraction of powder. Therefore, in addition to the mean particle size, each powder is characterized by dispersion (width of the

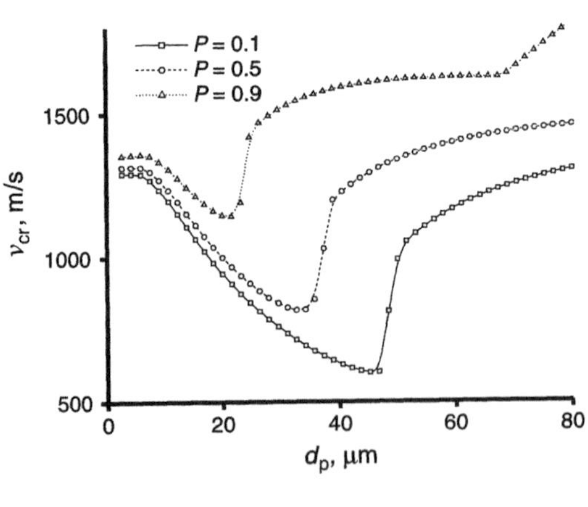

Fig. 2.38. Particle impact velocity versus the particle diameter for a prescribed particle-adhesion probability.

fraction). In the case of spraying of polydisperse powders, the total deposition efficiency is determined by the expression

$$k_d = \int_0^\infty f_p(x) P(v_p, x)\,dx = \sum n_i P(v_p, d_{pi}). \tag{2.87}$$

Here, n_i is the mass fraction of particles of size i, $P(v_p, d_{pi})$ is the probability of attachment of the particle of size i with a velocity v_p, $f_p(x)$ is the mass density of the particle-size distribution of the powder, and x is the particle diameter.

Figure 2.39 shows the curves of the deposition efficiency versus the particle velocity for a polydisperse aluminum powder with different fractions, ASD-1 with the mean particle diameter of approximately 30 μm, and ASD-4 ($d_{pm} \approx 25$ μm). Powders of similar compositions were used in experiments on studying the deposition efficiency and deformation of aluminum particles [2]. For comparison, Fig. 2.39 shows the experimentally measured values of deposition efficiency. The behavior of the deposition efficiency as a function of velocity is seen to be qualitatively identical in both cases. It should be noted that the deposition efficiency was calculated for the formation of the first (primary) layer, i.e., for the interaction of aluminum particles with a steel substrate. When the deposition efficiency presented here was measured in an experiment in the range of its low values (at $v_p \approx v_{cr}$), the coating thickness was less than 50 μm, which approximately corresponds to the first layer thickness. Therefore, a comparison of these data (experimental and calculated) is fairly reasonable for low values of deposition efficiency.

Without pretending to quantitative coincidence with the real pattern of particle–substrate interaction, the model proposed describes the character of the deposition process depending on the particle velocity and size. In addition, after model refinement, it can be used to solve optimization problems with allowance for particle-velocity and particle-size distributions available in practice.

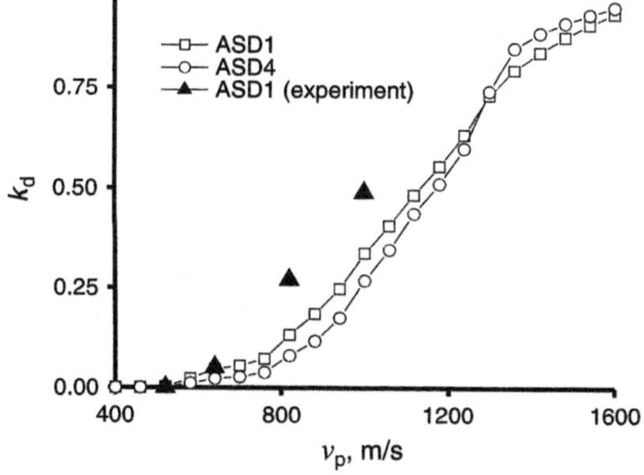

Fig. 2.39. Deposition efficiency of different aluminum fractions versus velocity.

Let us emphasize the main features of the model one more time. The impact involves a competition of two processes. On the one hand, bonds between the atoms of the particle and substrate materials are formed, which tend to attach the particle to the surface. On the other hand, part of kinetic energy is converted to elastic energy, which, vice versa, tends to tear the particle off from the surface; quenching this energy requires breakdown of a certain number of already formed bonds. The relation between the number of formed and broken bonds affects the probability of particle attachment (rebounding). We estimated the adhesion probability by extremely simple relations, which naturally have to be refined.

As a whole, we can state that the empirical statistical model described above offers some qualitative explanation for the cold spray phenomenon under a high-velocity impact of particles on the substrate. Quantitative data can be obtained on the basis of experiment.

2.5.4. Effect of surface activation on the cold spray process

In the previous Section 2.5.3, we proposed an empirical statistical model of adhesive interaction of particles with the substrate surface under a high-velocity impact. The results described in this section mainly refer to interaction of particles with the substrate that was not previously subjected to impacts of other particles. Therefore, the value of activation energy typical of the substrate material and identical for all impacting particles was used in calculations. In the real spraying process, however, particles impact on surface sections with different values of activation energy. As was experimentally demonstrated in Section 2.2.1, in the case of the impact of a flux of particles whose velocity is lower than a certain critical value v_{cr2} (v_{cr2} is the velocity at which particles start to adhere to a non-activated surface), particles start to adhere to the surface after a certain time, after the surface experiences a certain number of impacts. The effects can only be attributed to a change in the surface state due to impacts, which is described (including the degree of surface roughness), within the framework of the present theory by one parameter: activation energy. As the number of impacts at a surface point increases, the activation energy decreases, which increases the probability of particle attachment in the vicinity of this point.

The first impacting particles clean the surface (in the same manner as sandblasting or mechanical treatment) and create a specific microrelief. The mere surface cleaning should reduce the activation energy by a certain value. The next incident particles rebound but simultaneously increase the chemical activity of the surface, forming an elevated concentration of dislocations in the surface layer of the substrate during plastic deformation; the places where these dislocations reach the surface can serve as nucleation centers at which chemical interaction between the particle and the substrate begins[30]. In addition, these particles can leave a certain number of attached atoms of the particle substance on the surface. Obviously, these atoms should reduce activation energy to a value typical of the particle material. The thicker the layer of particle–material atoms the closer the value of activation energy to the activation energy of the particle material.

2.5.4.1. Activation energy

As the characteristic quantity that makes it possible to distinguish one surface material from another, we use the values of activation energy cited in [36]. The algorithm for calculating this quantity for various materials is also indicated there.

The value of activation energy at a certain point at a given time is given by the function [41]

$$E_a = k_{im} \frac{N_0 E_{aw} + N_{im} E_{ap}}{N_0 + N_{im}}. \tag{2.88}$$

It offers a qualitatively correct description of activation energy, which is determined by the state of the substrate surface at $N_{im} = 0$ and by the state of the deposited material as $N_{im} \to \infty$. Here, E_{aw} and E_{ap} are the activation energies typical of the substrate and particle materials, respectively (borrowed from [36]), and N_{im} is the number of impacts at the surface point (i.e., the number of particles hitting this surface point).

The constants k_{im} and N_0 should be chosen on the basis of experimental data. Thus, the factor k is found from the condition that the particles with the second critical velocity v_{cr2} are immediately attached (induction time equals zero). In the formula, this corresponds to the case $N_{im} = 0$, whence it follows that $E_a = k_{im} E_{aw}$. The experiment should be used to determine the value of the second critical velocity v_{cr2}, at which the particle-adhesion probability is close to unity (in the case of aluminum deposition, this velocity is about 900 m/s). After that, in calculations within the framework of the model, the value of k is chosen. For instance, for the case of interaction of aluminum particles with a copper substrate, the value of k should be 1.25. The second constant N_0 is determined, vice versa, at low impact velocities. For example, in the case of interaction of aluminum particles with a velocity of 600 m/s, approximately 50 impacts at one point are needed for one particle to become attached, as was shown in the experiment [8]. This fact allows us to choose the value of N_0 of the order of 400 to match the experimental and numerical data.

Thus, by matching the numerical and experimental data at two extreme points, one can model high-velocity adhesive interaction in all intermediate cases.

2.5.4.2. Numerical experiment

The numerical experiment was performed as follows. The matrix $M_{i,j}$ corresponds to the entire control surface. Each element of the matrix, $m_{i,j}$ (let us call it a "node"), corresponds to one point of the surface. In accordance with the Cartesian coordinate system, the nodes on the surface are located at the apices of a square $1\,\mu m \times 1\,\mu m$. To eliminate edge effects, the left edge of the surface is matched to the right edge, and the upper edge is matched to the lower edge (toroidal conditions of matching). Certain quantities characterizing the surface are associated with each node $m_{i,j}$. These are the total number of impacts at a given node, the number of particles attached at this node, and the current value of activation energy depending on the number of impacts at this node. The particle diameter and velocity are prescribed at the beginning of calculations. After that, the coordinates of the surface node containing the particle center are randomly chosen. In accordance with the particle size and velocity, the particle–substrate contact area is calculated, and hence, the nodes covered by the particle are found. In accordance with the activation energy, the adhesion energy at each node is calculated. As the nodes are located at a certain distance from the central node, the lower limit of integration (see formula (2.65)) has an individual value for each node, which is taken into account in calculations. The values of adhesion energy are summed, and the result is divided by the total number of nodes covered by the particle. Thus, the adhesion energy averaged over the particle–substrate contact area is determined. In accordance with this value of adhesion energy, the particle-adhesion probability is found. This value of probability is compared with a random quantity uniformly distributed on the segment from 0 to 1. The particle is assumed to be attached (if the calculated probability is greater than the random number $0 \leq \xi \leq 1$) or rebounded with the corresponding change in surface activation energy. Consecutively repeating the procedure many times, one can simulate the process of coating formation on the surface for a prescribed particle velocity and diameter.

2.5.4.3. Modeling results

It was further assumed in calculations that an aluminum particle was accelerated in a supersonic nozzle by a gas with a stagnation temperature of 300 K; the particle temperature at the impact was calculated; for example, for an aluminum particle 30 μm in diameter, this temperature is ≈220 K. Figure 2.40 shows the modeling results, as compared with

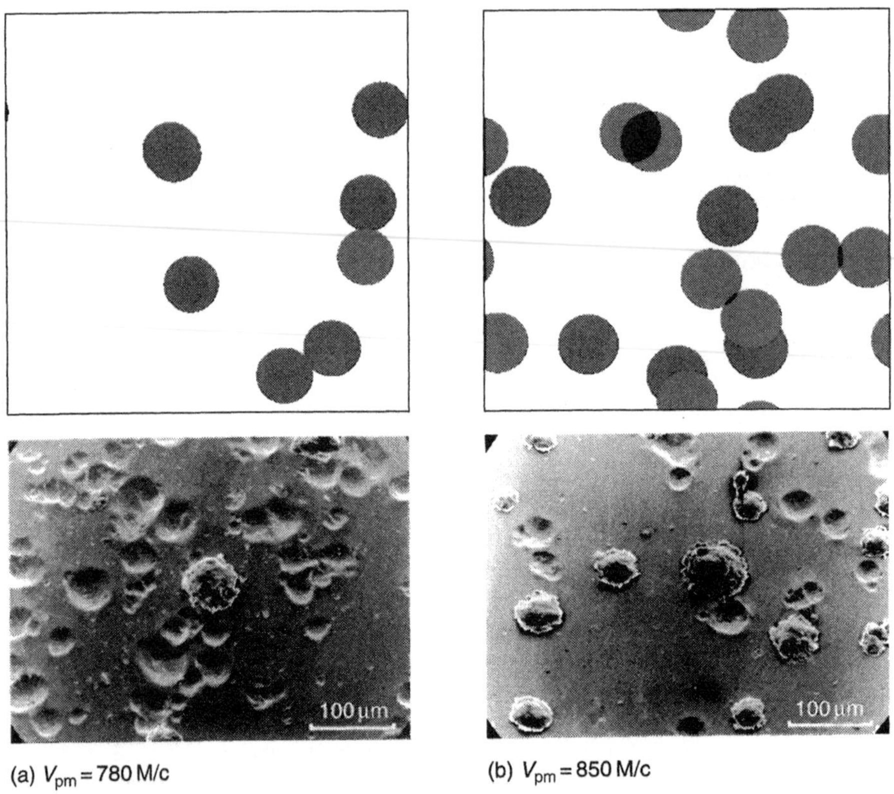

Fig. 2.40. Results of modeling compared with experimental photographs of the surface for similar conditions of deposition of aluminum particles on a copper substrate. The craters, attached particles, and places where two or more particles overlap are marked blue, red, and black, respectively.

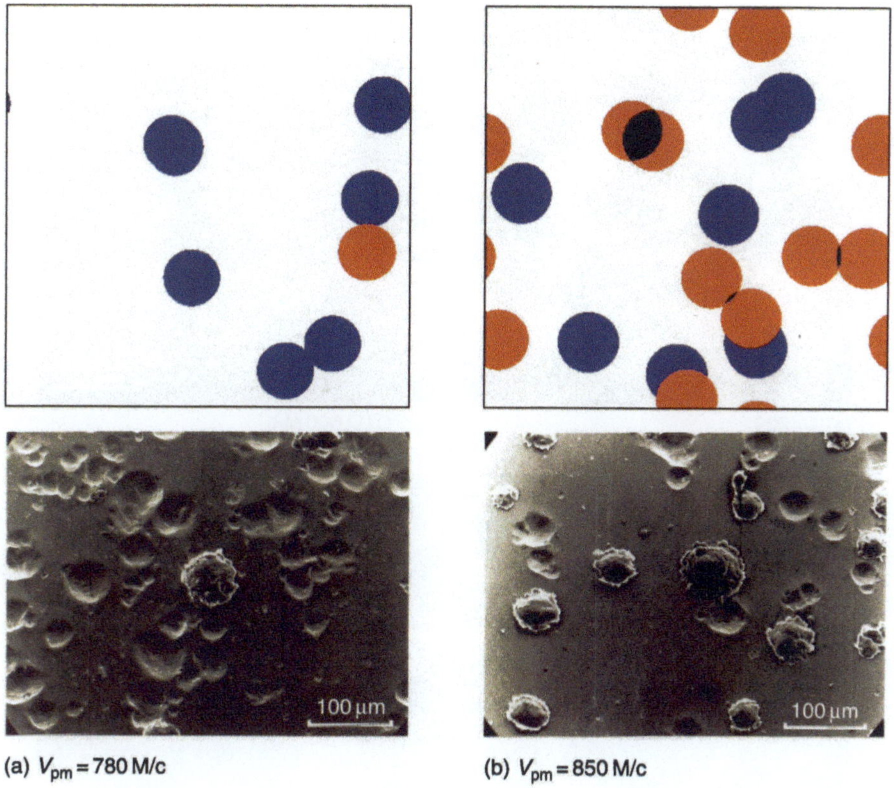

Fig. 2.40. Results of modeling compared with experimental photographs of the surface for similar conditions of deposition of aluminum particles on a copper substrate. The craters, attached particles, and places where two or more particles overlap are marked blue, red, and black, respectively.

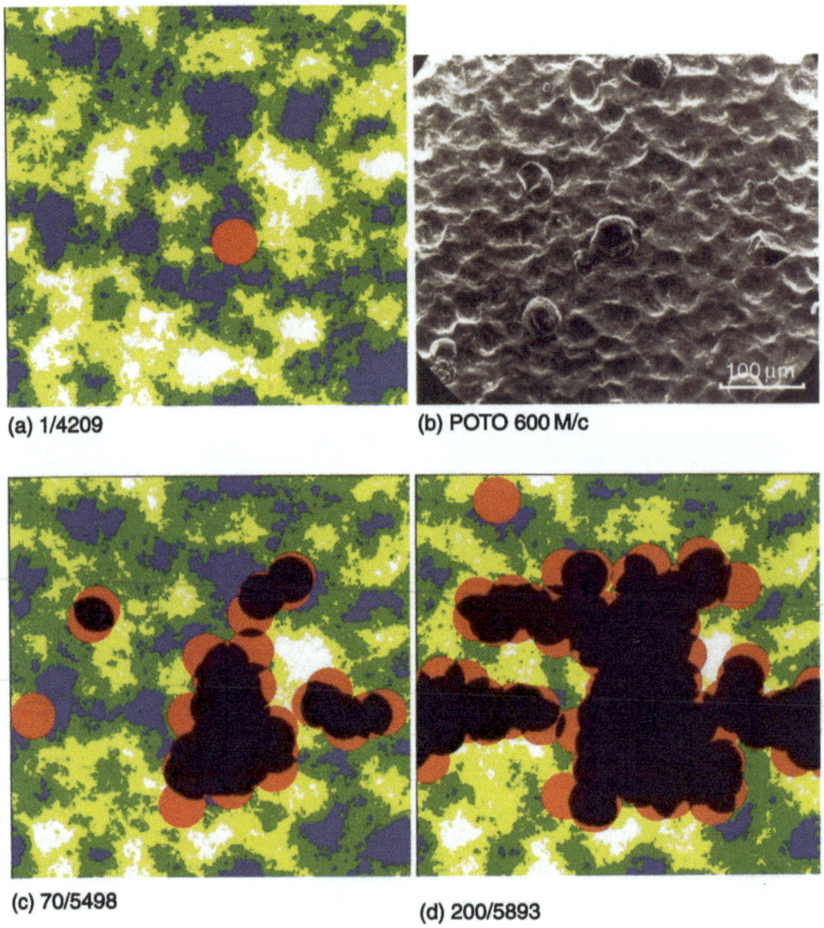

Fig. 2.41. Modeling of spraying with a velocity of 600 m/s. The white, yellow, green, and blue colors correspond to surface points subjected to a large number of impacts in increasing order. The numbers under the figures indicate the numbers of attached and incident particles, respectively. The red circles are attached particles; the places where two or more particles overlap are indicated by the black color.

experimentally obtained photographs of the surface for similar spraying conditions. A copper ($E_{aw} = 1.07 \times 10^{-19}$ J) substrate and aluminum ($E_{aw} = 0.5 \times 10^{-19}$ J) particles 30 μm in diameter (in the experiment, 30 μm was the mean particle size) were used in the calculations and experiments.

Both for the particle–substrate impact velocity of ≈780 m/s (where we see one attached particle and about 30 craters – the adhesion probability is 1/30) and for the impact velocity of ≈850 m/s (where the number of attached particles is approximately equal to the number of craters – the adhesion probability is 1/2), the results of the numerical experiment coincide with the data obtained experimentally.

Figure 2.41 shows the results of modeling of high-velocity adhesive interaction of aluminum particles 30 μm in diameter with a copper substrate for an impact velocity of 600 m/s. A surface segment 400 μm × 400 μm is shown.

The first particle is attached only after the substrate surface is sufficiently activated by preliminary impacts. In the present case, the number of preliminary impacts on the control surface was 4209 (Fig. 2.41a).

To have an idea about the distribution of the number of impacts at the surface point at the moment of attachment of the first particle, we constructed bar charts for impact velocities of 600 and 500 m/s, which are shown in Fig. 2.42.

Figure 2.42 shows the number of impacts at the surface point along the abscissa and the number of nodes experiencing the corresponding number of impacts along the ordinate. The same figure also shows the density functions of the normal distribution. For estimates, we can use the assumption of the normal distribution. For $v_p = 600$ m/s, the mean number of impacts at the surface point for the chosen conditions is approximately 45 in accordance with the experimental data [8]. For the impact velocity $v_p = 500$ m/s, the mean number of impacts at the point surface is 111. After the first particle is attached, the number of attached particles increases in an avalanche-type manner. The particles are attached predominantly as clusters. Thus, Fig. 2.41c shows formation of clusters, which increase in size, extend in width, and merge with each other (Fig. 2.41d). Coating formation has an obvious avalanche-type character confirmed by experiments.

Note that if the particles attached uniformly rather than as clusters, only approximately 3000 particles would suffice to cover the given area. Nevertheless, almost complete covering of the surface under conditions of the present numerical experiment occurs with an approximately threefold higher number of attached particles. The total number of incident particles reaches 6000 for $v_p = 600$ m/s and 17000 for $v_p = 500$ m/s. Note that such a mechanism of coating formation is typical only for those deposited materials whose activation energy is lower than the activation energy of the substrate material (e.g., as in the above-considered example of aluminum deposition onto copper).

2.5.4.4. Dependence of the coated area on the particle velocity

Figure 2.43 shows the increase in the covered area in the course of spraying modeling. To eliminate random effects, three calculations were performed for each impact velocity.

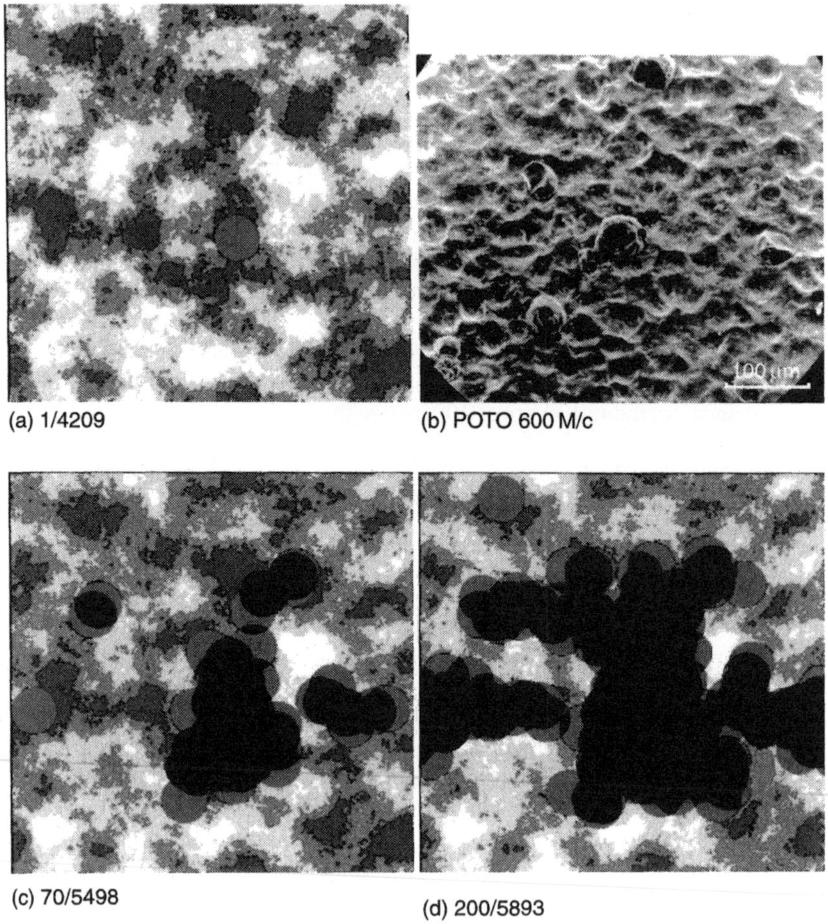

Fig. 2.41. Modeling of spraying with a velocity of 600 m/s. The white, yellow, green, and blue colors correspond to surface points subjected to a large number of impacts in increasing order. The numbers under the figures indicate the numbers of attached and incident particles, respectively. The red circles are attached particles; the places where two or more particles overlap are indicated by the black color.

The results show that the integral deposition on the surface occurs in a regular manner, though attachment of each individual particle is random, and the results calculated for an identical impact velocity almost coincide.

It is seen from Fig. 2.43 that the surface becomes completely coated after its treatment by a flux of particles, depending on their velocity. After that, the coating layer rapidly increases. The higher the particle velocity, the smaller number of particles is needed for complete coating to be formed on the surface. For a velocity $v_p = 800$ m/s, particles start to attach to the surface that was not subjected to preliminary impacts; therefore, a further increase in particle velocity does not change the dependence of S_c/S_{ex} on N_p.

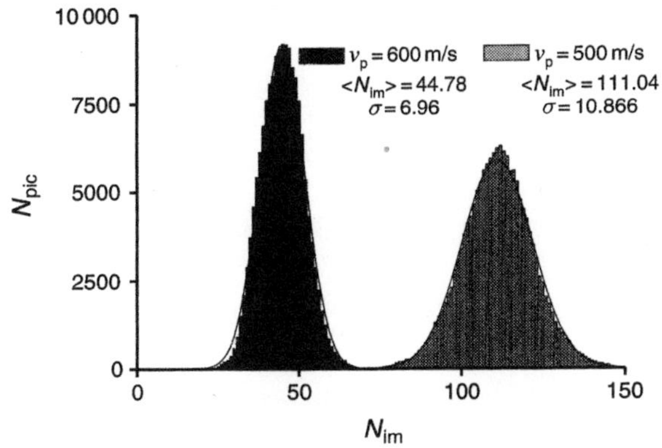

Fig. 2.42. Distribution of the number of impacts at the surface point at the moment of attachment of the first particle for two different impact velocities. The lines show the normal distribution curves.

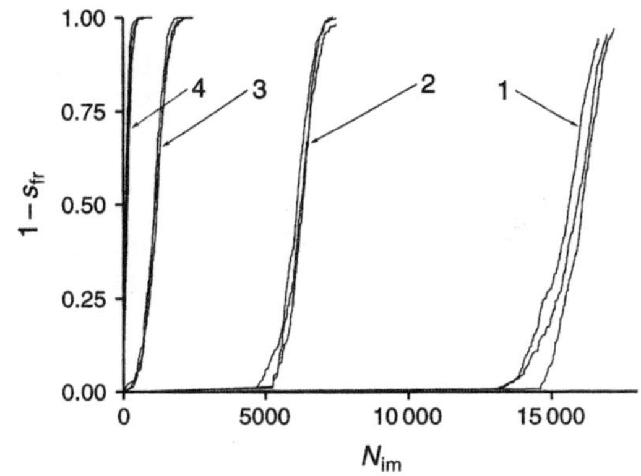

Fig. 2.43. Increase in the coated area in the course of spraying (numerical simulation) for different particle velocities. $T_p = 220\,\mathrm{K}$; $1 - v_p = 500\,\mathrm{m/s}$; $2 - v_p = 600\,\mathrm{m/s}$; $3 - v_p = 700\,\mathrm{m/s}$; $4 - v_p = 800\,\mathrm{m/s}$.

To compare the calculation results with the previously obtained experimental data [8], we pass from the variable N_p to the time t. The number of particles impacting on the surface of area S_{ex} can be determined as

$$N_p = \frac{6\varphi_p}{\pi d_p^3} S_{ex} v_p t,$$

Taking into account that

$$\varphi_p = \frac{G_{p1}}{\rho_p v_p}$$

where G_{p1} is the mass flow of particles through a unit area of the flow and ρ_p is the density of the particle material, we obtain

$$N_p = S_{ex}\frac{6}{\pi d_p^3}\frac{G_{p1}}{\rho_p}t. \tag{2.89}$$

Substituting $S_{ex} = 16\times 10^{-8}\,m^2$, $d_p = 30\times 10^6\,m$, and $\rho_p = 2700\,kg/m^3$, we obtain

$$N_p = 4\times 10^{-3}G_{p1}t,$$

and, naturally,

$$t = \frac{N_p}{4G_{p1}}10^{-3}. \tag{2.90}$$

Figure 2.6 shows the induction time t_i (time from the beginning of spraying to the beginning of particle attachment to the surface) as a function of the particle velocity: both the previously obtained experimental results [8] and the results obtained by analyzing the plots of Fig. 2.34 with $G_{p1} = 0.04\,kg/(m^2\,s)$. For such a specific mass flow, which is in good agreement with the experimental value, the experimental and numerical curves of the induction time versus the particle velocity almost coincide. This confirms that the model proposed gives an adequate description of the cold spray process.

During cold spray, it is possible to reach the value $G_{p1} \approx 30\,kg/(m^2\,s)$. For this specific mass flow, we have $t_i(500\,m/s) \approx 0.13\,s$, $t_i(600\,m/s) \approx 0.05\,s$, and $t_i(700\,m/s) \approx 8.3\times 10^{-3}\,s$. This time determines the maximum velocity of substrate motion relative to the nozzle, which is the ratio of the half thickness of the nozzle (if we want the deposition efficiency to be 0.5 or higher) to the induction time. Substituting the characteristic thickness of the nozzle $h = 3\,mm$, we find $v_{wmax}(500\,m/s) \approx 11.5\times 10^{-3}\,m/s$, $v_{wmax}(600\,m/s) \approx 30\times 10^{-3}\,m/s$, and $v_{wmax}(700\,m/s) \approx 0.18\,m/s$. The calculated velocities are also in good agreement with those used in real spraying processes.

2.5.4.5. Dependence of the coated area on the particle temperature

Calculations for different particle temperatures were also performed. Figure 2.44 shows the normalized coated area as a function of the number of impacts for different particle temperatures and an identical particle velocity $v_p = 500\,m/s$.

The character of dependences is similar to those in Fig. 2.43. By comparing Figs 2.44 and 2.43, we can see that an increase in particle temperature by 50 K in the examined range of particle velocities and temperatures approximately corresponds to an increase in particle velocity by 100 m/s. Note that the simulations do not include the possibility of rebounding of already attached particles due to an impact of another particle. Therefore, the real growth rate of the coating should be expected to be slightly lower than that in Figs 2.43 and 2.44.

Thus, results presented in this section should be considered as an attempt to construct a simple statistical model of adhesive interaction of particles with the substrate that allows

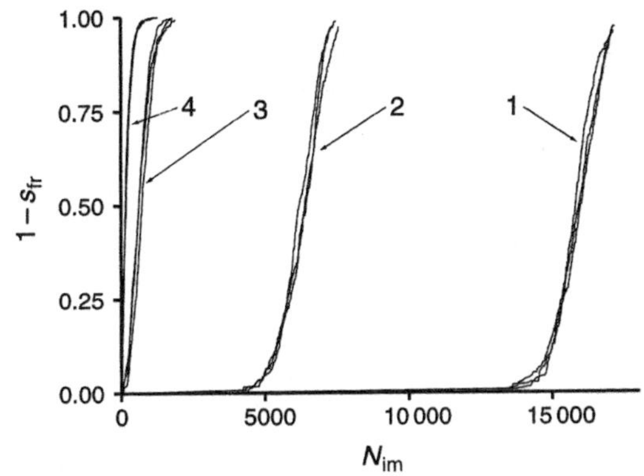

Fig. 2.44. Increase in the coated area in the course of spraying (numerical simulation) for different particle temperatures. $v_p = 500\,m/s$; $1 - T_p = 220\,K$; $2 - T_p = 270\,K$; $3 - T_p = 320\,K$; $4 - T_p = 370\,K$.

receiving some qualitative data related to the cold spray process. The objective was to study the influence of the governing parameters of spraying (first of all, the velocity and size of the deposited particles) on the process of particle adhesion onto the substrate surface. Quantitative estimates can be made on the basis of experiment when the values of some quantities are chosen to ensure the best fit with the experiment. Therefore, further improvement of the model and careful tests for its verification should be done.

2.6. Numerical Simulation of Self-organization Processes During the Particle–Surface Impact by the Molecular Dynamics Method

A new promising method of modeling various processes during the high-velocity impact of particles with the substrate is the molecular dynamics method whose detailed description can be found in [42, 43]. The current capabilities of advanced computers do not allow modeling of the impact of particles with sizes typical of cold spray by this method (in this book, the results for particles with $d_p \approx 5\,nm$ are presented). Nevertheless, the rapidly growing performance of computers allows us to hope that this will be possible in the near future. At the same time, qualitative investigation of strongly non-equilibrium processes, such as melting, disintegration, mechanical activation, and others, even at the currently available level can offer some progress in studying the physical aspects of the cold spray method. We believe that the molecular dynamics method can be useful for description of cold spraying nanostructured powders.

2.6.1. Impact of a spherical copper cluster on a rigid substrate

We considered an impact of three-dimensional spherical copper clusters with a potential barrier simulating a rigid wall. The atoms were positioned in nodes of a face-centered cubic lattice with a lattice constant $a = 3.615\,Å$ so that the distance from each atom to the cluster center was smaller than $23.5\,Å$; the number of atoms in the cluster N_{cl} was 4921.

To simulate the processes in macrobodies with a free boundary by the molecular dynamics method, we used the interaction potential for copper atoms proposed by Johnson [44], which was calculated within the framework of the embedded-atom method in the approximation of interaction of the nearest neighbors.

The potential barrier simulating the wall was the repulsive branch of the Lennard–Jones potential with the parameters $\varepsilon = 3 \times 10^{-14}$ erg and $d = 1$ Å:

$$W(x_i) = \varepsilon \left({}^{d}/_{x_i} \right)^{12}$$

The wall was located in the plane $x = 0$, the cluster impacted on the wall from the side of positive values of x, and the initial velocity of the cluster v_p was negative.

The trajectories were numerically calculated by the propagator modification of the molecular dynamics method described in [42, 43]. A second-order scheme in terms of the time step with the use of the "Verlet lists" was implemented. A large number of normalization parameters were used: the coordinates were measured in 10^{-10} m, the time in 10^{-13} s, the mass in 10^{-27} kg, the energy in 10^{-21} J, the velocity in 10^3 m/s, the force in 10^{-11} N, the pressure and stress in10^9 Pa. The time step was varied from 0.01 to 0.001 (from 10^{-15} to 10^{-16} s), so that the numerical error at the end of calculations, which amounted to 10^{-2}–1%, allowed for obtaining reliable values of the calculated macroparameters, the number of time steps in calculating one impact process was varied from 10^4 to 10^5.

The initial coordinates and impulses of the crystal at a temperature $T_p > 0$ K were simulated as follows [45]. First, the atoms were located in the positions of volume equilibrium with a lattice constant identical for all atoms and with zero impulses. After that, the dynamics of this system was numerically integrated with periodic equating of all particle impulses to zero. This procedure allows obtaining a crystal with a temperature $T_p = 0$. After that the system was heated by randomly directed impulses of a constant-amplitude force to an arbitrary prescribed value of temperature. The parameters of the acting random force were chosen in accordance with the requirement of the equilibrium Maxwellian distribution of impulses at each instant of the heating process.

The calculations were performed in the range of initial velocities $v_p = 100$–1000 m/s and initial temperatures of the crystal $T_p = 0$–300 K. To analyze the dynamics of the impact process, we calculated the following macroparameters of the system: velocity of the center of mass of the crystal v_c, force of interaction with the wall f_c, total internal energy of the crystal E_{in}, and its kinetic E_k and potential U components. The results presented below were obtained for the initial temperature $T_p = 0$ K. In terms of the character of cluster reflection from the wall, the entire range of velocities can be divided into three domains.

The first domain, $v_p < 300$ m/s, is the domain of a quasi-elastic impact. As an example, results for $v_p = 200$ m/s are given below. Figure 2.45 shows the time evolution of the velocity of the center of mass of the cluster and the force of interaction with the wall. One can clearly see the beginning and the end of interaction ($f_c = 0$ and $v_c = \text{const}$), which allows us to determine the contact time t_c.

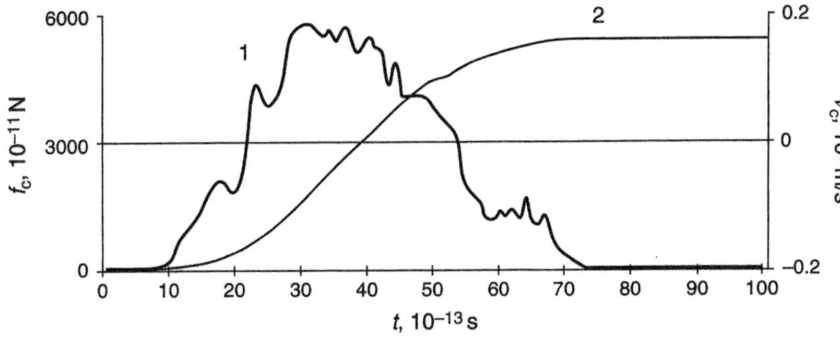

Fig. 2.45. 1 – Time evolution of the force of interaction with the wall f_c and 2 – the velocity of the center of mass of the cluster v_c. The initial velocity of the cluster is, $v_p = 200\,\mathrm{m/s}$.

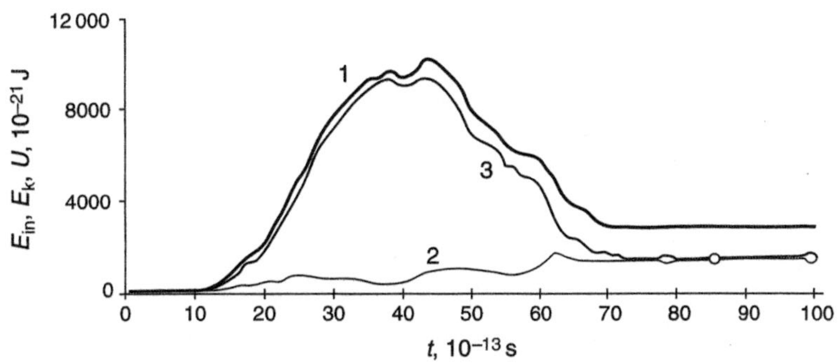

Fig. 2.46. 1 – Time evolution of the internal energy E_{in}, 2 – its kinetic component E_k, and 3 – its potential component U. The initial velocity of the cluster is $v_p = 200\,\mathrm{m/s}$.

The final velocity is somewhat lower than the initial value of 200 m/s, i.e., some part of the kinetic energy of the center of mass dissipates into the internal energy of the crystal (Fig. 2.46). The same figure shows the thermal energy E_k (kinetic energy of atoms in the system fitted to the center of mass of the crystal) and the change in the potential energy of atomic interaction $\Delta U = U - U\,(t = 0)$. After the impact, these energies acquire identical values, and each of them is equal to one half of the change in the internal energy $\Delta E_{in} = E_{in} - E_{in}\,(t = 0)$, which is a necessary condition of the final state equilibrium.

The second domain, $300\,\mathrm{m/s} < v_p < 500\,\mathrm{m/s}$, is the domain of moderately irreversible deformations. An impact of a cluster with $v_p = 400\,\mathrm{m/s}$ is analyzed below. Figure 2.47 shows the time evolution of the velocity of the center of mass of the cluster and the force of interaction with the wall.

In contrast to the first range of velocities, considerable dissipation of the kinetic energy of the center of mass is observed here, and the maximum value of the force increases by a factor of 2. The fraction of the thermal energy E_k after the impact (Fig. 2.48) significantly

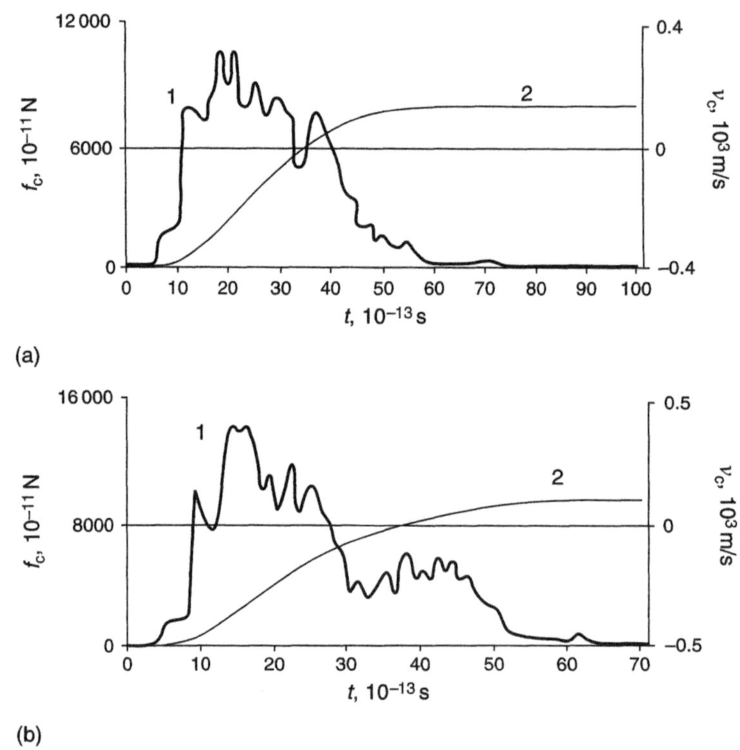

Fig. 2.47. 1 – Time evolution of the force of interaction with the wall f_c and 2 – the velocity of the center of mass of the cluster v_c. The initial velocity of the cluster is (a) $v_p = 400\,\text{m/s}$ and (b) $v_p = 500\,\text{m/s}$.

decreases, as compared to the accumulated potential energy ΔU, and the energy exchange between these two fractions is terminated.

Though the cluster shape is still close to spherical, its final structure (Fig. 2.49) becomes significantly different.

One can see typical boundaries of a cone approximately at an angle of 45° to the x axis, which separate the region with violations of the perfect FCC lattice from the "normal" structure at the "end" of the cluster. The most important qualitative information can be drawn from the energy analysis of atoms in the spherical layer (Fig. 2.50).

One can see the formation of conical boundaries with an elevated potential energy of atoms, caused by violations of the perfect structure.

The results for the initial velocity $v_p = 500\,\text{m/s}$ display the character of variation of the processes in the second range of velocities. For the time evolution of the cluster velocity and the force of interaction with the barrier (Fig. 2.47), we have results similar to those for the impact with a velocity of 400 m/s, whereas there are some new aspects in the

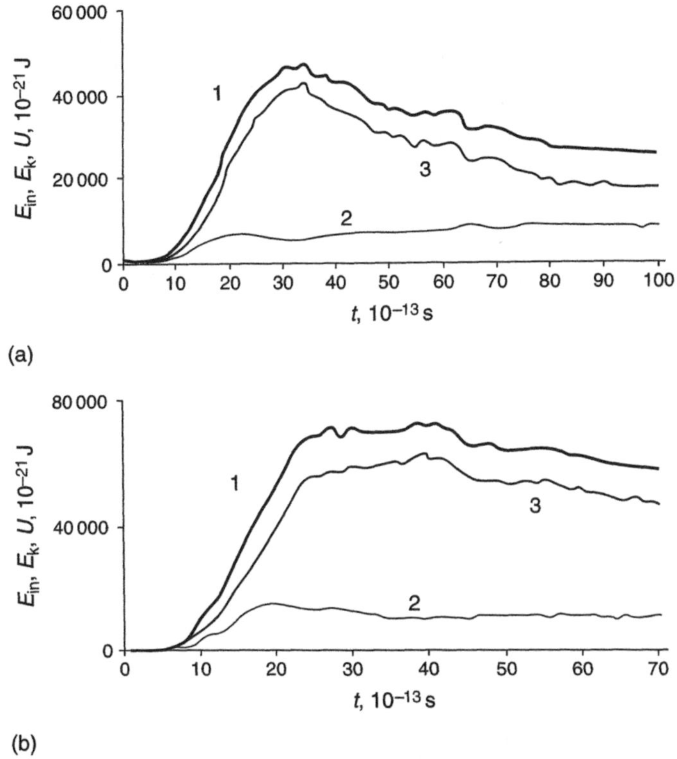

Fig. 2.48. 1 – Time evolution of the internal energy E_{in}, 2 – its kinetic component E_k, and 3 – its potential component U. The initial velocity of the cluster is (a) $v_p = 400\,m/s$ and (b) $v_p = 500\,m/s$.

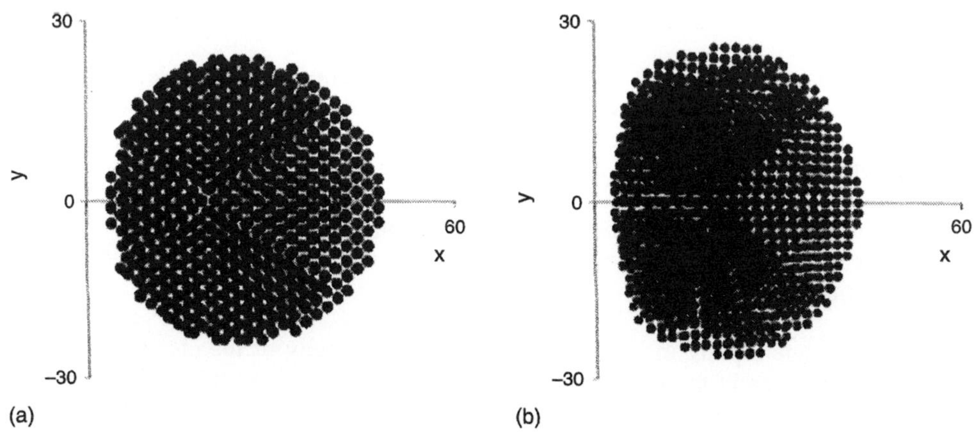

Fig. 2.49. Image of the cluster (projection onto the xy plane) cooled down after the impact with the wall with the initial velocity (a) $v_p = 400\,m/s$ and (b) $v_p = 500\,m/s$.

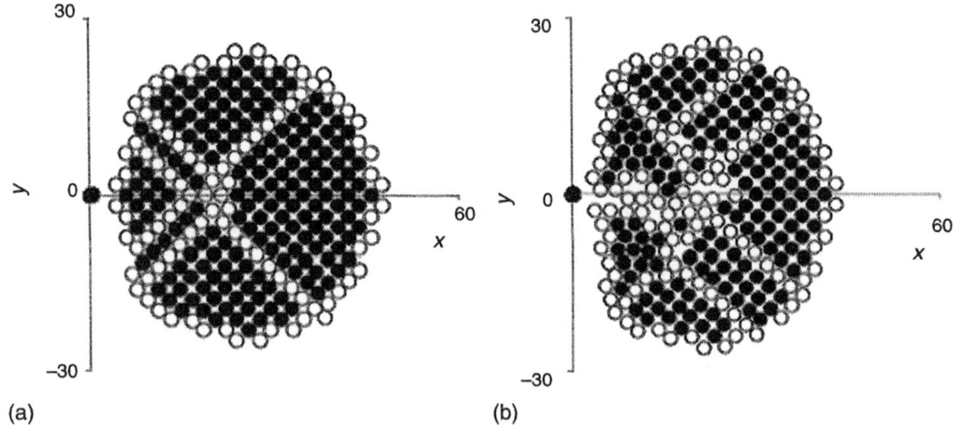

Fig. 2.50. Atomic cluster cooled down after the impact with the wall with the initial velocity (a) $v_p = 400\,m/s$ and (b) $v_p = 500\,m/s$ in the equatorial spherical layer of a height of 2 Å in the xy plane. The transparent circles correspond to atoms with potential energy higher than –550.

behavior of the energy characteristics (Fig. 2.48). First of all, it should be noted that the absolute value of the thermal energy of random motion changes weakly as compared with the increment of the potential component of internal energy, which indicates the increasing role of formation of crystal-structure defects in the course of dissipation of energy of ordered motion of the center of mass of the cluster. In addition, at the impact time $t = 25$, after a drastic decrease in the force of interaction with the barrier, a plateau is formed on the curve of the total potential energy of the cluster, i.e., the effect of the elastic component is not very strong. The shape of the cluster after rebounding is also close to spherical (Fig. 2.49). The energy analysis in the spherical layer (Fig. 2.50) shows that many complex-shaped microcrystallites with boundaries formed by the intersection of a number of crystallographic planes {111} are formed.

The third domain, $v_p > 500\,m/s$, is primarily characterized by almost complete dissipation of the initial kinetic energy of the center of mass. As an example, we show the dynamics of the impact with the initial velocity $v_p = 800\,m/s$. It is seen from Fig. 2.51 that the velocity of the center of mass of the cluster at the end of the impact is close to zero.

Despite the drastic decrease in the force of interaction with the barrier at time $t = 15$, a significant further increase in the potential energy of the cluster with plateau formation is observed (Fig. 2.52).

The rebound time rapidly increases because the final velocity of the cluster is close to zero, and it remains in the field of the potential barrier for a long time. The geometric shape of the cluster after the impact is significantly different from spherical and is close to cylindrical (Fig. 2.53).

An analysis of the crystal structure and energy in the spherical layer (Fig. 2.53b) shows that the entire central part is in the quasi-amorphous state with an elevated potential

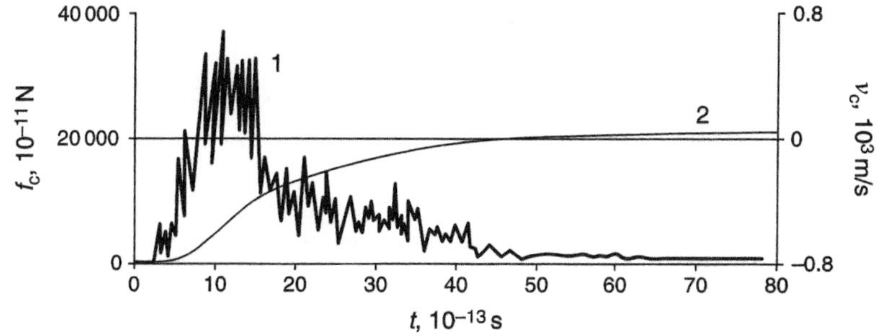

Fig. 2.51. 1 – Time evolution of the force of interaction with the wall f_c and 2 – the velocity of the center of mass of the cluster v_c. The initial velocity of the cluster is $v_p = 800\,m/s$.

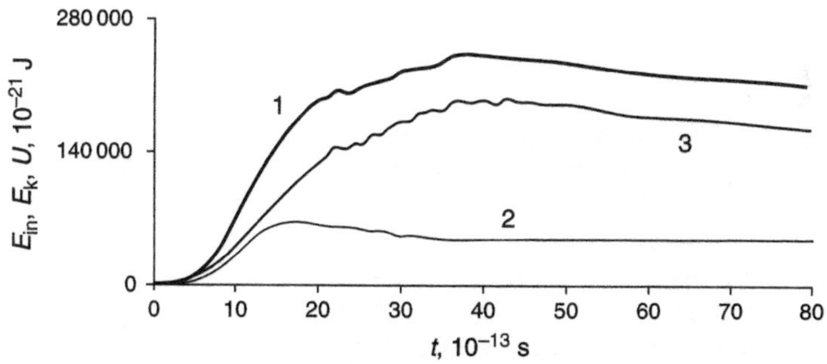

Fig. 2.52. 1 – Time evolution of the internal energy E_{in}, 2 – its kinetic component E_k, and 3 – its potential component U. The initial velocity of the cluster is $v_p = 800\,m/s$.

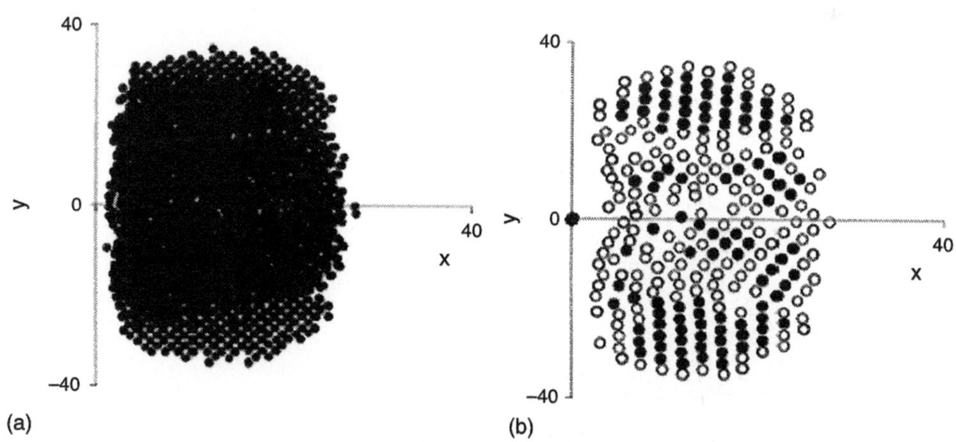

Fig. 2.53. Cluster cooled down after impact with the wall with initial velocity $v_p = 800\,m/s$. (a) projection onto the xy plane; (b) in the equatorial spherical layer of height of 2 Å in the xy plane; the transparent circles correspond to atoms with potential energy higher than –550.

energy of atoms, and the initial structure of the FCC lattice is retained in the shape of a thin-walled cylinder at the cluster periphery.

Of considerable interest is the analysis of the behavior of the most important macroparameters as functions of the initial velocity. First of all, this refers to identification of the domain of irreversible deformations. Physically, this phenomenon corresponds to the examined system in the final state being located in a local extremum of the potential energy U_f, which lies higher than the initial value U_0 at the temperature $T = 0\,\text{K}$, corresponding to the perfect crystal:

$$\Delta U_{irr} = U_f|_{T=0\,K} - U_0|_{T=0\,K}$$

To obtain the final energy $U_f|_{T=0\,K}$, the crystal rebounded from the wall was cooled down in the same manner as in obtaining the initial data. For $v_p < 300\,\text{m/s}$, the irreversible increment of the potential energy of the crystal ΔU_{irr} equals zero, i.e., the strains have a structurally reversible character, and the impact itself is quasi-elastic. The term "quasi-elastic" is used here because of the dissipation of some part of the initial kinetic energy of the center of mass to the thermal energy. The energy-dissipation factor $\Delta E_k = E_{k0} - E_{ka}/E_{k0} \times 100\%$, where E_{k0} and E_{kf} are the kinetic energy of the center of mass of the crystal at the beginning and at the end of the impact, respectively, reaches 66% for $v_p = 300\,\text{m/s}$. The second range of velocities from 300 to 500 m/s is characterized by an increase in the dissipation factor almost up to 100% as the fraction of the thermal energy in the total internal energy decreases. Hence, the increase in dissipation occurs owing to violations of the perfect structure of the crystal lattice. For velocities above $500\,\text{m/s}$, the final thermal energy starts to increase almost linearly, and the dependence of potential energy accumulated in irreversible deformations of the crystal lattice remains almost quadratic.

It seems of interest to qualitatively compare the impact time of the cluster t_c obtained within the framework of discrete-atomic mechanics with the results predicted by continuum mechanics (Fig. 2.54).

Dependences of the contact time of spherical aluminum and copper particles with a rigid substrate, calculated for elastic and elastoplastic particles, were given in Section 2.3. In the case of elastic particles, the results are in good agreement with those plotted in Fig. 2.14 in the first range of impact velocities $100\,\text{m/d} < v_p < 300\,\text{m/s}$ (with allowance

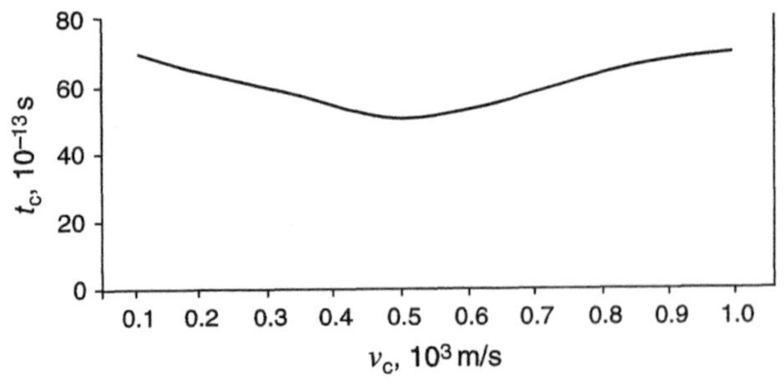

Fig. 2.54. Impact time of the cluster t_c with the wall versus the initial velocity.

for the linear dependence of t_c on the particle radius). These values of t_c are close to the analytical results obtained in the quasi-static approximation within the framework of Hertz's contact theory. In the case of elastoplastic particles, however, there are some differences in results. First of all, it is shown in Section 2.3 that particles experience plastic deformation already at the impact velocity of 100 m/s; as a result, the curve of the impact time versus the particle velocity has a minimum at a velocity approximately equal to 150 m/s (Fig. 2.14), and then the contact time starts to increase with increasing velocity, which differs from the dependence obtained in Section 2.3 (the contact time has a minimum at $v_p = 500\,\mathrm{m/s}$). These differences can be explained by significant differences in physical properties of nanocrystalline clusters and "massive" particles. Figure 2.15 shows that the minimum in the dependence of t_c on v_p is reached at higher initial velocities with increasing yield stress.

Thus, the dynamic study of the impact of the cluster on a rigid unstructured wall revealed three ranges of initial velocities v_p with principally different mechanisms of dissipation of the kinetic energy of the center of mass E_{c0}. In the range up to 300 m/s, the energy E_c is converted to the random energy of thermal motion of crystal atoms E_k and their potential energy of interaction U whose values correspond to the elastic approximation, as was shown by calculations. Indeed, in the case of reflection from the wall, conversion of the energy E_k to the energy of the center of mass E_c in accordance with the second law of thermodynamics is not observed, and the entire final energy E_c consists of the accumulated elastic component of the potential energy at the time E_c was equal to zero. With increasing velocity v_p (range of 300–500 m/s), the channel of energy conversion to random thermal motion is almost exhausted, and the entire energy E_k is accumulated in the potential energy of atomic interaction U. It has such a value that termination of cluster-wall interaction leads to the formation of selected planes with elevated residual potential energy of atoms. The system is positioned in local extremums whose values are significantly higher than the initial energy U_0. The final energy of the center of mass and the time of interaction with the wall monotonically decrease with increasing v_p in this interval, but the final shape of the cluster and of the FCC lattice structure are mainly retained. This is the domain of moderate elastoplastic deformations. Finally, for $v_p > 500\,\mathrm{m/s}$, the initial kinetic energy E_c reaches such a value that its complete dissipation at the moment the motion is terminated is accompanied by violations of the perfect crystal structure almost in the entire volume with simultaneous strong deformation of the initial shape. Thus, the system reaches very high local extremums of potential energy of the crystal. This is the domain of strong plastic deformations.

2.6.2. Melting at the contact plane in an impact of a nickel cluster on a rigid wall

One of the most important problems associated with cold spray is the study of the processes in surface regions at the cluster–substrate interface, responsible for generation of adhesion bonds. It was shown in Section 2.3 that a thin layer of melted metal can be formed in the near-contact region in the particle deformed by the impact with a certain velocity. Therefore, it is important to study the processes at the contact interface by the method of molecular dynamics based on fundamental principles.

Melting of spherical metal clusters was examined by the molecular dynamics method in numerous papers [46–47]. It was shown that melting of clusters proceeds from the surface toward the center, and both phases (solid and liquid) co-exist if the cluster possesses a certain energy [46]; the melting point decreases with decreasing cluster size [47, 48], and the temperature can decrease with increasing energy in the vicinity of the melting point at a certain level of energy [46].

2.6.2.1. Melting of spherical clusters

We considered melting of spherical nickel clusters of different sizes with the number of atoms $N_{cl} = 4921$, 1985, 959, 531, 225, and 87 under slow heating. We used the potential of inter-atomic interaction of nickel atoms, calculated by the embedded-atom method, which was proposed in [49]. Figure 2.55 shows the total energy E_m and temperature T versus the heating time for a system consisting of 4921 atoms.

The total energy increases almost linearly, whereas the temperature has a plateau in the vicinity of 1600 K and increases linearly after 1640 K. In addition, we calculated the mean distance between the central atom and the closest neighbors. This parameter in the crystalline state allows one to estimate the density in the central region; in the case of phase transition, this parameter behaves similar to the diffusion coefficient: namely, starts to increase rapidly at the time when the temperature curve changes its behavior from the plateau to linear growth. An important characteristic of the structural state of the substance, which is directly determined in experiments (diffraction of neutrons of x-ray radiation), is the structural factor $S(k)$ calculated by the formulas

$$S(k) = \frac{1}{N}\left\langle \left| \sum_{a=1}^{N} \sum_{i=1}^{3} \exp\left(ik^i r_a^i\right) \right|^2 \right\rangle,$$

where averaging is performed over the solid angle of the wave vector k^i, which makes the dependence $S(k)$ similar to that obtained in the case of diffraction of x-ray radiation on polycrystals. Normalization of the structural factor was chosen such that $S(k) \equiv 1$ for an ideal gas. Figure 2.56 shows the curves $S(k)$ for the cluster with $N_{cl} = 4921$

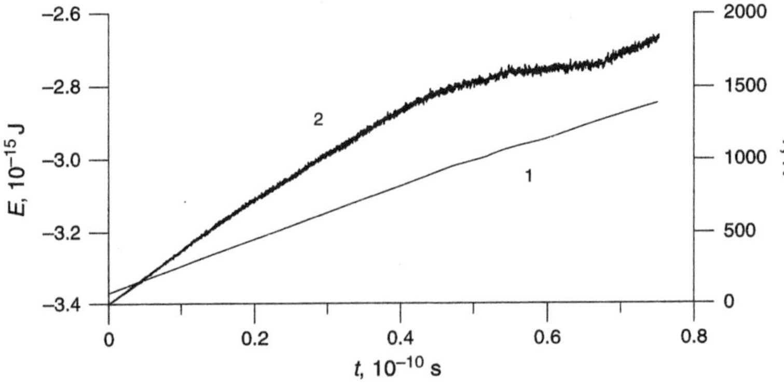

Fig. 2.55. 1 – Total energy E_m and 2 – temperature T as functions of the time of heating of a spherical nickel cluster with 4921 particles.

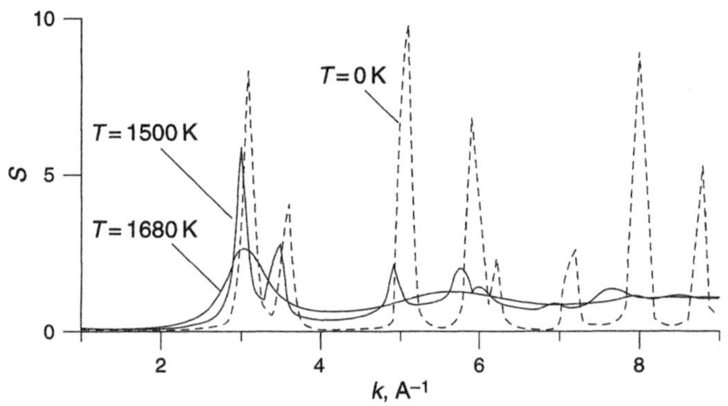

Fig. 2.56. Structural factor of the spherical nickel cluster with 4921 particles at temperatures $T = 0$, 1500 K, and 1680 K.

for different temperatures. At temperatures of 0 and 1500 K, one can clearly see the maximums corresponding to certain interplanar states in the crystal (the maximums k_{max} in the curve correspond to the interplanar distances $2\pi/k_{max}$). At a temperature of 1680 K, the dependence $S(k)$ corresponds to the liquid phase and is determined by short-range ordering.

The temperature T_m that ensures melting of the entire cluster decreases with decreasing number of particles in the cluster. Figure 2.57 shows the dependence of the logarithm $\Delta T_m = T_m^{exp} - T_m$, where $T_m^{exp} = 1726$ K is the experimental melting point, on the logarithm of the number of particles. This dependence is close to linear. Approximation of the curve by a straight line by the least squares technique yields $\Delta T_m \sim N_{cl}^{-0.66}$.

A further analysis shows that this method of heating yields an overpredicted melting point because of a significant increase in relaxation time near the phase-transition point. Nevertheless, the calculations with a permanent elimination of the random force and

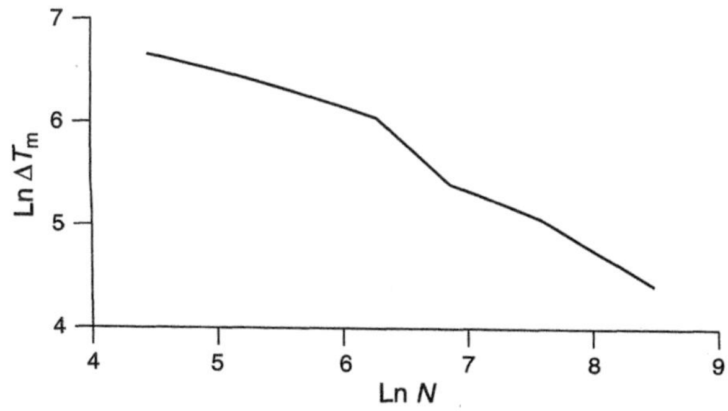

Fig. 2.57. Logarithm of the difference between the experimental melting point of nickel and the melting point of the cluster versus the logarithm of the number of particles in the cluster.

system relaxation during several thousands of time steps show that this excess in the value of T_m for the chosen heating parameters is smaller than 30 K. As a result, the refined value is $\alpha = 0.5$. This value differs from 0.33 obtained in phenomenological considerations, which take into account that the free surface energy of the liquid is smaller than the free surface energy of the crystal and yield the dependence $\Delta T_m \sim R_{cl}^{-1} \sim N_{cl}^{-1/3}$, where R is the cluster radius [47]. Possibly, this difference is related to a limited applicability of the classical thermodynamics to systems with a finite number of particles. As the number of particles decreases, fluctuations of temperature, pressure, and other thermodynamic parameters become greater–this can be the reason for a stronger decrease in the phase-transition temperature with decreasing radius than the dependence predicted by thermodynamics.

It is known that the melting point depends on pressure. For pressures close to the atmospheric values, this dependence can be neglected. As a further analysis shows, however, a cluster impact on a rigid wall generated local pressures in near-wall regions up to several dozens of GPa, which can significantly affect the value of the melting point. Therefore, we calculated melting of a cluster with the number of particles $N_{cl} = 1985$, which experienced an external pressure of 10 GPa. The pressure was simulated by a force directed to the cluster center and uniformly distributed over the surface. The pressure was calculated by the formula [50]

$$p = \frac{N_{cl} k_b T}{V_{cl}} - \frac{1}{3V_{cl}} \sum_{a=1}^{N} \sum_{i=1}^{3} r_a^{\,i} f_a^i,$$

where N_{cl}, V_{cl}, and T are the number of particles, cluster volume, and cluster temperature, and f_a^i is the i-th component of the force acting on the particle with the number a from the side of the remaining particles of the cluster. As a result, the melting point is close to 2100 K. This value is higher that T_m with zero external pressure approximately by 500 K. The estimate by the known Clapeyron–Clausius equation yields the difference in melting points close to 400 K. Thus, in further investigations of the processes in terms of reaching the thermal state of melting, we will use the condition

$$T > T_m^{exp} + 50p \tag{2.91}$$

where p is measured in GPa.

2.6.2.2. Analysis in the near-contact region of the cluster–rigid wall impact

As was shown above, in the case of a cluster impact on a rigid wall with the initial velocity higher than a certain value (500 m/s for copper), the cluster is subjected to considerable plastic strains, and its initial kinetic energy almost completely dissipates into internal energy. It is also known that velocities close to 500 m/s in cold spray are critical in terms of particle attachment to the substrate. To elucidate the mechanism of particle attachment, it seems of interest to consider whether the melting occurs in the near-contact region of the cluster with impact velocities above 500 m/s. The calculated distributions of local temperature over the cluster volume in the course of its impact on the wall show that the maximum temperatures are reached in the near-wall region, and they are significantly higher than the temperatures in other parts of the cluster, which are deformed less intensely. For further mesoanalysis in the near-contact region, the mesovolume was chosen to be a cylinder of height of 5 Å (1 Å $< x <$ 6 Å, the initial velocity being directed along the x axis); the radius from the contact center was 10 Å. The chosen mesoparameters were the mean internal energy of atoms, its kinetic and potential components (the kinetic component in equilibrium is proportional to temperature), pressure, and velocity of the center of mass.

We considered the impact of a nickel cluster with the number of particles $N_{cl} = 4921$ with the initial velocity $v_p = 600\,\text{m/s}$ on a rigid wall simulated by the repulsive branch of the Lennard–Jones potential [45]. The dissipation coefficient of the initial kinetic energy $\delta \bar{E}_k = (E_{k0} - E_{kf})/E_{k0}$, where E_{k0} and E_{kf} are the kinetic energy of the center of mass of the cluster before and after the impact, was 96%. This is the third domain of initial velocities in accordance with the above-given classification. In the course of the impact on the wall, the maximum temperature reached in the mesocell described above is approximately equal to 800 K. Hence, for this impact velocity, we cannot speak about melting.

The calculations for the initial velocity $v_p = 1000\,\text{m/s}$ show that the pressure–temperature relations in the chosen mesocell reach the values corresponding to the melting condition, Eq. (2.91). The temperature near the maximum fluctuates around T_m^{exp}, and the pressure does not exceed 3 GPa. Therefore, $v_p = 1000\,\text{m/s}$ is close to the critical value from the viewpoint of reaching the condition Eq. (2.91). It is of interest to consider an impact with a higher initial velocity of the cluster. For this purpose, the value of v_p was chosen to be 1200 m/s. Figure 2.58 shows the temperature and pressure in the near-wall region as functions of the impact time.

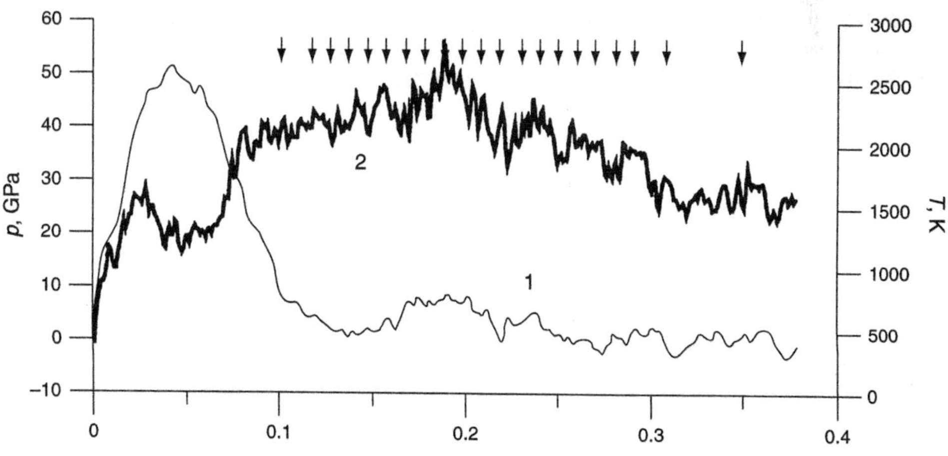

Fig. 2.58. 1 – Pressure and 2 – temperature in the near-wall region as functions of the time of impact on a rigid wall (the initial velocity of the cluster is 1200 m/s). The arrows indicate the time intervals where the melting condition (2.91) is satisfied.

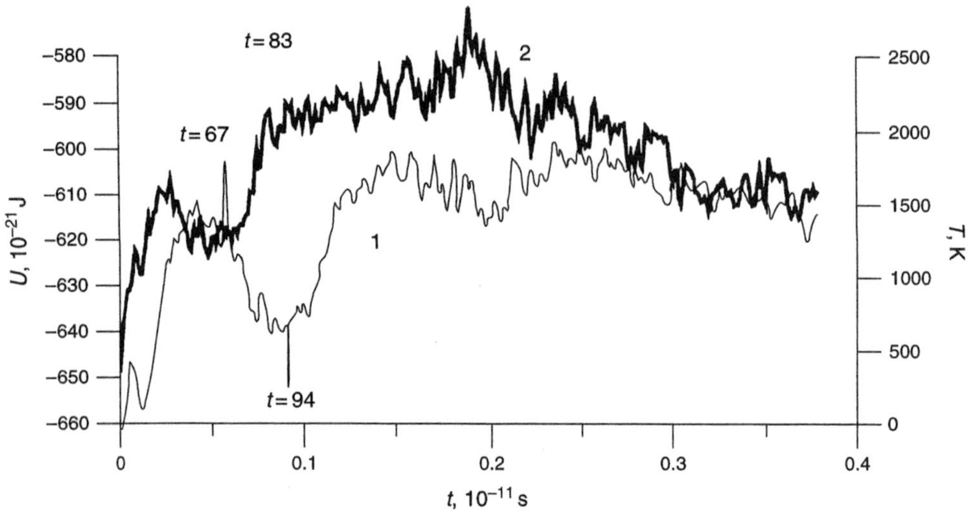

Fig. 2.59. 1 – Mean internal potential energy of atoms and 2 – temperature in the near-wall region as functions of the time of impact on a rigid wall (the initial velocity of the cluster is 1200 m/s).

The arrows indicate the time intervals where the melting condition Eq. (2.91) is satisfied. Figure 2.59 shows the time evolution of temperature and internal potential energy per atom in the mesovolume.

By the time $t = 67$, local thermodynamic equilibrium is reached, which is confirmed by the equalization of internal kinetic energy in all spatial directions and closeness of the Kolmogorov parameter to unity. In the interval $67 < t < 83$, the local temperature drastically increases and reaches approximately 2000 K. At $t = 83$, the drastic increase in temperature is terminated, and a dramatic increase in internal potential energy begins at $t = 94$; this energy increases by 25×10^{-21} J during a short time, and this value is close to the phase-transition enthalpy; after that, at time $t = 120$, the growth rate of internal energy sharply decreases. Figure 2.60 shows the structural factor in the near-wall region versus parameter k at times $t = 67$, 83, and 94.

In the interval $83 < t < 94$, a clear change of the crystalline structure by the liquid-phase structure is clearly seen. Thus, the analysis of thermodynamic, energy, and structural characteristics of the state of the substance in the region of contact with the rigid wall allows us to conclude that the cluster melts in the near-wall region in the course of the impact. Qualitatively, the phase transition does not differ from the case of slow heating. Rapid heating to a temperature close to the melting point occurs; then, the growth rate of temperature is rapidly decelerated; after that, the energy increases by a magnitude close to the latent heat of melting, and this increase occurs owing to the increase in the potential component of internal energy. After this moment, the energy-dissipation rate drastically decreases.

Thus, by an example of spherical nickel clusters, we performed a comparative analysis of the state of the cluster during its melting and during its impact on a rigid wall.

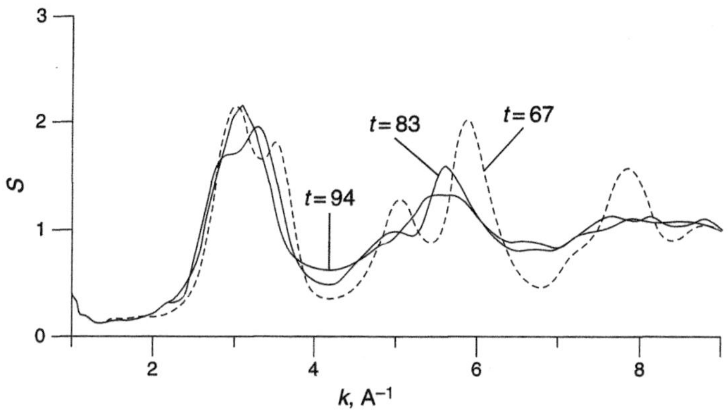

Fig. 2.60. Structural factor in the near-wall region at the times $t = 67$, 83, and 94.

The state diagrams for nickel clusters of different diameters being slowly heated were calculated. A mesoanalysis in the cluster-wall contact region in the course of the impact was performed. It was shown that thermodynamic parameters in the near-wall region reach values corresponding to melting if the impact velocity υ_p is greater than 1000 m/s, and the study of the structural changes of the cluster state in this region validate the assumption about melting of a thin layer of the cluster at the interface with the wall [51]. We believe that the molecular dynamics method can be useful for description of cold spraying nanostructured powders. The increasing performance and power of advanced computers allow us to hope that this method will be able to simulate the impact of particles whose size is typical of the cold spray method in the near future.

Symbol List

υ_p	Particle velocity
υ_{pm}	Mean particle velocity
ρ_p	Particle density
H_p	Dynamic hardness of particle
H_s	Dynamic hardness of substrate
ρ_s	Density of substrate material
D_p	Diameter of contact zone between particle and substrate surface
d_p	Particle size
d_{pm}	Mean particle size
h_p	Height of particle above surface
ε_p	Particle strain
$\varepsilon_{pm} = \frac{1}{N}\sum_{i=1}^{N}\varepsilon_i$	Mean value of particle strain
$sd = \sqrt{\frac{1}{N-1}\sum_{i=1}^{N}(\varepsilon_{pm} - \varepsilon_i)^2}$	Standard deviation of particle strain

$s = \mathrm{sd}/\sqrt{N}$	Confidence interval of mean value of particle strain
$s_{12} = \sqrt{\left(s_1^2 + s_2^2\right)}$	Confidence interval for two samples from general population
$\Delta\varepsilon_{\mathrm{pm}} = \left\lvert\varepsilon_{\mathrm{pm1}} - \varepsilon_{\mathrm{pm2}}\right\rvert$	Difference between two mean values of particle strain
v_{cr2}	Second critical velocity
t_{i}	Induction (delay) time of deposition
t	Time
$\dot{V}_{\mathrm{p}}$	Volumetric powder flow rate
$\dot{N}_{\mathrm{p}}$	Countable powder flow rate
N_{p}	Number of the particles that have impact about a surface
k_{p}	Packing coefficient of powder
$\dot{m}_{\mathrm{p}}$	Mass powder flow rate
m_{p}	Mass of the particles that have impact about a surface
S_{ex}	Square of exposing surface
$\dot{n}_{\mathrm{p}} = \frac{\dot{N}_{\mathrm{p}}}{S_{\mathrm{ex}}}$	Particle flow per surface square unit
$S_{\mathrm{c}} = \frac{\pi D_{\mathrm{p}}^2}{4}$	Square of contact between particle and substrate surface
$s_{\mathrm{c}} = \frac{S_{\mathrm{c}}}{S_{\mathrm{ex}}}$	Relative square of contact between particle and surface
P_{m}	Probability of exactly m particles impacting a given point of the surface during the time t
$\dot{n}_{\mathrm{im}}$	Mean number of impacts onto given point of surface per time unit
t_{ex}	Exposure time
$\langle N_{\mathrm{im}}\rangle_{\mathrm{i}} = \dot{n}_{\mathrm{im}} t_{\mathrm{i}}$	Mean number of impacts onto given point of surface during induction time
φ_{p}	Volume concentration of the disperse phase
v_{w}	Velocity of nozzle motion relatively substrate
S_{fr}	Free (i.e. non-occupied by particles) surface square
$s_{\mathrm{fr}} = S_{\mathrm{fr}}/S_{\mathrm{ex}}$	Relative free surface square
P_1	Probability of particle attachment onto free surface
P_2	Probability of particle attachment onto occupied surface
N_{c}	Total number of attached particles
m_{c}	Mass of deposited particles
t_0	Time of formation of primary layer of coating
m_{c0}	Mass of particles contained in primary layer of coating
h_{c}	Mean thickness of coating
$\delta h_{\mathrm{c}}/h_{\mathrm{c}} = \sqrt{\frac{d_{\mathrm{p}}\left(1-\varepsilon_{\mathrm{p}}\right)}{h_{\mathrm{c}}}}$	Relative value of roughness of coating
k_{d}	Deposition efficiency
k_{d0}	Theoretical value of deposition efficiency
m_{pi}	Mass of fallen particles during induction time
m_{pi}^*	Critical mass of fallen particles during induction time
t_{i}^*	Critical value of induction time
t_{im}	Mean time between impacts of particles into selected point of surface
m_{p0}	Mass of fallen particles during time of formation of primary layer of coating

L_c	Total length of nozzle passes over substrate
x	Coordinate along direction of velocity of nozzle motion relatively substrate
y	Coordinate perpendicular to x coordinate
D_j	Jet diameter
K	Compression modulus
μ_{sh}	Shear modulus
E	Elasticity (Yaung) modulus
ν_P	Poisson coefficient
Y_0	Dynamic yield stress
t_c	Contact time
t_{ce}	Contact time of elastic particle
t_{cp}	Contact time of elastic-plastic particle
$t'_c = \frac{t_{cp}}{t_{ce}}$	Ratio between contact times for elastic and elastic-plastic particles
f_c	Forth acting at boundary of contact
$e = c_V T$	Specific internal energy
e_m	Specific internal energy at melting point
v_{pr}	Velocity of particle after rebound
$s_c = \frac{s_{c\,max}}{s_m}$	Relative square of contact
$s_m = \pi \frac{d_p^2}{4}$	Square of middle section of particle
$e_r = \left(\frac{v_{pr}}{v_p}\right)^2$	Coefficient of restoration of kinetic energy of particle after rebound
c_V	Heat capacity at constant volume
c_p	Heat capacity at constant pressure
u	Velocity in radial direction
u_r	Velocity in radial direction at near wall layer
r	Distance from symmetric axis
δ_T	Thickness of temperature layer
δ_m	Thickness of molten layer
δ_μ	Thickness of viscous layer
Pr	Prandtl number
μ	Dynamic viscosity
u_R	Velocity at boundary of layer when $r = d_p/2$
T_m	Melting point
$Re_d = \frac{d_p u_R \rho_p}{\mu}$	Reynolds number
H_m	Specific heat of melting
$\mu\left(\frac{\partial u}{\partial z}\right)^2$	Volumetric sores of heat due to viscous friction
q	Heat flux
$\tau = t/t_c$	Relative time
$\zeta = r/d_p$	Relative radius of contact square
$T_c(\eta, \tau)$	Temperature of contact between particle and substrate
$T_c^0(\eta, \tau)$	Temperature of contact between two bodies at difference temperature
$T_v(\eta, \tau)$	Temperature of additional heating of contact due to heat generated during impact

$K_p = \sqrt{\frac{\lambda_p c_p \rho_p}{\lambda_s c_s \rho_s}}$	Criteria of heat activity of particle relatively substrate
T_s	Temperature of substrate before impact
T_p	Temperature of particle before impact
λ_s	Heat conductivity of substrate
λ_p	Heat conductivity of particle
c_s	Heat capacity of substrate
z^*	Characteristic size in direction perpendicular to contact plane
χ	Temperature conductivity of particle
β	Coefficient of localization of particle strain
$A(\eta', \tau')$	Heat generated per volume unit and per time unit
A_0	Heat generated per volume unit and time unit in case of uniform space-time distribution of generation intensity
Q_{s1}	Total heat generated at contact square unit
t^*	Characteristic time
δ_s	Substrate thickness
δ_H	Thickness of zone where heat is generated
N_σ	Number of bonds per contact square unit
$N_{\sigma 0}$	Maximal number of bonds per contact square unit
E_a	Activation energy
$t_c(r)$	Instant of appearance of contact between particle and substrate at distance r from center of contact
$k = 1.38 \times 10^{-23}\, m^2\, kg/s^2\, K$	Boltzmann constant
V_z	Particle volume heated during contact time
η	Coefficient of part of kinetic energy of particle transformed into heat of particle material
v_1	First impact velocity when melting point achieved
V_1	First volume where melting point achieved
v_2	Second impact velocity when melting of whole heated volume occurs
V_2	Second volume of molten material when melting of whole heated volume occurs
V_m	Volume of particle material where temperature is close to melting point
$q = \left\langle \frac{N_\sigma}{N_{\sigma 0}} \right\rangle$	Relative value of adhesion energy
E_{ad}	Adhesion energy
E^0_{ad}	Maximal value of adhesion energy
E_1	Energy of bond between two atoms
U_e	Elastic energy accumulated in particle
R	Energy of rebound
p_d	Contact stress at instance of rebound
E^*	Reduced elastic modulus
σ_s	Static yield stress
U_{100}	Value of rebound energy (elastic energy) at impact velocity 100 m/s
σ	Standard deviation of distribution of attachment probability

N_r	Number of dissociated bonds
P	Probability
E_{aw}	Value of activation energy characteristic for substrate material
E_{ap}	Value of activation energy characteristic for particle material
N_{im}	Number of impacting particles onto given point of surface
G_{p1}	Mass particle flow rate per flow cross section square unit
a	Lattice constant
N_{cl}	Number of atoms in cluster
v_p	Initial velocity of cluster
T_p	Initial temperature of crystal
v_c	Velocity of center of masses of crystal
f_c	Forth of interaction with substrate surface
E_{in}	Total internal energy of crystal
E_k	Kinetic energy of crystal
U	Potential energy of crystal
U_f	Loral extreme of potential energy
U_0	Initial value of potential energy at temperature 0 K
ΔU_{irr}	Inconvertible increment of potential energy of crystal
E_{k0}	Kinetic energy of center of masses of crystal before impact
E_{kf}	Kinetic energy of center of masses of crystal at the end of impact
$S(k) = \frac{1}{N}\left\langle \left\| \sum_{a=1}^{N} \sum_{i=1}^{3} \exp\left(ik^i r_a^i\right) \right\|^2 \right\rangle$	Structural factor
k^i	Corporal angle of wave vector
R_{cl}	Radius of cluster
V_{cl}	Volume of cluster
f_a^i	i-th component of forth acting onto particle with number a from side of other particles of cluster

References

[1] A.N. Papyrin, V.F. Kosarev, S.V. Klinkov, and A.P. Alkhimov, On the interaction of high speed particles with a substrate under the Cold Spraying, Intern. Thermal Spray Conf. 2002 (ITSC 2002), 2002 (Essen, Germany), Proceedings, pp. 380–384.

[2] A.P. Alkhimov, S.V. Klinkov, and V.F. Kosarev, *J. Appl. Mech. Tech. Phys.*, Vol. 41, No. 2, 2000, pp. 245–250.

[3] F.F. Vitman and N.A. Zlatin, *Zh. Tekh. Fiz.*, No. 8, 1963, pp. 982–989.

[4] L.V. Belyakov, F.F. Vitman, and N.A. Zlatin, *Zh. Tekh. Fiz.*, No. 8, 1963, pp. 990–995.

[5] N.A. Zlatin, A.P. Krasil'shchikov, G.I. Mishin, and N.N. Popov, *Ballistic Facilities and their Application in Experimental Research* [in Russian], Nauka, Moscow, 1974, 344 pp.

[6] D.J. Gardner, J.A.M. McDonnell, and I. Collier, *IJIE*, Vol. 19, No. 7, 1997, pp. 589–602.

[7] J.A.M. McDonnell, *IJIE*, Vol. 23, 1999, pp. 597–619.

[8] A.P. Alkhimov, V.F. Kosarev, A.N. Papyrin, *et al. New Materials and Technologies. Theory and Practice of Material Hardening in Extreme Processes*, eds M.F. Zhukov and V.E. Panin [in Russian], Nauka, Novosibirsk, 1992, 197 pp.

[9] S.V. Klinkov and V.F. Kosarev, *Fiz. Mezomekhanika*, Vol.5, No.3, 2002, pp. 27–35.

[10] S.V. Klinkov, V.F. Kosarev, and A.N. Papyrin, Modeling of particle-substrate adhesive interaction under the Cold Spray process, Int. Thermal Spray Conf., Thermal Spray 2003, Proceedings, *Advancing the Science and Applying the Technology*, eds C. Moreau and B. Marple, ASM International, Materials Park, OH, USA, 2003, pp. 27–35.

[11] G.A. Korn and T.M. Korn, *Mathematical Handbook for Scientists and Engineers*, McGraw Hill Book Company, New York, San Francisco, Toronto, Sydney, 1968.

[12] A.P. Alkhimov, V.F. Kosarev, and A.N. Papyrin, *Dokl. Akad. Nauk SSSR*, Vol. 315, 1990, pp. 1062–1065.

[13] V.M. Fomin, A.I. Gulidov, G.A. Sapozhnikov, *et al. High-Velocity Interaction of Bodies* [in Russian], Izd. Sib. Branch Ross. Akad. Nauk, Novosibirsk, 1999, 600 pp.

[14] A.I. Gulidov, V.M. Fomin, and R.V. Fursenko, Contact time in the impact of a spherical particle with a solid substrate, *XVI Conf. on Numerical Methods for Solving the Problems of the Theory of Elasticity and Plasticity* [in Russian], Proceedings, Novosibirsk, 1999, pp. 66–70.

[15] A.I. Gulidov, V.M. Fomin, and A.V. Seryakov, Numerical simulation of microparticle-substrate impacts, *XVII Conf. on Numerical Methods for Solving the Problems of the Theory of Elasticity and Plasticity* [in Russian], Proceedings, Novosibirsk, 2001, pp. 65–69.

[16] M.L. Wilkins, Calculation of elastoplastic flows, *Methods of Computational Physics*, eds B. Alder, S. Fernbach, M. Retenberg, Academic Press, New York, 1964.

[17] M.L. Wilkins, *Computer Simulation of Dynamic Phenomena*, Springer, 1999, 246 pp.

[18] N.A. Kil'chevskii, *Theory of Impacts of Solids* [in Russian], Naukova Dumka, Kiev, 1969, 247 pp.

[19] A.I. Gulidov and V.M. Fomin, *Prikl. Mekh. Tekh. Fiz.*, Vol. 21, No. 3, 1980, pp. 126–132.

[20] V.M. Boiko, A.I. Gulidov, A.N. Papyrin, *et al.*, *J. Appl. Mech. Tech. Phys.*, Vol. 23, No. 5, 1982, pp. 129–133.

[21] A.P. Alkhimov, A.I. Gulidov, V.F. Kosarev, and N.I. Nesterovich, *J. Appl. Mech. Tech. Phys.*, Vol. 41, No. 1, 2000, pp. 188–192.

[22] H. Schlichting, *Boundary Layer Theory*, McGraw-Hill, New York, 1955.

[23] A.P. Alkhimov, V.P. Gulyaev, A.F. Demchuk, V.F. Kosarev, V.P. Larionov, and V.P. Spesivtsev, Setup for coating deposition onto the inner surface of a tube, Russian Patent No. 2075535, *Bull. Izobr.*, No. 8, 1997, pp. 184–185.

[24] A.P. Alkhimov, A.F. Demchuk, V.F. Kosarev, and V.E. Kozhevnikov, Electrotechnical connector, Russian Patent No. 2096877, *Bull. Izobr.*, No. 32 (Part 2), 1997, pp. 376.

[25] A.P. Alkhimov, A.F. Demchuk, V.F. Kosarev, and V.P. Spesivtsev, Setup for deposition onto the inner surface of tubes, V Intern. Conf., *Films and Coatings-98*, St. Petersburg, 1998, Proceedings, pp. 117–120.

[26] A.P. Alkhimov, A.F. Demchuk, V.F. Kosarev, and V.V. Lavrushin, Technological processes of application of current-conducting corrosion-resistant coatings, V Intern. Conf., *Films and Coatings-98*, St. Petersburg, 1998, Proceedings, pp. 259–263.

[27] A.P. Alkhimov, V.F. Kosarev, and A.N. Papyrin, Spraying the current conducting coatings on electrotechnical unit by Cold Spray method, *United Thermal Spray Conf.*, Dusseldorf, 1999, Proceedings, pp. 288–290.

[28] V.V. Kudinov and V.M. Ivanov, *Plasma Application of Refractory Coatings* [in Russian], Mashinostroenie, Moscow, 1981, 192 pp.

[29] M.Kh. Shorshorov and Yu.A. Kharlamov, *Physical and Chemical Fundamentals of Detonation Gas Deposition of Coatings* [in Russian], Nauka, Moscow, 1978, 224 pp.

[30] V.V. Kudinov, P.Yu. Pekshev, V.E. Belashchenko, O.P. Solonenko, and V.A. Safiulin, *Plasma Application of Coatings* [in Russian], Nauka, Moscow, 1990, 408 pp.

[31] V.N. Danchenko, A.A. Milenin, and A.N. Golovko, *Poroshkovaya Metallurgiya*, Nos 7/8, 1998, pp. 10–15.

[32] A.P. Alkhimov, S.V. Klinkov, and V.F. Kosarev, *Fiz. Mezomekhanika*, Vol. 3, No. 1, 2000, pp. 53–57.

[33] A.N. Tikhonov and A.A. Samarskii, *Equations of Mathematical Physics* [in Russian], Nauka, Moscow, 1966, 724 pp.

[34] A.I. Zverev, S.Yu. Sharivket, and E.A. Astakhov, *Detonation Deposition of Coatings* [in Russian], Sudostroenie, Leningrad, 1979.

[35] M.Kh. Shorshorov and Yu.A. Kharlamov, *Physical and Chemical Fundamentals of Detonation Gas Deposition of Coatings* [in Russian], Nauka, Moscow, 1978, 224 pp.

[36] K.A. Osipov, *Some Activated Processes in Metals and Alloys*, Izd. Akad. Nauk SSSR, Moscow, 1962, 123 pp.

[37] Charles A. Wert and Robb M. Thomson, *Physics of Solids*, McGraw-Hill Book Company, New York, San Francisco, Toronto, London, 1964.

[38] K.L. Johnson, *Contact Mechanics*, Cambridge University Press, Cambridge, 1985.

[39] A.I. Celikov, A.D. Tomlenov, V.I. Zyuzin, *et al.*, Theory of rolling [in Russian], *Metallurgy*, Moscow, 1982, 355 pp.

[40] A.P. Alkhimov, S.V. Klinkov, and V.F. Kosarev, *J. Thermal Spray Technol.*, Vol. 10, No. 2, 2001, pp. 375–381.

[41] S.V. Klinkov and V.F. Kosarev, *Fiz. Mezomekhanika*, Vol. 6, No. 3, 2003, pp. 85–90.

[42] I.F. Golovnev, E.I. Golovneva, and V.M. Fomin, *Dokl. Akad. Nauk SSSR*, Vol. 356, No. 4, 1997, pp. 466–469.

[43] I.F. Golovnev, E.I. Golovneva, A.A. Konev, and V.M. Fomin, *Fiz. Mezomekhanika*, Vol. 1, No. 2, 1998, pp. 21–33.

[44] R.A. Johnson, *Phys. Rev. B*, Vol. 39, 1989, pp. 12554–12559.

[45] A.V. Bolesta, I.F. Golovnev, and V.M. Fomin, *Fiz. Mezomekhanika*, Vol. 3, No. 5, 2000, pp. 39–46.

[46] O.H. Nielsen, J.P. Sethna, P. Stoltze, *et al.*, *Europhys. Lett.*, Vol. 26, 1994, pp. 51–56.

[47] F. Ercolessi, W. Andreoni, and E. Tosatti, *Phys. Rev. Lett.*, Vol. 66, 1991, pp. 911.

[48] M.E. Fisher and A.N. Berker, *Phys. Rev. B*, Vol. 26, 1982, pp. 2507–2513.

[49] A.F. Voter and S.P. Chen, Accurate interatomic potentials for Ni, Al, and Ni3Al, *Mat. Res. Soc. Symp.*, Proceedings, 1987, p. 175.

[50] M.P. Allen and D.J. Tildesley, *Computer Simulation of Liquids*, Oxford University Press, 1987, 385 pp.

[51] A.V. Bolesta, I.F. Golovnev, and V.M. Fomin, *Fiz. Mezomekhanika*, Vol. 4, No. 1, 2001, pp. 5–10.

CHAPTER 3

Gas-dynamics of Cold Spray

Despite extensive investigations of jet gas-dynamics, some issues have not been adequately studied. There are some aspects of this problem, and one of the most important tasks is to increase the particle velocity as high as possible. Development of the boundary layer on the nozzle walls, the structure and stability of the jet in different exhaustion modes and interaction of a supersonic jet with the substrate, including the structure and time evolution of the high-pressure zone ahead of the substrate and heat transfer between the jet and the substrate, should be studied to obtain the optimal velocity and temperature of particles at the moment of its impact onto the substrate surface. The purpose of the present chapter is to discuss the above-stated gas-dynamic and thermal effects associated with a supersonic jet exhausting from the nozzle and its interaction with the substrate in the cold spray method.

To accelerate particles we suggested the use of two types of nozzles [33]: nozzles with circular and rectangular sections. Historically, gas-dynamics of jets exhausting from conical nozzles with circular cross sections, i.e., symmetrical-axis flows, was examined in more detail. An analysis of the features of such jets, as applied to the cold spray method, revealed that the use of nozzles with rectangular cross sections is also promising. With the same ratio of the nozzle-exit and throat cross sections, nozzles with a rectangular section can provide, on the one hand, a wider spray beam in the direction of the smaller size of the section and, on the other hand, a narrower beam (to 1–2 mm) in the direction of the larger size of the section. Such nozzles can also decrease the effect of particle deceleration in the compressed layer in front of the substrate by decreasing the thickness of the layer itself.

The issues of acceleration of finely dispersed particles in supersonic nozzles and formation of comparatively thin flat two-phase jets, which ensure high deposition efficiency over the area, are of significant interest in the process of cold spray and are important both for the theory and for applications. The experience in cold spray shows that the particle velocity reached immediately before the impact on the substrate plays the most important role in deposition of coatings by this method. The problem of estimating this velocity can be divided into four independent tasks:

1. character of injection of particles into the pre-chamber and their motion up to the nozzle throat;
2. acceleration of particles in the supersonic part of the nozzle;
3. motion of particles from the nozzle exit to the shock wave ahead of the substrate;
4. deceleration of particles in the compressed layer (between the shock wave and the substrate surface).

If the concentration of particles is moderate or low, the particle velocity can be calculated in the approximation of single particle motion, i.e., the effect of particles on the gas-flow parameters can be ignored. Such a calculation requires preliminary experimental and numerical investigations of gas flows in nozzles used in the cold spray method, the flow from the nozzle exit to the shock wave and the flow from the shockwave to the substrate. Figure 3.1 shows a schematic of the gas-dynamic duct of the acceleration of particles in a supersonic nozzle, their motion in the free jet, and their acceleration in the compressed layer.

The following gas-dynamic problems of cold spray are considered in the present chapter.

1. test-gas flow in a long supersonic nozzle with noticeable influence of boundary layers formed on the nozzle walls;
2. exhaustion of a supersonic jet with a rectangular cross section from such nozzles;
3. impact of a supersonic jet onto the substrate;
4. heat transfer between a supersonic jet and a substrate and determination of the substrate-surface temperature in the deposition spot.

These issues are important for optimization of particle acceleration in supersonic nozzles and, on this basis, optimization of the spraying technology.

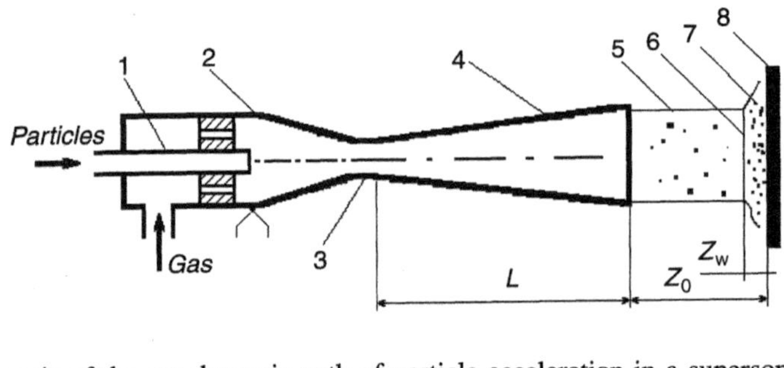

Fig. 3.1. Schematic of the gas-dynamic path of particle acceleration in a supersonic nozzle, their motion in the free jet, and their deceleration in the compressed layer. 1 – tube for injection of particles into the pre-chamber, 2 – pre-chamber, 3 – nozzle throat, 4 – supersonic part of the nozzle, 5 – free jet, 6 – bow-shock wave, 7 – compressed layer, and 8 – substrate.

3.1. Flow in a Supersonic Nozzle with a Large Aspect Ratio and a Rectangular Cross Section

An unusual nozzle shape (a greater value of the ratio between the length of the supersonic part of the nozzle and the minimum exit dimension $L/h = 20$–50) leads to the formation of jets that differ considerably from well-known symmetrical-axis jets with a uniform distribution of gas parameters at the nozzle exit. In particular, the boundary-layer effect can play an important role, which can make the gas-flow parameters in such nozzles differ from the parameters calculated for ideal nozzles [1]. It should be noted that many presented results of studying rectangular nozzles can also be used to examine nozzles with a conical supersonic part, which are more commonly used.

This section presents results of experiments and calculations on the influence of the nozzle geometry (length, thickness, cone angle of the supersonic part) on flow parameters.

3.1.1. Experimental determination of gas-flow parameters at the exit of a plane supersonic nozzle

3.1.1.1. Experimental setup

For effective acceleration of particles in the supersonic part of the nozzle, the length of the latter should be greater than the relaxation length of particles used for spraying. The relaxation length l_p of particles with a diameter $d_p = 50 \times 10^{-6}\,m$ accelerated in a supersonic nozzle with a Mach number $M^* = 2.0$–3.0 for characteristics values of the normalized velocity $\Delta v_p = v - v_p \sim 100\,m/s$ and density $\rho_p \approx 5 \times 10^3\,kg/m^3$ of particles, density $\rho \approx 3\,kg/m^3$ and viscosity $\mu \approx 10^{-5}\,kg/(m\,s)$ of the gas, and Reynolds number $Re = \Delta v_p d_p \rho/\mu \approx 10^3$ is estimated as $l_p = 4(e^{-2})\rho_p d_p/3\rho \approx 0.1\,m$ (the drag coefficient C_x of the particle for such values of Re is assumed to equal unity). Approaching the substrate, the particle is decelerated in the compressed layer formed by the supersonic jet incident onto the substrate. The estimate shows that the particle velocity ($d_p = 5 \times 10^{-6}\,m$ and $\rho_p = 5 \times 10^3\,kg/m^3$) decreases in the compressed layer by a factor of e over the thickness of $\sim 3 \times 10^{-3}\,m$. Taking this circumstance into account and the fact that the compressed layer thickness is mainly determined by the smaller transverse size of the jet, we used plane nozzle whose throat size was determined by the height b_{cr} and thickness of contoured inserts $h = (1$–$5) \times 10^{-3}\,m$. The output section of the Laval nozzle $H \times h$ corresponded to $M^* = 2.0$–3.0, the displacing action of the boundary layer being ignored.

The experiments were performed on a setup whose schematic is shown in Fig. 3.2. The main elements of the setup are a supersonic plane nozzle (1), a particle feeder (2), and a gas heater (3) with a temperature-control system (4). The test gas was air (5) or a compressed gas (helium or argon) from the gas holder (6), the pressures in the pre-chamber, at the nozzle exit, and in the feeder were monitored by standard manometers (7–9). The injection system of the setup allowed obtaining gas mixtures of different compositions, which made it possible to control the gas velocity at the nozzle exit within wide limits from the pure air velocity (560 m/s for $M^* = 2.6$) to the pure helium velocity (1400 m/s for $M^* = 2.6$) in the isobaric flow mode and also to vary the particle velocity in a wide range, as was demonstrated by further investigations. The setup allowed measurement of the gas-velocity distribution in the jet by a Pitot tube.

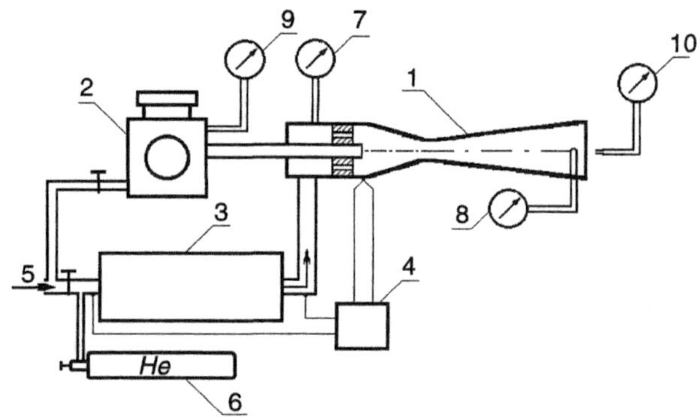

Fig. 3.2. Experimental setup for the determination of gas-flow parameters at the exit of a plane supersonic nozzle. 1 – plane supersonic nozzle, 2 – particle feeder, 3 – gas heater, 4 – controller of the gas-heater temperature, pre-chamber, 5 – input of high-pressure air, 6 – gas holder (helium, nitrogen, etc.), 7 – manometer for measuring the pressure in the pre-chamber p_0, 8 – manometer for measuring the static pressure near the nozzle exit p_c, 9 – manometer for measuring the pressure in the feeder, and 10 – manometer for measuring the total pressure behind the shock wave by the Pitot tube p_0'.

Table 3.1. Geometrical sizes of studied nozzles

Nozzle size mm	Nozzle number								
	1	2	3	4	5	6	7	8	9
L	50	75	100	110	110	120	130	150	200
h	1	2.9	2.4	3.0	3.0	2.9	3.0	4.5	5.0
b_{cr}	4.0	3.0	7.5	5.6	3.2	3.0	3.0	2.5	2.0
H	8.0	9.4	30.0	10.0	9.5	10.0	8.0	12.0	8.4

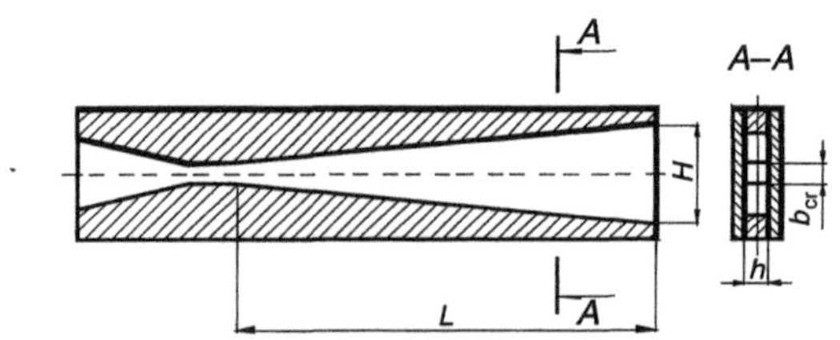

Fig. 3.3. Schematic of the nozzles; particular sizes are indicated in Table 3.1.

The geometric sizes of all nozzles considered are summarized in Table 3.1. The sizes listed in Table 3.1 are indicated in Fig. 3.3. For convenience and for brevity, all nozzles were enumerated, and the numbers are also listed in Table 3.1.

The total pressure behind the shock wave was measured in the experiments by a Pitot tube rigidly connected to a micrometric table, which allowed registration of coordinates in two

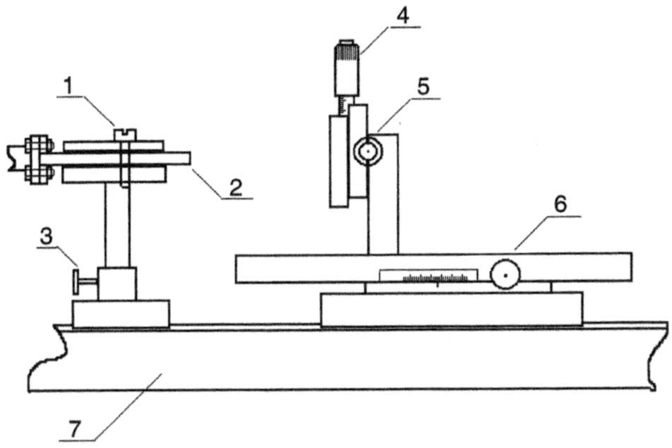

Fig. 3.4. Schematic of the nozzle and the micrometric table with the Pitot tube. 1 – hold-down bolt for nozzle fixation on the support, 2 – nozzle, 3 – screw for fixing the rod regulating the nozzle height above the rail, 4 – micrometric screw for vertical motion, 5 – micrometric screw for horizontal transverse motion, 6 – screw for horizontal longitudinal motion, and 7 – rail.

mutually perpendicular directions in the plane located at an angle of 90° to the nozzle centerline. For convenience of aligning the nozzle centerline and the Pitot tube axis, the nozzle and the micrometric table with the tube were mounted on an optical rail. The nozzle was mounted on a special support, which allowed variation of the nozzle height above the rail (Fig. 3.4). Such a system turned out to be very convenient for subsequent experiments with jets exhausting from nozzles.

3.1.1.2. Analysis of experimental results

The Mach number at the nozzle exit in the core flow can be determined by three methods on the basis of three measured pressures: stagnation pressure p_0, static pressure p_c, and dynamic pressure p'_0.

Method 1 (from the ratio p_c/p_0):

$$\frac{p_0}{p_c}=\left(1+\frac{\gamma-1}{2}M^2\right)^{\frac{\gamma}{\gamma-1}}, \quad \text{for air } \frac{p_0}{p_c}=\left(1+0.2M^2\right)^{3.5} \tag{3.1}$$

Method 2 (from the ratio p'_0/p_c). Using the known Rayleigh formula, we determine the Mach number from the ratio p'_0/p_c [2]:

$$\frac{p'_0}{p_c}=\left(\frac{\gamma+1}{2}\right)^{\frac{\gamma+1}{\gamma-1}}\left(\frac{2}{\gamma-1}\right)^{\frac{1}{\gamma-1}}\frac{M^{\frac{2\gamma}{\gamma-1}}}{\left(\frac{2\gamma}{\gamma-1}M^2-1\right)^{\frac{1}{\gamma-1}}}, \tag{3.2}$$

For air

$$\frac{p'_0}{p_c}=\frac{166.7M^7}{\left(7M^2-1\right)^{2.5}}$$

Method 3 (from the ratio p'_0/p_0). Assuming that stagnation pressure is constant along the nozzle, we determine the ratio of stagnation pressures on the shock wave and then calculate the Mach number [2]:

$$\frac{p'_0}{p_0} = \left(\frac{\gamma+1}{2}\right)^{\frac{\gamma+1}{\gamma-1}} \left(\frac{2}{\gamma-1}\right)^{\frac{1}{\gamma-1}} \frac{M^{\frac{2\gamma}{\gamma-1}}}{\left(\frac{2\gamma}{\gamma-1}M^2-1\right)^{\frac{1}{\gamma-1}}} \frac{1}{\left(1+\frac{\gamma-1}{2}M^2\right)^{\frac{\gamma}{\gamma-1}}}, \tag{3.3}$$

For air
$$\frac{p'_0}{p_0} = \frac{166.7M^7}{(7M^2-1)^{2.5}(1+0.2M^2)^{3.5}}.$$

The accuracy of determining the Mach number and other parameters by these methods depends on the magnitude of total pressure losses during gas motion along the nozzle. According to experimental data, the total pressure losses in the nozzles of the configuration examined is approximately 5%. An analysis of errors showed that the value of M is slightly underpredicted by Eq. (3.2), overpredicted by Eq. (3.3), and has the value intermediate between these two in Eq. (3.1), but the error is less than 5% anyway. The values of the thus-calculated Mach numbers at the nozzle exit M_{exp} and the Mach numbers corresponding to an ideal gas flow M_{id} are listed in Table 3.2.

The value of M_{exp} is significantly lower than M_{id} (by 10–20%). Such a difference cannot be attributed to the error in determining M_{exp} and M_{id}, because M_{exp} is determined within $\leq$5%, and the error in determining M_{id}, which is caused in inexact measurement of areas, is less than 2.5% if the accuracy of measuring linear dimensions is $\leq$0.1 mm. This means that the boundary layer on the nozzle walls has a rather strong effect on the core flow.

Based on the values of M_{exp} obtained, we estimated the effective cross-sectional area $(S^*/S_{cr})_{eff}$. Assuming that the effective area in the nozzle throat equals its geometric value because the boundary-layer thickness here is extremely small [3], we calculated the effective area in the exit cross section S_{eff}. Its relation with the geometric exit area is shown in Table 3.2.

Table 3.2. Data on Mach numbers and boundary layer

Parameter	Nozzle number								
	1	2	3	4	5	6	7	8	9
M_{id}	2.18	2.66	2.92	2.05	2.61	2.73	2.49	3.11	2.97
M_{exp}	1.75	2.4	2.6	1.75	2.25	2.3	2.1	2.75	2.55
M_{exp}/M_{id}	0.8	0.9	0.89	0.85	0.86	0.84	0.84	0.88	0.86
S_{eff}/S^*	0.7	0.78	0.74	0.79	0.72	0.67	0.70	0.71	0.67
$2\delta^*/h$	0.27	0.18	0.25	0.17	0.22	0.27	0.23	0.22	0.23
$2\delta/h$	1.27	0.64	0.85	0.78	0.86	1.02	0.95	0.74	0.8
M_{cal}	1.77	2.41	2.54	1.76	2.27	2.34	2.10	2.73	2.51

The boundary-layer displacement thickness at the nozzle exit was calculated by Eq. (3.4) under the assumption that this thickness is identical over the entire perimeter:

$$\delta^* = \frac{H+h-\sqrt{(H+h)^2-4\Delta S}}{4}. \qquad (3.4)$$

For $\delta^* \ll h$, we have

$$\delta^* \approx \frac{\Delta S}{P} = \frac{S^* - S_{\text{eff}}}{2\,(H+h)},$$

where $P = 2(H+h)$ is the nozzle-exit perimeter.

The boundary-layer thickness for known δ^* and M was estimated by the formula [2]

$$\frac{\delta^*}{\delta} = 1 - 7\int_0^1 \frac{\zeta^7 d\zeta}{1+0.2M^2\,(1-\zeta^2)}. \qquad (3.5)$$

where ζ is the formal integration variable.

The thus-calculated values of the boundary-layer thickness show (Table 3.2) that the boundary layers either converged (nozzles 1 and 6) or the situation was close to that.

Thus, the experimental studies showed that the boundary layer formed on the walls in the nozzles with a large aspect ratio $L/h = 20$–50 exerts a noticeable influence on the flow parameters inside the nozzle. This makes these parameters rather different from those calculated for an ideal gas. Therefore, it was necessary to develop a simple method for calculating gas parameters in such nozzles, whose results would not contradict experimental data.

3.1.2. Calculation of gas parameters inside the nozzle

3.1.2.1. Allowance for the displacing action of the boundary layer

If the boundary layer is not very thick, we can assume that stagnation pressure in the core flow remains unchanged, and variation of the gas parameters obeys the law of an ideal adiabat. The boundary-layer effect in the first approximation leads to a decrease in the channel cross section; thus, instead of the geometric ratio of areas, the calculations aimed at reconstructing the gas parameters in the core flow should involve the effective ratio, which is determined by the following formula if we assume that the boundary-layer displacement thickness is uniform over the perimeter: $S_{\text{eff}}(z) = (b(z)-2\delta^*(z))(h-2\delta^*(z))$. The most important reason for this consideration is the fact that stagnation pressure at the nozzle only slightly ($\leq 5\%$) differs from the pressure measured in the pre-chamber, which indicates that the losses due to friction in the core flow passing through the nozzles under study are low. According to [3], the boundary-layer growth can be assumed to start from the nozzle throat.

Based on the above-made assumptions, the flow at the nozzle centerline was calculated as follows. At the first step, the Mach number distribution along the axis was reconstructed from the known dependence of area along the nozzle. After that, all flow parameters were calculated with the help of isentropic formulas and known values of p_0 and T_0.

The boundary layer was calculated by the Karman equation under the assumption that it develops on a flat plate exposed to a flow without heat transfer, with a known pressure gradient along the centerline, and with a known velocity distribution [4]

$$\frac{d\delta^{**}}{dz} = \frac{c_f}{2} - \frac{\delta^{**}}{v}\frac{dv}{dz}\left(2 + H_1 - M^2\right), \tag{3.6}$$

$$\delta^* = \delta^{**} H_1,$$

where δ^{**} is the momentum thickness.

The ratio of the displacement thickness to the momentum thickness H_1 as a function of the Mach number was determined by the formula [5]

$$H_1 = 1.4(1 + 0.3M^2), \tag{3.7}$$

where c_f is the friction coefficient given by the expression [6]

$$c_f = 0.0263 Re_1^{-1/7} \frac{1-\xi}{\xi} \arcsin^2\sqrt{\xi}, \tag{3.8}$$

$$\text{where} \qquad \xi = \frac{\frac{\gamma-1}{2}M^2}{1 + \frac{\gamma-1}{2}M^2}.$$

Viscosity was calculated by Sutherland's law [2]

$$\mu = \mu_0 \left(\frac{T_c}{273}\right)^{1.5} \frac{273 + T_s}{T_c + T_s}, \tag{3.9}$$

where μ_0 is the viscosity at a temperature of 273 K and T_s is the Sutherland temperature (=122 K).

The next approximation takes into account the boundary-layer thickness, namely, the calculated displacement thickness is subtracted from the geometric size of the nozzle. In what follows, the calculations are performed in a similar manner with allowance for the changes in the nozzle shape because of the presence of the boundary layer. Several iterations (3–5) are sufficient for the process to converge. To speed up the convergence, $S_{eff}(x)$ in the first iteration was calculated as

$$S_{eff}(z) = (b(z) - 1.5\delta^*(z))(h - 1.5\delta^*(z)).$$

The calculated values of the Mach number M_{cal} are listed in Table 3.2. Good agreement is observed between experimental and numerical data, which allows us to use this method for estimating gas parameters in the core flow (if the boundary layers do not converge completely).

As an example, Fig. 3.5 shows the distribution of Mach numbers along the nozzle axis, with and without allowance for the displacing action of the boundary layer, for nozzles of different lengths with all other dimensions being identical ($b_{cr} = 3 \times 10^{-3}$ m, $h = 3 \times 10^{-3}$ m, and $H = 10 \times 10^{-3}$ m).

Based on results of these calculations, we plotted the dependence of M_{cal}/M_{id} on the aspect ratio of the nozzle h/L (see Fig. 3.6). The same figure also shows the experimental points M_{exp}/M_{id} for the examined nozzles. The calculations were performed for three different values $M_{id} = 2.18$, 2.72, and 3.45. For each value of M_{id}, a basic nozzle was chosen with $L = 0.1$ m, $b_{cr} = 3 \times 10^{-3}$ m, $h = 3 \times 10^{-3}$ m, and H corresponding to M_{id}($H = 6 \times 10^{-3}$ m for $M_0 = 2.18$, $H = 10 \times 10^{-3}$ m for $M_0 = 2.72$, and $H = 20 \times 10^{-3}$ m for $M_{id} = 3.45$). After that, the ratio h/L was changed by three different methods:

1. L was changed from 0.02 to 0.3 m, all other parameters being unchanged;
2. L was changed from 0.02 to 0.3 m with proportional changes in b_{cr} and H;
3. h was changed from 0.001 to 0.01 m, all other parameters being unchanged.

As a result, the results for the calculations were obtained for nozzles with $h = 0.001$–0.01 m, $L = 0.02$–0.3 m, $b_{cr} = 0.6 \times 10^{-3}$–$9 \times 10^{-3}$ m, and $H = 0.002$–0.03 m.

It is seen from Fig. 3.6 that the normalized Mach number in the considered range $M_{id} = 2.18$–3.45 mainly depends on h/L and starts rapidly decreasing from $h/L \leq 0.025$. The experimental points are in good agreement with the calculation results. The dashed

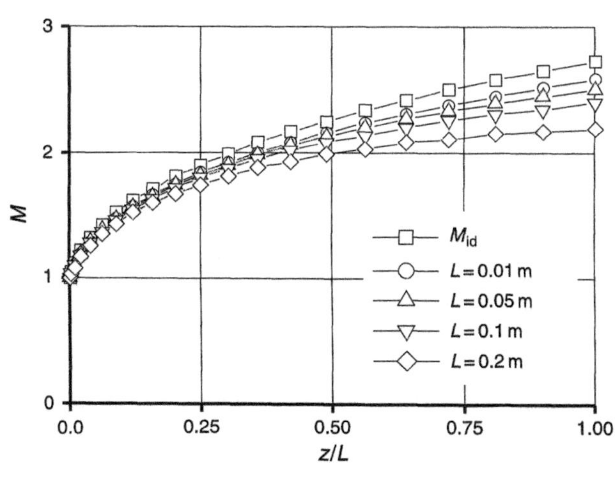

Fig. 3.5. Axial distribution of the Mach number for nozzles with different lengths of the supersonic part.

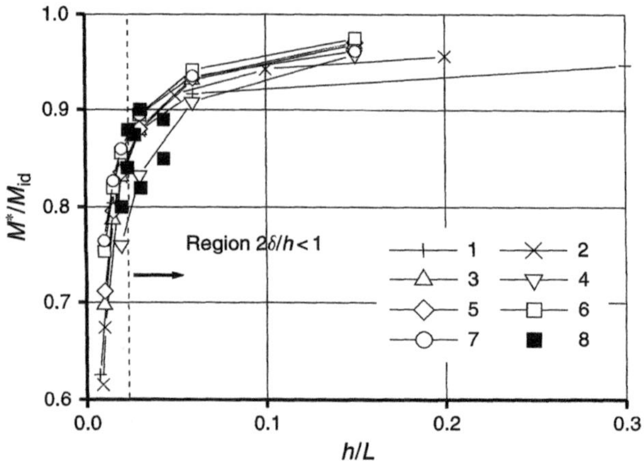

Fig. 3.6. Normalized Mach number on the nozzle axis versus the aspect ratio of the nozzle.
1 – $M_{id} = 2.72$, $p_0 = 1.5\,\text{MPa}$, $h = 3\,\text{mm}$, $b_{cr}/H = 0.3$; $b_{cr}/L = 0.03$;
2 – $M_{id} = 2.72$, $p_0 = 1.5\,\text{MPa}$, $L = 0.1\,\text{m}$, $b_{cr} = 3\,\text{mm}$, $H = 10\,\text{mm}$;
3 – $M_{id} = 2.72$, $p_0 = 1.5\,\text{MPa}$, $h = 3\,\text{mm}$, $b_{cr} = 3\,\text{mm}$, $H = 10\,\text{mm}$;
4 – $M_{id} = 2.18$, $p_0 = 0.6\,\text{MPa}$, $h = 3\,\text{mm}$, $b_{cr} = 3\,\text{mm}$, $H = 6\,\text{mm}$;
5 – $M_{id} = 3.45$, $p_0 = 1.5\,\text{MPa}$, $h = 3\,\text{mm}$, $b_{cr} = 3\,\text{mm}$, $H = 20\,\text{mm}$;
6 – $M_{id} = 3.45$, $p_0 = 4.0\,\text{MPa}$, $h = 3\,\text{mm}$, $b_{cr} = 3\,\text{mm}$, $H = 20\,\text{mm}$;
7 – $M_{id} = 3.45$, $p_0 = 4.0\,\text{MPa}$, $h = 3\,\text{mm}$, $b_{cr}/H = 0.15$, $b_{cr}/L = 0.03$; and
8 – $M_{id} = 2.0$–3.35, experimental results.

curve corresponds to the value $h/L \approx 0.025$, for which Eq. (3.5) predicts convergence of the boundary layers from the opposite sides of the nozzle, i.e., $2\delta/h = 1$. We have $2\delta/h < 1$ on the right of this curve and $2\delta/h > 1$ on the left. Thus, the drastic decrease in M_{cal}/M_{id} at $h/L \approx 0.025$ can be associated with convergence of the boundary layers, which start to intensely affect the core flow parameters. Correspondingly, the calculations by the method described above, which implies unchanged stagnation pressure in the core flow, become incorrect.

3.1.2.2. Calculation of flow parameters averaged over the cross section

The gas flow parameters averaged over the cross section were calculated in the one-dimensional approximation with allowance for the force of gas friction on the nozzle walls. The corresponding system of equations is

$$\begin{aligned} &G = \rho v S = const \\ &G\frac{dv}{dz} = -S\frac{dp}{dz} - F_f \\ &Gc_p\frac{dT}{dz} = \frac{G}{\rho}\frac{dp}{dz} + vF_f \\ &p = \rho RT \end{aligned}, \qquad (3.10)$$

The friction force F_f, the friction coefficient c_f, and the Reynolds number Re are determined as [2]:

$$F_f = \frac{1}{4} c_f \rho v^2 \left(b\left(z\right) + h\right) \tag{3.11}$$

$$c_f = \begin{cases} \dfrac{0.3164}{Re^{1/4}}, & 4 \times 10^3 \leq Re \leq 10^5 \\ \dfrac{1}{\left(2\lg\left(Re\sqrt{c_f}\right) - 0.8\right)^2}, & Re > 10^5 \end{cases}$$

$$Re = \frac{\rho v d_{eff}}{\mu}$$

$$d_{eff} = \frac{4S}{P} = \frac{2h}{1 + \frac{h}{b(z)}}$$

Resolving this system, we obtain the equation for the Mach number:

$$\frac{dM}{M} = \frac{1 + \frac{\gamma - 1}{2} M^2}{M^2 - 1} \left(\frac{dS}{S} - \frac{\gamma F_f dz}{\rho a^2 S} \right) \tag{3.12}$$

Knowing $S = f(z)$ and calculating the flow upstream of the nozzle throat by formulas for the gas without friction, we found the numerical values of the distribution of the Mach number and then all other parameters along the nozzle. Figure 3.7 shows the Mach number distribution along the nozzle, which was calculated for the core flow (1), with allowance for friction (2), and for an ideal gas (solid curve). For $L \geq 0.1$ m, the difference between the parameters averaged over the cross section from the parameters in the core flow is rather substantial.

The relation between the flow parameters averaged over the cross section and the parameters at the centerline can be obtained by assuming a certain law of their distribution over the nozzle cross section and performing averaging in the interval from 0 to $h/2$. In the first approximation, we can obtain an estimate for the two-dimensional problem ($H \gg h$), using the classical law of velocity distribution in the boundary layer [2]

$$\frac{v}{v_1} = \frac{1}{\kappa} \ln \frac{v_1 x}{\nu} + 5.5, \tag{3.13}$$

where x is the coordinate in the direction perpendicular to the side surfaces of the nozzle, $v_1 = \sqrt{\tau_w / \rho}$ is the velocity at the edge of the laminar sublayer, $\tau_w = c_f \rho v^2 / 2$ is the stress due to friction on the surface, c_f is the friction coefficient, $\kappa = 0.4$ is the universal constant of a turbulent flow, and $\nu = \mu / \rho$ is the kinematic viscosity.

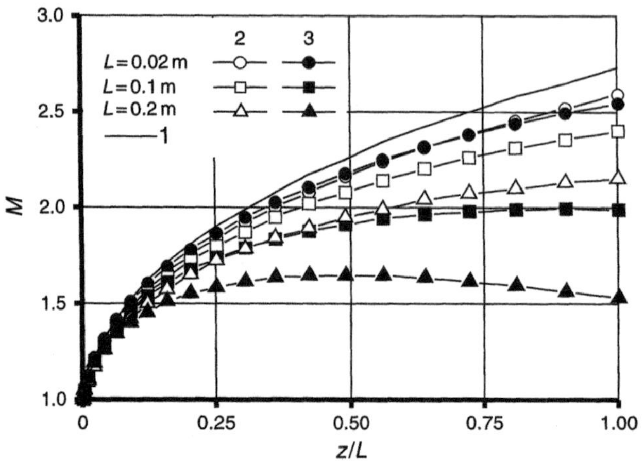

Fig. 3.7. Axial distribution of the Mach number for nozzles with different lengths of the supersonic part. The solid curve refers to an ideal gas, curve 1 refers to the core flow, and curve 2 is the one-dimensional calculation with allowance for friction.

Using the condition $v = v_0$ for $x = \delta$ if $\delta \le h/2$ and for $x = h/2$ if $\delta \ge h/2$, we obtain

$$\frac{v}{v_m} = \frac{\frac{1}{\kappa}\ln\frac{v_1 x}{\nu} + 5.5}{\frac{1}{\kappa}\ln\frac{v_1\delta}{\nu} + 5.5} \quad \text{for } \delta \le h/2, \tag{3.14}$$

$$\frac{v}{v_m} = \frac{\frac{1}{\kappa}\ln\frac{v_1 x}{\nu} + 5.5}{\frac{1}{\kappa}\ln\frac{v_1 h}{2\nu} + 5.5} \quad \text{for } \delta \ge h/2. \tag{3.15}$$

This law offers an accurate prediction of the distribution in plane nozzles used for spraying, which is illustrated in Fig. 3.8, where the experimentally measured distribution at the nozzle exit is compared with the distribution calculated by Eq. (3.13) with $\delta/h = 0.4$.

The gas velocities averaged over the cross section can be calculated by integrating Eqs (3.14) and (3.15).

For $\delta \le h/2$:

$$v_{av} = \frac{2}{h}\int_0^{h/2} v(x)\,dx = v_0\left(1 - \frac{2\delta}{h}\frac{1}{\ln\frac{v_1\delta}{\nu} + 5.5\kappa}\right).$$

For $\delta \ge h/2$:

$$v_{av} = \frac{2}{h}\int_0^{h/2} v(x)\,dx = v_0\left(1 - \frac{1}{\ln\frac{v_1 h}{2\nu} + 5.5\kappa}\right).$$

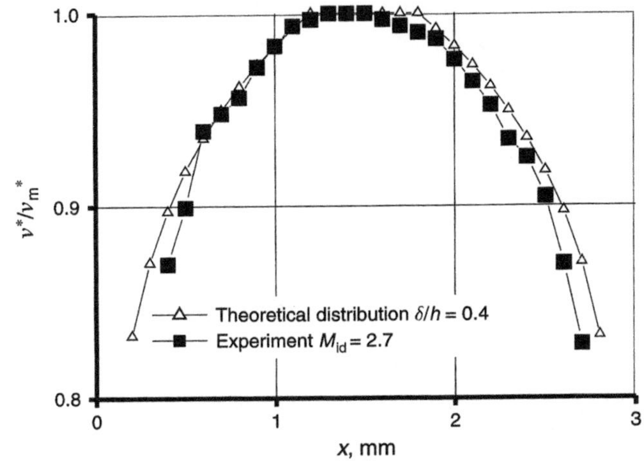

Fig. 3.8. Velocity distribution at the exit of a plane supersonic nozzle.

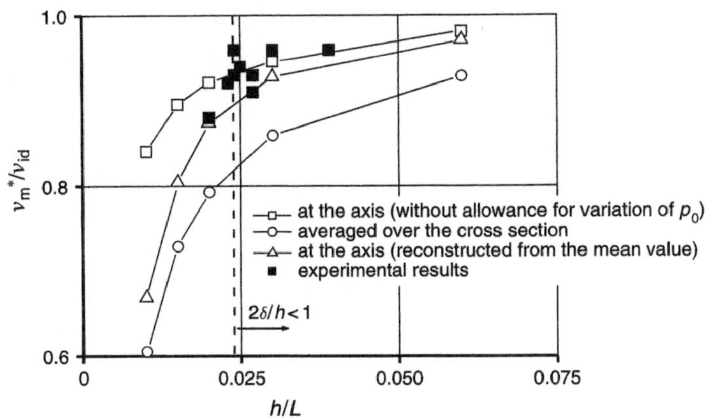

Fig. 3.9. Gas velocity on the nozzle axis, based on results of difference calculation methods and averaged over the cross section.

The influence of the boundary layers from two other surfaces can be ignored in the first approximation.

Figure 3.9 shows a comparison of the axial velocity normalized to the ideal-gas velocity, which was obtained with allowance for the displacing action of the boundary layer and with the use of results of the one-dimensional calculation with allowance for friction.

The small difference between the axial velocity calculations for $2\delta/h \leq 1$ allows us to use either of these methods. The significant difference in results for axial velocity in the region $2\delta/h > 1$ shows that the calculation method that implies unchanged stagnation pressure along the nozzle axis is invalid, which was already mentioned. The axial velocity should be reconstructed from the results of the one-dimensional calculation with allowance for friction.

Finally, we note that the good agreement of the calculated gas parameters in the core flow in a supersonic nozzle with a rectangular cross section with experimental results allows us to state that the method for calculating the gas parameters in a long supersonic nozzle is correct and we can pass to calculating particle acceleration in such nozzles.

3.2. Investigation of Supersonic Air Jets Exhausting from a Nozzle

Because of the unusual shape of studied nozzles, the jets formed differ from the well-examined symmetrical-axis jets or plane jets with a uniform distribution of parameters at the nozzle exit. In practice, one often has to estimate the possibility of using either these or those nozzles for successful spraying. One of the criteria used for comparing nozzles is the set of characteristics of jets exhausting from a given nozzle. Therefore, we performed experiments with jets whose characteristics were similar to the parameters of jets used for spraying [7–10]. As the axial velocity of the gas rapidly decreases behind the potential core, the initial supersonic part of the jet is of greatest interest for the spraying process. In some cases, it is necessary to vary the spraying distance, which involves the question about the limits of varying this distance without significant violations of the spraying process and changes in coating properties. To answer this question, we studied the supersonic part of the jet.

3.2.1. Experimental setup and research techniques

It is known that all parameters of the gas flow can be determined from known distributions of three quantities. Let us choose the Mach number as the first quantity, stagnation temperature as the second quantity, and static pressure as the third quantity. Thus, in studying isenthalpic ($T_0 = \text{Const}$) isobaric ($p = \text{Const}$) jets, one needs to find only one quantity, namely, the Mach number. It is convenient to calculate the Mach number by the Rayleigh formula from the measured stagnation pressures behind the normal shock wave formed on the tip of a thin tube (Pitot tube). In the first approximation, we can assume that p'_0 is proportional to M^2 and, hence, to the dynamic pressure ρv^2. Jets exhausting from three difference nozzles were considered (Table 3.3).

The angle of the nozzle in the direction of one transverse coordinate was roughly identical for all three nozzles, namely, 3×10^{-3}, and the angle in the direction of the other

Table 3.3. Parameters of gas flow at the nozzle exit

No.	M^*	$p_{0\text{cal}}$, MPa	h, mm	H/h
1	1.75	0.53	1	8
6	2.3	1.25	3	3.3
8	2.75	2.51	4.5	2.7

transverse coordinate, characterizing the smaller size of the nozzle, was equal to zero. The experimental setup was schematically shown previously (see Fig. 1.13).

The Schlieren method was used to study jet structure. The image of the jet illuminated by a parallel light beam with $\lambda = 0.69\,\mu m$ was registered on a photographic film through a red filter. The source of radiation was an upgraded OGM-20 laser with a standard control system. As the goal was to obtain one powerful light pulse, the modulator was a self-bleaching shutter on the basis of a vanadium phthalocyanide–nitrobenzene mixture. With the help of collimators, the laser beam was increased to 40–90 mm, which provided complete illumination of the jet with a sufficient light intensity and, as a result, reliable registration of the jet by photographing with magnification of the order of unity. We photographed the initial gas-dynamic part of the air jet exhausting from a rectangular nozzle. Pressure probes with an outer diameter of 0.5 mm were used in these experiments. A thermocouple was used as a temperature probe.

3.2.2. Profiles of parameters in jets

As argued in [11–13], it is known that the profiles of velocity (v) and dynamic pressure (ρv^2) are self-similar at the initial and main parts of the jet. It is convenient to present the dynamic pressure in the form $\gamma p_c M^2$; in the case of an isobaric flow, this leads to self-similarity of the profiles of M^2. Approximation formulas for velocity profiles are encountered in the literature, but it is rather difficult to find formulas for M^2 profiles. At the same time, it is the Mach number that is the most convenient quantity to be used in experiments because its determination requires only the knowledge of pressure field (and not temperature fields). In addition, it is convenient to express the law of conservation of excess momentum in terms of the Mach number. Thus, one of our tasks was to verify self-similarity of the M^2 profiles and to find an approximation function for them.

3.2.2.1. Mach number profiles

The profiles of M^2 were reconstructed from the experimentally obtained profiles of the static (p_c) and Pitot (p_0') pressures. The data gained in studying jets with different initial (indicated by the asterisk) parameters ($h = 1$–4.5 mm, $H/h = 2.7$–8, $M^* = 1.85$–3.1, and $T_0{}^* = 300$–600 K, where h and H are the small and large transverse sizes of the jet at the nozzle exit) and plotted in the coordinates $(M/M_m)^2$, x/δ_M are well fitted by one curve (Fig. 3.10).

With an insignificant scatter, this curve can be described by the expression

$$\varphi_M = \exp\left(-\left(\sqrt{\ln 2}\frac{x}{\delta_M}\right)^2\right), \tag{3.16}$$

where δ_M is the jet thickness along the smaller size (in the x direction), determined as the distance from the jet axis to the point where $M^2(\delta_M) = 0.5 M_m{}^2$.

It is worth noting that the stagnation temperature (T_0) and the jet-pressure ratio (n) in the examined range ($T_0 = 300$–600 K, $n = 0.5$–1) do not exert any substantial effect on the M^2 profile.

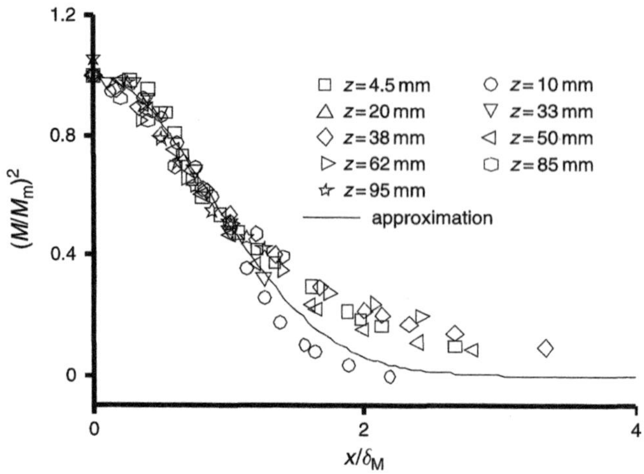

Fig. 3.10. Normalized M^2 profiles in an overexpanded jet exhausting from a nozzle with $h = 4.5$, $H/h = 2.7$, and $M^* = 3.1$.

3.2.2.2. Profiles of excess temperature

It is known from the jet theory that the profiles of the excess stagnation temperature ($\Delta T_0 = T_0 - T_a$) are also self-similar and admit the relation

$$\frac{T_0 - T_a}{T_{0m} - T_a} = \frac{\Delta T_0}{\Delta T_{0m}} = \left(\frac{v}{v_m}\right)^{\sigma},$$

where $\sigma = 0.5$ for plane jets, $\sigma = 0.75$ for symmetrical axis jets, v is the gas velocity, and T_a is the ambient temperature. Assuming that the profiles are described by functions of the same form, we can find the relation between the velocity-profile thickness (δ_v) and the temperature-profile thickness (δ_T):

$$\delta_v = \delta_T \sqrt{\sigma}.$$

A series of experiments was performed to validate self-similarity, to find the approximation function for excess stagnation temperature profiles, and to find the relation of thicknesses of M^2 and ΔT_0 profiles. Stagnation temperature was determined by a thermometric probe on the basis of a thermocouple. The profiles plotted in the coordinates $\Delta T_0/\Delta T_{0m}$, x/δ_T are fitted by the curve

$$\varphi_T = \exp\left(-\left(\sqrt{\ln 2}\frac{x}{\delta_T}\right)^2\right) \tag{3.17}$$

with an insignificant scatter (Fig. 3.11).

The experimentally found value of δ_T/δ_M for the examined range of parameters is close to 2.

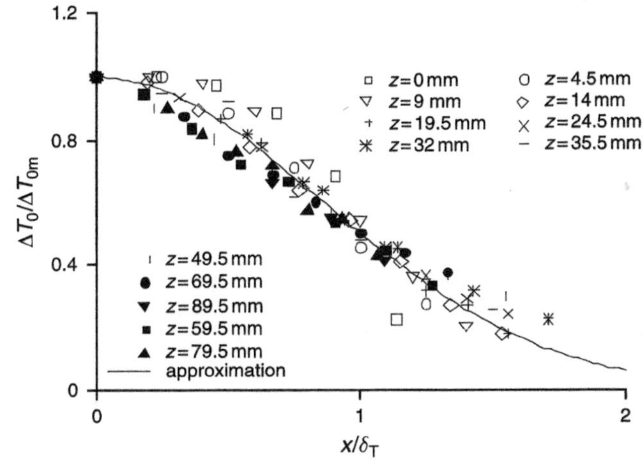

Fig. 3.11. Normalized profiles of excess stagnation temperature in an overexpanded jet exhausting from a nozzle with $h = 4.5$, $H/h = 2.7$, and $M^* = 3.1$.

3.2.3. Streamwise distribution of axial parameters

One of the problems of the jet theory is finding the axial values of parameters denoted here by the subscript m. Thus, Ginevskii [11] used the matching of two solutions for the initial and main parts; there was an inflection at the point of the matching (transitional part of the jet), which was not observed in our experiments. We made an attempt to find a smooth approximation function in the transitional region. Figure 3.12 shows the data borrowed from [12], and the results obtained in our experiments are plotted in Fig. 3.13.

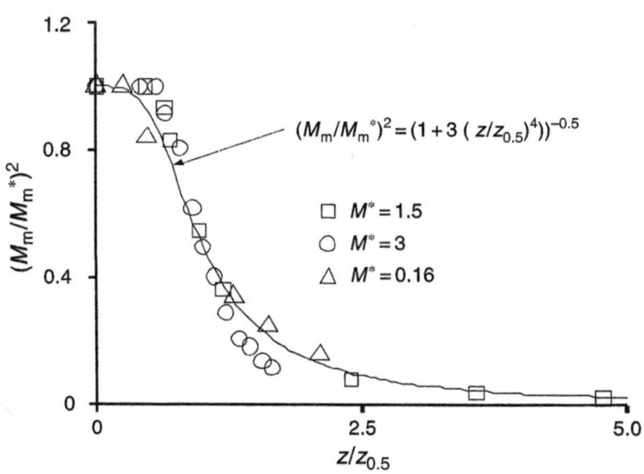

Fig. 3.12. Generalized distribution of the axial values of M^2 versus the streamwise coordinate [12].

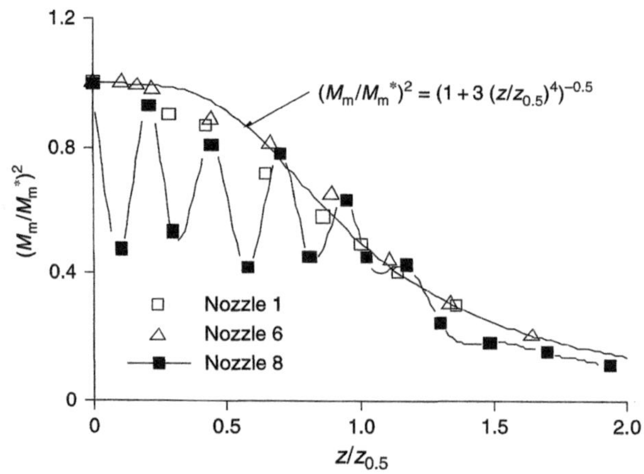

Fig. 3.13. Generalized distribution of the axial values of M^2 versus the streamwise coordinate.

All the data lie on one curve which is of the form

$$\left(\frac{M_{\mathrm{m}}}{M_{\mathrm{m}}^*}\right)^2 = \left(1+3\left(\frac{z}{z_{0.5}^M}\right)4\right)^{-0.5}, \tag{3.18}$$

where z is the streamwise coordinate of the jet, $z_{0.5}^M$ is the coordinate, and $M_{\mathrm{m}}^2(z_{0.5}^M) = 0.5M_{\mathrm{m}}^{*2}$.

The greatest deviation from this curve is observed for data obtained in studying an overexpanded jet, but the upper peaks lie on the curve even in this case, whereas the lower peaks at $z/z_{0.5}^M < 1$ lie approximately at one level. It should be noted that this function also yields a correct asymptotic value, because we have $M_{\mathrm{m}}^2 \sim 1/z^2$ for symmetrical-axis jets in accordance with the equation of conservation of momentum (all jets at large distances can be presented as a symmetrical-axis jet).

For moderate heating of the jets, the relation between the axial excess stagnation temperature and the axial value of M^2 should be close to the form

$$\Delta T_{0\mathrm{m}}/\Delta T_0^* = \left(M_{\mathrm{m}}^2/M_{\mathrm{m}}^{*2}\right)^{0.25}.$$

We used this circumstance to find the distribution function of the axial values of excess stagnation temperature (Fig. 3.14).

A comparison with experimental data allows us to assume that

$$\Delta T_{0\mathrm{m}} = \frac{\Delta T_0^*}{(1+15\bar{z}^{-3})^{0.25}} \qquad \bar{z} = z/z_{0.5}^T, \quad z_{0.5}^T \approx 2z_{0.5}^M. \tag{3.19}$$

The ratio $z_{0.5}^T/z_{0.5}^M$ obtained for three jets from the experiment is approximately equal to 2.

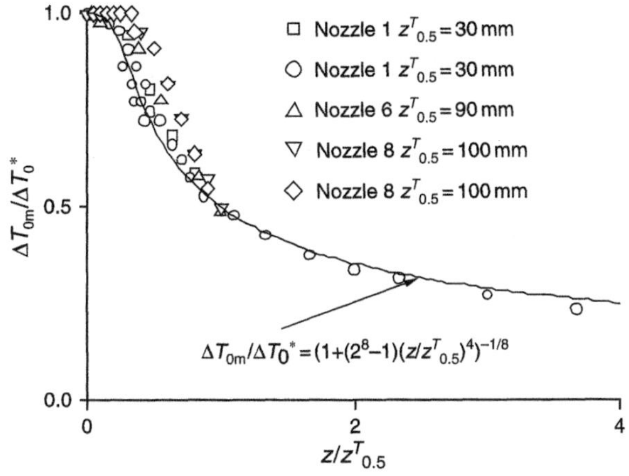

Fig. 3.14. Generalized dependence of normalized excess stagnation temperature on the streamwise coordinate.

3.2.4. Jet thickness

One important problem is to determine the jet-thickness growth as a function of the streamwise coordinate. It is known from the literature that the jet-thickness growth in the initial and main parts of the jet is linear but with different proportionality factors [12]. Thus, there is a transitional part where the jet-thickness growth is a nonlinear function. Since we studied jets with a non-uniform initial profile because of a noticeable boundary layer on the nozzle walls, we should expect that the potential core region is weakly expressed, and the entire region under study can be considered as transitional, with the jet thickness approximated by a nonlinear function. If we assume that the jet is plane, i.e., neglect its expansion in the direction of the larger size, we can obtain the relation between the jet thickness and the axial value of M^2 from the equation of conservation of momentum:

$$\delta_M = C^* h \left(1 + 3\left(\frac{z}{z^M_{0.5}}\right)^4\right)^{0.5}. \tag{3.20}$$

Here, C^* is a coefficient that takes into account, the jet thickness, in the very beginning (i.e., at the nozzle exit). It differs from the nozzle-exit thickness because the jet thickness is conventionally determined by the ratio of the boundary value of the squared Mach number to the value at the jet axis (here, we used the value of 0.5). Moreover, this coefficient changes, depending on the profile fullness (i.e., its closeness to the rectangular profile). Clearly, this coefficient cannot be rigorously equal to unity.

If we assume further that expansion along the larger size is exactly the same as expansion along the smaller size (quasi-symmetrical axis case), i.e., $\delta_y/\delta_M = H/h$ (δ_y is the jet thickness along the larger size) and use the expression

$$(M/M_m)^2 = \exp\left(-\left(\sqrt{\ln 2}\frac{x}{\delta_M}\right)^2\right)\exp\left(-\left(\sqrt{\ln 2}\frac{y}{\delta_y}\right)^2\right), \tag{3.21}$$

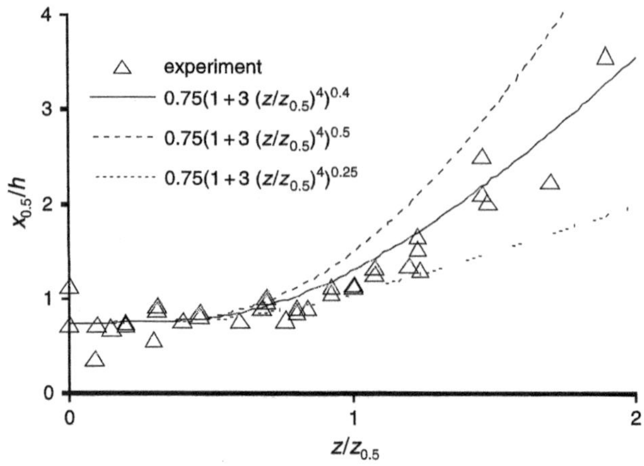

Fig. 3.15. Generalized dependence of the jet thickness on the streamwise coordinate.

we obtain

$$\delta_{\mathrm{M}} = C^* h \left(1 + 3\left(\frac{z}{z_{0.5}^{\mathrm{M}}}\right)^4\right)^{0.25}. \tag{3.22}$$

Based on experimental results, we can find a more exact curve (Fig. 3.15):

$$\delta_{\mathrm{M}} = 0.75h \left(1 + 3\left(\frac{z}{z_{0.5}}\right)^3\right)^{0.4}. \tag{3.23}$$

It is seen in Fig. 3.15 that the proposed formulas yield approximately identical results in the region $z/z_{0.5} < 1$. Significant differences are observed in the farther region $z/z_{0.5} > 1$.

Thus, as it could be expected, the examined jets can be referred neither to the plane case nor to the symmetrical-axis case.

3.2.5. Effect of the jet-pressure ratio

It is of interest to consider the dependence of the periodic structure of the non-isobaric jet on the jet-pressure ratio. It is convenient to use the distance from the nozzle exit to the shock wave as the characteristic distance. According to published data, this distance in the case of large pressure ratios ($n \gg 1$) should be proportional to $n^{0.5}$. The jet was visualized by the Schlieren technique. Figure 3.16 shows the photographs of the jet exhausting from a nozzle with $h = 3\,\mathrm{mm}$, $H/h = 3.3$, and $M^* = 1.5$ with different pressure ratios.

An analysis of the photographs obtained confirmed the proportionality to $n^{0.5}$. It is seen that a paraboloid shock wave originates at $n \sim 2.5$ and becomes straight at $n \sim 4.5$–4.8. It is worth noting that the straight shock wave originates at pressure ratios much higher than those in the case of symmetrical-axis jets ($n \approx 1.5$) [14].

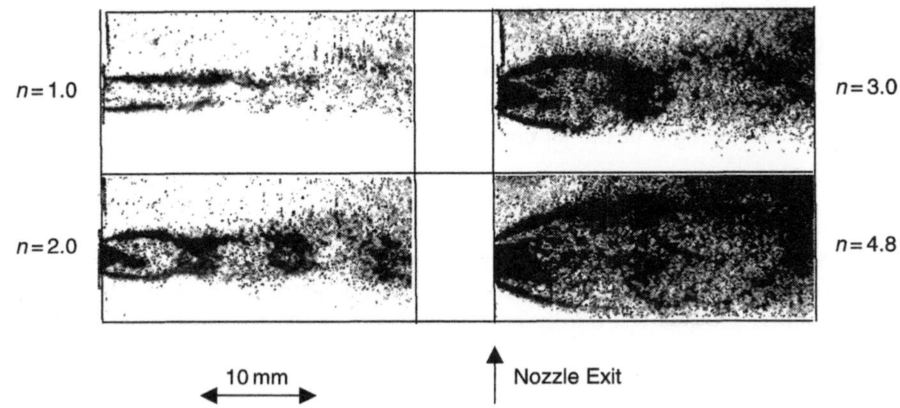

Fig. 3.16. Schlieren pictures of the jet exhausting from a nozzle with $h = 3\,\text{mm}$, $H/h = 3.3$, and $M^* = 1.5$ with different pressure ratios.

It is known that the number of barrels in the jet decreases with increasing pressure ratio, because of faster equalization of pressure. Therefore, we had to find the effect of the jet-pressure ratio on gas parameters far from the initial part of the jet, where the static pressure is already equal to the atmospheric value. This can be done by measuring the length of the supersonic part of the jet l_s, because the jet flow reaches the velocity of sound already in regions where the atmospheric pressure prevails, as was found experimentally. It is seen from Fig. 3.17, which shows these dependences, that the same law of proportionality with $n^{0.5}$ is observed with insignificant deviations.

It was found in the present study that the initial non-uniformity of gas parameters at the nozzle exit makes the transition in the streamwise distribution of M^2 from the initial to

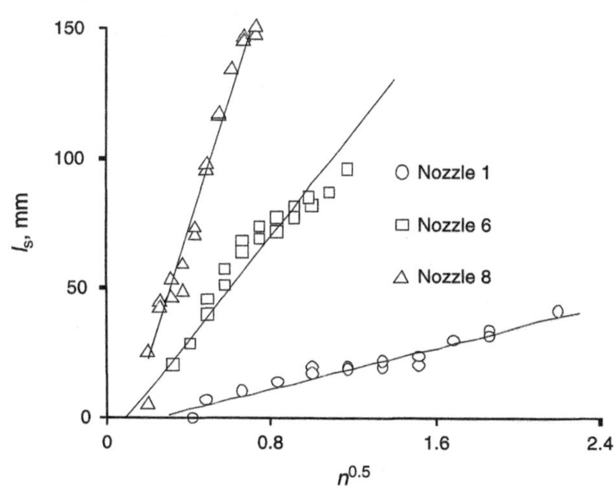

Fig. 3.17. Length of the supersonic part of the jet versus the jet-pressure ratio $n^{0.5}$.

the main part of the jet smoother. Observation of jet-thickness growth showed that the actually observed growth is smaller than that predicted for a plane jet, which seems to be attributed to tip effects arising in jets with a finite ratio of its sides. It was experimentally verified in the examined jets that the length of the element of the periodic jet structure and the supersonic length of the jet depend on the jet-pressure ratio as $\sqrt{n}$.

The study performed validated self-similarity of M^2, ΔT_0, and v profiles. The range of self-similarity starts at a certain distance from the nozzle exit and extends infinitely in the downstream direction. The transition through sonic lines has no effect on parameter profiles. Because of a significant thickness of the boundary layer formed on the nozzle walls, the initial profiles can hardly be distinguished from the self-similar profiles. For this reason, the range of self-similarity can be extended to the entire jet, beginning from the nozzle exit.

3.3. Impact of a Supersonic Jet on a Substrate

The present section describes the results on interaction of supersonic air jets with a rectangular cross section incident onto a flat infinite substrate at different impact angles [15, 16]. Though the shape of the coated part is not always a flat surface, the jet size is comparatively small, and the parameters of the gas, particles, and surface at the impact moment can be determined in the first approximation by solving the problem of interaction of supersonic rectangular jets with a flat infinite substrate. Particle concentrations typical for cold spray are normally much lower than the values at which the particles begin to noticeably affect the gas parameters. Therefore, in the first approximation, we can ignore the presence of particles in the flow and, thus, substantially simplify the problem.

A specific feature of studied nozzles is the large relative length, which leads to the formation of a jet with a non-uniform profile at the nozzle exit [10]. Most results published in the literature refer to symmetrical axis or plane jets with a uniform velocity profile at the nozzle exit. Therefore, it was necessary to study the impact of jets typical for cold spray onto a substrate.

The experiments were performed on a setup described in detail in the previous section and including a gas heater and a pre-chamber with attached nozzles of different geometry. A steel plate with an orifice 0.2 mm in diameter was used to measure the pressure on the substrate surface. The plate was mounted on the coordinate table, which made it possible to change the distance from the nozzle exit z_0, to move in the substrate plane into mutually perpendicular directions $x$and y to the nozzle centerline, and to vary the angle of inclination of the substrate plane φ to the nozzle centerline, corresponding to rotation of the substrate plane around the y axis.

The pressure profiles on the substrate surface was measured in two mutually perpendicular directions $x$and y. The origin was located at the center of the projection of the rectangular nozzle-exit section onto the substrate surface. The coordinate axes x and y were aligned parallel to the sides of the nozzle exit; the õ axis was parallel to the smaller side, the x axis was parallel to the larger side, and the z axis was normal to the substrate surface.

The values of the Mach number M in the region of the near-wall jet were determined by a Pitot tube with an inner diameter of 0.2 mm. The coordinate gear on which the Pitot tube was mounted allowed its motion in three mutually perpendicular directions.

3.3.1. Pressure distribution on the substrate surface and velocity gradient at the stagnation point

One of the tasks of experimental investigations of jet–substrate interaction was to determine the pressure distribution on the substrate surface. This information was necessary to reconstruct the character of the flow in the shock layer (based on the presence or absence of peripheral maximums) and to find the velocity distribution at the edge of the near-wall boundary layer with the use of Bernoulli integral. Figure 3.18 shows the normalized pressure profiles on the substrate for different impact angles of the jet φ_{im} and different distances between the nozzle exit and the substrate. Here, h is the smaller size of the nozzle exit, z_0 is the distance from the nozzle exit to the substrate, p_s is the pressure on the substrate surface, p_{sm} is the pressure on the substrate surface for $x = 0$, p_a is the ambient pressure, and $x_{0.5}$ is the half-width of the pressure profile ($p_s(x_{0.5}) - p_a = 0.5(p_{\mathrm{sm}} - p_a)$).

The points and the curve show the experimental data and the approximation. The experimental results are adequately approximated by the function

$$\frac{p_s - p_a}{p_{\mathrm{sm}} - p_a} = \left(1 + \left(\sqrt[4]{2} - 1\right)\left(\frac{x}{x_{0.5}}\right)^2\right)^{-4}, \tag{3.24}$$

borrowed from [17], where it is claimed that the pressure distribution on the substrate surface is self-similar. For $z_0 \leq 4h$, the value of $x_{0.5}$ is approximately one half of h. Figure 3.18 shows that self-similarity is observed in our case along the smaller size of the jet for angles $\varphi_{\mathrm{im}} = 50$–$90°$.

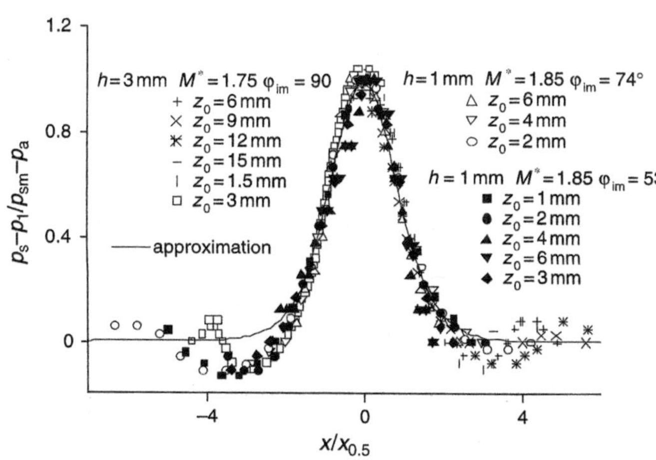

Fig. 3.18. Pressure profiles on the substrate surface for an isobaric jet.

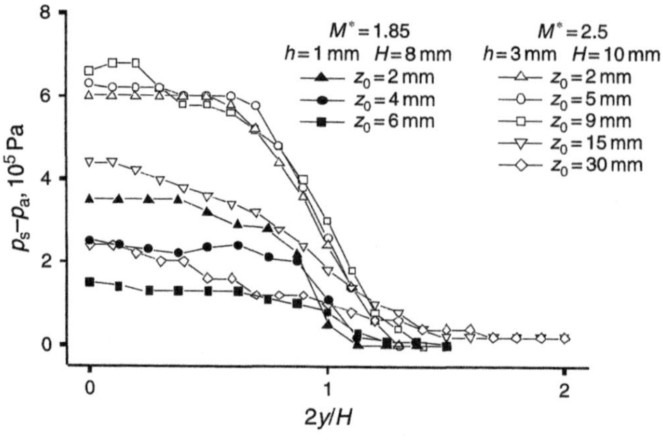

Fig. 3.19. Pressure profile on the substrate surface along the larger size of an isobaric jet exhausting from the nozzle.

Figure 3.19 shows the pressure profiles along the larger size of the nozzle exit H. The distribution (especially for small z_0) has a segment of roughly constant values of pressures, and the pressure practically vanished only at the ends of the curve. Thus, we can state that, on one hand, the pressure distribution along the y axis is not self-similar and, on the other hand, it can be assumed constant for rather large values of H/h.

3.3.1.1. Velocity gradient at the stagnation point

Based on the pressure profiles on the substrate surface, we can find the velocity gradient at the stagnation point along the x axis. For this purpose, we use the expression for pressure (Eq. (3.24)) and the isentropic relation between velocity (Mach number) and pressure. Finally, we obtain the expression for the velocity gradient at the stagnation point

$$\frac{du}{dx} = 2\frac{a_{cr}}{x_{0.5}}\sqrt{\frac{\gamma+1}{\gamma}\left(\sqrt[4]{2}-1\right)\left(1-\frac{p_a}{p'_0}\right)}, \quad (3.25)$$

where a_{cr} is the critical velocity of sound and p'_0 is the pressure measured by the Pitot tube. The value of the root in the right-hand part of the equation for typical Mach numbers $M = 1.8$–3.1 and $\gamma = 1.4$ equals 0.5 within 5%. Hence, the velocity gradient can be estimated by the following expression with accuracy sufficient for practical applications:

$$\beta = \frac{du}{dx} = \frac{a_{cr}}{x_{0.5}} \approx 2\frac{a_{cr}}{h}. \quad (3.26)$$

From Eq. (3.24), we find the ratio between the coordinate x_{cr} of the critical transition and the coordinate $x_{0.5}$. In the general case, this expression depends on the Mach number and jet-pressure ratio, but for an isobaric jet in the typical range, $M = 1.8$–3.1, it can be estimated within 5% as

$$\frac{x_{0.5}}{x_{cr}} = 0.87.$$

Thus, the value $x_{0.5}$ is fairly close to x_{cr}; hence, these two quantities can be estimated as $h/2$. The velocity in the accelerating flow region can be found by the formula [18]

$$\frac{u}{u_{ac}} = 1.5\frac{x}{x_{ac}} - 0.5\left(\frac{x}{x_{ac}}\right)^3, \tag{3.27}$$

where x_{ac} is the length of the acceleration region and u_{ac} is the velocity at the end of the acceleration region. Knowing the velocity gradient, we can find the relation between x_{ac} and u_{ac}:

$$x_{ac} = 1.5\frac{u_{ac}}{\beta}.$$

The value of u_{ac} is found from the condition of isentropic expansion of the gas with a stagnation pressure p'_0 to the atmospheric value:

$$u_{ac} = a_{cr}\sqrt{\frac{\gamma+1}{\gamma-1}}\left(1-\left(\frac{p_a}{p'_0}\right)^{\frac{\gamma-1}{\gamma}}\right)^{0.5}. \tag{3.28}$$

The value of p_a/p'_0 is determined by the Rayleigh formula. For typical conditions of an impact of an isobaric jet with $M^* = 2.5$ onto a substrate located in the region of the initial part of the jet, we obtain $M_{ac} = 2$, $u_{ac} = 1.62a_{cr}$, and $x_{ac} = 2.43\ x_{0.5}$, where $x_{0.5} \cong h/2$. Thus, the region of acceleration is slightly greater than the jet size h, counting from the stagnation point of the flow.

The above-made observations and estimates allow us to suggest a simple scheme of near-wall jet formation. The bow-shock wave can be conventionally replaced by a rigid wall, and the gas can be assumed to be accelerated in a nozzle formed by this wall and the substrate surface. The critical parameters of the gas are reached near the boundary of the incoming jet, i.e., the region from the stagnation to the critical point corresponds to the confuser part of the Laval nozzle. After that follows jet expansion and acceleration to supersonic velocities, which corresponds to the diffuser part of the Laval nozzle.

3.3.1.2. Comparison of pressure distributions in the jet and on the substrate surface

By comparing the pressure distributions in the free jet and on the substrate surface (Fig. 3.20), we can see that they are fairly close (z_0 is the distance from the nozzle exit to the substrate and to the input orifice of the Pitot tube).

Thus, to find the pressure distribution over the substrate surface, we have to know the pressure at the center and the thickness $x_{0.5}$, which depend only on z_0. In this case, the problem becomes one dimensional. It also follows from the data described above that the value of $x_{0.5}$ can be assumed to be equal to this value in the free jet. The same statement refers to the pressure at the substrate center: it can be estimated by the pressure at the centerline of the free jet behind the normal shock. We have to clarify the limits where these approximations can be used. For this purpose, we performed experiments whose results were compared with the distribution in the free jet.

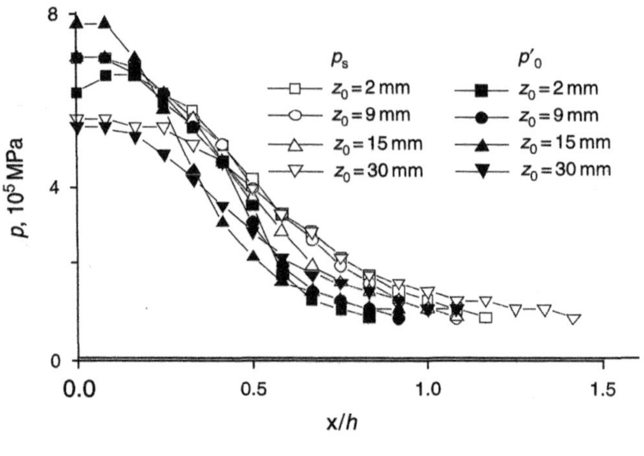

Fig. 3.20. Pressure profiles on the substrate surface p_s and behind the normal shock wave p'_0 along the smaller size of an isobaric air jet exhausting from the nozzle. $h = 3\,\text{mm}$, $H/h = 3.3$, $M^* = 2.5$, and $\varphi_{im} = 90°$.

3.3.2. Effect of the distance from the nozzle exit to the substrate on jet parameters. Oscillations of the jet

Figure 3.21 shows the distributions of the maximum pressure behind the shock wave in the free jet and on the surface of a substrate mounted at an angle of 90° to the jet axis.

The values of p'_0 and p_s initially coincide, but the pressure on the substrate decreases much more significantly with distance. Thus, at a distance $z_0 \approx 7h$, the pressure in the free jet

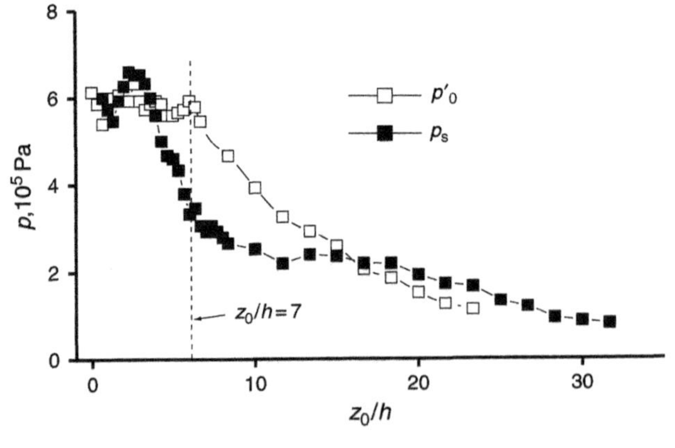

Fig. 3.21. Maximum pressure on the surface of a substrate mounted at an angle of 90° to the jet axis and behind the normal shock versus the distance to the substrate for an isobaric air jet ($T_0 = 300\,\text{K}$, $p_0^* = 1.4\,\text{MPa}$) exhausting from the nozzle ($h = 3\,\text{mm}$, $H/h = 3.3$, and $M^* = 2.5$).

does not yet decrease too much and equals, on the average, the pressure near the nozzle exit, whereas its value under impact conditions at the same distance is approximately twice lower than at the nozzle exit. Such a pattern is typical not only for isobaric but also for non-isobaric jets. Thus, the presence of the substrate involves some changes in the flow structure, though the values of p'_0 and p_s coincide in the regions $z_0 \leq 4h$ and $z_0 \geq 15h$. If the impact angles differ from 90° ($\varphi_{im} = 53$–$90°$), the behavior of the curves remains qualitatively the same as in the case of an impact onto a normally located substrate, and the pressure decrease is faster than that in the free jet. Apparently, this decrease is related to an emergence of oscillations of the jet incident onto the substrate, which increases the inflow of ambient air into the jet, and the total pressure at a certain part of the jet drastically decreases. Indeed, the photographs made with the help of a ruby laser (Fig. 3.22) show that the jet instability manifested in transverse oscillations is observed at certain distances from the nozzle exit to the substrate.

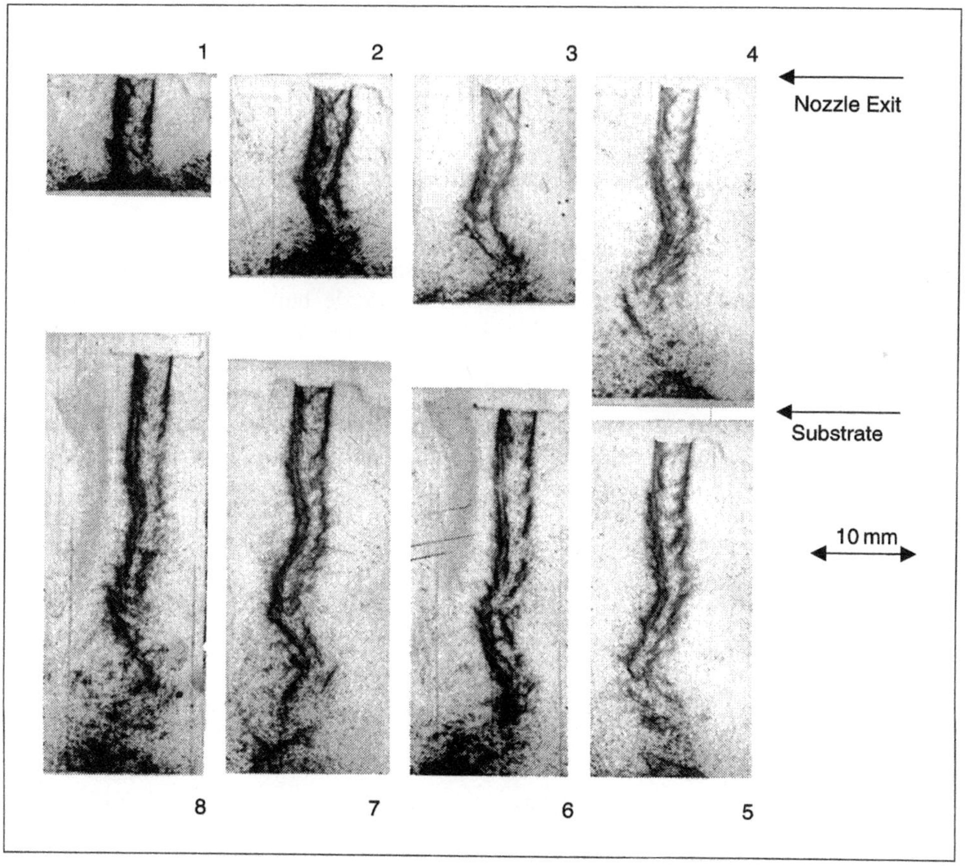

Fig. 3.22. Oscillatory impact of a rectangular supersonic jet onto a normally located substrate. The exposure time is $\tau = 30\,\text{ns}$, $M^* = 2.25$, $h = 3\,\text{mm}$, and $z_0/h = 3$ (1), 5 (2), 5.7 (3), 8 (4), 9 (5), 9.7 (6), 10.3 (7), and 11 (8).

Table 3.4. Characteristics of supersonic jet oscillations

Parameters	z_0/h	L_1/h	λ, mm
	7.7	1.4	9.9
$h = 3\,\text{mm}$	8.3	1.6–1.9	10.4–10.7
$v^* = 500\,\text{m/s}$	9.3	1.3	11.7
$M^* = 2.5$	9.7	2.9	10.7
$n = 1$	10	1.7–2.6	11.1–11.6
	10.6	1.7	11.7
$h = 1\,\text{mm}$	11.3	2.3	6.5
$v^* = 460\,\text{m/s}$	24	3.9	4.5
$M = 1.9$	31	3.9	5.2
$n = 1$	32	6.5	9.7
	$z_0 \gg h$	4.8	6.5–7.7–8.4

Here, L_1 is the length of the initial undisturbed section and λ is the wavelength determined as the distance between two neighboring apices.

The main parameters of oscillations gained from the photographs are summarized in Table 3.4.

The data from Table 3.4 and the form of the photographs indicate that disturbances do not develop immediately when the jet leaves the nozzle but at a certain distance L_1 from the nozzle exit. It is seen in Table 3.4 that the mean length of this undisturbed section is about 2–6 nozzle thicknesses. The frequencies based on the wavelength and gas velocity lie in the ultrasonic range (~50–100 kHz). It should be noted that the amplitude of oscillations increases in the downstream direction and reaches 2–3 nozzle thicknesses. Stability improves as the pressure in the pre-chamber increases and the flow regime becomes non-isobaric with $n > 1$.

In practice, the spraying distances are chosen such that instability does not have enough time to develop: in other words, from the condition $z_0 \leq L_1$.

3.3.3. Near-wall jet

One of the main goals of the present study was to obtain the M^2 profiles in the near-wall jet (Fig. 3.23).

In the region of the near-wall jet, where the static pressure was close to the ambient pressure, the value of M^2 was determined by the Rayleigh formula

$$\frac{p_0'}{p_a} = \left(\frac{\gamma+1}{2}\right)^{\frac{\gamma+1}{\gamma-1}} M^2 \left(\frac{M^2}{\gamma M^2 - \frac{\gamma-1}{2}}\right)^{\frac{1}{\gamma-1}}.$$

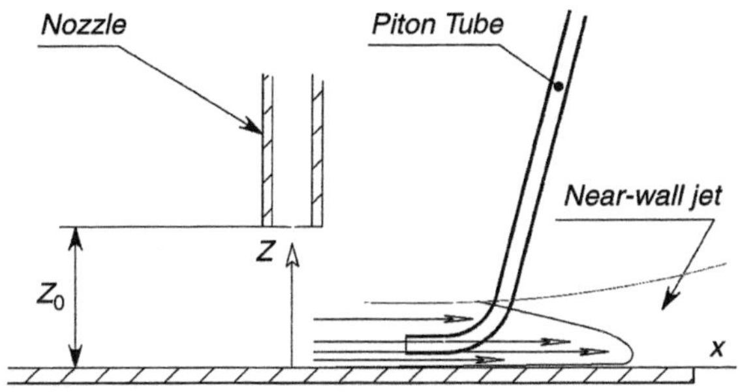

Fig. 3.23. Schematic of experimental investigation of the near-wall jet.

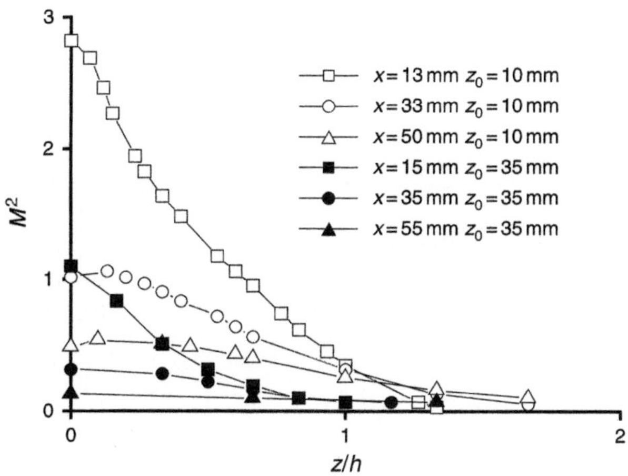

Fig. 3.24. Mach number profiles in the near-wall jet far from the critical point for a jet impacting on a normally located substrate. $h = 3\,\text{mm}$, $H/h = 3.3$, and $M^* = 2.5$.

The value of M^2 reconstructed from the measured pressures is plotted in Fig. 3.24. The values of the x coordinate were chosen rather large to avoid the region of the accelerating gas flow and reach the region of prevailing atmospheric pressure, which simplifies determination of M^2.

An analysis of Fig. 3.24 shows that the near-wall boundary layer on the substrate surface does not have enough time to develop (at least, it is thinner than the Pitot tube), and the boundary layer on the external side of the jet occupies the main part.

To verify self-similarity, we plotted the normalized M^2 profile in Fig. 3.25. There is some difference between these profiles, but they are rather adequately approximated by the function

$$\frac{M^2}{M_{\text{m}}^2} = \exp\left(-\left(\sqrt{\ln 2}\frac{z}{z_{0.5}}\right)^2\right). \tag{3.29}$$

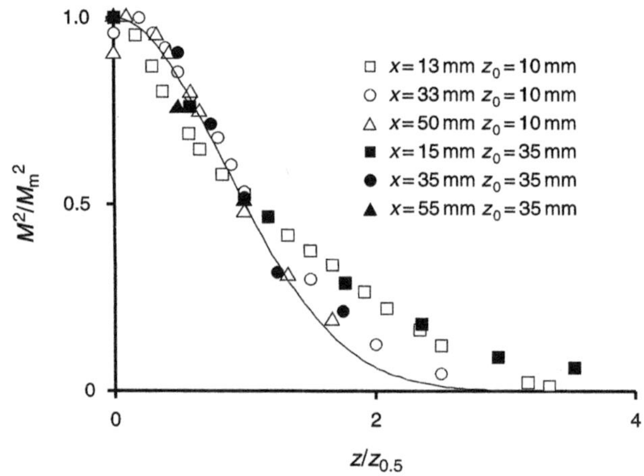

Fig. 3.25. Normalized Mach number profiles in the near-wall jet far from the critical point for a jet impacting on a normally located substrate. $h = 3\,\text{mm}$, $H/h = 3.3$, and $M^* = 2.5$.

To find the Mach number in the compressed layer (near the critical point), we used the values of pressure measured on the substrate surface p_s under the assumption of a constant total pressure, which allows us to use the isentropic formula

$$\frac{p_0}{p_s} = \left(1 + \frac{\gamma - 1}{2} M^2\right)^{\frac{\gamma}{\gamma-1}}.$$

After these procedures, we obtained the distributions of M_m^2 along the x axis of the substrate surface, corresponding to the maximum velocity in the near-wall jet (Fig. 3.26).

The gas is accelerated to supersonic velocities up to the distance $x_{ac} = 2h$–$3h$ and then decelerated.

Thus, it is shown that the pressure distribution over the substrate surface along the smaller size of the nozzle is self-similar in the case of the classical flow regime (i.e., in the absence of oscillations and circulation zones) and independent of the impact angle for $\varphi_{im} = 50$–$90°$. The critical parameters of the gas accelerated along the surface are reached in the vicinity of the boundary of the incident jet. The velocity gradient at the stagnation point can be determined by the formula $\beta = 2a_{cr}/h$. If the distance between the nozzle exit and the substrate is small ($z_0/h \leq 5$), the gas parameters can be assumed to be constant and equal to the parameters at the nozzle exit. The study of the near-wall jet showed that the velocity and Mach number profiles are self-similar, and the thickness of the near-wall boundary layer is negligibly small up to distances $x/h \approx 18$.

The results described above allow more detailed consideration of the processes of particle acceleration, including the specific features of particle motion within the jet, and the character of heat exchange between the jet and the substrate. Thus, these results ensure a

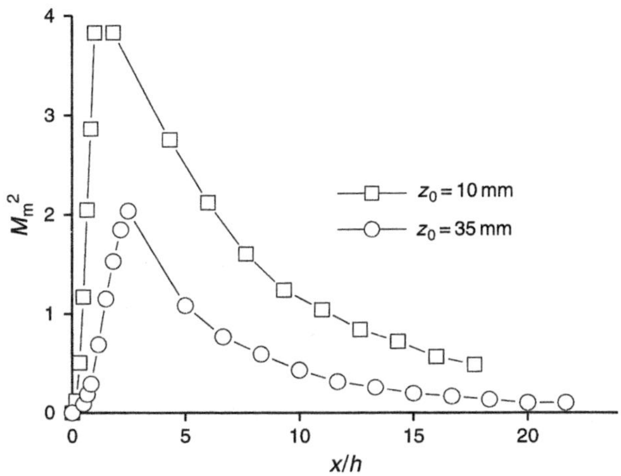

Fig. 3.26. Distributions of $M_m^2(x/h)$ along the surface of a normally located substrate. $h = 3$ mm, $H/h = 3.3$, and $M^* = 2.5$.

better insight into the physical background of the cold spray method and more profound development of the spraying technology.

3.3.4. Thickness of the compressed layer

An important problem is to determine the compressed layer thickness as a function of the jet parameters and the distance. We consider a supersonic jet impacting onto a normally located substrate (Fig. 3.27).

Deceleration and deflection of the gas flow occur ahead of the substrate surface. The transition from the high-velocity supersonic flow to the low-velocity subsonic flow occurs on the shock wave located at a certain distance z_w from the substrate surface. A high-pressure high-density gas layer is formed between the substrate surface and the shock wave. Obviously, fine particles of the deposited material passing through this layer are decelerated; the greater the compressed layer thickness, the greater the deceleration.

To determine the compressed layer thickness, we performed experiments with nozzles of different thicknesses and axial Mach numbers at the nozzle exit [15]. We used an experimental setup including an optical path for observation of the object. Photographs were taken, and the compressed layer thickness was estimated on the basis of the photographs obtained. These data are plotted in Figs 3.28 and 3.29; in addition to the data obtained for an isobaric jet, Fig. 3.28 shows the points obtained for $n = 3$. The compressed layer thickness and the distance from the nozzle exit to the substrate are normalized to the nozzle width.

For an isobaric jet, the compressed layer thickness in the first approximation can be assumed to be constant and equal to one half of the jet thickness. Figure 3.29 shows the data obtained for the non-isobaric flow mode ($n = 1.5$). Strong non-monotonicity within

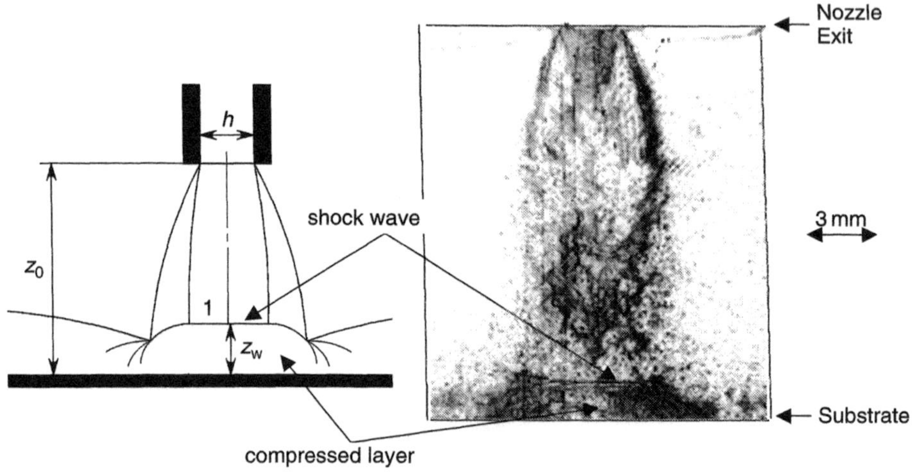

Fig. 3.27. Schematic and instantaneous photograph ($\tau \approx 30 \times 10^{-9}$ s, $n = 3$, $z_0 = 20$ mm) of the impact of a supersonic gas jet onto a flat infinite substrate. The detached shock wave is indicated by 1, h is the nozzle thickness, and z_0 is the distance from the nozzle exit to the substrate.

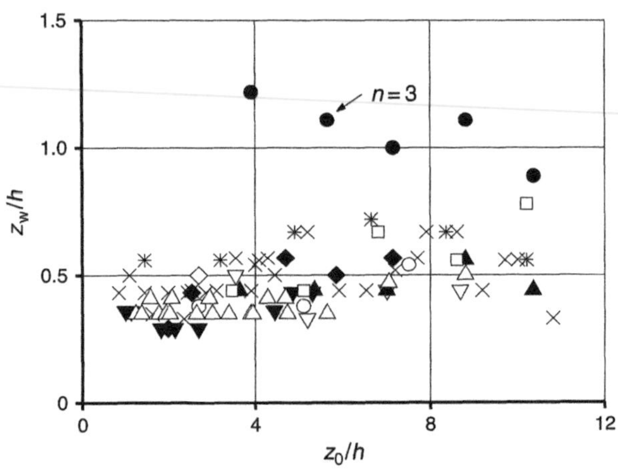

Fig. 3.28. Compressed layer thickness versus the distance. The parameters were varied in the following ranges: $h = 1$–5 mm, $H/h = 2.7$–8, and $M_{id} = 1.8$–3.1.

the first barrel can be noted. Such a behavior can be explained by interference of the wave structure of the jet with the bow-shock wave arising on the body. This is particularly noticeable for large jet-pressure ratios.

The compressed layer structure can be seen in the photographs in Fig. 3.30.

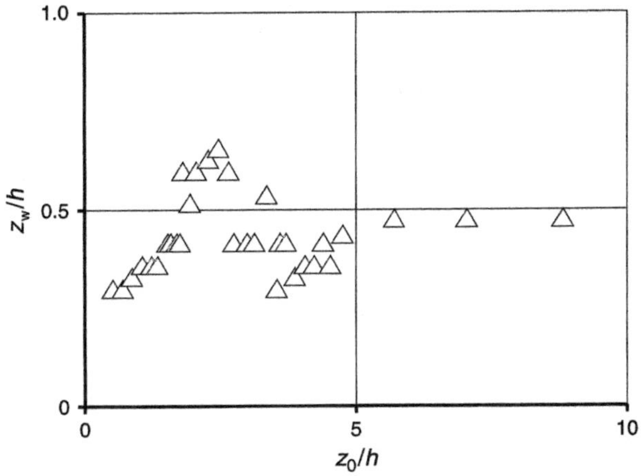

Fig. 3.29. Compressed layer thickness versus the distance for a supersonic non-isobaric ($n = 1.5$) jet exhausting from the nozzle ($h = 5, H/h = 1.68$, and $M_{id} = 2.55$).

We can give some simple considerations for estimating the compressed layer thickness. We write the equation of conservation of momentum of the jet with allowance for self-similarity of the dynamic pressure (or M^2) profiles

$$\frac{hH}{4}\rho_m v_m \int_0^1 \varphi(\xi)\,d\xi \int_0^1 \varphi(\eta)\,d\eta = z_w \frac{h+H}{2}\rho_k' u_m \int_0^1 \varphi(\zeta)\,d\zeta, \tag{3.30}$$

where $\varphi(\xi) = M^2/M_m{}^2, \varphi(\eta) = M^2/M_m{}^2$ along the x and y axes, $\xi = x/h, \eta = y/h, \varphi(\zeta) = M^2/M_m{}^2$ along the z axis, and $\zeta = z/z_w$. In the case of a uniform cross-sectional distribution of the gas parameters, we have

$$\int_0^1 \varphi(\xi)\,d\xi = \int_0^1 \varphi(\eta)\,d\eta = \int_0^1 \varphi(\bar{\zeta})\,d\bar{\zeta} = C = 1,$$

and the compressed layer thickness is

$$z_w = \frac{h}{2}\frac{1}{1+h/H}\left(\frac{\rho_m v_m}{\rho_k'}\right) = \frac{1}{2}\frac{h}{1+h/H}\Psi \tag{3.31}$$

$$\Psi = \frac{\left(1+aM_m{}^2\right)^{0.5}\left(\gamma M_m{}^2 - a\right)^{0.5/a}}{(cM_m)^b},$$

$$a = \frac{\gamma-1}{2}, \quad b = \frac{\gamma+1}{\gamma-1}, \quad c = \left(\frac{\gamma+1}{2}\right)^{0.5},$$

M_m is the Mach number at the axis of the incoming jet. The calculation of the function Ψ for Mach numbers of 1.8–3.1 yields 0.86–0.72, which can be approximated by a roughly

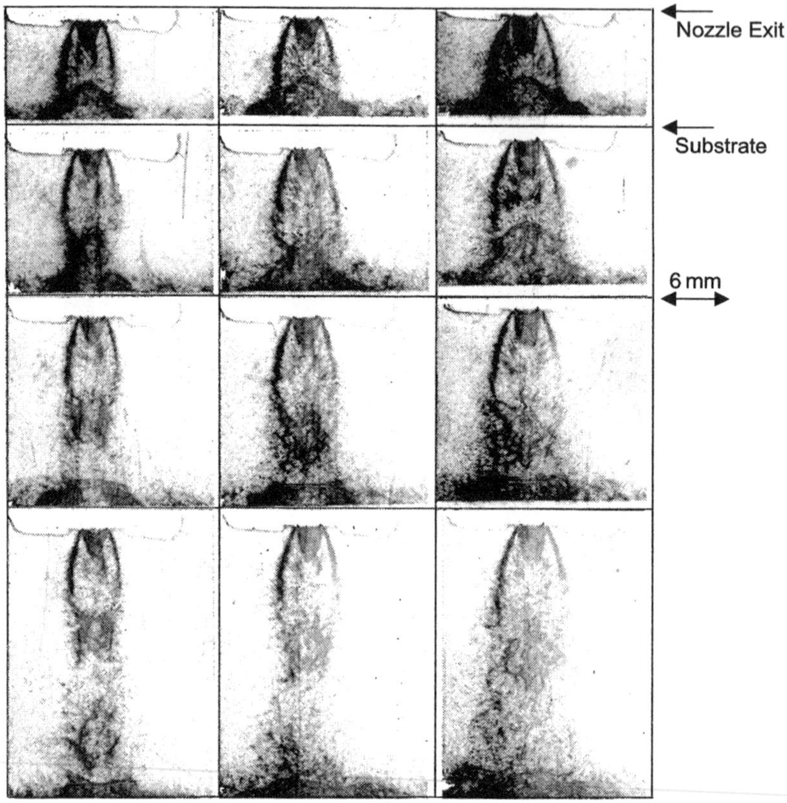

Fig. 3.30. Compressed layer structure. The different jet-pressure ratios are 2.5 (first column), 3 (second column), and 3.5 (third column). The distances are 10 mm (first row), 15 mm (second row), 20 mm (third row), and 30 mm (fourth row).

constant value of ~0.8. Thus, we can assume that the ratio of the compressed layer thickness to the jet thickness is approximately 0.4 for the plane jet. For the rectangular jet, a correction in accordance with Eq. (3.31) should be used.

It is seen from Eq. (3.31) that the compressed layer thickness tends to be approximately one half of the jet size for H much greater than h, i.e., for ideally plane nozzles and jets. After averaging all the data in Fig. 3.28 which refer to the isobaric air jet, we can estimate the compressed layer thickness as $\approx 0.45h$, independent of the distance within 0–$10h$.

3.4. Heat Transfer Between a Supersonic Plane Jet and a Substrate Under Conditions of Cold Spray

Investigation of heat transfer between a two-phase jet and a substrate under conditions of cold spray [19, 20] is important both for the theory and for applications. First, the processes of adhesive attachment of particles on the surface significantly depend on the surface temperature, as in the case of gas-thermal spraying [21, 22]. In addition, it is important to properly control the temperature of the coated part in many technological processes to ensure a required mode of coating formation and a required state of the part surface.

Heat transfer can be divided into two components: heat transfer between the particles and the surface and heat transfer between the carrier-phase gas jet and the surface. If the particle concentrations are low ($\varphi_p \leq 10^{-6}$), which is normally the case in cold spray, and the particle temperature is lower than the stagnation temperature of the jet, heat transfer between the particles and the surface is rather low, as compared to heat transfer between the surface and the gas flow. Therefore, in estimating the surface temperature, it is important to take into account heat transfer between the gas flow and the substrate.

3.4.1. Method for measuring the heat-transfer coefficient

The heat-transfer coefficient was measured by a calorimetric probe, which was a copper washer with an imbedded thermocouple. The probe was flush-mounted into a plate made of a heat-insulating material (Fig. 3.31). A shield (steel plate) reflecting the gas flow from the nozzle was placed between the nozzle and the substrate. When the registering equipment was ready for operation, the shield was rapidly removed, and the jet was impinging on the substrate with the calorimetric probe. For correct operation of this system, the time needed for the washer temperature to reach a steady level t_0 should be much greater than the time needed for stabilization of the gas flow; the latter can be estimated with the help of the velocity of sound a and the characteristic scale of the problem (e.g., distance between the substrate and the nozzle exit z_0) as $\tau_r \approx z_0/a$. For air, under our test conditions, we have $\tau_r \approx 10^{-4}$ s. For chosen parameters of the calorimetric probe, we obtain $t_0 = 1$–3 s. Based on the resultant dependences of temperature on time, we determined the heat-transfer coefficient by solving the one-dimensional heat-conduction equation.

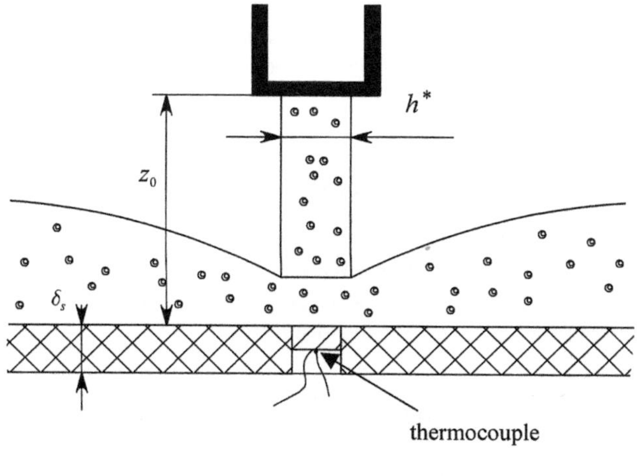

Fig. 3.31. Schematic of heat-transfer coefficient measurement for a supersonic jet impacting on the substrate.

Let us consider the heat transfer between the gas and an infinite plate of thickness δ_s. Figure 3.31 shows a schematic of the plane supersonic jet incident onto the substrate with indication of the coordinate axes and basic geometric parameters of the problem considered.

We assume that the heat-transfer coefficient α and the stagnation temperature of the gas T_0 are constant. At the initial time $t = 0$, there begins heat transfer at the interface $z = 0$ between the plate with the initial temperature T_{S0} and the gas. The second side of the plate is assumed to be thermally insulated. We introduce the dimensionless quantities

$$z = \xi\delta_s; \quad t = \tau\frac{\delta_s^2}{\chi}; \quad T_s = T_0(1-\theta),$$

to write the unsteady equation of heat conduction, and initial and boundary conditions in the following form:

$$\begin{aligned}
&\frac{\partial\theta}{\partial\tau} = \frac{\partial^2\theta}{\partial\xi^2}, \\
&\frac{\partial\theta}{\partial\xi} = \frac{\alpha\delta_s}{\lambda}\theta_w \qquad \text{at } \xi = 0, \\
&\frac{\partial\theta}{\partial\xi} = 0 \qquad \text{at } \xi = -1, \\
&\theta = \theta_0 = 1 - \frac{T_{s0}}{T_0} \qquad \text{at } \tau = 0
\end{aligned} \tag{3.32}$$

($\chi = \lambda/c\rho$ is the thermal diffusivity of the plate).

The solution is presented in the form of the series $\theta(\xi,\tau) = \sum_{i=1}^{\infty} f_i(\xi)\exp(-\varepsilon_i^2\tau)$, where $f_i(\xi)$ can be presented as the sum $A\cos(\varepsilon_i\xi) + B\sin(\varepsilon_i\xi)$. Using the boundary condition $f_i'(-1) = 0$, we obtain $B = Atg(\varepsilon_i)$. From the boundary condition $f_i'(0) = -\frac{\alpha\delta_s}{\lambda}f_i(0)$, we find the expression for determining ε_i:

$$\varepsilon_i tg(\varepsilon_i) = \frac{\alpha\delta_s}{\lambda} \tag{3.33}$$

For $Fo = \chi\tau/\delta_s^2 \geq 0.3$, which corresponds to $\tau \geq 0.3c\rho\delta_s^2/\lambda \approx 0.1$ s, we can cancel all terms of the series except for the first one, which yields a 1% error. In this case, it is convenient to present the temperature in a logarithmic form:

$$\ln\left(\frac{T_0 - T_s}{T_0}\right) = a + bt \tag{3.34}$$

$$b = -\frac{\varepsilon_1^2\chi}{\delta_s^2} \tag{3.35}$$

For experimental determination of α, we have to solve an inverse problem. Knowing the time evolution of temperature at a certain point of the plate, we can present it in the coordinates

$$\left(\ln\left(\frac{T_0 - T_s}{T_0}\right),\ t\right).$$

After that, we perform a root-mean-square approximation of all experimental points and construct a curve with coefficients a and b in accordance with Eq. (3.33). The value of ε_1 is found from the known value of b, by inverting Eq. (3.35):

$$\varepsilon_1 = \sqrt{(-b)\frac{\delta_s^2}{\chi}}.$$

The heat-transfer coefficient is found from Eq. (3.33):

$$\alpha = \frac{\lambda}{\delta_s}\varepsilon_1 tg(\varepsilon_1).$$

As an example, Fig. 3.32 shows the results of experiments on determining the coefficient of heat transfer between the jet ($p_0 = 1.45\,\text{MPa}$, $T_0^* = 330\,\text{K}$, which is the stagnation temperature at the nozzle exit) with the substrate at different distances x from the nozzle axis.

Figure 3.32a shows the experimental points of the temperature dependence on time, which was registered by the thermocouple at the back side of the probe. In Fig. 3.32b, the same data is plotted in the coordinates $\ln\frac{T_0(x)-T_s(x)}{T_0(x)}$, t together with the approximation curves passing through these experimental points. Heat-transfer coefficient corresponding to these cases and calculated on the basis of the curve slopes are also indicated.

A typical behavior of the normalized stagnation temperature $\bar{T}_0(x) = \frac{T_0(x)-T_a}{T_0^*-T_a}$ in the near-wall jet is shown in Fig. 3.33. In a wide range of z_0, the data are approximated by the function

$$f\left(\frac{x}{x_{0.5}}\right) = \left(1 + 15\left(\frac{x}{x_{0.5}}\right)^2\right)^{-0.25}. \tag{3.36}$$

It should be noted that the same distribution would be observed in the case of the jet impacting onto a non-heat-insulated surface (i.e., metallic surface) because heat transfer between the air jet and the substrate surface is only a small portion of the total amount of heat transferred by the jet (typical values of the Stanton number are $St \sim 0.01$). Thus, the decrease in stagnation temperature along the surface is mainly determined by the inflow of ambient air to the near-wall jet.

3.4.2. Heat-transfer coefficient

Using the above-described procedure, we measured the heat-transfer coefficients for the jet impacting on the substrate. Figure 3.34 shows the heat-transfer coefficient $\alpha(0)$ at the stagnation point of the flow versus the distance from the nozzle exit to the substrate.

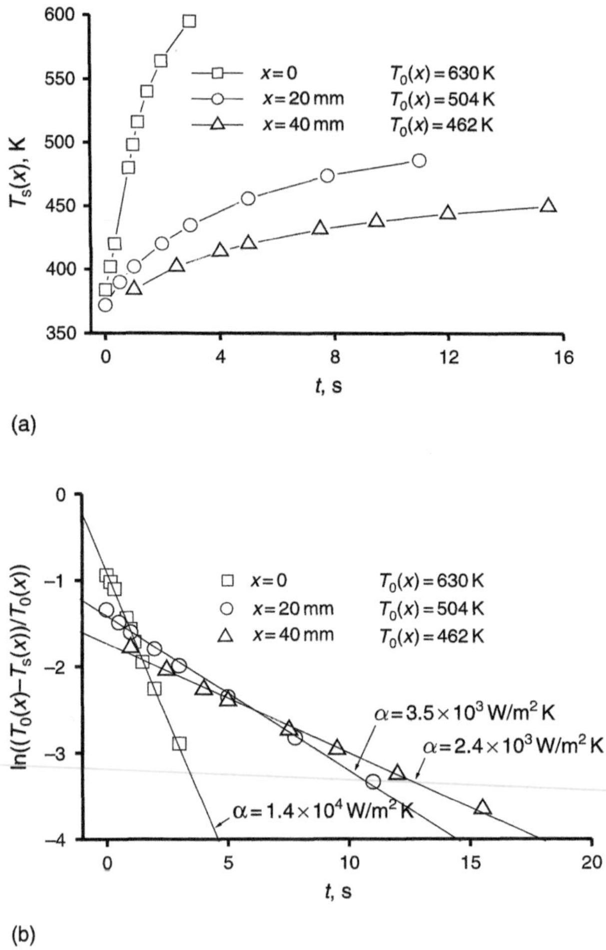

Fig. 3.32. Time evolution of temperature for an isobaric air jet. $p_0 = 1.45\,\text{MPa}$, $T_0^* = 330\,\text{K}$, $h^* =$ 3 mm (jet thickness at the nozzle exit), and $z_0 = 15\,\text{mm}$.

The heat-transfer coefficient is almost independent (in the range considered) of stagnation temperature of the jet at the nozzle exit; it reached the maximum value at a certain distance $z_0/h^* = 5$–7 and then decreases.

The experimentally measured Nusselt number (indicated by Δ) versus the Reynolds number Re_x, based on the distance from the stagnation point along the x coordinate, is shown in Fig. 3.35a. The dependence of the Nusselt number proportional to the heat-transfer coefficient is approximated by the formula

$$\frac{Nu\,(x)}{Nu\,(0)} = \left(1 + 15\left(\frac{Re_x}{Re_{0.5}}\right)^2\right)^{-0.25}, \tag{3.37}$$

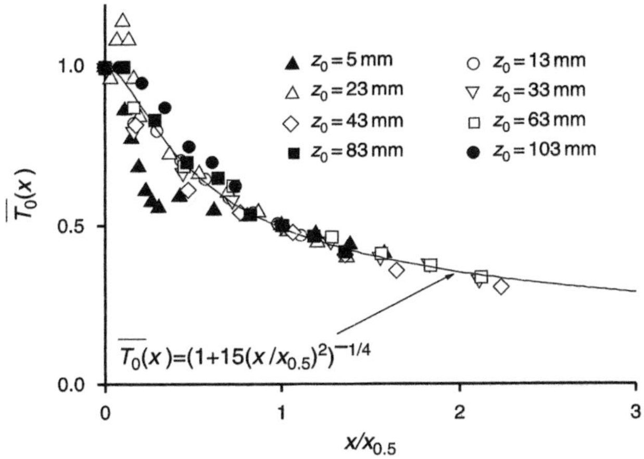

Fig. 3.33. Stagnation temperature in a near-wall air jet impacting on a normally located substrate, $T_0* = 550\,\mathrm{K}$, $T_a = 300\,\mathrm{K}$ (ambient air temperature).

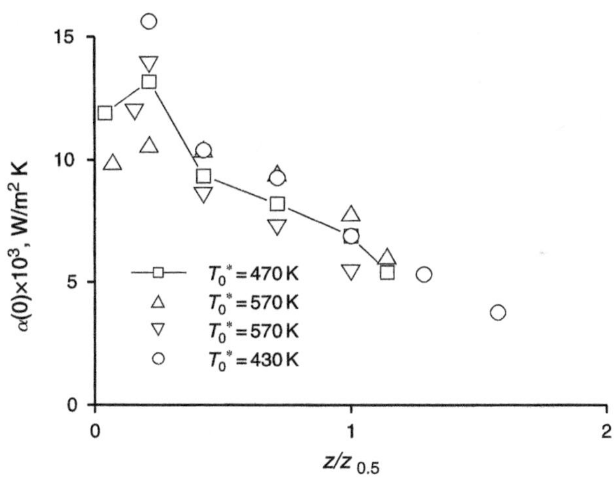

Fig. 3.34. Heat-transfer coefficient versus distance for the normal impact of an isobaric air jet, $z_{0.5} = 70\,\mathrm{mm}$, $\alpha_0 = 14 \times 10^3\,\mathrm{W/(m^2\,K)}$.

which covers the entire range of x, including the decay far from the impact point in the subsonic part of the near-wall jet, where $Nu \sim 1/x^{0.5}$ according to [23].

For comparison, we can calculate the heat-transfer coefficient as a function of Re_x, using the experimentally measured distributions of parameters at the outer edge of the near-wall jet $M_e^2(x)$, $u_e(x)$ [19], and $T_{0e}(x)$ by the formula from [24, 25]

$$\alpha = 0.04\ Pr^{-0.6} Re_{xe}^{-0.2} \rho_e u_e c_p \left(T_w / T_r\right)^{-0.16} \tag{3.38}$$

where ρ_e and u_e are the density and velocity at the outer edge of the near-wall jet.

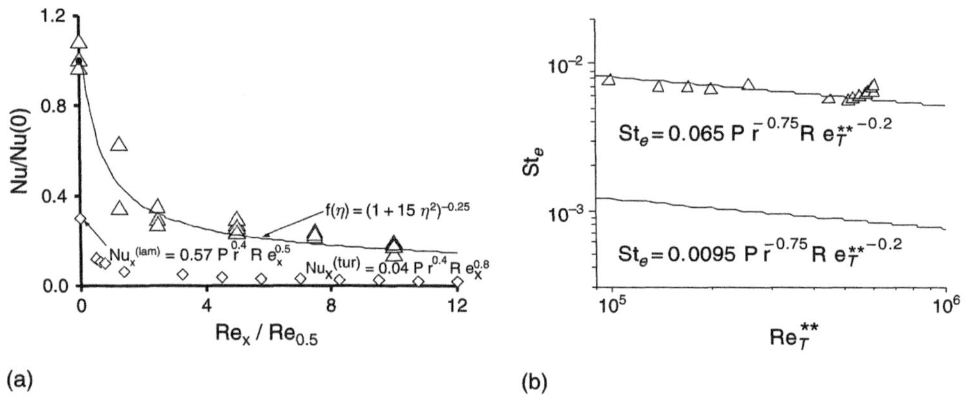

Fig. 3.35. (a) Nusselt number and (b) Stanton number versus Reynolds number. $z_0/h^* = 5$, $Re_{0.5} = 6.8 \times 10^4$, $Nu(0) = \alpha(0)h^*/\lambda_0 = 980$, $\lambda_0 \approx 0.04\,\mathrm{W/m\,K}$, and $\eta = Re_x/Re_{0.5}$.

Since $(T_w/T_r)^{-0.16}$ (T_w and T_r are the temperature of the substrate surface and the recovery temperature in the near-wall jet) has only a minor effect (for our test conditions, the maximum correction is about 1.1), it was replaced by unity. Formula 3.38 was derived on the basis of the theory of the turbulent boundary layer; a formula of the same form was derived in [26].

The heat-transfer coefficient in the vicinity of the stagnation point was calculated on the basis of the laminar boundary-layer theory for the jet impacting on the substrate with allowance for the velocity distribution in the vicinity of the stagnation point $u = \beta x$ [27]:

$$\alpha = 0.57/Pr^{0.6}\sqrt{\rho_0 \beta \mu_0 c_p^2}. \tag{3.39}$$

Typical values for test conditions obtained by Eq. (3.39) are $(3.8–4.2) \times 10^3\,\mathrm{W/m^2\,K}$ at the stagnation point for $\beta = 2a_{cr}/h^* = (2.4–3) \times 10^5\,\mathrm{s^{-1}}$.

The data calculated by Eqs (3.38) and (3.39) are plotted by diamonds in Fig 3.35a. The calculated values are substantially lower than the experimental results. This difference can be attributed to the influence of velocity fluctuations in the vicinity of the critical point and in the near-wall jet. For instance, in [17], the influence of fluctuations of velocity and other parameters is taken into account by the formula $Nu_t(0) = Nu(0)(1 + 0.75b^{0.54})$, $b = 0.18\varepsilon v^* \sqrt{\rho_0/\beta\mu_0}$, where $Nu(0)$ is the Nusselt number calculated with neglected turbulent oscillations, $\varepsilon = \sqrt{v'^2}/v^*$ is the degree of turbulence, ρ_0 is the density at the stagnation point, and μ_0 is the viscosity based on the stagnation temperature of the flow. For the results calculated by this formula to match the experimental data, we should use $\varepsilon = 0.25$. This value is within the range (0.04–0.5) of ε measured experimentally by independent methods [28].

Figure 3.35b shows the Stanton numbers $St_e = \alpha/\rho_e u_e c_p$ versus the Reynolds number based on the energy thickness δ_T^{**} calculated by the energy equation for a turbulent boundary layer, based on the postulate that the heat-transfer law in a turbulent flow is conservative [27]:

$$St_e = A\ Pr^{-0.75} Re_T{}^{**-m},\quad A = 0.0095, m = 0.2. \tag{3.40}$$

Then, we obtain the following expression for Re_T^{**}:

$$Re_T^{**} = \frac{1}{\Delta T}\left[\frac{A(1+m)}{Pr^{0.75}}\int \Delta T^{1+m}\frac{\rho_e u_e \mathrm{d}x}{\mu_e}\right]^{1/(1+m)},\qquad \Delta T = T_0(x) - T_w$$

Using the experimentally measured distributions of the parameters $M_e{}^2$, u_e, and T_{0e} on the upper edge of the near-wall boundary layer, we can integrate this expression and obtain the values of Re_T^{**}. As it follows from Fig. 3.35b, the experimental data are again higher than the calculated values. This suggests that heat transfer in the examined flow cannot be calculated by Eqs (3.38) and (3.39); apparently, the heat-transfer calculation model developed in [26, 27] is more accurate and promising. Nevertheless, there are some difficulties in calculating and measuring velocity fluctuations, and this problem, in many cases, is much more complicated than the determination of the heat-transfer coefficient itself.

3.4.3. Temperature of the substrate surface

The experimental results obtained allowed us to determine the temperature conditions on the substrate surface and inside the substrate. The temperature distribution in the substrate of length $2L_s$ and thickness δ_s were calculated by simultaneously solving the steady heat-conduction equation $\frac{\partial^2 T(x,z)}{\partial x^2} + \frac{\partial^2 T(x,z)}{\partial z^2} = 0$ ($T(x, z)$ is the temperature in the substrate) and the law of conservation of heat in the steady case $\int_0^{L_s} \alpha(x)\left[T_0(x) - T_s(x, 0)\right]\mathrm{d}x = 0$, using the experimental value of stagnation temperature and heat-transfer coefficient in the near-wall jet. The solution was sought in the form $T(x, z) = T_s(x) + a(x)z + b(x)z^2$, which is justified in the steady case with $\delta_s \ll L_s$ and low temperature gradients in the substrate. The boundary conditions on the surfaces $z = 0$ and $z = -\delta_s$ yield the relations

$$\lambda\frac{\partial T(x,z)}{\partial z}\bigg|_{z=0} = \alpha(x)\left(T_0(x) - T_s(x)\right) \Rightarrow a(x) = \frac{\alpha(x)}{\lambda}\left(T_0(x) - T_s(x)\right),$$

$$\lambda\frac{\partial T(x,z)}{\partial z}\bigg|_{z=-\delta_s} = 0 \Rightarrow b(x) = \frac{a(x)}{2\delta_s} = \frac{\alpha(x)\left(T_0(x) - T_s(x)\right)}{2\delta_s\lambda}.$$

Finally, we have

$$T(x,z) = T_s(x) + \frac{\alpha(x)}{\lambda}\left(T_0(x) - T_s(x)\right)\left(z + \frac{z^2}{2\delta_s}\right). \tag{3.41}$$

Substituting Eq. (3.41) into the heat-conduction equation and making the necessary transformations, we obtain the equation for the substrate-surface temperature:

$$\frac{\partial^2 T_s(x)}{\partial x^2} = \frac{\alpha(x)}{\delta_s}\left(T_0(x) - T_s(x)\right). \tag{3.42}$$

Solving it together with the integral equation of conservation of heat $\int_0^{L_s} \alpha(x)\left(T_0(x) - T_s(x,0)\right) \mathrm{d}x = 0$, we obtain the temperature distribution on the substrate surface for $0 \le x \le L$. After that, from the known $T_s(x)$, we calculate the coefficients $a(x)$ and $b(x)$ and find the temperature distribution in the substrate.

The results calculated for the case $L_s = 100 \times 10^{-3}$ m, $T_0^* = 1200$ K, and $\delta_s = 3$ mm are plotted in Fig. 3.36. Figure 3.36a shows the surface temperature for substrates made of different materials.

The calculations performed show that the noticeable decrease in surface temperature (for materials with $\lambda \ge 40$ W/m K), as compared to the stagnation temperature of the incoming jet, is caused by heat redistribution inside the substrate. As is seen from Fig. 3.36b, heat penetrates into the substrate at the beginning ($0 \le x \le 4h^*$), whereas the process is inverted at large distances: heat leaves the substrate and enters the near-wall jet. Based on the calculation results, we plotted the surface temperature in the deposition spot ($x = 0$) versus the substrate length for different substrate thicknesses δ_s (Fig. 3.37).

As the substrate length increases to (15–20)h^*, the surface temperature at the substrate surface decreases noticeably; the greater the value of δ_s, the greater the decrease. A further increase in the substrate length has practically no effect on the surface temperature at the substrate center. Experimental verification (symbols • and ■) showed that the measured surface temperature near the critical point is in good agreement with the calculated values, which confirms the validity of the assumptions made and allows the use of this heat-transfer model for practical estimates.

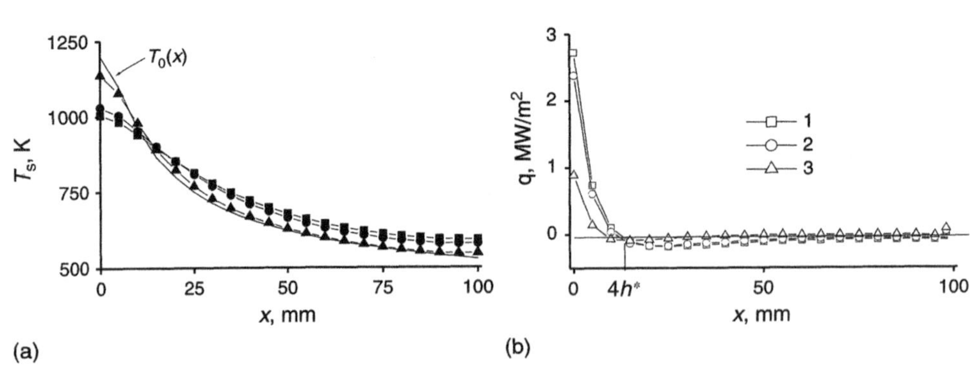

Fig. 3.36. Distributions of the (a) surface temperature and (b) heat flux on different substrates. 1 – Cu ($\lambda = 350$ W/m K), 2 – Al ($\lambda = 250$ W/m K), and 3 – Steel ($\lambda = 40$ W/m K).

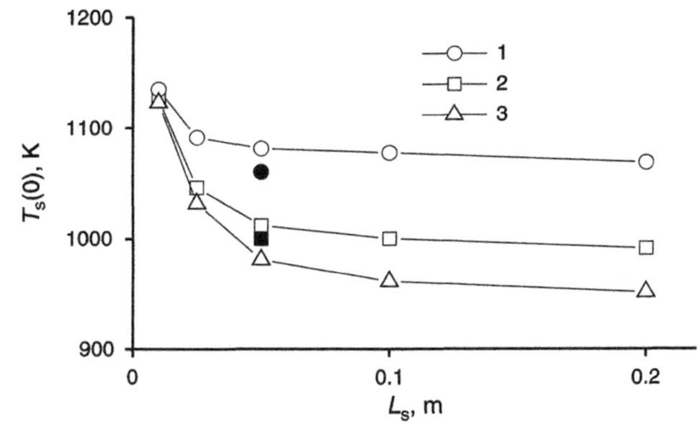

Fig. 3.37. Surface temperature in the deposition spot ($x = 0$) on a copper substrate versus its size. $1 - \delta_s = 1\,\text{mm}$, $2 - \delta_s = 3\,\text{mm}$, and $3 - \delta_s = 5\,\text{mm}$.

Using Eq. (3.41), we can estimate ΔT_{max} (the maximum difference in surface temperatures for $z = 0$ and $z = -\delta_s$). We find

$$\Delta T_{max} = \frac{\alpha(0)\,\delta_s}{2\lambda}\left(T_0(0) - T_s(0)\right),$$

and $\Delta T_{max} \approx 20\,\text{K}$ for calculation conditions in Fig. 3.36a. Hence, the surface temperatures for $z = 0$ and $z = -\delta_s$ are almost identical.

Thus, the distributions of stagnation temperature and heat-transfer coefficient in the near-wall jet at different distances from the exit of a rectangular supersonic nozzle to the substrate were obtained experimentally. The experimental values of the heat-transfer coefficient are substantially higher than the calculated results, and this difference can be explained by velocity fluctuations in the vicinity of the critical point and in the near-wall jet.

Using experimental data on stagnation temperature and heat-transfer coefficient, we calculated the substrate temperature in the steady case and showed that the surface temperature in the deposition spot is noticeably lower than the stagnation temperature. This is due to heat redistribution inside the substrate for heat-conducting materials ($\lambda \geq 40\,\text{W/m K}$). This effect should be taken into account, in particular, in testing spraying regimes with excitation of synthesis reactions directly on the surface, because the temperature in this case is an extremely important parameter affecting reaction initiation.

3.5. Optimization of Geometric Parameters of the Nozzle for Obtaining the Maximum Impact Velocity

Further development of the cold spray technology requires a systematic search for methods of improving its efficiency. The trial-and-error method does not satisfy the increasing requirements of basic and applied research. A comprehensive approach to solving the problem of optimization of coating application was first suggested in [29], as applied to the plasma spraying technique. Specific features of cold spray, however, necessitated additional investigations, which were not covered in [29]. In particular, it was necessary to develop a new formulation of the problem typical specifically of cold spray and including optimization of nozzle parameters in terms of particle velocities at the impact moment [30, 31].

3.5.1. Pattern of gas and particle motion

The particles and the gas leave the pre-chamber, where their velocities can be assumed to be identical (several dozens of meters per second), and enter the throat, where the gas velocity reaches the velocity of sound. Further, the gas is expanded and accelerated to supersonic velocities. The particles, because of their inertia, cannot be accelerated to the same velocities in a short time, and a two-phase flow non-equilibrium in terms of velocity is formed. For the particle velocity to approach the gas velocity, i.e., for the velocity equilibrium to be reached, the supersonic part of the nozzle should be extended. Yet, a large length of the nozzle involves the problem of thick boundary layers growing on the walls. If the nozzle is too long and its thickness is too small, supersonic motion can become impossible altogether. Therefore, there is some optimal nozzle length that ensures the maximum possible particle velocity at the nozzle exit.

Leaving the nozzle, the gas enters the ambient atmosphere, where it actively mixes with the ambient air. The mixing leads to a rapid decrease in gas velocity and temperature in the streamwise and transverse directions. Nevertheless, each jet has a short initial part where the axial velocity remains unchanged and retains the value at the nozzle exit. The length of this part depends on the initial non-uniformity of the jet, i.e., on the boundary-layer thickness at the nozzle exit and on the jet size, because the rapid decrease in jet parameters begins after the jet boundary layers induced by the contact of the moving gas from the nozzle and the quiescent air in the ambient atmosphere converge. Particles are also accelerated at this initial part of the jet, though the acceleration is less effective than that inside the nozzle. At this point, the acceleration process is terminated and the deceleration process begins.

When the supersonic gas jet hits the substrate, there arises a shock wave ahead of the substrate; a compressed gas layer is formed between the shock wave and the substrate (Fig. 3.27). In this compressed layer, the streamwise velocity of the gas decreases from the shock wave toward the substrate surface, and there appears a transverse component of velocity along the substrate surface, which increases from the shock wave toward the outer edge of the boundary layer developed because of gas motion along the substrate surface. The transverse vanishes again inside the boundary layer. The thickness of this boundary layer in the vicinity of the critical point is very small and can be neglected in practical applications. In addition, a very intense turbulent exchange by momentum is observed near the substrate surface inside the compressed layer, i.e., the fluctuating components of velocity are very high.

Again, because of its inertia, the particle passing through the shock wave does not change its velocity as a stepwise function but begins to decelerate; therefore, at the impact moment, the particle has a lower velocity than that upstream of the shock wave.

The velocity non-equilibrium is observed again, but now the particles move faster than the gas. To reach equilibrium, the particle should cover a certain distance, which is smaller than that during the particle motion in the nozzle, because the gas parameters inside the compressed layer are close to stagnation parameters, whereas the gas inside the nozzle is more rarefied. This raises the problem of decreasing the compressed layer thickness or decreasing the stand-off distance between the shock wave and the substrate.

The stand-off distance mainly depends on the transverse size of the jet: the thinner the jet, the thinner the compressed shock layer and the higher the particle velocity at the impact moment. We have already demonstrated, however, that thin nozzles cannot be very long. Hence, the nozzle thickness and length are the parameters that can be varied to reach the highest possible velocity of the impacting particle. These parameters will be called the optimal parameters, and the problem of finding these parameters will be called the problem of nozzle optimization.

Thus, to solve the nozzle-optimization problem, we need to construct a model of gas and particle motion over the entire gas-dynamic path. In solving this problem, we also need to clarify the influence of the particle size and density, distance from the nozzle exit to the substrate, and the ratio of the sides of the throat section on the optimal parameters, so that we could estimate the efficiency of this or that nozzle and ensure the possibility of choosing the most efficient nozzle in practice.

3.5.2. Model for calculating gas and particle parameters

In this section, we consider the model of gas and particle motion. We assume that the particle always moves along the centerline of the gas-dynamic path. This allows us to ignore the decrease in gas velocity in boundary layers and neglect the influence of the transverse component of the gas inside the compressed layer, because this component is assumed to be equal to zero along the axis. In addition, we perform the calculations under the assumption of motion of single particles, where the effect of the particle on the gas is negligibly small and can be ignored in calculating gas velocities. Thus, the problem is solved in two stages. First, we find the distributions of the gas parameters along the centerline of the entire gas-dynamic path and then calculate the particle motion by the following equation of motion with known gas parameters:

$$\rho_p \frac{\pi d_p^3}{6} v_p \frac{dv_p}{dz} = C_x \frac{\rho (v - v_p)^2}{2} \frac{\pi d_p^2}{4}. \tag{3.43}$$

Here, v and v_p are the gas and particle velocities, respectively, and the gas parameters are taken at the nozzle axis. We used Henderson's approximation for the drag coefficient:

$$M_p = \frac{v - v_p}{a}$$

$$Re_p = \frac{(v - v_p)\rho d_p}{\mu}$$

$$C_{x1} = \frac{24}{Re_p + 3.06\sqrt{M_p}} + \frac{4.5 + 0.0114\ Re_p + 0.1825\sqrt{Re_p}}{1 + 0.03\ Re_p + 0.48\sqrt{Re_p}} + 0.1M_p^2 + 0.2M_p^8$$

$$C_{x2} = 0.9 + \frac{0.34}{M_p^2}$$

$$C_x = \begin{cases} C_{x1}, & M_p < 1 \\ C_{x2}, & M_p > 1.75 \\ C_{x1}(M_p = 1) + 1.33\,(M_p - 1)\left[C_{x2}(M_p = 1.75) - C_{x1}(M_p = 1)\right], & 1 < M_p < 1.75 \end{cases}$$

The value of the Mach number in the compressed layer between the shock wave and the substrate surface was calculated by the cubic approximation formula derived from the boundary conditions:

$$\bar{z} = 1: \quad M = M'; \quad dM/d\bar{z} = 0$$

$$\bar{z} = 0: \quad M = 0; \quad dM/d\bar{z} = 0.5M'.$$

The last condition is borrowed from [17], where it is argued that this dependence coincides with experimental data. Finally, we have

$$M = M'\bar{z}\left(0.5 + 2\bar{z} - 1.5\bar{z}^2\right), \tag{3.44}$$

(M′ is the Mach number behind the shock wave, z_w is the distance between the shock wave and the substrate, and $\bar{z} = z/z_w$.

In the region of the free jet, the values of the gas parameters were chosen in accordance with the formula approximating the dependence obtained in experiments with jets and taking into account the decrease in jet parameters with distance from the nozzle exit. The distances in the calculations, however, were small, and the decrease in jet parameters was insignificant. We considered an isobaric gas jet, because the influence of the jet-pressure ratio on the compressed layer thickness was ignored. The gas flow inside the nozzle was calculated by the Karman equation, which allowed us to calculate the displacement thickness.

These assumptions allowed us to calculate the particle motion from the nozzle exit to the substrate surface and, thus, determine the particle velocities at the impact moment. In all calculations, the Mach number corresponding to the geometric ratio of the nozzle-exit and throat cross sections was assumed to be constant and equal to 2.75.

3.5.3. Computer application

The progress in computer engineering allows the development of user-friendly codes for creating new efficient units and setups used in various branches of industry. One of the codes is described in the present section; it serves to facilitate design of nozzle units for cold spray facilities [32].

The necessity in the development of software of this kind appeared long ago because the cold spray method has found its place and continues to gain more and more applications in industry [33–40]. With each new application, design of a new setup involves various questions dealing with gas dynamics, acceleration, and heating of particles of different sizes and made of different materials. To get a clear concept of the behavior of particles under varied gas-dynamic conditions, mathematical simulations of particle motion inside the nozzle unit from the point of particle injection in the pre-chamber to the nozzle exit are needed.

The main difficulties in simulations are caused by the necessity of taking into account the turbulent boundary layer developed on the nozzle walls. Involvement of the model of turbulent boundary-layer growth significantly complicates the computation process, which is rather expensive even in the simplified formulation. Nozzles designed for particle acceleration can have high values of the aspect ratio (ratio of the length of the supersonic part of the nozzle to the smaller size of the nozzle exit). In addition, to decrease the loss of particle velocity in passing through the compressed shock layer and to obtain more efficient coating on a given area of the part, cold spray nozzles can have a rectangular exit cross section with the ratio of sides equal to three and higher. All of these factors impose specific requirements to the model, which formed the basis for the **ProjectNozzleDirect_v1.1**, which is about code described below.

The main objective of the designer is to choose the necessary geometry and determine all geometric parameters required for nozzle manufacturing. It is important not to make mistakes and to retain the efficiency of the spraying device as a whole at a high level. For this purpose, the initial data should include the distributions of velocity and temperature of the gas and particles along the entire nozzle unit. Based on this data, the designer can adjust the geometry, operation mode of the setup, and the necessary parameters of the carrier gas for reaching the maximum deposition efficiency.

Thus, code development was based on all requirements mentioned above, including simple program management, i.e., the so-called "user-friendly interface".

Let us describe the code and some principles of its management. The code consists of one file **ProjectNozzleDirect_v1.1.exe**, which is about 300 kB, whose operation requires the operation system Windows 95/98 and higher versions. Double clicking the icon **ProjectNozzleDirect_v1.1.exe** initiates the code and displays the main window show in Fig. 3.38.

The first column on the left contains four basic functional buttons; the main of them (**Calculate**) starts calculations of gas and particle parameters along the nozzle unit with prescribed initial parameters listed in the next three columns. Let us consider this in more detail. The column **Nozzle** contains the main geometric parameters of the calculated nozzle in millimeters (Fig. 3.38): nozzle thickness h, nozzle-throat width b, and nozzle-exit width $h00$. Thus, the nozzle throat is described by the parameters h and b, and the exit section is described by h and $h00$, i.e., the nozzle is linearly expanded from the size b to the size $h00$, and the nozzle thickness h in the supersonic part of the nozzle remains constant.

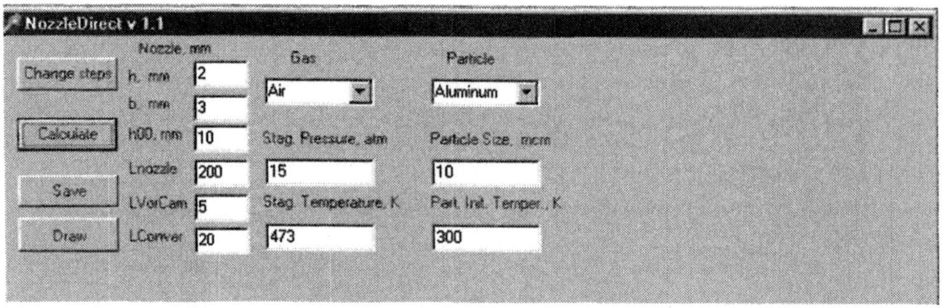

Fig. 3.38. Main window of the application.

The subsonic part of the nozzle is assumed to be conical with a cone length ***Lconver***. In addition, the subsonic cone of the nozzle is adjacent to the constant-diameter pre-chamber section of length ***Lvorcam***. The length ***Lvorcam*** is actually the distance from the beginning of the nozzle to the point where the particles are injected into the carrier-gas flow.

The next column **Gas** describes the carrier-gas parameters. The user can choose the gas from the pulldown menu in the upper field. Some parameters of the gas, such as viscosity, heat capacity, isentrope, etc., are automatically added to the calculation model. Two remaining fields allow the user to set the desired stagnation pressure and temperature of the gas in the pre-chamber. Note, the pressure is given in bars (1 bar = 0.1 MPa), and the temperature is given in Kelvin.

The last column of the input data contains the particle parameters: particle material, their size in micrometers, and initial temperature, which is normally close to room temperature under cold spray conditions.

After setting all necessary input values described above (the decimal comma is used instead of the decimal point), the user should click the **Calculate** button. After a certain time (normally, several seconds), the calculated values will be displayed (Fig. 3.39).

The extreme right column shows the Exit Pressure Ratio, i.e., the Ratio of the pressure in the jet to the ambient pressure, the Gas Flow Rate in grams per second, and the Gas Heat Rate necessary for gas heating from 273 K to the value given in the field Stagnation Temperature. The real power of the heater should be higher because the nozzle unit and the incoming pipeline are assumed to be thermally insulated, i.e., heat losses are ignored.

The table in the lower part of the main window of the code shows the gas and particle velocities at three reference points: at the entrance, in the throat, and at the exit.

The user can obtain a more detailed idea about particle acceleration and heating by using the **Draw** button. Clicking this button displays a figure, which shows three curves corresponding to the gas velocity, particle velocity, and particle temperature along the entire gas-dynamic path considered.

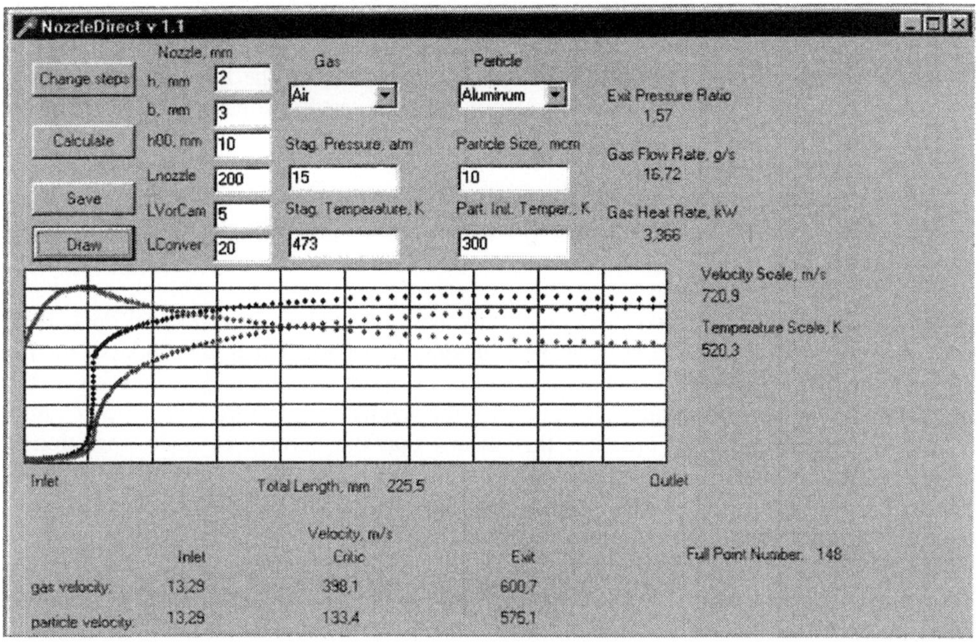

Fig. 3.39. Results of calculations shown in the main window of the application (Calculate and Draw).

The entire figure is conventionally divided by a grid of 10 × 10 cells. The total length of the gas-dynamic path in millimeters is indicated below as **Total Length**. The vertical axis combines the axis of velocities and temperatures. The scale interval for velocity is **Velocity Scale**/10, and the scale interval for temperature is **Temperature Scale**/10, i.e., in the case shown in Fig. 2.8, we have 72.09 m/s and 52.03 K, respectively.

The velocity and temperature curves are shown as individual points (in the so-called Scatter style). This was made deliberately. The user can visually find intervals where the calculation step is too large and reduce the latter to obtain a smaller computational error. This is made with the use of the **Change Steps** button. This button opens an additional window where the necessary corrections are made.

We comment only on those quantities that can be necessary for working with the program: nVorCam is the number of points over the length LVorCam, nConver is the number of points over the length Lconver, and n4 and n5 are the numbers of points in the supersonic part of the nozzle (it is recommended to vary only the value of n5 so that the step was uniform over the entire supersonic part of the nozzle). The total number of computational points is indicated in the right bottom corner of the main window of the program.

The last button **Save** allows the user to save the computed information in a file with the extension .dat in a specially allocated place on the hard disk or on a floppy disk with a possibility of subsequent editing of the graphs in editor system specially designed for this purpose. Currently, the Origin editor for scientific and technical graphs is widely used. Therefore, the code saves the dat-file in a standard that can be read by the Origin editor. To open the dat-file in the Origin editor, the user should click the File pulldown menu, choose import ASCII, and mark the necessary file. The result of this procedure is shown in Fig. 3.40.

Further processing of the calculated data is performed by tools of the Origin editor, which allows the user to employ the calculation results for composing parts, reports, presentations, etc.

Results calculated by this code were carefully verified against experimental data. Both gas and particle velocities were checked. It should be noted that the code has some restrictions. The model used in the code ignores origination of shock waves inside the nozzle under certain conditions. This occurs if the stagnation pressure in the pre-chamber is not sufficiently high. In practice, this means that the domain of code operation is bounded to jet-pressure ratios higher than 0.5 and aspect ratios lower than 150 (lower jet-pressure ratios or higher aspect ratios can lead to emergence of shock waves, which significantly distort the gas-dynamic pattern of the flow).

Thus, the code proposed is simple to use and allows the user to obtain a fast preliminary analysis of the nozzle-unit configuration for cold spray facilities to avoid rough mistakes in their design without expensive experiments. We hope that further applications of this kind will be developed to cover the flow pattern both inside and outside the nozzle unit.

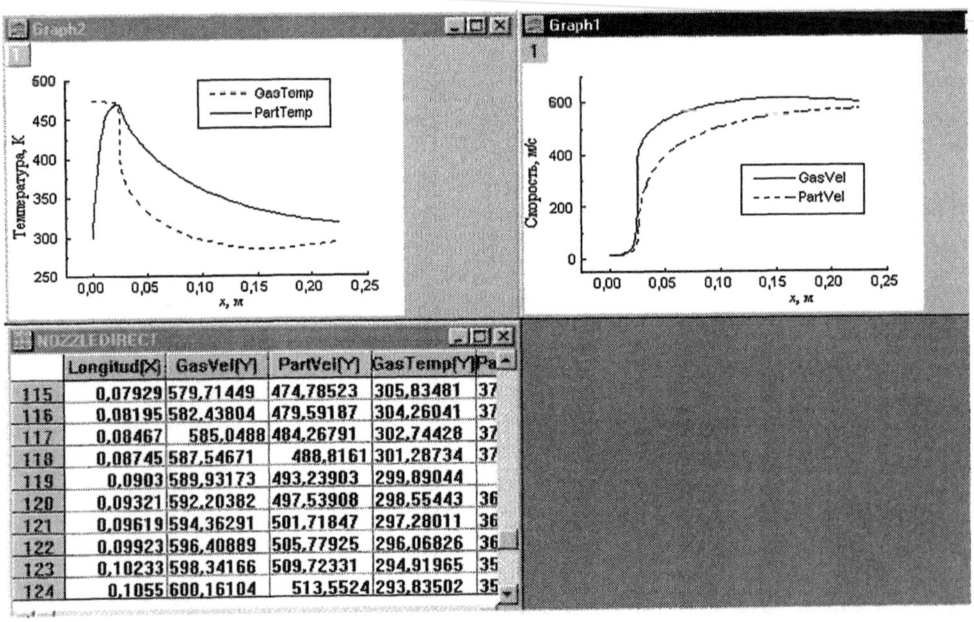

Fig. 3.40. Calculated data and graphs generated on their basis by the Origin editor.

3.5.4. Determination of impact temperature of particles

The most important parameter for particles in cold spray is the particle velocity. Therefore, optimization of nozzle parameters in terms of the impact velocity of particles is more relevant than optimization in terms of the impact temperature of particles. Nevertheless, it follows from simulation results that the impact temperature of particles plays an important role in adhesive attachment of particles on the substrate surface. Based on the results obtained, we calculated the nozzle used in the cold spray method. The particle temperature was calculated by the equation [41]

$$\rho_p v_p c_p \frac{dT_p}{dz} = Nu \frac{6\lambda}{d_p^2}\left(T_0 - T_p\right) \tag{3.45}$$

$$Nu = 2a + 0.459\ b\ Re_{p0}^{\ 0.55} Pr^{0.33}$$

$$a = \exp(-M_{p0})(1 + 17M_{p0}/Re_{p0})^{-1}$$

$$b = 0.666 + 0.333\exp(-17M_{p0}/Re_{p0})$$

To find the impact temperature of the particles incident onto the substrate surface, we apply the same approach used in the particle-acceleration problem. We assume that the particle moves along the axis of the gas-dynamic path, ignore the influence of particles on the gas, and divide the problem into two parts: finding the gas parameters at the axis and finding the particle velocity and temperature from the known values of gas parameters. The results calculated by this procedure are plotted in Fig. 3.41.

The values of parameters corresponding to exhaustion of air and particles of density of 2700 and 8900 kg/m^3 from nozzles of different lengths for the substrate located at a distance of 10, 20, or 30 mm were used in the calculations. Because of particle slipping, their temperature equals neither the stagnation temperature nor the static temperature of the gas

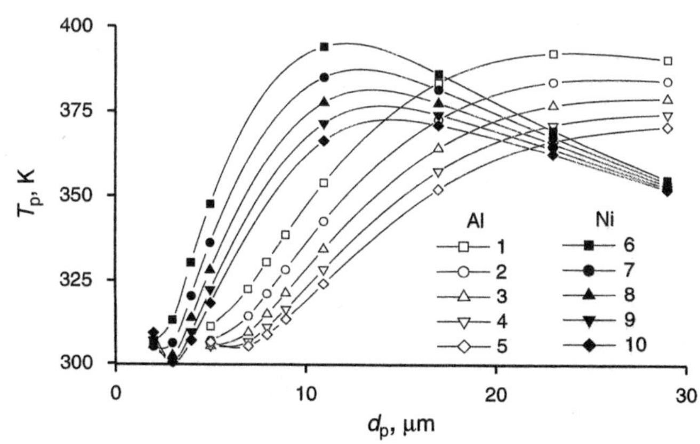

Fig. 3.41. Impact temperature of particles. $z_0 = 15$ mm; $T_0 = 500$ K, $M_{id} = 2.75$, $h = 3$ mm; $L =$ 60 mm (1 and 6); $L = 80$ mm (2 and 7); $L = 100$ mm (3 and 8); $L = 120$ mm (4 and 9); $L = 140$ mm (5 and 10).

flow at the nozzle exit. For the parameters considered, the axial Mach number at the nozzle exit depends weakly on the gas temperature: $M = 2.38$–2.41 for $T_0 = 600$–$1000\,\mathrm{K}$. The ratio of the static to the stagnation temperature for $M = 2.4$ is close to 0.46. It is seen from Fig. 3.41 that the impact temperature of particles, normalized to the stagnation temperature of the gas, depends on the particle size and density and reaches 0.6–0.8 of the stagnation temperature of the gas (for optimal nozzles), which is significantly higher than 0.46.

3.5.5. Optimization of nozzle parameters in terms of the impact velocity of particles

Let us now consider the results calculated by the model described above. Figure 3.42 shows the isolines of the impact velocity of particles near the maximum in the plane h, L. This maximum is fairly shallow.

The curves in Fig. 3.42 were obtained for an aluminum particle $10\,\mu\mathrm{m}$ in diameter under conditions where the ratio of the nozzle-throat sides was constant and equal to unity. The distance from the nozzle exit to the substrate was 15 mm, and the stagnation temperature of the gas in the pre-chamber was $T_0 = 500\,\mathrm{K}$. The presence of a shallow peak significantly simplifies the problem of choosing the optimal nozzle, because this is the case where one nozzle can rather efficiently accelerate particles of different sizes.

Figure 3.43 shows the calculation results for self-similar nozzles with a constant ratio of the nozzle-throat sides. The data obtained for 1:1 and 1:2 are plotted here. The distance

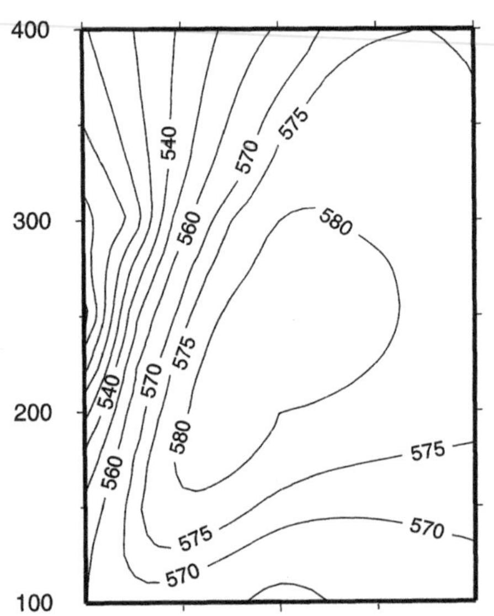

Fig. 3.42. Isolines of the impact velocity of aluminum particles $d_p = 10\,\mu\mathrm{m}$ (the ratio of the nozzle-throat sides is 1:1, $z_0 = 15\,\mathrm{mm}$). The abscissa and ordinate have the scale of $100h$ (mm) and L (mm), respectively.

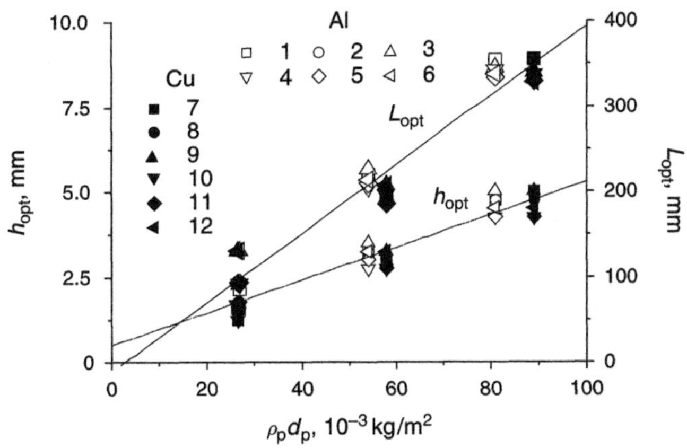

Fig. 3.43. Optimal parameters versus $\rho_p d_p$. The ratio of the nozzle-throat sides is 1:1 (1, 2, 3, 7, 8, and 9) and 1:2 (4, 5, 6, 10, 11, and 12); $z_0 = 10$ mm (1, 4, 7, and 10); $z_0 = 20$ mm (2, 5, 8, and 11); $z_0 = 30$ mm (3, 6, 9, and 12).

between the nozzle exit and the substrate was rigorously set and was equal to 10, 20, or 30 mm.

The optimal values corresponding to acceleration of particles of the same size are almost independent of the ratio of the nozzle-throat sides and of the distance to the substrate. The reason is that the gas and particle velocities are mainly affected by the boundary layer growing on the nozzle walls separated by the minimum gap, and the parameters in the free jet change little for the chosen values of the distance between the nozzle exit and the substrate. The dependences of L_{opt} and h_{opt} on the value of $\rho_p d_p$ in the examined range, as is clearly seen from Fig. 3.43, are adequately approximated by the linear dependences (in millimeters):

$$L_{opt} = 4.06 \times 10^3 \rho_p d_p - 11.7$$

$$h_{opt} = 0.048 \times 10^3 \rho_p d_p + 0.49$$

The values of v_{pmax} are almost independent of $\rho_p d_p$ (Fig. 3.44).

We should say a few words about the influence of particle density. In the equation of motion of particles, the most profound effect is produced by the combination $\rho_p d_p$. Hence, we can expect some similarity in motion of particles of greater density but of smaller size if this product remains unchanged. The calculations confirmed the validity of this assumption. For particles of density of 8900 kg/m^3 (copper, nickel), the calculated points lie on the same line, with the only difference that the particle size is smaller, i.e., the point for the copper or nickel particle 10 μm in diameter lies approximately at the same place as the point for the aluminum particle 30 μm in diameter.

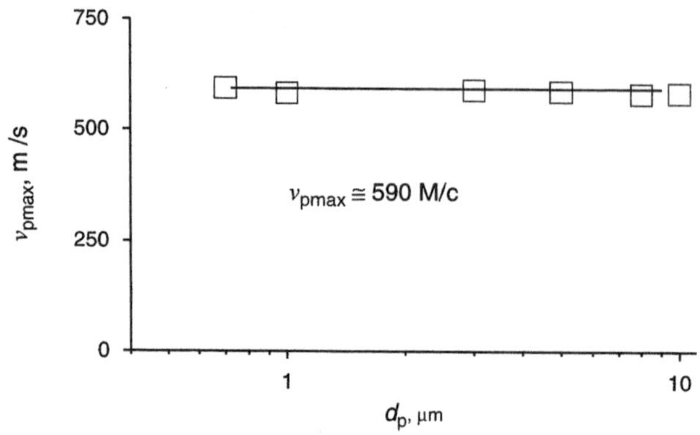

Fig. 3.44. Maximum impact velocity of the particle as a function of the particle size.

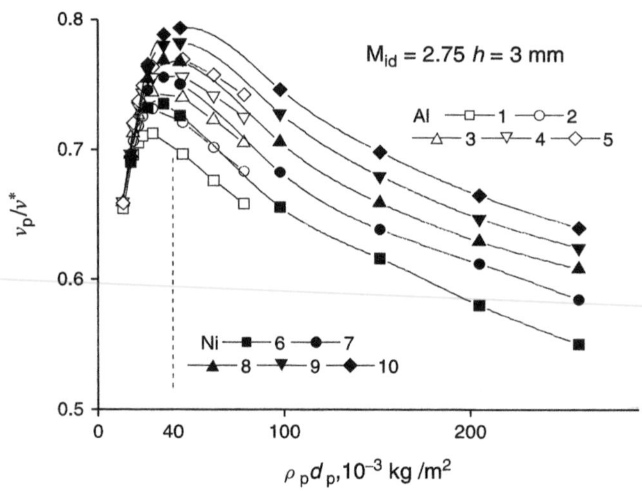

Fig. 3.45. Impact velocity of particles versus their diameter and nozzle length. $L = 60$ mm (1 and 6); $L = 80$ mm (2 and 7); $L = 100$ mm (3 and 8); $L = 120$ mm (4 and 9); $L = 140$ mm (5 and 10); $z_0 = 15$ mm; $T_0 = 500$ K.

To estimate the efficiency of using the nozzle with specified parameters (h, L), Fig. 3.45 shows the calculated results for acceleration of particles with densities of 2700 and 8900 kg/m^3 by an air jet from a typical nozzle used in the cold spray method.

The vertical axis shows the aluminum and nickel (copper) particle velocity normalized to the gas velocity at the nozzle exit, and the horizontal axis shows the combination $\rho_p d_p$. The influence of the nozzle length is shown by different curves. The range of motion of coarse particles is located to the right of the maximum. It is seen that the impact velocity of particles depends on the nozzle length, whereas deceleration in the compressed layer has a minor effect. The range of motion of fine particles is located to the left of the maximum. In this case, the nozzle length has no influence at all, and the main effect is produced by the compressed layer thickness. As the length L changes by more than a factor of 2, the maximums of the curves are shifted insignificantly, indicating that the impact velocity of particles is weakly affected by the nozzle length near the maximum.

The calculations performed verified the high efficiency of the nozzles used to accelerate aluminum particles 5–30 μm in diameter. Nevertheless, successful acceleration of heavier particles (copper, nickel) requires, strictly speaking, the development of another nozzle, because the present nozzle can ensure effective acceleration of heavy particles 3–10 μm in diameter. On the other hand, the present nozzle can be effectively used with finer particles of heavy substances.

The present chapter described the results of research whose ultimate goal was to develop the technique and obtain results on optimization of gas dynamics in the cold spray process. The problems of optimization of the supersonic flow are important in cold spray and allow for improvement of cold spray equipment and technological processes of coating application by this method.

Symbol List

z_0	Distance from nozzle exit up to substrate surface
z_w	Distance from shock wave to substrate surface
L	Length of supersonic part of nozzle
h	Minimum exit dimension of nozzle
l_p	Length of particle relaxation
d_p	Particle diameter
M	Mach number
M^*	Mach number at the nozzle exit
$\Delta v_p = v - v_p$	Relative particle velocity
v	Gas velocity
v_p	Particle velocity
ρ_p	Particle density
ρ	Gas density
μ	Gas viscosity
$Re = \Delta v d_p \rho / \mu$	Reynolds number
C_x	Drag coefficient of particle
b	Breadth of nozzle
b_{cr}	Breadth of nozzle at critical section
H	Maximum exit dimension of nozzle
p_0'	Stagnation pressure behind shock wave
p_0	Stagnation pressure
p_c	Static pressure
p_0'	Dynamic pressure
M_{exp}	Experimental Mach number at nozzle exit
M_{id}	Mach number of ideal (perfect) gas flow
$(S^*/S_{cr})_{eff}$	Effective ratio between exit and critical sections of nozzle
S^*_{eff}	Effective square of nozzle section at exit

δ	Thickness of boundary layer
δ^*	Displacement thickness of boundary layer at nozzle exit
δ^{**}	Momentum thickness
T_0	Stagnation temperature
c_f	Friction coefficient
μ_0	Viscosity at temperature 273 K
T_s	Sutherland Temperature (for air $T_s = 122\,K$)
M_{cal}	Calculated Mach number
F_f	Friction forth
a	Sound velocity
z	Longitudinal coordinate in jet
x	Coordination perpendicular to nozzle walls
$v_l = \sqrt{\tau_w/\rho}$	Velocity at boundary of laminar sublayer
$\tau_w = c_f \rho v^2/2$	Friction stress at surface
$\kappa = 0.4$	Universal constant of turbulent flow
$\nu = \mu/\rho$	Dynamical viscosity
v_{av}	Gas velocities averaged over the cross section of the nozzle
v_m	Gas velocity on the axis
v^*	Gas velocity at the nozzle exit
$v_m{}^*$	Gas velocity at the nozzle exit on the axis
v_{id}	Velocity of ideal (perfect) gas flow
δ_M	Jet thickness along minor size (in direction of x coordinate) defined as distance from jet axis up to point where $M^2(\delta_M) = 0.5M_m{}^2$.
n	Non-isobarity factor
T_a	Ambient temperature
δ_v	Thickness of velocity profile
δ_T	Thickness of temperature profile
$z^M{}_{0.5}$	Coordinate where $M_m{}^2(z^M{}_{0.5}) = 0.5M^{*2}$
$z^T{}_{0.5}$	Coordinate where $T_m(z^T{}_{0.5}) = 0.5T^*$
δ_y	Jet thickness along major size
l_s	Length of supersonic part of jet
p_s	Pressure at substrate surface
p_{sm}	Pressure at substrate surface at $x = 0$
$x_{0.5}$	Half-thickness of pressure profile ($p_s(x_{0,5}) - p_a = 0.5(p_{sm} - p_a)$)
φ_{im}	Angle of impingement
a_{cr}	Critical sound velocity
x_{cr}	Coordinate of the critical transition
x_{ac}	Length of acceleration part
u_{ac}	Velocity at exit of acceleration part
M_{ac}	Mach number at the end of acceleration region
τ	Exposure time
L_1	Length of initial undisturbed part of jet
λ	Wave length between two neighboring tops of jet disturbation
$\beta = 2a_{cr}/h$	Velocity gradient at stagnation point
φ_p	Particle concentration
t_0	Time of probe temperature growth to steady state
$\tau_r \approx z_0/a$	Time of relaxation of gas flow
δ_s	Thickness of plate

α	Heat exchange coefficient
T_{S0}	Initial temperature of plate
$\chi = \frac{\lambda}{c\rho}$	Temperature conductivity of plate
$Fo = \frac{\chi\tau}{\delta_s^2}$	Fourier number
$\bar{T}_0(x) = \frac{T_0(x)-T_a}{T_0^*-_a}$	Relative stagnation temperature
St	Stanton number
$\alpha(0)$	Heat exchange at stagnation point
$Nu = \alpha h/\lambda_0$	Nusselt number
λ_0	Heat conductivity
ρ_e	Density of wall jet at external boundary
u_e	Velocity of wall jet at external boundary
T_w	Temperature of substrate surface
T_r	Temperature of restitution
$\varepsilon = \sqrt{v'^2}/v_1$	Turbulence factor
$St_e = \alpha/\rho_e u_e c_p$	Stanton number
L_s	Length of the substrate
ΔT_{max}	Maximal difference of surface at $z = 0$ and $z = -\delta_s$
M'	Mach number behind shock wave
L_{opt}	Optimal value of nozzle length
h_{opt}	Optimal value of nozzle thickness
v_{pmax}	Maximal impact particle velocity

References

[1] A.P. Alkhimov, S.V. Klinkov, and V.F. Kosarev, *Teplofiz. Aeromekh.*, Vol. 6, No. 1, 1999, pp. 51–58.

[2] G.I. Abramovich, *Applied Gas Dynamics* [in Russian], Nauka, Moscow, 1969.

[3] D.R.Bartz, *Trans. ASME*, Vol. 77, No. 8, pp. 1235–1245.

[4] H. Schlichting, *Boundary Layer Theory*, McGraw-Hill, New York, 1955.

[5] M.E. Deich and A.E.Zaryankin, *Gas Dynamics of Diffusers and Exhaust Nozzles of Turbomachinery* [in Russian], Energiya, Moscow, 1970.

[6] L.G. Loitsyanskii, *Fluid Mechanics* [in Russian], Nauka, Moscow, 1970.

[7] A.P. Alkhimov, S.V. Klinkov, V.F. Kosarev, and A.N. Papyrin, Gas-dynamic spraying. Investigation of a plane supersonic two-phase jet, *Jet and Unsteady Flows in Gas Dynamics*, Novosibirsk, 1995, Abstracts, pp. 8–9.

[8] A.P. Alkhimov and V.F. Kosarev, Laser diagnostics of supersonic two-phase jets, *8th Intern. Conf. on the Methods of Aerophys. Research,* Novosibirsk, 1996, Proceedings, Pt 2, pp. 3–8.

[9] A.P. Alkhimov, S.V. Klinkov, V.F. Kosarev, and A.N. Papyrin, *J. Appl. Mech. Tech. Phys.*, Vol. 38, No. 2, 1997, pp. 324–330.

[10] A.P. Alkhimov, S.V. Klinkov, and V.F. Kosarev, A study of supersonic air jets exhausted from a rectangular nozzle, *9th Intern. Conf. on the Methods of Aerophys. Research,* Novosibirsk, 1998, Proceedings, Pt 3, pp. 41–46.

[11] A.S. Ginevskii, *Theory of Turbulent Jets and Wakes. Integral Methods of Calculation* [in Russian], Mashinostroenie, Moscow, 1969.

[12] G.I. Abramovich, *Theory of Turbulent Jets* [in Russian], Nauka, Moscow, 1984.

[13] L.A. Vulis and V.P. Kashkarov, *Theory of Viscous Fluid Jets* [in Russian], Nauka, Moscow, 1965.

[14] V.S. Avduevskii, E.A. Ashratov, A.V.Ivanov, and U.G. Pirumov, *Supersonic Non-Isobaric Gas Jets* [in Russian], Mashinostroenie, Moscow, 1985.

[15] A.P. Alkhimov, S.V. Klinkov, and V.F. Kosarev, *Teplofiz. Aeromekh.*, Vol. 7, No. 2, 2000, pp. 255–232.

[16] A.N. Papyrin, A.P. Alkhimov, V.F. Kosarev, and S.V. Klinkov, Experimental study of interaction of supersonic two-phase jet with a substrate under cold spray, *Intern. Thermal Spray Conf. and Exposition "Advancing Thermal Spray in the 21st Century"*, Singapore, 2001, Proceedings, pp. 423–431.

[17] I.A. Belov, *Interaction of Nonuniform Flows with Targets* [in Russian], Mashinostroenie, Moscow, 1983.

[18] B.N. Yudaev, M.S. Mikhailov, and V.K. Savin, *Heat Transfer During Interaction of Jets with Targets* [in Russian], Mashinostroenie, Moscow, 1977.

[19] A.P. Alkhimov, S.V. Klinkov, and V.F. Kosarev, *Teplofiz. Aeromekh.*, Vol. 7, No. 3, 2000, pp. 389–396.

[20] A.P. Alkhimov, S.V. Klinkov, and V.F. Kosarev, Research of heat exchange of a supersonic jet of a rectangular cut with a surface for cold gasdynamic spraying, *10th Intern. Conf. on the Methods of Aerophys. Research,* Novosibirsk, 2000, Proceedings, Pt 2, pp. 3–8.

[21] M.Kh. Shorshorov and Yu.A. Kharlamov, *Physical and Chemical Fundamentals of Detonation Gas Deposition of Coatings* [in Russian], Nauka, Moscow, 1978.

[22] V.V. Kudinov, P.Yu. Pekshev, V.E. Belashchenko, O.P. Solonenko, and V.A. Safiulin, *Plasma Application of Coatings* [in Russian], Nauka, Moscow, 1990.

[23] B.N. Yudaev, M.S. Mikhailov, and V.K. Savin, *Heat Transfer During Interaction of Jets with Targets* [in Russian], Mashinostroenie, Moscow, 1977.

[24] I.A. Belov and B.N. Pamadi, *IIT-AERO-TN*, Bombay Inst. of Technology, No. 3, 1970.

[25] I.A. Belov, I.G.Ginzburg, V.A. Zazimko, and V.S. Terpigor'ev, Effect of turbulence of the jet on its heat exchange with the target, *Heat and Mass Transfer* [in Russian], ITMO, Minsk, Vol. 2, 1969, pp. 167–183.

[26] O.I. Gubanova, V.V. Lunev, and L.I. Plastinina, *Izv. Akad. Nauk SSSR, Mekh. Zhidk. Gaza*, No. 2, 1971, pp. 135–138.

[27] E.P. Volchkov and S.V. Semenov, *Fundamentals of the Boundary-Layer Theory* [in Russian], ITP SB RAS, Novosibirsk, 1994.

[28] G.T. Kalghatgi and B.L. Hunt, *Aeronaut. Quarterly*, Vol. 27, 1976, pp. 169–185.

[29] M.F. Zhukov and O.P. Solonenko, *High-Temperature Dusty Jets in Processing of Powder Materials* [in Russian], V.E.Nakoryakov, ed., ITP SB RAS, Novosibirsk, 1990.

[30] A.P. Alkhimov, S.V. Klinkov, and V.F. Kosarev, The features of acceleration of particles in supersonic nozzles of a rectangular cut for cold gasdynamic spraying, *10th Intern. Conf. on the Methods of Aerophys. Research*, Novosibirsk, 2000, Proceedings, Pt 2, pp. 9–15.

[31] A.P. Alkhimov, S.V. Klinkov, and V.F. Kosarev, *J. Thermal Spray Technology*, Vol. 10, No. 2, 2001, pp. 375–381.

[32] S.V. Klinkov and V.F. Kosarev, Computer application for design of COLD SPRAY nozzle units, 6th Intern. Conf.*Films and Coatings – 2001*, St. Petersburg, 2001, Proceedings, pp. 226–231.

[33] A.P. Alkhimov, V.F. Kosarev, N.I. Nesterovich, A.N. Papyrin, and M.M. Shushpanov, Gas-dynamic spraying method for applying coatings, United States Patent No. 5,302,414, *Official Gazette*, Vol. 1161, No. 2, 1994.

[34] A.P. Alkhimov, V.F. Kosarev, N.I. Nesterovich, A.N. Papyrin, and M.M. Shushpanov, Method and device for coating, European Patent No. 0 484 533 A1, *Europian Patent Bullitin,* No. 20, 1992.

[35] A.P. Alkhimov, V.F. Kosarev, and A.N. Papyrin, Prospects of using the COLD SPRAY method for recovery and hardening of parts, *Activities in the Field of Recovery and Hardening of Parts*, Workshop Proceedings, Moscow, Pt. II, 1991, p. 3.

[36] A.P. Alkhimov, A.F. Demchuk, V.F. Kosarev, and A.N. Papyrin, Possibility of using the COLD SPRAY method for anticorrosion protection and recovery of parts, *State and Prospects of Recovery and Hardening of Machine Elements*, Moscow, 1994, Abstracts, pp. 77–78.

[37] A.P. Alkhimov, A.F. Demchuk, V.F. Kosarev, and A.N. Papyrin, Gas-dynamic coatings in power engineering, Regional Workshop *New Technologies and Scientific Developments in Power Engineering*, Novosibirsk, 1994, Abstracts, pp. 19–22.

[38] A.P. Alkhimov, V.F. Kosarev, and A.N. Papyrin, COLD SPRAY method for creating structurally inhomogeneous materials, 4th Intern. Conf. *Computer Design of Promising Materials and Technologies*, Tomsk, 1995, Abstracts, pp. 143–144.

[39] A.P. Alkhimov and V.F. Kosarev, Compaction of new materials by the COLD SPRAY method, Ist Conf. of the Siberian Association of Material Scientists *Materials of Siberia*, Novosibirsk, 1995, Abstracts, pp. 114–115.

[40] A.P. Alkhimov, A.F. Demchuk, V.F. Kosarev, and V.V. Lavrushin, Deposition of current-conducting coatings preventing electrochemical corrosion, Workshop

Automation of Technological Processes on Fuel Engineering, Power Engineering, and Pipeline-Transportation Enterprises in Russia, Design and Technology Institute of Computational Engineering SB RAS, Novosibirsk, 1998, p. 4, Internet journal (http://www.kti.nsc.ru/seminar1998/index2.htm).

[41] S.P. Kiselev, G.A. Ruev, A.P. Trunev, V.M.Fomin, *et al.*, *Shock-Wave Processes in Two-Component and Two-Phase Media* [in Russian], Nauka, Novosibirsk, 1992.

CHAPTER 4

Cold Spray Equipments and Technologies

Based on the results of research conducted at many research centers over the world, several types of equipment have been developed by different companies including ITAM SB RAS (Russia), Ktech Corporation (USA), Cold Gas Technology (Germany), and others. This chapter presents a description of this equipment as well as some technologies as an example of using this equipment.

4.1. Equipment and Technologies Developed by ITAM SB RAS (Russia)

Using results of studies conducted at the Institute of Theoretical and Applied Mechanics of Siberian Branch of the Russian Academy of Sciences (ITAM SB RAS) and presented in Chapters 1–3, number of technical solutions related to development of cold spray equipment and technologies were suggested; these solutions are patented in USA, Europe, and Russia [1–13] and presented in this section.

4.1.1. Development of the main elements of the equipment

The main elements of the cold spray setup are the spraying unit consisting of a pre-chamber and a supersonic nozzle, powder feeder, gas heater, source of a compressed gas, spraying chamber with a motion system, and system for monitoring and controlling spray parameters. The setup should ensure:

- wide-range variation (200–1200 m/s) of the impact velocity of particles $d_p = 1\text{–}50\ \mu m$ with the substrate;
- uniform concentration of particles in the jet with a varying concentration within wide limits;
- constant technological parameters (stagnation pressure and temperature).

4.1.1.1. Nozzle unit

Among the elements of the cold spray setup listed above, the main unit responsible for setup operation is the supersonic nozzle. Based on the research performed, two types of the nozzles were developed at ITAM SB RAS: nozzles with rectangular (Fig. 4.1) and circular (Fig. 4.2) cross sections of supersonic part. As was mentioned in Chapter 3, with the same ratio of the nozzle-exit and throat cross sections, nozzles with a rectangular section can provide, on one hand, a wider spray beam in the direction of the smaller size of the nozzle and, on the other hand, a narrower beam (to 1–2 mm) in the direction of the larger size of the section. Such nozzles can also decrease the effect of particle deceleration in the compressed layer in front of the substrate by decreasing the thickness

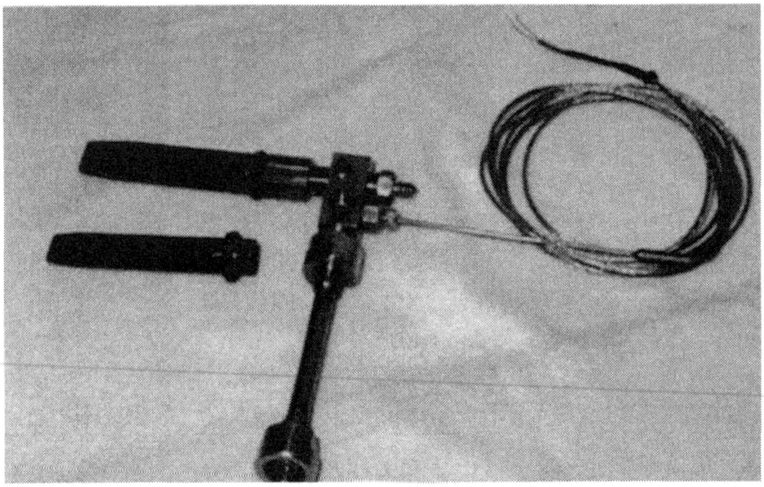

Fig. 4.1. Photograph of the nozzle unit consisting of a pre-chamber with a thermocouple and a nozzle with a rectangular cross section of the supersonic part.

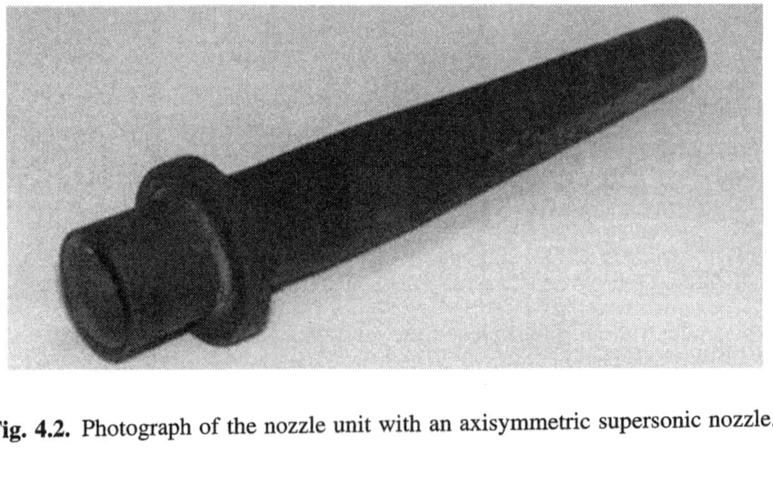

Fig. 4.2. Photograph of the nozzle unit with an axisymmetric supersonic nozzle.

of the layer itself. The typical dimensions: smaller size of the exit for rectangular nozzle was $h = 2\text{–}3\,\text{mm}$, the length of the supersonic part $L = 80\text{–}120\,\text{mm}$, and Mach numbers $M = 2.0\text{–}3.0$.

Some practical applications require nozzle units with high performance in terms of the area covered (m^2/h). In particular, this refers to high-performance application of corrosion-resistant coatings on metal sheets and pipes.

The relation between the parameters of the main elements (feeder, gas heater, and nozzle unit) and the efficiency in terms of mass can be written as

$$P_{\text{m}} = v_{\text{w}} H \delta_{\text{c1}} \rho_{\text{c}}, \tag{4.1}$$

where v_{w} is the velocity of motion of the coated surface with respect to the nozzle exit, m/s, H is the width of the band sprayed in one pass, which is equal to the larger size of the nozzle-exit section, δ_{c1} is the thickness of the coating sprayed in one pass, and ρ_{c} is the coating density, kg/m^3.

The maximum possible flow rate of the powder through the nozzle $G_{\text{p max}}$ is such a flow rate for which the influence of the disperse phase on the flow parameters inside the supersonic nozzle is not very substantial yet. The study shows that this flow rate is approximately equal to one half of the flow rate $G_{\text{p max}} = 0.5G$ determined for a supersonic nozzle by the formula

$$G = p_0 S_{\text{cr}} \left(\frac{2}{\gamma + 1} \right)^{\frac{\gamma+1}{2(\gamma-1)}} \sqrt{\frac{\gamma}{RT_0}}. \tag{4.2}$$

For air:

$$G = \frac{0.04 p_0 S_{\text{cr}}}{\sqrt{T_0}}. \tag{4.3}$$

As a result, the maximum flow rate of the powder through the nozzle:

$$G_{\text{p max}} = 0.5G = \frac{0.02 p_0 S_{\text{cr}}}{\sqrt{T_0}}. \tag{4.4}$$

The efficiency in terms of mass equals the maximum flow rate of the powder multiplied by the deposition efficiency k_{d}

$$v_{\text{w}} H \delta_{\text{c1}} \rho_{\text{c}} = k_{\text{d}} \frac{0.02 p_0 S_{\text{cr}}}{\sqrt{T_0}}. \tag{4.5}$$

Based on this expression, the efficiency in terms of the deposition area is

$$P_{\text{s}} = v_{\text{w}} H = k_{\text{d}} \frac{0.02 p_0 S_{\text{cr}}}{\delta_{\text{c1}} \rho_{\text{c}} \sqrt{T_0}}. \tag{4.6}$$

It is seen that P_{s} can be increased only by increasing the nozzle-throat section S_{cr}, because p_0 and T_0 are technological parameters of the spraying process, δ_{c1} is prescribed, and ρ_{c} is mainly determined by the density of the coating material.

Let us estimate the maximum possible velocity of motion of the coated surface with respect to the nozzle in the case of spraying a coating of certain thickness in one pass for rectangular nozzle. For $S_{cr} = b_{cr} \times h$, $h = 3\,\text{mm}$, $k_d = 0.8$, $p_0 = 1.5\,\text{MPa}$, $\delta_{c1} = 50\,\mu\text{m}$, $T_0 = 200\,°\text{C}$, $\rho_c \approx 2700\,\text{kg/m}^3$ (for Al), and $H/b_{cr} \approx 3$, expression (4.6) yields

$$v_{w\,max} = k_d \frac{0.02 p_0 h}{\delta_{c1}\rho_c\sqrt{T_0}} \frac{b_{cr}}{H} \approx 8\,\text{m/s}. \tag{4.7}$$

The specific feature of the supersonic nozzle is one constant size h of its pneumatic duct over the entire nozzle length from the throat to the exit. As the nozzle-duct width increases, the thickness of the compressed gas layer ahead of the coated surface also increases and, hence, the impact velocity of particles on the substrate decreases. The value of h found experimentally should not exceed 3 mm for finely dispersed powders used in cold gas-dynamic spraying. Therefore, it is necessary to increase the size b_{cr} and, proportionally, the value of H (in order to retain the technological regime, i.e., the Mach number and, correspondingly, the particle velocity).

Yet, a significant increase in b_{cr} and H is not feasible because this will lead to an increase in the angle of expansion of the nozzle duct β_n, which is determined as $\beta_n = 2\text{arctg}\,\frac{H-b_{cr}}{2L}$ for a constant length of the supersonic part of the nozzle. Beginning from a certain critical angle β_{cr}, the effect of the non-uniform distribution of particles over the nozzle-exit section becomes noticeable. It was experimentally demonstrated that this effect becomes substantial for $\beta_n = 10\text{–}15°$.

Thus, it is obvious that the nozzle-throat area S_{cr} is limited and, hence, the efficiency of equipment is also limited. Let us use expression (4.6) to estimate the maximum possible efficiency in terms of area for a single-nozzle setup. The critical angle is related to the nozzle geometry as follows:

$$\frac{H_{max} - b_{cr\,max}}{2L} = \text{tg}\frac{\beta_{cr}}{2}. \tag{4.8}$$

From this expression, with allowance for $H \approx 3b_{cr}$, $L \approx 0.1\,\text{m}$, and $\beta_{cr} = 15°$, $b_{cr\,max} \approx 13.2\,\text{mm}$. Substituting $b_{cr\,max} \approx 13.2\,\text{mm}$, $h = 3\,\text{mm}$, $k_d = 0.5$, $p_0 = 1.5\,\text{MPa}$, $\rho_c \approx 2500\,\text{kg/m}^3$ (for Al), $\delta_{c1} = 200\,\mu\text{m}$, and $T_0 = 200\,°\text{C}$ into expression (4.6), the results are $P_{s\,max} = 0.07\,\text{m}^2/\text{s} = 250\,\text{m}^2/\text{h}$.

For higher efficiency to be reached, the nozzle should have several pneumatic ducts with individual channels for injection of the gas–powder mixture and with a common pre-chamber, so that the exits of the supersonic parts of the ducts formed a common flat duct exit (see Fig. 4.3) with an expansion angle β_{n1} smaller than β_{cr} and with an exit-section width equal to the width of each duct. The angle of expansion of the supersonic part of individual ducts should not exceed the critical angle β_{cr1} determined by the expression $\beta_{cr1} = (M-1)\,26.5°$, where M is the Mach number at the nozzle exit.

The number of individual ducts is determined by the efficiency of the setup and by the width of the coating applied in one pass.

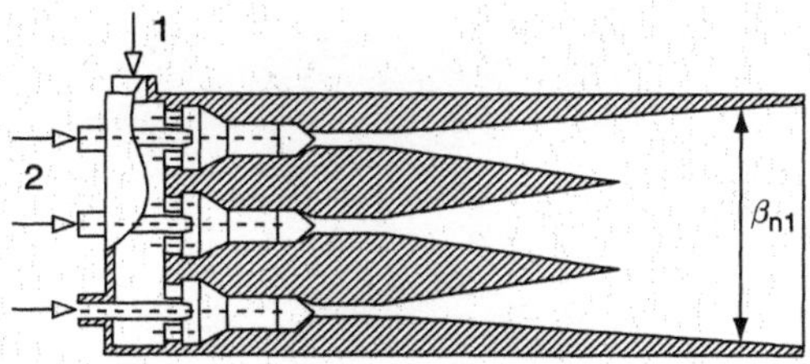

Fig. 4.3. Schematic of a multiduct nozzle. 1 – working gas and 2 – gas–powder mixture.

4.1.1.2. Powder feeder

Another element important for the cold spray setup is the particle feeder, which should provide a uniform controlled supply of the powder into the nozzle pre-chamber. Most powders used in cold spraying have sizes from 1–10 to 40–50 μm and it is difficult to provide a uniform powder feed rate because of its agglomeration. Many traditional powder feeders become ineffective under working with such fine powders.

Based on the research performed, we have developed a drum-type powder feeder (Fig. 4.4). The powder located in a tank (4) falls under its own weight onto the feeder drum (2) rotating clockwise, being set into motion by an electric drive (the latter is not shown in the schematic). The powder is captured by grooves on the cylindrical surface of the drum and falls into the mixing chamber (6) where it is mixed with air (or another gas) and it further entrained into the output branch pipe (7) and then into the supersonic nozzle. The gas moving from the input branch pipe (5) to the mixing chamber removes the powder stuck to the drum teeth. The by-pass pipe (3) equalizes the pressure in the tank containing the powder and in the casing, and the manometer monitors pressure. The drive operating on the basis of a dc electric engine allowed us to change the velocity of revolution of the feeder drum from 0.03 to 0.1 rounds per second and, correspondingly, the flow rate of the powder. A set of drums with different depth of grooves being available, the flow rate of the powder can be changed within wide limits (0–5 g/s). Testing of the mixers–feeders showed their high reliability and the absence of noticeable fluctuations of the particle concentration in the jet. An important factor, especially in experiments aimed at technology improvement, is the possibility of using a small amount of the powder (50–100 g) in this feeder and the possibility of rapid replacement of the powder without substantial disassembling of the feeder. This feeder has a drum with a small number of grooves and ensures an extremely low flow rate of particles, which allows, in particular, its use in experiments on interaction of single particles with the substrate surface.

In some cases, a proportioning feeder was used (Fig. 4.5), which allowed injection of a prescribed (≤ 0.2 g) amount of the powder or a certain amount of particles into the gas flow during a short (≤ 1 s) time. This powder feeder is very convenient under the study of interaction of individual particles with substrate.

It operates on the following principle. When the radial channels of the barrel of the feeder (4) are matched with the radial holes drilled in the casing (5), the compressed

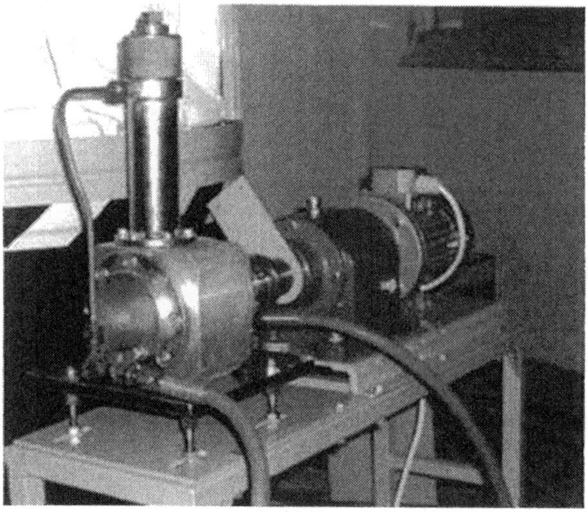

(a)

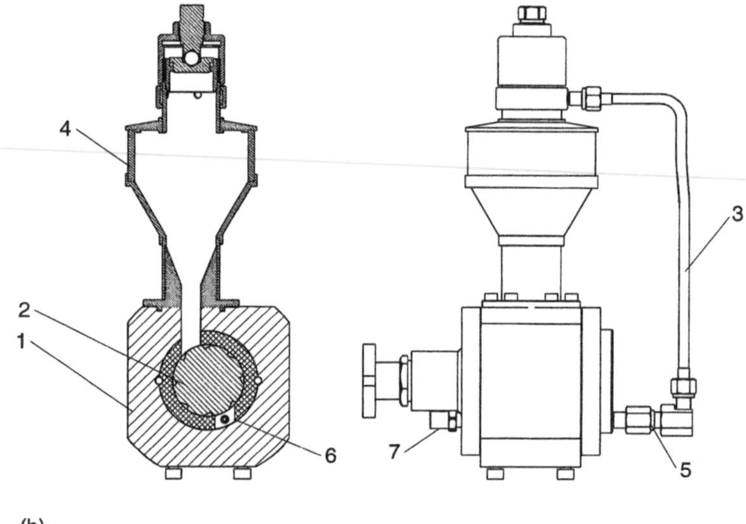

(b)

Fig. 4.4. Photograph (a) and Schematic (b) of the drum-type powder feeder. 1 – body, 2 – feeder drum, 3 – by-pass pipe, 4 – tank, 5 – input branch pipe, 6 – mixing chamber, and 7 – output branch pipe.

gas partly deviates into the channel of the barrel and captures the powder placed there beforehand, when the holes are not matched with the channels and the gas cannot enter the channel. The barrel is turned manually after the operation mode of the setup is set.

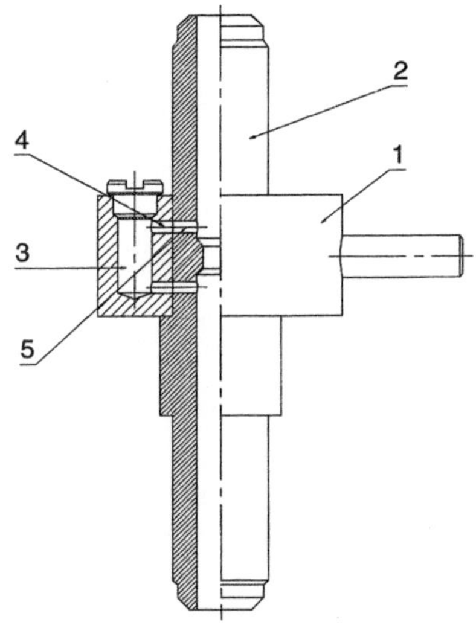

Fig. 4.5. Schematic of the structure of the proportioning powder feeder. 1 – Ring of feeder, 2 – body, 3 – powder hopper, 4 – radial channels, 5 – radial holes.

The proportioning feeder allows a significant decrease in time of each particular experiment. Moreover, as was already mentioned, the amount of the powder sufficient for one experiment is only ~0.1–0.2 g, and this is important in working with expensive powders. In addition, this structure allows rapid replacement of the powder if the mere possibility of applying different powders onto the substrate is checked.

4.1.1.3. Gas heater

The gas heater is used to heat the working gas with a certain flow rate G to a necessary temperature. The heater should satisfy the following requirements:

- it should be simple to manufacture, reliable, and convenient in exploitation;
- it should not introduce significant hydrodynamic resistance into the pipeline;
- it should have the minimum possible dimensions, and the number of energy-intense units should not be too large.

In one of the simplest and most reliable schemes of the heater, air passes through tubes heated by electric current. The tubes (made of nichrome, stainless steel, etc.) are mounted in parallel in a sealed casing and are connected into an electric circuit in series. Cold air from the input fitting first enters the primary contour formed by the casing and the screen and then enters the secondary contour consisting of parallel tubes. This scheme allows reaching a necessary ohmic (dc) resistance of the heater and a substantial decrease in its hydrodynamic resistance. A particular case is a heater consisting of one tube. Such a heater can have the primary contour or be devoid of the latter. Nevertheless, the technique for heater calculations described below is applicable in both cases, because the main heat release occurs inside the tube. Some recommendations on calculating the above-described tubular heater are given below.

Formulation of the problem

The heater was calculated under the following conditions and assumptions.

1. The maximum temperature of heating equals a chosen value (e.g., 250 °C)

$$\Delta T_{\mathrm{hmax}} = (T_{\mathrm{hex}} - T_{\mathrm{hin}})_{\mathrm{max}} = 250\,°\mathrm{C}, \tag{4.9}$$

   where T_{hin} and T_{hex} are the gas temperatures at the inlet and exit of the heating element, respectively.

2. The tube surface (this primarily refers to the heater exit) should not be heated above a temperature determined by the structural strength of the heating element material (e.g., 700 °C), i.e.,

$$T_{\mathrm{wex}} - T_{\mathrm{hex}} \leq 450\,°\mathrm{C}, \tag{4.10}$$

   where T_{w} is the temperature of the inner surface (wall) of the heating element.

3. To provide intense heat transfer from the tube walls to the gas, it is necessary to ensure a developed turbulent gas flow in the tubes, which is reached with

$$Re_{\mathrm{h}} = \frac{\rho v d}{\mu} = \frac{4G}{\pi N_{\mathrm{h}} d_{\mathrm{h}} \mu} \geq 10^4,$$

   where $Re_{\mathrm{h}} = \frac{\rho v d_{\mathrm{h}}}{\mu} = \frac{4G}{\pi N_{\mathrm{h}} d_{\mathrm{h}} \mu}$ is the Reynolds number of the gas flow inside the tube; ρ, v, μ, and G are the density, velocity, viscosity, and flow rate of the gas inside the tube; d_{h} is the inner diameter of the heating element, and N_{h} is the number of heating elements (tubes).

4. The hydrodynamic resistance of the heater (pressure losses) should be low, e.g., $\Delta p_{\mathrm{h}} \leq 0.1\,\mathrm{MPa}$.

5. The total cross-sectional size of the heating elements should be at least two times greater than the nozzle-throat cross section, i.e., $N_{\mathrm{h}} \frac{\pi d_{\mathrm{h}}^2}{4} \geq 2S_{\mathrm{scr}}$.

Law of conservation of power during heat transfer

The necessary maximum power of the heater is expressed in terms of the flow rate, maximum temperature of heating, and heat capacity c_{p} of the gas:

$$P_{\mathrm{h}} = Gc_{\mathrm{p}}(T_{\mathrm{hex}} - T_{\mathrm{hin}}) \tag{4.11}$$

Equating the power and the heat transfer from a unit length of the tube, the results are

$$\alpha \pi d_{\mathrm{h}}(T_{\mathrm{w}} - T_{\mathrm{h}}) = \frac{Gc_{\mathrm{p}}(T_{\mathrm{hex}} - T_{\mathrm{hin}})}{N_{\mathrm{h}} L_{\mathrm{h}}}, \tag{4.12}$$

where L_h is the length of the heating element and $\alpha = \frac{\lambda Nu}{d_h}$ is the heat-transfer coefficient.

For air with $Re_h \geq 10^4$, the Nusselt number can be estimated by the formula [14] $Nu \approx 0.018Re^{0.8}$.

The thermal conductivity λ for air is estimated by the expression [15]

$$\lambda = \mu c_p \frac{9\gamma - 5}{4\gamma} \approx 1.425 \times 10^3 \mu.$$

The dependence of viscosity μ of air on temperature is determined by the Sutherland formula (see, e.g., [16])

$$\mu = \mu_0 \left[\left(\frac{T_h}{T_0} \right)^{\frac{3}{2}} \frac{T_0 + T_s}{T_h + T_s} \right],$$

where $T_0 = 273\,\text{K}$, $T_s = 124\,\text{K}$, $\mu_0 = 17.08 \times 10^{-6}\,\text{kg/m s}$, and $c_p = 1.05 \times 10^3\,\text{J/kg deg}$ (for air).

After all substitutions, from Eq. (4.12):

$$T_w - T_h = \left(\frac{G}{N_h \mu_0} \right)^{0.2} \frac{c_p (T_{hex} - T_{hin})\, d_h^{0.8}}{96.7 L_h} \left[\left(\frac{T_h}{T_0} \right)^{\frac{3}{2}} \frac{T_0 + T_s}{T_h + T_s} \right]^{0.8} \tag{4.13}$$

Condition on the surface temperature of the heating element
With allowance for Eq. (4.13), condition (4.10) is written in the form

$$\left(\frac{G}{N_h \mu_0} \right)^{0.2} \frac{c_p (T_{hex} - T_{hin})\, d_h^{0.8}}{96.7 L_h} \left[\left(\frac{T_h}{T_0} \right)^{\frac{3}{2}} \frac{T_0 + T_s}{T_h + T_s} \right]^{0.8} \leq 450\,^\circ\text{C} \tag{4.14}$$

Substituting numerical values of these quantities, one of the criteria is obtained:

$$N_h \geq \frac{3.125 \times 10^8 G d_h^4}{L_h^5}. \tag{4.15}$$

For a heater with one heating element, the relation between the length and diameter of the heating element is obtained:

$$L_h \geq 50 G^{0.2} d_h^{0.8}. \tag{4.16}$$

Condition on the Reynolds number
Considering the criterion $Re_h \geq 10^4$ in a similar manner, we obtain

$$N_h \leq \frac{7.45 G}{d_h}. \tag{4.17}$$

For a heater with one heating element, we have

$$d_h \leq 7.45 G. \tag{4.18}$$

Condition on hydrodynamic resistance
The hydrodynamic resistance of the gas in the tube is determined by the formula [16]

$$\Delta p_{\mathrm{h}} = \xi \frac{L_{\mathrm{h}}}{d_{\mathrm{h}}} \rho \frac{v^2}{2}, \tag{4.19}$$

where ξ is the specific friction resistance; for $Re = 8 \times 10^3$–10^7, we have $\xi = 0.188 Re^{-0.2}$. Local hydraulic resistance at the tube entrance and exit, determined as $\Delta p_{\mathrm{in}} = 0.5 \rho \frac{v^2}{2}$ and $\Delta p_{\mathrm{ex}} = 1.0 \rho \frac{v^2}{2}$, respectively, can be neglected, as compared to Eq. (4.19).

Substituting all values into Eq. (4.19) and performing the necessary transformations, we obtain

$$\Delta p_{\mathrm{h}} = 0.145 \frac{L_{\mathrm{h}} G^{1.8} \mu^{0.2}}{\rho d_{\mathrm{h}}^{4.8} N_{\mathrm{h}}^{1.8}}. \tag{4.20}$$

For example, formula (4.20) predicts that the hydrodynamic resistance of a tubular heater ($L_{\mathrm{h}} = 5\,\mathrm{m}$, $d_{\mathrm{h}} = 8 \times 10^{-3}\,\mathrm{m}$) heating 0.03 kg/s of air with a total pressure of 1.6 MPa is 0.06 MPa.

Based on the criterion $\Delta p_{\mathrm{h}} \le 0.1\,\mathrm{MPa}$, for an operating pressure of 1.6 MPa, expression (4.20) yields

$$N_{\mathrm{h}} \ge \frac{4.04 \times 10^{-5} G L_{\mathrm{h}}^{5/9}}{d_{\mathrm{h}}^{8/3}}. \tag{4.21}$$

For a heater with one heating element, we obtain

$$L_{\mathrm{h}} \le 8.1 \times 10^7 \frac{d_{\mathrm{h}}^{4.8}}{G^{1.8}}. \tag{4.22}$$

Condition on the open-flow area
With allowance for expression (4.3), condition 5 of Formulation of the problem (at the beginning of this section) can be written as

$$N_{\mathrm{h}} \ge \frac{200 G \sqrt{T_{\mathrm{hex}}}}{\pi p_0 d_{\mathrm{h}}^2}. \tag{4.23}$$

For a heater with one heating element, we obtain

$$d_{\mathrm{h}}^2 \ge \frac{200 G \sqrt{T_{\mathrm{hex}}}}{\pi p_0}. \tag{4.24}$$

Flow rate of the gas in a supersonic nozzle
The flow rate of the gas through a supersonic nozzle is determined by the pressure p_0 and the temperature T_{hex} of the gas in the pre-chamber as well as by the cross-sectional area of the nozzle throat S_{cr} (see Sections 4.2 and 4.3). For operating pressures $p_0 = 1.2$–$1.6\,\mathrm{MPa}$ and temperatures $T_{\mathrm{hex}} = 0$–$250\,^\circ\mathrm{C}$, the flow rate of air through the nozzle with the throat area $S_{\mathrm{cr}} = 9 \times 10^{-6}\,\mathrm{m}^2$ varies within $G = 0.018$–$0.033\,\mathrm{kg/s}$. In the regime with transfer of

the maximum power from the heater to the gas ($p_0 = 1.6\,\text{MPa}$, $T_{\text{hex}} = 250\,°\text{C}$), the flow rate of air is $G = 0.0245\,\text{kg/s}$.

Analysis of compatibility of criteria
For this flow rate of air, criteria (4.15), (4.17), (4.21), and (4.23) are rewritten in the form

$$N_h \geq \frac{7.66 \times 10^6 d_h^4}{L_h^5} \tag{4.25}$$

$$N_h \leq \frac{0.183}{d_h} \tag{4.26}$$

$$N_h \geq \frac{9.97 \times 10^{-7} L_h^{5/9}}{d_h^{8/3}} \tag{4.27}$$

$$N_h \geq \frac{2.29 \times 10^{-5}}{d_h^2}. \tag{4.28}$$

The hatched region in Fig. 4.6 for $L_h = 0.25\,\text{m}$) shows the range of the values of N_h and d_h with which the designed heater simultaneously satisfies conditions (4.25), (4.26), (4.27), and (4.28).

It is seen from Fig. 4.6 that the curves that refer to conditions (4.25), (4.27), and (4.28) intersect approximately at one point. Conditions (4.27) and (4.25) are stronger than the condition (4.28) on the left and on the right of the intersection point, respectively. An analysis of the formulas (4.15), 4.21), and (4.23) shows that this situation is observed for all lengths of heating elements. Therefore, condition (4.28) can be ignored in what follows. Heaters with arbitrary efficiency can be calculated in a similar manner. As an example, Fig. 4.7 shows the ranges of admissible values of N_h and d_h for a gas heater designed for heating 1.0 kg/s of air to a temperature of 200 °C for heating element lengths $L_h = 1.0$ and 1.5 m.

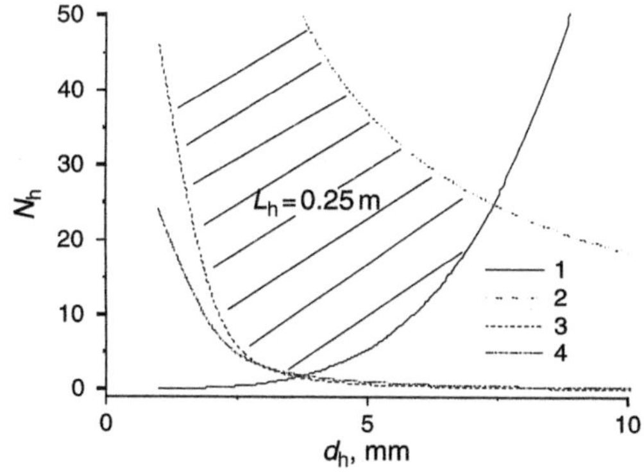

Fig. 4.6. Range of admissible values of N_h and d_h of the gas heater. $G = 0.0245\,\text{kg/s}$, $L_h = 0.25\,\text{m}$. Curves 1, 2, 3, and 4 refer to conditions (4.25), (4.26), (4.27), and (4.28), respectively.

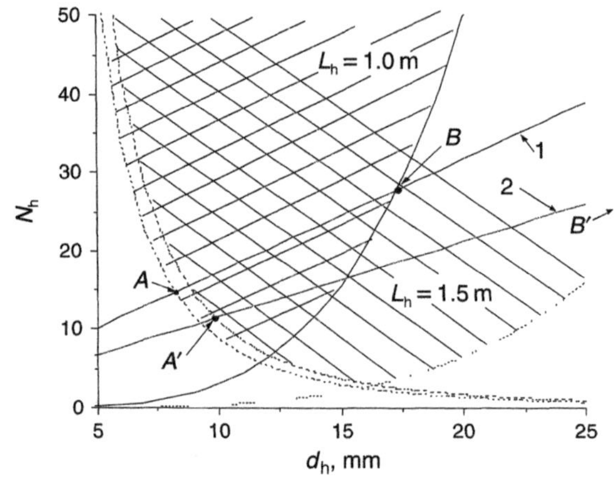

Fig. 4.7. Range of admissible values of N_h and d_h for gas heaters. $G = 1.0\,\text{kg/s}$, $L_h = 1.0$ and 1.5 m.

Condition on voltage applied

The power necessary for heating air to a temperature $T_{hex} = 250\,°\text{C}$ is determined by the expression

$$P_h = Gc_p\left(T_{hex} - T_{hin}\right). \tag{4.29}$$

On the other hand, the power released in heating elements is determined by the ohmic resistance of the heater R and by the operating voltage U of the source

$$P_h = \frac{U^2}{R_h}. \tag{4.30}$$

The resistance of heating elements connected in series is

$$R_h = \rho_h \frac{4N_h L_h}{\pi\left(D_h^2 - d_h^2\right)} = \rho_h \frac{N_h L_h}{\pi\delta_h\left(d_h + \delta_h\right)}, \tag{4.31}$$

where ρ_h is the specific ohmic resistance of the material of the heating elements, Ω m, and δ_h is the thickness of the heating element wall, m.

Equations (4.29) and (4.30) yield the relation between N_h and d_h:

$$N_h = \frac{\pi\delta_h\left(d_h + \delta_h\right)U^2}{\rho_h L_h G c_p\left(T_{hex} - T_{hin}\right)}. \tag{4.32}$$

The straight lines $1'(L_h = 1.0\,\text{m})$ and $2'(L_h = 1.5\,\text{m})$ in Fig. 4.7 show the dependence of N_h on d_h for the following values of parameters: $U = 220\,\text{V}$, $\rho_h = 10^{-6}\,\Omega\,\text{m}$, $G = 1.0\,\text{kg/s}$; $c_p = 1.05 \times 10^3\,\text{J/kg deg}$, $\delta_h = 2 \times 10^{-3}\,\text{m}$, and $T_{hex} - T_{hin} = 200\,°\text{C}$. Thus, for these values of parameters, the relation between the number of heating elements and their inner diameter is determined by the plot in Fig. 4.7: for $L_h = 1.0$ m, the relations between N_h and d_h lie on the segment AB; for $L_h = 1.5$ m, the relations between N_h and d_h lie on the segment A′B′ (the point B′ is located rather far and is not shown in the figure).

Analysis of the single-tube heater

For a heater with one heating element, relations (4.16), (4.18), and (4.22) yield the range of admissible lengths and inner diameters of the heating element. Figure 4.8 shows an example of such a calculation for a heating temperature of 200 °C and gas flow rate equal to 0.0245 kg/s.

It is seen that the admissible tube diameter for chosen conditions is always greater than the diameter predicted by condition (4.24) ($d_h = 4.8$ mm). This demonstrates once again that condition (4.23) can be ignored in calculating the heater.

Practical application

Using the above-described technique, we designed and manufactured various tubular heaters. A schematic and the photograph of one of these heaters, which has one tube coiled into a spiral, are shown in Figs. 4.9 and 4.10 respectively.

The experience of working with these heaters proves their simplicity, safety, and high reliability. In addition (this is particularly important for obtaining chemically pure coatings), ohmic heating does not introduce any admixtures into the working gas and, correspondingly, into the coating.

Development of the basic units of the cold gas-dynamic spraying setup made it possible to pass to design and manufacturing of a wide range of facilities; some of them are described below.

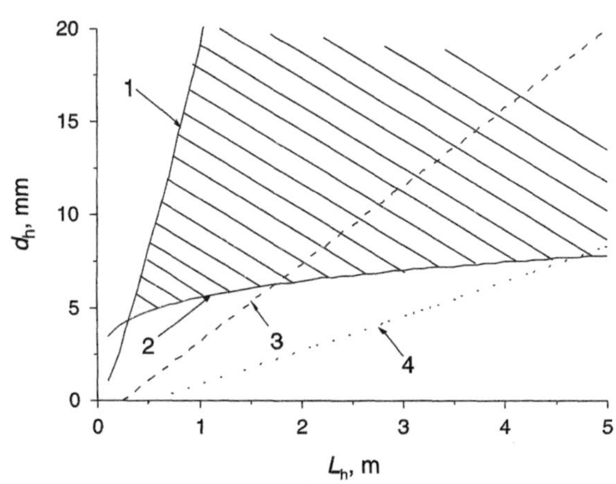

Fig. 4.8. Range of admissible values of L_h and d_h of the gas heater with one heating element. $G = 0.0245$ kg/s. Curve 1 refers to criterion (4.16), curve 2 refers to criterion (4.22), and curves 3 and 4 refer to criterion (4.29) for $U = 20$ and 30 V, respectively.

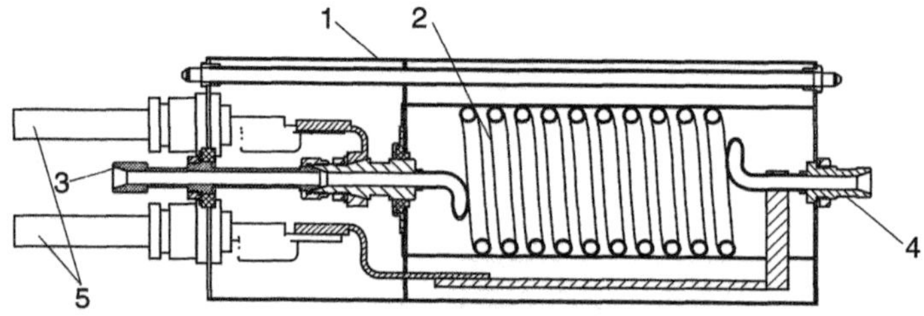

Fig. 4.9. Schematic of a tubular ohmic heater of the working gas. 1 – body, 2 – Nichrome tube, 3 – input branch pipe, 4 – output branch pipe, and 5 – power supply.

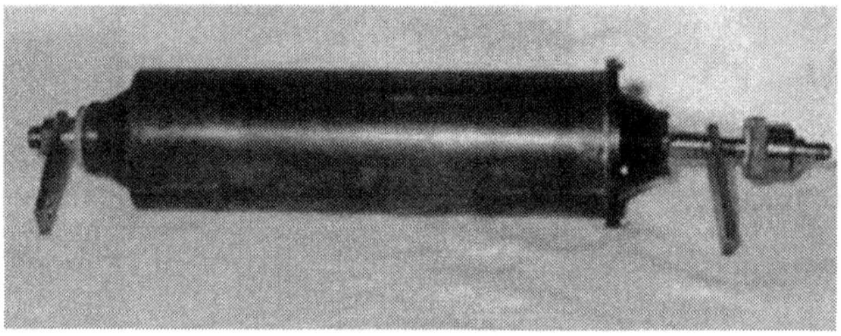

Fig. 4.10. Photograph of the ohmic heater of the working gas.

4.1.2. Facilities for applying corrosion-resistant coatings onto pipes

Development of efficient technologies aimed at protecting steel pipes against corrosion is of significant interest for practice. The comprehensive character of the results described above made it possible to develop the technological processes and to pass to design and manufacturing of equipment for applying corrosion-resistant coatings onto the inner and outer surfaces of long (up to 12 m) pipes.

4.1.2.1. Facility for applying corrosion-resistant coatings onto the outer surface of long pipes

One of the widespread methods of protection against corrosion is applying coatings by various methods: chemical and electrochemical deposition, thermal spraying, etc. The efficient technology is hot zinc and aluminum cladding of the outer surface of steel pipes. Its essential drawbacks (restrictions) are related to complexity and high requirements to surface-preparation processes (including chemical etching), limited possibility of changing the coating thickness, and high expenses on environmental safety of the processes. In addition, this technology has a long response time, i.e., requires much time for launching and, correspondingly, terminating the process (it is necessary to bring a large mass of metal used for the coating to the melted state). The transition from one type of the coating to another requires several hours.

The cold spray technology is devoid of these drawbacks and restrictions. In addition, available technological solutions provide a necessary sequence and continuity of the basic technological operations, including loading of pipes onto the roller conveyer, surface preparation (mechanical and thermal), applying coatings with controlled thickness, rejection and off-loading of the coated pipes into a storage unit. Figures 4.11 and 4.12 show the layout and photo of the setup for cold spraying applying protective coatings onto the outer surface of long pipes.

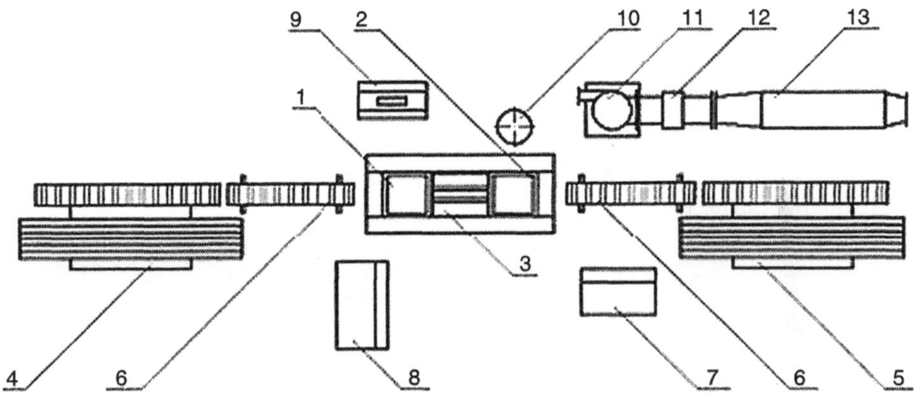

Fig. 4.11. Layout of the cold spray setup. 1 – chamber for surface preparation, 2 – spraying chamber, 3 – drive, 4 – rack, 5 – storage unit, 6 – roller conveyer, 7 – control panel, 8 – electric cabinet, 9 – transformer, 10 – heater, 11 – cyclone separator, 12 – fan, and 13 – filter.

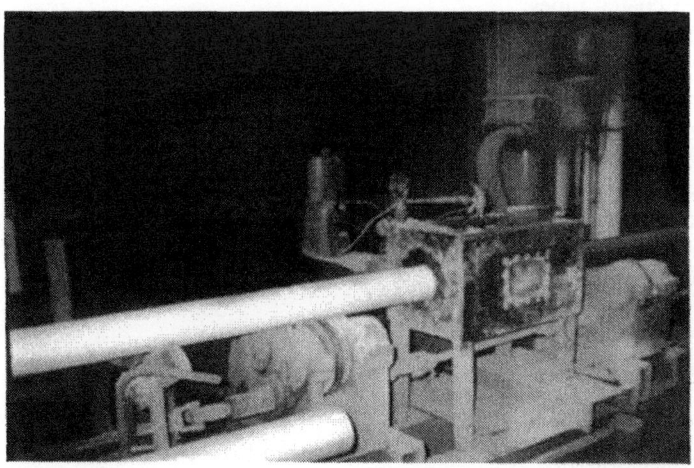

Fig. 4.12. Photograph of the cold spray setup corresponding to the schematic shown in Fig. 4.11.

The setup operates as follows: a pipe 100–250 mm in diameter and up to 12 m long from the storage unit is fed to the roller conveyer and the following devices are consecutively triggered from the control panel:

- dust-removing (exhaust) device;
- drives of needle cutters;
- drive of pipe transportation.

The pipe is set into rotational and translational motion simultaneously (the rotation velocity is set by the drive of pipe transportation and the translational velocity is defined by the angle of rotation of transportation units). When the pipe passes through transportation units with upper rollers, the pipe is clamped by the upper rollers, thus, providing forced transportation of the pipe consecutively through cleaning and spraying chambers. In the cleaning chamber, the pipe surface is cleaned by needle cutters. Particles formed during surface processing by needle cutters are removed (coarse particles deposit to the lower box of the chamber under their own weight, and fine particles are removed by the dust-removing device).

After the cleaning chamber, the pipe enters the spraying chamber with appropriate spraying parameters (stagnation pressure p_0 and temperature T_0) being already set. When the pipe approaches the nozzle unit, the feeder drive is switched on, and the powder enters the pre-chamber of the nozzle, where it is mixed with the main gas flow. After that, the flow with the particles is accelerated and moves toward the nozzle exit, where its spraying onto the pipe surface occurs. When the end of the pipe passes under the nozzle unit, the feeder drive is switched off. Powder particles not deposited onto the pipe surface are removed by the dust-removing system.

Parameters of the setup

1. Efficiency, pipes/h	1–2
2. Size of coated pipes:	
length, m	6–12
outer diameter, mm	100–250
3. Thickness of the deposited layer, max, μm	100–300
4. Deposition rate, m^2/h	3–5
5. Gas pressure in the gas source, MPa	1.6
6. Working gas pressure, MPa	1.2–1.6
7. Working gas temperature, K	300–570
8. Flow rate of the powder, kg/h	2.0–5.5
9. Coating material	Al, Zn, Al + Zn
10. Flow rate of the gas, m^3/h	60–90
11. Required electric power, less than, kW	12
12. Deposition efficiency, %	50–80

The above-described variant of the setup with open-flow chambers ensures the minimum delay between the processes of surface preparation and coating application (from several seconds to tens of seconds). Universal elements of the setup allow its upgrading with an increase in pipe diameter to ~1 m and the possibility of using open-flow chambers of thermal (annealing for elimination of fatty films and pipe heating) and pneumatic-abrasive processing. Moreover, cold spray setups can be readily implemented into available lines of pipe reduction, which allows an effective use of thermal energy and applying coatings onto already heated pipes with different surface temperatures; hence, the coating quality, in particular its adhesion, is improved.

4.1.2.2. Facility for applying corrosion-resistant coatings onto the inner surface of long pipes

It is more difficult to spray coatings on the inside surface of pipes. Currently available thermal spray methods do not allow applying metallic coatings onto the inner surface of long pipes with diameters 100–250 mm. Other methods (electrostatic sedimentation, galvanic method, submerging into a solution, etc.) require large-size expensive equipment, and implementation of these methods involves significant expenses on ensuring environmental safety.

The technology and equipment developed at ITAM [10] allow implementation of low-temperature (with working gas temperatures of 100–200 °C for aluminum, zinc, and their mechanical mixtures) processes of applying economical and environmentally safe coatings possessing wide technological possibilities owing to the use of novel technological solutions based on specific features of the cold spray method. In particular, the basic spraying units are mounted in a moving hollow rod. The gripping-rotating mechanism connecting the sprayed pipe with the dust collector and dust-removing system forms a dust-collecting channel, which allows collecting and repeated using of the non-deposited powder. Coupling of the functions of heating elements and pneumatic pipelines in the gas heater ensures compact location of the spraying unit in the rod and expands technological capabilities of spraying in small-diameter pipes.

The use of this technology and equipment is most promising for corrosion protection of pipes for heat and water supply, oil pipelines, etc., because the service life of unprotected pipes used for these purposes in some regions of Russia is approximately three years. After that, the pipes should be replaced, which leads to significant material and financial expenses including not only the cost of new pipes but also the cost of recovery activities.

A photograph and a schematic of the setup are shown in Figs 4.13 and 4.14, respectively.

The setup consists of the spraying unit with assembly elements providing relative displacement of the sprayed pipe and nozzle unit (1), control panel (2), source of power of the gas heater (3), and the device for removal and collection of the unused powder (4). The spraying unit consists of the frame (5) with the carriage (6) moving along the guides of the frame. The motion of the carriage and rotation of the sprayed pipe are ensured by the drive (7). The nozzle unit is mounted at the end of the rod (8), which enters inward the sprayed pipe. The air pressure at the entrance, in the pre-chamber, and in the powder feeder (9) is controlled from the control panel (10).

The rod (Fig. 4.15) consists of the casing (1), which contains the tubular ohmic heater of the gas (2) and the ball bearing (3), and the nozzle unit consisting of the pre-chamber (4)

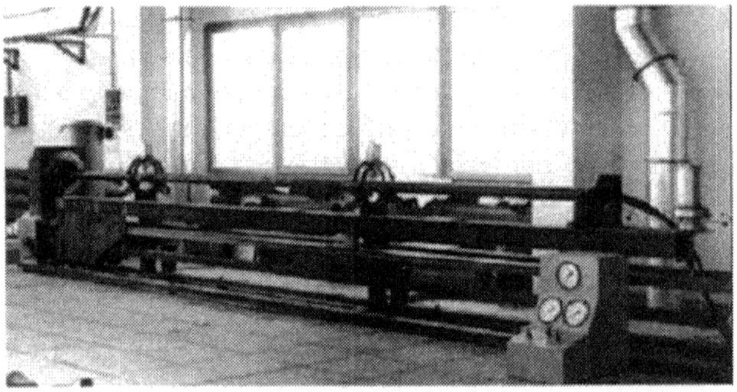

Fig. 4.13. Photograph of the Cold Spray setup corresponding to the schematic shown in Fig. 4.14.

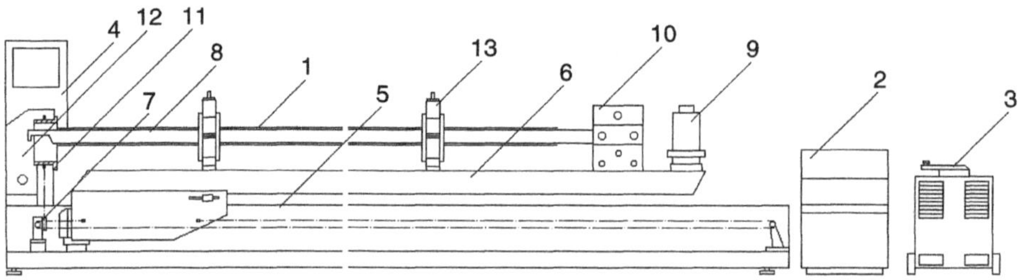

Fig. 4.14. Schematic of the Cold Spray setup. 1 – sprayed pipe, 2 – control panel, 3 – source of power of the gas heater, 4 – system of removal and collection of the unused powder, 5 – frame, 6 – carriage, 7 – drives, 8 – rod, 9 – powder feeder, 10 – panel for monitoring gas parameters, 11 – gripping-rotating mechanism of the tunnel, 12 – dust collector, and 13 – steadyrests.

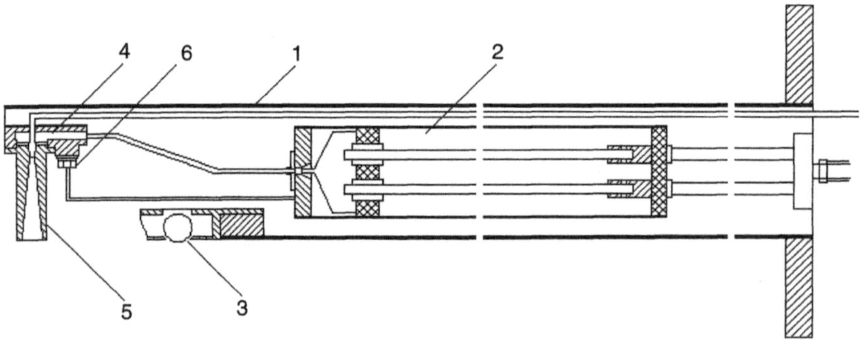

Fig. 4.15. Rod with the spraying unit and gas heater. 1 – casing of the rod, 2 – tubular ohmic heater of the gas, 3 – ball bearing, 4 – pre-chamber of the nozzle unit, 5 – plane supersonic nozzle, and 6 – thermocouple.

and the plane supersonic nozzle (5). The temperature in the pre-chamber was monitored by the thermocouple (6).

The setup is designed for cold spray applying coatings onto the inner surface of long (up to 12 m) pipe with allowance for ecological requirements. This problem is solved owing to the fact that the spraying unit, consisting of the nozzle, pre-chamber, and heater, is mounted in a moving hollow rod and is connected with the pneumatic pipeline, with the powder feeder, and with the panel mounted on the carriage of the traversing gear. The gripping–rotating mechanism (11) connecting the sprayed pipe with the dust collector (12) and with the dust-removing system forms a dust-removing channel, which prevents powder dissemination in the room and allows collecting and repeated using of the non-deposited powder.

The ball bearing mounted at the end of the rod and resting on the inner surface of the coated pipe improves the quality of the deposited coatings owing to a fixed distance from the nozzle exit to the sprayed surface.

Coupling of the functions of heating elements and pneumatic pipelines in the gas heater ensures compact location of the spraying unit in the rod and expands technological capabilities of spraying in small-diameter (100–250 mm) pipes.

The setup operates as follows. The sprayed pipe is placed onto the support rollers of the steadyrests; the rod and the spraying unit are in the extreme right position. The pipe is moved into the orifice of the gripping–rotating mechanism and fixed there. The dust collector with the system of powder removal and collection forms a channel with the inner space of the pipe. By means of the drive of the traversing gear, the rod is moved to the extreme left position in the coated pipe. After that, the system of removal and collection of the remaining powder is switched on, a necessary processing regime is set, compressed air is fed into the powder feeder, and its drive is initiated. The gas–powder mixture follows the pneumatic pipeline and enters the pre-chamber of the nozzle unit; the working gas (compressed air) is also supplied into the pre-chamber through pneumatic pipelines, which play the role of the heater. Simultaneously, the drive of pipe rotation and the drive of translational motion of the carriage and the rod are switched on. The mixture is accelerated in the supersonic nozzle and, owing to the ball bearing providing a necessary controlled gap between the nozzle exit and the pipe wall, is uniformly applied onto the surface over the entire length of the pipe.

Parameters of the setup

1. Efficiency, pipes/h	1–2
2. Size of coated pipes:	
length, m	6–12
inner diameter, mm	100–250
Thickness of the deposited layer, max, μm	100–300
3. Deposition rate, m^2/h	3–5
4. Gas pressure in the gas source, MPa	1.6
5. Working gas pressure, MPa	1.2–1.6
6. Working gas temperature, K	300–570

7. Flow rate of the powder, kg/h 2.0–5.5
8. Flow rate of the gas, m^3/h 60
9. Required electric power, less than, kW 12
10. Deposition efficiency, % 50–80

The use of the above-described setup allows obtaining corrosion-resistant aluminum and zinc coatings 100–300 μm thick and possessing prescribed properties on the inner surface of long pipes. For instance, the powder efficiency is normally 50–70% and can reach 90–95% in the case of the repeated use of the powder collected by the dust-removal system. In this case, the adhesion of the deposited layer to the pipe surface is 20–40 MPa, which is sufficient for many practical applications. The porosity (closed porosity, as the open porosity is almost absent) of coatings is 2–5%, depending on the spraying regime, and this is one of the factors that ensure good protective properties of such coatings.

It follows from the above-given information that the cold sprayed coatings obtained on the setup with the use of air as a working gas, which makes this setup fairly economical, are rather promising for protection of pipes against corrosion in acids and salt media.

4.1.3. Portable setup for cold spraying

The wide use of powder-spraying methods is hindered to a large extent by limited capabilities of setups and equipment as a whole. Therefore, an important R&D problem is improvement of technological equipment for powder spraying and development of multifunctional setups.

The present section describes the results of development of a mobile (portable) setup for the application of powder coatings by the cold spray method. The main objective was to expand the functional and technological capabilities of the cold spray method, including applying coatings onto open areas, in places with difficult access, inside reservoirs, in semi-closed volumes, and for repair and recovery activities.

The setup shown in Fig. 4.16 consists of two portable units and powder feeder (3) connected by flexible pneumatic pipelines and electric cables. One of them (spraying unit (1) is made in the form of a portable handheld tool with remote control and includes the nozzle unit (5), the unit for gas heating (4), and auxiliary elements, such as the thermal sensor (6) and the button (7) for remote initiation of the powder-feeder drive.

The second unit (unit for spraying control and monitoring (2)) includes the system (8) (fed from the mains 220/380 V) connected by an electric cable with electric heating elements, locking-control systems fed from the compressed gas source and connected by pneumatic pipelines with the gas heater, powder feeder, and manometers, and also the gas-temperature indicator (9) connected to the thermal sensor.

Technical parameters

1. Thickness of the deposited layer, μm 20–2000
2. Gas pressure in the pneumatic pipeline, less than, MPa 2.5

3. Operating pressure of the gas, MPa	1.5–2.0
4. Operating temperature of the gas, K	300–700
5. Flow rate of the gas, less than, m^3/min	1.3
6. Flow rate of the powder, kg/h	2.0–10
7. Power mains:	
Voltage, V	220 ± 10%
Frequency, Hz	50 ± 1
Number of phases	1
8. Consumed power, less than, kW	15
9. Dimensions, mm	
length	480
width	750
height	1060
10. Weight, less than, kg	65

To obtain a required (prescribed) coating thickness, it is necessary to form a two-phase (gas-powder) jet with a constant powder feed rate and with a uniform distribution of particles over the nozzle cross section. Experiments performed with laser diagnostics showed that the optimal variant is injection of the gas–powder mixture (from the feeder) along the nozzle centerline. Significant parallel displacements of the injection point lead only to partial filling of the cross-sectional area of the nozzle, to separation of particles (in terms of their size), and, as a result, to uncontrolled changes in the spraying-band width. At the same time, injection along the nozzle centerline allows uniform filling of the nozzle cross section by either fine (1–10 μm) or coarser (10–50 μm) powder. Lateral injection into the supersonic part of the nozzle distorts the flow structure and substantially decreases the efficiency of particle acceleration and, as a consequence, the deposition efficiency.

The small size and weight of the spraying unit are caused by the structural solution of the gas heater, namely, by the presence of several short pneumatic channels in the heat insulator, which ensures low losses of the working gas pressure. The choice of the number of pneumatic channels and their diameter (with allowance that part of the nozzle cross section is filled by heating elements) allows setting the most appropriate parameters of the flow around the heating elements and, thus, significant intensification of heat removal by ensuring a transitional or turbulent flow.

Effective heat removal from the heating elements to the gas allows one to sustain a fairly low temperature of the surface of the heating elements and to supply (if necessary) a higher power to these elements and, consequently, to the gas, i.e., to operate under conditions of an elevated heat flux removed from a unit area. This improves the efficiency and reproducibility of the system as a whole.

The device operates as follows. The control and monitoring system is fed by compressed gas and electric power. The control system defines a required temperature of the working gas, the locking-control system supplies the compressed gas to the gas heater and powder feeder, and a necessary value of the gas pressure is set. When a required pressure is reached in the powder feeder and gas heater, electric power is supplied to the latter. The working gas passes through the pneumatic channels, is heated there, enters the supersonic nozzle,

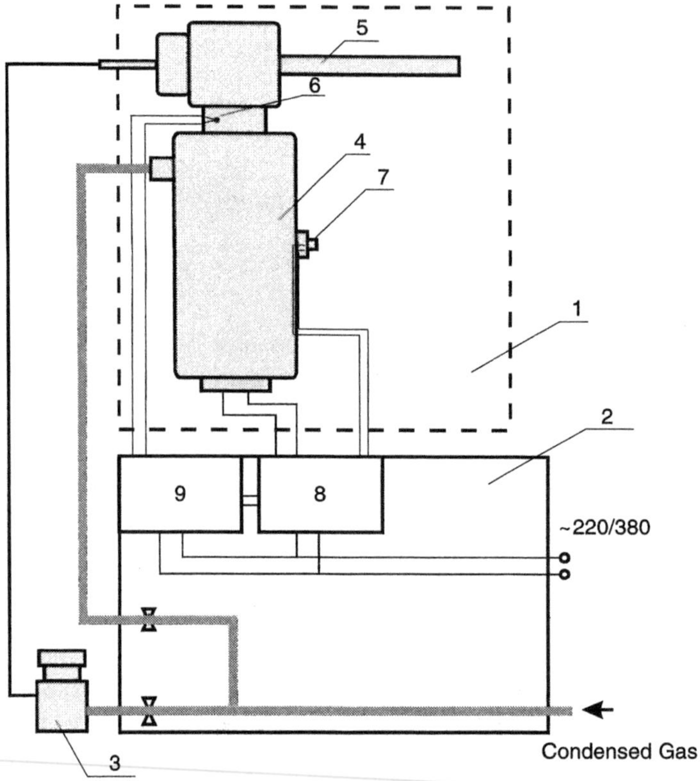

Fig. 4.16. Schematic of the pistol-type device for gas-dynamic spraying. 1 – spraying unit, 2 – unit for spraying control and monitoring, 3 – powder feeder, 4 – gas-heating unit, 5 – supersonic nozzle, 6 – thermocouple, 7 – button of remote initiation of the feeder drive, 8 – electron system feeding the gas-heating unit, and 9 – gas-temperature indicator.

is accelerated to a supersonic velocity, and exhausts into the atmosphere. When the setup reaches a steady-state regime in terms of the working gas temperature and pressure, the button of remote initiation is used to switch on the electric drive of the powder feeder, and the gas–powder mixture is injected into the nozzle along the centerline. The sprayed powder is accelerated in the nozzle, heated by the gas flow from the heater, and deposited onto the treated part. The control system automatically sustains the working-gas temperature.

A photograph of the pistol-type device for gas-dynamic spraying and a statuary element with a nickel coating applied by such a device are shown in Figs 4.17 and 4.18, respectively.

As a whole, the structure of this device made in the form of two units functionally connected by flexible elements makes it possible to operate with a significant distance between the units and from the sources of the compressed gas and electric power and to apply coatings to structural elements with difficult access including repair and restoration activities.

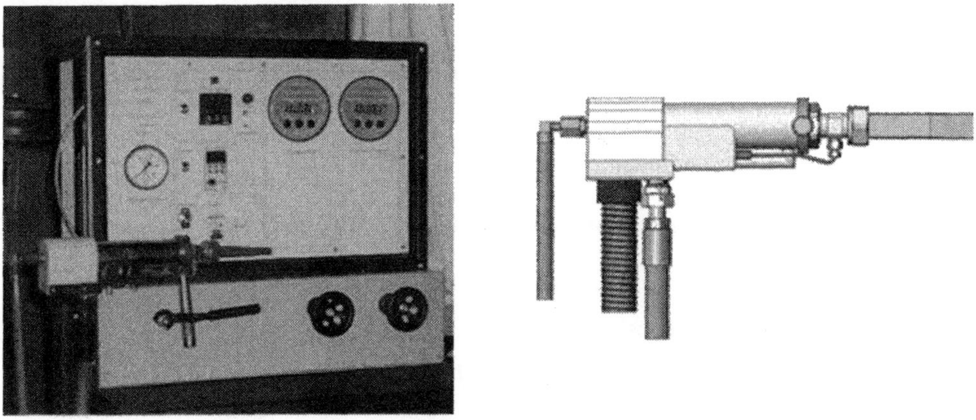

Fig. 4.17. Pistol-type device for gas-dynamic spraying.

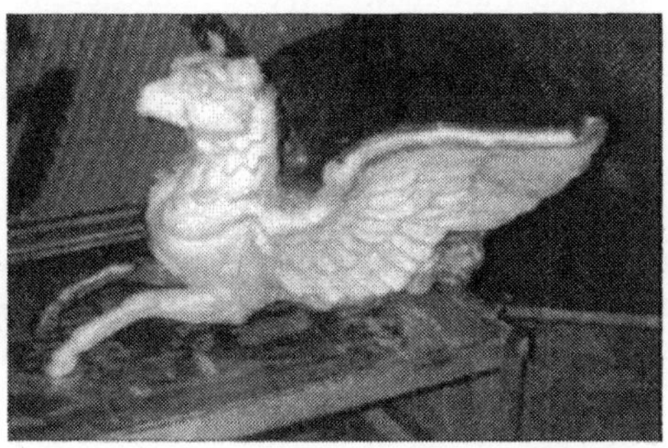

Fig. 4.18. Statuary element coated by nickel with the use of the pistol-type device.

4.1.4. Technologies

As an example of using the above described equipment two technologies are presented below:

1. spraying electro-conductive corrosion-resistant coatings
2. spraying metal-polymer coatings

4.1.4.1. Electro-conductive corrosion-resistant coatings onto electro-technical part

Important structural elements of power engineering systems are tips of connecting cables and connecting plates. In the course of exploitation, the contact of different materials is a frequent phenomenon. For instance, aluminum tips are normally connected to copper buses, etc. The contact between the copper wire of the transformer and the aluminum tip of the cable of the electric mains is a typical situation as well. Under the action of atmospheric moisture and electric current, intense electrochemical oxidation processes occur in such a contact pair, which increases the resistance of the contact and leads to contact and circuit breakdown. Aqueous solutions of acids, alkali, and salts are electrolytes, i.e., liquids capable of conducting the electric current. All types of natural (sea, river, rain, and atmospheric) water and, moreover, technical water contain dissolved salts and, therefore, are electrolytes. To prevent oxidation of contacting elements, it is necessary to avoid the presence of different materials in contacts.

Cable tips and connecting plates are normally made of three types:

1. aluminum (light and comparatively inexpensive)
2. copper (heavy and expensive)
3. hybrid (copper + aluminum, complicated in manufacturing and rather expensive).

Hybrid cable tips and connecting plates are often unsuitable because of their low mechanical strength. The latter is the reason for their damage at the point of welding of aluminum and copper elements, which, in turn, can lead to severe accidents. Tips and connecting plates made completely of copper are rather expensive because of the high cost of copper. Therefore, aluminum tips and connecting plates are most often used, though they cannot ensure the required characteristics in exploitation.

Description of the technology

ITAM SB RAS has developed the technological process and equipment [11], which allows applying a thin (0.05–0.2 mm) and strong layer of copper, nickel, or zinc onto the operating surface of the tip by cold spraying, which eliminates conditions that favor electrochemical corrosion. In this case, there is no need to switch off the mains for replacing or preventive stripping of the tips, the probability of accidents and energy losses are reduced, and 50-fold saving of expensive copper is reached, as compared to hybrid tips. Figure 4.19 shows a schematic of the cable tip with a deposited layer and a photograph of such tips.

Technique for testing tips

Cable tips and connecting plates were tested by a laboratory of the company "Industrial Electric Engineering" in St. Petersburg, Russia. The objective was to verify that the contact joints of the TA 70-10-12 aluminum cable tips and aluminum connecting plates with copper, zinc, and nickel coatings applied by the cold spray method satisfy the requirements of the Russian Standard No. 10434 "Electric contact joints. Classification. General Technical Requirements" in terms of the initial contact resistance (Clause 2.2.1), temperature of contact joints being heated by a nominal current (Clause 2.2.4), and increase in electric resistance after an accelerated test in the regime of electric heating (Clause 2.2.3). The test technique was in agreement with the Russian Standard No. 17441 "Electric contact joints. Acceptance and test techniques."

To determine the initial electric resistance, the contact joints were connected in series; for comparison, this circuit contained a cable conductor equal in length to the contact joint. Contact joints were assumed to pass the test if the mean value of the sampling did not exceed the resistance of the cable conductor whose length was identical to the contact-joint length.

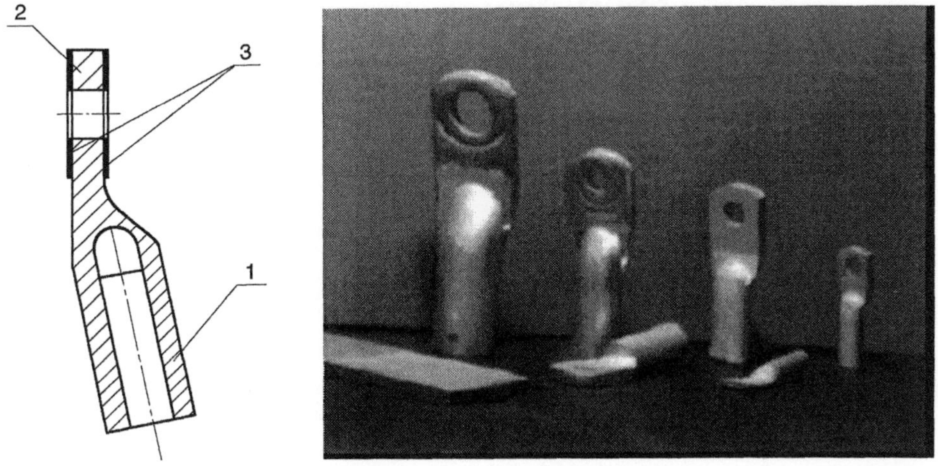

(a) (b)

Fig. 4.19. Cable tips with coatings applied by the Cold Spray method. (a) Schematic: 1 – tail part, 2 – clamped part, and 3 – deposited layer: (b) Photograph of the general view of tips of various types and sizes.

Joints that passed the tests on determining the initial contact resistance were subjected to heating by a nominal current. In the present tests, the heating current was 255 A. Contact joints were assumed to pass the test if their steady-state temperature was lower than 95 °C.

Joints that passed the tests by heating by the nominal current were subjected to accelerated testing in the cyclic heating regime. The accelerated tests were performed at a temperature and humidity of a heated workroom. The testing implied alternating (cyclic) heating of the contact joints to 120 ± 5 °C by the electric current and subsequent cooling to 25 ± 5 °C. The magnitude of the current was established in an empirical manner from the condition that the heating time should be 2–10 min. The number of heating–cooling cycles was 500. Periodically, every 100 cycles, the resistance of the contact joints was measured after they were cooled to room temperature, and the mean resistance of the sampling was determined. Contact joints were assumed to pass the test if the growth of the mean resistance from the initial value was within 50%.

Test results

The results of testing the initial electric resistance R_0, temperature of contact joints T_{rc} after heating by the nominal current, resistance after heating by the nominal current R_{rc}, and resistance after cyclic heating R_c averaged for eight samples for each metallic coating at room temperature equal to 19 °C are listed in Table 4.1.

Contact connecting plates with a cross-sectional size of 50×6 with a deposited copper layer and 50×5 with a deposited zinc layer were tested by the technique described above. The test results are listed in Table 4.2.

Table 4.1. Electrical properties of joints

Contact joint	R_0, μΩ	T_{rc}, °C	R_{cI}, μΩ	R_c after cyclic treatment, μΩ				
				100	200	300	400	500
copper	9.16	41.6	8.7	7.8	8.0	8.4	8.5	8.1
nickel	7.5	43	7.3	7.3	7.7	7.6	8.2	8.2
zinc	7.0	41	6.8	6.9	7.1	7.2	7.7	7.8
cable conductor	12.0							

Table 4.2. Electrical properties of connecting plates

Contact joint	R_0, μΩ	T_{rc}, °C	R_{cI}, μΩ	R_c after cyclic treatment, μΩ				
				100	200	300	400	500
copper	6.9	74	7.5	7.6	8.0	7.9	7.9	7.8
zinc	5.0	76	5.7	5.8	6.0	6.0	6.1	6.1
cable conductor	7.0							

The tests showed that the contact joints of aluminum cable tips with copper, nickel, and zinc coatings and the contact joints of aluminum plates with copper and zinc coatings satisfy the requirements of Clause 2.2.1 in terms of the initial electric resistance, Clause 2.2.4 in terms of temperature under the action of the nominal current, and Clause 2.2.3 in terms of electric resistance after cyclic heating tests of the Russian Standard No. 10434.

Metallographic research with the use of an electron-scanning microscope was performed in a laboratory of the French Department of the TAFA Corp. The conclusions made in the laboratory indicate that the coating is characterized by high quality with minimum porosity similar to that of plasma coatings obtained under conditions of dynamic vacuum. In addition, the contact surface between the basic material and coating is intact and unbroken. There are no visible signs of oxidation.

The materials presented show that cold spray application of a thin copper layer onto aluminum tips reduces copper consumption by a factor of 50, the technical characteristics are close to those of copper tips, and the net cost is close to that of aluminum tips.

4.1.4.2. Metal–polymer coatings and their properties

Metal–polymer composites refer to promising objects of advanced material science. By changing the fraction of the interphase component, it becomes possible to affect the electro-physical, physicomechanical, and chemical parameters of materials. This is the path to creating new materials with unique controlled characteristics.

This section presents some features of cold spray applying coatings made of specially prepared composite powders (copper + polytetrafluoroethylene (PTFE)) and the basic properties of such coatings. The objective was to develop coatings [17] that have low friction and simultaneously high conductivity, which allows the use of these coatings as antifriction current-conducting coatings.

Experimental setup
The experimental studies on application of metal–polymer (copper + PTFE) coatings were performed on a cold spray setup shown schematically in Fig. 4.20. The setup was equipped by feeders forming multispecies powder mixtures and ensured a wide range of dynamic and temperature parameters.

At the first stage, we considered the behavior of fine PTFE of the "Forum" brand: its separation into portions and feeding into the pneumatic pipeline, formation of a subsonic and then supersonic gas–powder flow, and interaction of the latter with the substrate surface under conditions of shock loading.

The experiments showed that physicochemical activation caused by shock interaction of PTFE particles with the substrate is insufficient for formation of strong-adhesion coatings of practical interest. Yet, it was noted that formation of PTFE-containing gas–powder jets becomes much simpler if such a two-phase jet is supplemented by particles of metals, alloys, or composites. This means that a realistic possibility appeared to experimentally study the interaction of multispecies gas–powder flows with the substrate and the formation of metal–polymer coatings and materials.

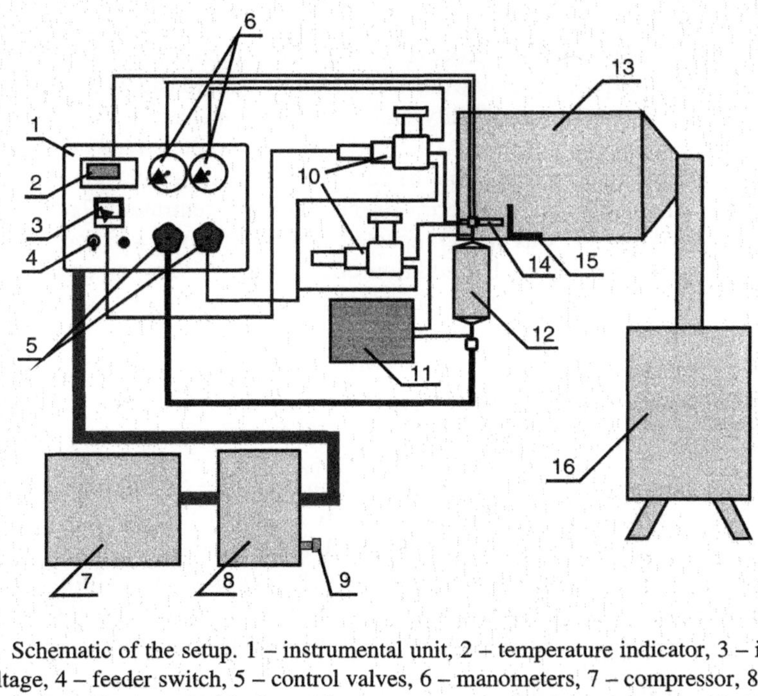

Fig. 4.20. Schematic of the setup. 1 – instrumental unit, 2 – temperature indicator, 3 – indicator of feeder voltage, 4 – feeder switch, 5 – control valves, 6 – manometers, 7 – compressor, 8 – receiver, 9 – safety valve, 10 – powder feeders, 11 – power source for the gas heater, 12 – gas heater, 13 – spraying chamber, 14 – pre-chamber-nozzle unit, 15 – traversing gear, and 16 – dust-removal system.

The main experiments were performed with metal–polymer (metal + PTFE) particles obtained by joint mechanical treatment of initial metallic powders (Cu, Al, etc.) and PTFE. In addition to these powders, multispecies composite powders, e.g., with addition of hard materials, such as tungsten carbide, and more complicated mechanical mixtures were used in some cases.

Research results

The metal–polymer composite particles of a particular size, prepared by the technology of joint mechanochemical activation [18, 19], were prior selected (griddled through a 45 μm sieve). The experiments showed that the deposition (compacting) efficiency k_d of particles on the substrate is mainly determined by the PTFE content in the composite. For the PTFE content of ≤ 1 wt%, the compacting process did not involve any technological difficulties. It was possible to apply coatings of thickness $\delta_c \geq 100$ μm with the deposition efficiency $k_d \geq 0.5$. As the normalized weight of PTFE increased to 3%, the coefficient k_d decreased almost by a factor of 1.5 and was close to zero for the PTFE mass fraction above 10%.

For composite powders consisting of aluminum particles (high-purity Al powder (HPAP) and fine Al powder (FAP) and PTFE with an initial concentration ranging from 1 to 6 wt%), the qualitative pattern of the compacting process was almost identical to that for the previously considered materials.

Special experiments were performed to prove that the PTFE concentration is the main factor affecting the compacting process in a given temperature-dynamic regime. An industrially produced (in Russia) powder was added to a composite powder with a known composition and compacting capability and formed the matrix of the coating material. For example, the powder composite Al + 5% PTFE was supplemented by 5 wt%, 10 wt%, etc., of HPAP, which made it possible to vary the PTFE concentration in a wide range with a limited set of composites in terms of the PTFE concentration. The powder of the Al + 5% PTFE composite was not compacted and no coating was formed on various metallic and ceramic substrates, but addition of 5% of HPAP led to persistent formation of coatings. The compacting efficiency increased with increasing HPAP amount. Similar features of the effect of the HPAP concentration were observed both for two-species composite powders such as Cu + PTFE with addition of the copper powder PMS-2 and for multispecies powders such as ($Cu + TiB_2 + PTFE$) + PMS and (WC + Cu + PTFE) + PMS.

Thus, we found definite confirmation of the strong influence of the fluorocarbon concentration on formation of adhesion-cohesion bonds in composite metal–polymer powders upon their shock interaction with the substrate. Moreover, the study performed allowed us to determine the physicochemical conditions of compacting (coating formation), namely, to choose the temperature-dynamic regime and PTFE concentration limits that ensure compacting of multispecies composite PTFE-containing powder materials.

Thus, lots of samples with cold spray coatings with different types and contents of initial components were manufactured to study their physicotechnical properties; some of them are described below.

Physicotechnical properties of metal–polymer thin layers and compacted powder materials

As was noted above, the raw powders of metals, oxides, and fluorocarbon polymer were subjected to various physicochemical actions for preparing composite powders and materials. Therefore, we could expect changes in the chemical composition and other properties of the final product. In particular, joint mechanochemical activation in the ball mill could yield a material including the material of this equipment (steel walls and balls). Changes in the initial crystalline lattice, including partial amorphization, are also possible in cold gas-dynamic spraying. Therefore, a chemical analysis of the above-mentioned substances was performed in addition to optical research (microscopy).

Results of investigations by the method of synchrotron radiation diffraction

The samples were diagnosed by the method of synchrotron radiation (SR) diffraction at the Budker Institute of Nuclear Physics of the Siberian Branch of the Russian Academy of Sciences [20]. Figures 4.21–4.23 show the diffractograms of the raw PTFE powder (Fig. 4.21), copper–PTFE composite made by the technology of joint mechanochemical grinding and cladding of the initial copper and PTFE powders (Fig. 4.22), and coating compacted by the cold spray method from a copper–PTFE powder composite (Fig. 4.23).

A comparative analysis of these data showed that the same PTFE peak (2.45–2.46) is clearly visible on the graphs for the raw PTFE powder (Fig. 4.21) and the composite powder (Fig. 4.22). Figure 4.22 also shows a more intense copper peak (2.09). The diffractogram of the sprayed coating (Fig. 4.23) shows that the initial substances (copper and PTFE) are retained in the coating; no other substances are observed.

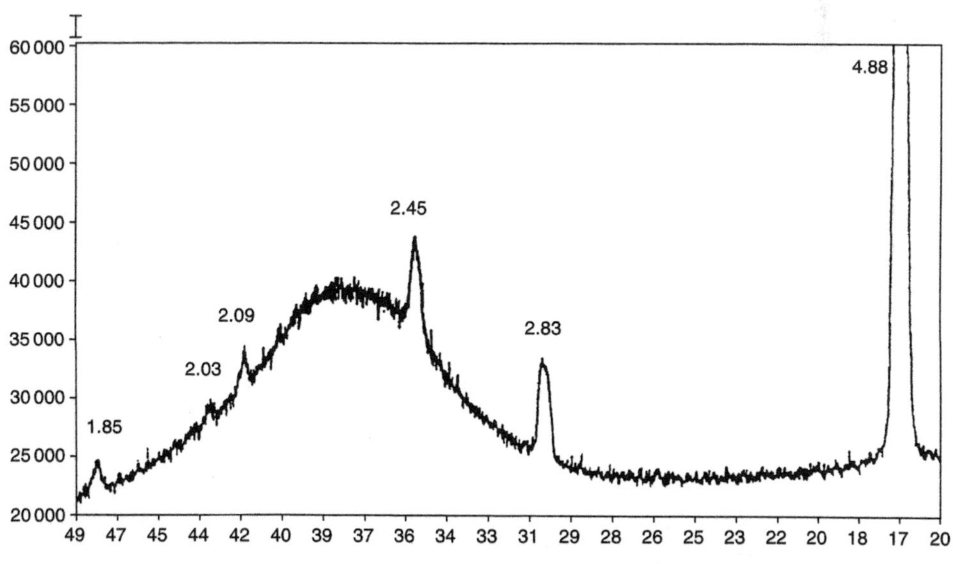

Fig. 4.21. Diffractogram of the raw PTFE powder.

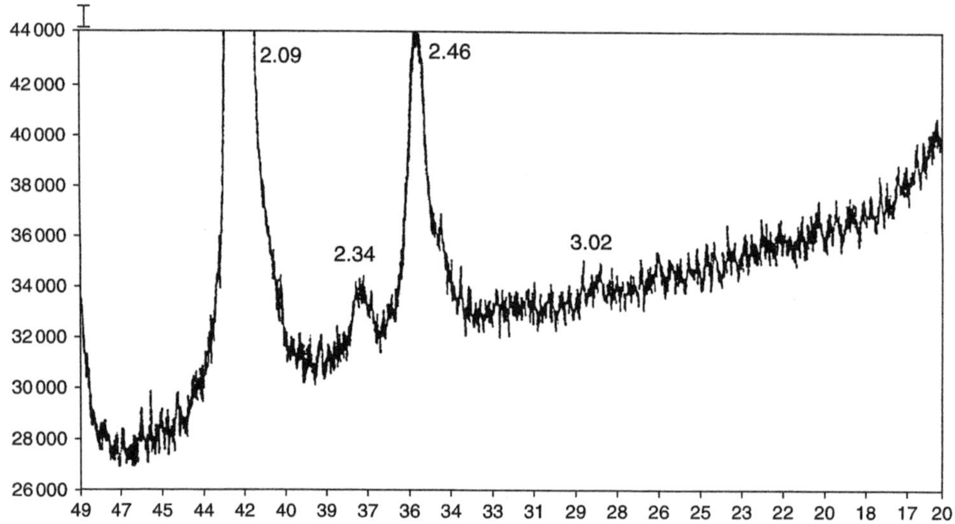

Fig. 4.22. Diffractogram of the copper–PTFE composite.

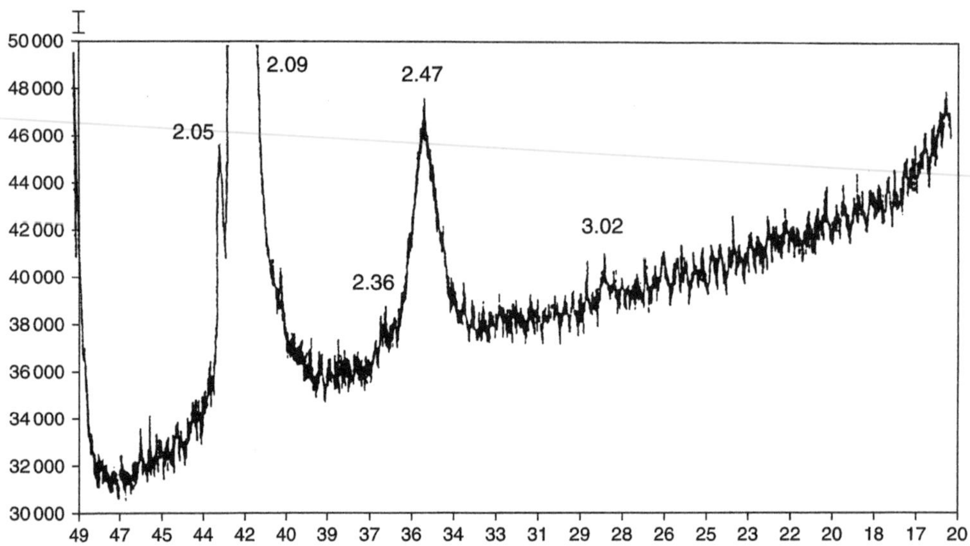

Fig. 4.23. Diffractogram of the cold spray-compacted coating from the copper–PTFE powder composite.

Similar data for other combinations show that the actions applied to raw powder materials and composites do not introduce any foreign inclusions, which could exert a substantial effect on the final product. In addition, a comparative analysis of Figs 4.22 and 4.23 shows that the intensities of the copper and PTFE peaks in the composite powder and in the compacted coating are almost identical.

Thus, we can conclude that cold spray compacting does not result in any degradation of the sprayed powder and does not involve any significant changes in the ratio of the initial components in composite powders. It allows one to create composite materials with particular compositions compacted in the form of coatings and, hence, change the physicotechnical properties of materials.

Some of these properties of particular interest are described below, namely, the adhesion-cohesion, electroconducting, and tribotechnical properties.

Adhesion-cohesion strength
To estimate the strength properties of comparatively thin layers (films), we used the cross-cut adhesion test (grid test) in accordance with the Russian Standard No. 15140-78. Adhesion was estimated by a four-point system. Except for rare cases, no spalling was observed in all grid cells for coatings materials Cu + (1–5)% PTFE and Al + (1–5)% PTFE on substrates made of copper, aluminum, and some of their alloys. For thicker layers reaching hundreds of microns and more (compacted materials), we used the known methods, such as the pin method, the glue method, etc.

Typical values of adhesion and cohesion strength are listed in Table 4.3.

The data in Table 4.3 describe the dependence of the adhesion-cohesion strength on the PTFE content. The strength drastically increases as the PTFE content decreases from 5 to 1% but then remains almost unchanged with a further decrease in the PTFE content. This is typical for both two-species and multispecies composites. Summarizing these results, we should note that copper- or aluminum-based metallic matrices with the addition of PTFE (approximately 1% or less) have a fairly high strength and can be used in friction pairs.

Table 4.3. Adhesion strength of PTFE-containing coatings

Material		Adhesion Strength, MPa	Comment
Coating	Substrate		
(Al + 5% PTFE)	D16	10–15	The powder composition is indicated in brackets.
(Al + 3% PTFE)	–	15–20	
(Al + 1% PTFE)	–	25–30	
(Al + 1% PTFE) + 50% HPAP	–	30–35	Aluminum of the HPAP type was added.
(Al + 1% PTFE) + 90% HPAP	–	30–35	
(Cu + 5% PTFE)	Copper	15–20	Cohesion breakdown, thick layers
(Cu + 1% PTFE)	–	20–25	
(Cu + TiB_2 + 1% PTFE)	–	20–25	Copper of the PMS-2 type was added
(WC + Cu + 0.1% PTFE)	–	30–35	
(Cu + TiB_2 + 1% PTFE) + 40% Cu	–	25–30	Cohesion breakdown, thick layers
(Cu + TiB_2 + 0.1% PTFE) + 40% Cu	–	30-40	

Electric resistance of composite materials

The electric conductivity of the powder compositions Al + PTFE and Cu + PTFE was measured by a micrometer on samples whose substrate was Al_2O_3 ceramics. To reduce the relative measurement error (the error was $\pm 2\,\mu\Omega$), we used coatings shaped as rectangular stripes with small thickness $\delta_c = 30$–$100\,\mu m$, length of 80–100 mm, and width of 5 mm. These geometric parameters were chosen so that we could expect the electric conductivity of the samples to be in the interval 5–$10 \times 10^{-3}\,\Omega$ and higher. The specific resistance of composite coatings (Al + 1% PTFE) + 90% HPAP at 20 °C was 2.9 $\mu\Omega$ cm, which almost coincides with the specific electric conductivity of the raw material such as A5 used to prepare the Al powder (equal to 2.8 $\mu\Omega$ cm at 20 °C). For PTFE-containing copper composites with a standard PMS-2 powder containing 99.6% of copper, (Cu + 1% PTFE) + 90% Cu, (Cu + TiB_2 + 0.1% PTFE), and (WC + Cu + 0.1% PTFE) + 40% Cu, the specific resistance was 1.75–1.8 $\mu\Omega$ cm. The specific resistance of copper used to prepare the powder PMS-2 was 1.73 $\mu\Omega$ cm at 20 °C.

It follows from the data presented that PTFE addition ($\approx$1%) to current-conducting powders increases the specific electric resistance insignificantly, within 1–4% and less, and is mainly determined by the type of the material of the metallic matrix. Hence, we can conclude that composite materials compacted by the gas-dynamic method in the form of coatings can be used in various systems of sliding current contacts.

Tribotechnical properties of PTFE-containing coatings

As was already noted, PTFE has one of the lowest coefficients of dry friction. Therefore, it is of interest to study the possibility of using this material in composite coatings.

Testing of samples of composite powders containing copper, tungsten carbide, and PTFE of the "Forum" brand proved their high resistance to wear. For this reason, they were chosen as a basis for obtaining coating samples with the addition of the industrially produced copper powder and determining the friction coefficient.

As an example, Fig. 4.24 shows the friction coefficient as a function of loading in the case with minimum PTFE content, $\approx$1%, for composite powders of tungsten carbide WC, copper Cu, PTFE, and addition of the copper powder such as PMS-2.

It is shown that the PTFE concentration of 0.06–0.1% is already sufficient to obtain the minimum friction coefficient equal to 0.05–0.07 and commensurable with a value typical of friction between pure PTFE and metal. Such a behavior can be attributed to structural non-uniformity of PTFE and its capability of plastic deformation and spreading into thin films, including molecular films.

Modeling of friction of a metal-polymer composite

We consider a metal-based composite consisting of a metal (copper) with grains of a substance with a lower friction coefficient than that of the main bulk of the material; the grains are uniformly distributed over the sample with a volume concentration φ_t. If the PTFE inclusions are uniformly distributed over the composite, PTFE will be uniformly transferred to the surface as soon as the friction surface is worn out.

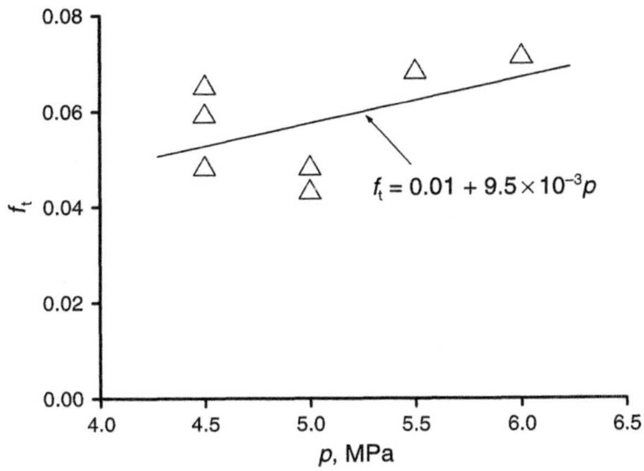

Fig. 4.24. Friction coefficient versus loading for (WC–Cu + 0.1% PTFE) 60% + Cu (PMS) 40%.

Basic principles of simulation

We simulate a composite material sample in the form of a disk of diameter D_m and thickness h_m with a cylindrical inclusion at the center; the inclusion has a diameter d_t and a thickness equal to the disk thickness h_m (see Figs 4.25 and 4.26).

To obtain the volume concentration φ_t of PTFE in the deposited coating, the inclusion diameter should be related to the composite diameter as

$$d_t = D_m\sqrt{\varphi_t}.$$

The dimensionless area occupied by PTFE inclusions in an arbitrary cross section of the sample is φ_t, both in the model and in the real sample.

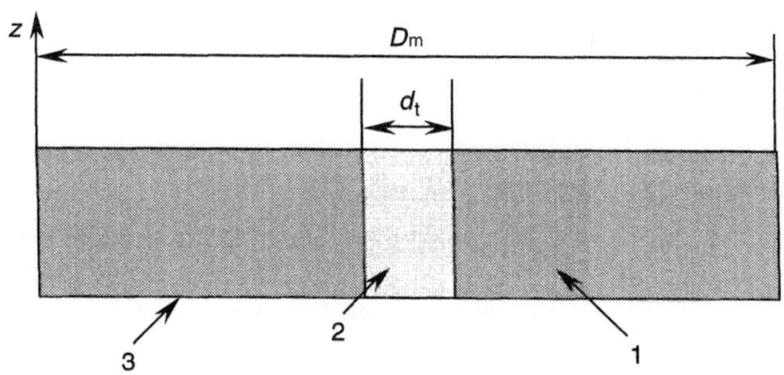

Fig. 4.25. Elementary cell of the composite material. 1 – basic material, 2 – PTFE inclusion, and 3 – friction surface.

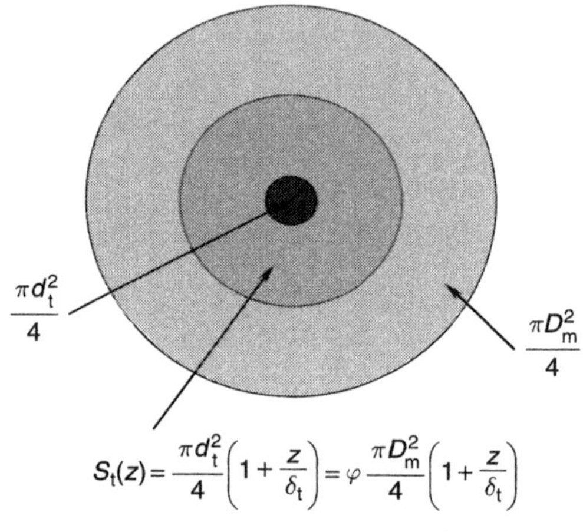

Fig. 4.26. Elementary cell of the composite material.

In the case of linear wear of the composite sample z_{wear}, the PTFE output to the surface is

$$V_t(z) = z_{\text{wear}}\frac{\pi d_t^2}{4} = z_{\text{wear}}\frac{\pi D_m^2}{4}\varphi_t,$$

correspondingly, for a spreading film thickness δ_t, the surface occupied by PTFE is

$$S_t(z) = \frac{\pi d_t^2}{4} + z_{\text{wear}}\frac{\pi d_t^2}{4}\frac{1}{\delta_t} = \frac{\pi d_t^2}{4}\left(1+\frac{z_{\text{wear}}}{\delta_t}\right) = \varphi_t\frac{\pi D_m^2}{4}\left(1+\frac{z_{\text{wear}}}{\delta_t}\right).$$

The dimensionless area of the sample surface occupied by PTFE can be written as

$$s_t(z_{\text{wear}}) = \begin{cases} \varphi_t\left(1+\frac{z_{\text{wear}}}{\delta_t}\right) \text{ for } z_{\text{wear}} \le \delta_t\frac{1-\varphi_t}{\varphi_t}, \\ s_t(z_{\text{wear}}) = 1 \text{ for } z_{\text{wear}} > \delta_t\frac{1-\varphi_t}{\varphi_t}. \end{cases} \quad (4.33)$$

The main assumptions for simulations are as follows:

1. The material wear rate without PTFE inclusions is v_{z0}.
2. As the wear proceeds, an inclusion grain enters the composite surface 3 and spreads over the surface in the form of a film, of thickness δ_t.
3. The friction coefficient of the composite at an arbitrary time is presented as

$$\eta_c = s_t\eta_t + (1-s_t)\eta_m,$$

where η_c is the friction coefficient of the composite, η_t is the friction coefficient of PTFE, η_m is the friction coefficient of the basic material, and s_t is the dimensionless area occupied by the spread PTFE.

4. The current wear rate of the composite material is proportional to the friction coefficient. The PTFE film thickness δ_t is determined by the properties of the material and by the friction conditions (loading, temperature, etc.) and should be prescribed in simulations. In what follows, we assume it to be $\delta_t = 10 \times 10^{-9}$ m.

It follows from expression (4.33) that PTFE will cover the entire surface of the metal-containing composite at a certain value of wear depending on the volume concentration of PTFE and thickness of the PTFE film, and conditions of the minimum friction coefficient and, hence, the minimum wear rate typical of friction of pure PTFE on a metallic surface will be reached. It is necessary in practice, however, that this situation should be reached for the value of wear not exceeding a certain value z^*_{wear}. This, in turn, imposes a restriction on the minimum concentration of PTFE in the composite, which is determined by the formula

$$\varphi_{t_{min}} = \frac{1}{1+z^*_{wear}/\delta_t} \approx \frac{\delta_t}{z^*_{wear}} \tag{4.34}$$

From assumption 4, we obtain

$$v_{z0} = \alpha\eta_m \Rightarrow \alpha = \frac{v_{z0}}{\eta_m}.$$

Moreover,

$$\frac{dz_{wear}}{dt} = v_z\left(z_{wear}\right) = \alpha\eta_c = \frac{v_{z0}}{\eta_m}\left[s_t\eta_t + (1-s_t)\,\eta_m\right].$$

By introducing the characteristic time $t_t = (z^*_{wear})/v_{z0}$ and passing to dimensionless variables $\tau = t/t_t$, $\zeta = z_{wear}/z^*_{wear}$, and $\eta'_t = \eta_t/\eta_m$, we obtain the expression

$$\frac{d\zeta}{d\tau} = s_t(\zeta)\,\eta'_t + [1 - s_t(\zeta)] = 1 - s_t(\zeta)\,(1-\eta'_t). \tag{4.35}$$

Substituting (4.33) into (4.35), we have

$$\frac{d\zeta}{d\tau} = \begin{cases} 1 - \varphi_t\left(1 + \frac{z^*_{wear}}{\delta_t}\zeta\right)(1-\eta'_t) \text{ for } \zeta \le \frac{\delta_t}{z^*_{wear}}\frac{1-\varphi_t}{\varphi_t} \\ \frac{d\zeta}{d\tau} = \eta'_t \text{ for } \zeta > \frac{\delta_t}{z^*_{wear}}\frac{1-\varphi_t}{\varphi_t} \end{cases} \tag{4.36}$$

Solving this equation, we find the time evolution of all quantities of interest: linear wear, linear wear rate, friction coefficient, and dimensionless area of friction of the composite material covered by the PTFE film. Introducing the notation $\tau_0 = \frac{\delta_t}{\varphi_t z^*_{wear}(1-\eta'_t)}$ and $\tau^* = \tau_0 \ln\frac{1}{\eta'_t}$ (corresponding to the time when the friction surface is completely covered by PTFE) and integrating relation (4.35) with ζ replaced by $s_t(\zeta)$, we obtain the dependence of the dimensionless area of the friction surface occupied by PTFE on the dimensionless time:

$$s_t(\tau) = \begin{cases} 1 - \frac{\exp(-\tau/\tau_0) - \eta'_t}{1-\eta'_t} \text{ for } \tau \le \tau^* \\ s_t(\tau) = 1 \text{ for } \tau > \tau^* \end{cases} \tag{4.37}$$

It follows from Eq. (4.33) that

$$\zeta(\tau) = \tau_0 (1 - \eta_e')(s_t - \varphi_t);$$

correspondingly, the dependence of the dimensionless linear wear on the dimensionless time can be re-written in the form

$$\zeta(\tau) = \begin{cases} \tau_0 [1 - \varphi_t (1 - \eta_e') - \exp(-\tau/\tau_0)] & \text{for } \tau \le \tau^* \\ \zeta(\tau) = \tau_0 (1 - \eta_e')(1 - \varphi_t) + \eta_t' (\tau - \tau^*) & \text{for } \tau > \tau^* \end{cases} \quad (4.38)$$

The dependences of the dimensionless friction coefficient $\eta_c' = \eta_c/\eta_m$ and dimensionless wear rate $v_z' = v_z v_{z0}$ on the dimensionless time are identical and can be written as

$$\eta_c(\tau), v_z' = \begin{cases} \exp(-\tau/\tau_0) & \text{for } \tau \le \tau^* \\ \eta_c(\tau), v_z' = \eta_t' & \text{for } \tau > \tau^* \end{cases} \quad (4.39)$$

Results of simulations and discussion

We use the following values of quantities necessary for simulations: friction coefficient of the basic material $\eta_m = 0.3$; friction coefficient of PTFE on metal $\eta_t = 0.03$; initial linear wear rate typical of metal-on-metal friction $v_{z0} = 10^{-6}\,\text{m/s}$; thickness of the PTFE film on the friction surface $\delta_t = 10 \times 10^{-9}\,\text{m}$; critical linear wear $z^*_{\text{wear}} = 100 \times 10^{-6}\,\text{m}$; characteristic time $t_t = 100\,\text{s}$; the volume concentration of PTFE inclusions in the course of simulations will be varied around the value of $\varphi_{t\,\text{min}}$ determined by Eq. (4.34).

Figures 4.27–4.29 show the effect of the dimensionless time on the dimensionless area of the friction surface occupied by PTFE (Fig. 4.27), linear wear rate and friction coefficient

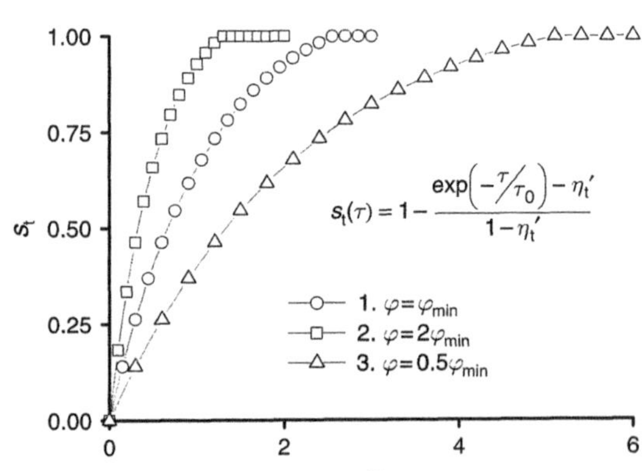

Fig. 4.27. Dimensionless area of the friction surface of the composite material occupied by PTFE versus dimensionless time. 1 – $\varphi_t = \varphi_{\text{tmin}}$, $\tau_0 = 1.1$, $\tau^* = 2.56$, $t^* = 256\,\text{s}$; 2 – $\varphi_t = 2\,\varphi_{\text{tmin}}$, $\tau_0 = 0.55$, $\tau^* = 1.28$, $t^* = 128\,\text{s}$; and 3 – $\varphi_t = 0.5\,\varphi_{\text{tmin}}$, $\tau_0 = 2.2$, $\tau^* = 5.12$, $t^* = 512\,\text{s}$.

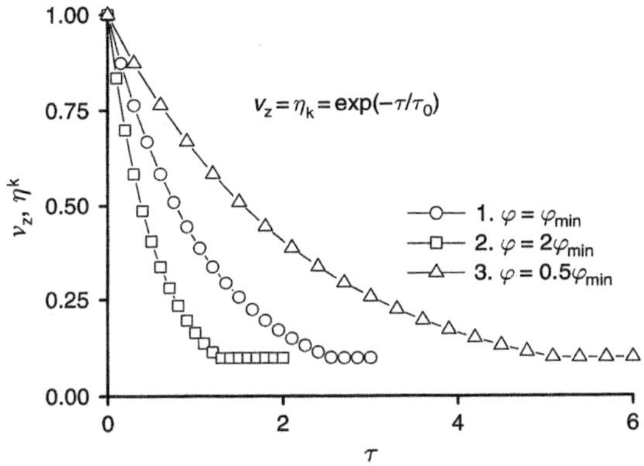

Fig. 4.28. Dimensionless linear wear rate and friction coefficient of the composite material versus dimensionless time. 1 – $\varphi_t = \varphi_{tmin}$, $\tau_0 = 1.1$, $\tau^* = 2.56$, $t^* = 256$ s; 2 – $\varphi_t = 2\ \varphi_{tmin}$, $\tau_0 = 0.55$, $\tau^* = 1.28$, $t^* = 128$ s; and 3 – $\varphi_t = 0.5\ \varphi_{tmin}$; $\tau_0 = 2.2$, $\tau^* = 5.12$, $t^* = 512$ s.

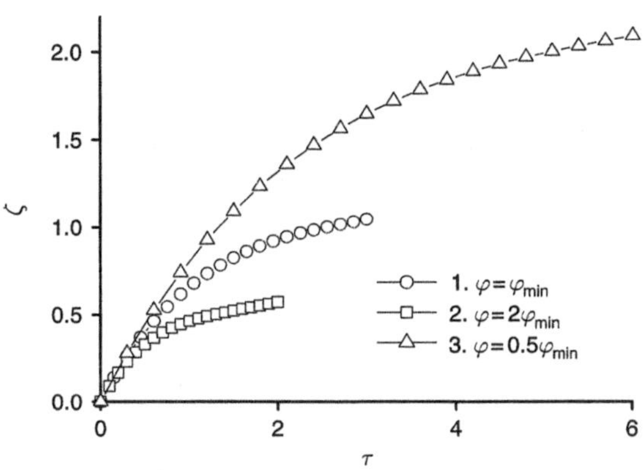

Fig. 4.29. Dimensionless linear wear of the composite material versus dimensionless time. 1 – $\varphi_t = \varphi_{tmin}$, $\tau_0 = 1.1$, $\tau^* = 2.56$, $t^* = 256$ s; 2 – $\varphi_t = 2\ \varphi_{tmin}$, $\tau_0 = 0.55$, $\tau^* = 1.28$, $t^* = 128$ s; and 3 – $\varphi_t = 0.5\ \varphi_{tmin}$, $\tau_0 = 2.2$, $\tau^* = 5.12$, $t^* = 512$ s.

(Fig. 4.28), and linear wear (Fig. 4.29) of the composite material for different volume concentrations of PTFE inclusions.

It is seen from Figs. 4.27–4.29 that conditions for reaching very low values of linear wear of the metal–polymer material and its friction coefficient η close to the PTFE friction coefficient (see Fig. 4.28) are obtained with a sufficiently low volume concentration of PTFE in the composite material, $\varphi \approx 0.5 \times 10^{-4}$, and after a certain time (delay or induction time) from the beginning of the friction process.

The results show (Fig. 4.27) that the tribotechnical parameters are time-dependent because the portion of the friction surface covered by a thin PTFE film increases in the course of friction. A comparison of results plotted in Figs 4.27–4.29 shows that the highest tribotechnical properties are reached in several minutes, when the friction surface is almost completely covered by the PTFE film.

The minimum volume concentration determined in simulations, which is sufficient for high tribotechnical properties to be reached, is in good agreement with experimental data.

Summarizing the results of simulations and data on physicotechnical properties of powder metal–polymer thin layers and materials compacted by the gas-dynamic method, we should note that these material possess rather high adhesion-cohesion and strength properties, which allow the use of these materials in friction pairs, high electric conductivity close to the electric conductivity of the raw metals, and low coefficient of dry friction close to the PTFE friction coefficient. Addition of small amounts of finely dispersed powders of metal carbides, borides, and similar materials to the powder mixtures offers significant expansion of the range of reachable technical parameters, including wear resistance, hardness, etc., without changing the electric conductivity and friction coefficient of the parts.

4.2. Eqiupment and Technologies Developed by Ktech Corporation (USA)

4.2.1. Equipment and performance data

Ktech's cold spray system consists of the following major components:

- prechamber and supersonic nozzle assembly
- resistive coil gas heater and power supply
- gas control module
- laboratory powder feeder
- process control and data acquisition system.

Ktech has elected to manufacture its components in a modular configuration rather than in a single cabinet to facilitate convenience of installation at the facility. Ktech also designed a compact and lightweight pre-chamber and nozzle assembly and coil heater so that they can be easily attached to motion control equipment to spray complex shapes [21]. Next, the system layout is described followed by a description of the equipment and provide some performance data.

4.2.1.1. System layout

Cold spray systems require the same supporting equipment as typical thermal spray operations, such as an acoustic room, fumehood, dust collection equipment to capture the overspray, gas supply systems, and motion control systems. Outside of the acoustic room

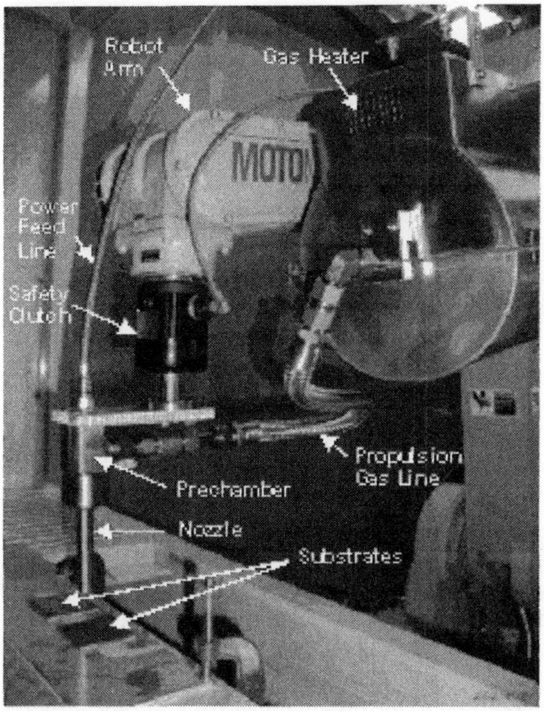

Fig. 4.30. Close-up view of the pre-chamber and supersonic nozzle assembly and resistive coil mounted onto the end effector of a six-axis robot.

are the LabVIEW process control and data acquisition system, the robot controller, and the gas control module (GCM). This system controls all the cold spray process equipment.

Figure 4.30 shows a closer view of the position of the pre-chamber and the nozzle assembly above a planar substrate mounted for spraying inside the fumehood. The pre-chamber and the nozzle assembly are mounted to the end effector of the robot just below the safety clutch. The lightweight coil gas heater is shown mounted to the robot arm above and to the right of the nozzle assembly. A high pressure, high temperature, flexible braided stainless steel hose connects the heater to the pre-chamber and the nozzle assembly. This short distance minimizes heat losses between the exit of the heater and entrance to the pre-chamber. Power is delivered to the coil heater from the power supply located on top of the acoustic enclosure using high current braided copper leads penetrating the roof just above the heater coil. Powder is delivered to the pre-chamber of the nozzle utilizing Ktech's drum type, laboratory powder feeder (not shown) through a 0.125-inch diameter high pressure, flexible braided stainless steel hose.

4.2.1.2. Pre-chamber and supersonic nozzle assembly

Ktech's cold spray system incorporates a lightweight pre-chamber/nozzle (gun) configuration with a supersonic (de Laval) nozzle for spraying through either rectangular or

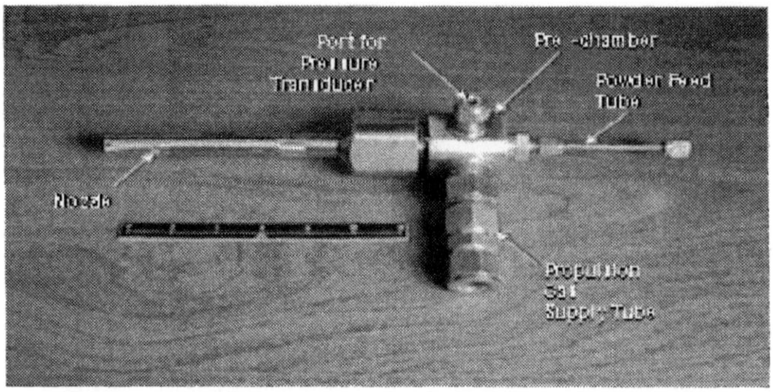

Fig. 4.31. Ktech's compact nozzle and pre-chamber assembly.

circular exit geometry. The pre-chamber and nozzle assembly only weigh approximately 1.4 kg, and are shown in Fig. 4.31. The unit is designed to conveniently attach to the end effector of a multi-axis robot or other motion control systems for versatility.

The pre-chamber contains the inputs for mixing the powders and propulsion gas as well as ports for a thermocouple and pressure transducer for monitoring the temperature and pressure respectively, of the propulsion/powder feed gas within the chamber.

The connection of the nozzle to the pre-chamber is by a conical flange, using a single large nut. The throat diameter of the nozzles is 2 mm. The circular nozzles are of one-piece construction, made of either stainless steel or tungsten carbide, and are machined using standard fabrication practices. The rectangular exit geometry is fabricated in two pieces to achieve the rectangular geometry and welded and machined to the final configuration.

The performance of the nozzles, i.e., particle velocity of copper sprayed for a given set of gas pressures and temperatures, have been benchmarked and compared with data acquired for nozzles used at Sandia National Laboratories (SNL), USA. The performance of Ktech's rectangular and circular nozzles is characterized by measuring the particle velocity profile across the exit of the nozzle using helium and spraying 20.5 μm copper powder at 2.1 MPa, 325 °C at a 25 mm standoff distance. The measured particle velocity profiles plotted as a function of position from the axis of the nozzle are shown in Fig. 4.32. The particle velocity for an SNL rectangular nozzle is also plotted for comparison and, as can be seen, agrees quite well with Ktech's rectangular nozzle. The particle velocity profiles are quite different comparing the circular and rectangular exit geometries. The rectangular nozzles provide a more uniform particle velocity across the exit of the nozzle. The circular exit is parabolic in shape. Both profiles are characteristic of their respective exit geometries. A particular desired spray profile may be obtained by changing the nozzle exit geometry.

4.2.1.3. Gas heater

The gas heater consists of a tubular stainless steel coil resistively by a 480 V, single phase, 25 kVA power supply. The 25 kVA transformer is typically mounted on the

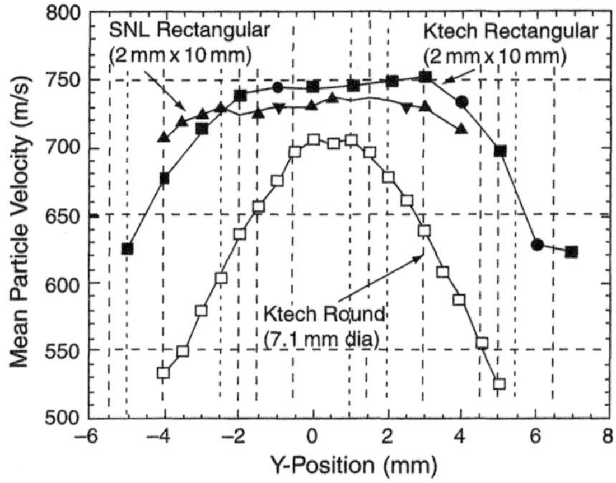

Fig. 4.32. Comparison of particle velocities for round and rectangular spray nozzles.

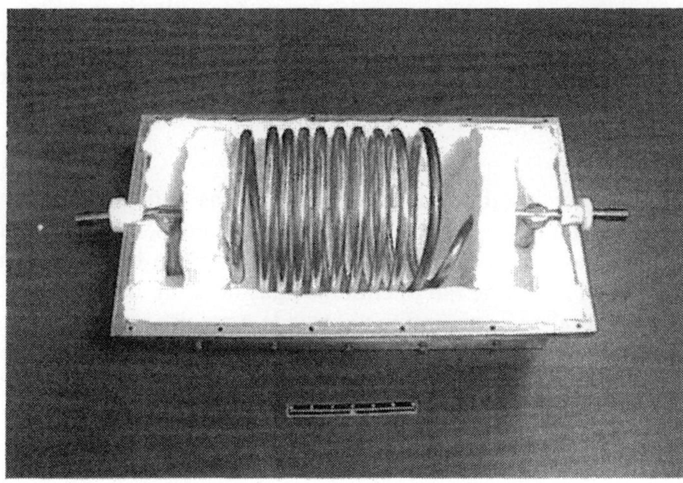

Fig. 4.33. 25 kW resistive coil gas heater assembly.

roof of the acoustic enclosure to minimize the length of the power leads and thus power losses. The tubular heating coil shown in Fig. 4.33 is housed in a thermally insulated aluminum enclosure. The unique feature of this heater is that it only weighs approximately 11 kg. This lightweight allows it to be conveniently mounted onto a Cartesian X-Y system or the end effector of a robot. The heater is capable of delivering 0.15–7 m^3/min of high-pressure gas up to 3.4 MPa at temperatures of up to 500 °C. The propulsion gas is transported from the gas control module to the coil heater via a flexible non-conductive high-pressure hose connected to the stainless steel tubing leading into the sound enclosure. The desired gas temperature is entered through the LabVIEW graphical user interface on the control console. The gas is automatically heated to the set point temperature through instrumentation providing feedback and process control. The temperature at the nozzle is controlled by the data acquisition and control system. A thermocouple installed in the pre-chamber provides a feedback signal to the process control unit that internally compares the feedback signal with the set point temperature. The process controller then provides a signal to a silicon control rectifier to control the current to the coil. A thermocouple is also located on the heater coil near the exit for temperature monitoring.

The heater takes between 60 and 160 s to achieve the process temperature. For a set point temperature of 500 °C, it takes approximately 160 s to reach the process temperature. The temperature can be controlled within 2% of the set point temperature after the system reaches steady-state operation.

4.2.1.4. Gas control module

The Gas Control Module (GCM) is designed to provide accurate gas flow to the nozzle through the main gas line and also to the powder gas line to drive the powder from the powder feeder to the pre-chamber of the nozzle. Gas flow is controlled using high-pressure electronic regulators and solenoid valves to regulate the flow of the main and the carrier gases through the process control and data acquisition system.

The GCM can be controlled to deliver different gases (nitrogen or helium) to the coil heater and powder feeder during the spray process. Table 4.4 illustrates the combinations available.

Pressure transducers are installed in both the main gas and powder gas lines. Check valves are installed for safety. The GCM has two exit ports, one for the main gas and one for the powder gas. The enclosure is configured with a blow-out panel in case of overpressurization and a cooling fan to eliminate gas build-up inside the enclosure. Mass flow meters can be installed as an option to provide a precise measure of the flow rate to the nozzle for main and powder feed gases. The GCM can control the flow of nitrogen or helium gas via the process control system at any time during the spray process. This thereby allows the use of nitrogen to be used for establishing the heater temperature then switching to helium for the actual spray process.

The GCM also houses the OPTO 22 I/O rack containing 15 slots for analog or digital control input and output to the various instrumentation used to control the process functions. The OPTO 22 communicates with the process control and data acquisition system through an Ethernet connection. This helps minimize wire runs.

Table 4.4. Gas combinations available with gas control module

Gas Selection				
Propulsion Gas	N_2	N_2	He	He
Powder Gas	He	N_2	N_2	He

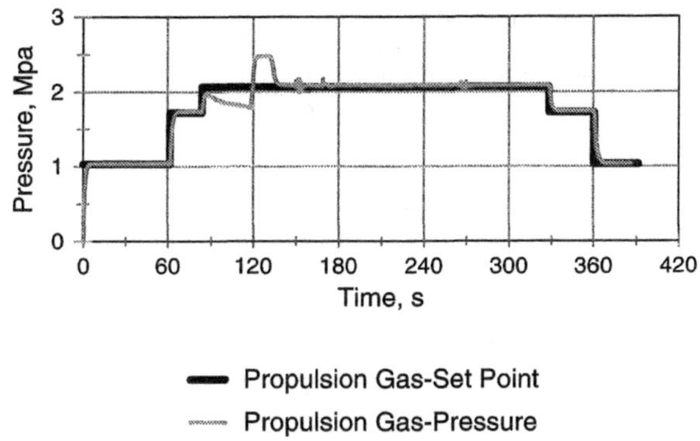

Fig. 4.34. Propulsion gas response to set point pressures.

The process control system very accurately controls the pressure of the propulsion gas. Figure 4.34 shows a plot comparing the set point pressure at 1, 1.75, and 2.1 MPa and the actual propulsion gas pressure for nitrogen as a function of time. As can be seen in the figure, the actual gas pressure responses almost instantaneously to the set point pressure. The perturbation in pressure between 75 and 140 s is caused when the GCM was switched from flowing nitrogen to helium. The pressure can be controlled within 1% of the set point pressure when the pressure reaches steady-state operation.

4.2.1.5. Laboratory powder feeder

With the emergence of cold spray technology, there have been numerous applications that have come to the forefront requiring the spraying of fine (<10 microns) powders, providing more uniform coatings, and improving the reliability in measuring deposition efficiency. The performance of high-pressure commercial feeders on the market today lacks one or more of these desired performance characteristics. Further, researchers are interested in spraying many powders of different materials where the feeder can be quickly and easily cleaned and the new powder installed to facilitate productivity. The laboratory powder feeder (Fig. 4.35) described is specifically designed for processes requiring extremely high operating gas pressures.

The feeder delivers a continuous flow of powder at mass rates between 5 and 10 kg/h to processes requiring up to 3 MPa operating backpressure. The feeder has a variable volume canister design, thus, facilitating short run research and development applications, or higher volume extended run time dispensing. The design features uniform delivery of fine powders with minimal pulsing, easy cleaning, quick turnaround of different powders, and convenience for measuring deposition efficiency without incorporating expensive balance scales or measuring powder flow rates external to the process. A variable frequency electronic vibrator mounted to the base of the main body facilitates uniform delivery of the powder from the canister to the powder feed drum.

The feeder incorporates electronically controlled, pneumatically actuated flow control valves that start and stop the feed of powder instantaneously, and a bypass to depressurize

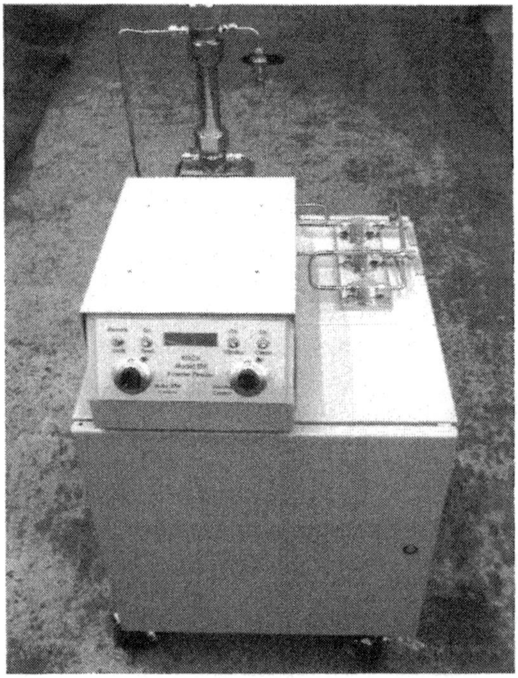

Fig. 4.35. High pressure laboratory powder feeder.

the feeder after each run. This eliminates any spewing of residual powder through the nozzle. The feeder is designed to operate either locally or remotely through an Ethernet connection to the control system. For local operation, a variable potentiometer is provided to adjust the speed of the d.c. motor coupled to the feed drum from 0 to 9.9 rpms. The feeder is an excellent tool for high-pressure cold spray processes requiring the delivery of fine powders with minimal or no pulsing depositing uniform coatings.

4.2.1.6. Process control and data acquisition system

The process control and data acquisition consists of a 500 MHz, Pentium III processor, 17-inch monitor, control and communication hardware, LabVIEW source software, and required programming for controlling the laboratory powder feeder, gas heater, and gas control module. The LabVIEW control system interfaces with the OPTO 22 control instrumentation located in the gas control module through an Ethernet connection. The control system can also provide remote control of optional devices such as Cartesian *XY* system, robot, dust collector, spindle motor, turn table, etc. All the process data can be logged and printed on an Excel spreadsheet or other format and can be plotted graphically. Up to two process functions can be selected by the operator to be viewed real time. This facilitates decision-making during spray operations.

Figure 4.36 shows the graphical user interface with all the numerous control functions (top of screen) that can be managed by the operator. Process algorithms and safety limits

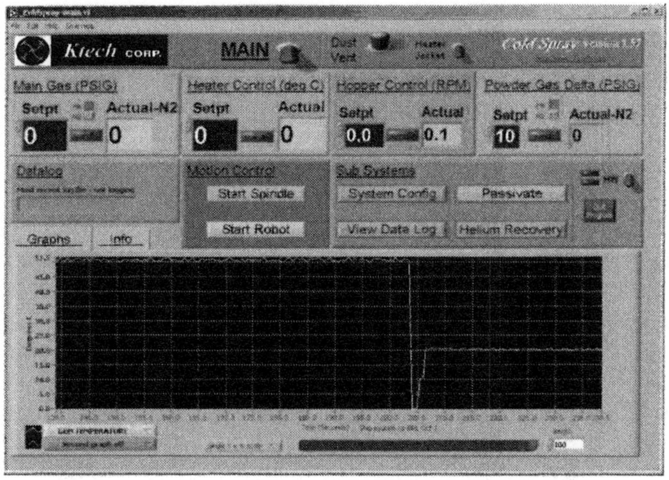

Fig. 4.36. LabVIEW cold spray graphical user interface (control panel).

prevents the operator from damaging the system. In the lower section of the screen is the real time display of process data that can be selected and viewed by the operator.

4.2.2. Spray forming titanium alloys

Based on this equipment different technologies were developed. As an example some results on spray forming titanium alloys are presented below.

Development of new, low-cost methods for spraying near net shapes of titanium and titanium alloys is critical for many industries and applications. Direct fabrication technologies would have an impact on many industries because of the potential to quickly manufacture complex parts or additive features with minimal waste. However, currently used high temperature spray technologies (Lasform, thermal spray methods, etc.) involve melting and solidification. When thermal-spraying titanium, problems occur because of its high susceptibility to oxygen and nitrogen contamination. To avoid oxidation, special equipment and processes such as inert gas chambers (Lasform, deposition in vacuum, etc.) must be used. However, such equipment is expensive to build and operate, thus making the process less attractive to the industry.

More promising for spraying titanium alloys is a cold spray process [22–24]. In the cold spray process the jet temperature is always lower than the melting temperature of the sprayed material providing fabrication of parts from particles in solid state. As a consequence, the deleterious effects of high temperature oxidation, evaporation, melting, crystallization, residual stresses, gas release, and other common problems associated with high temperature methods can be avoided or minimized.

This section presents some results of studies to develop a technology for spraying near net shapes of titanium alloys based on using the cold spray process. Several types of

Ti-6Al-4V powder were tested in experiments. Microstructure, hardness, and porosity of sprayed materials as well as their mechanical properties were evaluated. The effect of post-treatment (heat-treatment and HIPing) on material properties was studied and is reported.

4.2.2.1. Experimental setup

Experiments to test various titanium powders and to develop process parameters were performed using chemically pure (CP) titanium substrates 25 mm × 50 mm × 3.1 mm thick. Prior to spraying the substrates, they were cleaned with methanol to remove any residual grease or oils on the surface. Then the substrate was grit blasted with SiC powder at 125 psi to roughen the surface to improve the bonding of the powders when sprayed. Then the sample was cleaned again with methanol. The sample was then securely mounted in the fumehood. The robot path was programmed with the teach pendent overlapping each spray path to ensure the surface of each substrate was completely coated.

4.2.2.2. Powder materials

This section describes the selection and analysis performed on the powders used in this project. Unlike thermal spray processes, for cold spray, coating formation is more sensitive to powder manufacturer, powder fabrication technique, chemical composition, morphology, and hardness. For this reason three manufacturers of Ti-6Al-4V powders and one manufacturer of Ti-CP powders were selected for testing. The powders were analyzed for morphology, chemical composition, hardness, and particle size distribution. Table 4.5 summarizes the manufacturer and the characteristics of the four powders tested.

Particle morphology

Powder morphology was performed using the Hitachi S-2300 Scanning Electron Microscope (SEM). The Ti-6Al-4V powders manufactured by Crucible Research and Pyrogenesis, Inc. are produced by an atomization process yielding a spherical morphology. The HDH powders (Ti-6Al-4V and Ti-CP) produced by Affinity, Inc. consist of particles with a very irregular (angular) shape and sharp edges. This is typical for HDH powders because they are produced by a grinding process and then sieved to size. There were a high percentage of fine particles resident in both HDH powders.

Table 4.5. Characteristics of tested powders

Powder Type	Manufacturing Technique	Morphology	Manufacturer	Mean Size, μm	Hardness (VHN)
Ti-6Al-4V	Gas Atomized	Spherical	Crucible Research USA	29	291
Ti-6Al-4V	Plasma Atomized	Spherical	Pyrogenesis Canada	27	280
Ti-6Al-4V	Hydride-DeHydride	Angular	Affinity China	30.7	351
Ti-CP	Hydride-DeHydride	Angular	Affinity China	21	153

Chemical composition
The chemical analysis for the powders was performed on mechanically polished samples using a Jeol Scanning Electron Microscope with an electron microprobe analysis attachment. The weight percent of the elements in all cases is typical of what would be expected of Ti-6Al-4V and Ti-CP materials.

Hardness
The hardness of the powders can affect the deposition efficiency and porosity. Therefore, microhardness measurements were performed on each powder for comparison. The powder samples were mounted in epoxy similar to the technique for mounting samples for metallography analysis. The surface was polished producing a flat cross-section for each particle. Microhardness measurements were then made using a Leco M-400-G hardness tester applying a 200 g load for 20 s. Five readings were taken for each powder and then averaged. The results are presented in Table 4.5 as Vickers Hardness numbers (VHN).

Particle size analysis
Particle size distribution analysis was performed using a Coulter Particle Size Analyzer. The analysis of each powder yielded the differential volume percent as a function of particle size.

As seen in Table 4.5, a mean particle size for all types of Ti-6Al-4V powders is very close ranging from 27 to 30.7 μm. The largest spread in particle size is for Affinity Ti-6Al-4V HDH powder, which contains more fine and coarse particles. The Ti-CP HDH powder had a mean size of 21 μm; 6–10 μm smaller than the Ti-6Al-4V powders.

4.2.2.3. Parameter development tests with helium

Parameter development tests were performed using helium, which provides higher particle velocities and as a consequence higher deposition efficiency and better coating properties. To provide high density coatings and from past experience, all the powders were sprayed at a pressure of 2.4 MPa and at two different temperatures 450 °C and 550 °C. Coatings were deposited on 25 mm × 50 mm × 3.1 mm thick Ti-CP substrates between 1 and 1.5 mm thick. Table 4.6 summarizes the process parameters used to deposit the coatings.

Table 4.6. Process parameters for coatings deposition

Spray Parameters	Value
Gas	Helium
Pressure	2.4 MPa
Temperature	450 °C and 550 °C
Nozzle Transverse Velocity	100 mm/s
Substrate Materials	Ti-CP
Nozzle Raster Index	2 mm
Nozzle Standoff Distance	25 mm

Deposition efficiency measurements

Deposition Efficiency (DE) measurements were conducted with helium at the highest spray parameters used in the parameter development tests (pressure 2.4 MPa, temperature 550 °C). The deposition efficiency for each powder was determined in separate tests by measuring the mass of powder deposited onto the planar Ti-CP substrate (spraying inside the boundaries of the 50 mm × 100 mm × 3 mm substrate) to the mass of powder (~30–40 g) loaded into the laboratory powder feeder. Results of measurements are present in Table 4.7.

The highest DE was measured for Ti-6Al-4V (Pyrogenesis) at 86%. This was greater than the more ductile Ti-CP (Affinity) registering a value of 85%. The lowest DE was measured for HDH Ti-6Al-4V (Affinity Inc.) at 66%. However, there are many factors that can affect DE, and one of these factors is the ductility of the powder. Comparing the DE for the various powders with their hardness in Table 4.7, Section 3 shows the harder the powder the lower the DE.

Metallography analysis

Figure 4.37 shows a micrograph of the coating formed by the Pyrogenesis Ti-6Al-4V plasma atomized powder at 530 °C. This micrograph is also typical of that observed for the Crucible Research powder.

Table 4.7. Results of deposition efficiency measurements

Powder Type	Deposition Efficiency, %
Ti-6Al-4V, Gas Atomized, made by Crucible Research	78
Ti-6Al-4V, Plasma Atomized, made by Pyrogenesis	86
Ti-6Al-4V, HDH type, made by Affinity Int.	66
Ti (chemically pure), HDH type, made by Affinity Int.	85

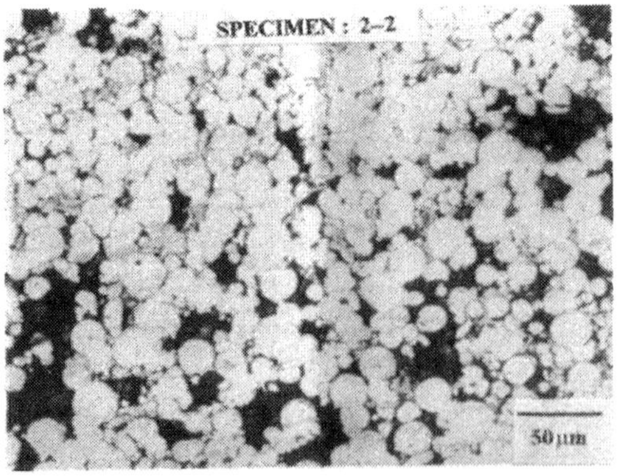

Fig. 4.37. As-sprayed Ti-6Al-4V (PA) Pyrogenesis, Helium @ 530 °C, Porosity 18%.

Figure 4.38 shows a micrograph of the coating formed by the Affinity Ti-6Al-4V HDH powder at 530 °C. This micrograph is also typical of that observed for the Affinity Ti-CP powder.

Table 4.8 shows a summary of the porosity of the as-sprayed coatings with helium at various temperatures.

Except for the porosity measured for the Crucible Ti-6Al-4V the porosity decreased with increased temperature for all the powders tested. The porosity for the gas and plasma atomized powders ranges between 18 and 26% considering all sprayed temperatures. The Ti-6Al-4V from Affinity Inc. exhibited the lowest porosity of 4 and 7% sprayed at

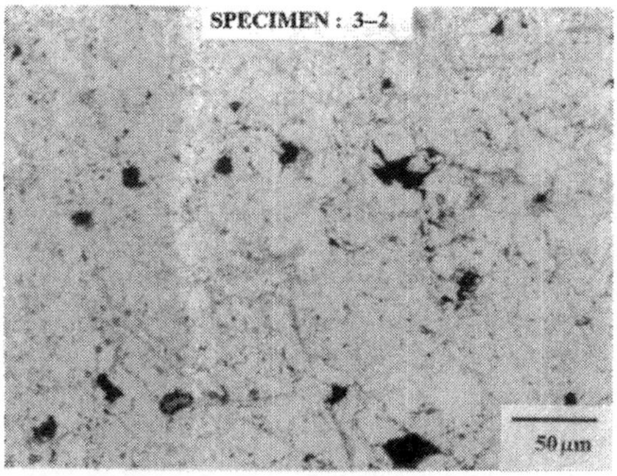

Fig. 4.38. As-sprayed Ti-6Al-4V (HDH) Affinity, Helium @ 530 °C, Porosity 4%.

Table 4.8. Data on sample porosity measurements

Manufacturers	Percent Porosity	Sprayed Parameters
Ti-6Al-4V (GA)		
Crucible Research	18	Helium @ 450 °C
	26	Helium @ 530 °C
Ti-6Al-4V (PA)		
Pyrogenesis	21	Helium @ 450 °C
	18	Helium @ 530 °C
Ti-6Al-4V (HDH)		
Affinity Int'l.	7	Helium @ 450 °C
	4	Helium @ 530 °C
Ti-Cp (HDH)		
Affinity Int'l.	12	Helium @ 450 °C
	9	Helium @ 530 °C

530 and 450 °C respectively. Similar results have been observed for Ti-CP. The porosity sprayed with helium is 12% when sprayed at 450 °C but decreases to 9% at 530 °C.

It is believed that better consolidation of the (HDH) powders occurs because of the large number of fine particles available when compared to the gas and plasma atomized particles to fill the voids during the spray process and reduce the porosity. For the as-sprayed gas and plasma atomized powder coatings, it does not appear that the particles undergo much deformation resulting in large voids, interconnecting porosity, and low cohesion.

Hot isostatic pressing analysis

Based upon the porosity results of the coatings, a sample of each material was sent to Bodycote IMT (USA) for Hot Isostatic Pressing (HIPing) to determine if this technique could be used to reduce or eliminate the porosity observed in the as-sprayed coatings.

For the HIPing process the samples were encapsulated in a low carbon steel can with 3.5 mm thick covers. The cans were helium leak checked and were hot off gassed at 290 °C overnight, then sealed. The HIP cycle was 900 ± 15 °C for 2 h at 103 MPa.

After HIPing the samples, they were analyzed by metallography to measure porosity. In addition to being sectioned and polished the samples were etched for 8 s using a solution containing 96 ml distilled water, 2 ml hydrofluoric acid (HF) and 3 ml of nitric acid (HNO_3) to reveal the grain structure. A Hitachi S-2300 scanning electron microscope was used to examine both the microstructure of the as-sprayed and HIPed coatings. The porosity of the as-sprayed samples was measured by the lineal intercept method.

After HIPing, the porosity of all the coatings was reduced to zero regardless of the initial porosity. Figures 4.39 and 4.40 show the grain structure for the polished and etched HIPed coating deposited with the Pyrogenesis and Affinity Ti-6Al-4V powders, respectively. Similar results were observed for the Crucible Research gas atomized and Affinity HDH Ti-CP powders. The as-sprayed micrographs are shown in Figs 4.37 and 4.38, respectively for comparison.

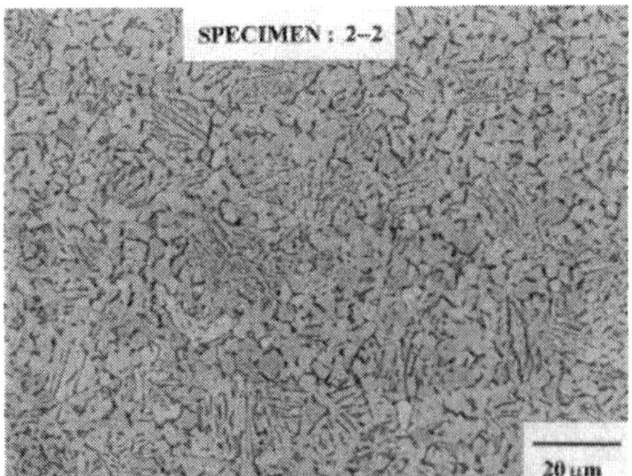

Fig. 4.39. HIPed Ti-6Al-4V (PA) Pyrogenesis, Helium @ 530 °C.

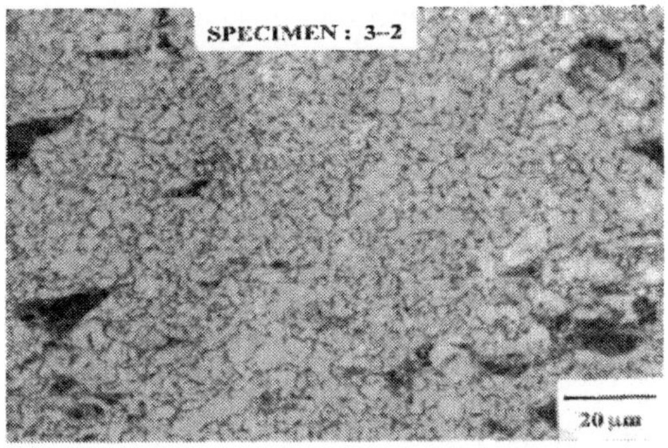

Fig. 4.40. HIPed Ti-6Al-4V (HDH) Affinity, Helium @ 530 °C.

Metallography analysis for the Crucible and Pyrogenesis coatings HIPed samples shows predominantly equiaxed alpha structure resulting from the re-crystallization of the alpha phase due to the heavy deformation occurring during spray deposition. Small regions of intergranular beta are observed. Additionally, for the samples sprayed with the Pyrogenesis powder few areas of non-recrystallized elongated lamellar alpha-beta are present.

For the Ti-CP samples the microstructure reveals recrystallized single-phase alpha. No beta phase is present. The dark areas observed in the polished and etched microstructure of the Ti-6Al-4V (HDH) Affinity coating (Figure 4.40) also raises a question because they are not observed in the as-sprayed coating. An electron microprobe analysis was performed on the dark areas and the results did not show the presence of any other elements except titanium, vanadium, and aluminum. In general the microstructures of HIPed samples are the same as what would be observed in cast and wrought deformed and recrystallized material.

4.2.2.4. Spray forming tests

The objective of the spray forming tests was to spray rectangular prisms of the selected powders at thicknesses of up to 12.5 mm on flat Ti-CP substrates for post processing (heat treating and HIPing) and fabrication of tensile specimens to evaluate the material properties (hardness, yield strength (YS) and ultimate strength (UTS), modulus of elasticity (E), percent elongation (e), and reduction in area (Ra)). Additionally, a couple symmetrical axis geometries were sprayed on thin-walled substrates to demonstrate that this process can be used for direct fabrication, rapid prototyping, developing forging performs, and depositing spray form shapes. Preliminary tests have shown that spraying with helium provides higher values of density and deposition efficiency. Based on these results and the parameters optimized in the preliminary tests, thick samples were sprayed with helium at the spray parameters previously developed (Table 4.6).

Heat treating and HIPing

As-sprayed cold sprayed coatings are typically hard because of the work hardening the powder material experiences through the high velocity impact and deformation to build up the coating. Therefore, a set of samples were heat treated in an attempt to anneal the as-sprayed coating and possibly get some grain boundary migration to reduce the porosity and improve material properties compared to the as-sprayed coatings. The heat-treating process involved placing the samples in a tube furnace purged with argon. The samples were solution treated at 840 °C for four hours and then air cooled to room temperature. The same HIPing procedures were used to HIP thick samples as the 25 mm × 50 mm screening samples (see Section 4.2.2.3).

4.2.2.5. Material property results

Tensile data

For analysis of mechanical properties mini-tensile specimens were machined from as-sprayed, heat-treated, and HIPed coatings. Tensile tests were conducted per ASTM standard (E8-96a) on an MTS servo hydraulic test machine. The specimens were tested at a stroke rate of 2.5 mm/min. A 25 mm gauge length extensometer was used to measure strain.

Selected tensile data comparing as-sprayed, heat-treated, and HIPed stress versus strain curves are shown for specimens machined from coating sprayed using Crucible, Pyrogenesis, Affinity Ti-6Al-4V (HDH), and Affinity Ti-CP (HDH) powders in Figs 4.41 and 4.42, respectively.

Table 4.9 shows typical material property data for wrought Ti-6Al-4V and Ti-CP annealed rod.

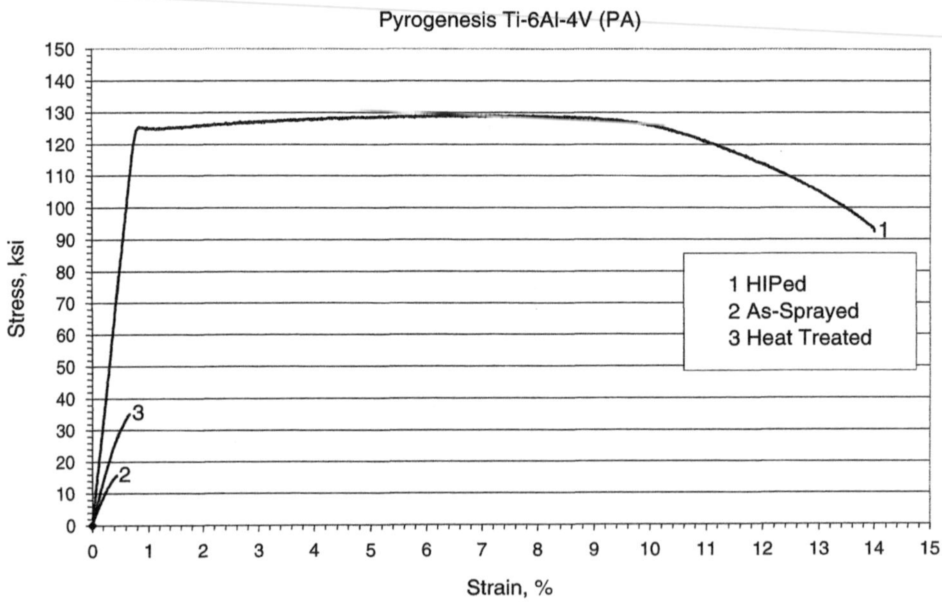

Fig. 4.41. Stress versus strain curve comparing the as-sprayed, heat-treated and HIPed properties for Ti-6Al-4V (PA), Pyrogenesis specimens.

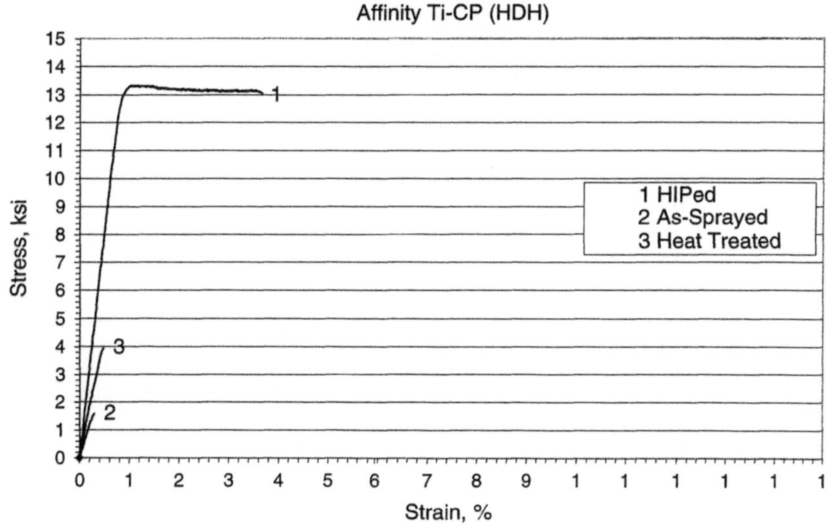

Fig. 4.42. Stress versus strain curve comparing the as-sprayed, heat-treated and HIPed properties for Ti-CP (HDH), Affinity specimens.

Table 4.9. Material property data for wrought Ti-6Al-4V and Ti-CP annealed rod

Material	Yield Strength, MPa	Ultimate Strength, MPa	Elastic Modulus, MPa	Percent Elongation, %	Percent Reduction In Ave., %	Hardness VHN
Ti-6Al-4V	828	924	105	14	45	360*
Ti-CP	248	345	103	35	70	150*

Data were taken from *Metals Reference Book*, 5th edn, C.J. Smithells, 1978, Butterworth & Company (Publishing) Ltd. 1976; *Hardness data REMBAR Titanium Fabrication web page, www.rembar.com/titan.htm.

There are numerous comparisons that can be made by analyzing this material data and most are obvious. Therefore, below are presented the primary results of importance for the material property data acquired separating Ti-6Al-4V and Ti-CP.

Ti-6Al-4V material property analysis

As-sprayed materials have shown poor performance for all powders tested. Values of YS and UTS are one order of magnitude less than for wrought material.

Low values of E, e, and Ra show that the as-sprayed materials are very brittle because of high porosity and cold worked particles. All the as sprayed samples failed in a brittle mode at low strains $<0.48\%$. Heat-treatment improves the material properties in comparison to the as-sprayed samples. Values of YS, UTS, and *e* are 2–4 times greater. However, these properties are still 3–4 times lower than for wrought annealed materials.

The strongest effect on material properties takes place after HIPing. For the Ti-6Al-4V (GA) and (PA) powders manufactured by Crucible and Pyrogenesis respectively, data for YS, UTS, *E*, *e*, and Ra meet or exceed corresponding data for wrought materials.

Ti-CP material property analysis

The tensile specimens machined from the as-sprayed coatings fail in a brittle mode with little ductility. The yield strength is about half and UTS is 1/3 than expected for wrought annealed material. Heat treatment improved the YS and UTS by a factor of 2.5 but the tensile specimens failed in a brittle mode with very little elongation, $<0.47\%$. Elasticity improved by a factor of 2 but is half the value for wrought annealed titanium.

HIPing significantly improved the properties. YS and UTS increase a factor of 3.5 over the heat treated samples and *e* increased by a factor of 14 to 4%. The strength properties exceed those of wrought annealed by a factor of 3.7 and 2.6 respectively, and the modulus is higher by about 10%. Conversely, the percent elongation is a factor of 8 and 17 respectively, lower than wrought annealed material.

Hardness measurements were made on the end of the tensile samples after testing. Table 4.10 shows the average Vickers Hardness Number compared with the hardness of the respective powder particles before spraying.

The hardness values for the as-sprayed and heat-treated materials are probably not accurate due to the amount of porosity resident causing the readings to be lower than what they actually are. In reality, because of the cold worked structure, the hardness should be higher than the particles sprayed. However, it is interesting to note that the hardness of the Ti-6Al-4V HIPed material is nearly the same as the hardness of the respective particle material. HIPing restores the as-sprayed coating properties near to that of the original powder materials. Conversely, for Ti-CP the hardness of the HIPed coating is 52% greater than the original particle.

Table 4.10. Vickers hardness data for samples and respective powder particles before spraying

Powder	Powder Hardness (VHN)	Coating Hardness (VHN)		
		As Sprayed	Heat Treated	HIPed
Ti-6Al-4V (GA) Crucible	291	215	189	288
Ti-6Al-4V (PA) Pyrogenesis	280	272	178	290
Ti-6Al-4V (HDH) Affinity	351	258	304	381
Ti-CP (HDH) Affinity	153	142	218	279

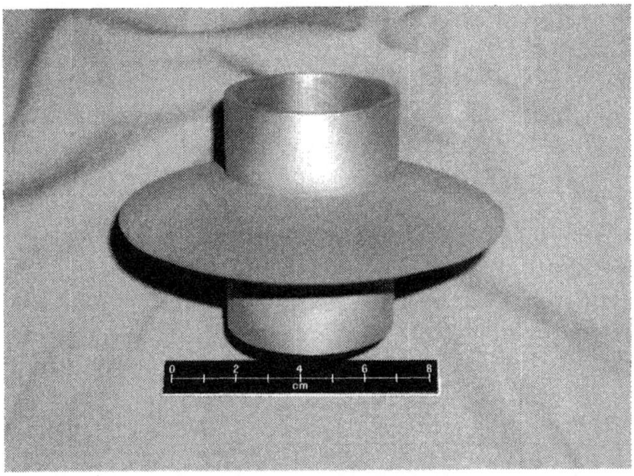

Fig. 4.43. Ti-6Al-4V fin sprayed onto 2 in. diameter aluminum cylinder.

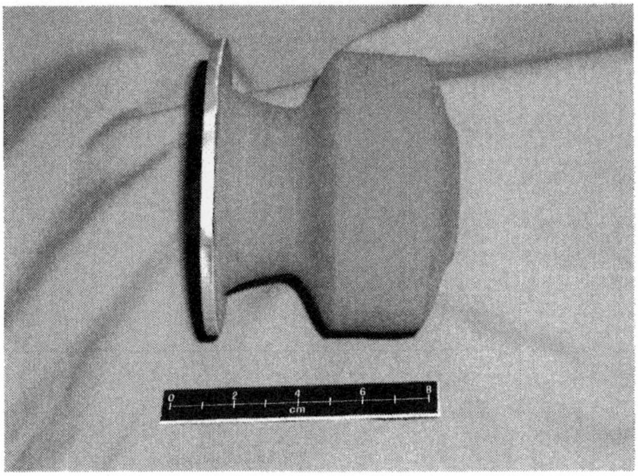

Fig. 4.44. Ti-6Al-4V axisymmetric shape sprayed onto flat 1/8 in. aluminum substrate.

4.2.2.6. Spray formed shapes

In order to demonstrate the ability of the process to spray form shapes, the parameters in Table 2 were taken and a series of tests were set up to spray Ti-6Al-4V symmetrical axis shapes with several centimeters in dimension using Pyrogenesis powder. Figures 4.43 and 4.44 show the shapes generated proving that cold spray can be used for rapid prototyping and production of high value parts. The parts shown were sprayed at a deposition efficiency of 80%, powder feed rate of 5 kg/h, and spray beam size of 7 mm. The time to spray these shapes took a few minutes (2–5 min.). No post machining was performed on the sprayed shapes.

Thus, it is shown that various types of Ti-6Al-4V powder (gas and plasma atomized, HDH) can successfully be sprayed with cold spray. Metallography analysis has shown that after HIPing, the density of all the coatings was close to 100% regardless of initial density and the interconnecting porosity was eliminated. The microstructure of the HIPed samples is the same as it is obtained in cast and wrought deformed and recrystallized material.

Presented results have shown that as-sprayed and HIPed parts provide high mechanical properties that are close or exceed those for wrought material and, as a consequence, can meet requirements for commercial applications. This clearly demonstrates that the cold spray process can be used for direct fabrication, rapid prototyping, developing forging performs, and depositing spray form shapes.

4.3. Cold Spray System Kinetic 3000 Developed by Cold Gas Technology (Germany)

This section presents the cold spray equipment – Kinetic 3000 developed by Cold Gas Technology (CGT), Germany [25]. The cold spray system Kinetic 3000 is designed as a commercial system for the industrial use. The first version was introduced in 2001. Today this is the first cold spray system that is used for development of many industrial applications. In author's opinion this is the best stationary cold spray equipment in the world that can be used for different applications.

4.3.1. Brief description of equipment

The system consists of a control cabinet with integrated power supply and gas control, a gas heater, a high pressure powder feeder, and the spray gun. The process parameters – gas pressure up to 30 bar and gas temperature up to 700–800 °C at the gun – can easily be adjusted via an user-friendly touch screen panel. The latest improvement is the high pressure powder feeder PF 4000 Comfort, developed by CGT. The development of the whole spray system is the result of a close collaboration between experts in automation technology and gas engineering from CGT and Linde AG and experts in fluid dynamics and material science from the University of the Federal Armed Forces in Germany.

This section provides some details about the individual components and about the performance of the system in extended time tests and in industrial production.

4.3.1.1. Control unit

The control panel consists of the micro controller, the power electronics and the gas distribution panel. This is the module where all the temperature, pressure, and flow values as well as safety signals come together. The system operates 16 digital inputs, 10 digital outputs, 9 analog inputs, and 5 analog outputs. Also the 20 kW heat source is built in this panel, Fig. 4.45.

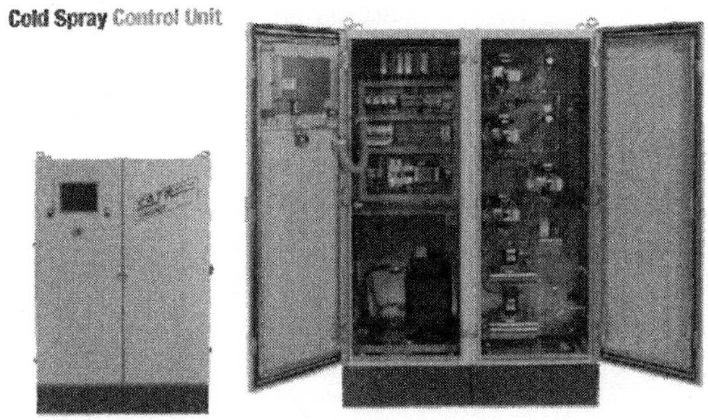

Fig. 4.45. Control Unit.

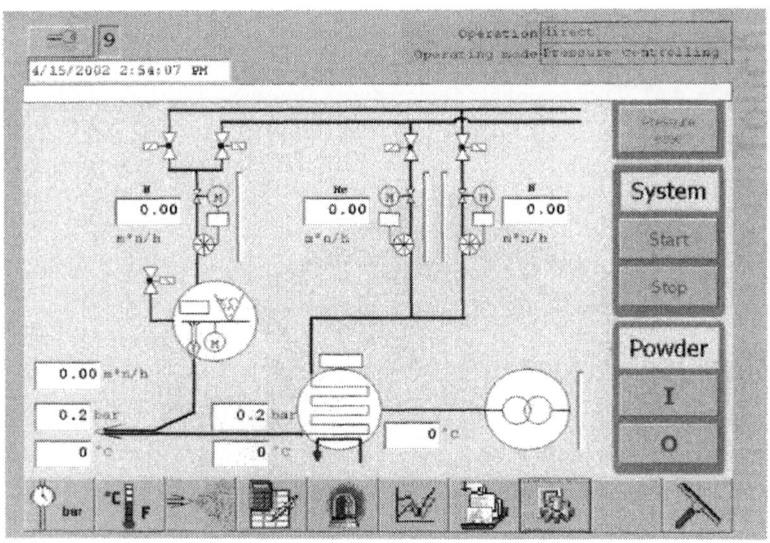

Fig. 4.46. MP370 Touch Screen.

The parameters are set and stored within frames on the MP 370 Touch Screen Monitor, Fig. 4.46. All the user has to do is to START and STOP the system. Even a handshake mode with a robot system or an external controller for process automation is already realized.

On the right side of the screen there is the START and STOP for the system as well as the ON and OFF buttons for the powder feeder. The system graphic in the center is used to display the status and important values of the process. The process values can be automatically stored on memory card or via Ethernet data transfer. In Fig. 4.47 you can see a production period of 3 h and 40 min.

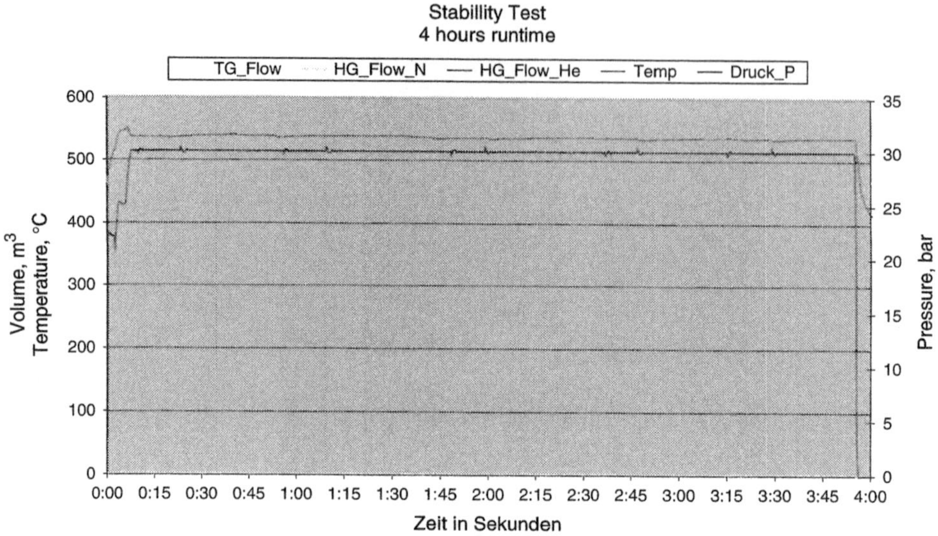

Fig. 4.47. Data recording: Temperature – Pressure – Gas consumption.

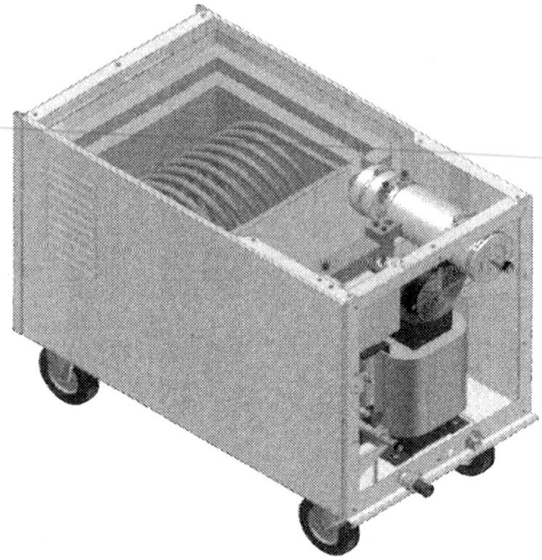

Fig. 4.48. Gas heater.

4.3.1.2. LINSPRAY® gas heater

A first prototype of the heater was developed by Linde. The experience gained at this state was used to develop a robust heater for the industrial use, Fig. 4.48.

The heating coil can be operated up to a material temperature of 800 °C at a pressure of 35 bar. The design allows gas temperatures close to 800 °C at the outlet of the heater.

Heat losses are minimized by employing appropriate insulation. Material and gas temperature are monitored and used to prevent the coil from overheating. This guarantees a safe and reliable operation. Extensive tests have shown no signs of material fatigue after 1000 operating hours.

4.3.1.3. Powder gun

The powder gun is the front end of the technology, Fig. 4.49. The gun is connected to the heater via a flexible high temperature hose. This allows a maximum of flexibility for handling any process. A robot system needs only 16 kg load for operation.

The gun body has inputs for the heated process gas and for the feeder gas what is carrying the powder, as well as ports for the temperature and the pressure sensor. The Laval nozzle is fixed with a spigot nut. Today there are two nozzles for the industrial use available, Fig. 4.50. Those nozzles are made from Tungsten Carbide what makes them excellent and long-lasting.

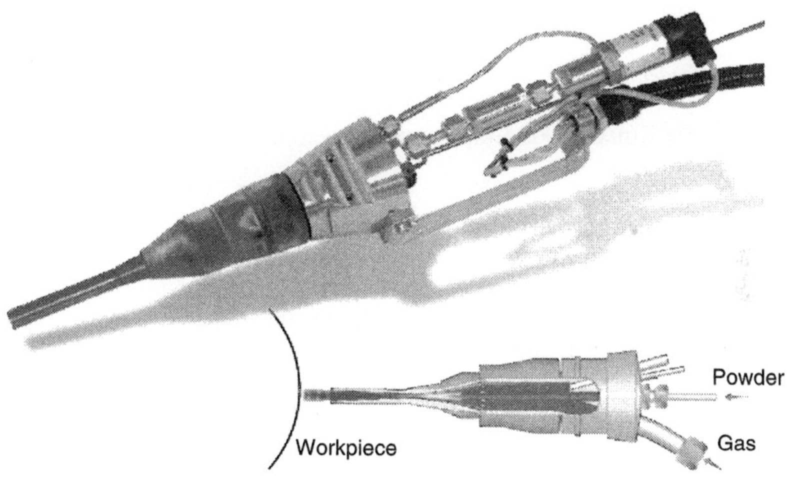

Fig. 4.49. Powder gun body with sensors and nozzle.

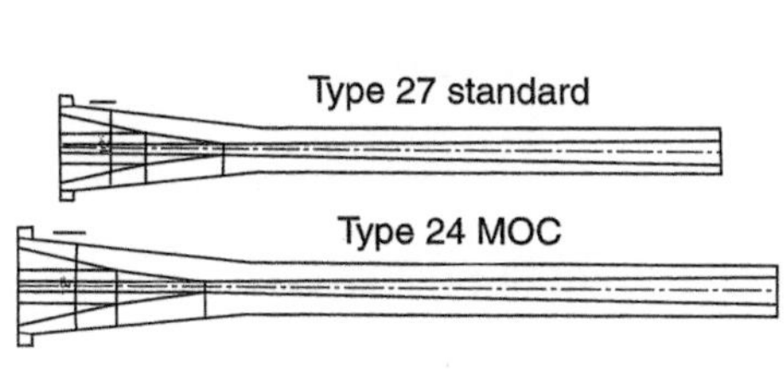

Fig. 4.50. Industrial nozzle geometries.

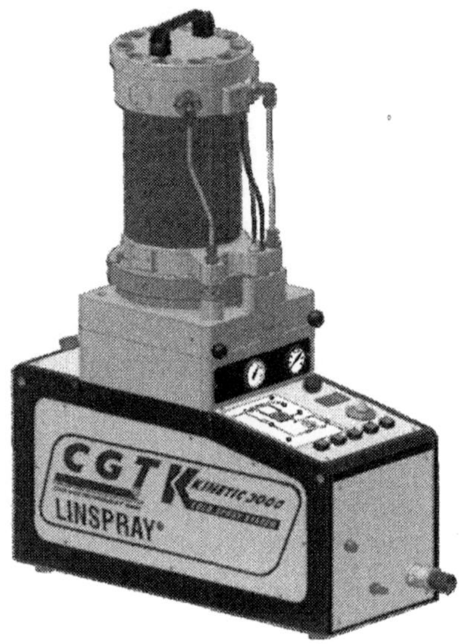

Fig. 4.51. Kinetic 4000 Comfort.

4.3.1.4. Powder feeder

The powder feeder Kinetic 4000 Comfort was developed for high pressure spray systems, Fig. 4.51.

The first process to use has been cold spraying with pressures up to 35 bar. However it is also applicable with plasma or HVOF system. There are no tools needed to disassemble the feeder, Fig. 4.52. Refilling can be done within 2–3 min. Cleaning for the use of a different powder material takes 10–15 min. Using the integrated bypass system those operations can be done while the spray system is in stand mode.

The feeder can load up to 4 dm^3 of powder which enables production periods longer then 4 h. Using 3 kg/h copper, 8 hours are possible.

So, the Kinetic 3000 cold spray system is the first one for industrial cold spray applications [25]. The system has proved its reliability and performance in many installations around the world. A lot of different technologies were tested and developed on the basis of this system. The ongoing research and development work within the Cold Spray Competence Group will further push the technology to become an excellent tool for specific applications.

4.4. Low Pressure Portable Cold Spray System

Development of portable low pressure cold spray systems is of prime importance because such systems allow applying coatings to structural elements with difficult

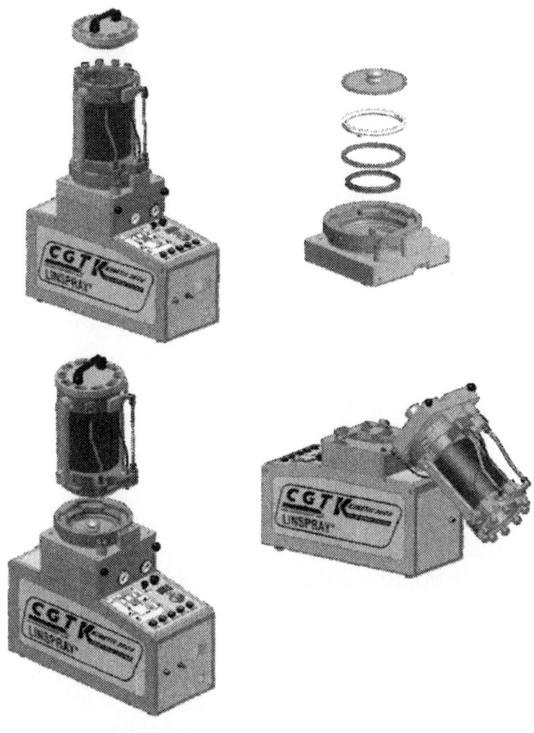

Fig. 4.52. Disassembling without tools.

access, surfaces of semi-closed volumes, and reservoirs, including repair and restoration activities.

Understanding the dependence of the microstructure of spray coatings on operating conditions of the low pressure system is of practical interest. To obtain good quality coatings the portable system and spray technology parameters should be selected carefully, and due to the large variety in process parameters, much trial goes into optimizing the process for each specific coating and substrate combinations. A brief description of low pressure portable cold spray system is presented below.

4.4.1. Process history

The first original prototype of such equipment was developed in Russia at the Obninsk Center for Powder Metallurgy at the end of 1980s. Further this Russian company was focused mostly on the development of particular device and technology for repair and maintenance applications in various Russian industries. In 1997 this portable device was introduced in North America by the R&D company "Technologies Decision Management Inc" (Windsor, Ontario) as an equipment which can be applied for various automotive and aircraft industrial applications. The first project was related to the implementation of cold spray technology for specific needs of auto manufacturing. This particular project started in 1998, was supported by DaimlerChrysler Corp., and was successfully realized in 2001.

Further R&D activities on the emerging low pressure gas-dynamic spray technology with portable apparatus were primarily conducted by the University of Windsor and "Technologies Decision Management Inc" (Windsor, Ontario) [26]. Today University of Windsor established an R&D Center, supported by Canadian Federal Government with various North American industrial Partners which lead R&D activity in this direction. Based on results of these studies, one of the leading weld manufacturers in North America "Centerline Windsor Ltd." started manufacturing portable cold spray equipment.

4.4.2. Description of portable equipment

The two main clear-cut distinctions of the low and high pressure cold spray technologies are the following:

1. low gas pressure utilization (0.5–1 MPa instead of 2.5–3 MPa)
2. radial injecting powder instead of axial injecting in the most of cases.

At closer examination of these differences one can note that the particle content in gas-particle jet is considerably increased because of a decrease of gas flow rate. The dependences of the particle volume concentration on powder and gas mass flow rate are shown in Fig. 4.53. Both of these variables are being changed in the case of low pressure system as compared with axial injection for high pressure system.

Decreasing gas flow rate due to diminishing gas pressure causes the increase of particle concentration in gas–particle jet. The volume solid content of the gas–particle jet in high pressure system is in the range of 10^{-5}–10^{-6} while the volume content in low pressure system is in the range of 10^{-4}–10^{-5}. For this reason parameters of gas–powder flow vary considerably depending on the type of cold spray system.

The industrial low pressure equipment produced by "Centerline Windsor Ltd." is shown on Figs 4.54 and 4.55.

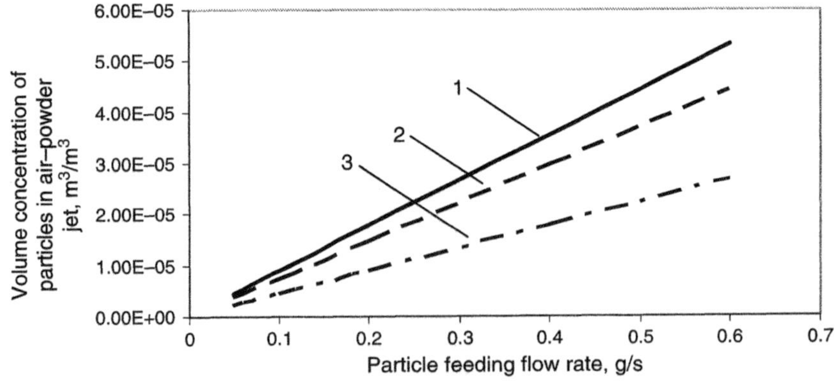

Fig. 4.53. The particle volume concentration in powder laden jet for low pressure GDS. 1 – air flow rate 0.25 m^3/min, 2 – air flow rate 0.3 m^3/min, and 3 – air flow rate 0.5 m^3/min.

During very short time the rugged and flexible design of the portable supersonic spray technology (SST) machine was developed by Centerline Windsor Ltd. and successfully presented at different international exhibitions (Fig. 4.54) [27, 28]. All-metal enclosure provides with outstanding durability and can be moved from worksite to worksite easily and quickly. A touch screen display panel provides convenient and precise control while monitoring the machine's settings and diagnostics. Through the use of electronics, the digital controller ensures peak system performance by monitoring air pressure, air temperature, powder feed rates, etc. The SST spray gun incorporates an ergonomic and durable design intended to promote operator control and feel. With two mode selection buttons and an easy-to-operate trigger, it is comfortable for both right and left handed operators. The hopper and powder delivery system are equipped with programmable feed control and is sure to provide a long time of trouble-free performance. Dual 400 ml hoppers feed custom powder and abrasive compounds which are supplied in convenient hopper refills that can be easily replaced when replenishment of material is required. An integrated "explosion-proof rated" system is used to provide quick and easy worksite clean-up. An easy to dispose feature allows for the disposal of collected residual material safely and quickly. The touch screen control provides precise control of vacuum system (Fig. 4.55) [29].

The low pressure system was analyzed in [30] with respect to the effects of air temperature and powder jet composition. The air temperature influences the air and particle velocity, which are to be as high as possible. As an example Fig. 4.56 shows some features of powder mixtures sprayed at low air pressures. Deposition efficiency (DE) is found to be low in the range of temperatures 100–500 °C, but sharply increases at temperatures higher

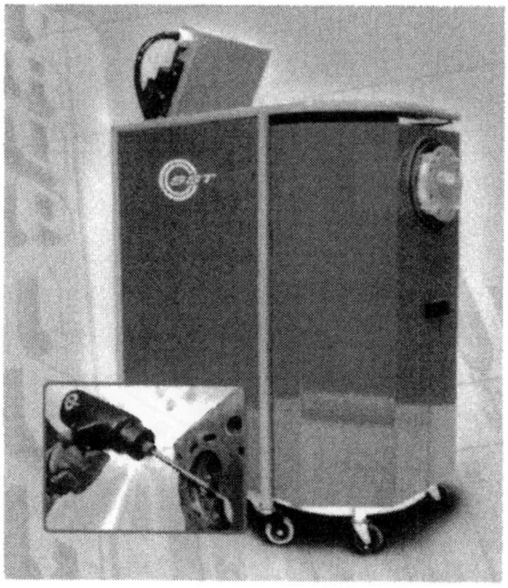

Fig. 4.54. Portable cold spray machine using the configuration where the powder is directly injected into the downstream of the DeLaval nozzle. This particular design uses regular 80–90 psi. compressed air for carrier gas (Courtesy of SST, a Division of Centerline Windsor Ltd.).

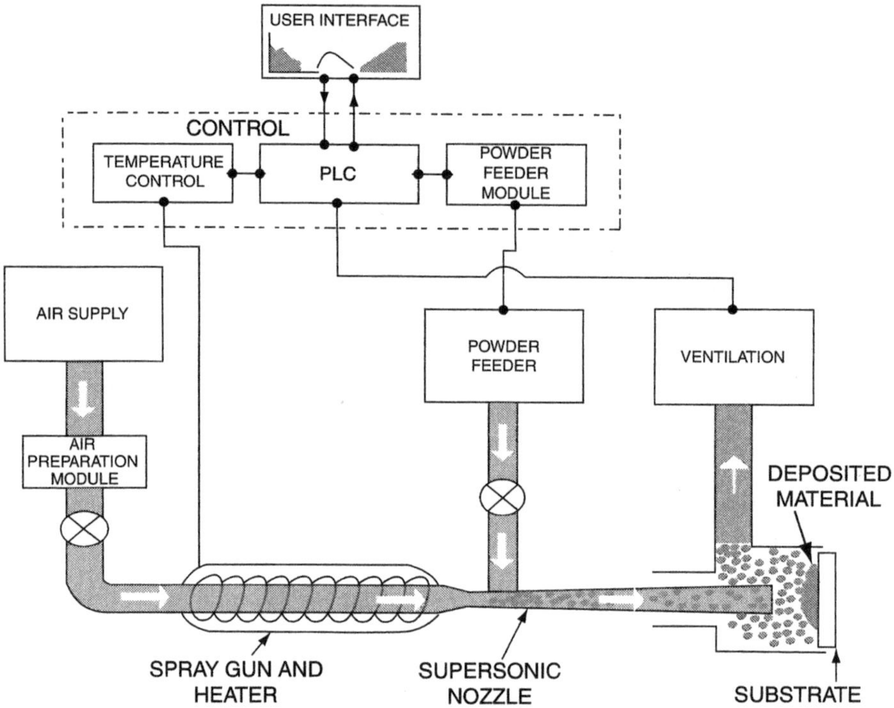

Fig. 4.55. Schematic diagram of the cold spray SST Centerline system, where the powder is injected downstream in the DeLaval nozzle.

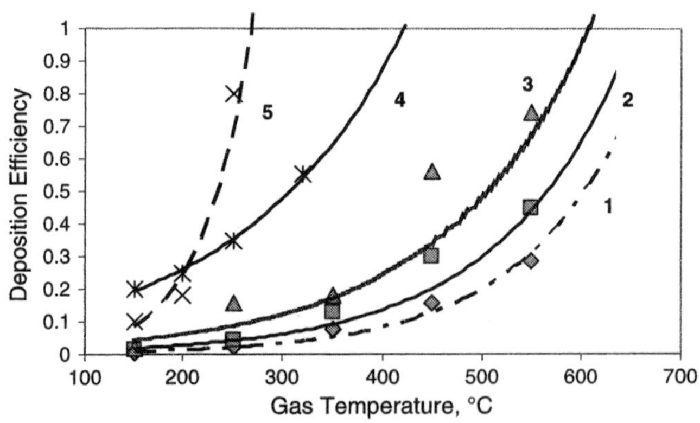

Fig. 4.56. Deposition efficiency for powder mixtures: 1 – Powder mixture with weight concentration $0.25Al_2O_3 + 0.5Al + 0.25Zn$, 2 – Powder mixture with weight concentration 0.5Ti + 0.25Al + 0.25Zn, (to remove) 3 – Powder mixture with weight concentration 0.5W + 0.25Al + 0.25Zn, 4 – Cu [11], and 5 – Ti [12].

than 600 °C and becomes comparable with the values of DE for Ti and Cu (around 0.6) sprayed with high pressure system at temperature 300–350 °C [31, 32].

The low pressure system has proved its reliability in many installations. Many technologies were tested and developed on the basis of this system allowing applying coatings to structural elements with difficult access, surfaces of semi-closed volumes, and reservoirs, including repair and restoration activities.

Symbol List

L	Length of the supersonic part of the nozzle
h	Minimum exit dimension of the nozzle
d_p	Particle diameter
M	Mach number
$P_m = v_w H \delta_c \rho_c$	Performance (deposition efficiency) in terms of mass
v_w	Velocity of the coated surface with respect to the nozzle exit
H	Width of the band sprayed during one stroke, equal to the larger size of the nozzle-exit section
δ_c	Thickness of the deposited coating
δ_{c1}	Thickness of the coating deposited during one stroke
ρ_c	Density of the coating
G_{pmax}	Maximum flow rate of the powder through the nozzle
G	Flow rate of the gas through the nozzle
p_0	Stagnation pressure
S_{cr}	Area of the supersonic nozzle throat
T_0	Stagnation temperature
k_d	Deposition efficiency
P_s	Performance (deposition efficiency) in terms of area
b_{cr}	Width of the nozzle throat
β_n	Angle of expansion of the pneumatic channel
β_{cr}	Critical angle of expansion of the pneumatic channel
β_{cr1}	Critical angle of expansion of the supersonic part of individual pneumatic channels
ΔT_{hmax}	Maximum heating temperature
T_{hin}	Gas temperature at the inlet of the heating element
T_{hex}	Gas temperature at the exit of the heating element
T_w	Temperature of the inner surface of the heating element
$Re_h = \frac{\rho v d_h}{\mu} = \frac{4G}{\pi N_h d_h \mu}$	Reynolds number of the gas flow inside the tube
ρ	Gas density
v	Gas velocity
μ	Gas viscosity
d_h	Inner diameter of the heating element
N_h	Number of heating elements (tubes)

Δp_h	Hydrodynamic resistance of the heater (pressure losses)
P_h	Power of the heater
L_h	Length of the heating element
$\alpha = \frac{\lambda Nu}{d}$	Heat-transfer coefficient
c_p	Heat capacity of the heated gas
λ	Thermal conductivity of the gas
μ_0	Viscosity at a temperature of 273 K
T_s	Sutherland temperature (for air, T_s = 122 K)
ξ	Specific friction resistance
$\Delta p_{in} = 0.5\rho\frac{v^2}{2}$	Local hydraulic resistance at the tube inlet
$\Delta p_{ex} = 1.0\rho\frac{v^2}{2}$	Local hydraulic resistance at the tube exit
U	Operating voltage of the source
R_h	Ohmic resistance of the heater
ρ_h	Specific ohmic resistance of the heating element material
δ_h	Wall thickness of the heating element
R_0	Initial electric resistance
T_{rc}	Nominal current
R_{cI}	Resistance after heating by the nominal current
R_c	Resistance after cyclic heating
f_{fr}	Friction coefficient
p_{fr}	Load
D_m	Diameter of the composite material sample
h_m	Thickness of the composite material sample
d_t	Diameter of the cylindrical inclusion
φ_t	Volume concentration of PTFE
z_{wear}	Linear wear of the composite sample
$V_t(z_{wear})$	Volume of PTFE entrained onto the surface
δ_t	Thickness of the PTFE film
$S_t(z_{wear})$	Area occupied by PTFE
v_{z0}	Wear rate of the material without PTFE inclusions
η_c	Friction coefficient of the composite
η_t	Friction coefficient of PTFE
η_m	Friction coefficient of the basic material
s_t	Dimensionless area of the surface occupied by the PTFE film
φ_{tmin}	Minimum concentration of PTFE in the composite
z^*_{wear}	Characteristic wear
$t_t = \frac{z^*_{wear}}{v_{z0}}$	Characteristic time
$\tau = \frac{t}{t_t}$	Dimensionless time
$\zeta = \frac{z}{z^*_{wear}}$	Dimensionless wear
$\eta'_t = \frac{\eta_t}{\eta_m}$	Dimensionless friction coefficient of PTFE
$\tau_0 = \frac{\delta_t}{\varphi_t z^*_{wear}(1-\eta'_t)}$	Characteristic dimensionless time
$\tau^* = \tau_0 \ln\frac{1}{\eta'_t}$	Dimensionless time of complete coverage of the friction surface by PTFE
$\eta'_c = \frac{\eta_c}{\eta_m}$	Dimensionless friction coefficient of the composite
$v'_z = \frac{v_z}{v_{z0}}$	Dimensionless wear rate
$t^* = \tau^* t_t$	Time of complete coverage of the friction surface by PTFE

References

[1] A.P. Alkhimov, V.F. Kosarev, N.I. Nesterovich, A.N. Papyrin, and M.M. Shushpanov, Gas-dynamic spraying method for applying coatings, United States Patent No. 5,302,414, *Official Gazette*, Vol. 1161, No. 2, 1994.

[2] A.P. Alkhimov, V.F. Kosarev, N.I. Nesterovich, A.N. Papyrin, and M.M. Shushpanov, Method and device for coating, European Patent No. 0 484 533 A1, *European Patent Bulletin*, No. 20, 1992.

[3] A.P. Alkhimov, V.F. Kosarev, N.I. Nesterovich, A.N. Papyrin, and M.M. Shushpanov, Gas-dynamic spraying method for applying coating, Reexamination Certificate, United States Patent No. 5,302,414, *Official Gazette*, 25 Feb. 1997.

[4] A.P. Alkhimov, V.F. Kosarev, N.I. Nesterovich, A.N. Papyrin, and M.M. Shushpanov, Device for coating application, Patent No. 1618777 of the Russian Federation, *Bull. Izobr.*, No. 1, 1991, p. 77.

[5] A.P. Alkhimov, V.F. Kosarev, and A.N. Papyrin, Device for coating application by spraying, Patent No. 1674585 of the Russian Federation, *Bull. Izobr.*, No. 18, 1993, p. 195.

[6] A.P. Alkhimov, V.F. Kosarev, N.I. Nesterovich, and A.N. Papyrin, Method for coating application, Patent No. 1618778 of the Russian Federation, *Bull. Izobr.*, No. 1, 1991, p. 77.

[7] A.P. Alkhimov, V.F. Kosarev, N.I. Nesterovich, and A.N. Papyrin, Device for coating application, Patent No. 1603581 of the Russian Federation, *Bull. Izobr.*, No. 23, 1996, p. 196.

[8] A.P. Alkhimov, V.F. Kosarev, N.I. Nesterovich, and A.N. Papyrin, Method for application of metal-powder coatings, Patent No. 1773072 of the Russian Federation, *Bull. Izobr.*, No. 7, 1995, p. 262.

[9] A.P. Alkhimov, V.F. Kosarev, and A.N. Papyrin, Device for coating application, Patent No. 2010619 of the Russian Federation, *Bull. Izobr.*, No. 7, 1994, p. 32.

[10] A.P. Alkhimov, V.P. Gulyaev, A.F.Demchuk, V.F. Kosarev, V.P. Larionov, and V.P. Spesivtsev, Setup for coating application onto the inner surface of a pipe, Patent No. 2075535 of the Russian Federation, *Bull. Izobr.*, No. 8, 1997, pp. 184–185.

[11] A.P. Alkhimov, A.F. Demchuk, V.F. Kosarev, and V.E.Kozhevnikov, Electrotechnical connector, Patent No. 2096877 of the Russian Federation, *Bull. Izobr.*, No. 32 (Part II), 1997, p. 376.

[12] A.P. Alkhimov, V.F. Kosarev, N.I. V.V. Lavrushin, and O.A. Alkhimov, Device for gas-dynamic spraying of powder materials, Patent No. 2190695 of the Russian Federation, *Bull. Izobr. Pol. Mod.*, No. 28 (Part II), 2002, p. 317.

[13] V.F. Kosarev, V.V. Lavrushin, V.P. Spesivtsev, Sun Tyanin, U. Tsze, and Zin Huanzu, Device for gas-dynamic spraying of powder materials, Patent No. 2247174 of the Russian Federation, *Bull. Izobr.Pol. Mod.*, No. 6, 2005.

[14] A.V. Lykov, *Heat mass exchange. Hand-book* [in Russian], Energy, Moscow, 1978, 480 p.

[15] *Physical encyclopedic dictionary* [in Russian], Soviet encyclopedia, Moscow, 1984, 944 p.

[16] G.I. Abramovich, *Applied Gas Dynamics* [in Russian], Nauka, Moscow, 1969, 824 p.

[17] V.M. Buznik, A.K. Tsvetnikov, A.P. Alkhimov, V.V. Lavrushin, O.I. Lomovskii, and E.Yu. Belyaev, Composition for coatings and method for its application, Patent No. 2149218 of the Russian Federation, *Bull. Izobr.*, No. 14, 2000.

[18] O.I. Lomovskii, Mechanical sintering and mechanochemical synthesis for obtaining metallic micro- and nanoncomposite materials, in *Physicochemistry of Finely Disperse Systems, Proc. V All-Russia Conf.*, Moscow, 2000, pp. 158–159.

[19] Yu.V. Baikalova and O.I. Lomovsky, *J. Alloys Comp.*, Vol. 297, 2000, pp. 87–91.

[20] F.V. Bolesta, V.M. Fomin, M.R. Sharafutdinov, and B.P. Tolochko, Investigation of interface boundary occurring during cold gas-dynamic spraying of metallic particles, *Nuclear Instruments and Methods in Physics Research*, Vol. 470, 2001, pp. 249–252.

[21] R.E. Blose, T.J. Roemer, *et al.*, Automated Cold Spray System: Description of Equipment and Performance Data, Proceedings of ITSC 2003, Orlando, USA, pp. 103–111.

[22] Papyrin, A.N., *et al.*, A Cold-gas Spray coating process for enhancing titanium, *JOM*, Vol. 50, No. 9, 1998, pp. 52–54.

[23] J. Karthikeyan, *et al.*, *Cold Spray Processing of Titanium Powder, Thermal Spray: Surface Engineering via Applied Research*, 2000, pp. 255–262.

[24] J. Vlcek, H. Huber, H. Voggenreiter, A. Ficher, E. Lugscheider, H. Hallen, and G. Pache, Kinetic Powder Compaction Applying the Cold Spray Process. A Study on Parameters. Presented at the International Thermal Spray Conference, Singapore, 2001.

[25] W. Kroemmer, P. Heinrich, and P. Richter, Cold Spraying – Equipment and Application Trends, Proceedings of ITSC 2003, Orlando, USA, pp. 97–103.

[26] R.G. Maev, E. Strumban, V. Leshchynsky, and M. Beneteau, Supersonic Induced Mechanical Alloy Technology and Coatings for Automotive and Aerospace Applications, Cold Spray 2004: An Emerging Spray Coating Technology, 27–28 Sept. 2004 (Akron, Ohio), Proc. ASM International (CD), 2004.

[27] Kashirin *et al.*, Apparatus for gas-dynamic coating. US Patent 6,402,050, 11 June 2002.

[28] Julio Villafuerte, Cold Spray: A new technology, *Welding Journal*, Vol. 84, No. 5, May 2005, pp. 24–29.

[29] http://www.supersonicspray.com/

[30] R. Gr. Maev and V. Leshchynsky, Air Gas Dynamic Spraying of Powder Mixtures: Theory and Application, *J. Thermal Spray Technol.*, Vol. 15, No. 2, 2006, pp. 379–391.

[31] C. Borchers, F. Gartner, T. Stoltenhoff, H. Assadi, and H. Kreye, Microstructural and macroscopic properties of cold sprayed copper coatings, *J. Appl. Phys.*, Vol. 93, No. 12, pp. 10064–10070.

[32] Chang-Jiu Li and Wen-Ya Li, Deposition characteristics of titanium coating in cold spraying, *Surface and Coating Technology*, Vol. 167, 2003, pp. 278–283.

CHAPTER 5

Current Status of the Cold Spray Process

In previous Chapters 1–3 we presented results of original studies conducted at the Institute of Theoretical and Applied Mechanics of Siberian Branch of the Russian Academy of Sciences that led to the development of the cold spray process.

At the present time the cold spray method is recognized by world leading scientists and specialists and a wide spectrum of research is being conducted at many research centers and companies over the world, including the Institute of Theoretical and Applied Mechanics of the Russian Academy of Sciences; Sandia National Laboratories; the Pennsylvania State University; ASB Industries Inc., Ford Motor Company, Pratt & Whitney, Rutgers University, Army Research Laboratory, Delphi Automotive Systems, Galaxy Sprayed Metals, Exxon Mobil Upstream Research Company (USA); University of Nottingham, University of Liverpool, Yasaki Europe, BOC Gases (England); University of the Federal Armed Forces, Cold Gas Technology, Linde Company, Siemens, EADS Corporate Research (Germany); Shinshu University, Plasma Gigen (Japan), CRISO (Australia), Mahle Metal Leve (Brazil); companies in South Korea, China, India, and many others. The cold spray propagates over the world so fast that it is difficult to mention all the companies and institutions involved in this activity. There has been a great surge in publications on the cold spray process. Many high level studies have been conducted at these centers and many interesting and important results for further developments and improvements of cold spray have been obtained.

The present chapter is an attempt to make a brief overview of the studies conducted at most of the research centers over the world. Results of research in the following basic areas are presented: gas-dynamics of cold spray, interaction of high-speed particle with the substrate and bonding mechanism, and technologies and applications. The overview includes most of publications made until year 2006 including papers presented at ITSC-2005 (Basel, Switzerland).

5.1. Gas-dynamics of Cold Spray

Obtaining coatings by the cold spray method involves the use of a high-velocity gas flow for accelerating and heating of particles. Therefore, first we will consider some general features of gas flows and motion of particles in nozzles and jets, as well as the jet impact onto a substrate.

As the cold spray process is primarily determined by the particle velocity, it is important to understand how this parameter is affected by the process parameters (pressure and temperature of the gas in the pre-chamber) and nozzle geometry. The particle velocity that can be reached in a cold spray facility is limited by the gas velocity. Owing to the use of high gas pressures, long nozzles, and fine particles, the particles move with a velocity close to the gas velocity that can be increased by using gases with low molecular weights and by gas heating. In practice, it is desirable to reach a sufficient particle velocity with pre-chamber and nozzle units being compact for the smallest flow rate of the gas. It is also desirable to avoid the use of high pressures and temperatures of the gas.

The isentropic model of the gas flow is described in detail, e.g., in [1–3]. This approximation implies that the gas flow in a converging/diverging nozzle (Laval nozzle) is isentropic (the flow is adiabatic and has no friction) and one dimensional. The gas is perfect and has a constant ratio of specific heats. Equations that describe the flow of such a gas can be taken, e.g., from [4, 5]. The isentropic model ignores the presence of the boundary layer on the nozzle walls, where the gas moves slower than near the nozzle centerline, and the calculated gas velocity is somewhat higher than that measured experimentally. The gas parameters are functions of the nozzle geometry, total temperature of the gas, and stagnation pressure. The flow is accelerated or decelerated when the cross-sectional area of the flow is changed. The stagnation temperature and pressure of the gas are measured in the source of the gas, where the latter is at rest. As the gas is accelerated in the nozzle, its pressure and temperature decrease and its velocity increases. In this case, the gas parameters are usually written as functions of the local Mach number (gas velocity divided by the local velocity of sound), and the Mach number depends on the cross-sectional area of the flow. The optimal variation of the cross-sectional area in the stream-wise direction (shape of the nozzle contour) is one of the sought quantities, which can be obtained by means of an analysis.

The stagnation temperature of the gas is normally set higher than the ambient temperature. If a particle moves slowly, it is surrounded by the gas with a temperature close to the stagnation temperature. If the particle velocity is close to the gas velocity, however, the particle is cooled down. If the particle concentration in the flow is not very high, the heat transfer between the particles and the gas does not violate the assumption about the adiabatic gas flow. The gas exhausts from a large volume where the pressure equals the stagnation pressure, the temperature equals the stagnation (total) temperature, and the velocity equals zero. In practice, this situation is similar to conditions upstream of the nozzle throat (critical cross section) where the cross-sectional area of the flow is at least three times greater than that of the cross-sectional area of the nozzle throat (in this case, the error is less than 3% in terms of pressure and 1% in terms of temperature).

The prescribed parameters in [1] are the total temperature and the flow rate of the gas (but not the stagnation pressure). For the gas to reach the velocity of sound in the nozzle throat (i.e., the Mach number equal to unity), a rather high stagnation pressure of the gas is necessary, which is usually provided in experiments. The gas pressure at the nozzle exit can differ from the pressure in the spraying chamber. If the pressure at the nozzle exit is lower than the pressure in the chamber, the flow is overexpanded; otherwise, the flow is underexpanded. In such flow regimes, the flow outside the nozzle (in the jet) cannot be described by simple one-dimensional equations of gas dynamics. The results of one-dimensional modeling inside the nozzle are applicable until overexpansion leads to origination of a normal shock at the nozzle exit. If the ratio of areas of the nozzle-exit and throat cross sections is set, it is possible to determine the Mach number at the nozzle exit and then all other gas parameters on the basis of this Mach number.

Particle acceleration is usually described by the equation

$$\frac{d\vec{v}_p}{dt} = C_D \frac{\rho}{2m_p} S_p \left|\vec{v} - \vec{v}_p\right| \left(\vec{v} - \vec{v}_p\right), \tag{5.1}$$

where $\vec{v}$ and $\vec{v}_p$ are the gas and particle velocities, m_p is the particle mass, ρ is the gas density, S_p is the particle mid-section area, and t is the time. The drag coefficient C_D can be borrowed from [6].

It follows from Eq. (5.1) that, first, the particle velocity is bounded by the gas velocity and, second, the particle velocity monotonically increases with increasing time of particle residence in the gas flow. As the distance covered by the particle increases with time, the longer the particle path, the higher its velocity. Third, the particle acceleration increases with increasing gas density. The optimal conditions of acceleration are determined by the condition of the maximum drag force in the right side of Eq. (5.1). The calculations performed in [1] show that the optimal density and velocity of the gas, which ensure the maximum acceleration of the particle, are obtained with a dimensionless Mach number close to $M \approx 1.4$. The optimal shape of the nozzle contour is obtained if the dimensionless Mach number (the difference between the gas and particle velocities divided by the velocity of sound in the gas) in each cross section is close to this value. Thus, a change in stagnation parameters of the gas leads to a change in the optimal geometry of the nozzle. To simplify the analysis, it is often assumed that the drag force reaches its maximum if the dimensionless Mach number equals 1 rather than 1.4. The particle density and size also affect the particle-acceleration process.

The effect of the nozzle geometry (three types of the nozzle contour: converging + barrel, converging and diverging (Laval type), and converging and diverging + barrel) was considered in [2]. The particles were assumed to have a spherical shape and have no temperature gradient inside. The effect of gravity, interaction of particles with each other, and effect of particles on the gas were ignored. The calculations were performed for a fixed total length of the nozzle equal to 300 mm, length of the converging section equal to 50 mm, and nozzle-throat diameter equal to 2 mm. The particle velocity at the exit of the Laval-type nozzle turned out to be higher than that in other nozzles. The highest temperature of particles was reached at the exit of the "converging nozzle + barrel" combination.

The velocity profiles for helium-accelerated copper particles (diameter 20.5 μm, stagnation pressure of the gas 2.1 MPa, and stagnation temperature 600 K) at the exit of rectangular and conical nozzles were compared in [7]. It was shown that a rectangular nozzle provides a more uniform distribution of particle velocity across the jet. The velocity profiles given in that paper demonstrate that the particle velocity at the jet boundary does not vanish but only decreases by 13–21%.

The study described in [8] employs a comparative simple analysis based on the isentropic model [9, 10] and the FLUENT program [11]. In both cases, the computations first deal with the gas flow and then with the particle motion [12, 13].

Based on isentropic computations, it was demonstrated that the particle temperature is almost independent of pressure, but the particle velocity increases by 15% if the pressure is doubled (from 1.5 to 3 MPa). A change in the gas temperature at a constant pressure of 2.5 MPa increases the particle velocity by 25% if the temperature is doubled (from 300 to 600 K). At high temperatures (above 793 K), the increase in particle velocity is less pronounced because of the decrease in gas density. Finer particles have higher velocities, but they are more intensely cooled, in contrast to coarser particles, which have an almost constant temperature if their diameter exceeds 30 μm. A comparison with FLUENT computations shows that the particle velocity is 10% lower than in the isentropic model. As the FLUENT program contains a stochastic model for particle tracks, their velocities differ by several meters per second. Thus, the critical velocity is somewhere between 530 and 550 m/s. The particle temperature is higher than that in the isentropic model. The experiments and FLUENT computations yield the optimal distances of 20–50 mm. The adverse effect of addition of the ambient air is manifested at larger distances.

The experiments and calculations were performed for four different nozzles. Nozzle A of a conical shape has the length of the expanding section equal to 65 mm and the ratio of the nozzle-exit to the throat section area (the so-called expansion ratio) equal to 6. Nozzle B has the same length and shape, but the expansion ratio equal to 9. Nozzle C is the version of nozzle A extended by a factor of 1.5 with a bell-shaped contour. The bell-shaped nozzle D is the version of nozzle B extended by a factor of 1.8. All nozzles were used to deposit copper particles onto an aluminum substrate. Only particles that reached the critical velocity were assumed to attach; for the measured distribution function of the particle size, only those particles were assumed to attach whose size was smaller than the diameter for which the cumulative mass fraction is equivalent to deposition efficiency. This diameter is 12.2 μm for nozzle A, 14.3 μm for nozzle B, 15.8 μm for nozzle C, and 17.5 μm for nozzle D; the velocities for all these sizes are calculated within 550–570 m/s. The effect of the nozzle geometry on particle velocity was considered in more detail by one-dimensional calculations. Nozzle B was compared with a nozzle designed by the method of characteristics and possessing the length of the expanding section equal to 130 mm. To accelerate particles 10, 15, and 20 μm in diameter to a velocity of 560 m/s, the gas temperature and pressure were varied within 373–673 K and 1.5–3.5 MPa. For instance, a 10 μm particle reaches the critical velocity at a temperature of 593 K and a pressure of 1.8 MPa or at a temperature of 450 K and a pressure of 3.5 MPa. In accordance with the previously made assumptions, deposition of all particles with diameters up to 10 μm corresponds to the deposition efficiency of 22%. Acceleration of 15 μm particles to the critical velocity is possible at a temperature of 593 K and a pressure of 3.3 MPa. In this case, the deposition efficiency is 58%. An increase in length and contouring of the nozzle by the method of characteristics yields similar particle velocities for lower temperatures and pressures of the gas. Such a nozzle can accelerate larger particles (u to 20 μm and more) to the critical velocity and provide the deposition efficiency equal to 80%.

Similar optimization was described in [14, 15]. The problem of optimization of the gas-dynamic path with allowance for motion of particles in the nozzle and their deceleration in the compressed shock layer immediately ahead of the substrate was solved in [14]. Simple analytical estimates for the particle velocity at the nozzle exit and at the impact moment were found. Two-dimensional modeling of the gas–particle flow in the nozzle with allowance for turbulence was performed in [15]; the influence of particles on the gas was neglected. If the aluminum particle size was smaller than 5 μm, the particle velocity drastically decreased because of the shock wave ahead of the substrate.

The calculated particle velocities at the nozzle exit were compared with experimental values obtained by the PIV method in [16] (see Fig. 5.1). The measurements were performed at a distance of 16 mm from the nozzle exit, the particles being accelerated by nitrogen and helium. The stagnation temperature and pressure were varied independent of each other within 573–773 K and 2.0–2.4 MPa. A nickel powder (with the mean particle size of 19 μm) with the flow rate of 3.7×10^5 kg/s was used. The Laval nozzle with the throat diameter of 2.6 mm, exit diameter of 8.4, and the length of the supersonic section of 125 mm allows accelerating particle by nitrogen up to 540–590 m/s for 2.0 MPa and to 570–600 m/s for 2.4 MPa and by helium up to 725–775 m/s for 2.0 MPa and to 760–800 m/s for 2.4 MPa. The figures refer to the extreme values of stagnation temperature. In the considered range of parameters, the increase in velocity is almost linear. The predictions are in good agreement with the experiments for helium and yield lower values (approximately by 40 m/s) for the case of using nitrogen.

In addition, the calculations reveal a shock wave inside the nozzle, very close to the nozzle exit, in the case of a helium flow with the stagnation parameters of 2.4 MPa and 773 K.

The impact velocity of copper and platinum particles ranging from 0.1 to 50 μm was calculated in [17] (see Fig. 5.2). In a nozzle with a very large expansion ratio (ratio of the

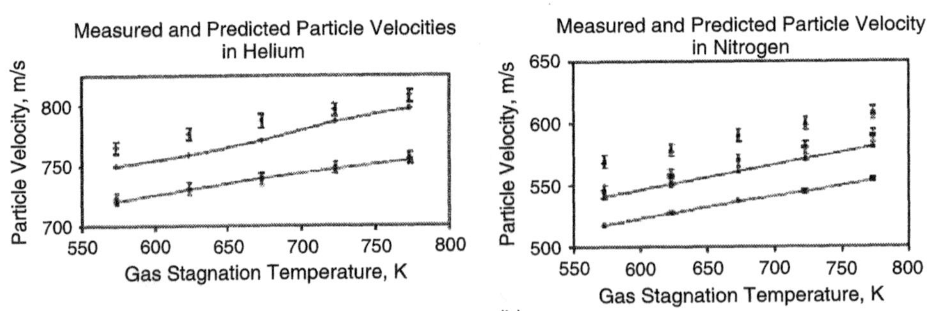

(a) (b)

Fig. 5.1. Comparison between the measured average particle velocity in the first 16 mm of the jet and predicted average particle velocity [16]. The predicted values are connected with a line. (a) Helium and (b) Nitrogen.

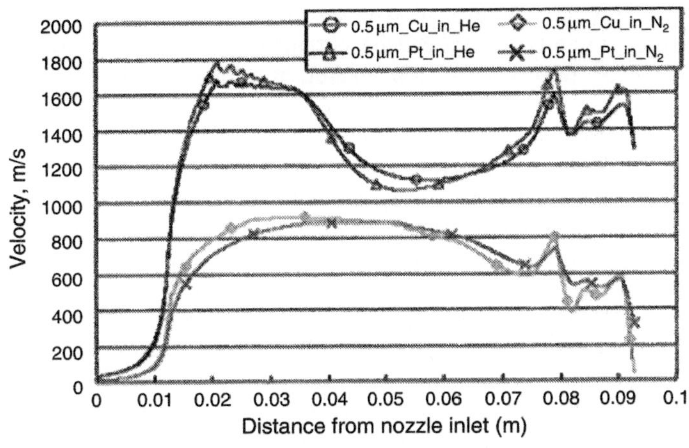

(a)

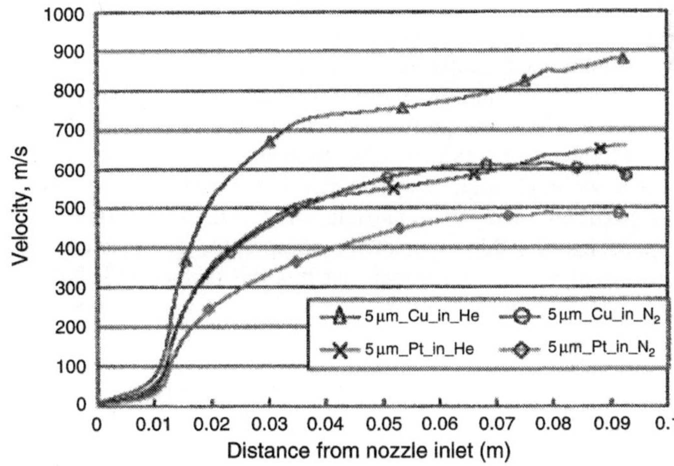

(b)

Fig. 5.2. Comparison of velocity of copper and platinum particles [17]. (a) $d_p = 0.5\,\mu m$ and (b) $d_p = 5\,\mu m$.

nozzle-exit to the throat area equal to 28.4), a nitrogen flow with stagnation parameters of 2.0 MPa and 773 K could ensure the maximum velocity (600 m/s) for 5 μm particles of copper and the minimum velocity (50 m/s) for 0.5 μm particles of copper. The use of a helium flow with the same stagnation parameters yields the maximum velocity (1400 m/s) for 0.5–1 μm and the minimum velocity (200 m/s) for 50 μm particles of copper. It was noted that 0.1 μm particles could not reach the substrate because they were entrained by the gas.

It was argued in [18] that the particle velocity, being the most important cold spray parameter, is not the only factor that determines the state of the particle before and after the impact. It is seen from a simple analysis that the particle momentum for an unchanged velocity and size depends on the density of the particle material, whereas the impact force and pressure, in turn, depend on momentum. The estimates showed that a pressure of approximately 3 GPa can be obtained in an impact. The critical velocity is 560 m/s for copper, 600 m/s for iron, nickel, and their alloys, and 680–700 m/s for aluminum (20% higher than for copper). The experience shows that a high deposition efficiency for an identical set of parameters and, hence, identical velocities of the gas can be obtained for aluminum and iron powders with identical size distribution functions. It should be noted that the particle velocities are different in these cases. The measurements of velocities of spherical iron and aluminum particles of a commensurable size show that their acceleration agrees with the theoretical estimates. Iron particles reach the maximum velocity at a distance of 75–100 mm from the nozzle exit, and aluminum particles reach the maximum velocity at a distance of 25–50 mm from the nozzle exit, the velocities of aluminum and iron particles being approximately 620 and 450 m/s, respectively.

The optimal size of particles as a function of the input parameters (type of the gas, its pressure and temperature, density of particles, nozzle geometry, etc.) is analytically estimated in [19]. The optimal size is understood as a particle size at which the particles impact onto the substrate with the maximum velocity and/or maximum temperature. Obtaining the highest possible velocities is necessary because many experiments show that the quality of coatings is improved with increasing particle size. Moreover, for a given powder/substrate combination, there exists a critical velocity (increasing for an oblique impact) above which the particles start attaching to the substrate [20, 21]. The study [22] showed that the factors providing high impact velocities are the use of gases with low molecular weights, high temperatures and pressures of the gas, long nozzles, low densities of particles, and small particle sizes. The factor ignored, however, was deceleration of particles in a thin layer of the compressed gas between the substrate and the shock wave formed when a supersonic jet hits the surface [23, 24]. Passing through this layer, the particles lose their velocity; the higher the gas pressure and the lower the particle density and size, the greater the decrease in velocity.

The powder is usually inserted into the flow upstream of the supersonic nozzle throat along the nozzle centerline, which facilitates a comparison of experimental data with the results of one-dimensional modeling of particle acceleration. As it follows from [19], the experimentally measured distribution of particle velocity (25 mm from the nozzle exit) is in reasonable agreement with the distribution calculated for a given powder (mean size 15 μm and standard deviation 5 μm), though the model does not take into account collisions between the particles and with the nozzle wall. The following empirical relation, which generalizes the data on particle-velocity measurements at the exit of a supersonic nozzle with a rectangular cross section, was derived in [25]:

$$\frac{v_p^*}{v^*} = \left(1 + 0.85\sqrt{\frac{d_p}{L}\frac{\rho_p v^{*2}}{p_0}}\right)^{-1} \tag{5.2}$$

Deceleration of particles in the stagnant region is studied by using analytical relations. The stagnant region can include a recirculation flow [26–28]. It was demonstrated in experiments that the thickness of this region is approximately one half of the minimum thickness of the jet [25] and varies depending on the pressure at the nozzle exit and on the distance between the nozzle exit and the substrate. Oscillations of the bow shock wave are frequently observed as well. Assuming that the gas velocity in the stagnant region is low as compared with the particle velocity, we can integrate the equation of motion of the particle to obtain an analytical solution, which, however, ignores the lateral flow (along the substrate surface) entraining the particle along the surface. Obviously, small particles lose their velocities significantly in the stagnant region, whereas large particles do not have enough time to be accelerated to sufficient velocities in the nozzle. Thus, for each set of gas parameters and nozzle geometry, there is an optimal diameter of particles that gives the highest velocity. The calculations show that the maximum impact velocities are identical, despite the differences in particle densities and sizes. The optimal particle size is different for different types of the accelerating gas: the optimal size for nitrogen is greater than that for helium. At the same time, it should be taken into account that powders are characterized by a certain distribution in size, which is usually described by the normal distribution with a known mean particle size and standard deviation. If the powder is chosen such that the mean size coincides with the optimal value, some of these particles (whose size is much smaller or much larger than the optimal value) have very low impact velocities. Therefore, powders with the impact velocities of the smallest and the largest particles being higher than the critical velocity should be chosen.

It often happens that the deposition efficiency measured for typical experimental parameters is lower than the theoretical value (which is determined as the fraction of the powder whose velocity is higher than the critical value). The theoretical deposition efficiency can be reached only under the condition of the minimum growth of the coating during one pass to be sure that the impact occurs at an angle of 90° to the surface (the critical velocity concept implies the normal impact). To check the statement that the maximum impact velocity is necessary to obtain coatings with the best characteristics, experiments on copper deposition onto aluminum under different conditions were performed [19]; the results of these tests proved the validity of this statement. An increase in velocity increases the deposition efficiency and adhesion and decreases the porosity and roughness of the coating. Moreover, the higher the particle (and/or substrate) temperature, the higher the adhesion and deposition efficiency and the lower the coating porosity. Thus, the analytical and experimental results show that the best quality of coatings is obtained with the maximum particle velocity. For this purpose, deposition should be performed with the maximum pressure and temperature of the gas and with the optimal size of particles. High temperatures of the gas also offer other advantages, e.g., lower flow rates of the gas.

It was shown in [29] that the size, shape, and the method of powder production affect the characteristics of the process, whereas the type, temperature, and the pressure of the gas influence the deposition efficiency. In turn, the process parameter affects the coating microstructure, which alters the mechanical and thermal properties of the coating. The results can be summarized as follows:

- metals, composites, and alloys readily form coatings with good adhesion and density;
- metallic matrix composites can be obtained with good adhesion between the matrix and the disperse material;
- coatings of different stainless steels have significantly different microstructures under identical process conditions.

One-dimensional modeling of particle acceleration during cold spraying with the use of the Navier–Stokes equations, including the $\kappa - \varepsilon$ model of turbulence, which was verified experimentally, was performed in [30]. It was demonstrated that fine particles are affected by the shock wave ahead of the substrate, which decelerates the flow. The computations were performed with two programs: the first one involved a finite-difference scheme [31], and the second one was the FLUENT program. The advantage of the first program is the possibility of controlling artificial viscosity, aimed at stabilizing the solution. A comparison of the computational time showed that the computations with the second program are 30% faster. The computational domain is divided into two sub-domains: one is the region inside the nozzle and the other is the region of the jet and the impact onto the substrate. The no-slip and adiabatic conditions were set on the nozzle walls. The distance from the nozzle exit to the substrate was 10 mm. The solution for the flow at the nozzle exit was used as the boundary condition for a free supersonic jet. The static pressure at the jet boundary was 0.1 MPa. The no-slip condition was set on the substrate surface, which was assumed to have a constant and uniform temperature of 20 °C.

A comparison between the measured pressure distribution and the numerical estimates shows that they are very close, though there are certain differences caused by two factors. First, it is difficult to exactly establish the substrate position with respect to the nozzle exit, as there is some positioning error; the second factor is the error in modeling of turbulence of such flows by the $\kappa - \varepsilon$ model. The flow characteristics were computed for a stagnation pressure of 0.493 MPa, stagnation temperature of 22 °C, and an ambient pressure of 0.1 MPa. The distance to the substrate was varied from 10 to 70 mm with a step of 10 mm. For a distance of 10 mm, the computations predicted a shock wave ahead of the substrate; in passing through this shock wave, the flow velocity at the jet axis decreases instantaneously from 650 to 200 m/s, and then it smoothly decreases to zero at the stagnation point. The shock wave in the vicinity of the jet axis is straight, but it becomes oblique toward the jet edges. The oblique shock wave is formed because the normal shock does not change the flow direction, in contrast to oblique waves. As the flow turns sharply to move along the substrate surface, the presence of an oblique shock wave at the jet edges is required. The oblique shock wave does not reduce the velocity to an extent the normal shock does: the flow turned by the oblique shock wave still has a velocity of approximately 350 m/s. After turning, the flow is again accelerated to a supersonic velocity. Significant velocity gradients arise near the substrate surface, which lead to high shear stresses, and the latter can be sufficiently high to cause spalling of the newly formed coating. It should be noted that these results are in good agreement with the experimental data obtained in [32].

The results obtained at a distance of 50 mm differ from those obtained at a distance of 10 mm. There is no shock wave in the flow: at such a distance, viscous forces reduce the flow velocity to subsonic values. Thus, the flow is subsonic in the vicinity of the substrate, and no shock wave is needed to reduce the velocity and turn the flow parallel to the surface. For a distance of 10 mm, the pressure drastically increases in passing through the shock wave and the gas density increases to $2.45\,\mathrm{kg/m^3}$, whereas the flow is decelerated. For a distance of 50 mm, the pressure increases gradually, and the gas density increases to $2.17\,\mathrm{kg/m^3}$.

The motion of copper particles 10 and 1 μm in diameter was calculated in [30]. It was found that the distance has a pronounced effect on the impact velocity of fine particles, which increases from 420 to 550 m/s with the distance increased from 10 to 50 mm. This occurs because of shock-wave attenuation, because the influence of viscous forces becomes more significant with increasing distance, which leads to a decrease in the Mach number in the vicinity of the substrate, and the lower the Mach number, the weaker the shock wave is needed for the flow to pass to a subsonic regime. The results are lower densities of the gas behind the shock wave and a smaller difference in velocities. The drag force decreases thereby, and the impact velocity increases. This favorable effect disappears if the distance becomes greater than 50 mm and the shock wave vanishes. A similar behavior is typical for particles 10 μm in diameter, though the difference in velocities for distances of 10 and 50 mm is less than 5%. Coarser particles have a greater momentum and experience less significant deceleration by the shock wave; such a behavior was predicted in [22]. Higher impact velocities at a distance of 50 mm should have provided higher deposition efficiency, but this is not confirmed by the experiments [30], which showed that the deposition efficiency decreases with increasing distance. It was argued in [30] that the main reason for this contradiction being the allowance for particles moving only along the axis made in computations. In reality, most particles do not move strictly in the axial direction. Particles moving outside the close vicinity of the axis cross the oblique shock wave, which reflects the particles. Therefore, these particles hit the substrate at an angle different from 90°, which decreases the deposition efficiency. In addition, as the gas velocity is lower at the jet boundaries than that in the jet core, the impact velocity of peripheral particles is lower than the predicted value. Note that a decrease in the substrate and particle temperatures can also reduce the deposition efficiency.

A simple empirical formula for the particle velocity at the nozzle exit, which was obtained by modifying Eq. (5.2), was obtained in [33]. The Al12Si powder with the mean particle size of 25 μm was deposited onto a soft steel substrate. The distributions of particles in terms of their velocity and size at the nozzle exit versus gas temperature and pressure were obtained in experiments. The particle-velocity distributions can be approximated by the upper part of the Gaussian curve. Particle velocities close to zero could not be registered in the experiment: thus, e.g., the minimum particle velocity for the jet temperature of 400 °C and pressure in the pre-chamber of 2.5 MPa is approximately 400 m/s, while the maximum particle velocity is 800 m/s (see Fig. 5.3).

The distribution of particles over the jet cross section has a clearly expressed Gaussian character with a dramatic decrease in the particle concentration at the jet boundaries (see Fig. 5.4).

The coating-growth kinetics depending on the gas temperature (150–500 °C) and pressure (2.5 and 2.9 MPa) and on the number of passes (1 and 2) was studied in detail. Figure 5.5 shows the experimentally measured distributions of particle velocity, concentration, and coating thickness.

Based on these comparisons, the critical deposition velocity for these conditions was determined: approximately 580 m/s for the interaction of particles with the substrate

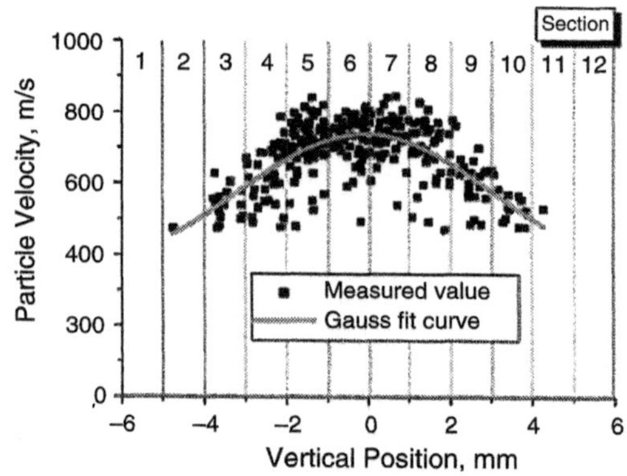

Fig. 5.3. Distribution of particle velocity at the exit of an axisymmetric nozzle for the gas (helium) temperature of 400 °C and stagnation pressure of 2.5 MPa [33].

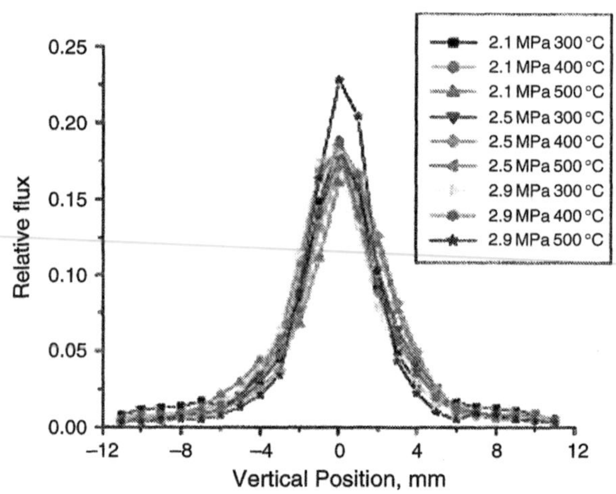

Fig. 5.4. Concentration of particles in the jet at the exit of an axisymmetric nozzle for different stagnation pressures and temperatures of helium [33].

surface and 700 m/s for the interaction of particles with the surface formed by previously deposited particles.

The effect of the particles of sizes from 10 to 100 μm and the diameter of the tube for powder insertion on deposition with the use of a nozzle with a rectangular cross section, the throat diameter of 3 mm, and the exit size of 3 mm × 10 mm was considered in [34]. A decrease in the powder-tube diameter (from 2.54 to 0.9 mm) and an increase in particle size from (a) 10% of particles smaller than 9 μm, 50% of particles smaller than 20 μm, and 90% of particles smaller than 40 μm to (b) 10% of particles smaller than 45 μm, 50% of particles smaller then 62 μm, and 90% of particle smaller than 80 μm for aluminum

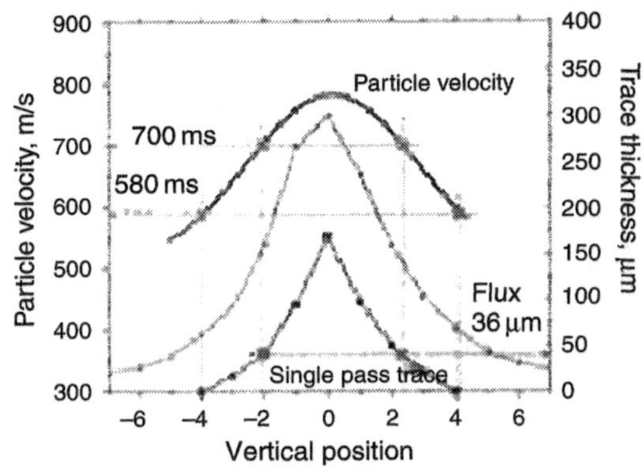

Fig. 5.5. Particle velocity, concentration, and coating thickness versus the jet radius [33].

and from (a) smaller than 45 μm to (b) 10% of particles smaller than 34 μm, 50% of particle smaller than 62 μm, and 90% of particles smaller than 112 μm for copper lead to a higher deposition efficiency. If the tube was moved inward the pre-chamber, the deposition efficiency of coarse particles decreased to the value typical of fine particles. A possible explanation for this effect proposed in [34] is an increase in residence time of particles in a hot gas, and this factor increases the thickness of the oxide film on the particle surface, which interferes with particle attachment.

The structure of the nozzle with radial injection of powder downstream of the Laval nozzle throat was described in [35]. The main reason for this study was the possibility of decreasing the pressure in the feeder. The computations showed that the performance of such a structure is not worse than that of the traditional one (axial supply of powder at the entrance of the Laval nozzle), but such a structure also provides a higher impact velocity of particles. Thus, the particle velocity in the conventional structure with a stagnation pressure of 0.7 MPa is 742 m/s; in the structure with radial injection further downstream, the particle velocity for a stagnation pressure of 2 MPa (in this case, the pressure in the feeder is 0.7 MPa) reaches 900 m/s. If the stagnation pressure in the conventional structure is also set to 2 MPa, the velocity turns out to be higher (981 m/s). It was demonstrated in computations that the optimal length of the expanding part of the nozzle should be 270 mm for the nozzle-throat diameter of 2 mm and nozzle-exit diameter of 6.3 mm. In such geometry the powder should be inserted at a distance of 35–40 mm downstream of the throat cross section.

Experimental and computed velocities of nickel particles with the mean size of 20 μm at the exit of an axisymmetric Laval nozzle are compared in [36]. The model takes into account turbulence via the $\kappa - \varepsilon$ turbulence model, and the influence of particles on the gas is neglected. The parameters varied in computations and experiments were stagnation temperature (573–873 K) and pressure (2.0 and 2.4 MPa). Good agreement was reached between experimental and numerical data. It is of interest to note that the computations revealed the formation of oblique shock waves shortly upstream of the nozzle exit. The computations predict that the gas velocity behind these waves significantly decreases (from 2530 to 1800 m/s for helium, 773 K, 2.4 MPa and from 1100 to 500 m/s for nitrogen, 773 K, 2.4 MPa). The authors did not indicate the reasons for wave formation and did not propose any method to avoid it.

Advantages of a contoured nozzle over the conventional conical nozzle are considered in [37]. Nozzle contouring allows obtaining a more uniform profile of particle velocity and expanding the range of size of particles reaching the critical deposition velocity. The technology of sintering of solid alloys (e.g., WC-Co) for manufacturing contoured nozzles is fairly beneficial because it facilitates manufacturing, prevents powder deposition on the nozzle walls, and thus increases the gas temperature. Data are presented on spraying of a composite coating $Al + Al_2O_3$, which maintains high electrical and thermal conductivity but its wear resistance is twice higher than that of a pure aluminum coating.

Experimental aspects of determining the critical deposition velocity are discussed in [38]. The velocities of the incident particles and the number of rebounded particles were determined by the time-of-flight optical method with three-exposure filming. The critical deposition velocity can be determined on the basis of the decrease in the number of rebounded particles. The method is not sufficiently accurate, however, because of the distributions of particles in terms of size and velocity, fluctuations in material properties, selectivity of the method, etc. The effect of selectivity in deposition is also noted in the paper, namely, whereas the mean size of the initial copper powder is 16.2 μm, the mean size of particles in the coating is 6.5 μm. The authors of the paper do not give any comments on this phenomenon.

To conclude this section, we should note that models with an adequate description of the motion of the gas and particles inside the Laval nozzle with circular and rectangular cross sections, a large aspect ratio, and a small (several millimeters) thickness for low concentrations of particles are currently available. With allowance for the decelerating effect of the compressed layer ahead of the substrate, one can calculate the impact velocity and the temperature of particles before the impact. Still insufficient attention is paid to optimization of loading the gas flow by the powder and to investigations of unconventional schemes of flow formation (e.g., ejector scheme, etc.). The substrate geometry is usually plane, there are no experimental measurements of the gas and particle velocities inside the compressed layer, and unsteadiness of the bow shock wave is ignored. Influence of particles on the shock-wave structure of the flow in the vicinity of the substrate is not considered, and the substrate temperature is given little attention (in experiments as well). These and some other issues in the field of cold spray gas-dynamics require additional studies.

5.2. Interaction of High-speed Particles with the Substrate. Bonding Mechanism

The mechanism of formation of bonds between the particle and the substrate owing to a high-velocity impact is the topic of many discussions in the field of cold gas-dynamic spraying.

Based on a brief analysis of the impact of particles and investigations of compression phenomena in the shock wave, an attempt was made in [39] to systematize the suitability of materials for cold gas-dynamic spraying. It is commonly recognized that a material to be used for cold spray should have features of plasticity ensuring pressing, shear of surfaces, and fixation. According to the theory of impact dynamics, the pressure wave and the resulting plastic shock wave lead to significant deformations of the particle. The estimates made on the basis of the equation of state show that the peak shock pressure in the velocity regime typical of cold spray reaches 40–50 GPa for materials based on iron and copper. The deformation kinetics (determined by material properties, mainly by the crystal and grain structure and by the type of bonding inside the material) and the time evolution of the shock pressure were modeled for a particle 20 μm in diameter made of the 316L material with allowance for its properties depending on the strain rate and temperature in accordance with the data of [40]. The computations implied that the deformation is adiabatic (as a consequence of the short time of the process) and that 90% of the plastic work is transformed to heat. The substrate was modeled by a cylinder with the diameter and height equal to 3 and 5 particle sizes, respectively. The grid was generated with the cell size decreasing in regions of high strains. A detailed analysis of the increase in particle and substrate deformation with increasing velocity can be found in [41, 42]. It was shown that the contact pressure in the impact direction depends on the particle velocity, and its maximum is observed at the first stage of the impact (13 and 25 GPa for impact velocities of 700 and 1200 m/s, respectively). The further change in pressure with time is determined by the increase in the contact area between the particle and the substrate.

The fundamental description of the behavior of metals subjected to compression in the shock wave (SW) is provided by the Hugoniot equation of state [43–45]. The Hugoniot curve shows the final states reachable during SW transition and depends on material properties. The line connecting the first and last points is called the "Rayleigh line" and characterizes the SW velocity. The area under the Rayleigh line reproduces the increase in internal energy, which increases with increasing temperature up to the shock temperature. After the SW has passed, the unloading follows the isentrope, and the material is heated to a certain temperature (the so-called residual temperature). The Hugoniot curve and the curve of adiabatic unloading (isentrope) deviate from each other insignificantly; therefore, the residual temperature is low, in contrast to the shock temperature. For the majority of metals, the Hugoniot curve reflects the fact of continuous compression with increasing SW pressure. A typical feature of iron is the non-monotonic behavior at a pressure of 13 GPa at which the transformation of alpha- to gamma-iron occurs.

The reachable residual temperatures are insufficient for material melting. At the boundary with high strains, however, melting is possible owing to shear processes and high SW pressures. An analysis of samples with deposited coatings of the TiAl6V4 alloy shows that local melting occurs [41]. The authors of [39] believe that melting is possible (at least theoretically) if the particle temperature before the impact is about 500 °C.

The SW behavior in the material is described by the laws of conservation of mass, momentum, and energy at the SW front. A linear relation between the mass velocity and SW velocity for moderate pressures is applicable for most metals. The proportionality factor depends on the Grueneisen parameter and describes the relation between the internal energy and pressure at constant volume. The flow of the material is determined by the Mises–Tresca criterion: at this limiting stress, the elastic SW passes to the plastic state.

Depending on characteristics of the materials, the equiaxial description of the dynamic yield stress allows one to estimate the ultimate stresses. A simple estimate of this ultimate value by a quantity proportional to the Brinell hardness was given in [44].

The particle impact proceeds in two stages: an increase in pressure and elastic deformation of particles up to the dynamic yield stress and plastic deformation with significant deformation of the material structure and material heating. If the impact velocity is sufficient and the yield stress is exceeded, the elastic phase is negligibly short. The impact pressure is determined by material properties included into the Grueneisen parameter [46].

The computations [39] show that the contact pressure of 2.5 GPa acts for 3×10^{-8} s if the velocity is 700 m/s. The impact kinetics is terminated here. After that, the pressures are much lower, though still higher, than the dynamic yield stress. The strain rate is very high, above $10^5\ s^{-1}$, which is the reason for the hardening effect due to accumulation of dislocations. Correspondingly, it is difficult to obtain a dense coating from the strain-hardening 316L alloy. Strain hardening of the TiAl6V4 alloy at temperatures below the beta-transition is insignificant; moreover, it poorly yields to cold working, and this can explain high porosity and cracks in coatings [47, 48].

In cold spray, the form of the dependence of material properties on the strain rate plays the governing role. The deformation process is determined by mobility of dislocations and their interaction [49]. This implies, in particular, that the crystal structure and the type of bonds, the structure and size of grains, and foreign atoms and phases determine the resistance to strains. A comparison of deformation properties of various materials shows that metals with the same crystal structure and type of bonds have an identical mechanism of deformation [50].

Polycrystalline solids are classified into isomechanical groups, i.e., groups that possess similar mechanical properties. The most important isomechanical groups of metals are: aluminum, copper, silver, gold, platinum, nickel, and gamma-iron (face-centered cubic (FCC) lattice); tungsten, tantalum, molybdenum, niobium, vanadium, chromium, alpha-iron, and beta-titanium (bulk-centered cubic (BCC) lattice); and cadmium, zinc, cobalt, magnesium, and titanium (hexagonal lattice, which is the densest packing).

Metals with the FCC lattice have the greatest number of slipping planes, which is responsible for their high plasticity; metals with the hexagonal structure have much fewer slipping planes, which yield a lower plasticity; and metals with the BCC lattice have the lowest plasticity among the three types. Groups of tetragonal or trigonal crystalline systems include oxides that are not suitable for cold spray because of their low plasticity (this issue has not been adequately addressed to definitely state inapplicability of all oxides and ceramics for cold spray).

If we plot the homological temperature (ratio of temperature to the melting point) on the x axis and the product of the shear modulus and compression modulus on the y axis and mark points corresponding to various metals in the diagram, it turns out that more plastic materials are located in the right side of the diagram close to the x axis, whereas less plastic materials can be found in the left side of the diagram close to the y axis. This positioning allows us to classify materials from the viewpoint of their suitability for cold spray. Copper is considered as an almost ideal material, which has a low resistance to strain and a melting point below 1100 °C. Materials with a low melting point can be readily compacted. In general, cold spray treatment of BCC metals involves more difficulties, because the mobility of spiral dislocations under strains with high rates is limited by Peierls stresses [51].

A high impact pressure forms a plastic shock wave responsible for strain hardening of the material. An extremely rapid increase in pressure during the impact is an important characteristic of the process. It was demonstrated numerically and experimentally [52] that a certain time of pressure growth and duration of the plastic wave can cause melting. The time of pressure growth should be shorter than the time needed for the SW-induced heat to dissipate. The calculations show that the peak pressure is reached in less than 10^{-8} s. For titanium-containing materials, insignificant dissipation of heat occurs during this time, and melting can start on the contact area.

Deformation of the entire particle is impossible because the plastic SW is rapidly attenuated as the SW front surface increases. When the stress decreases to a value equal to the Hugoniot elastic limit (limiting pressure at which a bilateral transition from elasticity to plasticity and back occurs), a plastic SW transforms to an elastic SW. Simple estimates show that the pressure acting during the impact exceeds the Hugoniot elastic limit (HEL). It can turn out, however, that the HEL is not reached at the first instant of the contact (depending on the material). For titanium-containing materials, the ultimate stresses are high, and the impact pressures are lower than those for, e.g., copper. This testifies that it is more difficult to obtain coatings from titanium-containing materials by the cold spray than coatings from copper. Copper-containing materials have extremely low ultimate stresses and high impact pressures; as a result, there are plastic deformations until the end of the process. Aluminum forms cold spray coatings rather easily [53–55] because its typical features are high impact temperatures, low dynamic limits of the flow, and low values of the yield criterion, which significantly depends on temperature in the range above 150 °C [56]. For some particular aluminum-containing alloys, a dense coating can hardly be formed, which is due to a high HEL and a low impact pressure.

It is difficult to deposit materials with the BCC lattice by the cold spray method, even if helium is used as an accelerating gas. Under moderate strain rates, some BCC metals can be deformed similar to FCC metals; for strain rates typical of cold spray, however, the necessity of activating the motion of spiral dislocations (which require 200 times more energy that dislocations in the FCC matrix) makes this type of metals much more difficult for plastic deformation. Metals with a hexagonal structure and low melting point can be readily deposited. Therefore, some other parameters should be taken into account in addition to mechanical characteristics, e.g., such as the bonding strength.

From the viewpoint of material science, the suitability of materials for cold spray could be related to Peierls stress, but available publications are insufficient to draw this conclusion. The material characteristic, such as phonon mobility, plays the governing role at high strain rates, but no data that confirm this assumption were found in the literature. Because of its low strength, magnesium could be expected to easily form coatings by the cold spray; nevertheless, because of its low density and, correspondingly, low impact momentum, it requires high particle velocities for necessary impact pressures to be reached. The low melting point of magnesium restricts the deposition process by low temperatures of the gas (correspondingly, by low impact velocities), which necessitates the use of lighter gases (helium) for magnesium compacting. Hence, in addition to strength characteristics of the material, one should also consider whether the required particle velocity and impact temperature can be reached in practice.

The particle impact leads in most cases to high plastic strains as soon as the dynamic ultimate strength is exceeded. Elastic strains can be negligibly small in the first approximation. The mobility of dislocations in the crystal lattice is classified by the lattice type: FCC, BCC, and hexagonal types. The deformability (plasticity) and, hence, the possibility of deposition by the cold spray also depend on the lattice type. The type of bonding of molecules characterized in the first approximation by the melting point can be used as a criterion for the estimate. Materials with the melting point approximately at 1600 °C or higher are usually poorly compacted by the cold spray method. Zinc, aluminum, and copper are ideal materials because they have a low ultimate strength and become softened with increasing temperature. For most iron- and nickel-containing materials, vice versa, low temperatures of the process do not allow obtaining high-quality coatings [39]. It should be emphasized, nevertheless, that the features considered offer only an approximate idea about the capability of materials to form coatings in the cold spray. There some exceptions: experiments with nanostructured oxide ceramics (e.g., from the ZrO_2 oxide) [57] show that these materials can be deposited by the cold spray, though the resultant coating can be only one layer thick.

The effect of the substrate material on deposition was considered in [58]. An experiment with an impact of aluminum particles displays associated phenomena: substrate-melting, deformation of the substrate and particles, and evidence of formation of a metal jet (similar to a jet formed in explosive welding). It is difficult to initiate aluminum deposition onto non-metals (where the substrate/particle metallic bond cannot be formed) and onto soft metals (where substrate melting was observed in the case tin was used). As a whole, metal substrates possessing a higher hardness than aluminum particles are favorable for deposition. In this case, initiation proceeds easily, even if there is no substrate deformation.

There is a certain analogy between the particle impact and explosive welding. A distinctive feature of explosive welding is formation of a metal jet [59]. This jet is formed under the action of high static pressures provided by an HE explosion. Explosive welding depends on the formation of a pure surface owing to ejection of the metal contained in the jet and, as a consequence, on the close contact. An impact of a plastic particle onto a non-deformable substrate with velocities typical of SGC conditions was simulated [60] with the use of results of experimental investigations of aluminum particles sprayed onto non-deformable substrates. The predicted distribution of the radial component of velocity showed that an ejection of the metal jet is possible. At the same time, it was established that melting in the contact zone in a very thin layer can occur under certain conditions. Other researchers (see, e.g., [10, 61]) also tend to assume that both surface melting and formation of pure metal surfaces in the metal jet similar to explosive welding can contribute to formation of adhesive bonds.

Some papers, e.g., [22], display the evidence of metal-jet formation and show that the particle or the substrate need not be in the melted state to obtain high adhesion in the cold spray process. Deposition of coarse aluminum particles (greater than 50 μm) onto a brass substrate was described in [62]; it was argued there that particle melting does not occur, and adhesive bonds arise as a result of significant deformation and fracture of oxide films on metal particles, which allows pure metals to contact each other. The stages of coating formation were described, which allows better understanding of the cold spraying kinetics (see Fig. 5.6).

There are some investigations that support the fact of melting in the case of spraying aluminum particles onto a nickel substrate [63]. X-ray diffraction revealed the formation of an intermetallide zone 200–500 Å in the particle/substrate contact region. This was an indication of possible melting of aluminum, as the temperature at the beginning of the reaction where aluminum nickelides are formed is higher than the melting point of aluminum.

Some researchers study the influence of surface topography on the formation of bonds between the particle and the substrate. It was assumed in [64] that the first incident particles activate the substrate by generating roughness on it, and the subsequent particles are attached to the thus-prepared surface.

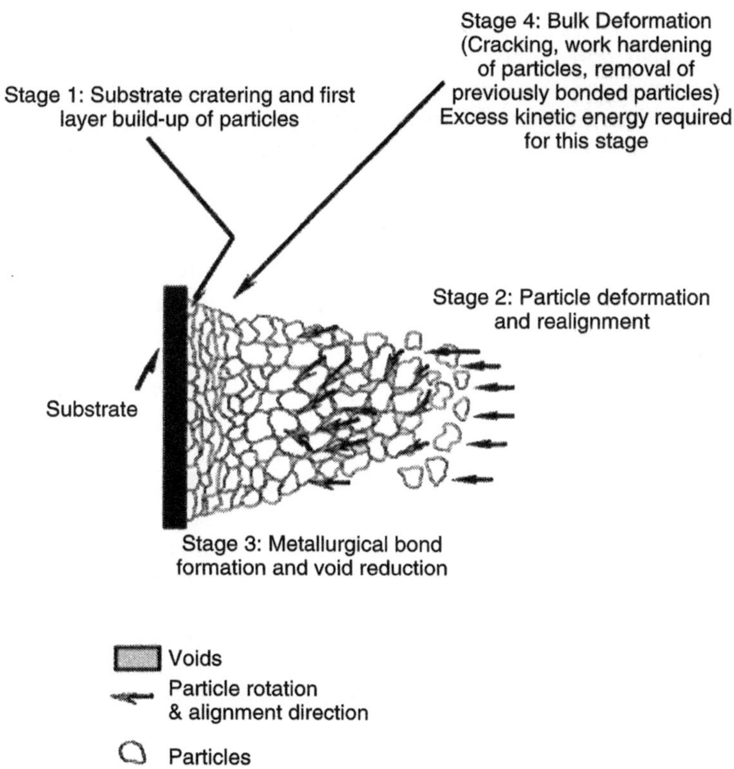

Fig. 5.6. Stages of coating formation in the kinetic spray process [62].

The impacts of particles of various powders on various substrates were considered in [18]. The difference in the capability of particles to deposition was described in terms of mechanical properties of the substrate and the specific impulse of the impact. Particle adhesion is primarily related to the readiness of the substrate and particle to deform, and adhesion is assumed to be possible if the particle is substantially more plastic than the substrate.

It was shown in [58] that the degree of the adhesive bond depends on the nature of the substrate material rather than on its mechanical properties only. The evidence of metal-jet formation was presented simultaneously with the evidence that melting can occur in some particular cases. Aluminum powder with a particle size of $75 \pm 15\,\mu m$ and Vickers microhardness of 0.315 GPa was used in the experiments of [58]. The surface of substrates made of different materials was polished by diamond paste with a grain size of $1\,\mu m$. The particles were accelerated by helium at room temperature and at a stagnation pressure of 2.5 MPa. Coatings of best quality were obtained on metal substrates whose hardness was higher than 2 GPa. Spraying onto non-metals formed a very thin layer with bald patches. As the growth of the coating thickness implies that particles are attached to particles that have already attached to the substrate, the difference in spraying onto different substrates can be expected to refer mainly to the stage of interaction of particles with the substrate surface: in other words, to formation of the first layer of the coating.

Among all materials tested, only tin was softer than aluminum particles. An insignificant amount of aluminum particles were deposited onto the tin surface: only particles less than $5\,\mu m$ in diameter. The fraction of fine particles in the powder used was rather small. The estimates of [65] show that more than 80% of the kinetic energy of the impact transforms to heat. The occurrence of melting depends on the heat capacity of the volume where heat dissipates, on thermal conductivity, and on melting point of the substrate material. The apparent reason for tin melting is its low melting point; no melting was observed for other materials. Because of an extremely low mutual solubility of two metals and a short period during which melting occurs, there is no evidence of the presence of aluminum in melted structures.

Deposition of aluminum onto a tin substrate is very difficult. Tin melts in an impact, and the strength of the contact is very low; hence, aluminum particles readily rebound from the surface. It is only very small particles that are attached. It is not clear whether they really form a bond or simply penetrate into the surface [58].

In the case of deposition onto an aluminum alloy, there is a large number of fine particles and some coarse particles attached to the surface. It is not clear, however, whether coarse particles are attached directly to the substrate or on tops of fine particles already attached to the surface. Though the aluminum alloy is harder than aluminum particles, significant deformation of the surface is observed. Ejection of the material around the edges of coarse particles is also observed, which implies an intense shear flow. Deposition of aluminum particles on aluminum-alloy substrates is worse than that on brass or copper substrates, though all these materials have the same hardness. The aluminum alloy has the lowest modulus of elasticity and a strong oxide film, which can be responsible for the observed differences in deposition initiation [58].

Interaction of aluminum particles with hardened steel differs from interaction with iron-non-containing materials. First, the deposition can be most easily initiated for steels. No deformation of substrates made of hardened or tempered steel was observed (i.e., it is the particle deformation that occurs in most cases). In deposition onto steel, coarse particles are attached, which are substantially deformed and have corona-shaped protuberances at the periphery. It is of interest that fine aluminum particles were not found on the steel surface, whereas fragments of iron-containing materials were observed. The most probable reason is that this material is related to the impact of aluminum particles onto the substrate. If it were related to interaction of aluminum particles with the steel nozzle, such particles would have been observed in all cases. Fragments of the material are iron-containing and form as part of the process of metal-jet formation, similar to that observed in explosive welding [58]. Direct observations of the products of metal ejection shows why initiation of particle attachment is so easy for steels with so small deformation of the substrate and suggests that this is actually a metallurgical bond. It is the hardness of steel that facilitates localization of deformation of aluminum particles and favors the metal-jet formation.

In deposition onto the ABC polymer (ABC in what follows), the polymer is destroyed because of its low hardness; thus, no deformation of aluminum particles necessary for bond formation occurs. The authors found that experiments with deposition onto glass (the hardness of the substrate of the same order as that of steels), no small particles resulting from jet formation are observed on the glass surface, because no ejection of the metal jet occurs. The glass is substantially damaged, which leads to adhesion of some particles (apparently, mechanical cohesion). A similar behavior is observed during deposition onto a polished corundum surface. Thus, though glass and corundum favor the concentration of deformation predominantly in the particle, adhesion initiation is difficult. Apparently, this occurs because the particle is not capable of forming a metallic bond with the surface [58]. Hence, we can conclude that a metal surface whose hardness is greater than the hardness of particles is needed for successful initiation of adhesion of aluminum particles on the surface with small roughness by the cold spray. In this case, significant deformation at high pressure leads to adhesion, like in explosive welding. Metal ejection cleans the surface, and a metallurgical bond is formed. Bond formation does not require substrate deformation but is hindered by the presence of oxide layers on the substrate surface [58].

Calculations and microscopy methods were used in [66] to study the microstructure evolution at the particle/substrate interface. It was found that adhesion of particles during cold spray is accompanied by intense plastic deformation at the interface [60, 67].

Results of a numerical analysis of the impact of particles with a description of the strain field and temperature distribution in the particle and the substrate are presented in [22]. The authors believe that successful adhesion is related to phenomena similar to explosive welding and explosive compacting [68–70].

Researchers offer a concept of a critical velocity, focusing their attention on relations between the measured deposition efficiency and particle velocity, which are estimated by semi-empirical and numerical methods [21, 54, 71]. The results show that successful adhesion requires a certain particle velocity, which mainly depends on thermal and mechanical properties of materials. In estimating the critical velocity, one should take into account the influence of the particle temperature. Therefore, the most appropriate method for a comprehensive analysis of critical velocities implies the use of an identical set of spraying parameters for different nozzle geometries [72]. The particle-velocity distribution for a given set of parameters is first calculated and then compared with the measured values of deposition efficiency, which yields the size and velocity of the largest particles capable of adhering to the substrate. The velocity calculated for these largest (hence, slowest) deposited particles is assumed to be the critical velocity. Spraying of high-purity materials (copper and aluminum with nitrogen used as a working gas) yielded velocities of 570 and 680 m/s, respectively. These results are in good agreement with the data of other researchers [53, 73].

An analysis was performed with allowance for strain hardening, strain-rate-depending hardening, thermal softening, friction-induced heating, and plastic and viscous dissipation of kinetic energy into heat. Heating was assumed to be adiabatic, i.e., heat transfer was not considered. To experimentally study the impact of single particles, a thin layer (less than a monolayer) of the coating was deposited by moving the substrate with a high velocity perpendicular to the flow of particles [66]. The calculations for copper particles 25 μm in diameter impacting onto a flat copper substrate with a velocity of 570 m/s and at room temperature revealed very localized heating at the contact boundary and formation of a jet-type flow of the material at early stages of the impact. An impact of two 5 μm particles with a velocity of 600 m/s and temperature of 200 °C was also calculated. The initial distance between the particles admitted penetration of the first particle prior to the impact of the second particle onto the substrate. Jet-type ejection of the material was observed in both cases. Jet formation for the second particle, however, is subjected to the influence of the changed morphology and properties of the substrate owing to the first impact [66].

Plastic strains increase with a rate of $0.5 \times 10^9\,s^{-1}$ until they reach the final value approximately equal to 4 for velocities lower than 580 m/s and 10 for a velocity of 580 m/s. An increase in strain at this velocity can be the result of the transition from the plastic to the viscous flow mechanism.

The behavior of temperature is similar to the behavior of strain. The heating rates for all impact velocities are approximately 10^9 K/s. For a velocity of 580 m/s, the temperature reaches the melting point for copper, whereas this is not the case for lower temperatures. The resistance of the material to the shear flow near the condition of thermal softening is rather low. This means that the material ceases to resist shear stresses when approaching the melting point and is subjected to considerable strains with insignificant applied stresses. On the other hand, such significant strains generate resistance of the viscous type, which prevents further deformation at high pressures. Rapid changes in strain, temperature, and stress show that the transition from the plastic to the viscous flow occurs within a narrow range of impact velocities between 550 and 580 m/s [66].

An analysis performed in [66] shows that the transition from the plastic to the viscous flow is mandatory only for particles and does not necessarily occur in the substrate. On the other hand, modeling of an impact of copper particles onto an aluminum substrate shows that the strain rates on the surfaces of copper spheres are too small to reach temperatures necessary for the viscous flow. Nevertheless, weak adhesion can be achieved if the substrate material reaches the critical conditions. In any case, if coatings thicker than two layers are deposited, it is the particle material that determines the adhesion mechanism.

More that 80% of particles are attached if the copper substrate is impacted by copper particles 5–25 μm in diameter with impact velocities of 550−670 m/s, respectively. Adhesion of particles is accompanied by formation of a ring of jet-type ejection around the contact zone. Particles that are not attached leave craters in the substrate without any signs of ejection. A microscopic analysis of the surface of different substrates subjected to an impact of a single particle of copper shows that the critical conditions are reached in regions close to the crater edge.

Adhesion of particles depends on many factors: area of the contact surface, crater depth, plastic strain, yield stress, pressure and temperature at the contact boundary, etc. In turn, these factors are affected by the impact velocity of the particle. Therefore, it seems logical to assume that these parameters reach their critical values at velocities close to the critical one or their dependence on velocity becomes different. Postulating of some adhesion criterion requires these critical values and conditions to be determined. In explosive welding, for instance, jet formation at the boundary is often considered as a criterion of successful adhesion [74]. The jet flow of the material, however, proceeds in a wide range of impact velocities, which makes this criterion ineffective. Thus, the mere fact of formation of a metal jet (or, correspondingly, a corona around the particle) does not guarantee adhesion, because jets are also formed at lower impact velocities, where no adhesion occurs.

If the contact time is too small or the tensile stresses at the contact boundary are too high, the particle can reflect from the surface before the adhesion conditions are reached. A particle obliquely incident onto the substrate can serve as an example of such a situation. In an oblique impact, the additional increase in temperature can occur at the boundary owing to friction-induced dissipation. The tangential component of the particle momentum, however, generates tensile forces at the contact boundary, which can be sufficiently high to separate the particle from the substrate [66].

The experimental value of the critical velocity of 570 m/s for the copper powder used is in good agreement with the transition velocity of 580 m/s obtained in modeling. The calculated strain field obtained in axisymmetric and three-dimensional simulations corresponds to the morphology observed, in particular, to formation of a jet of the material. The modeling results and the microscopic analysis show that plastic strains and adhesion at the critical velocity are limited to the external zone of the particle/target contact plane. This means that softening of the entire contact requires the particles to possess a higher kinetic energy. A good correlation between the calculated and experimentally observed critical velocities implies that, to reach successful adhesion, a high strain rate is needed in a localized region only. Rough estimates show that only 15–25% of the total area of the contact has high strain rates for impact velocities of 580 m/s. Moreover, the critical conditions in this case can be reached at one boundary only: either the particle or the substrate boundary. This coincides with the transmission electron microscopy (TEM) results [66].

The properties of a copper coating on a copper substrate were considered in [67]. In particular, it was shown that the coating has residual compressive stresses of 33 MPa on the average. A similar effect was obtained for a steel coating on an aluminum substrate: residual compressive stresses of 469 MPa on the average. The residual stresses are uniformly distributed in the coating, beginning from the external side of the coating to a distance of approximately 400 μm to the coating/substrate interface. In the transitional zone between the coating/substrate interface and the distance of approximately 400 μm, the stresses rapidly decrease. The zero value of stresses, however, is reached at different points: inside the coating in the case of a copper coating on a copper substrate and inside the substrate in the case of a steel coating on an aluminum substrate.

The mechanism of adhesion due to cold spray is considered in more detail in [75]. Particle deformation during the impact was analyzed by the ABAQUS program, which takes into account strain hardening, strain-rate-induced hardening, friction-induced heating, thermal softening, and plastic and viscous dissipation. An example of such a calculation is illustrated in Fig. 5.7.

In most cases, heating was assumed to be adiabatic, i.e., heat transfer was ignored. This approach is justified in modeling processes with high strain rates owing to the dimensionless parameter $x^2/\chi t$, where x is the characteristic size, χ is the thermal diffusivity,

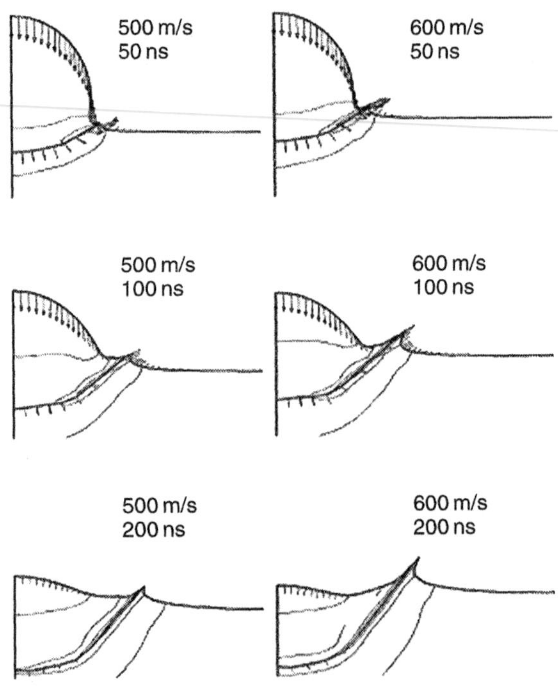

Fig. 5.7. Simulated impact of a copper particle onto a copper substrate for the initial velocities of 500 and 600 m/s. The arrows represent the velocities of modes at the respective surfaces of the particle and the substrate, and the contours indicate the temperature distribution [75].

and t is the time [76]. The value of this parameter equal to unity or higher is indicative of adiabatic heating. The authors argued that the value of this parameter is much higher than unity for the particle impact in cold spray if typical values $\chi = 10^{-6}$ and $t = 10^{-8}$ s are used for the size of an element in a particle 10^{-5} in diameter equal to 10^{-6}. It should be noted, nevertheless, that the arguments presented above are based on solving the heat-conduction equation. Heat transfer at very small scales is determined by the mechanism of wave propagation rather than by diffusion [77, 78]. This implies that, as the particle size decreases, the velocity of heat propagation approaches the velocity of propagation of plastic waves and, in any case, is limited by the velocity of sound in the particle material. In other words, heat transfer for high-velocity impacts of very small particles is slower than that predicted by the heat-conduction (diffusion) equation. Therefore, adiabatic heating can be reasonably assumed for impacts, including impacts of very small particles for which this parameter is smaller than unity. It was also assumed that dissipation of kinetic energy into heat depends on the strain rate, i.e., the portion of the plastic work dissipating into heat should be higher for high values of strain rates [79]. This again supports the assumption about adiabatic heating of particles in the cold spray. Not to completely exclude the possibility of heat conduction and energy accumulation, nevertheless, only 90% of kinetic energy was assumed to dissipate into heat. The modeling was performed for particles made of copper, which is a material convenient for comparisons. Copper was chosen as a reference material because of the clearly expressed formation of coatings and availability of data on material constants in the literature (e.g., [80–83]). In most cases, the plastic response of copper was assumed to obey the Johnson—Cook model. The elastic response of copper was assumed to follow the linear model. The linear model turned out to be fairly adequate for low and medium impact velocities. The Mie–Grueneisen equation of state was used as an alternative for comparisons with the linear model of elasticity. The method of semi-empirical determination of the critical velocity, which was described in detail in [72], yielded the value of 570 m/s for copper particles (5–22 μm) and 660 m/s for aluminum particles (smaller than 45 μm), which agrees with the data of other researchers. The results of an experimental study of spraying of copper particles 5–25 μm onto a copper substrate with impact velocities of 550–670 m/s, respectively, showed that more than 80% of impacting particles become attached to the surface. The attached particles have a ring around the contact zone, which is related to formation of a cumulative jet. The rebounded particles leave craters without any signs of formation of the cumulative jet. The mean ratio of the spot diameter to the particle diameter is 1.3.

The paper [84] continues the discussion started in [75], where the authors relate the beginning of adhesion in the cold spray with the onset of adiabatic shear instability. The phenomenon of adiabatic shear instability (ASI) and the associated formation of shear bands was first considered in [85, 86]. To give an idea of this phenomenon, Fig. 5.8 shows the typical stress—strain curves obtained in experiments.

For a typical material with strain hardening, the stress–strain curve monotonically increases under non-adiabatic (isothermal) plastic strain. In the case of an adiabatic flow of the material, the plastic strain energy dissipates into heat, which leads to an increase in temperature and thermal softening. The rate of hardening decreases with increasing strain, and the stress reaches a maximum value and then starts decreasing. Because of inhomogeneity of real materials, the shear and heating are localized in a comparatively small volume, whereas the strain and heating are almost terminated in the remaining

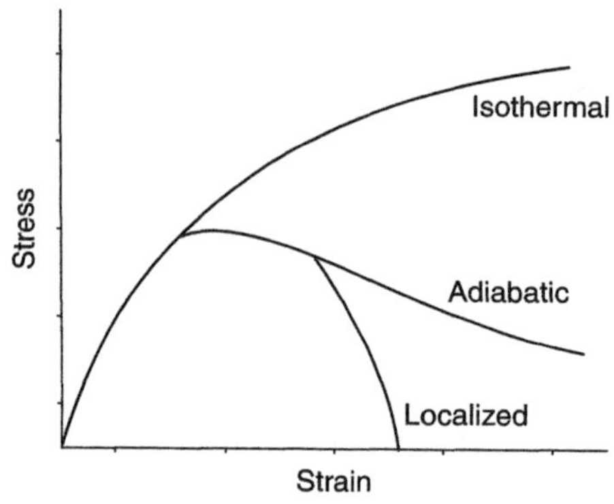

Fig. 5.8. Stress-strain curves in isothermal, adiabatic, and localized deformation of materials [84].

(larger) part of the material volume. Strain localization favors more intense heating and, as a consequence, thermal softening of the material inside the localization zone, which finally yields rapid vanishing of stress in the entire sample. Beginning from this moment, the flow of the material is no longer plastic; it becomes viscous (i.e., the stress becomes proportional to the strain rate).

Modeling of the particle impact under cold spray conditions, which was performed in [84], made it possible to draw the following conclusions.

- With increasing impact velocity, the size of the localization region (i.e., the thickness of the layer with an intense flow near the particle/substrate contact surface) decreases.
- For softer (i.e., with a lower modulus of elasticity) and denser materials of particles, the size of the localization region is smaller.
- Beginning from the critical impact velocity, at a certain moment of evolution of the impact process, the localization zone displays a rapid increase in strain, strain rate, and temperature and a decrease in stress almost to zero. These critical velocities for different materials are close to critical velocities of cold spray observed in experiments.

Hence, it is clear that softening and shear localization play an important role in formation of bonds between the particle and the substrate in the cold spray. It was assumed in [84] that atomic diffusion does not play any important role because of the very short time of contact (the diffusion distance is much smaller than the distance between the atoms in the lattice) and cannot lead to particle adhesion. Shear localization and associated formation of the near-contact jet result in formation of pure contact surfaces. Additional softening in the contact zone together with a high contact pressure favors the formation of mutually conformal contact surfaces. Therefore, as soon as the conditions for shear localization are reached, the conditions for extensive adhesion of the particle and substrate surfaces are also achieved, which leads to formation of bonds.

The initial stage of formation of a coating from copper particles (20 μm) on aluminum and aluminum particles (20 μm) on copper in the range of velocities 400–1000 m/s at

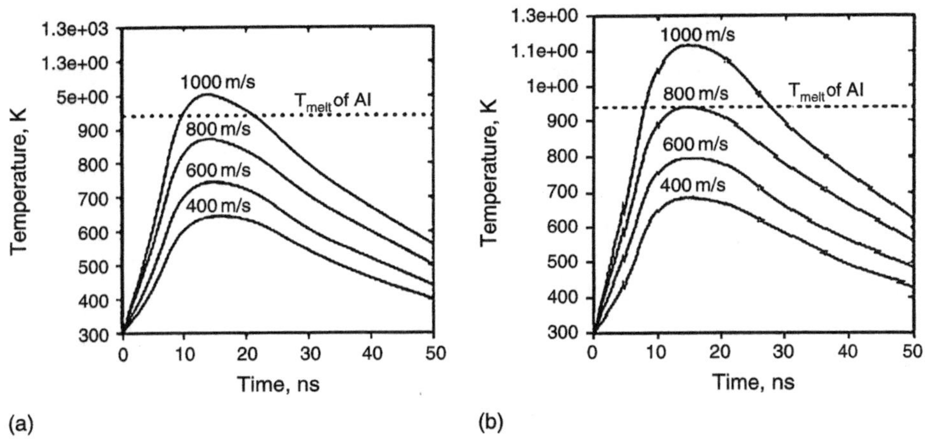

Fig. 5.9. Evolution of the maximum temperature at the particle/substrate interface during the deposition of aluminum on copper (a) and copper on aluminum (b) for four particle velocities [87].

room temperature prior to the impact was modeled in [87]. The calculations show that the melting point of aluminum in both combinations can be reached at comparatively high impact velocities (800–900 m/s) (see Fig. 5.9).

It was noted that heat conduction can be important. Plastic strains are localized over the contact periphery. As one of the adhesion mechanisms in the cold spray, the authors propose micromixing (by analogy with the motion of two fluids at the interface) owing to formation of vortices and other wave instabilities. Another mechanism can be the formation of a crater of such a shape that prevents particle rebounding.

The effect of temperature, size, and purity of particles on the critical velocity of adhesion was also considered in [88, 89]. The impact was modeled by the ABAQUS/Explicit software system. Heat conduction was taken into account in these papers. It should be noted that the heat conduction (diffusion) equation becomes inapplicable if the particle size is very small or if the heat-propagation velocity reaches the velocity of sound. In this case, the mechanism of wave propagation of heat dominates [75]. Yet, this case was not calculated. The metal used for calculations was copper. The authors used the Johnson–Cook model, though they noted that the data for copper were determined for a strain rate of 10^6. For $10\,\mu$m particles with impact velocities of 600 m/s, however, the strain rates reach 10^9, and it is fairly probable that this model cannot be applied. The lack of experimental data for such a level of strain rates does not allow yet a more accurate model to be developed. The authors give the following formula for the critical velocity of copper deposition (in SI measurement units):

$$v_{\text{crit}} = 667 - 0.014\rho + 0.08(T_{\text{m}} - T_{\text{R}}) + 10^{-7}\sigma_{\text{u}} - 0.4(T_{\text{i}} - T_{\text{R}}). \tag{5.3}$$

Here T_{i} is the impact temperature, T_{m} is the melting temperature, $T_{\text{R}} = 293\,\text{K}$, ρ is the density of the particle material, and σ_{u} is the yield stress.

The experimental study was performed with copper and 316L steel powders with different distributions of particles in size and with acceleration in nozzles of different lengths with nitrogen and helium used as working gases. Metal spheres 20 mm in diameter accelerated to velocities from 200 to 1500 m/s were used to study individual impacts. The results of these tests showed that adhesion begins from a velocity of approximately 350 m/s, but the adhesion zone is extremely narrow. The optimal adhesion zone is obtained at velocities of 600–750 m/s, and the loss of the material is observed above these velocities. Adhesion is terminated at a velocity of 1150 m/s, and erosion reaches 140% of the initial mass of the copper sphere at a velocity of 1450 m/s. The authors do not inform, however, if attachment of large spheres took place or there were only traces of bonding inside the zones.

Immediately after the impact, the high pressure extends into the particle and the substrate from the point of the primary contact. The pressure gradient in the gap between the colliding boundaries generates a shear load, which accelerates the material and, hence, is the reason for localized shear strain. If the impact pressure and strain are high enough, then shear strain leads to shear instability. This means that thermal softening locally dominates over hardening, which results in a drastic increase (in a jumplike manner) of strain and temperature and in an immediate decrease in stress. The viscous flow in this region generates a jet of the material with a temperature close to the melting point. The phenomenon of jet formation was also observed in explosive welding. The oxide layers are broken at the boundaries subjected to high strains, and the hot surfaces are pressed together, which results in their welding. This model can yield the basic requirements necessary for successful adhesion in the cold spray. The material should be plastic for deformation to proceed without cracking and for the coating to be dense. In the contact zone, the material should withstand a localized plastic flow with strain rates of 10^9 and strains about 10 or even higher without formation of cracks. The rate of cooling in the contact zone should be, on one hand, sufficiently low to ensure shear instability and, on the other hand, sufficiently high for the boundaries to be able to become solidified and for a bond to be formed before the particle rebounds. Moreover, the adhesion force should be sufficient to withstand elastic rebound and separation of the particle.

For very small sizes, origination of shear instability can be difficult because of high cooling rates arising owing to high gradients of temperature inside a small particle. The strain rate is high, and the associated hardening is more significant for fine particles. The viscous shear stress in the jet region is also higher for fine particles. These dynamic effects prevent localized deformation and, thus, increase the critical velocity of deposition. Moreover, finer particles are subjected to higher hardening velocities during powder production and possess higher static characteristics of the material because of their finer structure (e.g., because of the Hall-Patch effect). Owing to a greater area/volume ratio, finer particles often have higher contamination. Surface contamination, such as oxide layers, also has a significant effect on adhesion. All these effects lead to an increase in the critical velocity for finer particles.

It was found by calculations that shear instability does not arise for particles 5 μm in diameter with impact velocities of 400–600 m/s. The impact of particles 15–50 μm with the same velocities leads to shear instability. For coarse particles (25–50 μm), the temperature reaches a value close to the melting point (see Fig. 5.10).

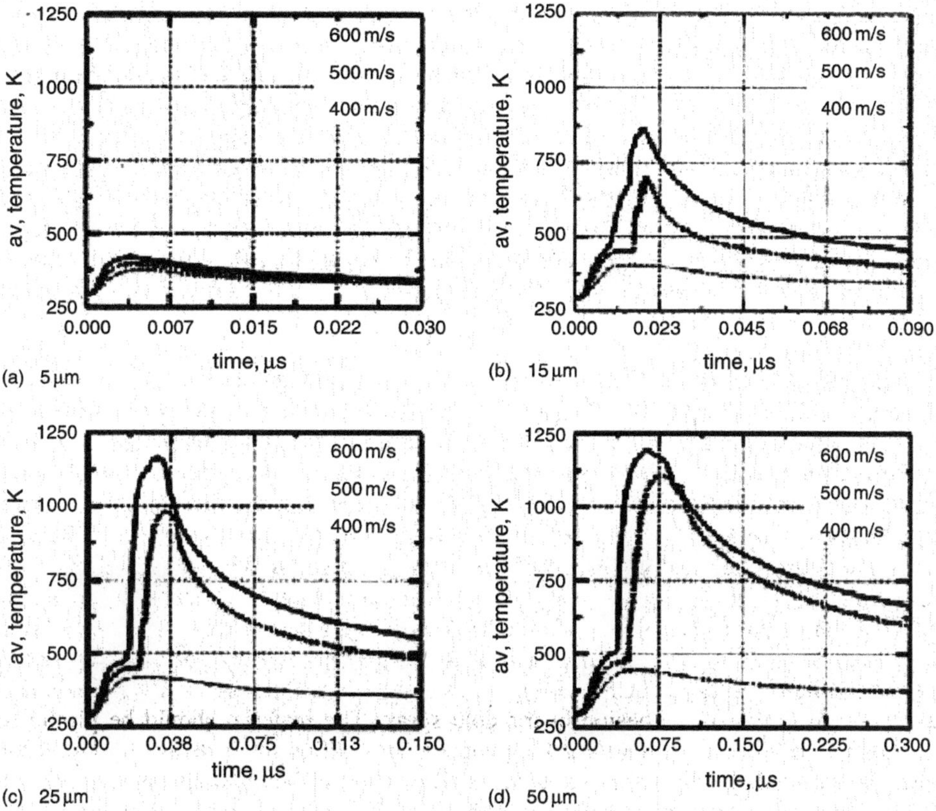

Fig. 5.10. Temporal evolution of the temperature at the monitored volume (sheared interface) of copper particles of different size and for different impact velocities [89].

If bond formation is considered as a diffusion process, the quality of bonding should depend on the thermal history of the contact zone and, probably, on the contact pressure. A 5 μm particle is attached with low adhesion, a 15 μm particle is attached at a velocity of 600 m/s, a 25 μm particle is attached at 500 m/s, and a 50 μm particle is attached at 450 m/s. The quality of bonding is expected to increase with increasing particle size at an unchanged velocity because of the increase in contact temperature and time. Higher initial temperatures of particles reduce the critical velocity of deposition because of the more pronounced effect of thermal softening. Moreover, heat conduction becomes less effective because of the lower temperature gradient, which increases the time for diffusion and bond formation. Thus, the quality of bonding can be improved by increasing the initial temperature of particles. These effects were verified experimentally in tensile tests of copper coatings obtained under different spraying conditions and from powders with different distributions of particles in size. The calculated critical velocities are in good agreement with the experimental values. The calculations show that heat conduction can exert a significant effect on adhesion in the cold spray. Qualitative analytical modeling of heat conduction yielded the minimum particle size at which shear instability occurs

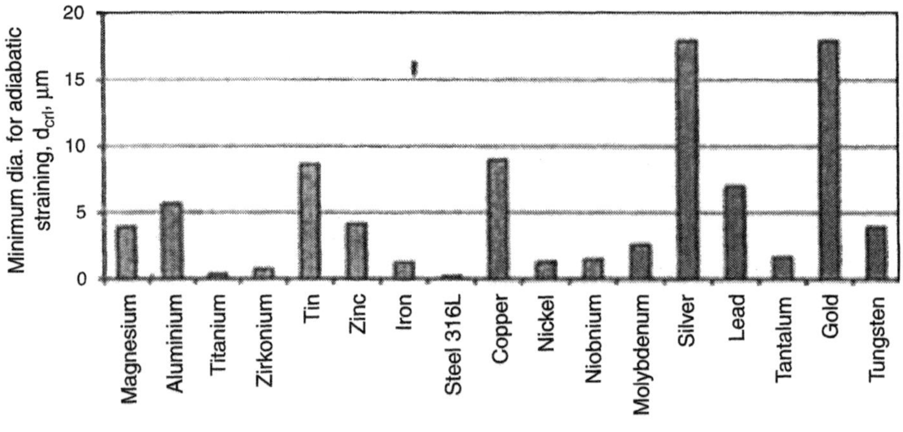

Fig. 5.11. Minimum particle diameter for localized adiabatic deformation during an impact, calculated for different materials with semi-empirical Eq. (5.3) [89].

for various metals. This means that particles of this or smaller diameter do not reach conditions for adhesion (see Fig. 5.11).

A qualitative analysis performed in [89] made it possible to derive a formula for the critical velocity of deposition for various metals on substrates of the same material:

$$v_{\text{crit}} = \sqrt{\frac{4F_1\sigma_{\text{TS}}}{\rho}\left(1 - \frac{T_i - T_R}{T_m - T_R}\right) + F_2 c_p (T_m - T_i)}. \tag{5.4}$$

In this formula, F_1 and F_2 are the fitting coefficients for reaching agreement with the experiment ($F_1 = 1.2$ and $F_2 = 1.2$), σ_{TS} is the yield stress at the temperature T_R, other conditions being identical, ρ is the density of the particle (substrate) material, T_i is the initial temperature of the particle, T_m is the melting point, and c_p is the heat capacity.

It is argued that Eq. (5.4) is in better agreement with experimental data than Eq. (5.3) (see Fig. 5.12).

In addition, the limiting high velocities are given for various metals, above which erosion occurs. For instance, the limiting velocities for tin and lead are very low (about 250 m/s); for zinc, copper, and silver, it reaches 750–1000 m/s; for remaining metals, this velocity exceeds 1000 m/s, in particular, for aluminum it ranges between 1250 and 1500 m/s. The following formulas derived from experimental data are given in [89] for calculating the critical velocity of deposition as a function of the particle size (within the range of 5–200 μm at a temperature of 20 °C):

$$v_{cr} = 900 d_p^{-0.19} \text{ for copper,} \tag{5.5}$$

$$v_{cr} = 950 d_p^{-0.14} \text{ for steel.} \tag{5.6}$$

It was experimentally demonstrated in [89] that the quality of coatings depends on the particle size. For instance, in obtaining coatings from 316L steel, the optimal powder

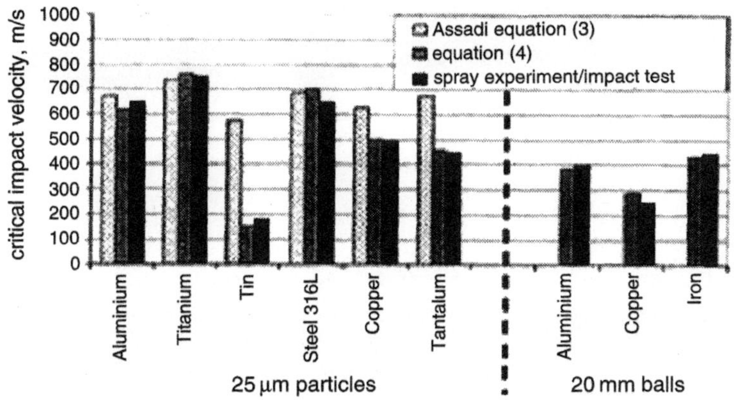

Fig. 5.12. Comparison of calculated v_{crit} with experimental results of spray experiments and impact tests [89].

(with a high deposition efficiency and coating density) turned out to be the powder with a particle size of 15–45 μm for both nitrogen and helium used as an accelerating gas (Fig. 5.13).

To optimize the microstructure of coatings and their properties, the cold spray conditions are chosen for each powder experimentally. This process requires systematic variations of deposition conditions and an analysis of coatings, which is rather expensive in terms of time and funding. Therefore, it is necessary to develop alternative methods for testing whether particular powders are suitable for cold spray. High strain rates can be readily reached in explosive compacting, where the conditions of adhesion (cohesion) of particles are similar to cold spray conditions. The use of a special structure can ensure that the shock-loading conditions cover a wide range of energy in one experiment. To estimate the capabilities of this method, the microstructural properties of the contact boundaries in explosive compacting were considered and compared with similar data in the cold spray in [68].

Dense hard compacts of metals and ceramics can be obtained with appropriately chosen impact pressure and impact duration [90, 91]. The shock wave is generated either by detonation of a high explosive in direct contact with the powder-containing system or by an impact of a high-velocity projectile. Nonequilibrium alloys and AISI 304 L stainless steel were successfully obtained in [92–94] with the use of a specially designed pistol for accelerating the projectile by compressed air. The presence of a melting zone between the particles was considered to be a necessary condition for the compacting process. A powder of a heat-resistant alloy designed for operation at temperatures of 760–1100 °C was used in [91] to study shock-wave compacting. The main element of this powder was nickel and then (in order of decreasing percentage) zirconium, cobalt, chromium, aluminum, and titanium. The greater fraction of the powder contained particles 37–74 μm in diameter. The particles were mainly spheres with a microdendrite structure formed if the metal is cooled more slowly than it is needed for the formation of the microcrystalline structure. Therefore, we can conclude that the cooling rate of the examined powder during its production was insufficient for the microcrystalline structure to form.

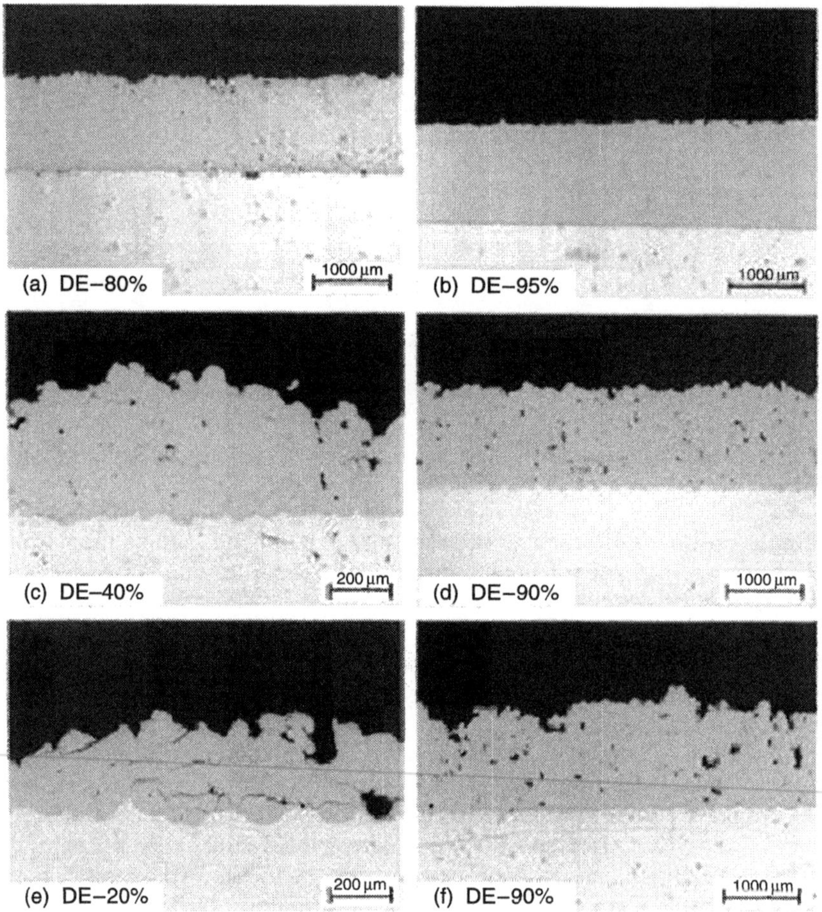

Fig. 5.13. 316L steel sprayed with nitrogen (a, c, e) and helium (b, d, f). Size distribution: $-45+15\,\mu m$ (a, b), $-88+45\,\mu m$ (c, d), $-177+53\,\mu m$ (e, f) [89].

For explosive compacting, the powder is placed into a cylindrical cavity inside the high explosive charge located in a sufficiently long steel or cardboard tube. The detonation is initiated by a small explosive charge. The compacting process depends on the ratio of the high explosive mass to the tube mass: a higher value of this ratio ensures better adhesion between the particles and a larger zone of melting between the particles. The melting zone at the boundary between the particles in the compact has a microcrystalline structure with a very small grain size (less than $0.3\,\mu m$). This microcrystalline morphology is related to extremely high cooling rates: about $10^8\,K/s$. In any case, it is higher than the cooling rate at which the particles of the powder were initially obtained (10^4–$10^5\,K/s$) [91].

In explosive welding, the metal surfaces are attached to each other owing to an impact, the typical impact velocity is 200–1000 m/s, and the impact angle is 5–25°. The impact ensures a plastic flow with high strain rates at the contact boundary. A metal jet is formed, which cleans the surfaces and removes the oxide layers, which results in strong adhesion between the impacting plates [95]. Substantially deformed extended grains, re-crystallized grains, and sometimes structures of repeated solidification are observed within several millimeters from the contact boundary, though melting and re-solidification are often observed only in a zone less than 1 μm thick at the interface [96]. By analogy with explosive welding, successful adhesion during powder compacting [97] and in the cold spray is related to critical conditions for intense plastic deformation at the contact boundaries. The evidence for the formation of a rapidly moving metal jet at the boundary is known both for powder compacting [93, 98] and in the cold spray.

Shock compacting is determined by compression and consolidation of particles. During compression, the powder is compressed by a weak shock wave without any significant effect of consolidation of particles. A strong wave ensures consolidation of particles; hence, the compact properties are close to those of a cast material [99]. Shock consolidation requires very rapid compression of particles and rapid input of energy at the boundaries between the particles. If the wave is too strong, however, melting and cracking occur owing to the unloading wave propagating in the compact. The shock pressure necessary for consolidation is often related to the powder hardness [43]. Other factors, such as density, melting temperature, shape, size, and contamination of the surface, also affect the process [100]. It should be noted that there are some differences between cold spray and compacting. The main difference is that the particles during compacting are heated and remain compressed by a high pressure during a comparatively long time, which improves bonding between the particles.

In cold spray, the compressive stresses and strains are limited in space by a size of the order of one particle size. The results of [68] show that individual impacts in the cold spray lead to lower deformation of particles than those in explosive compacting of the powder. According to modeling and experiments on explosive compacting of the powder, however, the critical velocity for successful deposition of 316L steel in the cold spray is 700 m/s. The study shows that explosive compacting of the powder is applicable in determining the critical conditions for adhesion of materials in the cold spray method [68].

The mechanism of adhesion in the cold spray with the use of the so-called acceleration by a laser impact was considered in [101]. The essence of the technique is as follows. Copper foil 25 μm thick is place parallel to a flat plate made of aluminum at a distance of 470 μm. A laser pulse with a duration of 29 ns from a neodymium solid-state laser focused on the copper foil into a spot 4 mm in diameter accelerates it to an impact velocity of 830 m/s. It is assumed that the impact and adhesion mechanisms coincide with those in the cold spray. It should be noted that intermetallides were found in the contact zone; their origin is associated with melting of metals in the contact zone.

The effect of temperature and composition of the powder mixture on deposition efficiency was considered in [102]. It was found that the deposition efficiency as a function of temperature for the examined compositions of powders can be described by the Arrhenius law

$$k_{\rm d} = k_{\rm d0} \exp(-E_{\rm a}/RT_0), \tag{5.7}$$

where $E_{\rm a}$ is the activation energy, which depends on the powder composition and on the gas type.

The cross section of single particles of the Al12Si alloy (25 μm) attached to soft steel in a characteristic range of velocities (measured experimentally) from 585 to 755 m/s was examined in [103]. The formation of ejections and the presence of craters of insignificant (hardly measurable) depth are confirmed. The crater surface contains fine particles of the aluminum melt (about 1–2 μm in size) (see Fig. 5.14).

Scanning laser microscopy data confirm that the envelope of the particle cross section can be approximated by a paraboloid of revolution. The final strain of particles depends only slightly on velocity: 0.7 for 585 m/s and no more than 0.75 for 755 m/s (see Fig. 5.15). The particles were accelerated by nitrogen at a temperature of 400 °C. The velocity was varied by changing the stagnation pressure.

The existence of an optimal velocity was demonstrated in [104] by an example of spraying of the same aluminum alloy (25 μm) onto soft steel with the use of nitrogen and helium at a temperature of 400 °C. The authors counted the number of attached particles and divided it by the sum consisting of the number of attached particles and the number of craters; it turned out that the maximum of this quantity (70%) is reached at an impact velocity of 700 m/s (see Fig. 5.16).

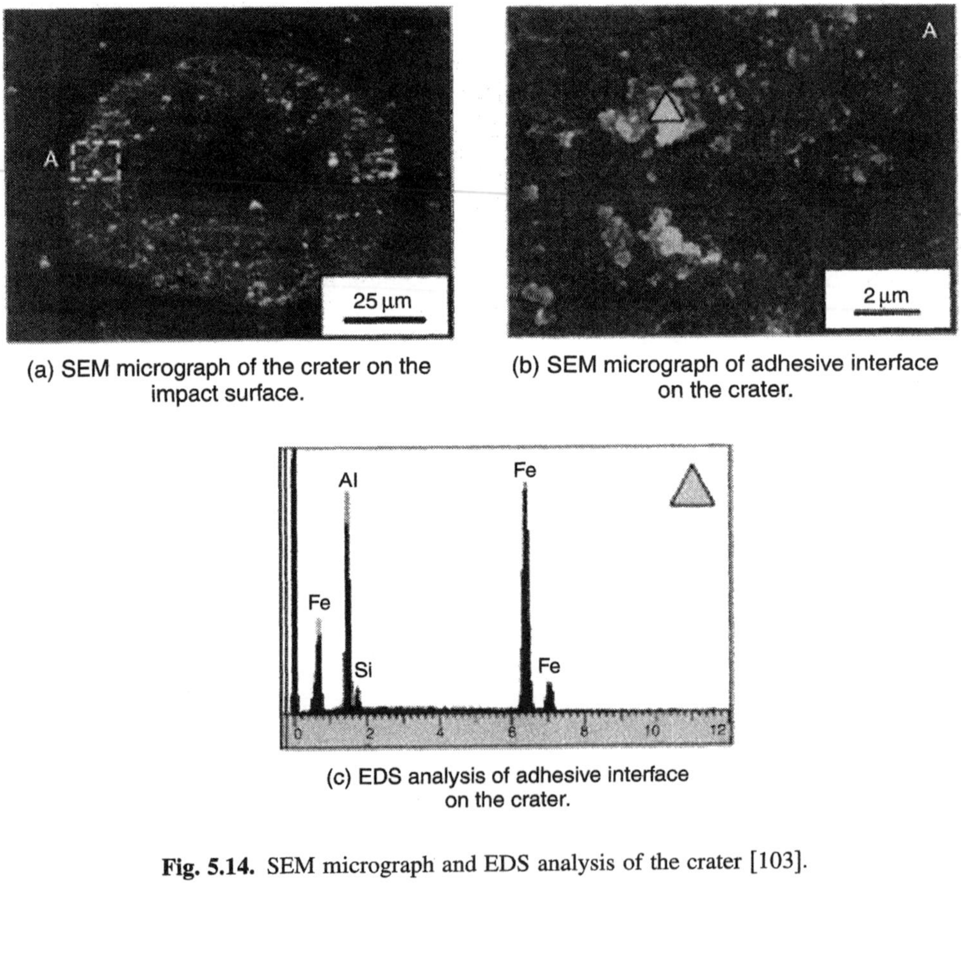

(a) SEM micrograph of the crater on the impact surface.

(b) SEM micrograph of adhesive interface on the crater.

(c) EDS analysis of adhesive interface on the crater.

Fig. 5.14. SEM micrograph and EDS analysis of the crater [103].

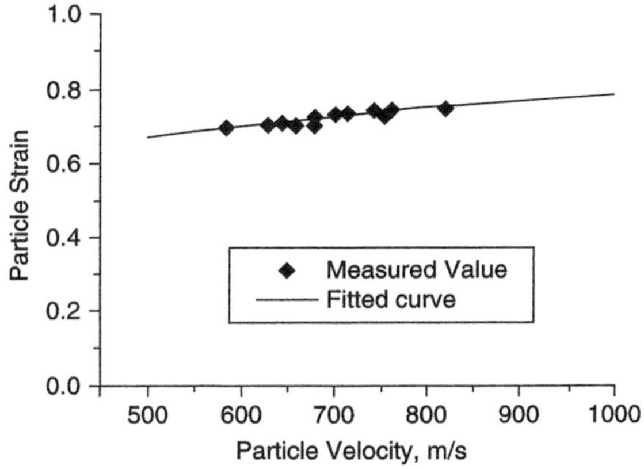

Fig. 5.15. Particle strains as obtained from impact modeling and measurement of LSM data [103].

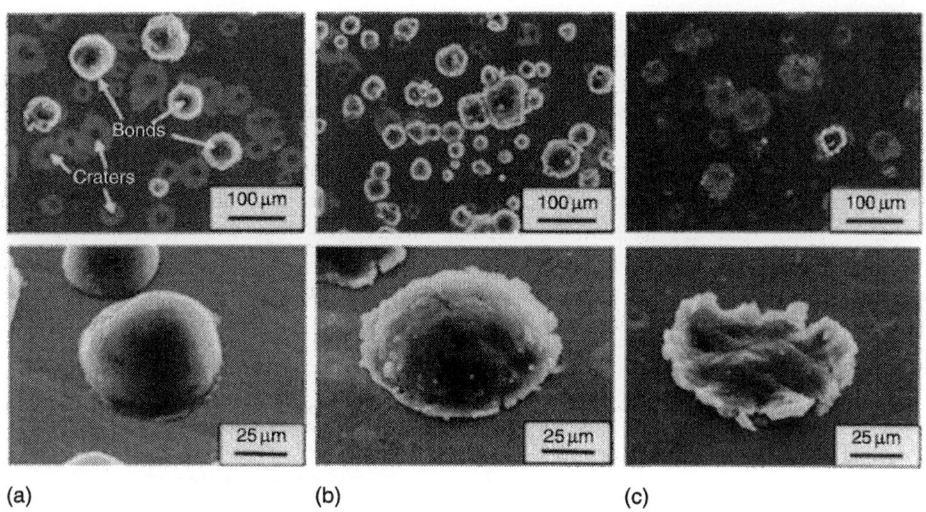

Fig. 5.16. SEM micrograph of the contact surfaces (top view) and the attached Al–Si particles (45° angle view). Impact with a mean particle velocity of (a) 500 m/s; (b) 700 m/s; and (c) 1000 m/s [104].

The velocity was measured experimentally. To explain this effect, the authors used the theory of competition between the adhesion energy and the elastic rebound energy. According to the estimates, indeed, there is a velocity range where the adhesion energy is higher than the elastic rebound energy; the opposite situation is observed outside this range. It was shown that the experimental curve is qualitatively similar to the curve representing the difference between the adhesion energy and the elastic rebound energy.

A semi-empirical method for determining the critical velocity in the cold spray was proposed in [105] by the example of copper deposition onto stainless steel; the method involves approximation of the real distribution of the particle size by a function of the form

$$f_m = \left\{1 - \exp\left[-\left(\frac{d_p - d_{min}}{d_0}\right)^m\right]\right\} \times \left\{1 - \exp\left[-\left(\frac{d_{max} - d_{min}}{d_0}\right)^m\right]\right\} \times 100\%$$

with the parameters $d_0 = 27.5\,\mu m$, $m = 1.8$, $d_{max} = 89.5\,\mu m$, and $d_{min} = 2.0\,\mu m$.

After that, the experimentally obtained particle velocity as a function of the particle size is approximated by a function of the form

$$v_p = \frac{k}{d_p^n}$$

with the parameters $k = 1287$, $n = 0.36$ for N_2 and $k = 1962$, $n = 0.36$ for He.

The particles that reach the critical velocity are assigned the critical size. Thus, the fraction of the powder with sizes smaller than the critical value is assumed to contribute to coating formation; the remaining particles rebound; this relation determines the deposition efficiency. The authors presented data on the deposition efficiency as a function of the deposition angle and concluded that the experimental data are adequately described if the critical velocity is assumed to be 550 m/s both for nitrogen and helium.

The coating-formation kinetics in the cold spray was experimentally examined in [106] by the example of double and triple mixtures of powders and alloys (Zn (45–90 μm), Al (53–75 μm), AlSi (53–75 μm, 10–32 μm), and Si (40–50 μm) in weight proportions Zn + 40 Al, Zn + 60 Al, Zn + 68 Al + 15 Si, Zn + 34 Al + 15 Si, 6–70 Zn + AlSi). The existence of the induction time and the nonlinear character of the kinetic curve (see Fig. 5.17) are confirmed; the latter is explained by the fact that the first particles interact

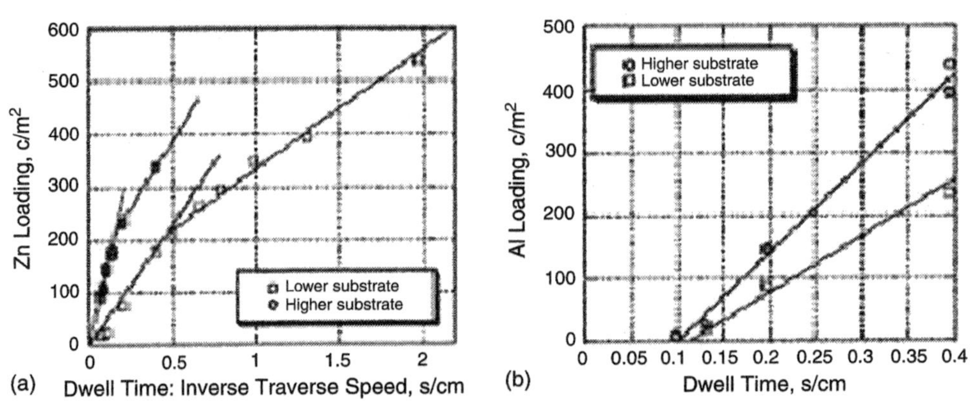

Fig. 5.17. (a) Mass loadings of the Zn coatings as functions of dwell time, i.e. the inverse of traverse speed (the two powder rates for Zn were 0.4 g/s and 1.2 g/s, respectively). (b) Mass loadings of the Al coatings as functions of dwell time (the two powder rates for Al were 0.3 g/s and 0.5 g/s, respectively) [106].

with the substrate surface, whereas the later particles interact with the surface formed by previously attached particles.

The photographs of the surface and cross section of the coatings formed display a typical cluster structure (the size of clusters is much greater than the size of particles). In the case of spraying of triple alloys, the residual content of components in the coating is given (Zn + 78 Al + 3 Si and Zn + 38 Al + 2 Si for the first and second mixture, respectively). Inspection of the latter mixture shows that the content of zinc in the coating increases nonlinearly with increasing its content in the initial mixture (see Fig. 5.18). Approximately at the 20% content in the initial powder (70% in the coating), the curve has an inflection and becomes less steep, reaching 90% in the coating for 70% in the initial mixture.

To conclude this section, we should note that bonding mechanism is not adequately understood. In authors opinion the most important contribution in this area is made by H. Kreye and his colleagues on the basis of adiabatic shear instability approach. In several papers the concept of the critical velocity is discussed; formulas for calculating the critical velocity as a function of some material properties and deposition parameters are proposed. The presence of mechanical, metallurgical, and chemical bonds is assumed. It was found that there is a viscoplastic transition and the melting point is sometimes reached in the contact, which allows us to assume that adhesion can also be ensured by micromixing. The significance of the impact velocity, size and temperature of the particles and substrate, heat conduction, and SW loading is discussed. An analogy with explosive welding and explosive compacting of powdered materials is mentioned. It is clear that more research should be done in this field to understand and describe the nature of bonding mechanism and influence of various parameters on the process of coating formation.

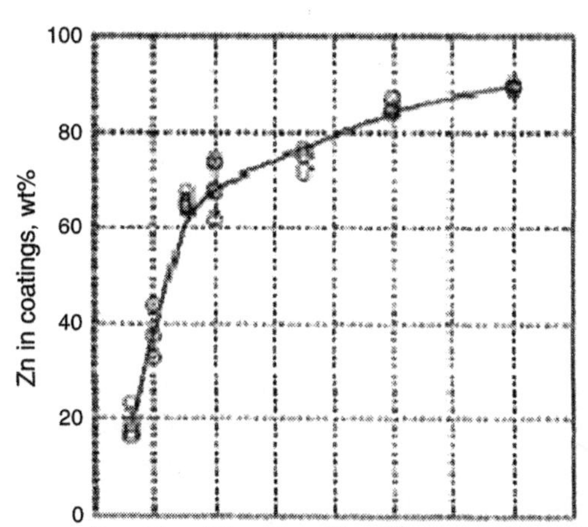

Fig. 5.18. Composition of the composite coatings of Zn + (Al . . . Si) deposited from the starting powders with varying compositions [106].

5.3. Cold Spray Technologies and Applications

A large number of publications deal with engineering aspects of the cold spray method, which involve development of different technologies, investigation of coating properties, etc.

5.3.1. Aluminum-containing coatings

The anticorrosive properties of an aluminum coating (from the 1100 A1 powder with a particle size of 1–40 μm accelerated by helium and by a mixture of helium and 20% of nitrogen at a temperature of 500–800 K and a pressure of 2.07 MPa on the substrate of the same material) were considered in [107]. The coating obtained with the use of the gas mixture was more porous but also more corrosion-resistant. The authors believe that a greater number of active centers that initiate corrosion are formed because of more intense deformation of particles in the impact in the case of acceleration by helium. At the same time, the corrosion resistance of both coatings was higher than that of the substrate.

Coatings from nanocrystalline (nanostructured) aluminum powders with a particle size of 20 μm were compared with those of conventional aluminum in [35]. Nanocrystalline coatings are used to improve material properties, such as electrical conductivity, corrosion resistance, and high yield strength. The cold gas-dynamic spraying method is preferable for application of such powders because the nanocrystalline structure is retained in the course of deposition. The coatings were applied with the use of helium at room temperature and a pressure of 3.7 MPa on an aluminum substrate prior subjected to sandblasting. Because of the radial injection of the powder downstream of the nozzle throat, the pressure in the feeder was 0.675 MPa. It was found that the nanocrystalline coating possesses higher hardness than the coating from the commonly used powder.

The aluminum coating on an aluminum substrate obtained in [108] has a low level of the oxygen content and porosity, which is the reason for expecting high corrosion resistance of this coating. The Vickers 0.3 hardness of the coating was 45.

A coating formed from aluminum particles 1–50 μm in diameter (20 μm on the average) accelerated by helium and deposited onto an aluminum substrate was analyzed in [109]. The boundary between the particles in the coating was visualized with the use of the Krolls etching agent (3:6:100 $HF/HNO_3/H_2O$), which allowed the authors to conclude that the main mechanism of adhesion is mechanical clamping, though there are also some places with metallurgical bonding.

Deposition of Al 1100 by a mixture of helium and nitrogen (20 wt%) onto the substrate of the same material was considered in [110]. It was noted that the structure of the helium-processed coating almost coincides with the structure of the cast material (of the substrate). Coatings obtained with the use of a mixture of gases have a different structure and an elevated porosity. The hardness of helium-processed coatings is higher than that of coatings obtained with the use of a mixture of gases (see Fig. 5.19).

It was noted thereby, however, that the corrosion resistance of the coating obtained with the use of a mixture of gases is higher than that of the helium-processed coating. This

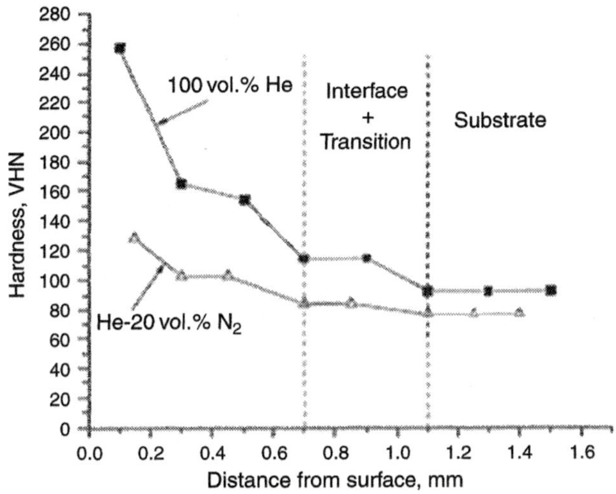

Fig. 5.19. Relative evaluation of mechanical properties of 1100 Al coatings in terms of hardness value [110].

fact can be attributed to higher plastic strains in the helium-processed coating and, as a consequence, a greater number of active centers. The corrosion resistance of both coatings is higher than that of the substrate (i.e., cast aluminum).

The effect of thermal treatment of aluminum coatings obtained with the use of helium at a temperature of 350–400 °C was examined in [111]. Three different powders were used (with mean sizes of 11.8, 25.9, and 26.4 μm). It was noted that the coatings after thermal treatment reach the values of the elasticity modulus, ultimate strength, etc., which are commensurable with those of cast aluminum. The coating produced from a finer powder is more dense and plastic than the coatings produced from coarser powders.

Application of coatings by the cold spray from the 2618 aluminum alloy (Al-Cu-Mg-Fe-Ni) with the addition of Sc (metallurgical, powder fraction with a particle size of 5–40 μm, the mean size of 22 μm, spherical particles), which significantly strengthens the basic alloy, was studied in [112, 113]. The coating has a low porosity and very good bonding with the aluminum substrate. Application of this alloy mainly refers to aeronautics and car building.

The influence of surface preparation on formation of a coating from an Al (6.9 wt%) Mg with a mean particle size of 50 μm was considered in [114]. This powder was grinded with liquid nitrogen (i.e., cryogenically grinded) to obtain a nanocrystalline structure. The resultant powder had a wide range of particle sizes (17–80 μm) with a mean value of 40 μm and an angular shape. The powder was sprayed onto an aluminum substrate with the use of a helium flow at a pressure of 1.7 MPa in one pass and with a constant flow rate of the powder from the feeder. The substrate was subjected to different types of preliminary processing: by silica sand with a mean particle size of 686 μm and glass sand with a mean particle size of 254 μm. Substrates 6.35 and 1 mm thick were used in the experiments. The experiments showed that the coating mass increases approximately by 10% owing to pre-processing by silica sand (which is coarser and has higher hardness than glass sand). One theory of particle adhesion involves mechanical attachment. Therefore, it can be reasonably assumed that elevated surface roughness improves particle adhesion because there are many hole (recesses) where the particles can deposit and stick. These particles are then subjected to additional compacting by subsequent incident particles. The presence of very large particles in the initial powder implies that larger recesses on the substrate surface are needed for these particles to attach. Larger recesses (related to the high roughness of the surface) yield a larger contact area between the deformable particle and the substrate. As it was expected, the microstructure of the coatings was almost identical (independent of surface preparation) because there was no more influence of the surface as soon as the first layer of the coating is formed.

The coating from the Al12Si alloy (5–25 μm) obtained in [115] has a low porosity and strong adhesion to the substrate; the coating composition coincides with the composition of the initial powder.

5.3.2. Copper-containing coatings

Pratt & Whitney used deposition of a copper coating by the cold spray to improve the structure and functioning of a new aircraft engine [116, 117]. A thick layer of the copper coating was necessary to improve heat removal from the combustion-chamber zone. If the coating thicker than 1 mm is applied by the traditional electrolytic technology, the adhesion is very low; in addition, the process takes a long time (two weeks). Application of a copper coating applied by the cold spray allows one to significantly reduce the time of the process, improve adhesion, and avoid the use of hazardous chemicals necessary in the conventional electrolytic method.

The requirements to the coating are rather severe: it has to withstand cyclic thermal loads, including connection (welding) of tubes, etc. The highest thermal load is the heating up to 1200 K in vacuum, and the coating has to be still operational under these conditions (have no bubbles and exfoliation). High temperature gradients arise when the engine is started and shut down; therefore, the coating has to withstand high thermal impacts without exfoliation. To check the coating operation in this regime, the coated samples were cooled in liquid nitrogen and water.

An analysis of various methods for coating application showed that it is possible to obtain a copper coating with prescribed parameters by the electrolytic method, vacuum plasma deposition, and cold spray. The researchers from Pratt & Whitney first decided to use the electrolytic technology to obtain the required coating. It turned out, however, that this method requires several processes of treatment to obtain a high-quality coating and that this method should be significantly upgraded.

The plasma coating satisfied the tests [118], but the process was too long and too expensive. Moreover, masking and mechanical post-processing (improvement of accuracy to a necessary level) are rather labor-consuming, because the article to be coated has a very intricate shape, which makes it difficult to reach the necessary dimensions within admissible margins.

A preliminary analysis of the cold spray showed that it is possible to obtain dense coatings without inclusions and with a low content of oxides (in some cases, even lower than in the initial material) [119]. Moreover, obtaining very thick coatings with good adhesion during a short time [120] and with acceptable expenses is the advantage of the cold spray, which evoked the interest in this method.

A series of experiments [116] were performed with copper spraying onto stainless steel under different conditions: the varied parameters were the surface roughness, spraying parameters (pressure and temperature), etc. Initially, the coatings exfoliated from most samples. A microstructural study showed that the coating behavior during the tests are affected, in addition to spraying parameters, by the powder purity and the state of the surface. Therefore, an attempt was made to obtain coatings from powders of higher purity and with precise control of the spraying parameter (stagnation pressure and temperature of the gas). Testing of the samples obtained showed that they can withstand thermal cycles without exfoliation of coatings.

A metallographic analysis of coatings applied with optimized parameters revealed good adhesion and low porosity. After this encouraging result was obtained, an engine mockup was fabricated, and a copper coating more than 2.5 mm thick was applied. Then the coating was treated by grinding and drilling holes to demonstrate that the coating can withstand stresses caused by machining. After this treatment, the coated articles successfully passed the thermal tests. Thus, it was demonstrated that the cold spray can be used to obtain dense, phase-pure, and thick coatings with good adhesion, which can withstand significant thermal loads. In addition, the cold spray was shown to be promising for production of Hi-Tech articles/elements. In the latter activity, the cold spray advantages are the high production efficiency, acceptable cost, environmental safety, etc. [116] over other methods.

Obtaining an aluminum-bronze coating on a stainless-steel substrate from aluminum–bronze powder with a particle size smaller than 40 μm was considered in [121]. Detailed inspection of the element composition in the vicinity of the coating/substrate interface showed that copper and aluminum in the coating migrate to the substrate material. At the same time, iron and chromium from the substrate migrate to the coating material. Moreover, the farther from the interface, the lower the diffusion of copper and aluminum to the substrate and the lower the diffusion of iron and chromium to the coating. The width of the diffusion zone is several microns.

The effect of the spraying parameters (stagnation pressure and temperature, velocity of substrate motion) on the properties of copper coatings (from a copper powder with a particle size of $-22+5\,\mu$m) on an aluminum substrate was examined in [122]. Prior to spraying, the substrate was cleansed by ethyl alcohol denatured by methyl alcohol. Spraying was performed with the use of helium. An increase in deposition efficiency with increasing stagnation pressure was noted, as well as a certain (from 90 to 85%) decrease in deposition efficiency with increasing flow rate of the powder from 45 g/min (21 wt% of the gas flow rate) to 76 g/min (36 wt% from the gas flow rate). It was noted that the coating starts exfoliating from the surface after it reaches a certain thickness owing to compressive stresses. The tendency to exfoliation can be prevented or significantly reduced in many cases by means of gas heating. The coating hardness increases with increasing pressure from 1.1 to 2.2 MPa and then stabilizes with a further increase in pressure to 2.9 MPa. An increase in temperature (from 300 to 700 K) leads to a decrease in hardness.

Obtaining coatings from a copper powder (5–25 μm) on aluminum, copper, steel, and stainless steel pre-processed by sandblasting was considered in [123]. Coatings approximately 600 μm thick were applied onto samples 20 mm in diameter; before the tensile tests by the glue method, however, the coating was polished off to a thickness of 300 μm. The experiments showed that the adhesion of a copper coating applied with the use of nitrogen was higher on the aluminum substrate than on the copper substrate. In spraying the particles onto the carbon steel and stainless steel substrates, the coating exfoliated from the substrate in the course of spraying, as soon as the coating thickness reached approximately 500 μm, whereas no exfoliation occurred if helium was used. In addition, the adhesion was much higher than that in the case of spraying by nitrogen. The authors also noted that the adhesion force depends on the working gas pressure (in the range of 1–3 MPa): the higher the pressure, the higher the adhesion. If the threshold pressure is exceeded, the coating starts separating along the epoxy resin/coating interface rather than along the coating/substrate interface. Depending on the substrate material, the adhesion force is distributed as follows (in increasing order): stainless steel, steel, aluminum, and copper.

The influence of the spraying angle on application of coatings of copper particles was considered in [124]. The deposition efficiency increases with increasing spraying angle from zero at a critical angle to 100% at 90°. The size of this region depends on the particle-velocity distribution. The most important parameter, however, is the velocity of the impact onto the substrate. The critical velocities for copper are given in [53]: approximately 560–580 m/s. The critical velocity is affected by the particle size, the particle-size distribution [62], and the substrate material. On the other hand, the particle velocity for a certain material is determined by the type of the accelerating gas, its pressure and temperature, and the nozzle structure. The particle properties (density, size, and shape) also affect the acceleration of particles and, correspondingly, the spraying process [61].

If the particles hit the substrate surface at an angle other than 90°, the normal component of the particle velocity is smaller than that in the normal impact. As the particle deformation depends on the normal velocity, the angle can be assumed to affect the spraying process and the coating microstructure. Though the influence of the angle on the microstructure and properties of coatings obtained by thermal spraying are known, such effects have different features in the cold spray, because the sprayed particles are in a non-melted state. There are only a few papers where the influence of the spraying angle in cold gas-dynamic spraying was considered [21, 124].

Commercial copper powders (with a particle size of 15–37 μm) were used in experiments. These copper powders were obtained by atomization and contained spherical particles. Stainless steel was used as a substrate material. The substrate was subjected to sandblasting by a corundum powder to study the process of copper deposition and was polished to study the copper-coating microstructure. The nozzle had a throat diameter of 2 mm, an exit diameter of 6 mm, and a length of the supersonic section of

100 mm; the powder was injected along the nozzle centerline. Nitrogen with a pressure of 2.0 MPa and a temperature of 220 °C was used to accelerate copper particles. The distance between the nozzle exit and the substrate was 15 mm, and the velocity of substrate motion was 80 mm/s. The microstructure was analyzed with the use of a scanning electron microscope (JEOL, JSM5800). It was demonstrated that the dimensionless deposition efficiency has a maximum at angles of 80–90°. This means that the spraying angle has an insignificant effect within these limits. With a further decrease in spraying angle, however, the dimensionless deposition efficiency rapidly decreases and vanishes at an angle of 40°. Thus, there is an angle below which no deposition occurs. As the particles in the normal impact are attached at a velocity higher than the critical value, the normal component of velocity can be assumed to be the main factor. As the spraying angle decreases, the normal component of the impact velocity also decreases; when the normal velocity component becomes lower than the critical velocity, the particle is not attached.

The cold spray method simultaneously involves deposition of particles and erosion of the substrate. Adhesion of particles occurs when they reach a velocity higher than the critical value, while erosion occurs because there are particles whose velocity is lower than the critical value. As there is some distribution of particles in terms of their velocity, the critical velocity can turn out to be inside this distribution, and only some portion of particles attach to the substrate. On the other hand, particles with lower velocities rebound and destroy the coating. If the particle hits the substrate at a certain angle, the impact velocity of the particle can be divided into the normal component and the tangential component with respect to the substrate surface. If the effect of the tangential component is assumed to be small, the deposition is mainly determined by the normal component of velocity. Correspondingly, the dimensionless deposition efficiency changes insignificantly as the angle decreases from 90° to an angle at which the normal component reaches the critical velocity. With a further decrease in spraying angle, the dimensionless deposition efficiency decreases from 100 to 0%. The experimental results obtained support the validity of this model. Following this model, we can assume that the range of transitional angles depends on the particle-velocity distribution. The transitional region in terms of the spraying angle is wide for particles with a wide velocity distribution and narrow for particles with a narrow velocity distribution. The transitional region for copper is approximately 40°. A wide distribution of the particle size leads to a wide distribution of the particle velocity. The copper powder used in the experiments had a relatively wide distribution responsible for a wide transitional region in terms of the spraying angle.

The effect of various parameters of the substrate, such as the substrate thickness, surface roughness, substrate temperature, number of passes, and velocity of substrate motion, was considered in [125] by an example of copper coatings (mean particle size of 8 μm) on soft steel. Nitrogen with a pressure of 3 MPa and a temperature of 623 K was used as a working gas. The deposition efficiency for copper increases (from 60 to 70%) with increasing substrate thickness (from 6 to 32 mm). The deposition efficiency also slightly increases with increasing substrate roughness (from 0.2 to 7 μm R_a). Pre-heating of the substrate from room temperature to 450 K and an increase in the number of passes (from 1 to 3) exert the same effect as an increase in the substrate thickness. The deposition efficiency significantly decreases (from 70 to 55%) with increasing velocity of substrate motion (from 20 to 100 mm/s). Unfortunately, the authors did not give any comments on these effects.

The copper coating on an aluminum substrate (polished or etched) obtained in [108] displays a low level of porosity. Moreover, the content of oxygen in the coating is approximately 0.1%, which coincides with the content in the initial material of the powder. It follows from here that cold spray does not oxidize the initial material. The electrical conductivity of coatings is approximately 90% of the electrical conductivity of copper proper, which is much higher than the electrical conductivity of coatings obtained by gas-thermal methods, such as the gas-plasma and the electric-arc methods (only 30–40% of the electrical conductivity of copper proper). The Vickers 0.3 hardness of the cold spray coating is 150, and the coating/substrate interface does not contain defects. Mechanical tests were performed for two types of coatings: immediately after spraying and after annealing at 400 °C during 1 hour to examine the influence of annealing on mechanical properties. After annealing, the coating becomes more plastic. The coating sample without annealing after spraying broke under a load of 66 MPa and a strain of 0.06%, whereas the annealed sample could withstand a load of 195 MPa with a total strain of 1.04%. A comparison with characteristics of copper shows that Young's moduli differ insignificantly, but the coating strength is lower. Composite coatings from copper and aluminum were also dense and, which is especially important, had a uniform distribution of materials. Thus, the cold spray allows obtaining composite coatings consisting of mixtures of materials [108].

The properties of the copper coating on an aluminum substrate and the degree of the influence of spraying parameters on the coating density were considered in [126]. In the examined range, the greatest effect on the coating quality is exerted by the stand-off distance, and then there follow the gas temperature and pressure. The influence of voltage on the powder feeder (of the drum type), which occupies the last position, is also noted. Yet, the authors commented that the degree of the influence of temperature and pressure could be prevailing if the range of parameters is expanded. Thus, the tests performed are primarily useful for optimization of a particular cold spray setup rather than for optimization of the cold spray process proper. A decrease in microhardness with increasing coating annealing temperature from 160 to 90 ($H_{v0.2}$) is noted (the latter figure corresponds to the hardness of the cast material). Coating adhesion turned out to be 18 MPa. The authors assumed that the basic mechanisms of adhesion are submelting and mechanical adhesion. The experiments aimed at determining the thermal and electrical conductivity of coatings showed that these quantities reach approximately 70% of the corresponding values for the cast material. This ratio is almost unaffected by annealing.

The effect of thermal treatment of copper coatings on their structure and properties was considered in [127]. The grain size increases from 60 to 120 nm with increasing annealing temperature from 25 to 200 °C. The microhardness of copper coatings remains roughly unchanged. As the annealing temperature increases to 300 °C and higher, recrystallization with a further increase in the grain size occurs (dislocations related to microstrains form new strain-free grains), which impairs the hardness of coatings. It was assumed in [128] that grains of an approximately identical size are formed under conditions of dynamic recrystallization (i.e., under high strains and strain rates), but the recrystallization itself is initiated at temperatures above $0.4T_m$. Dynamic recrystallization can occur in the course of deposition because of the formation of a high density of dislocations and a local increase in temperature owing to adiabatic shear and heating of the substrate. The grain size in the deposited coating is too small for optical microscopy; annealing at 200 °C reveals several very small grains, and annealing at 500 °C leads to noticeable recrystallization with a grain size from 1 to 5 μm. The feature most frequently encountered in tensile tests of coatings is the plastic fracture in the case of annealing at 600 °C. This indicates that there exists a clear boundary with good adhesion between the particles already during the spraying process, and the microstructure is improved during annealing. Directly after deposition, the coatings display fracture close to brittle fracture. The tensile force, however, is very high, which again confirms the hypothesis about high-quality adhesion of particles.

The influence of thermal treatment on electrical resistance and hardness of copper coatings (spherical particles 24 μm in diameter on the average) on tough copper substrates, which were obtained with the use of nitrogen at a temperature of 150 °C and a pressure of 2 MPa, was considered in [129]. It turned out that the coating resistance immediately after deposition in the direction parallel to the substrate surface is approximately half its value in the perpendicular direction (47% against 81% of the value for the cast material). After annealing, however, they become very close and reach 95–96% of the value for the cast material. The coating hardness decreases with increasing annealing temperature.

The effect of thermal treatment of coatings obtained from copper powders (10–36 μm) on electrical resistance and coating hardness was examined in [130]. It was noted that annealing of the copper coating at a temperature of 300 °C or higher decreases the coating hardness (from 140 to 80 $H_{v0.1}$). The electrical resistance of the entire composition (steel substrate and copper coating) also decreases with increasing annealing temperature. At an annealing temperature of approximately 200 °C and higher, the resistance reaches the value of $1.8 \times 10^{-8}\,\Omega$m (the resistance of the cast material is $1.6–1.7 \times 10^{-8}\,\Omega$m) against $2.3 \times 10^{-8}\,\Omega$m in the coating without thermal treatment. The resistance of the coating proper without the substrate is $3.7 \times 10^{-8}\,\Omega$m.

The influence of the flow rate of the powder was examined in [131]. Significant concentrations of the powder in the gas flow reduce the impact velocity of particles. If the powder concentrations are insufficient, the coating formed has some holes. In both extreme cases, the quality of coatings is not as good as that desired. The effect of the copper-powder concentration in a helium flow with deposition onto an aluminum substrate on the coating thickness and microstructure and on deposition efficiency was considered. A copper powder with angular particles (similar to crushed stone) with a mean size of 25–30 μm was used in the experiments. The aluminum substrates were prior subjected to sandblasting and cleaning. An axisymmetric nozzle with an exit diameter of 6.3 mm was used. The stagnation temperature of helium was equal to room temperature, its stagnation pressure was 1.7 MPa, and the difference in pressure between the feeder and the pre-chamber was 35 kPa. During the deposition, the flow rate of the powder was changed (from 0.9 to 5.0 g/min), whereas the substrate velocity was constant; one pass was made. The modeling showed that the particle velocity should be higher than the critical velocity (equal to 450 m/s for copper); therefore, the deposition efficiency was expected to be fairly high. In addition, the influence of particles on the gas can be neglected even for the highest concentrations of the powder. Interesting results were obtained. The coating thickness and mass (per unit length of the deposition band) increase if the flow rate of the powder is low, but their values decrease if the flow rate of particles exceeds 4.1 g/min. Moreover, the coating starts exfoliating. The deposition efficiency thereby remains approximately unchanged (about 85–90%). If the substrate velocity is increased, however, no exfoliation occurs, and the coating is as dense as that obtained with lower flow rates of the powder. The authors attribute exfoliation to more intense cold working owing to enhanced bombardment of the surface, i.e., residual stresses in the coating become higher, which is the reason for exfoliation. Unfortunately, the authors did not comment the observed decrease in coating mass and thickness.

The influence of the temperature and impact angle of copper particles with a mean particle size of 56 μm on the critical velocity of adhesion on a copper substrate was studied experimentally and theoretically studied in [132]. Nitrogen and helium was used for acceleration in an axisymmetric nozzle with the supersonic section 100 mm long. The motion of the gas and particles is modeled by the FLUENT + DPM software; the particle deformation during the impact was modeled by the LS-DYNA program [133], which takes into account the effects of hardening and thermal softening but ignores heat transfer. The theoretical value of the critical deposition velocity is related to the emergence of adiabatic shear instability. Experimentally, the critical deposition velocity is determined on the basis of the measured deposition efficiency. Reasonable agreement was achieved between numerical and experimental results. The values obtained, however, were slightly lower (from 295 to 355 m/s) than those mentioned in other publications (about 410 m/s). This difference was attributed to the presence of an oxide film, but this phenomenon was not modeled.

The properties of cold spray produced copper coatings were examined in [134] and compared with copper coatings obtained by various gas-thermal methods. It was found that the electrical resistance of the coatings is commensurable with that of the cold-drawn cast material (1.7 μΩ cm), which turned out to be lower than the resistance of gas-thermal coatings. The hardness of cold spray produced copper coatings was estimated as 140–160 $H_{V0.3}$, which coincides with the hardness of cold-drawn copper; the adhesion of cold spray produced copper coatings was estimated as 30–40 MPa, which coincides with the adhesion of coatings obtained by gas-thermal methods (HVOF, HVCW (combustion wire)).

Copper coatings obtained by the cold spray and plasma methods were compared in [135] (see Fig. 5.20): porosity 0.5% against 9%; surface roughness R_a 8 μm against 13 μm; roughness of the coating/substrate boundary R_a 1.3 μm against 13 μm (the first and second values in each pair refer to cold spray and plasma-produced coatings, respectively). The coating was produced by the cold spray with the use of nitrogen with stagnation parameters of 2.8 MPa and 823 K and spheroidized copper powder with a particle size of −22 + 5 μm on a 2017 Al substrate.

Restrictions of thermal spraying in the automobile industry are often related to a comparatively low quality of electroconducting elements with coatings applied by conventional methods. The cold spray method can find its application for contact joints, etc. The study of the microstructure of copper coatings [136, 137] showed that their properties depend on the powder characteristics and on the spraying regime and that the coating becomes more plastic after annealing.

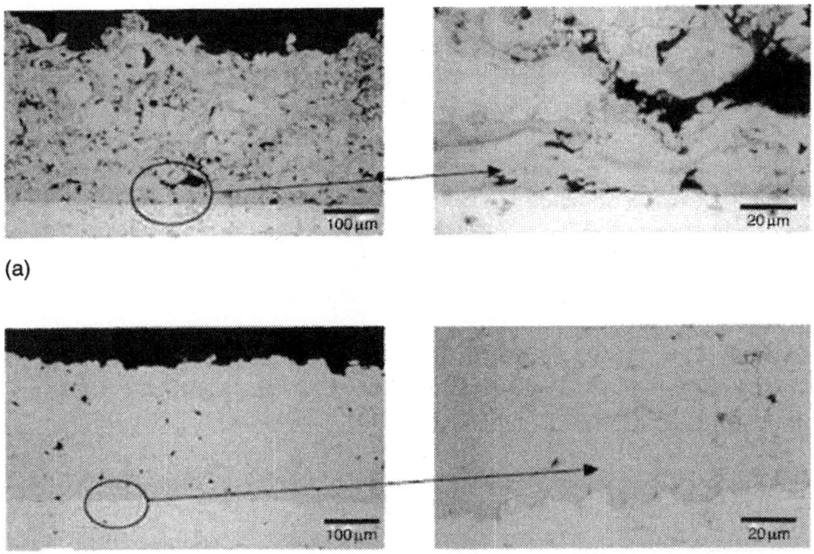

(a)

(b)

Fig. 5.20. Optical cross-sections of (a) APS P and (b) CS P coatings [135].

5.3.3. Nickel-containing coatings

Some results obtained in a Ford research laboratory in studying the possibility of cold spray application in car industry were considered in [138]. Though thermal spraying is not a dominating technology in preparing car surfaces, it still plays a certain role in production of various elements of cars [139, 140].

The study of properties of nickel coatings without a posteriori treatment [141] revealed comparatively high values of Young's modulus of the coating (76–95% of Young's modulus of nickel proper). Such comparatively high values of Young's modulus of coatings obtained by the cold spray, as compared with the metal proper, in contrast to lower values of Young's modulus (typically 25–35%) of coatings obtained by conventional methods (e.g., electrometallization or plasma technology), imply that the microstructure of materials obtained by the cold spray is more dense. Similarly, the high purity of material obtained by the cold spray implies a much improved structure at the atomic level. The strength characteristics of coatings are often insufficient, as compared with the cast material, because of cold hardening and the granulated nature of coatings. Post-processing of coatings, such as annealing, can turn out to be beneficial for recovering coating plasticity to a certain level [138].

The cold spray method has the following advantages: coatings can be rather thick, without contamination and oxides; the spraying process has a high degree of spatial localization (small size of the deposition spot). At the same time, the cold spray setup and cold spray coating properties have some adverse features: the use of helium for obtaining high-quality coatings; coatings have a granular-type structure at the point of their fracture, which requires annealing; incorporation of gases into coatings and subsequent liberation; injection of the powder at high pressures, which makes the setup more complicated; strong dependence of the process on powder parameters. Some problems can be solved by organizing recirculation of the powder and helium, injection of the powder downstream of the nozzle throat, etc. [138].

Iron-containing coatings obtained by the cold spray are extremely pure, can be annealed, are magnetically active, and have a number of advantages (e.g., in terms of density and purity) over coatings obtained by thermal spraying [142, 143]. This property of cold spray coatings can find its application in electrical machinery. The studies showed that it is possible to obtain composites of hard materials such as NdFeB in a soft metallic matrix of Fe by the cold spray [54]. Elements of electrical machines, which involve metallization, and also soft and hard magnets can find application in fabrication of magnetos, compact motors, sensors, etc.

Electrolytic nickel plating can be used to fabricate miniature components, such as pinions, junctions, and other two-dimensional mechanical structures. This process provides excellent coatings, but it has low efficiency and is highly expensive. Materials that can be now obtained by the electrolytic method are copper, nickel, permalloy, and gold. The development of alternatives to the electrolytic method will allow designers to choose other materials, including ceramics and nonmetals, for structural design. As the cold spray allows obtaining dense coatings with a low content of oxides and is highly efficient, it can become an alternative to electrolytic nickel plating. In addition, the cold spray can be used for materials (such as stainless steel and aluminum), which are never applied by the electrolytic method. Cold gas-dynamic spraying proceeds at temperatures close to room temperature, which offers potential advantages, such as the absence of stresses due to cooling, undesirable phases, oxidation, and grain growth during the deposition process.

The mechanical properties of nickel coatings obtained by the cold spray were studied in [144] immediately after deposition and after thermal treatment and were compared with the properties of cast and electrolytic nickel. The nickel coatings were obtained with the use of helium at a temperature of 325 °C and a powder with a mean particle size of 14 μm, standard deviation of 9 μm, and flow rate of 25 g/min. The particle velocity was 880 m/s with a standard deviation of 80 m/s; the deposition efficiency was 20%. Nickel was sprayed onto a copper substrate moving with a velocity of 25 mm/s; the coating was grown until it became 3.5 mm thick. After spraying, the coating surface was processed by milling. Half of the sample was then subjected to thermal treatment at 600 °C during one hour in an inert atmosphere of argon [145] and then was slowly tempered.

Tensile tests of the coating without annealing revealed the absence of the plastic behavior. Young's modulus and the yield stress were close to values typical of the electrolytic coating. The coating without annealing displayed 53% of the ultimate strength of the electrolytic coating. Some plastic features appeared after thermal treatment. Young's modulus was similar to that of the electrolytic coating. The yield stress was 68% of the electrolytic coating, and the ultimate strength was 54% of that of the electrolytic coating. Scanning electron microscopy (SEM) revealed some features of brittle fracture of the coating without annealing and plastic fracture after thermal treatment.

Compressive tests of the coating without annealing showed that the samples have a high yield stress and ultimate strength. A high value of the yield stress was observed if there were a large number of dislocations present in the material. Young's modulus was close to that of the electrolytic coating. The yield stress was 322% of that of the electrolytic coating, and the ultimate strength was 226% of that of the electrolytic coating. Young's modulus of the processed coating was close to that of the electrolytic coating. The yield stress was 76% of that of the electrolytic coating, and the ultimate strength was 73% of that of the electrolytic coating [144].

The study of the microstructure showed that the nickel coating without annealing has weak bonds between the particles. Wide peaks on X-ray diffraction curves showed that nickel was subjected to intense cold hardening [146]. The nickel coating experienced brittle fracture under a stress much higher than the yield stress of nickel proper. The compressive strength of the coating was four times the compressive strength of nickel proper.

After thermal treatment, the nickel coating behaved as a fine-grained material. Metallography and X-ray diffraction showed that nickel recrystallized and had a grain size smaller than 10 μm. A typical feature of the nickel coating is its plastic behavior, and its failure strain is one third of the failure strain of cast nickel. Thus, the nickel coating produced by the cold spray is brittle, but thermal treatment makes its properties approach the properties of nickel proper.

Coatings of nickel and nickel-containing alloys NiCrAlY 1 (Cr 31%), NiCrAlY 2 (Cr 22%), CoNiCrAlY, and Hastelloy C (Ni 59%, Cr 15%, Mo 16.5%, Fe 5%, W 4%) with spherical particles whose size ranged from 5 to 30 μm were considered in [147] with the use of the Kinetic 3000 cold spray System. The materials obtained have high density, hardness, and Young's modulus. Spraying was performed with the use of a helium flow at a pressure of 2.4 MPa and a temperature of 500 °C onto 316L stainless steel. A nickel coating 715 μm thick with 2% porosity was obtained; the deposition efficiency was 82%. The deposition efficiency and porosity of the CoNiCrAlY alloy were 19% and 4%, respectively. The corresponding values for the Hastelloy C alloy were 23% and 7%. The NiCrAlY alloys do not form a thick coating, though attempts were made to increase the helium temperature and pressure; yet, only the so-called monolayer was formed. Another alloy from this family, however, NiCrAlY 2 (produced by another company) was successfully deposited with a deposition efficiency of 22%. The hardness of the nickel coating is close to that of nickel proper. In the case of CoNiCrAlY and Hastelloy C alloys, the coating hardness is much higher than the hardness of the initial material. The authors put forward a hypothesis that the probability of adhesion decreases because of the increase in hardness in the course of coating growth. This could also be the reason for monolayer formation in the case the NiCrAlY 1 alloy was used. It was also noted that this alloy has the lowest Young's modulus among all powders tested. Though its hardness is close to that of the Hastelloy C alloy, the yield stress is higher, which, in the authors' opinion, leads to a higher probability of rebound for particles of the NiCrAlY 1 alloy.

Nickel coatings clad by aluminum (with 5 wt% of aluminum), which were obtained by four different methods: air-plasma method, metallization (arc between wires), high-velocity oxy-fuel method (HVOF), and cold spray, were compared in [148]. A preliminary inspection of the flows revealed the following mean parameter of particles (droplets) before their impact onto the surface: 120 m/s and 2600 K in the plasma method, 90 m/s and 2600 K in metallization, 600 m/s and 2100 K in the HVOF method, and 700 m/s in the cold spray. Figure 5.21 shows the photographs of the coatings obtained.

The plasma and metallization coatings had a high porosity, whereas the coatings obtained by the high-velocity gas-plasma and cold spray methods were very dense. Though the cold spray coating was denser than the HVOF coating, the hardness and thermal conductivity of the cold spray coating were lower. The elasticity modulus of the coatings along and across the coating was examined in detail. The results of this examination are listed in Table 5.1.

The elasticity modulus of the HVOF coating reached the value of cast nickel. Special attention was paid to residual stresses. Residual stresses are developed in to stages: during

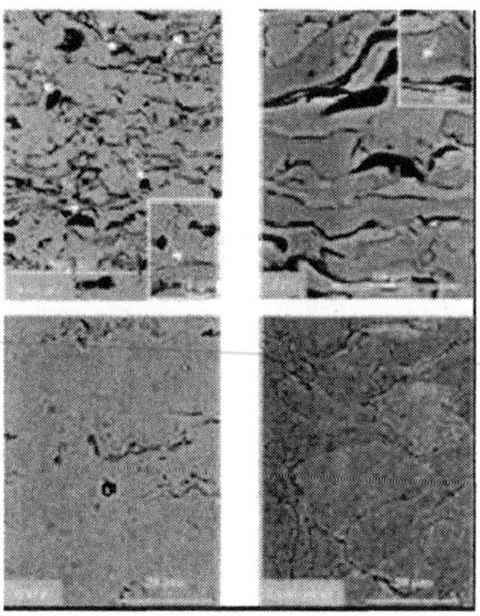

Fig. 5.21. Cross-sectional micrographs of four different deposits (the substrate is at the bottom; the arrows in the wire-arc sprayed coating point to metallurgical bonding areas) [148].

Table 5.1. Comparison of mechanical properties of coatings produced by different methods

Process	Method		
	Spherical indentation		Four-point bending
	E(GPa)—in plane	E(GPa)—cross-section	E(GPa)—cross-section
APS	105 ± 17	83 ± 5	78 ± 6
TWA	80 ± 21	110 ± 23	103 ± 25
HVOF	172 ± 17	178 ± 10	166 ± 5
Cold spray	110 ± 31	58 ± 7	–

spraying and during cooling after spraying. Hardening stresses arise at the spraying stage owing to rapid cooling and solidification of melted particles during the impact. As the solidified particles are attached to the surface, they can no longer be in free contact (i.e., contact with slipping), and tensile hardening stresses are developed. In the HVOF method, a high-velocity impact leads to plastic deformation of the surface layer and generates compressive stresses of the so-called cold hardening. It is this type of stresses that is typical of the cold spray method. At the end of spraying, the substrate/coating system has usually an elevated temperature, and cooling to room temperature generates thermal stresses because of the difference in thermal expansion coefficients of the substrate and coating materials. This stress shifts the initial level of stresses toward extension or compression, depending on the ratio of the thermal expansion coefficients. The final residual stress is a superposition (addition) of stresses generated by these two mechanisms. The residual stresses in coatings measured by the method of neutron diffraction [149] are plotted in Fig. 5.22.

The surface stresses in coatings obtained by low-velocity methods are compressive and then gradually transform to tensile stresses at the coating/substrate interface. Numerical simulations were performed for these coatings [150], which coincided with the experimental data. Coatings obtained by high-velocity methods display the opposite situation: the stresses are compressive in the coating.

The effect of the substrate hardness (reached by hardening to 316L 42 CrMo4 steel to different values) on deposition of Ni and NiCrAlY powders by helium at a temperature of 773 K was considered in [151]. The particle size of the nickel and nichrome powders ranged from 10 to 33 μm and from 5.7 to 29 μm, respectively. The deposition efficiency turned out to decrease with increasing substrate hardness for the examined powders. The influence of hardness is more significant for nichrome than for nickel (as the hardness increases from 200 to 600 units H_{v30}, the deposition efficiency decreases by 13% for nickel and by 41% for nichrome). In absolute value, the deposition efficiency for nickel is 15 times higher than that for nichrome. The coating thickness varied between 92 and

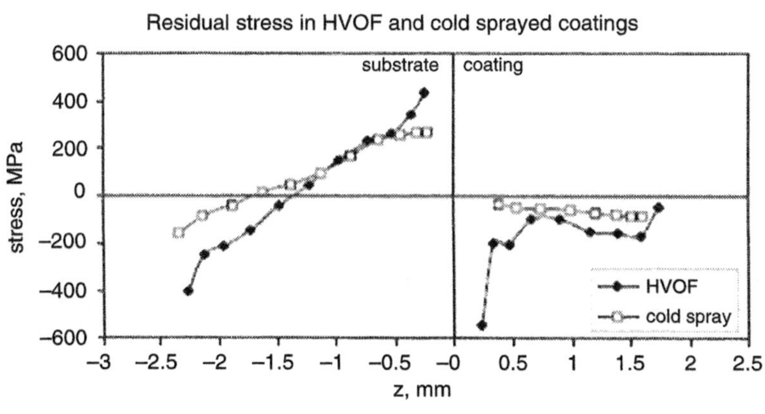

Fig. 5.22. Through-thickness profile of the residual stress in HVOF sprayed and cold-sprayed Ni… 5% Al deposit and steel substrate [148].

206 μm. The authors estimated the monolayer thickness (minimum coating thickness at which the substrate material affects the deposition process) to be 1% for nickel and 10% for nichrome, because the nichrome coating thickness was smaller. The authors did not give any comments on the phenomenon observed. The properties of the coatings themselves (porosity and hardness), however, remain unaffected by the substrate hardness.

The properties of coatings on light weight alloys containing aluminum AA1050, AA3005, AA5754, AA7022, magnesium AZ91, and titanium TiAl6V4 from a mixture of the powders Cu +50% Ni, Cu + 70% Ni, and Cu + 90% Ni were considered in [152]. The particle size in copper and nickel powders was 5–25 μm. Nickel-copper mixtures form dense coatings. It was noted that the coating exfoliates at low pressures and temperatures of spraying, i.e., it has weak adhesion to the substrate.

To obtain a nanostructured powder, the authors of [153] used a mixture of the iron power with 10 wt% of silicon with a particle size of 75 μm, which was prepared in a ball mill. Such alloys are widely used for magnetic components in electrical industry owing to their soft magnetic properties with low coercion and high saturation threshold. Normally, the content of silicon is limited to 3–4% because the resultant alloy is brittle, which prevents material rolling into sheets. Therefore, an urgent challenge is to develop alternative methods for obtaining materials of this type with a high content of silicon. The methods currently used are the formation of fibers from the melt [154], method of rapid cooling [155], spraying from the melt [156], and mechanical method of alloy production [157]. A possibility of obtaining coatings from such an alloy by cold gas-dynamic spraying was also considered. Nitrogen was used to accelerate the particles, and the velocity of substrate motion was 80 mm/s. When the powder was prepared in the ball mill, the mean size of particles, which had an angular shape, was several micrometers. After deposition of a simple mechanical mixture at a temperature of 250 °C, the coating structure was obviously layered and porous; silicon entered this structure in the form of inclusions in an iron matrix. The powder obtained in the ball mill produced a dense coating deposited at temperatures of 290 and 400 °C, and the microstructure of the initial powder remained unchanged.

Deposition of the 57Ni18Ti20Zr3Si2Sn alloy (with a mean particle size of 15–30 μm) by the cold spray was considered in [158]. A specific feature of the cold spray setup in that work was the use of an additional heater for heating the powder to temperatures of 623 and 723 K (see Fig. 5.23).

With the use of nitrogen, the coating could not be obtained even at a temperature of 873 K. With the use of helium (the measured particle velocities reached 800–1000 m/s), the coating was successfully obtained and its properties were examined. It was noted that the phase and microstructural compositions of the coating coincided with the characteristics of the initial powder. Additional heating led to higher strains, lower porosity (down to 4%), higher adhesion (up to 90 MPa), higher hardness (up to 700 $H_{V0.3}$), and higher deposition efficiency (see Fig. 5.24).

The coating obtained in [108] from 316L steel was dense, and the content of oxides was low. The Vickers 0.3 hardness of the coating was 275. The MCrAlY coating deposited onto a steel substrate with the use of helium had a low porosity. As the main application

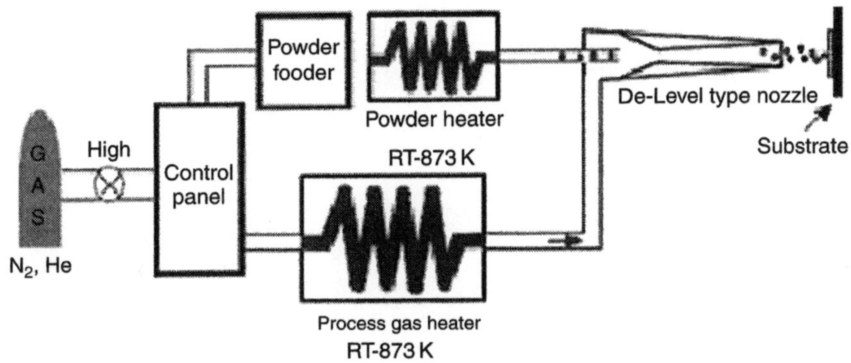

Fig. 5.23. Layout of the modified kinetic spraying system [158].

of such coatings is anticorrosion protection, the use of the cold spray for these purposes is fairly justified. The Vickers 0.3 hardness of the coating was 575.

The results of studying the deposition of an amorphous material, the so-called metallized glass (NiTiZrSiSn powder with particles 5–45 μm with a mean size of 25 μm) onto a substrate of SS41 soft steel with the use of nitrogen and helium and additional heating of the powder (i.e., in addition to the accelerating gas, the powder is additionally heated to increase the initial temperature of the powder at the nozzle entrance) are described in [159]. Submelting of particles is noted, which is the reason for their adhesion. The use of helium allows obtaining more dense coatings and ensures a higher deposition efficiency. The coating composition did not display any significant differences from the composition of the initial powder.

5.3.4. Zinc-containing coatings

Deposition of zinc particles (smaller than 48 μm) by a nitrogen flow onto a stainless steel substrate subjected to sandblasting was considered in [160]. The modeling results revealed the possibility of melting of zinc particles in a local contact region. The experimental data support this conclusion: an amorphous phase was found at the interface between the zinc particles in the coating; the formation of this phase is associated with rapid solidification of the melted material.

The interface between the coating obtained from the zinc powder and the substrate of the AZ91 magnesium alloy and between the coating obtained from the zinc powder with addition of the aluminum powder (5 wt%) and the substrate of the AA7022 alloy was examined in [161]. Mechanical alloys were observed at the interface. The interface contains vortex zones of mixing of the coating and substrate materials. Phases obtained as a result of the reaction were also observed, which is indicative of short-time melting. These phases were found inside the transitional zone in the vicinity of the vortices. Several submicron and nano-sized intermetallide inclusions with different compositions were also observed. Their exact compositions could not be identified because of their small size. Both effects, i.e., mechanical alloy formation in zones of vortex mixing of

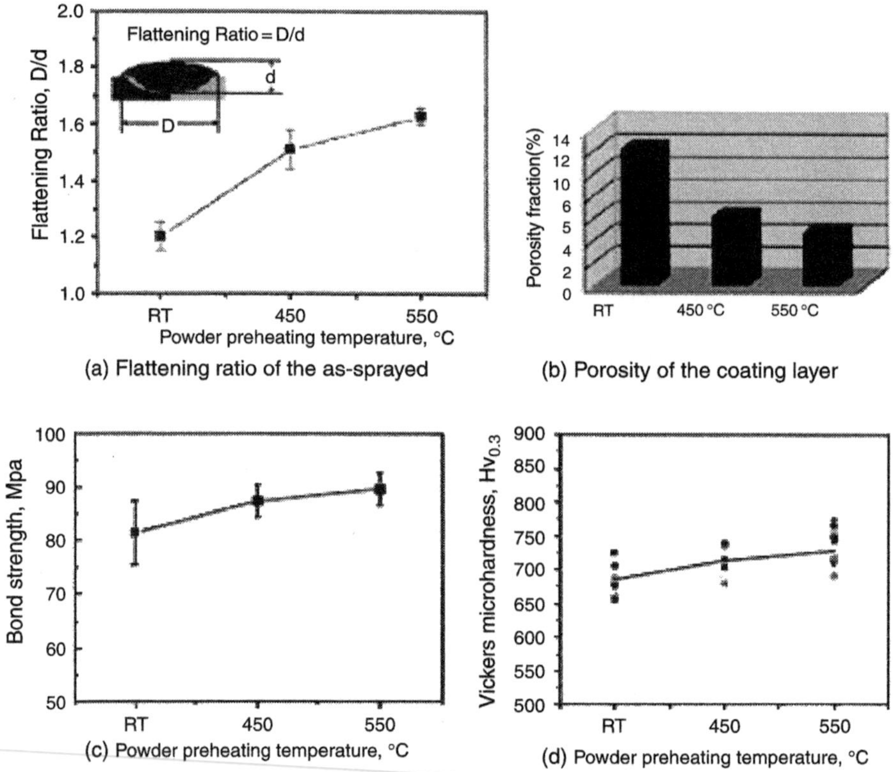

Fig. 5.24. (a) Strain, (b) porosity, (c) bond strength, and (d) microhardness of the coating layer according to the powder preheating temperature [158].

materials and metallurgical reactions in the vicinity of these zones, are responsible for strong adhesion between the coating and the substrate in the cold spray. The oxide layers found at the coating/substrate interface appeared most probably as a consequence of corrosion processes during preparation of the samples.

Formation of coatings on DH-36 steel substrates with the use of helium and nitrogen from the powders of aluminum (mean size 25 μm, angular shape), zinc (spherical particles with a mean size of 30 μm), and their mixtures (Zn + 15% Al and Zn + 55% Al) was studied in [162]. The measured deposition efficiency is summarized in Table 5.2.

An analysis of components in the coating for the mixture of powders showed that the content of zinc is smaller than that in the initial powder. Thus, for the initial mixture Zn + 15 Al, the coating contained Zn + 29 Al in the case of spraying by nitrogen and Zn + 49 Al in the case of spraying by helium; for the initial mixture Zn + 55 Al, the coating contained Zn + 85 Al in the case of spraying by nitrogen and Zn + 74 Al in the case of spraying by helium. The authors argued that this phenomenon can be attributed to different deposition efficiencies of the Zn and Al powders individually, as if they were sprayed independently, i.e., there is no mutual influence of the powders on each other. In

Table 5.2. Results of deposition efficiency measurements

Powder	Gas	Deposition efficiency
Zn	N_2	16.5%
	He	29%
Al	N_2	24.1%
	He	94.6%
Zn + 15Al	N_2	18.8%
	He	33.3%
Zn + 55Al	N_2	22.4%
	He	68%

addition, the coating porosity was determined, which varied within 0.5–3% in the case of spraying by nitrogen and 0.5–1% in the case of spraying by helium. Determination of coating adhesion did not reveal any significant dependence on spraying parameters. Adhesion of almost all tested coatings lies within 6.89–13.78 MPa; in the case of spraying of pure aluminum by helium, it was slightly lower: 2.445 MPa. The authors noted that the data on adhesion were obtained by testing three samples for each combination. Thus, this deviation should be considered as rather substantial. Special attention was paid to corrosion resistance of coatings for protecting vessels. It was noted that all coatings prevent corrosion of steel; the coating from the mixture Zn + 15 Al was particularly noted.

The properties of coatings on light weight alloys of aluminum AA1050, AA3005, AA5754, AA 7022, magnesium AZ91, and titanium TiAl6V4 from the mixtures of powders Zn + 5% Al and Zn + 15% Al were studied in [163]. The size of the aluminum and zinc particles was 5–20 μm and 20–45 μm, respectively. Zinc-containing coatings have a low porosity and good adhesion to the substrate. The coating composition differs from the initial composition of the powder (the content of aluminum is roughly doubled). Intense mechanical alloy formation at the particle/substrate interface was noted. The main objective of the study was to check the possibility of welding plates of above-mentioned materials, the coatings being used as an intermediate layer. As a whole, the coatings turned out to be suitable for these purposes.

5.3.5. Titanium-containing coatings

The process of formation of coatings from titanium and titanium-containing materials is somewhat different from that for materials more typical of cold spray (aluminum, copper, nickel, and zinc) considered above. Therefore, information that gives an idea about the character of the spraying process and titanium-based coatings is presented below.

Obtaining coatings from the titanium powder (10–70 μm) on aluminum, copper, steel, and stainless steel substrates pre-processed by sandblasting was considered in [164]. Coatings approximately 600 μm thick were applied onto samples 20 mm in diameter; before the tensile tests by the glue method, however, the coating was polished off to a thickness of 300 μm.

At a pressure of 2 MPa, the coating adhesion to the stainless steel substrate was identical, independent of the working gas, whereas it became substantially higher in the case of spraying by helium at a pressure of 3 MPa. Moreover, the strength of adhesion between the coating and the aluminum substrate, which was obtained at a pressure of 2 MPa in the helium flow, was close to the strength of adhesion to the stainless steel substrate. With the use of nitrogen, however, it was not possible to obtain continuous titanium coatings on the aluminum substrate: erosion with small islands of titanium was observed. To explain the results obtained, the authors considered the ratio of the particle and substrate materials in terms of hardness. It was argued that deposition is extremely difficult or impossible if the particle is harder than the substrate (as in the case of deposition of titanium onto aluminum). As the mechanism of bonding, the authors suggested the formation of metallic bonds, but do not exclude the anchor effect either.

The effect on the spraying angle on the process of application of titanium coatings was examined in [124]. Commercial titanium powders (37–44 μm) were used in experiments. The titanium powder with particles of angular shape was obtained by hydrogenization and subsequent dehydrogenization. Stainless steel was used as a substrate material. The substrate was polished to study the titanium-deposition process. The nozzle had the following parameters: throat diameter 2 mm, exit diameter 6 mm, and length of the supersonic section 100 mm; the nozzle was injected along the nozzle centerline. The accelerating gas was nitrogen with a pressure of 2.0 MPa and a temperature of 240 °C. The distance between the nozzle exit and the substrate was 15 mm, and the velocity of substrate motion was 80 mm/s. The spraying process was characterized by a dimensionless deposition efficiency determined as the ratio of the weight increment to the maximum weight increment among all samples obtained with different spraying angles in one pass. The microstructure was analyzed by a scanning electron microscope (JEOL, JSM5800). The following dependence of the dimensionless deposition efficiency for titanium on the spraying angle was obtained: almost unchanged from 70 to 90° and no deposition at 50° and smaller angles. The titanium powder had a comparatively narrow fraction of 37–44 μm, which provided a narrow distribution of velocities and, correspondingly, a narrow transitional zone. Moreover, acceleration of particles depends on the particle density. A low density of titanium yields high mean velocities with a narrow distribution. As a result, the dimensionless deposition efficiency of titanium reaches 100% in wider ranges in terms of the spraying angle, whereas the transitional zone is rather narrow.

The effect of various parameters of the substrate, such as the substrate thickness, surface roughness, substrate temperature, number of passes, and velocity of substrate motion, on the process of obtaining titanium coatings (mean particle size of 25 μm) on soft steel was considered in [125]. Nitrogen with a pressure of 3 MPa and a temperature of 623 K was used as a working gas. A weak decrease in titanium deposition efficiency (from 20 to 15%) was noted with increasing substrate thickness (from 6 to 32 mm). The deposition efficiency slightly increases with increasing substrate roughness (from 0.2 to 7 μm R_a). Pre-heating of the substrate from room temperature to 450 K and an increase in the number of passes (from 1 to 3) exerts the same effect as the increase in substrate thickness. The deposition efficiency substantially decreases (from 20 to 0%) with increasing velocity of substrate motion (from 20 to 100 mm/s).

It was noted in [108] that porous titanium coatings can be used for biomedical prosthetic devices where a high-porosity and pure titanium implant is needed to ensure a tight connection with bones and tissues. Therefore, the cold spray can be of interest for production of implants of this kind. Composite coatings from titanium and aluminum (50:50 wt%) turned out to be dense and, which is especially important, had a uniform distribution of materials. Thus, the cold spray allows obtaining composite coatings from mixtures of different materials [108].

Obtaining coatings from the titanium powder (5–50 μm) with addition of 25 vol.% of hydroxyapatite nanopowder (this composition is used in medicine as a material for implants) pre-processed in a ball mill was studied in [165]. Coatings on a titanium substrate were obtained with the use of air with a pressure of 5.5 MPa and a temperature of 315 °C. It was noted that thick coatings could not be obtained under these conditions and that the bonding between the particles and the substrate was mechanical and no traces of melting were observed.

The influence of the particle-size distribution, surface conditions, and stagnation pressure of the gas on formation of titanium coatings was considered in [166]. Titanium powders (particles of angular shape obtained by the method of hydrogenization and subsequent dehydrogenization) with a mean size of 28 μm and with a mean size of 47 μm, which were sprayed onto substrates of the Ti6Al4V alloy and conventional soft steel, were used in the experiments. Helium at room temperature was used as a working gas. The velocity of substrate motion was fixed at 100 mm/s, and the necessary coating thickness (about 900 μm) was reached in a required number of passes. The following glue method was used for adhesion tests of the coatings. Coatings in the form of discs were applied onto a substrate of a larger size with the help of a mask (8.16 mm in diameter). After that, the second element necessary for testing was glued to the coating by epoxy glue. Before gluing, the surface of the second element was sandblasted and degreased by methyl alcohol. The particle velocity was determined by one-dimensional calculations. The deposition efficiency of the finer powder was approximately twice the deposition efficiency of the coarser powder. The lowest porosity (about 13%) of the coating was obtained by spraying the coarser powder at the maximum examined pressure of 2.9 MPa. The minimum porosity of the coating from the finer powder was higher (14% at a pressure of 2.0 MPa). Neither the change in pressure nor the treatment of the substrate surface made it possible to reduce the porosity. It was noted that the same level of porosity of titanium coatings (10–30%) was declared in [167]. Adhesive tests did not reveal any significant dependence on the particle size; there is a weak dependence on pressure (adhesion increases with increasing pressure from 20 MPa at a pressure of 1.5 MPa to 24 MPa at a pressure of 2.9 MPa) and a significant dependence on the method of substrate-surface treatment. Adhesion on the sandblasted surface was approximately two times lower than that on the polished and non-treated surfaces (10 MPa against 20 MPa), and this feature is observed both for the substrate from the Ti6Al4V alloy and for the soft steel substrate! The authors attributed such an unusual behavior for the titanium powder (comparatively high porosity and low adhesion on the sandblasted surface) by the hexagonal structure of titanium but did not clarify how the structure can affect the characteristics observed.

Coatings from mixtures of titanium (−45 μm) and 50% aluminum (+10 − 45 μm) on an aluminum substrate were obtained in [168] with the use of helium with stagnation parameters 1.6 MPa and 300–500 K. The coating was obtained in several passes. An elevated content of aluminum was observed at the boundaries of the layers corresponding to one pass. The coating experience brittle fracture, and no traces of the plastic flow were observed at the interfaces between the particles, which allowed the authors to conclude that the predominant adhesion mechanism is mechanical clamping (interlocking). The content of aluminum in the coating decreased to 44%. The porosity of the coatings was approximately 20%, and the porosity of purely aluminum and purely titanium coatings was 2–12% and 10–30%, respectively. The hardness of the aluminum component of the coating was close to the corresponding value for the cast material: 24 against 30 $H_{V0.1}$; the hardness of the titanium component was 50 against 160 $H_{V0.1}$, which was attributed to the initial porosity of the titanium powder used. No changes in the phase and structural composition in the coatings were observed. Emergence of intermetallide components after thermal treatment (up to 1473 K in the argon atmosphere) was noted.

5.3.6. Coatings with brittle components

The studies of cold gas-dynamic spraying of coatings from mixtures containing brittle materials (oxides, ceramics, etc.) deserve special attention. The interest is stimulated both by the possibility of obtaining new unique coatings and by expansion of knowledge on the cold spray nature because the conventional theories based on particle plasticity are inapplicable in this case and, in addition, the erosion/adhesion competition is manifested especially clearly. According to the classical concepts of erosion, addition of erosive particles into the powder of a plastic material (aluminum, copper, zinc, or nickel) should have led to erosion of the growing coating and, as a consequence, to a decrease in deposition efficiency or to complete erosion of the substrate. Nevertheless, this is not the case. The brittle component is present in coatings to a certain extent; moreover, addition of the brittle component sometimes improves the deposition efficiency and strength of adhesion of the basic plastic material and also the coating properties (e.g., wear resistance).

The paper [169] describes obtaining a photocatalyst on the basis of titanium dioxide, which is a promising material owing to its potential applications in environmental purification, production of solar arrays, application in cancer therapy, and obtaining antifog agents [170, 173]. The initial powders (10–45 μm) were prepared by agglomeration of ultrafine particles with the use of polyvinyl alcohol as a binder and had a particle size of 200 and 7 nm. After agglomeration, the particles had a spherical shape. The substrate was a stainless steel plate. Before spraying, the substrate was subjected to sandblasting by corundum. The cold spray scheme developed at the Xi'an Jiaotong University (Japan) was used [174]. The working gas was nitrogen with a pressure of 2 MPa and a temperature of 300 °C. During spraying, a robot moved the nozzle with a velocity of 0.5 m/s at a distance of 10 mm from the substrate. The microstructure of the resultant coatings was inspected by SEM, an X-ray diffraction system, etc. The coatings had a rough and porous surface, which was desirable in this case because the activity of the catalyst depends on the state of the surface. It was argued that the microcrystalline structure of the powders was retained. The surface was completely covered without any bald spots, but the coating thickness was rather small: 10–15 μm (attempts to apply a thicker coating failed). Coatings from two different powders displayed an identical photocatalytic activity, though initial powders of significantly different sizes were used to obtain them. It turned out that the coating thickness depends on the size of the initial powder (a finer powder produces a thinner coating).

A coating 2–10 μm thick from oxides of tungsten WO_3 and yttrium Y_2O_3 on a silicon crystal was obtained in [175]; the particles were accelerated by air with a stagnation temperature of 600 K. The initial size of oxide particles was 30–50 μm for tungsten oxide and 10 μm for yttrium oxide. The deposition efficiency was lower than 10%. An analysis showed that oxide particles are destroyed by the impact in a brittle manner, so that only very small fragments remain on the surface; no crystallographic or chemical changes in the initial material occur thereby. The coating in the vicinity of the surface is densely packed. No craters due to the impact on the silicon surface were observed in that work, which could be caused by the major part of kinetic energy of the particles being spent on particle disintegration. The authors indicated mechanical clamping (interlocking) as the main mechanism of bonding. Unfortunately, the authors did not give any data on the level of coating adhesion.

The coating from the tungsten/copper composite obtained by the plasma and cold spray methods was inspected in [176]. The powder was prepared in a ball mill from a mixture of the tungsten powder (75 wt%, particle size smaller than 1 μm) and the copper powder (25 wt%, particle size smaller than 45 μm). The sieved fraction used consisted of spherical particles (see Fig. 5.25) consisting of a large number of fine particles (smaller than 1 μm) with the following size distribution: 50% smaller than 20 μm, 27% within 21–44 μm, and 23% within 47–75 μm.

Spraying was performed with the use of nitrogen with a mean temperature of 730 K. A coating 600 μm thick was obtained and analyzed in terms of the tungsten content and porosity. According to the data obtained, the tungsten content in the coating was 35–40 wt% on the average, and the porosity was 0.5–1% (see Fig. 5.26). It was noted that most of the pores were located in the vicinity of tungsten-rich regions.

The characteristics of WC-Co coatings on stainless steel were considered in [177]. Four types of powders were used with acceleration by nitrogen and helium with temperatures of 900–1200 K. The powders were agglomerates consisting of nanoparticles. The spraying conditions and the coating parameters are summarized in Table 5.3. It is seen that the parameters indicated by B were the best ones.

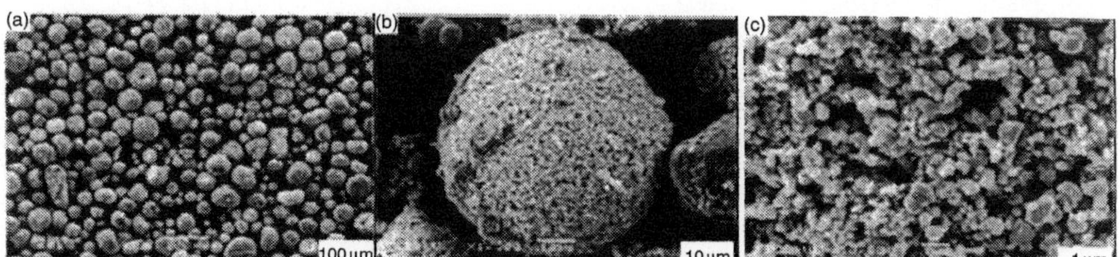

Fig. 5.25. SEM images of agglomerated W/Cu composite feedstock (a) ×150, (b) ×1300, and (c) ×10 000 [176].

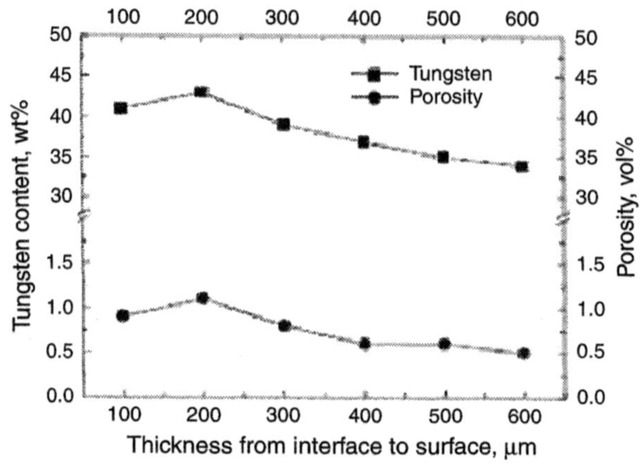

Fig. 5.26. Tungsten content and porosity versus location in the deposited layer [176].

Table 5.3. Spray conditions and coatings properties

Conditions	A	B	C	D
Powder composition, wt%	WC-15% Co	WC-12% Co	WC-12% Co	WC-17% Co
Powder size, μm	1–20	5–45	15–45	15–45
WC size	nano	nano	micro	micro
Gas	nitrogen	helium	nitrogen	helium
Distance, mm	10	15	10	15
Feeder rotation frequency, rpm.	30	30	40	30
Gas temperature, °C	800	600	700	600
Powder heating, °C	250	500	250	200
Pressure, atm	45	31	45	35
Nozzle motion velocity, mm/s	10	10	10	10
Number of passes	4	2	2	2
Coating thickness, μm	300	900	250	200
Hardness, HV 500 g	1480	2053	984	918
Content of carbon, powder/coating, wt%	5.67/5.62	5.52/5.88		

The possibility of obtaining coatings from the WC + Co composition with the use of additional heating of the powder (i.e., increasing its initial temperature at the nozzle entrance) accelerated by helium was considered in [178, 179]. Powders with the following compositions were used: WC nanopowders (particle size 100–400 nm) with addition of 17% Co (the powder particles were agglomerated to 5–45 μm), micropowder with a particle size of 15–45 μm, and the so-called multimodal powder consisting of a mixture of carbide particles 1–2 μm and 100–300 nm agglomerated to a particle size of 5–45 μm. Spraying was performed onto SUS 304 stainless steel. It was noted that the composition of the coatings almost coincided with the composition of the initial powders. As a whole, the quality of coatings was very good, with a low porosity and high hardness reaching the hardness of cast WC. The drawback is the brittleness of the coatings.

Obtaining coatings from the WC + 12% Co nanopowder on soft steel was studied in [180]. To be accelerated to high velocities, the powder was agglomerated to a particle size of 10–43 μm, and heated nitrogen was used (up to 540 °C). These conditions made it possible to obtain dense coatings with good adhesion and with a hardness of $1225 \pm 282\,\text{kgf/mm}^2$. It was noted that coatings of approximately identical hardness are obtained by gas-thermal spraying techniques.

Obtaining coatings from zinc-clad iron (the iron core was surrounded by zinc (39.8 wt%)) with addition of the TiO_2 nanopowder and subsequent treatment of the resultant coating by laser radiation was considered in [181]. The clad powder has the following size distribution: smaller than 180 μm (0.4%), 180 μm (11.5%), 250 μm (21.9%), 300 μm (56.7%), 500 μm (9.4%), and larger than 710 μm (0.1%), i.e., the powder was rather coarse. Preliminary experiments were aimed at clarifying the influence of the air pressure and the substrate material on the deposition efficiency for the Zn–Fe powder. In spraying onto the SS400 soft steel, the deposition efficiency increases almost linearly with increasing mass of the powder used; in addition, the slope of the curves increases with increasing pressure of the working gas, see Fig. 5.27.

The use of a different substrate material reveals the nonlinear character of the kinetic curve. In this case, the highest deposition efficiency was obtained on an aluminum substrate, and the kinetic curve has a noticeably nonlinear character (see Fig. 5.28).

It should be noted that thus-obtained coatings are not typical for the cold spray because they are very thin, as compared with the initial size of particles in the powder; the coating thickness is approximately 60 μm. If a titanium–oxide powder (4.8 – 2.4 wt%) is added

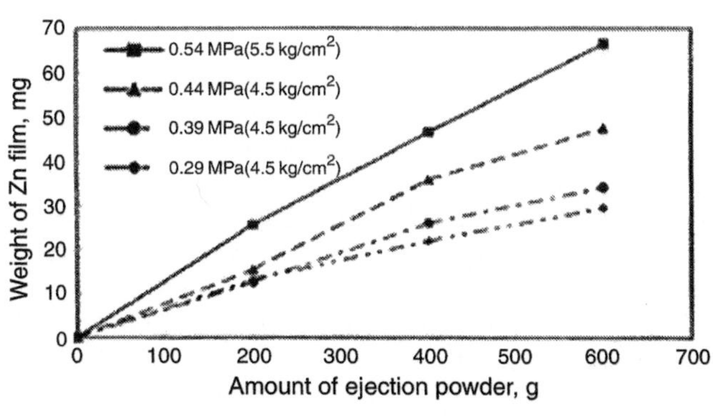

Fig. 5.27. Relationship between deposited Zn coating weight and air pressure (SS400) [181].

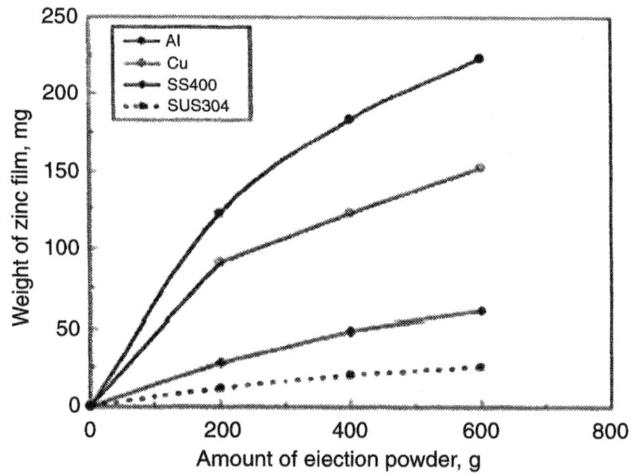

Fig. 5.28. Effect of substrates on the deposited Zn coating (4.5 kg/cm^2) [181].

to the Zn–Fe powder, the content of titanium oxide in the resultant coating is close to its content in the initial powder. The TiO_2-Zn-Fe coatings were treated by focused laser radiation with a power of 100–200 W with a displacement velocity of 1.5 m/min. It was noted that the coating properties (hardness, density, adhesion-cohesion) are improved by this treatment. The main objective was to compare the photocatalytic properties of the pure titanium–oxide powder, coating from titanium oxide with addition of zinc-clad iron, and the same coating after laser treatment. This comparison revealed applicability of the coating and treated coating along with the pure powder.

Obtaining composite coatings from mixtures of powders of aluminum and diamond, carborundum, aluminum nitride, and tungsten on bronze, stainless steel, aluminum, and corundum was considered in [182].

For better understanding of composite properties, the properties of the aluminum coating were first examined. The coating density was 90% of the density of cast aluminum. The thermal conductivity of the aluminum coating in the direction perpendicular to the direction of spraying at room temperature is almost twice as low as the thermal conductivity of cast aluminum (114 W/m K against 240 W/m K). After annealing, however, it increases to 168 W/m K (70% of the value for the cast material). The decrease in thermal conductivity owing to porosity was estimated by the formula borrowed from [183] as 205 W/m K. Thus, the decrease in thermal conductivity of coatings can be explained by the joint effect of the coating porosity and, which is even more important, by imperfection of the contact between the particles composing the coating. By inspecting the curve of the thermal conductivity as a function of temperature, the authors concluded that scattering of electrons on the grain boundary plays the dominating role in the thermal conductivity in pure aluminum, which increases at low temperatures. The dominating process restricting the thermal conductivity in pure aluminum is scattering of electrons by photons. As the temperature decreases, this scattering becomes less intense, which leads to an increase in the thermal conductivity of pure aluminum. Obviously, this process is concealed in the coating by stronger, temperature-independent thermal resistance of grain boundaries. The thermal conductivity of the aluminum coating parallel to the spraying direction is close to the thermal conductivity perpendicular to the spraying direction.

Composite coatings were obtained from the following mixtures of powders: 70 vol.% Al (51–63 μm) + diamond (51–90 μm), 70 vol.% Al (51–63 μm) + SiC (51–63 μm), 50 vol.% Al (63–90 μm) + AlN (51–63 μm), and 50 vol.% Al (63–90 μm) + W (63–90 μm). All composites except for Al/AlN form coatings several millimeters thick.

The aluminum/diamond mixture forms a coating with the diamond content equal to 56 vol.% (higher than in the initial mixture). Its thermal conductivity was 168 W/m K, but it increased to 202 W/m K after annealing. The authors of that book believe that such a composite had not been obtained previously by any of the methods. In the resultant composite coating Al/SiC, the content of SiC was 12 vol.% (lower than in the initial mixture). The coating from the Al/W mixture contains 53 wt% (17 vol.%) of tungsten (smaller than in the initial powder).

The Al/AlN composite has the lowest growth rate of the coating thickness. A coating 0.8 mm thick was obtained in [182]. The microphotographs of the coating testify that AlN particles experience fragmentation due to the impact. The authors did not comment whether there are any changes in the AlN content in the coating as compared with that in the initial mixture.

To improve adhesion, deposition efficiency, and density of Al and Cu coatings, it was proposed [184] to add ceramic powders (Al_2O_3, SiC, or their mixtures) and Zn powder to the basic powder. These mixtures are to be introduced into the supersonic section of the nozzle with an air flow, which has a stagnation temperature of 400–700°C and a pressure that ensures sufficient rarefaction at the injection point (about 0.1 MPa and lower).

It is clear that presented above analysis does not cover many aspects related to different technologies and coating properties and more detailed overview and analysis should be made in this field. However, as we can see from the presented above data the cold spray process allows to apply wide spectrum of various coatings made of metals, alloys, composites, etc. This area (coating properties and technologies and applications) probably is the most intensely developed area of the cold spray because of its important advantages that include avoiding oxidation and undesirable phases, retaining properties of initial particle materials, spraying thermally sensitive materials, working with highly dissimilar materials, etc. Eliminating the effects of high temperature on coatings and substrates makes cold spray promising for producing and repairing a wide range of industrial parts. Examples include turbine blades, pistons, cylinders, valves, rings; bearing components, pump elements, sleeves, shafts, and seals for many industries. Various coatings may add strengthening, hardening, wear resistance, corrosion resistance, electro-magnetic conductivity, thermal conductivity, and other properties. The process is also suitable for production of compact powder materials and for direct fabrication of parts.

References

[1] R.C. Dykhuizen, and M.F. Smith, Gas dynamic principles of cold spray // *Journal of Thermal Spray Technology*, 1998, Vol. 7, No. 2, pp. 205–212.

[2] K. Sakaki, N. Huruhashi, K. Tamaki, and Y. Shimizu, Effect of nozzle geometry on cold spray process // Tagungsband Conference Proceedings / Ed. E. Lugssheider, Deutscher Verband Für Schweiβen, Dusseldorf, Germany, 2002, pp. 385–389.

[3] K. Sakaki, Y. Shimizu, Y. Guoda, and A. Devasenapathi, Effects of gun nozzle geometry on high velocity oxygen-fuel (HVOF) thermal spraying process // *Thermal Spray: Meeting the Challenges of 21st Century* / Ed. C. Coddet, ASM International, Materials Park, OH, USA, 1998, pp. 445–450.

[4] A.H. Shapiro, The dynamics and thermodynamics of compressible fluid flow, Ronald Press, 1953.

[5] R.H. Sabesky, A.J. Acosta, and E.G. Hauptmann, Fluid Flow, Macmillan, 1971.

[6] C.B. Henderson, Drag coefficients of spheres in continuum and rarefied flows // *AIAA J.* 1976, Vol. 14, pp. 707–708.

[7] R.E. Blose, T.J. Roemer, A.J. Mayer, D.E. Beatty, and A.N. Papyrin, Automated cold spray system: Description of equipment and performance data // *Thermal Spray 2003 Advancing the Science and Applying the Technology* / ed. B.R. Marple, C. Moreau, ASM International, Materials Park, OH, USA, 2003, pp. 103–111.

[8] T. Stoltenhoff, J. Voyer, and H. Kreye, Cold spraying – state of the art and applicability // Tagungsband Conference Proceedings / ed. E. Lugssheider, Deutscher Verband Für Schweiβen, Dusseldorf, Germany, 2002, pp. 366–374.

[9] T. Stoltenhoff, H. Kreye, W. Kroemmer, and H.J. Richter, Cold spraying – from thermal spraying to high kinetic energy spraying // HVOF Colloquium 2000 / ed. P. Heinrich, Gemeinschaft thermisches Spritzene, 2000, pp. 29–38.

[10] T. Stoltenhoff, H. Kreye, H.J. Richter, and H. Assadi, Optimization of the cold spray process // *Thermal Spray 2001: New Surfaces For A New Millennium* / ed. C.C. Berndt, K.A. Khor, and E. Lugscheider, ASM International, Materials Park, OH, 2001, pp. 409–416.

[11] Fluent, Inc. Lebanon NH, USA, 1999.

[12] G.B. Wallis, One-dimensional two phase flow, New York, NY: Mc Graw Hill, 1969.

[13] M.J. Walsh, Drag coefficient equation for small particles in high speed flows // *AIAA J.*, 1975, Vol. 13, pp. 1526–1528.

[14] M. Grujicic, C.L. Zhao, C. Tong, W.S. DeRosset, and D. Helfritch, Analysis of the impact velocity of powder particles in the cold-gas dynamic-spray process // *Materials Science and Engineering* A368, 2004, pp. 222–230.

[15] E.H. Kwon, J.W. Han, C.H. Lee, and H.J. Kim, Computer simulation of injected particle behavior during cold spray process // Proc. Thermal spray conference. Thermal spray connects: Explore its surfacing potential!, Basel, Swizerland, May 2–4, 2005, ed. E. Lugscheider, pp. 1345–1348.

[16] B. Jodoin, F. Raletz, and M. Vardelle, Cold spray modeling and validation using an optical diagnostic method // *Surface and Coating Technology*, Vol. 200, Nos 14–15, 10 April 2006, pp. 4424–4432.

[17] T.-Ch. Jen, L. Li, W. Cui, Qi. Chen, and X. Zhang, Numerical investigations on cold gas dynamic spray process with nano- and microsize particles // *Int. J. Heat and Mass Transfer* 48, 2005, pp. 4384–4396.

[18] J. Vlcek, H. Huber, H. Voggenreiter, A. Fischer, E. Lugscheider, H. Hallen, and G. Pache, Kinetic power compaction applying the cold spray process. A study on parameters // *Thermal Spray 2001: New Surfaces For A New Millennium* / ed. C.C. Berndt, K.A. Khor, and E. Lugscheider, ASM International, Materials Park, OH, 2001, pp. 417–422.

[19] R.C. Dykhuizen and R.A. Neiser, Optimizing the cold spray process // *Thermal Spray 2003: Advancing the Science and Applying the Technology* / ed. B.R. Marple and C. Moreau, ASM International, Materials Park, OH, USA, 2003, pp. 19–26.

[20] D.L. Gilmore, R.A. Neiser, R.C. Dykhuizen, and M.F. Smith, Analysis of the critical velocity for deposition in the cold spray process // MRS Fall Meeting, Boston, Mass, 1999.

[21] D.L. Gilmore, R.C. Dykhuizen, R.A. Neiser, T.J. Roemer, and M.F. Smith, Particle velocity and deposition efficiency in the cold spray process // *Journal of Thermal Spray Technology*, 1999, Vol. 8, pp. 576–582.

[22] R.C. Dykhuizen, M.F. Smith, D.L. Gilmore, R.A. Neiser, X. Jiang, and S. Sampath, Impact of high velocity cold spray particles // *Journal of Thermal Spray Technology*, 1999, Vol. 8, No. 4. pp. 559–564.

[23] V. Shukla and G. Elliott, The fluid dynamics of cold gas dynamic spray // Proc. ASM International Materials Solutions Conf., St. Louis, Missouri, USA, 2000.

[24] V. Shukla, Laser diagnostic in cold gas dynamic spray // ASM Thermal Spray Society, cold spray, New Horizons in Surface Technology, Albuquerque, New Mexico, USA, 2002.

[25] A.P. Alkhimov, V.F. Kosarev, and S.V. Klinkov, The features of cold spray nozzle design // *Journal of Thermal Spray Technology*, 2001, Vol. 10, No. 2. pp. 375–381.

[26] F.S. Alvi, J.A. Ladd, and W.W. Bower, Experimental and computational investigation of supersonic impinging jets // *AIAA J*, 2002, Vol. 40, pp. 599–609.

[27] A. Krothapalli, E. Rajakuperan, F.S. Alvi, and L. Lourenco, Flow field and noise characteristics of a supersonic impinging jet // *J. Fluid Mechanics*, 1999, Vol. 393, pp. 155–181.

[28] A. Powell, The sound producing oscillations of round underexpanded jets impinging on normal plates // *J. Acoustical Society of America*, 1988, Vol. 83, pp. 515–533.

[29] J. Karthikeyan, and C.M. Kay, cold spray technology: An industrial perspective // *Thermal Spray 2003: Advancing the Science and Applying the Technology* / ed. B.R. Marple and C. Moreau, ASM International, Materials Park, OH, USA, 2003, pp. 117–121.

[30] B. Jodoin, Effects of shock waves on impact velocity of cold spray particles // *Thermal Spray 2001: New Surfaces For A New Millennium* / ed. C.C. Berndt, K.A. Khor, and E. Lugscheider, ASM International Materials Park, OH, 2001, pp. 399–407.

[31] B. Jodoin, P. Proulx, and Y. Mercadier, Numerical study of supersonic direct current plasma nozzle flow // *AIAA J.* Vol. 36, No. 4, pp. 578–584.

[32] V. Shukla, G.S. Elliot, and B.H. Kear, Nanopowder deposition by supersonic rectangular jet impingement // *Journal of Thermal Spray Technology*, 2000, Vol. 9, No. 3, pp. 394–398.

[33] J. Wu, H. Fang, S. Yoon, H.J. Kim, and Ch. Lee, Measurement of particle velocity and characterization of deposition in aluminum alloy kinetic spraying process // *Applied Surface Science*, Vol. 252, No. 5, Dec. 2005, pp. 1368–1377.

[34] T. Van Steenkiste and J.R. Smith, Evaluation of coating produced via kinetic and cold spray processes // *Thermal Spray 2003: Advancing the Science and Applying the Technology* / ed. B.R. Marple and C. Moreau, ASM International, Materials Park, OH, USA, 2003, pp. 53–61.

[35] J. Mondoux, B. Jodoin, L. Ajdelsztain, J.M. Schoenung, and G.E. Kim, Nanostructured aluminum coatings produced using cold spraying technology // *Thermal Spray Solutions. Advances in Technology and Application* / Verband Für Schweißen and verwandte Verfahren DVS-Verlag GmbH, Dusseldorf/Germany, 2004.

[36] B. Jodoin, F. Raletz, and M. Vardelle, Cold spray flow modeling and validation // Proc. Thermal spray conf. Thermal spray connects: Explore its surfacing potential!, Basel, Switzerland, May 2–4, 2005, ed. E. Lugscheider, pp. 165–169.

[37] F. Gartner, T. Stoltenhoff, T. Schmidt, and H. Kreye, The Cold spray process and its potential for industrial applications // Proc. Thermal spray conf. Thermal spray connects: Explore its surfacing potential!, Basel, Switzerland, May 2–4, 2005, ed. E. Lugscheider, pp. 158–164.

[38] F. Raletz, M. Vardelle, and G. Ezo'o, Fast determination of particle critical velocity in cold spraying // Proc. Thermal spray conf. Thermal spray connects: Explore its surfacing potential!, Basel, Switzerland, May 2–4, 2005, ed. E. Lugscheider, pp. 684–692.

[39] J. Vlcek, L. Gimeno, H. Huber, and E. Lugscheider, A systematic approach to material eligibility for the cold spray process // *Thermal Spray 2003: Advancing the Science and Applying the Technology* / ed. B.R. Marple and C. Moreau, ASM International, Materials Park, OH, USA, 2003, pp. 37–44.

[40] H. Dell, and G. Oberhofer, Simulation zur Deformation eines spharischen Pulverpartikels beim Kaltkinetischen Kompaktieren // Report Ingenieurburo MATFEM, Munich, 12/2000.

[41] J. Vlcek, H. Huber, H. Voggenreiter, and E. Lugscheider, Melting upon particle impact in the cold spray process // Materials Week 2002, Int. Congress on Advanced Materials, their Processes and Applications, 2002.

[42] J. Vlcek, *et al.* Characteristics of kinetic powder compaction with the cold spray process // Materials Week 2001, Int. Congress on Advanced Materials, their Processes and Applications, 2001.

[43] R. Prummer, Explosivverdichtung pulveriger Supstanzen Springer Verlag, Berlin/Heidelberg, 1987.

[44] A. Zukas, High velocity impact dynamics, New York: John Wiley and Sons, 1990.

[45] J.R. Asay, and M. Shahinpoor, *High Pressure Shock Compression of Solids*. New York: Springer Verlag, 1993, pp. 7–113.

[46] M.A. Meyer, and L.E. Murr (eds), Appendix F – Tabulation of shock wave parameters, shock waves and high strain rate phenomena in metals // Plenum Press, New York, 1981, p. 1061ff.

[47] G. Welsch, R. Boyer, and E.W. Collings, *Materials Properties Handbook: Titanium Alloys*, 2nd edition: ASM International, Materials Park, OH, 1998. pp. 483–636.

[48] Y.V. Prasad, and S. Sasidhara, Hot working guide: A compendium of processing maps. ASM International, Materials Park, OH, USA, 1997, pp. 1–24.

[49] Y.V. Prasad, and S. Sasidhara, Hot working guide: A compendium of processing maps. ASM International, Materials Park, OH, USA, 1997, pp. 1–24.

[50] H.-J. Frost and M.F. Ashby, Deformation mechanism maps – the plasticity and creep metals and ceramics, Pergamon Press, Oxford, 1982.

[51] P.O. Kettunen, *Physical Metallurgy*. IMS Tampere University, 1995.

[52] D. Raybould, The cold welding of powders by dynamic compaction, // *Int. J. of Powder Metallurgy and Powder Technology*, 1980, Vol. 16, No. 1, pp. 9–19.

[53] A.P. Alkhimov, V.F. Kosarev, and A.N. Papyrin, A method of cold gas dynamic deposition // Sov. Phys. Dokl. 1990. Vol. 35, No. 12, Dec., pp. 1047–1049, American Institute of Physics, 1991.

[54] R.C. McCune, A.N. Papyrin, J.N. Hall, W.L. Riggs II, and P.H. Zajchowski, An exploration of the cold gas dynamic spray method for several material systems // *Thermal Spray Science and Technology* / ed. C.C. Berndt and S. Sampath, ASM International, Materials Park, OH, 1995, pp. 1–5.

[55] A.P. Alkhimov, A.I. Gulidov, V.F. Kosarev, and N.I. Nesterovich, Specific features of microparticle deformation upon impact on a rigid barrier // *J. Appl. Mech. and Tech. Phys.* 2000, Vol. 41, No. 1. pp. 188–192.

[56] H. Lippmann, and O. Mahrenholtz, Plastomechanik der Umformung metallischer Werkstoffe. Berlin: Springer Verlag, 1967.

[57] J. Vlcek, *et al.* Where are the limits of cold spray? – Ceramic Deposition // cold spray Horisons in Surfacing Technology, Albuquerque, New Mexico, 2002.

[58] D. Zhang, P.H. Shipway, and D.G. McCartney, Particle-substrate interactions in cold gas dynamic spraying // Thermal Spray 2003 Advancing the Science and Applying the Technology / ed. B.R. Marple, C. Moreau, ASM Imternational, Materials Park, OH, USA, 2003, pp. 45–52.

[59] B. Crossland, Exposive welding of metals and its application. Oxford: Clarendon Press, 1982.

[60] A.N. Papyrin, V.F. Kosarev, S.V. Klinkov, and A.P. Alkhimov, On the interaction of high speed particles with a substrate under the cold spraying // Tagungsband Conference Proceedings / ed. E. Lugssheider, Deutscher Verband Für Schweiβen, Dusseldorf, Germany, 2002, pp. 380–384.

[61] T.H. Van Steenkiste, J.R. Smith, R.E. Teets, J.J. Molrski, *et al.* Kinetic spray coatings // *Surf. Coat. Technol.* 1999, Vol. 111, No. 1, pp. 107–115.

[62] T.H. Van Steenkiste, J.R. Smith, R.E. Teets, J.J. Moleski, *et al.* Aluminum coating via kinetic spray with relatively large powder particles // *Surf. Coat. Technol.* 2002, Vol. 154, No. 2–3, pp. 237–252.

[63] A.V. Bolesta, V.M. Fomin, M.R. Sharafutdinov, and B.P. Tolochko, Investigation of interface boundary occurring during cold gas-dynamic spraying of metallic particles // *Nuclear Inst. and Methods in Phys. Res. A*, 470, 2001, pp. 249–252.

[64] A.O. Tokarev, Structure of aluminum powder coatings prepared by cold gas dynamic spraying // *Metal Sci. and Heat Treatment.* 1996. Vol. 38, pp. 136–139.

[65] I.M. Hutchings, A model for the erosion of metals by spherical particles at normal incidence // *Wear.* 1981, Vol. 70, pp. 269–281.

[66] F. Gaertner, C. Borchers, T. Stoltenhoff, H. Kreye, and H. Assadi, Numerical and microstuctural investigations of the bonding mechanisms in cold spraying // *Thermal Spray 2003: Advancing the Science and Applying the Technology* / ed. B.R. Marple, C. Moreau, ASM International Materials Park, OH, USA, 2003. pp. 1–8.

[67] R.C. McCune, W.T. Donlon, E.L. Cartwright, A.N. Papyrin, E.F. Rybicki, and J.R. Shadley, Characterization of Copper and steel coatings made by the cold gas dynamic spray method // *Thermal Spray: Practical Solutions for Engineering Problems* / ed. C.C. Berndt, ASM International, Materials Park, OH, USA, 1996, pp. 397–403.

[68] T. Schmidt, H. Kreye, F. Gaertner, High strain rate deformation phenomena in explosive powder compaction and cold spraying // *Thermal Spray 2003: Advancing the Science and Applying the Technology* / ed. B.R. Marple, C. Moreau, ASM International Materials Park, OH, USA, 2003, pp. 9–18.

[69] V.F. Nesterenko, Dynamic loading of porous materials: potential and restrictions for Novel materials applications // Proc. Int. Conf. on metallurgical and materials application of shock wave and high strain rate phenomena "EXPLOMET 95" / ed. L.E. Murr, K.P. Staudhammer, M.A. Meyers, Elsevier, Amsterdam, 1995, pp. 3–28.

[70] R.B. Schwarz, P. Kasiraj, T. Vreeland, and T.J. Ahrens, A theory for the shock wave consolidation of powders // *Acta Metall.* 1984, Vol. 32, pp. 1243–1252.

[71] A. Papyrin, Cold Spray technology // *Advanced materials and processes.* 2001, Vol. 159, pp. 49–51.

[72] T. Stoltenhoff, H. Kreye, H.J. Richter, An analysis of the Cold Spray process and its coatings // *Journal of Thermal Spray Technology.* 2002, Vol. 11, pp. 1–9.

[73] C. Borchers, T. Stoltenhoff, F. Gaertner, H. Kreye, and H. Assadi, Deformation microstructure of Cold Sprayed coatings studied by electron microscopy // *Mat. Res. Soc. Symp. Proc. 673*, 2001, pp. 7–10.

[74] A.A. Deribas and I.D. Zakharenko, Surface effects with oblique collisions between metallic plates // *Fisika Goreniya I Vzryva*. 1974, Vol. 10, pp. 409–421.

[75] H. Assadi, F. Gaertner, T. Stoltenhoff, H. Kreye, Bonding mechanism in Cold Spraying // Acta Materiala 2003; Vol. 51, No. 15, Sept. pp. 4379–4394.

[76] G.B. Olson, J.F. Mescall, and M. Azrin, Adiabatic deformation and strain localization, in M.A. Meyers, L.E. Murr, eds, Shock waves and high straing rate phenomena in metals. Plenum Press, New York. 1981. pp. 22–1.

[77] D.Y. Tzou, *ASME J Heat Transfer*. 1995. pp. 117–118.

[78] G.S. Prakash, S.S. Reddy, S.K. Das, T. Sundararajan, and K.N. Seetharamu, *Num Heat Transfer A*. 2000. 38 513.

[79] R. Kapoor and S. Nemat-Nasser, *Mech Mater.*, 1998, 28 1.

[80] G.R. Johnson, *Prog Astronaut Aeronaut.*, 1993, 155 165.

[81] R.R. Karpp, *Prog Astronaut Aeronaut.*, 1993, 155 223.

[82] F. Kamler, P. Niessen, R.J. Pick, *Can J Phys.*, 1995, 73 295.

[83] S. Nemat-Masser and Y. Li, *Acta Mater.*, 1998, 46 565.

[84] M. Grujicic, C.L. Zhao, W.S. DeRosset and D. Helfricht, Adiabatic shear instability based mechanism for particle/substrate bonding in the cold – gas dynamic-spray process // *Materials and Design*. Vol. 25, No. 8, Dec. 2004, pp. 681–688.

[85] T.W. Wright, Shear band susceptibility: work hardening materials // *Int J Plasticity* 1992; Vol. 8, No. 2. pp. 583–602.

[86] T.W. Wright, Toward a defect invariant basis for susceptibility to adiabatic shear bands // *Mech Mater*. 1994, Vol. 17, No. 1, pp. 215–222.

[87] M. Grujicic, J.R. Saylor, D.E. Beasley, W.S. DeRosset, and D. Helfritch, Computational analysis of the interfacial bonding between feed-power particles and the substrate in the cold-gas dynamic-spray process // *Applied Surface Sci* 219, 2003, pp. 211–227.

[88] T. Schmidt, F. Gartner, T. Stoltenhoff, H. Kreye, and H. Assadi, High velocity impact phenomena and coating quality in cold spraying // Proc. Of Thermal spray conf. Thermal spray connects: Explore its surfacing potential!, Basel, Switzerland, May 2–4, 2005, ed. E. Lugscheider, pp. 232–238.

[89] T. Schmidt, F. Gartner, H. Assadi, and H. Kreye, Development of a generalized parameter window for cold spray deposition // *Acta Mater* 54, 2006, pp. 729–742.

[90] R.G. O' Donnel, Parameter describing the cylindrical explosive consolidation technique // *Propellants, Explosives, Pyrotechnics*. 1993, Vol. 18, pp. 230–236.

[91] M.A. Meyers and L.E. Murr, Shock wave consolidation of rapidly solidified superalloy powders // *J. Metals*. 1981, Vol. 33, pp. 21–26.

[92] D. Raybould, The production of strong parts and non-equilibrium alloys by dynamic compaction // *Shock Waves and High-Strain-Rate Phenomena in Metals: Concept and Applications* / ed. M.A. Meyers and L.E. Murr, Plenum Press, NY, 1981, pp. 895–911.

[93] D. Raybould, The properties of stainless steel compacted dynamically to produce interparticle, Welding, *J. Metals Sci.* 16, 1981, pp. 589–598.

[94] D. Raybould, D. Morris, and G.A. Cooper, A new powder metallurgy method // *J. Metals. Sci.*, 1979, Vol. 14, pp. 2523–2526.

[95] T.Z. Blazynski, *Explosive Welding, forming and Compaction*. Applied Science Publishers, London, UK, 1983, 17–82, pp. 189–287.

[96] M. Hammerschmidt, Mikrostruktur und Eigenschaften von Explosivschweissungen, VDI Verlag GmbH Dusseldorf, Germany, 1983.

[97] S.S. Batsanov, Effects of explosion on materials. Springer Verlag, New York, USA. 1994. pp. 1–90.

[98] D.G. Morris, Bonding processes during the dynamic compaction of metallic powders // Materials Science and Engineering. 1983, Vol. 57, pp. 187–195.

[99] E.P. Carton, Dynamic compaction of ceramics and composites. Delft University Press, Delft, Netherlands, 1997.

[100] L.E. Murr, Shock waves for industrial applications. Noyes Publications, Park Ridge, New Jersey, USA, 1988, pp. 237–333.

[101] S. Barradas, R. Molins, M. Jeandin, M. Arrigoni, M. Boustie, C. Bolis, L. Berthe, and M. Ducos, Laser shock flier impact simulation of particle-substrate interaction in cold spray // Proc. Thermal spray conf. Thermal spray connects: Explore its surfacing potential!, Basel, Switzerland, May 2–4, 2005, ed. E. Lugscheider, pp. 343–351.

[102] R. Maev, A. Aczel, V. Leshchynsky, G. Salloum, and M.-Ui Islam, Air gas dynamic spraying of powder mixtures: Theory and application // Proc. Thermal spray conf. Thermal spray connects: Explore its surfacing potential!, Basel, Switzerland, May 2–4, 2005, ed. E. Lugscheider, pp. 1121–1127.

[103] J. Wu, H. Fang, H. Kim, and Ch. Lee, High speed impact behaviors of Al alloy particle onto mild steel substrate during kinetic deposition // *Mater Sci and Eng A*, Vol. 1, 417 2006, pp. 114–119

[104] J. Wu, H. Fang, S. Yoon, H. Kim, and Ch. Lee, The rebound phenomenon in kinetic spraying deposition // *Scripta Materialia*, Vol. 54, 2006, pp. 665–669.

[105] Ch.-J. Li, W.-Y. Li, Y.-Y. Wang, G.-J. Yang, and H. Fukanuma A theoretical model for prediction of deposition efficiency in cold spraying // *Thin Solid Films*, Vol. 1, 489, 2005, pp. 79–85.

[106] Z.B. Zhao, B.A. Gillispie, J.R. Smith, Coating deposition by the kinetic spray process // *Surface and Coatings Technology*, Vol. 200, Nos 16–17, 27 April 2006, pp. 4746–4754.

[107] J. Karthikeyan, T. Laha, K. Balani, A. Agarwal, and N. Munroe, Microstructural and electrochemical characterization of cold-sprayed 1100 aluminum coating //

Thermal Spray Solutions. Advances in Technology and Application/Verband Für Schweiβen and verwandte Verfahren DVS-Verlag GmbH, Dusseldorf, Germany, 2004.

[108] J. Voyer, T. Stoltenhoff, and H. Kreye, Development of cold gas sprayed coatings // *Thermal Spray 2003: Advancing the Science and Applying the Technology* / ed. B.R. Marple and C. Moreau, ASM International Materials Park, OH, USA, 2003, pp. 71–78.

[109] R. Morgan, P. Fox, J. Pattison, C. Sutcliffe, and W. O'Neill, Analysis of cold gas dynamically sprayed aluminum deposits // *Materials Letters*, Vol. 58, 2004, pp. 1317–1320.

[110] K. Balani, T. Laha, A. Agarwal, J. Karthikeyan, and N. Munroe, Effect of carrier gases on microstructural and electrochemical behavior of cold-sprayed 1100 aluminum coating // *Surface and Coatings Technology*, Vol. 195, Nos. 2–3, 31 May 2005, pp. 272–279.

[111] A.C. Hall, D.J. Cook, R.A. Neiser, T.J. Roemer, and D.A. Hirschfeld, The effect of a simple annealing heat treatment on the mechanical properties of cold sprayed aluminum // Proc. Thermal spray conf. Thermal spray connects: Explore its surfacing potential!, Basel, Switzerland, May 2–4, 2005, ed. E. Lugscheider, pp. 251–253.

[112] L. Ajdelsztajn, A. Zuniga, B. Jodoin, and E.J. Lavernia, Cold spray of Al-Cu-Mg-Fe-Ni alloy with Sc addition // Proc. Thermal spray conf. Thermal spray connects: Explore its surfacing potential!, Basel, Switzerland, May 2–4, 2005, ed. E. Lugscheider, pp. 245–250.

[113] L. Ajdelsztajn, A. Zuniga, B. Jodoin, and E.J. Lavernia, Cold gas dynamic spraying of a high temperature Al alloy // *Surface and Coating Technology*, 2005, in press.

[114] P. Richer, B. Jodoin, K. Taylor, E. Sansoucy, and M. Johnson, Effect of particle geometry and substrate preparation in cold spray // Proc. Thermal spray conf. Thermal spray connects: Explore its surfacing potential!, Basel, Switzerland, May 2–4, 2005, ed. E. Lugscheider, pp. 193–198.

[115] B. Wielage, T. Grund, S. Ahrens, A. Wank, and F. Trommer, CGS sprayed filler coatings for brazing of light weight alloys // Proc. Thermal spray conf. Thermal spray connects: Explore its surfacing potential!, Basel, Switzerland, May 2–4, 2005, ed. E. Lugscheider, pp. 1245–1249.

[116] J. Haynes and J. Karthikeyan, Cold Spray copper application for upper stage rocket engine design // *Thermal Spray 2003: Advancing the Science and Applying the Technology* / eds. B.R. Marple and C. Moreau, ASM International Materials Park, OH, USA, 2003, pp. 45–52.

[117] C. Cooley, S. Fentress, and T. Jennings, Hot firing of a full scale copper tubular combustion chamber // AAAF 2002-S.18.02, 6th Int. Symp. Propulsion for Space Transportation of the XXIst Century, Versailles, France, 2002.

[118] R. Hickman, T. McKechnie, Plasma Processes, Inc., and R. Holmes, NASA-Marshall Space Flight Center, Material properties of vacuum plasma sprayed

Cu-8Cr-4Nb for liquid rocket engines // 37th AIAA/ASME/SAE/ASEE/ Joint propulsion Conf., Salt Lake City, Utah, 2001.

[119] M.F. Smith, J.E. Brockmann, R.C. Dykhuizen, D.L. Gilmore, R.A. Neiser, and T.J. Roemer, Cold Spray direct fabrication – high rate, solid state, material consolidation // Materials Research Society Proc. 542, 1999, pp. 65–76.

[120] J. Karthikeyan, Cold Spray processing of metals, alloys, and composites // ASM Thermal spray Society Workshop on Cold Spray, 2002.

[121] T. Xiong, Ch. Gu, W. Zhang, M.-J. Wu, J. Wu, H. Jin, and T. Li, Study of aluminum bronze coating by cold spray process // *Thermal Spray Solutions. Advances in Technology and Application* / Verband Für Schweißen and verwandte Verfahren DVS-Verlag GmbH, Dusseldorf, Germany, 2004.

[122] E. Galla, D.G. McCartney, and P.H. Shipway, Deposition of copper by cold gas dynamic spraying: an investigation of dependence of microstructure and properties of the deposits on the spraying conditions // *Thermal Spray Solutions. Advances in Technology and Application* / Verband Für Schweißen and verwandte Verfahren DVS-Verlag GmbH, Dusseldorf, Germany, 2004.

[123] H. Fukanuma, and N. Ohno, A study of adhesive strength of cold spray coatings // *Thermal Spray Solutions. Advances in Technology and Application* / Verband Für Schweißen and verwandte Verfahren DVS-Verlag GmbH, Dusseldorf, Germany, 2004.

[124] C.-J. Li, W.-Y. Li, Y.-Y. Wang, and H. Fukanuma, Effect of spray angle on deposition characteristics in cold spraying // *Thermal Spray 2003: Advancing the Science and Applying the Technology* / eds. B.R. Marple and C. Moreau, ASM International Materials Park, OH, USA, 2003, pp. 91–96

[125] K. Sakaki, T. Tajima, H. Li, S. Shinkai, and Y. Shimizu, Influence of substrate conditions and traverse speed on cold sprayed coatings // *Thermal Spray Solutions. Advances in Technology and Application* / Verband Für Schweißen and verwandte Verfahren DVS-Verlag GmbH, Dusseldorf, Germany, 2004.

[126] T. Xiong, Z. Bao, T. Li, and Z. Li, Study on cold-sprayed copper coating's properties and optimizing parameters for the spraying process // Proc. Thermal spray conf. Thermal spray connects: Explore its surfacing potential!, Basel, Switzerland, May 2–4, 2005, ed. E. Lugscheider, pp. 178–184.

[127] E. Calla, D.G. McCartney, and P.H. Shipway, Effect of heat treatment on the structure and properties of cold sprayed copper // Proc. Thermal spray conf Thermal spray connects: Explore its surfacing potential!, Basel, Switzerland, May 2–4, 2005, ed. E. Lugscheider, pp. 170–176.

[128] M.A. Meyers, L.W. Meyers, J. Beatty, U. Andrade, K.S. Vecchio, and A.H. Choksi, High strain, high strain rate deformation of copper, in *Shock-wave and High-strain-rate Phenomenon in Materials*, eds. M.A. Meyers, L.E. Murr, and K.P. Staudhammer, Marcel Dekker, New York, 1992, pp. 529–542.

[129] W.-Y. Li, and C.-J. Li, Effect of annealing treatment on the microstructure and properties of cold-sprayed Cu coating // Proc. Thermal spray conf. Thermal spray

connects: Explore its surfacing potential!, Basel, Switzerland, May 2–4, 2005, ed. E. Lugscheider, pp. 1258–1263.

[130] J. Lagerbom, H. Makinen, and P. Vuoristo, Effect of heat treatment on properties of cold sprayed coatings // Proc. Thermal spray conf. Thermal spray connects: Explore its surfacing potential!, Basel, Switzerland, May 2–4, 2005, ed. E. Lugscheider, pp. 240–244.

[131] K. Taylor, B. Jodoin, J. Karov, and P. Richer, Particle loading effect in cold spray // Proc. Thermal spray conf. Thermal spray connects: Explore its surfacing potential!, Basel, Switzerland, May 2–4, 2005, ed. E. Lugscheider, pp. 186–190.

[132] C.-J. Li and W.-Y. Li, Examination of the critical velocity for deposition of particles in cold spraying // Proc. Thermal spray conf. Thermal spray connects: Explore its surfacing potential!, Basel, Switzerland, May 2–4, 2005, ed. E. Lugscheider, pp. 217–224.

[133] Livermore Software Technology Corporation, LS-DYNA theoretical manual, 1998.

[134] C. Borchers, F. Gartner, T. Stoltenhoff, H. Assadi, and H. Kreye, Microstructural and macroscopic properties of cold sprayed copper coatings // *J. of Appl. Phys.* Vol. 93, No. 12, 2003, pp. 10064–10070.

[135] S. Barradas, R. Molis, M. Jeandin, M. Arrigoni, M. Boustie, C. Bolis, L. Berthe, and M. Ducos, Application of laser shock adhesion testing to the study of the interlamellar strength and coating-substrate adhesion in cold-sprayed copper coating of aluminum // *Surf and Coat Techn*, Vol. 197, 2005, pp. 18–27.

[136] R.C. McCune, W.T. Donlon, O.O. Popoola, and E.L. Cartwright // *J. Thermal Spray Technol.*, 2000, Vol. 9, No. 1, pp. 73–82.

[137] R.C. McCune, R.P. Cooper, and O.O. Popoola, Post-processing of cold spray deposits of copper and iron // *Thermal Spray: Surface Engineering via Applied Research* / ed. C.C. Berndt, ASM International, Materials Park, OH, 2000, pp. 905–908.

[138] R.C. McCune, Potential applications of cold-spray technology in automative manufacturing // *Thermal Spray 2003: Advancing the Science and Applying the Technology* / eds. B.R. Marple and C. Moreau, ASM International Materials Park, OH, USA, 2003, pp. 63–70.

[139] P.M. Nakagawa, F. Kawakami, and T. Kudoh, Trends in automative applications of thermal spray technology in Japan // *Thermal Spray Industrial Application* / eds. C.C. Berndt and S. Sampath, ASM International, Materials Park, OH, 1994, pp. 1–4.

[140] R.C. McCune, Thermal spraying: an enabling technology in automobile manufacturing // Proc. Int. Conf. advances in welding technology: the joining of high-performance materials, Edison Welding Institute, Columbus, OH, 1996, pp. 181–189

[141] M.K. Decker, H.D. Tran, and Y.-L. Shen, Mechanical properties of cold gas-dynamic spray nickel // Sandia National Laboratories Report SAND2000-2679, Sandia National Laboratories, Albuquerque, NM, 2000.

[142] D.L. Ohmann, MS Thesis, University of Wisconsin, Madison, WI, 1998.

[143] R.E. Chalmers, Rapid tooling technology from Ford Country // *Manufacturing Engineering*, 2001, Vol. 127, No. 5. pp. 36–41.

[144] M.K. Decker, R.A. Neiser, D. Gilmore, and H.D. Tran, Microstructure and properties of Cold Spray nickel // *Thermal Spray 2001: New Surfaces for a New Millennium* / eds. C.C. Berndt, K.A. Khor, and E. Lugscheider, ASM International, Materials Park, OH, 2001, pp. 433–439.

[145] J.R. Davis, Metals handbook, Desk Edition, Second Edition, 1044–6, ASM International, Materials Park, OH, 1998, p. 118.

[146] M.K. Decker, Mechanical properties of cold gas-dynamic spray nickel, Master's thesis, University of New Mexico, Albuquerque, NM, 2000.

[147] F. Raletz, G. Ezo' o, M. Vardelle, and M. Ducos, Characterization of cold-sprayed nickel-base coatings // *Thermal Spray Solutions. Advances in Technology and Application*/Verband Für Schweiβen and verwandte Verfahren DVS-Verlag GmbH, Dusseldorf, Germany, 2004.

[148] S. Sampath, X.Y. Jiang, J. Matejicek, L. Prchlik, A. Kulkarni, and A. Vaidya, Role of thermal spray processing method on the microstructure, residual stress and properties of coatings: an integrated study for Ni-5wt.%Al bond coats// *Material Science and Engineering A*, Vol. 364, No. 1–2, 15 January 2004, pp. 216–231.

[149] J. Matejicek, Materials science and engineering, PhD Thesis, State University of New York, Stony Brook, 1999.

[150] Y.C. Tsui and T.W. Clyne, *Thin Solid Films*, Vol. 306, No. 1, 1997, p. 23.

[151] F. Raletz, G. Ezo'o, P. Brenot, and M. Vardelle, On the influence of the substrate hardness on cold-sprayed nickel coating // Proc. Thermal spray conf. Thermal spray connects: Explore its surfacing potential!, Basel, Switzerland, May 2–4, 2005, ed. E. Lugscheider, pp. 1244–1249.

[152] B. Wielage, T. Grund, S. Ahrens, A. Wank, and F. Trommer, CGS sprayed filler coatings for brazing of light weight alloys // Proc. Thermal spray conf. Thermal spray connects: Explore its surfacing potential!, Basel, Switzerland, May 2–4, 2005, ed. E. Lugscheider, pp. 1245–1249.

[153] Ch.-J. Li, W.-Y. Li, and W.-H. Ma, Characterization of microstructure of nanostructured Fe-Si coating deposited by cold spraying // *Thermal Spray Solutions. Advances in Technology and Application* / Verband Für Schweiβen and verwandte Verfahren DVS-Verlag GmbH, Dusseldorf, Germany, 2004.

[154] M. Manivel Raja, K. Chattopadhyay, B. Majumdar, and A. Narayanasamy, Structure and soft magnetic properties of Finemet alloys // J. of Alloys and Compounds. 2000. Vol. 297. pp. 199–205.

[155] G. Herzer, Grain size dependence of coercivity and permeability in nanocrystalline ferromagnets // IEEE Transactions on Magnetics, 1990, Vol. 26, No. 5. pp. 1397–1402.

[156] M. Miyazaki, M. Komatsu, and K. Matusita // *J. of Applied Physics*, 1992, Vol. 71, pp. 2368–2374.

[157] N. Stevulova, A. Buchal, P. Petrovic, K. Tkacova, and V. Sepelak, Structural investigation of the high-energy milled Fe-Si system // *J. of Magnetism and Magnetic Materials*, 1999, Vol. 203, No. 1–3, pp. 190–192.

[158] S. Yoon, H. J. Kim, and Ch. Lee, Deposition behavior of bulk amorphous NiTiZr-SiSn according to the kinetic and thermal energy levels in the kinetic spraying process // *Surface and Coatings Technology*, Vol. 200, Nos 20–21, 22 May 2006, pp. 6022–6029.

[159] S. Yoon, C. Lee, H.J. Kim, and H. Choi, Kinetic spraying deposition behavior of bulk amorphous NiTiZrSiSn feedstock // Proc. Thermal spray conf. Thermal spray connects: Explore its surfacing potential!, Basel, Switzerland, May 2–4, 2005, ed. E. Lugscheider, pp. 1254–1257.

[160] Ch.-J. Li, W.-Y. Li, and H. Fukanuma, Impact fusion phenomenon during cold spraying of zinc // *Thermal Spray Solutions. Advances in Technology and Application* / Verband Für Schweiβen and verwandte Verfahren DVS-Verlag GmbH, Dusseldorf, Germany, 2004.

[161] B. Wielage, H. Podlesak, T. Grund, and A. Wank, High resolution microstructural investigations of interfaces between light weight alloy substrates and cold sprayed coatings // Proc. Thermal spray conf. Thermal spray connects: Explore its surfacing potential!, Basel, Switzerland, May 2–4, 2005, ed. E. Lugscheider, pp. 154–158.

[162] R.E. Blose, D. Vasquez, and W. Kratochvil, Metal passivation to resist corrosion using the cold spray process // Proc. Of Thermal spray conf. Thermal spray connects: Explore its surfacing potential!, Basel, Switzerland, May 2–4, 2005, ed. E. Lugscheider, pp. 126–135.

[163] B. Wielage, T. Grund, S. Ahrens, A. Wank, and F. Trommer, CGS sprayed filler coatings for brazing of light weight alloys // Proc. Of Thermal spray conf. Thermal spray connects: Explore its surfacing potential!, Basel, Switzerland, May 2–4, 2005, ed. E. Lugscheider, pp. 1245–1249.

[164] H. Fukanuma, and N. Ohno, A study of adhesive strength of cold spray coatings // *Thermal Spray Solutions. Advances in Technology and Application* / Verband Für Schweiβen and verwandte Verfahren DVS-Verlag GmbH, Dusseldorf, Germany, 2004.

[165] V. Shukla, G.S. Elliott, B.H. Kear, and L.E. McCandlish, Hyperkinetic deposition of nanopowders by supersonic rectangular jet impingement // *Scripta mater*, Vol. 44, 2001, pp. 2179–2182.

[166] T. Marrocco, D.G. McCartney, P.H. Shipway, and A.J. Sturgeon, Production of titanium deposits by cold gas dynamic spray // Proc. Thermal spray conf. Thermal spray connects: Explore its surfacing potential!, Basel, Switzerland, May 2–4, 2005, ed. E. Lugscheider, pp. 225–231.

[167] J. Karthikeyan, C.M. Kay, J. Lindeman *et al.* Cold spray processing of titanium powder // *Thermal Spray: Surface Engineering via Applied Research*, ed. C.C.

Berndt, May 8–11, 2000, Montreal, Quebec, Canada, ASM International, 2000, pp. 255–262.

[168] T. Novoselova, P. Fox, R. Morgan, and W.O'Neill, Experimental study of titanium/aluminum deposits produced by cold gas dynamic spray // *Surf and Coat Techn.* Vol. 200, 2006, pp. 2775–2783.

[169] Ch.-J. Li, Gu.-J. Yang, Xi.-Ch. Huang, and W.-Y. Li, Formation of TiO2 photocatalyst through cold spraying // *Thermal Spray Solutions. Advances in Technology and Application* / Verband Für Schweißen and verwandte Verfahren DVS-Verlag GmbH, Dusseldorf, Germany, 2004.

[170] A. Fujishima, and K. Honda, Electrochemical photolysis of water at a semiconductor electrode // Nature, 1972, Vol. 238, pp. 37–38.

[171] D.F. Ollis, and H. Al-Ekabi, Photocatalytic purification and treatment of water and air // Elsevier, Amsterdam, 1993.

[172] M.R. Hoffman, S.T. Martin, W. Choi, and D.W. Bahnemann, Environmental application of semiconductor photocatalysis // Chem. Rev., 1995, Vol. 95, pp. 69–96.

[173] A. Fujishima, T.N. Rao, and D.A. Tryk, Titanium dioxide photocatalysis // *J. Photochem. Photobio.*, 2000, C 1, pp. 1–21.

[174] C.-J. Li, and W.-Y. Li, Deposition characteristics of titanium coating in cold spraying // *Surf. Coat. Technol.*, 2003, Vol. 167, pp. 278–283.

[175] H.Y. Lee, Y.H. Yu, Y.C. Lee, Y.P. Hong, and K.H. Ko, Interfacial studies between cold-sprayed WO_3, Y_2O_3 films and Si substrate // *Applied Surface Science*, Vol. 227, 2004, 244–249.

[176] H.-K. Kang and S.B. Kang, Tungsten/copper composite deposits produced by a cold spray // *Scripta Materialia*, Vol. 49, 2003, pp. 1169–1174.

[177] H.-J. Kim, C.-H. Lee, and S.-Y. Hwang, Fabrication of WC-Co coatings by cold spray deposition // *Surf. Coat. Technol.*, Vol. 191, Nos. 2–3, 21 February 2005, pp. 335–340.

[178] H.J. Kim, S.Y. Hwang, and C.H. Lee, Characterization of nano WC-Co coatings produced by dynamic powder deposition // Proc. Thermal spray conf. Thermal spray connects: Explore its surfacing potential!, Basel, Switzerland, May 2–4, 2005, ed. E. Lugscheider, pp. 1489–1494.

[179] H.-J. Kim, Ch.-H. Lee, and S.-Y. Hwang, Superhard nano WC-12%Co coating by cold spray deposition // *Mat. Sci. Eng. A*, Vol. 391, 2005, pp. 243–248.

[180] R.S. Lima, J. Karthikeyan, C.M. Kay, J. Lindemann, and C.C. Berndt, Microstructural characteristics of cold-sprayed nanostructured WC-Co coatings // *Thin Solid Films*, Vol. 416, 2002, pp. 129–135.

[181] J. Morimoto, T. Onoda, Y. Sasaki, and N. Abe, Improvement of solid cold sprayed TiO2-Zn coating with direct diode laser // *Vacuum*, Vol. 73, 2004, pp. 527–532.

[182] D.T. Morelli, A.A. Elmoursi, T.H. VanSteenkiste, D.W. Gorkiewicz, and B. Gillispie, Kinetic spray of aluminum metal matrix composites for thermal man-

agement applications // *Thermal Spray 2003: Advancing the Science and Applying the Technology*, eds. C. Moreau and B. Marple, Published by ASM International, Materials Park, OH, USA, 2003 pp. 85–90.

[183] A.L. Geiger, D.P.H. Hasselman, and P. Welsh, *Acta Mater.*, Vol. 45, No. 391, 1997.

[184] Kashirin *et al.*, US Patent No. 6,756,073, Method for applying sealing coating with low gas permeability.

Index

FSC
www.fsc.org
MIX
Papier | Fördert gute Waldnutzung
FSC® C083411

Kolibri 360 GmbH
Ferdinand-Jühlke-Straße 7
99095 Erfurt, Deutschland
produktsicherheit@kolibri360.de